MANAGEMENT OF ISCHEMIC STROKE

NOTICE

MANAGEMENT OF ISCHEMIC STROKE

EDITOR

Stanley N. Cohen, M.D.

Department of Neurology
UCLA School of Medicine and Medical Center and
Veterans Affairs Greater Los Angeles Healthcare System
Los Angeles, California

McGraw-Hill
HEALTH PROFESSIONS DIVISION

New York   St. Louis   San Francisco   Auckland   Bogotá
Caracas   Lisbon   London   Madrid   Mexico City   Milan   Montreal
New Delhi   San Juan   Singapore   Sydney   Tokyo   Toronto

McGraw-Hill

*A Division of The **McGraw·Hill** Companies*

MANAGEMENT OF ISCHEMIC STROKE

1234567890 DOCDOC 99

ISBN 0-07-0120455

This book was set in Times Roman by The PRD Group, Inc.
The editors were John Dolan and Peter McCurdy.
The production supervisor was Catherine H. Saggese.
The project was managed by Hockett Editorial Service.
The cover designer was Dorothy Wachtenheim.
The index was prepared by Alexandra Nickerson.
RR Donnelley & Sons Company was printer and binder.

This book is printed on acid-free paper.

**Cataloging-in Publication Data is on file for this title at the Library
of Congress.**

CONTENTS

v

A color insert falls between pages 368 and 369.

CONTRIBUTORS

Gregory W. Albers, M.D.
Stanford Stroke Center
Stanford University Medical Center
Palo Alto, California

Andrei V. Alexandrov, M.D.
Stroke Program and Program in Humanities and
Technology in Health Care
University of Texas/Houston Medical School
Houston, Texas

Jeffrey R. Alger, Ph.D.
Department of Radiology
UCLA School of Medicine and
Medical Center
Los Angeles, California

José Biller, M.D.
Department of Neurology
Indiana University School of Medicine
Indianapolis, Indiana

Askiel Bruno, M.D.
Department of Neurology
Indiana University School of Medicine
Indianapolis, Indiana

John C. M. Brust, M.D.
Department of Neurology
Harlem Hospital Center and
Columbia College of Physicians and
Surgeons
New York, New York

Marc I. Chimowitz, M.D.
Department of Neurology
Emory University School of Medicine
Atlanta, Georgia

Helena C. Chui, M.D.
Department of Neurological Sciences
Rancho Los Amigos Medical Center
Downey, California and
University of Southern California School of Medicine
Los Angeles, California

Benjamin J. Cohen, M.D., F.A.C.C.
Veterans Affairs Greater Los Angeles Healthcare
System and
University Cardiovascular Medical Group
Los Angeles, California

Stanley N. Cohen, M.D.
Department of Neurology
UCLA School of Medicine and Medical Center and
Veterans Affairs Greater Los Angeles Healthcare
System
Los Angeles, California

Bruce H. Dobkin, M.D.
UCLA Neurologic Rehabilitation and Research
Program
Reed Neurologic Research Center
Los Angeles, California

Andre Duerinckx, M.D., Ph.D.
UCLA School of Medicine and
Veterans Affairs Greater Los Angeles Healthcare
System
Los Angeles, California

Suzie M. El-Saden, M.D.
Department of Neuroradiology
UCLA School of Medicine and Medical Center and
Veterans Affairs Greater Los Angeles Healthcare
System
Los Angeles, California

ix

Pierre B. Fayad, M.D.
Department of Neurology
Yale University School of Medicine
New Haven, Connecticut

Glenn M. Fischberg, M.D.
Department of Neurology
University of Southern California School of Medicine
Los Angeles, California

Mark Fisher, M.D.
Department of Neurology
University of California at Irvine
Los Angeles, California

John G. Frazee, M.D.
Division of Neurosurgery
UCLA School of Medicine and Medical Center
Los Angeles, California

Marc Garant, M.D.
Department of Neuroradiology
UCLA School of Medicine and Medical Center and
Veterans Affairs Greater Los Angeles Healthcare
System
Los Angeles, California

Peter A. Glassman, M.D.
Veterans Affairs Greater Los Angeles Healthcare
System
UCLA School of Medicine and Medical Center
Los Angeles, California

Y. Pierre Gobin, M.D.
Division of Interventional Neuroradiology
UCLA School of Medicine and Medical Center
Los Angeles, California

David Lee Gordon, M.D.
Department of Neurology
The University of Mississippi Medical Center
Jackson, Mississippi

Lynn K. Gordon, M.D.
Department of Ophthalmology
UCLA School of Medicine and Medical Center and
Veterans Affairs Greater Los Angeles Healthcare
System
Los Angeles, California

Philip B. Gorelick, M.D.
Department of Neurological Sciences
Center for Stroke Research
Rush Medical Center and Rush Medical College
Chicago, Illinois

Edward G. Grant, M.D.
UCLA School of Medicine and
Veterans Affairs Greater Los Angeles Healthcare
System
Los Angeles, California

James C. Grotta, M.D.
Stroke Program and Program in Humanities and
Technology in Health Care
University of Texas/Houston Medical School
Houston, Texas

Linda A. Hershey, M.D.
Departments of Neurology and Pharmacology
Veterans Affairs Western New York Healthcare
System and
State University of New York at Buffalo
Buffalo, New York

Marion Ho, M.D.
Veterans Affairs Greater Los Angeles Healthcare
System
Los Angeles, California

Darryl L. Kaelin, M.D.
Department of Physical Medicine and Rehabilitation
Indiana University School of Medicine
Indianapolis, Indiana

Mary A. Kalafut, M.D.
Department of Neurology
UCLA Stroke Center
UCLA School of Medicine and Medical Center
Los Angeles, California

Sangeeta Rao Kashyap, M.D.
Department of Endocrinology and Metabolism
Veterans Affairs Greater Los Angeles Healthcare
System
Los Angeles, California

Vikram S. Kashyap, M.D.
Department of Surgery
UCLA Center for the Health Sciences
Los Angeles, California

Chelsea S. Kidwell, M.D.
Department of Neurology
UCLA Stroke Center
UCLA School of Medicine and Medical Center
Los Angeles, California

David Lefkowitz, M.D.
Department of Neurology
Wake Forest University School of Medicine
Winston-Salem, North Carolina

Seymour R. Levin, M.D.
Department of Endocrinology and Metabolism
Veterans Affairs Greater Los Angeles Healthcare System
Los Angeles, California

David S. Liebeskind, M.D.
Department of Neurology
UCLA Stroke Center
UCLA School of Medicine and Medical Center
Los Angeles, California

Alfred M. Lopez-Yunez, M.D.
Department of Neurology
Indiana University School of Medicine
Indianapolis, Indiana

Betsy Love, M.D.
Department of Neurology
Indiana University School of Medicine
Indianapolis, Indiana

Timothy G. Lukovits, M.D.
Neurosurgical and Neurological Group
Springfield, Massachusetts

Helmi L Lutsep, M.D.
Oregon Stroke Center
Oregon Health Sciences University
Portland, Oregon

Patrick D. Lyden, M.D.
Department of Neurology
Veterans Affairs Medical Center
San Diego, California

Amir Mohammadi, M.D.
Department of Neurology
University of Southern California School of Medicine
Los Angeles, California

Wesley S. Moore, M.D.
Department of Surgery
UCLA School of Medicine and Medical Center
Los Angeles, California

David M. Pelz, M.D., F.R.C.P.C.
Departments of Diagnostic Radiology and Clinical Neurological Sciences
The University of Western Ontario
London, Ontario, Canada

Stanley J. Reiser, M.D., M.P.A., Ph.D.
Stroke Program and Program in Humanities and Technology in Health Care
University of Texas/Houston Medical School
Houston, Texas

William A. Rock, Jr., M.D.
Department of Pathology
The University of Mississippi Medical Center
Jackson, Mississippi

Hamid R. Salari-Namin, M.D.
Veterans Affairs Greater Los Angeles Healthcare System
Los Angeles, California

Owen B. Samuels, M.D.
Department of Neurosurgery
Emory University School of Medicine
Atlanta, Georgia

Jeffrey L. Saver, M.D.
Department of Neurology
UCLA Stroke Center
UCLA School of Medicine and Medical Center
Los Angeles, California

Freddi Segal-Gidan, P.A., Ph.D.
Department of Neurological Sciences
Rancho Los Amigos Medical Center
Downey, California
University of Southern California School of Medicine
Los Angeles, California

Elyse J. Singer, M.D.
Department of Neurology and
Center for AIDS Research and Education (CARE)
UCLA School of Medicine
Los Angeles, California

Ravinder Singh, M.D.
Department of Neurosciences
Marin Luther King-Drew Medical Center
Charles R. Drew University of Medical Sciences
Los Angeles, California

George J. So, M.D., M.S.E.
Department of Radiological Sciences
UCLA School of Medicine and Medical Center
Los Angeles, California

Sidney Starkman, M.D.
Departments of Neurology and Emergency Medicine
UCLA Stroke Center
UCLA School of Medicine and Medical Center
Los Angeles, California

Daniel A. Streja, M.D., F.R.C.P.C., F.A.C.P
UCLA School of Medicine and Medical Center
Los Angeles, California

Shuichi Suzuki, M.D.
Department of Neurology
University of Southern California School of Medicine
Los Angeles, California

Hartmut Uschmann, M.D.
Department of Neurology
The University of Mississipi
Medical Center
Jackson, Mississippi

Panayiotis N. Varelas, M.D.
Department of Neurology
Yale University School of Medicine
New Haven, Connecticut

Fernando Viñuela, M.D.
Division of Interventional Neuroradiology
UCLA School of Medicine and Medical Center
Los Angeles, California

Engin Y. Yilmaz, M.D., Ph.D.
Department of Neurology
Indiana University School of Medicine
Indianapolis, Indiana

Justin A. Zivin, M.D.
Department of Neurology
Veterans Affairs Medical Center
San Diego, California

PREFACE

It was not that long ago that the role of a physician treating a stroke victim was limited to diagnosis and prognosis. The texts from that era had limited sections on stroke therapy with the recommendations based on anecdotal experience or consensus opinion. Therapeutic dogma was passed from generation to generation.

In the past few years, there has been an explosion of knowledge in stroke therapeutics. Many clinical trials have been published. Some are well-designed prospective, controlled, double-blinded trials and others are retrospective reports of sequential patients. Even some of the large prospective trials with statistically significant results are surrounded with controversy. The interpretation of these reports and implementation of the results into day-to-day practice are not easy tasks.

This text is an evidence-based practical guide to managing the ischemic stroke patient. Management of the stroke patient depends on when the patient is seen in relation to the onset of symptoms. Problems faced in the first 2 hours after stroke onset are very different from those faced 2 days post onset. These are different still from those 2 weeks after stroke onset. The text is organized to address this time progression. The chapters in Part 1 guide the physician according to when the patient's symptoms begin, starting with the 911 call, through the acute and subacute periods, and ending with the issues involved in management of the chronic problems facing the stroke survivor. Recognizing that stroke intervention is rapidly changing, Part 2 deals with evolving and controversial therapies. Part 3 deals with diagnosing some of the more common as well as some of the uncommon, nonatherosclerotic causes of ischemic stroke, and an evidence-based approach to treating them. Other issues in stroke management are the subject of Part 4, and Part 5 features an amply illustrated discussion of diagnostic testing and the uses and limitations of the imaging modalities commonly used in ischemic stroke management decision making.

This is not a reference text intended for only occasional use to look up an obscure topic. This text is written for use in day-to-day management decisions by emergency department physicians, internists, family physicians, neurologists, and neurology residents who care for complex patients with ischemic stroke.

The authors selected for this text are all nationally and internationally respected experts in the areas about which they are writing. Each is a physician-scientist who is actively involved in patient care as well as clinical research. I thank them for the timely preparation of the manuscripts and putting up with my frequent e-mails, faxes, and phone calls. I also thank my wife and family for tolerating my use of family time for the preparation of this text. And finally, I thank Dr. Wallace Tourtellotte, my mentor and friend, for teaching me to fish.

MANAGEMENT OF ISCHEMIC STROKE

Part 1
DIAGNOSIS AND MANAGEMENT OF ACUTE, SUBACUTE, AND CHRONIC STROKE

Chapter 1

THE ACUTE STROKE PATIENT: PREHOSPITAL STROKE IDENTIFICATION AND TREATMENT

Chelsea S. Kidwell
Jeffrey L. Saver
Sidney Starkman

INTRODUCTION, HISTORICAL BACKGROUND, AND ORGANIZATION OF EMERGENCY MEDICAL SERVICES

Emergency medical services (EMS) is the expansion of emergency medical care into the community, providing prehospital management for victims of sudden and serious illness or injury. This system relies on the accessibility and coordination of many elements, including an educated public capable of recognizing a medical emergency, a communications network, prompt dispatch of appropriate vehicles and personnel, hospital notification, and transfer to a medical center for definitive care. The universal 911 emergency telephone number, search and rescue teams, and prehospital and emergency department personnel are key ingredients required for the system to function.

A historical look at prehospital care demonstrates the dramatic evolution of the EMS response capabilities. In 1966, a National Academy of Sciences report, *Accidental Death and Disability: The Neglected Disease of Modern Society*, revealed that the average U.S. citizen, when injured, had a higher chance of survival in a Korean or Vietnamese combat zone than on the nation's highways.[1] At this time, few hospitals had emergency departments staffed by physicians, and patients were commonly transported to hospitals in vehicles operated by mortuary services. This report, documenting widespread deficiencies in emergency care, catalyzed the creation of the modern EMS system. In addition, Congress passed the 1966 National Highway Safety Act enabling the U.S. Department of Transportation to finance ambulances, communications, and training programs for prehospital medical services.

In 1973, public law 93-154 was created with the intent of improving emergency medical care and EMS on a national scale. This law described the 15 factors to be addressed in an EMS system: (1) manpower, (2) training, (3) communications, (4) transportation, (5) facilities, (6) critical care units, (7) public safety agencies, (8) consumer participation, (9) access to care, (10) transfer of care, (11) standardization of patient records, (12) public information and education, (13) independent review and evaluation, (14) disaster linkage, and (15) mutual aid agreements.[2] Individual state legislatures provide laws that define levels of ambulance service capability and requirements for training, equipment, physician leadership, and accountability. In most communities, the fire department coordinates emergency medical services, although other types of EMS organizations exist or may work in conjunction with the fire department (third service, private providers, volunteer services, hospital-based services). As the EMS has strong ties with both the police and fire departments, public safety officials have input into EMS councils, and EMS providers have input into public safety decisions that impact emergency medical care.

Emergency physicians are involved in providing medical control to ensure that the medical care provided is safe, effective, and in accordance with accepted standards. This control is characterized as either immediate "on-line" or "off-line," also called organizational control. On-line control involves the provision of medical orders to paramedics in the field either in person or by radio or telephone communication. The EMS medical director is responsible for staffing the emergency department (ED) with physicians that are familiar with the protocols that the paramedics use to administer care. Off-line medical control is assumed by the medical director and involves the development of standards, standing field protocols, quality assurance, and training programs for the ongoing educational needs of the prehospital care providers.[3]

Ground vehicles that are constructed and equipped according to federal standards deliver emergency patients to the nearest appropriate facility. Depending on the situation, dispatchers within tiered EMS systems can select from a variety of response modes, sending advanced life support (ALS) or basic life support (BLS) ambulances, sirens on or off, with or without first responders, supervisors, or physicians.[4] Responding personnel also vary in training level, from emergency medical technician-basics (EMT-Basics) to paramedics, distinguished by expanded knowledge base, their ability to utilize drugs, and additional emphasis on airway management.[5] Occasionally, air transport via helicopter or plane is used for transporting patients over long distances, decreasing total prehospital time and reaching patients in inaccessible locations, such as rural areas.[6] Designation of a facility as a trauma center or pediatric critical care center requires local political and logistic considerations, including availability of appropriate level of care, competing facilities, resources affecting transport time and distances, and ability to provide care to the next critically ill patient within the paramedic catchment area. In the 30 years since the establishment of the first federal EMS standards, efforts by the EMS providers have helped make the U.S. EMS highly advanced. As a result of this remarkable accomplishment, there is great opportunity to incorporate EMS personnel into present and future stroke management.

Recent advances in stroke research have now clearly demonstrated that "time is brain," and early stroke recognition and intervention is critical. The EMS is often the first medical contact for stroke patients, thereby playing a crucial part in the identification and treatment of acute stroke patients. Further, the recent availability of thrombolytic therapy for stroke patients presenting within 3 h of symptom onset has served to emphasize the significance of EMS response. Many more potential acute stroke treatments are on the hori-

zon. However, few stroke patients qualify for treatment because they present beyond the narrow therapeutic time window available for salvaging ischemic brain tissue. EMS organizations can reduce delays by alerting emergency stroke response teams and hospital personnel to expedite care for the stroke patient. The role of the EMS will involve rapid identification of acute stroke patients, expeditious transport to a definitive care facility, prenotification of the receiving hospital leading to activation of the stroke team, and, potentially, initiation of treatment in the field with neuroprotective agents. However, optimal utilization of the EMS for the treatment of acute stroke will necessitate many changes, requiring a fresh approach to stroke among prehospital personnel.

These changes are under way in many communities and include identifying methods to facilitate rapid transport and reduce delays, development of new tools or instruments devised to help EMS personnel recognize stroke, and large scale education of prehospital personnel. Although these changes pose logistic challenges, the reward would be well justified; for example, in acute myocardial infarction (MI), 33 percent of patients are treated with acute interventions (thrombolytics or reperfusion methods).[7] Moreover, prehospital identification of MI and early notification of the receiving hospital reduces time to initiation of thrombolytic therapy by 20 to 75 min.[8–10] Currently, however, prehospital programs lack sufficient instruction for the identification and treatment of stroke. A survey of paramedic education programs in the U.S. revealed that up to now the length of didactic, practical skills, laboratory, hospital clinical, and field internship portions of paramedic programs varies widely.[11] Furthermore, prehospital personnel training textbooks in the past have provided minimal stroke training (4 to 5 pages out of a 1000-page text) and have not stressed the time urgency of rapid evaluation and transport.[12–14]

Nevertheless, increasing the number of stroke patients eligible for thrombolytic treatment from current levels of 0.5 to 4 percent to that achieved in patients with acute MI is a worthy and achievable goal. Adapting from the approach used in acute MI, the emergency cardiac care *chain of survival,* Hazinski, Pepe, and others have proposed implementing a *stroke chain of survival or recovery.*[15–17] Using a seven-step approach, coined the "seven Ds," Hazinski's stroke chain of survival includes (Fig. 1-1): (1) detection of the onset of stroke signs and symptoms, (2) dispatch through activation of the EMS system and prompt EMS response, (3) delivery of the victim to the receiving hospital while providing appro-

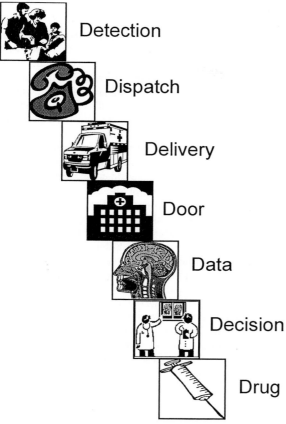

Detection

Dispatch

Delivery

Door

Data

Decision

Drug

Figure 1-1.
Stroke chain of survival: The seven "Ds."

priate prehospital assessment and care and pre-arrival notification, (4) door (emergency department triage), (5) data (emergency department evaluation, including head computed tomographic (CT) scan), (6) decision about potential therapies, and (7) drug therapy.[15] To be successful, each link in the chain must function efficiently; most significantly, acute stroke must be viewed by both patients and all medical personnel as an emergency similar to major trauma and acute MI. This chapter will focus on the first four "Ds," whereas later chapters will address the last three "Ds."

DELAYS TO PRESENTATION AND ACCESS TO STROKE MEDICAL CARE

The critical factor that prevents the majority of stroke patients from receiving thrombolytic therapy or partici-

pating in clinical trials of other acute stroke treatments is delayed time to presentation. In the National Institute of Neurologic Disease and Stroke (NINDS) study that led to Food and Drug Administration (FDA) approval of tissue plasminogen activator (tPA) for treatment of acute stroke, less than 4 percent of stroke patients that were screened actually qualified for treatment with thrombolytic therapy. The main reason for exclusion was presentation beyond the 3-h window for treatment.[18] Chiu and colleagues reported that only 6 percent of university hospital stroke patients and 1.1 percent of community hospital stroke patients received tPA in Houston during a 1-year period since thrombolytic therapy has been FDA approved. Delayed presentation was again the most common disqualifying reason for not being treated.[19]

Multiple studies have evaluated emergency department arrival times and reasons for delays to presentation in stroke patients. Median time to arrival to the ED from the time of symptom onset ranges from 4 to 10 h in various United States studies.[20,21] As few as 24 percent of patients arrive within 3 h of symptom onset,[22] increasing to 59 percent with public education campaigns.[23] Only 40 to 76 percent of stroke patients present within 6 h[23,24] and 42 to 88 percent within 24 h.[25,26] A study conducted in 36 academic U.S. medical centers in the current tPA era demonstrated that only 52 percent of ischemic stroke patients present within the first 24 h.[24] Similar studies conducted in other countries have also shown a wide variation in presentation times with 60 percent of patients presenting within 3 h in an Italian study[27] compared with 27 percent within 3 h in a study from the United Kingdom.[26] Across these studies, significant factors associated with delayed presentation included ischemic (vs. hemorrhagic) stroke, living alone, onset at night, private vehicle transport (vs. use of 911), first contact with personal physician, being retired, Caucasian race, female gender, and having a milder stroke.[21,24,28–45]

Currently, only 35 to 70 percent of all stroke patients are transported to the emergency department by emergency medical services.[23,34,46,47] This number approaches 60 percent for patients enrolled in hyperacute stroke studies who may have more severe strokes and may therefore be more likely to activate 911.[48] Porteous and co-workers found that of the 50 percent of acute stroke patients transported by 911 systems to two San Francisco hospitals, the most frequent presenting symptoms were language difficulty (30 percent), weakness (30 percent), and decreased ability to stand or walk (25 percent).[49] Approaches to increasing use of the 911 system and minimizing delays to presentation are discussed in the following sections.

DETECTION OF THE ONSET OF STROKE SIGNS AND SYMPTOMS

Background and Evidence

The first "D" in the stroke chain of survival or recovery is detection of stroke signs and symptoms by the patient, a family member, friend, or other bystander. Detection not only requires awareness of the signs and symptoms of stroke but also an understanding of the urgency for rapid medical attention and the importance of activating the 911 system. However, the majority of studies performed to date demonstrate that the public in general, and stroke patients in particular, have little knowledge about stroke.

Pancioli and colleagues performed a telephone survey of the general population in the greater Cincinnati area with a total of 1880 respondents.[49a] They found that only 57 percent of respondents correctly listed at least one of the five established stroke warning signs identified by the NINDS (sudden weakness or numbness of the face, arm, or leg; sudden dimness or loss of vision; sudden difficulty speaking or understanding speech; sudden severe headache with no known cause; unexplained dizziness, unsteadiness, or falls). Older patients (who are at the greatest risk for stroke) tended to be less knowledgeable about stroke. Kothari and colleagues interviewed 163 possible stroke patients admitted to the emergency department and found that 39 percent did not know a single sign or symptom of a stroke.[50] Of interest, Kothari et al also reported that patients with knowledge of signs and symptoms were *not* more likely to call 911 than those without stroke knowledge. In another study, over 48 percent of patients presenting with stroke did not recognize that they were having a stroke.[51] Williams and colleagues interviewed 67 stroke patients and found that only 25 percent correctly interpreted their symptoms.[22] Perhaps most astounding were the findings of a Gallup survey performed by the National Stroke Association in which 40 percent of the public did not know that a stroke occurs in the brain, and 42 percent could not identify weakness, numbness, or paralysis in the face, arm, or leg as a stroke symptom.[52]

Stroke awareness and knowledge has also been shown to be surprisingly deficient in patients at elevated risk for stroke and even with a personal history of cerebrovascular events. Samsa and colleagues surveyed 1253 patients at-risk for stroke and found that fewer than half (41 percent) were aware of their stroke risk.[53] Chaturvedi and Femino found that a group of patients with first-ever stroke (aphasic and demented patients were excluded) or transient ischemic attack (TIA) in an urban medical center scored worse on a stroke knowledge questionnaire than did a group of control patients.[54] Moreover, they seemed unfamiliar with the concept of a TIA. They also found that although patients with prior stroke were more likely to correctly interpret their symptoms, they were not more likely to present early.

Both small- and large-scale campaigns have been undertaken to educate the public about stroke. In the prethrombolytic era, Alberts and colleagues demonstrated that a community public education program could improve presentation within 24 h from 42 to 86 percent.[25] In the current thrombolytic era, Dornan and colleagues performed a baseline survey of stroke knowledge followed by a public stroke education campaign.[55] Following the campaign, they found a significant increase in public knowledge of stroke warning signs (ability to name one stroke warning sign increased from 57 to 78 percent). Women were found to be more knowledgeable about stroke at baseline and more likely to improve knowledge with education. The National Stroke Association Clinical Trials Accelerated Program found that centers provided with the tools for a public education program were more successful in enrolling patients in the trials.[56] In the NINDS tPA trial, study coordinators used a variety of educational techniques to increase public awareness about stroke. Anecdotal observations suggested a trend toward improved stroke awareness, and all participating centers were remarkably successful in recruiting patients within the narrow time windows.[57,58]

In the last few years, large-scale public stroke education programs have been sponsored by the National Stroke Association, the American Heart Association, and the National Institutes of Health. These programs emphasize recognition of stroke warning signs and stroke risk factors and the critical message that stroke is a medical emergency or "brain attack" (and that the 911 system should be activated if a stroke is suspected). The effect of these national educational programs is not yet clear, and simply increasing stroke awareness and knowledge may not necessarily translate into changing behavior with decreased delays to presentation. Although several large-scale education programs have been effective in changing behavior in the past (50 percent reduction in smoking in U.S., increased use of seatbelts, increased use of condoms with AIDS education),[59] educational campaigns geared to earlier response to chest pain have been largely unsuccessful at decreasing delays to seeking medical care with median time to arrival remaining at 3 h after symptom onset.[60]

Recommendations

Public education campaigns to increase public stroke knowledge and awareness should be continued. Physicians should take particular care to educate all at-risk patients and their families. These campaigns should include education regarding stroke risk factors as well as stroke warning signs and symptoms. The message should emphasize the time urgency for immediate medical attention, the availability of treatment for patients if given within a few hours, and the importance of activating the 911 system at the onset of a stroke. The NINDS consensus conference guidelines recommend large comprehensive programs with simple, clear messages delivered through a variety of communication techniques appropriately tailored to individual groups.[61]

DISPATCH

Background and Evidence

The second "D" in the stroke chain of survival is dispatch through activation of the EMS system and prompt EMS response. The importance of using the 911 system to optimize rapid transport for patients with acute stroke has been demonstrated in several studies. Barsan and colleagues found that patients who contacted their primary care physician arrived with a mean time of 379 min as compared with 179 min for patients who contacted 911 first.[23] Kothari et al reported that patients transported to the hospital by 911 were more likely to arrive within 3 h vs. those transported by private vehicle (47 vs. 19 percent, $p = .001$).[50] Another study by Zweifler et al reported data on the first 100 patients that triggered a stroke code system implemented in Mobile, AL. Forty-five percent of patients were transported by EMS, and these patients arrived nearly twice as quickly as those who used other means of transport.[36] Although Bratina and colleagues found no difference in arrival time between patients arriving by ambulance vs. private vehicle, they did find that ambulance arrivers were evaluated by ED personnel more rapidly.[34]

Once a 911 call is placed, the dispatcher becomes the first medical contact for the patient. Enhanced 911 systems (that automatically display the caller's address) have been adopted in many communities and may be of particular benefit to stroke patients who are dysarthric or aphasic. The dispatcher assesses the type and nature of the complaint, and based on this information makes the decision regarding dispatch priority and level of expertise (e.g., ALS or BLS), decisions which will impact hospital arrival time. The general medical supervision, training, and expertise among dispatchers varies from one community to another. Most EMS systems do not have an algorithm in place to help dispatchers identify acute stroke patients, and many communities continue to dispatch potential stroke patients at a lower level of emergency than patients with acute MI or trauma. In a study of 61 "911" calls for patients with a final diagnosis of stroke in San Francisco, Porteous and colleagues found that the dispatch code was "CVA (cerebrovascular accident)" in only 31 percent of calls, and the majority (59 percent) of ambulances were dispatched at low priority.[49] Even when the caller used the word "stroke," only half of these cases were dispatched as such. In addition to identifying potential stroke calls, dispatchers may play an important role in optimizing rapid transport by initiating pre-arrival instructions to the caller (confirm time of onset, prepare patient for transport, collect medical records and medications). The effectiveness of these techniques in reducing delays and increasing the number of patients eligible for acute treatment will require further study in the future.

Recommendations

911 operators and dispatchers should be educated to recognize the signs and symptoms of stroke. Medical supervision should be encouraged whenever possible. Enhanced 911 systems automatically displaying caller's address and telephone number should be adopted whenever feasible. Algorithms should be developed and validated to help dispatchers identify and prioritize potential stroke patients. Communities should recognize the urgency for rapid transport and upgrade acute stroke calls to high priority for rapid transport (particularly if the patient may be a candidate for thrombolytic therapy). Finally, pre-arrival instructions to help expedite rapid transport once prehospital personnel arrive should be developed for the dispatcher to provide to the caller and include confirming time of onset, preparing patient

for transport, and collecting medical records and medications.

DELIVERY

The third "D" in the stroke chain of survival is delivery of the patient to the receiving hospital while providing appropriate prehospital assessment and evaluation. For the stroke patient, optimal delivery requires (1) accurate stroke recognition by prehospital personnel, (2) appropriate in-field treatment, (3) notification of the receiving hospital, and (4) patient transport. Each phase of delivery provides opportunities to minimize delays and optimize rapid transport.

Stroke Identification

Background   As acute therapies are now available, prehospital personnel will likely play an increasingly important role in the initial evaluation and care of stroke patients. Accurate identification of stroke patients by prehospital personnel is important for a variety of reasons; appropriate treatment can be initiated in the field (and potentially detrimental or inappropriate treatment avoided), the receiving hospital can be notified, and rapid transport can be initiated. In the future, prehospital personnel may divert identified acute stroke patients from local hospitals to dedicated stroke critical care centers and may administer neuroprotective agents in the field. It should be emphasized that accurate identification requires not only a high degree of sensitivity but also a high positive predictive value.

Studies performed to date have demonstrated that the accuracy of stroke identification by prehospital personnel is variable from one community to another. Smith and colleagues found a sensitivity of only 61 percent for stroke recognition by prehospital personnel in San Francisco with a positive predictive value of 77 percent.[62] Hanson and colleagues collected data on two EMS ambulances transporting patients to two Minneapolis hospitals over a 6-month period.[63] They reported a 77 percent sensitivity and 88 percent specificity for ischemic stroke, improving to 94 percent sensitivity and 80 percent specificity if transient ischemic attacks and intracerebral hemorrhages were included. They found that posterior circulation events were more likely to be misdiagnosed. Zweifler and colleagues reported an even higher degree of accuracy for paramedics transporting patients to a university hospital in Alabama.[47] Prior to

an educational program, prehospital personnel correctly identified 29 of 32 (91 percent sensitivity) stroke patients and incorrectly identified 15 nonstroke patients as having a stroke (71 percent positive predictive value) prior to education. Following the educational intervention, sensitivity improved to 97 percent, yet positive predictive value remained modest at 78 percent. Finally, in a study from a suburban area of Reading, OH, Kothari and colleagues reported a positive predictive value of 72 percent.[64]

These results likely reflect variations in the stroke educational programs provided to prehospital personnel. However, in each of these studies, the positive predictive values remained modest, suggesting a tendency for prehospital personnel to overdiagnose stroke and not recognize stroke mimics. Improved rates of positive predictive values will be necessary in the future if stroke teams are activated based on prehospital evaluations to avoid "burn-out" or if neuroprotective agents are to be administered in the field. Several research groups have been developing programs designed specifically to aid paramedics and EMTs in identification of acute stroke patients in the field. These programs offer promising means of improving the ability of prehospital personnel to accurately and rapidly identify acute stroke patients in the field.

Evidence

Cincinnati Prehospital Stroke Scale   The Cincinnati Prehospital Stroke Scale (initially called the Out-of-Hospital National Institutes of Health Stroke Scale) is a three-item exam designed to aid prehospital personnel identify acute stroke patients. Kothari and colleagues derived the scale by analyzing National Institutes of Health Stroke Scale (NIHSS) findings in a retrospective stroke cohort.[65] These findings were recorded by physicians in the emergency department on 74 patients with acute ischemic stroke and compared with 225 nonstroke patients. The three components of the NIHSS found to be the most discriminating predictors of stroke were facial palsy, arm motor testing, and dysarthria. The investigators modified the third item to combine dysarthria and aphasia into a single item called "best language." In development of the scale, Kothari and colleagues found that the instrument retrospectively had a sensitivity of 100 percent and specificity of 88 percent when performed by a physician in the emergency department. In a subsequent report, physician vs. paramedic/EMT use of the scale was compared on 171 patients. The patients were examined by the physician while the paramedics/EMTs watched, and all recorded their findings. There was good correlation between prehospital providers and physicians on arm weakness but only fair correlation for facial droop and speech.[66] A prospective in the field validation study for the Cincinnati Prehospital Stroke Scale is needed.

Los Angeles Prehospital Stroke Screen The Los Angeles Prehospital Stroke Screen (LAPSS) was designed not only to identify acute stroke patients by exam but also to exclude likely stroke mimics and provide critical information required for the rapid evaluation and triage of acute stroke patients. The LAPSS (Fig. 1-2) is a one-page instrument that takes approximately 3 min to perform and consists of four history items, a blood glucose measure, and three exam items. The four history items and serum glucose measure exclude potential stroke mimics (history of seizure, hyperglycemia or hypoglycemia, patients wheelchair bound or bedridden with baseline deficits) or patients unlikely to qualify for acute stroke interventions or trials (onset >24 h, wheelchair bound or bedridden at baseline). The exam, intended to identify the most obvious and common types of stroke, tests for unilateral face, arm, and/or hand weakness. Eighty to ninety percent of stroke patients have unilateral motor weakness. The instrument is designed to emphasize not only sensitivity but also specificity and positive predictive value to identify the best candidates for prehospital activation of the stroke team and, in the future, in-field treatment. The LAPSS investigators reported that paramedics and EMTs-in-training can quickly and accurately be trained to use the LAPSS and can significantly improve general stroke knowledge with a brief LAPSS-based video training session.[67,68]

In a retrospective study, the LAPSS exam was applied to patients enrolled in hyperacute neuroprotective drug studies at three university-associated hospitals over 3 years.[48] LAPSS results were derived from NIHSS exams performed by physicians in the emergency department. Of the 48 total stroke patients arriving by ambulance, 44 were correctly identified by the LAPSS (92 percent sensitivity). The authors reported a calculated theoretical time-savings for paramedic initiation of a neuroprotective drug in the field ranging from 1 h and 32 min (for patients treated pre-CT) to 1 h and 59 min (for patients treated post-CT). In a prospective validation study, paramedics performed the LAPSS screening in the field on 1298 consecutively transported patients with neurologic complaints (36 strokes). Paramedic performance employing the LAPSS demonstrated sensitivity of 91 percent and positive predictive value of 86 percent. The positive predictive value improved to 97 percent after correction of documentation.[69]

TeleBAT An integrated mobile telecommunications system called TeleBAT is being researched as an aid in prehospital acute stroke evaluation.[70] This system has been pioneered by stroke investigators at the University of Maryland and uses wireless digital cellular communication. While en route to the emergency department, ambulance paramedics provide a hospital neurologist with real-time visual access to a patient's neurologic exam as well as transmission of vital signs. Prospective studies using the TeleBAT system are under way. This approach may not only shorten time to treatment but may also become an important component of stroke treatment in rural communities where early access to tertiary hospitals and stroke expertise is limited.

National Institutes of Health Stroke Scale In San Francisco, Smith and colleagues have reported results of a prehospital stroke education curriculum incorporating training and use of the NIHSS by prehospital personnel. Following a 4-h training session, stroke knowledge examination scores increased from 56 to 80 percent ($p < .01$).[71] Although paramedics' NIHSS ratings of video vignettes of stroke patients often differed from neurologists' ratings, scores generally fell within a 3-point range of each other. Gordon and colleagues have also trained paramedics to use the NIHSS.[71a] Because current stroke examination instruments such as the NIHSS are designed for physicians to document the type and severity of neurologic deficits in patients already diagnosed with stroke rather than for initial stroke identification, they may lack appeal for widespread use in the prehospital setting because of their relative complexity and long (>3 min) duration of administration. Stroke exam measures will likely be important for field treatment studies, however, to characterize the baseline pretreatment deficit. The utility and feasibility of their in-the-field administration awaits further study.

Recommendations All EMS systems should develop a stroke education protocol for prehospital personnel that includes education about common stroke signs and symptoms, common stroke mimics, and the need for urgent transport. The importance of determining the time of symptom onset should be emphasized. Prehospital stroke recognition instruments are in evolution. EMS

Los Angeles Prehospital Stroke Screen (LAPSS)

1. Patient Name: _____   _____
                              Last   *First*

2. Information/History from:
   [ ] Patient
   [ ] Family Member _____   Phone: _____
   [ ] Other   *Name*

3. Last known time patient was at baseline or deficit free and awake: *Military Time:* _____
                                                                          Date: _____

SCREENING CRITERIA:

		Yes	Unknown	No
4.	Age > 45	[ ]	[ ]	[ ]
5.	History of seizures or epilepsy **absent**	[ ]	[ ]	[ ]
6.	Symptom duration **less than** 24 hours	[ ]	[ ]	[ ]
7.	At baseline, patient is **not** wheelchair bound or bedridden	[ ]	[ ]	[ ]

		Yes	No
8.	Blood glucose between 60 and 400:	[ ]	[ ]

9. Exam: **LOOK FOR OBVIOUS ASYMMETRY**

	Normal	Right	Left
Facial Smile/Grimace:	☐	☐ Droop	☐ Droop
Grip:	☐	☐ Weak Grip	☐ Weak Grip
		☐ No Grip	☐ No Grip
Arm Strength:	☐	☐ Drifts Down	☐ Drifts Down
		☐ Falls Rapidly	☐ Falls Rapidly

Based on exam, patient has **only unilateral** (and not bilateral) weakness: Yes [ ]   No [ ]

10. ***Items 4,5,6,7,8,9 all YES's (or unknown) → LAPSS screening criteria met:***   Yes [ ]   No [ ]

11. If LAPSS criteria for stroke met, call receiving hospital with a "code stroke", if not then return to the appropriate treatment protocol. (Note: the patient may still be experiencing a stroke even if LAPSS criteria are not met.)

Figure 1-2.
Los Angeles Prehospital Stroke Screen (LAPSS).

organizations should consider use of a specific, prospectively validated stroke recognition instrument to improve prehospital stroke identification in the field.

Treatment in the Field

Background and Evidence The primary role of emergency medical services is to ensure that a patient is medically stable and transported to a medical facility for definitive care. Prehospital personnel generally take a rapid history including past medical history and current medications and then perform an abbreviated exam with emphasis on stabilizing the ABCs (airway, breathing, circulation).[17] Many EMS systems have developed standing field protocols individualized for different medical conditions that allow for basic medical interventions (e.g., starting peripheral intravenous (IV) access). Although these protocols vary from one community to another, in-field stroke treatments may include serum glucose measure, supplemental oxygen, or placement of a peripheral intravenous line. No data are available demonstrating the utility of supplemental oxygen in acute stroke patients, and the optimal oxygen saturation is not known. Increased oxygen may benefit ischemic regions but may also cause vasoconstriction and/or formation of oxygen-derived free radicals. Glucose should only be administered if serum glucose is measured and is <60–80. Supplemental glucose may otherwise lead to formation of lactic acid in ischemic zones, which has been demonstrated to worsen ischemia in animal stroke models.[72,73] Duldner and colleagues reported that implementation of an out-of-hospital stroke protocol improved evaluation and management of patients (increased initiation of IV access, pulse oximetry, and blood glucose measures).[74] Further studies will be necessary to determine if significant time-savings and improved patient outcomes result from these interventions.

Recommendations In-field evaluation and treatment by prehospital personnel may include (1) medical stabilization (ABCs), (2) recognition that a patient is having an acute stroke, (3) determining time of onset, (4) monitoring vital signs, (5) blood glucose measure, and (6) placement of peripheral intravenous access.

Hospital Notification and Transport

Background and Evidence Prehospital personnel may help minimize delays by notifying the receiving hospital that a stroke patient is being transported. This allows the receiving hospital to clear and ready a CT scanner (and call in technicians if needed) and to activate the stroke team in advance. No studies have been conducted in stroke patients to determine the time-savings of using this approach. However, in patients with acute myocardial infarction, significant reductions in time to treatment (from 130 min to 81 min) with thrombolytic agents were achieved by prehospital transmission of the electrocardiogram and prenotification to the receiving hospital.[75]

After the patient is evaluated and stabilized in the field, stroke patients should be rapidly transported to the emergency department. Upgrading potential thrombolytic candidates to a more rapid, higher level of transport (e.g., use of lights and/or sirens during ground transport) may decrease both transport and emergency department triage delays. However, use of lights and sirens and speedier transport increases risk of traffic accidents or injuries, which may outweigh any benefit achieved.

Recommendations Once an acute stroke patient has been identified, prehospital personnel should notify the receiving hospital, which in turn should ready the CT scanner and alert the stroke team. The patient should be immediately, safely, and expeditiously transported to the emergency department. The use of lights and sirens by ground transport ambulances has not been adequately studied to make specific recommendations.

DOOR

Background and Evidence

The fourth "D" in the stroke chain of survival is "Door," which stresses the role of rapid triage, evaluation, and early mobilization of resources once the patient has arrived to the emergency department. Historically, stroke patients were triaged in the ED as low priority as there was little that could be done acutely besides supportive care. Delays, therefore, occurred at many levels from triage, to nursing, to physician evaluation, to obtaining laboratory and other diagnostic tests, and to evaluation by a neurologist. To change this established pattern of response and sense of therapeutic nihilism, emergency departments are developing comprehensive plans for rapid evaluation and treatment of the stroke patient. These plans need to include ongoing education of personnel and establishment of designated stroke teams and protocols.[76]

Optimizing the care of the acute stroke patient in the emergency department requires a team approach. The team concept is of established value for treatment of patients with trauma and acute myocardial infarction[77–79] and can be appropriately applied to patients with stroke to shorten delays to treatment and potentially improve patient outcome. Bratina and colleagues demonstrated that implementation of a stroke team did in fact decrease interval delays (e.g., interval from ED arrival to CT completion was reduced from 139 to 50 min).[34] Similarly, Gomez and colleagues found that activation of the stroke team led to earlier neurologic consultation.[80] Englander and colleagues reported similar reductions in delays after implementation of a stroke team in a community hospital while employing continuous quality improvement methods for studying and identifying causes of delay and measuring improvement.[81] Finally, Davalos and colleagues demonstrated that, in their experience, early involvement of a neurologist (within 6 h) led to better patient outcome.[82]

Because the emergency department plays such a critical role in the initial evaluation and treatment of acute stroke patients in the current era of thrombolytic therapy, it has been suggested that patients only be transported to hospitals that have stroke expertise or at a minimum are capable of delivering tPA in a rapid and safe manner. The NINDS issued a consensus conference statement detailing the level of expertise needed for delivery of thrombolytic therapy.[83] These recommendations include (1) physician evaluation within 10 min of patient arrival in the emergency department, (2) notification of the stroke team within 15 min of arrival, (3) initiation of a head CT within 25 min of arrival, (4) interpretation of the CT scan within 45 min of arrival, (5) ensuring a door-to-drug (needle) time of 60 min from arrival in 80 percent of patients, and (6) transferring the patient to an in-patient setting within 3 h of arrival. Additionally, stroke expertise should be available within 15 min of hospital arrival for patients who meet thrombolytic treatment criteria and neurosurgical expertise within 2 h. In hospitals where a neurologist is not available within 15 min of arrival, emergency physicians may develop stroke expertise and successfully administer tPA.[84]

The concept of "stroke critical care centers" is gaining momentum in some communities. Similar to the "trauma center" model, stroke patients would be diverted from the closest medical facility to hospitals designated as stroke centers with proven capability of delivering thrombolytic therapy. Advantages of stroke centers include ensuring minimal level of expertise (such that all eligible patients who are candidates for thrombolytic therapy may be appropriately treated), improved methods of monitoring and measuring outcomes, standardized care, and access to research and newly emerging interventions including acute endovascular procedures. Disadvantages may include delays in transport, decreased access to care in rural areas, and logistic and political constraints. Another option involves linking community and rural hospitals to stroke centers using telemedicine (including phone). Alternatively, helicopter and air rescue services may be used in remote areas to rapidly transport acute patients to stroke centers. Individual communities and EMS systems will need to develop methods of designating which hospitals have minimal requirements for stroke care and devise plans for rapid transport to these hospitals for potential thrombolytic candidates. The concept of stroke critical care centers has not been widely or routinely implemented, and no data are available evaluating patient outcome using such a model.

Recommendations

The core stroke team should be identified and include emergency department nurses, emergency physicians, a neurologist, a radiologist trained in stroke CT interpretation, and a neurosurgeon. One of these members should be identified as the team leader. The extended team may include triage personnel, radiology technicians, pharmacists, and laboratory personnel. The core team members should either be available at all times in the emergency department or carry a "code stroke" or "brain attack" beeper. Suggested stroke protocols, flow charts, or algorithms may be developed and implemented, particularly for thrombolytic candidates. Each aspect of emergency department stroke care from triage, to nursing, to physician evaluation, to laboratory testing and head CT should be addressed. Triage for early identification of potential thrombolytic candidates is especially important. Members of the team should be provided with frequent stroke education updates. Figure 1-3 is a sample algorithm for outlining critical events in the emergency department evaluation and treatment of a stroke patient. Continuing medical education programs to re-enforce key messages as well as methods of quality assessment and reviews should be developed to evaluate the effectiveness of this approach and methods of improvement.

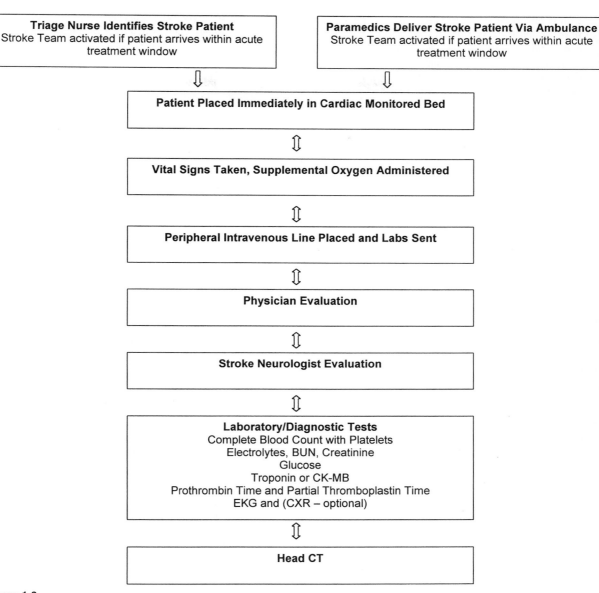

Figure 1-3.
Emergency department stroke patient evaluation and treatment (events often occur simultaneously).

CONCLUSION

Emergency medical services and prehospital personnel are assuming increasingly important roles in the evaluation and treatment of the acute stroke patient. A critical focus of this care is minimizing delays to presentation, which remain a significant stumbling block for treating the majority of stroke patients with thrombolytic therapy. Large-scale campaigns are under way to educate the public about stroke warning signs and the need for emergent medical care and activation of the 911 system. Emergency medical services should focus on educating dispatchers, EMTs, and paramedics about stroke and incorporate stroke recognition instruments and algorithms into their systems. New-onset, acute stroke patients should be transported at an appropriate high priority and to medical facilities capable of delivering optimal stroke care. Individual hospitals and emergency departments should develop stroke teams and stroke critical care pathways for rapid and appropriate treatment and evaluation. Emergency department and other involved personnel need continued stroke education. Finally, methods of outcome and quality assessment will need to be developed on a local and national level to monitor the effectiveness of various approaches to stroke care.

REFERENCES

1. National Academy of Sciences NRC: *Accidental Death and Disability: The Neglected Disease of Modern Society.* U.S. Dept. of Health, Education and Welfare, 1966.
2. US Senate, 93rd Congress, 1st Session. *Emergency Medical Services Act of 1973,* Report No. 93-397. Washington: US Government Printing Office, 1973.
3. Lilja GP, Swor R: Emergency Medical Services, in Tintinalli JE, Ruiz E, Krome RL (eds): *Emergency Medicine: A Comprehensive Study Guide.* New York, McGraw-Hill, 1997.
4. Zachariah BS, Dunford J, Van Cott CC: Dispatch life support and acute stroke patient: Making the right call, in Marler JR, Jones PW, Emr M (eds): *The National Institute of Neurological Disorders and Stroke: Proceedings of a National Symposium on Rapid Identification and Treatment of Acute Stroke: 1996.* Bethesda, MD, National Institute of Neurologic Disorders and Stroke, 1996.
5. Sayre MR, Swor RA, Honeycutt LK: Prehospital identification and treatment, in Marler JR, Jones PW, Emr M (eds): *The National Institute of Neurological Disorders and Stroke: Proceedings of a National Symposium on Rapid Identification and Treatment of Acute Stroke: 1996.* Bethesda, MD, National Institute of Neurologic Disorders and Stroke, 1996.
6. Benson NH, Prasad NH, Rural EMS: in Tintinalli JE, Ruiz E, Krome RL (eds): *Emergency Medicine: A Comprehensive Study Guide.* New York, McGraw-Hill, 1997, pp 7–10.
7. Genentech I: *National Registry of Myocardial Infarction II (NMRI II).* Quarterly Data Report, 1996.
8. Linderer T, Schroder R, Arntz R, et al: Prehospital thrombolysis: Beneficial effects of very early treatment on infarct size and left ventricular function. *J Am Coll Cardiol* 22:1304, 1993.
9. Weaver WD, Cerqueira M, Hallstrom AP, et al: Prehospital-initiated vs hospital-initiated thrombolytic therapy: The Myocardial Infarction Triage and Intervention Trial. *JAMA* 270:1211, 1993.
10. Foster DB, Dufendach JH, Barkdoll CM, Mitchell BK: Prehospital recognition of AMI using independent nurse/ paramedic 12-lead ECG evaluation: Impact on in-hospital times to thrombolysis in a rural community hospital. *Am J Emerg Med* 12:25, 1994.
11. Margolis GS, Stoy WA: The length of paramedic education programs in the United States. *JEMS* S21, 1998.
12. Crosby LA, Lewallen DG: American Academy of Orthopaedic Surgeons: *Emergency Care and Transportation of the Sick and Injured.* 6th ed. Rosemont, IL, American Academy of Orthopaedic Surgeons, 1997.
13. Bledsoe BE, Cherry RA, Porter RS: *Brady Intermediate Emergency Care.* Upper Saddle River, NJ, Brady Prentice Hall, 1991.
14. Grant HD: *Brady Emergency Care.* 7th ed. Englewood Cliffs, NJ, Brady Prentice Hall Education Career & Technology, 1995.
15. Hazinski MF: Demystifying recognition and management of stroke. *Curr Emerg Cardiac Care* 7:8, 1996.
16. Pepe PE, Zachariah BS, Sayre MR, Floccare D: Ensuring the chain of recovery for stroke in your community. *Acad Emerg Med* 5:352, 1998.
17. American Heart Association: Acute stroke, in *Advanced Cardiac Life Support.* Dallas, TX, 1997.
18. The National Institute of Neurological Disorders and Stroke rt-PA Stroke Study Group: Tissue plasminogen activator for acute ischemic stroke. *N Engl J Med* 333:1581, 1995.
19. Chiu D, Krieger D, Villar-Cordova C, et al: Intravenous tissue plasminogen activator for acute ischemic stroke: Feasibility, safety, and efficacy in the first year of clinical practice. *Stroke* 29:18, 1998.
20. Feldmann E, Gordon N, Brooks JM, et al: Factors associated with early presentation of acute stroke. *Stroke* 24:1805, 1993.
21. Kwiatkowski T, Silverman R, Palano R, Libman R: Delayed hospital arrival in patients with acute stroke (Abstract). *Acad Emerg Med* 3:538, 1996.
22. Williams LS, Bruno A, Rouch D, Marriott DJ: Stroke patients' knowledge of stroke: Influence on time to presentation. *Stroke* 28:912, 1997.
23. Barsan WG, Brott TG, Broderick JP, Haley EC, Levy DE, Marler JR: Time of hospital presentation in patients with acute stroke. *Arch Intern Med* 1993:2558, 1993.
24. Kennedy B, Lichtman JH, Fayad PB, Cerese J, Krumholz HM, Brass LM: Clinical factors influencing time to admission (Abstract). *Stroke* 29:313, 1998.
25. Alberts MJ, Perry A, Dawson DV, Bertels C: Effects of public and professional education on reducing the delay in presentation and referral of stroke patients. *Stroke* 23:352, 1992.
26. Harper GD, Haigh RA, Potter JF, Castleden CMI: Factors delaying hospital admission after stroke in Leicestershire. *Stroke* 23:835, 1992.
27. Pistollato G, Ermani M: Time of hospital presentation after stroke: A multicenter study in northeast Italy. Italian SINV (Societa Interdisciplinare Neurovascolare) Study group. *Ital J Neurol Sci* 17:401, 1996.

28. Kay R, Woo J, Poon WS: Hospital arrival time after onset of stroke. *J Neurol Neurosurg Psychiatry* 55:973, 1992.
29. Lago A, Geffner D, Temble J, Vilar C: Hospital arrival time after acute stroke: A study in Valencia (Spain). *Cerebrovasc Dis* 6:32, 1996.
30. Anderson NE, Broad JB, Bonita R: Delays in hospital admission and investigation in acute stroke. *Br Med J* 311:162, 1995. Erratum: *Br Med J* 311:545, 1995.
31. Kolominsky PL, Heuschmann P, Ellul J, Barer DH, on behalf of the European Stroke Database Collaboration: Delays in admission to hospital for acute stroke: An international comparison (Abstract). *Cerebrovasc Dis* 6:178, 1996.
32. Eriksson S, Asplund K, Hägg E, Lithner F, Strand T, Wester PO: Clinical profiles of cerebrovascular disorders in a population-based patient sample. *J Chronic Dis* 40:1025, 1987.
33. Fogelholm R, Murros K, Rissanen A, Ilmavirta M: Factors delaying hospital admission after acute stroke. *Stroke* 27:398, 1996.
34. Bratina P, Greenberg L, Pasteur W, Grotta JC: Current emergency department management of stroke in Houston, Texas. *Stroke* 26:409, 1995.
35. Kothari RU, Sauerback L, Jauch EC, et al: Acute stroke: Delays to presentation and the patient's perceptions (Abstract). *Stroke* 29:314, 1998.
36. Zweifler RM, Drinkard R, Cunningham S, Brody ML, Rothrock JF: Implementation of a stroke code system in Mobile, Alabama: Diagnostic and therapeutic yield. *Stroke* 28:981, 1997.
37. Duncan P, Lai SM, Keigly J, Rymer R: Time to medical attention after a mild to moderate stroke (Abstract). *Stroke* 29:312, 1998.
38. Morris DL, Gorton RA, Hinn AR, Hohenhaus SM, Rosamond WD: Delay in seeking care for stroke-demographic determinants: The delay in accessing stroke (Abstract). *Acad Emerg Med* 3:539, 1996.
39. Foulkes MA, Wolf PA, Price TR, Mohr JP, Hier DB: The Stroke Data Bank: Design, methods, and baseline characteristics. *Stroke* 19:547, 1988.
40. Streifler JY, Davidovitch S, Sendovski U: Factors associated with the time of presentation of acute stroke patients in an Israeli community hospital. *Neuroepidemiology* 17:161, 1998.
41. Smith MA, Doliszny KM, Shahar E, McGovern PG, Arnett DK, Luepker RV: Delayed hospital arrival for acute stroke: The Minnesota Stroke Survey. *Ann Intern Med* 129:190, 1998.
42. Azzimondi G, Bassein L, Fiorani L, et al: Variables associated with hospital arrival time after stroke: Effect of delay on the clinical efficiency of early treatment. *Stroke* 28:537, 1997. Erratum: *Stroke* 28:1092, 1997.
43. Menon SC, Pandey DK, Morgenstern LB: Critical factors determining access to acute stroke care. *Neurology* 51:427, 1998.
44. Ferro JM, Melo TP, Oliveira V, et al: An analysis of the admission delay of acute strokes. *Cerebrovasc Dis* 4:72, 1994.
45. Saver JL, Bruno A, Feldmann E, et al: Time from stroke onset to arrival in the hospital (Abstract). *J Stroke Cerebrovasc Dis* 6:146, 1996.
46. Tirshwell DL, Longstreth WT, Kukull WA, Beekly DL, Cobb LA, Copass MK: Prehospital care of stroke in Seattle, Washington: A population-based study (Abstract). *Stroke* 29:313, 1998.
47. Zweifler RM, York D, U TT, Mendizabal JE, Rothrock JF: Accuracy of paramedic diagnosis of stroke. *J Stroke Cerebrovasc Dis* 7:446, 1998.
48. Kidwell CS, Saver JL, Schubert GB, Eckstein M, Starkman S: Design and retrospective analysis of the Los Angeles Prehospital Stroke Screen (LAPSS). *Prehosp Emerg Care* 2:267, 1998.
49. Porteous FH, Corry M, Smith WS: Emergency medical dispatcher identification of stroke and TIA victims (Abstract). *Stroke* 29:314, 1998.
49a. Pancioli AM, Broderick J, Kothari R, et al: Public perception of stroke warning signs and knowledge of potential risk factors. *JAMA* 279:1288, 1998.
50. Kothari R, Sauerbeck L, Jauch E, et al: Patients' awareness of stroke signs, symptoms, and risk factors. *Stroke* 28:1871, 1997.
51. Barsan WG, Brott TG, Olinger CP, Adams HP, Jr, Haley EC, Jr, Levy DE: Identification and entry of the patient with acute cerebral infarction. *Ann Emerg Med* 17:1192, 1988.
52. National Stroke Association. Stroke remains a deadly mystery to many Americans. *Be Stroke Smart* 13:2, 1996.
53. Samsa GP, Cohen SJ, Goldstein LB, et al: Knowledge of risk among patients at increased risk for stroke. *Stroke* 28:916, 1997.
54. Chaturvedi S, Femino L: A pilot study regarding knowledge of stroke risk factors in an urban community. *J Stroke Cerebrovasc Dis* 6:426, 1997.
55. Dornan WA, Stroink AR, Pegg EE, et al: Community Stroke Awareness Program increases public knowledge of stroke (Abstract). *Stroke* 29:288, 1998.
56. Todd HW: Lessons from current and previous stroke public education campaigns, in Marler JR, Jones PW, Emr M (eds): *Proceedings of a National Symposium on Rapid Identification and Treatment of Acute Stroke: 1997.* Bethesda, MD, National Institute of Neurologic Disorders and Stroke, 1997.
57. Barsan WG, Brott TG, Broderick JP, Haley EC, Jr, Levy DE, Marler JR: Urgent therapy for acute stroke: Effects of a stroke trial on untreated patients. *Stroke* 25:2132, 1994.
58. Daley S, Braimah J, Sailor S, et al: Education to improve stroke awareness and emergent response: The NINDS rt-PA Stroke Study Group. *J Neurosci Nurs* 29:393, 1997.
59. Maibach EW: Lessons for success in public education campaigns, in Marler JR, Jones PW, Emr M (eds): *Proceedings of a National Symposium on Rapid Identification and Treat-*

ment of Acute Stroke: 1997. Bethesda, MD, National Institute of Neurologic Disorders and Stroke, 1997.

60. Ho MT, Eisenberg MS, Litwin PE, Schaeffer SM, Damon SK: Delay between onset of chest pain and seeking medical care: The effect of public education. *Ann Emerg Med* 18:727, 1989.

61. Spilker JA: The importance of patient and public education in acute ischemic stroke, in Marler JR, Jones PW, Emr M (eds): *Proceedings of a National Symposium on Rapid Identification and Treatment of Acute Stroke: 1997*. Bethesda, MD, 1997.

62. Smith WS, Isaacs M, Corry MD: Accuracy of paramedic identification of stroke and transient ischemic attack in the field. *Prehosp Emerg Care* 2:170, 1998.

63. Hanson S, Adlis S, Weaver A, Porth K, Koller R: Accuracy of prehospital stroke diagnosis: Treatment implications (Abstract). *Stroke* 26:157, 1995.

64. Kothari R, Barsan W, Brott T, et al: Frequency and accuracy of prehospital diagnosis of acute stroke. *Stroke* 26:937, 1995.

65. Kothari R, Hall K, Brott T, Broderick J: Early stroke recognition: Developing an out-of-hospital NIH stroke scale. *Acad Emerg Med* 4:986, 1997.

66. Kothari RU, Pancioli A, Liu T, Brott T, Broderick J: Cincinnati prehospital stroke scale: Validity and reproducibility (Abstract). *Stroke* 29:313, 1998.

67. Kidwell CS, Saver JL, Revels S, Kolodaro G, Starkman S: High accuracy of emergency medical technician identification of stroke using the Los Angeles prehospital stroke screen (LAPSS) (Abstract). *Stroke* 29:313, 1998.

68. Kidwell CS, Saver JL, Eckstein M, Kalafut M, Weems K, Starkman S: Improving paramedic recognition of stroke in the field: A Los Angeles prehospital stroke screen (LAPSS) training program (Abstract). *Neurology* 50:157, 1998.

69. Kidwell CS, Starkman S, Eckstein M, Weems K, Saver JL: Identifying stroke in the field: Prospective validation of the Los Angeles Prehospital Stroke Screen (LAPSS) *Stroke* 1999 (*in press*).

70. LaMonte MP, Xiao Y, Mackenzie CF, Cullen JS, Gagliano DM: Tele-BAT: Mobile telemedicine for the brain attack team (Abstract). *Stroke* 29:312, 1998.

71. Smith WS, Corry MD, Fazackerley J, Isaacs M: Paramedic accuracy in the application of the NIH stroke scale to victims of stroke (Abstract). *Acad Emerg Med* 4:379, 1997.

71a. Gordon DL, Issenberg SB, LaCombe DM, et al: Prehospi-

tal provider training in management of acute stroke. *Stroke* 30:265, 1999.

72. Wass CT, Lanier WL: Glucose modulation of ischemic brain injury: Review and clinical recommendations. *Mayo Clin Proc* 71:801, 1996.

73. Li PA, Kristián T, Shamloo M, Siesjö K: Effects of preischemic hyperglycemia on brain damage incurred by rats subjected to 2.5 or 5 minutes of forebrain ischemia. *Stroke* 27:1592, 1996.

74. Duldner JE, Burlle AM, Costello MS, et al: Effect of a stroke protocol on management of out-of-hospital stroke patients (Abstract). *Acad Emerg Med* 5:440, 1998.

75. Kereiakes DJ, Gibler WB, Martin LH, Pieper KS, Anderson LC: Relative importance of emergency medical system transport and the prehospital electrocardiogram on reducing hospital time delay to therapy for acute myocardial infarction: A preliminary report from the Cincinnati Heart Project. *Am Heart J* 123:835, 1992.

76. McDowell FH, Brott TG, Goldstein M, et al: Stroke: The first six hours. National Stroke Association consensus statement. *Stroke Clin Updates* 14:1, 1993.

77. Petrie D, Lane P, Stewart TC: An evaluation of patient outcomes comparing trauma team activated versus trauma team not activated using TRISS analysis: Trauma and injury severity score. *J Trauma* 41:870, 1996.

78. Driscoll PA, Vincent CA: Organizing an efficient trauma team. *Injury* 23:107, 1992.

79. Markel KN, Marion SA: CQI: Improving the time to thrombolytic therapy for patients with acute myocardial infarction in the emergency department. *J Emerg Med* 14:685, 1996.

80. Gomez CR, Malkoff MD, Sauer CM, Tulyapronchote R, Burch CM, Banet GA: Code stroke: An attempt to shorten inhospital therapeutic delays. *Stroke* 25:1920, 1994.

81. Englander EN, Morich DH, Minniti MM: Accelerating the evaluation of acute stroke patients in a community hospital (Abstract). *Neurology* 50:A114, 1998.

82. Davalos A, Castillo J, Martinez-Vila E: Delay in neurological attention and stroke outcome. Cerebrovascular Diseases Study Group of the Spanish Society of Neurology. *Stroke* 26:2233, 1995.

83. Bock BF: Response system for patients presenting with acute stroke, in Marler JR, Jones PM, Emr M (eds), *Proceedings of a National Symposium on Rapid Identification and Treatment of Acute Stroke: 1997*. Bethesda, MD, 1997.

84. Broderick JP: Logistics in acute stroke management. *Drugs* 54(Suppl 3):109, 1997.

Chapter 2

THE ACUTE STROKE PATIENT: THE FIRST SIX HOURS

Mary A. Kalafut
Jeffrey L. Saver

INTRODUCTION

The time window for effective therapy in acute ischemic stroke is all too brief. The period of reversibility of ischemic brain injury varies from patient to patient, reflecting interindividual variations in the severity of blood flow compromise. In all but the most exceptional patient, however, threatened tissue is no longer salvageable much beyond 6 h after symptom onset. Actions taken in the first few hours of stroke will determine the quality of patients' existences for the rest of their lives. In these critical hours, prompt, efficient diagnosis and management can tip the balance between mild impairment and devastation.

In the past, stroke was not considered a medical emergency, and intervening to change the course of patients functional outcome was considered impossible. As a result, effective treatment remained elusive. Recently, several centers have shown that stroke patients can be reliably diagnosed and treated as rapidly as within 90 min of onset.[1–3] This chapter will focus on the critical interventions for the acute ischemic stroke patient within the first few hours.

THE PATHOPHYSIOLOGY OF BRAIN ISCHEMIA

Because the brevity of the time window for salvage of ischemic tissue is of such paramount importance in designing acute treatment strategies, it is worthwhile to briefly review physiologic data that have defined this duration.

Changes in cerebral blood flow result in a continuum of metabolic and ionic disturbances that occur in a predictable order. Studies in animal models of focal stroke suggest that as blood flow declines initially, protein synthesis begins to decrease at values that are close to normal (40 to 50 mL/100 g/min), followed by anaerobic glycolysis (35 mL/100 g/min), loss of synaptic transmission (20 mL/100 g/min), and finally anoxic depolarization of cell membranes (15 mL/100 g/min).[4] These observations in stroke animal models have been supported by human positron emission tomography (PET) studies of the relationship between blood flow and neuronal compromise. Regional cerebral blood flow (rCBF) below 12 mL/100 g/min results in necrosis, whereas only transient deficits occur when rCBF remains above 22 mL/100 g/min.[5] Tissue with rCBF between 12 and 22 mL/100 g/min represents the ischemic penumbra, an area of stunned parenchyma surrounding the ischemic core, which has the potential for recovery, but only if reperfusion is rapidly established.

In addition to the magnitude of blood flow reduction, the length of time cells are ischemic also determines viability. Numerous studies indicate the threshold for metabolic and ionic disturbance increases as the duration of ischemia increases.[4] For example, studies have shown that during the first 2 h of vascular occlusion the threshold for irreversible suppression of spontaneous neuronal unit activity rises from 5 to 12 mL/100 g/min.[6] Other studies have shown that when ischemia lasts only a few hours, brain tissue is able to survive flows as low as 12 mL/100 g/min. However, if the ischemia is permanent, brain necrosis occurs in regions with flows as high as 24 mg/100 g/min.[4] Thus, the viability of the ischemic area is in flux in the first few hours after stroke onset, its fate determined by the extent and duration of impaired blood flow. However, this dynamic period of potential reversibility is evanescent. Studies in a large number of rodent and nonhuman primate stroke models demonstrate that, in general, significant volumes of neuronal tissue can be salvaged by reperfusion only within the first 4 to 6 h of ischemia onset.[7]

STROKE RAPID RESPONSE SYSTEMS/ STROKE TEAMS/CODE STROKE

Background

Time is of the essence in acute ischemic stroke care. In the often hectic environment of an emergency receiving facility, multiple diagnostic procedures must be performed and interpreted, and several therapeutic interventions must be carried out as rapidly as possible. Several hospital programs must work in smooth coordination, including emergency medicine, neurology, primary care medicine, radiology, pharmacy, nursing, and the clinical laboratories. To marshal these forces efficiently requires forethought, planning, and an organized approach to care. Many terms have been applied to acute stroke care protocols, including "stroke teams," "brain attack teams," "code stroke," "rapid response systems," and acute stroke care "clinical pathway" or "care map."[2,8–14] Under whatever rubric, the essence of the process is to bring key representatives of all participating hospital programs together, draw up protocols for rapid response, establish process targets of care, continuously monitor performance, identify areas of delay, and iteratively innovate to improve response efficiency. This approach is modeled after the successful acute care systems that have been developed to care for patients with trauma and myocardial infarction.[15,16]

The most important aspects of a well-run stroke team are communication and education. Communication is facilitated by establishing a stroke code beeper system that alerts team members through interconnected beepers that are united by one common access number. When the access number is dialed, all pagers in the network are activated simultaneously. This allows for early notification of all stroke team members.[9]

The stroke team includes not only physicians but also prehospital personnel and members of the ancillary staff. In the field, the medical personnel who first encounter the patient are paramedics and emergency medical technologists. Participation by these members of the team is of paramount importance because their advance notice allows other team members to prepare for the patient's arrival.[17] Ideally, stroke team members will be notified far enough in advance so they can meet the patient upon arrival in the emergency room and clear the CT scanner for rapid imaging. Hospital-based members of the stroke team include triage nurses, emergency department nurses, emergency department physicians, neurologists, radiologists, and interventional neuroradiologists. Ancillary personnel including CT technologists, pharmacists, and laboratory personnel are also essential in delivering streamlined care.

The development of an effective management protocol begins with participation by all members of the team. Each hospital is unique, with its own set of strengths and weaknesses that must be taken into account when building a protocol.[18] Nevertheless, certain universal strategies are important in implementing a well-run protocol. First, it is important to involve team members early in the process by asking them what aspects of the protocol may be problematic and how these difficulties could be avoided.

Once a protocol has been completed, it is useful to organize it in flow-chart form, making it easy to follow in an emergency situation. Several in-service meetings may be necessary for team members to modify and become familiar with the protocol. Because of the small number of acute stroke patients, the protocol may not be carried out often enough for team members to remain familiar with it. This makes periodic retraining essential for maintaining a well-run stroke team.

As the protocol is utilized, alterations are usually required to improve upon the system. These changes may require extra resources, such as a dedicated person to deliver blood work. One of the most common administrative difficulties surrounds the CT scan. Setting up guidelines for weekend and night coverage by the CT technician prevents unnecessary delays. In addition, it is imperative to establish a policy that acute stroke patients are to be treated emergently and must be given top priority for the scanner.

Providing feedback to all team members after each code is essential to improving response time. This is the time to reinforce the parts of the protocol that were run well and to brainstorm about ways to improve on deficiencies.

Evidence

No randomized trials have compared stroke rapid response team care with conventional care of acute ischemic stroke. Relevant data are available from observational series reporting experience with stroke rapid response teams, often with historical control comparator data.

In a study of eight Houston-area hospitals, the presence of a stroke team was associated with a reduction in the time from Emergency Department (ED) arrival to physician exam from 28 min to 15 min, and in elapsed time from ED arrival to CT scan from 100 min to 37 min.[8] In St. Louis, implementation of a code stroke beeper system shortened the mean time from ED arrival to physician evaluation from 25 min to 4.8 min ($p < .05$) and from ED arrival to treatment initiation from 42 min to 30 min ($p = .06$).[9] The successful hyperacute therapy National Institute of Neurological Disorders and Stroke (NINDS)-TPA trials were undergirded by a study-wide systematic protocol for early patient evaluation.[2]

Consensus time guidelines for the evaluation and treatment of acute stroke patients have been proposed by the NINDS-sponsored National Symposium on the Rapid Identification and Treatment of Acute Stroke.[19] These guidelines recommend the following time intervals between stroke patient arrival and action: physician evaluation of patient, 10 min; consultation with a specialist with stroke expertise, 15 min; CT scan obtained, 25 min; CT scan interpreted, 45 min; if indicated, thrombolytic therapy initiated, 60 min; hospital admission to a closely monitored unit, 3 h. The door to needle time of 60 min for thrombolytic stroke therapy, and each of the other intervals, is to be obtained at least 80 percent of the time (Table 2-1).

Table 2-1.
NINDS recommended time guidelines for acute ischemic stroke management

Time from ED arrival to task completion	
Door to physician	10 min
Door to neurologic expertise[a]	15 min
Door to CT completion	25 min
Door to CT interpretation	45 min
Door to thrombolytic treatment, if appropriate	60 min
Door to neurosurgical expertise[a]	2 h
Door to monitored bed	3 h

[a]By phone or in person.

CT, computed tomography.

Recommendations

Every hospital should develop a stroke rapid response evaluation and treatment plan that takes into account local resources, strengths, and limitations. Goals that should be universal across all hospitals are (1) obtaining a CT within 25 min of patient arrival and (2) a door to needle time for thrombolytic therapy of 60 min. A continuous performance improvement process should monitor the achievement of time interval targets and the quality of delivered therapies and promote serial improvement in treatment algorithms. A designated "stroke team" and a "code stroke" beeper system may be helpful in accelerating changes in care and rapid response.

EVALUATION OF THE ACUTE STROKE PATIENT

The goals of the initial evaluation are to (1) determine if an immediate complication is likely, (2) confirm that ischemic stroke and not a mimic is the cause of the focal deficit, (3) assess the reversibility of the pathology, (4) obtain clues to the likely vascular mechanism and etiology, and (5) institute appropriate treatment.[19,20]

The first step in the evaluation is not different than with any other critically ill patient. The ABCs (airway, breathing, circulation) should be rapidly assessed to ensure patient stability.[19–21] The first priority is to provide resuscitation if there is any airway, ventilatory, or hemodynamic compromise. Once these essential areas are assessed, and treated if necessary, the patient can be specifically evaluated for cerebral ischemia.

History

Obtaining an accurate history in a rapid fashion is an important skill in treating acute stroke patients. Often, the history will need to be obtained serially. A brief 5-min synopsis from the most cogent observer is sufficient to guide ordering of initial diagnostic and therapeutic studies. When these are under way, a more thorough history can be elicited from the patient and all other available witnesses.

Establishing the time of stroke onset is especially important because it determines available treatment options. Information should be sought from the patient, family members, and anyone who was with the patient at the time of ictus. It may be necessary to call witnesses who did not accompany the patient to the hospital. Asking pointed questions can help witnesses more accurately pinpoint the onset time. For instance, members of the NINDS TPA trial found it helpful to ask if the patient was watching television at the time of onset and kept a listing of TV program times in the Emergency Department as a guidepost to determine stroke onset (personal communication, P. Lyden, 1997). When onset cannot be specified precisely, the ischemia duration clock is started from the time the patient was last known to be well. This convention applies to patients who awake with their deficits, who are found down and uncommunicative, or who simply are unable to clearly communicate when their deficit started. For example, time of onset for patients who awake from sleep with new deficits is assumed to be the time they went to sleep. Consequently, the 31 percent of ischemic stroke patients who awake from sleep with their deficit are generally not candidates for thrombolytic stroke therapy.[22]

Other essential history questions focus on ruling out stroke mimics and provisionally characterizing the stroke mechanism. Seizures, intoxications, head trauma, and acute systemic infections must be ruled out.[23] The presence of cervical trauma and neck pain may point toward a diagnosis of dissection. Headaches and nausea raise the possibility of intracerebral hemorrhage or brainstem infarction. The tempo of deficit onset is ascertained. Registry studies suggest that strokes with maximum disability at onset but without headache are most often found to be embolic whether cardiac or artery-to-artery, whereas those with a fluctuating course are more likely owing to thrombosis.[24–27] A history of multiple prior transient ischemic attacks (TIAs) in the same circulation suggests an atherothrombotic mechanism. A steadily expanding deficit over 5 to 20 min is typical of intracerebral hemorrhage.

Inquiring about previous medical conditions also sheds light on the stroke mechanism. Patients suffering from cardiac disease including arrhythmia, valvular disease, ventricular aneurysm, patent foramen ovale, and congestive heart failure are prone to cardioembolic events. A history of hypertension, coronary artery disease, tobacco use, diabetes, or claudication is associated with large vessel atherothrombosis. Hypertension and to a lesser degree tobacco use and diabetes also are often seen in lacunar infarcts.[28]

In addition, the ethnic background of the patient can point to a possible stroke etiology. African-American, Chinese, and Japanese populations have a relatively high incidence of intracerebral hemorrhage and intracranial atherosclerotic disease.[29] White populations are more likely to have extracranial atherosclerotic disease and cardiac disease.[30,30a]

Physical Examination

The initial physical examination should be strategic rather than exhaustive and need not exceed 10 min. The goals of the initial exam are to determine patient level of consciousness, stroke severity, stroke localization, and stroke etiology.[19,23,31]

Careful neurovascular examination includes auscultating the heart for the presence of gallops, murmurs, or dysrhythmias. The peripheral vascular system is interrogated by palpating the radial, femoral, and pedal pulses to determine strength and regularity. The carotid artery is palpated and the neck auscultated for bruits. It should be borne in mind that bruits are caused not only by local narrowing of the internal carotid artery but also by stenosis of the external and common carotid artery, by hyperdynamic states, and by other causes of turbulant flow.

The fundoscopic exam provides a unique opportunity to visualize blood vessels. Signs of internal carotid artery disease include cholesterol crystals, retinal infarctions, and venous stasis retinopathy. When compared with the fellow unaffected eye, the involved side may have reduced artery caliber and less severe hypertensive changes.[28] Subretinal hemorrhages and papilledema suggest raised intracranial pressure.

Unexplained fever or nuchal rigidity raise the possibility of other diagnoses such as meningitis or other infection, or subarachnoid hemorrhage. Coma is extremely uncommon in acute ischemic stroke and suggests intracerebral or subarachnoid hemorrhage or metabolic and other nonstroke processes.

The neurologic examination includes rapid screening of mental state, including tests of aphasia and neglect, cranial nerve evaluation including visual field and ocular motility testing, motor, coordination, sensory, and reflex examination.[32] The pattern of findings permits localization to the anterior or posterior circulations and their subdivisions[33] (Table 2-2). Use of a formalized exam scale permits quantification of stroke severity. In widest use in North America is the National Institutes of Health Stroke Scale (NIHSS), which has been incorporated into formal guidelines for thrombolytic therapy decision-making[34–36] (Table 2-3). An efficient practice is to perform an NIHSS exam in all patients supplemented by key additional neurologic exam elements relevant to the patient's complaints and findings.

General Diagnostic Testing   Table 2-4 lists recommended tests that should be ordered on all stroke patients on an emergent basis.[19,23] The frequent coexistence

Table 2-2.
Localization of ischemia according to neurologic findings

Left anterior hemisphere (ICA, MCA, and/or ACA)
Aphasia, right hemiparesis, right hemisensory loss, right visual field defect, left gaze preference, acalculia

Right anterior hemisphere (ICA, MCA, and/or ACA)
Left visuospatial neglect, left visual field defect, left hemiparesis, left hemisensory loss, right gaze preference double simultaneous extinction, visuospatial impairment

Left posterior hemisphere (PCA)
Right visual field defect, visual agnosia, alexia without agraphia, aphasia, right hemisensory loss or dysesthesia

Right posterior hemisphere (PCA)
Left visual field defect, left hemisensory loss or dysasthesia, color agnosia

Brainstem, cerebellum, and/or posterior hemisphere (vertebrobasilar)
Vertigo, diplopia, crossed sensory and motor findings, motor or sensory loss in all four limbs, dysarthria, nystagmus, ataxia, bilateral visual field defects, amnesia

Subcortical or brainstem (small vessel penetrators)
Pure hemiparesis without deficits in higher cortical function, sensory function, or level of consciousness
Pure hemisensory loss without deficits in higher cortical function, sensory function, or level of consciousness

of heart disease with ischemic stroke mandates concern in all patients for acute myocardial infarction, congestive heart failure, arrhythmias, and sudden death, dictating the need for cardiac enzymes, electrocardiography, and chest radiograph. The possibility of early aspiration and pneumonitis also supports chest radiography. Cardiac monitoring should be maintained continuously throughout the first 24 h to detect potentially lethal arrhythmias.[37–40] Glucose measurement is essential as hypo- and hyperglycemia may mimic or exacerbate stroke deficits.[41] Electrolyte and renal dysfunction may also exacerbate stroke impairments. Tests of blood cell counts, platelet counts, and the clotting system identify abnormalities that may have contributed to the acute stroke and that will influence urgent management.

Neuroimaging   Neuroimaging strategies for the acute ischemic stroke patient are rapidly evolving. This state of creative flux is driven on the demand side by urgent calls from clinicians for more precise measures of patient-specific cerebral physiology to aid decision making regarding an effective, but risky, treatment (thrombolysis), and on the supply side by a steady stream of technologic advances across a variety of imaging modalities.

The ideal acute neuroimaging battery would provide images of large vessels, perfusion, and tissue energetic state. Imaging of cervicocephalic vessels would permit identification of stroke mechanism and likely etiology and direct vascular intervention strategies. Imaging of perfusion and tissue state would permit definition of the region of already irreversibly infarcted tissue, the region of threatened but salvageable tissue, and the degree of current blood flow impairment. In addition, the imaging battery would be inexpensive, rapid, widely available, easy to interpret, free of adverse effects, compatible with close patient monitoring, and easily tolerated. No such imaging system is yet available. In current actual practice, imaging protocols mix the practical and the ideal, depending on the available imaging alternatives in local facilities.

Noncontrast CT Scan

Background   Widely available, noncontrast CT scans are the most valuable diagnostic test in the management of the acute stroke patient. A standard cranial CT scan can be obtained in 3 to 6 min of table time with minimal x-ray exposure and is well-tolerated by even gravely ill patients. More than 90 percent of hospitals with 200 or more beds in the United States have CT scanners.[23]

Evidence   When obtained within 3 h of symptom onset, CT aids the diagnosis of acute ischemic stroke most reliably by exclusion, ruling out other entities. Stroke mimics such as tumor or infection are readily identified on CT scan.[42] CT identifies nearly 100 percent of parenchymal brain hemorrhages and subdural hemorrhages and 85 to 97 percent of subarachnoid hemorrhages.[43,44]

In addition, CT can demonstrate subtle signs of early ischemic injury in up to 50 to 60 percent acute ischemic stroke patients scanned within 6 h of onset. Detecting early ischemic insult requires close attention to subtle parenchymal changes.[45,46] These changes include loss of gray–white differentiation, development

Table 2-3.
National Institutes of Health Stroke Scale

1a. Level of consciousness
0 = Alert; keenly responsive
1 = Not alert but arousable by minor stimulation to obey, answer, or respond
2 = Not alert, requires repeated stimulation to attend, or is obtunded and requires strong or painful stimulation to make movements (not stereotyped)
3 = Responds only with reflex motor or autonomic effects or totally unresponsive, flaccid, areflexic

1b. Level of consciousness
Patient is asked the month and age.
0 = Answers both questions correctly
1 = Answers one question correctly
2 = Answers neither question correctly

1c. Level of consciousness
Patient is asked to open and close eyes and to grip and release nonparetic hand.
0 = Performs both tasks correctly
1 = Performs one task correctly
2 = Performs neither task correctly

2. Best gaze
0 = Normal
1 = Partial gaze palsy, when gaze is abnormal in one or both eyes, but where forced deviation or total gaze paresis is not present
2 = Forced deviation, or total gaze paresis not overcome by oculocephalic maneuver

3. Visual
0 = No visual loss
1 = Partial hemianopia
2 = Complete hemianopia
3 = Bilateral hemianopia

4. Facial palsy
0 = Normal symmetric movement
1 = Minor paralysis
2 = Partial paralysis
3 = Complete paralysis of one or both sides

5. Motor arm
Scored for right and left arm
0 = No drift, arm holds 90 degrees if sitting (or 45° if supine) for full 10 s
1 = Drift, arm holds 90 degrees if sitting, (or 45° if supine) but drifts down before full 10 s; does not hit bed or other support
2 = Some effort against gravity, arm cannot get to or maintain 90 degrees if sitting (or 45° if supine), drifts down to bed, but has some effort against gravity
3 = No effort against gravity, arm falls
4 = No movement
X = Amputation, joint fusion

Table 2-3.

National Institutes of Health Stroke Scale (Continued)

6. Motor leg

Scored for right and left leg

0 = No drift, leg holds 30 degrees position for full 5 s

1 = Drift, leg falls by the end of the 5-s period but does not hit bed

2 = Some effort against gravity; leg falls to bed by 5 s but has some effort against gravity

3 = No effort against gravity, leg falls to bed immediately

4 = No movement

X = Amputation, joint fusion

7. Limb ataxia

0 = Absent

1 = Present in one limb

2 = Present in two limbs

8. Sensory

0 = Normal; no sensory loss

1 = Mild to moderate sensory loss; patient feels pinprick is less sharp or is dull on the affected side, or there is loss of superficial pain with pinprick but patient is aware of being touched

2 = Severe to total sensory loss; patient is not aware of being touched in the face, arm, and leg

9. Best language

0 = No aphasia; normal

1 = Mild to moderate aphasia; some obvious loss of fluency or facility of comprehension, without significant limitation of ideas expressed or form of expression; reduction of speech and/or comprehension makes conversation about provided material difficult or impossible

2 = Severe aphasia; all communication is through fragmentary expression; great need for inference, questioning, and guessing by the listener; range of information that can be exchanged is limited; listener carries burden of communication

3 = Mute, global aphasia; no usable speech or auditory comprehension

10. Dysarthria

0 = Normal

1 = Mild to moderate; patient slurs at least some words and at worst can be understood with some difficulty

2 = Severe; patient's speech is so slurred as to be unintelligible in the absence of or out of proportion to any dysphasia, or is mute/anarthric

X = Intubation or other physical barrier

11. Extinction and inattention

0 = No abnormality

1 = Visual, tactile, auditory, spatial, or personal inattention or extinction to bilateral simultaneous stimulation in one of the sensory modalities

2 = Profound hemi-inattention or hemi-inattention to more than one modality. Does not recognize own hand or orients to only one side of space.

Table 2-4.

Emergency laboratory examination for patients with acute ischemic stroke

Initial tests for all patients

CT of brain without contrast

Electrocardiogram and initiation of continuous cardiac monitoring

Chest x-ray

Complete blood count

Platelet count

Prothrombin time

Partial thromboplastin time

Electrolytes

Blood glucose

Blood urea nitrogen/creatinine

Pulse oximetry

Additional tests in select patients

Lateral cervical spine x-ray (if trauma is suspected)

Lumbar puncture (if subarachnoid hemorrhage suspected and CT negative)

Electroencephalogram (if seizure suspected)

Pregnancy test (in women of child-bearing age)

Liver function tests (if altered level of consciousness)

Troponin or CK/MB (if myocardial infarction suspected)

Arterial blood gas (if hypoxia suspected)

Urine toxicology (if substance abuse suspected)

Blood cultures and erythrocyte sedimentation rate (if endocarditis or other infection suspected)

of sulcal effacement, blurring of margins between basal ganglia and internal capsule and/or external capsule (lenticular obscuration), loss of the insular ribbon (insular ribbon sign), and hyperdensity of the middle cerebral artery indicating acute clot lodged in the artery (hyperdense MCA sign)[47-49] (see Chapter 34). Lacunar and posterior fossa infarctions may be impossible to detect on the acute CT.

As the infarction ages, the involved parenchyma becomes more hypodense. This progression of hypodensity allows estimation of the age of the infarction so that the CT findings can provide corroborative evidence regarding time of stroke onset.[50] Sometimes, the CT will provide an important clue to an inaccurate history. When patients or other witnesses place the onset of symptoms within the last 3 h but the CT depicts an obvious area of hypodensity, reeliciting the history scrupulously often reveals an earlier time of onset.

The initial CT may also provide an early glimpse of stroke etiology. An infarction confined to the cortex or involving multiple vascular territories is most consistent with an embolic source, whereas combined MCA/ACA ischemia suggests ICA occlusion. These early clues to the stroke pathogenesis can help direct the subsequent workup and guide treatment options in the acute stroke setting.

Findings on the acute CT have been associated with subsequent outcome. In a study of CTs performed within 14 h of ictus, Moulin and colleagues found that scans exhibiting two of three parenchymal findings (attenuation of the lentiform nucleus, loss of the insular ribbon, and hemispheric sulcus effacement) were associated with eventual extended infarction and poor outcome.[45] In addition, they reported that a hyperdense MCA sign, the radiographic evidence of clot lodged in the MCA, was always accompanied by all three signs of acute ischemic injury and invariably indicated poor outcome. In the NINDS-TPA trials, in which all patients had CTs performed under 3 h, 5 percent had evidence of early ischemic injury. These findings were associated with poor outcome at 3-month follow up, regardless of treatment group.[51]

Accurately interpreting the acute CT for hemorrhage or signs of early infarction is imperative, especially if the patient is being considered for anticoagulant or thrombolytic therapy.[35,36] However, many physicians do not perform optimally at discriminating hemorrhages and major infarcts on early CTs. For example, in one study overall accuracy in recognition of hemorrhages and infarctions was 67 percent for emergency physicians, 83 percent for neurologists, and 83 percent for radiologists.[52]

Recommendations Noncontrast cranial CT should be performed as soon as possible after patient arrival in all suspected acute ischemic stroke patients. The scan should be read by a physician familiar with acute stroke CT interpretation; training in a particular specialty is not an adequate proxy for such expertise.[52]

Conventional Magnetic Resonance Imaging

Background Conventional MRI includes T1-weighted, T2-weighted, and proton density images (see Chapter 33). Conventional MRI has several advantages over CT, including better contrast resolution of brain parenchymal structures, finer spatial resolution, generally better sensitivity to tissue abnormalities, multiplanar imaging, and the lack of ionizing radiation. Although

MRI is widely employed in the subacute workup of stroke patients, its use in the acute stage has been limited. MRI disadvantages include lack of universal availability, contraindications for patients with pacemakers, metal implants and severe claustrophobia, greater susceptibility to motion artifacts, longer scan times than CT on machines not equipped with echo-planar hardware, and difficulty monitoring a seriously ill patient during the examination. Ischemic injury produces signal hyperintensities evident on sequences with T2 weighting, but these alterations take time to develop. In addition, the loss of normal signal voids in fast flowing arteries or contrast enhancement of slowly flowing obstructed arteries may be seen within the first minutes to hours of stroke onset, but their frequency and diagnostic utility in the hyperacute stage have not been systematically investigated.

Evidence   The sensitivity of MRI in the detection of ischemic stroke is reported to be 82 to 95 percent in the first 72 h.[53] Early studies comparing CT and MRI in the detection of ischemic stroke within 24 h found MRI generally to be superior to CT.[54-56] MRI may especially surpass CT in identifying brainstem and cerebellar infarcts and small deep cerebral infarcts.[55,57,58] The first signal change observed in these studies was generally the development of hyperintensity on T2-weighted images. However, a majority of the subjects in these studies were not imaged until 8 h after stroke onset, and MRI was usually performed after CT. Later studies examining subjects within the first 6 h of symptoms have found no difference in the ability of CT or MRI to reliably characterize infarction in the acute stage.[57,59] Changes on T2-weighted images generally do not reliably begin to appear until 4 to 8 h after symptom onset. Fluid attenuated inversion recovery (FLAIR) sequences slightly heighten MRI ability to discriminate acute ischemic stroke but still are often unrevealing in the first 2 to 6 h after onset.[60] A major concern that has hindered adoption of MRI as the initial imaging study in stroke patients is that hyperacute hemorrhage is more readily appreciated on CT than MRI. Although one small series has suggested that early parenchymal hemorrhage may be adequately detected by MRI, especially if gradient-refocused echo sequences sensitive to hemorrhage are employed,[61] further demonstration of adequacy in ruling out parenchymal hemorrhage is required. Conventional MRI is highly insensitive to subarachnoid hemorrhage; however, preliminary studies have shown FLAIR sequences are able to detect blood in the subarachnoid space.[62,63] Because subarachnoid hemorrhage may generally adequately be distinguished from ischemic stroke patients on the basis of history and physical exam alone, MRI insensitivity to this entity is not crucial.

Recommendation   Conventional brain MRI is generally not recommended in place of CT scan in the evaluation of acute ischemic stroke in the first 6 h of onset owing to its potential insensitivity to the presence of hemorrhage. MRI should be considered as a second imaging study when initial CT is negative and when time lost in obtaining the study will not interfere with an acute intervention. MRI may be considered as the initial acute imaging when initial imaging is being obtained more than 6 h after onset, by which time hemorrhage will more easily be detected. MRI may also be advantageous as the initial imaging study when thrombolytic and anticoagulant therapies are not being contemplated in patients with suspected brainstem, cerebellar, or small, deep hemispheric infarcts.

Magnetic Resonance Angiography

Background   Magnetic resonance angiography (MRA) provides images of large cervical and cerebral arteries. A variety of noncontrast MRA techniques have been developed, including black blood, two-dimensional time of flight, and three-dimensional time of flight. Most take advantage of the fact that flowing blood within a vessel lumen will carry an excitation input pulse out of the field of view, so the lumen will yield a distinctive void of return of signal. Through this technique, MRA can provide visualization of blood flow without the use of contrast agents. However, MRA without contrast has a tendency to overestimate the degree of stenosis and the incidence of occlusion. Newer MRA techniques that employ contrast enhancement reduce this tendency[64,65] but have not been investigated in the hyperacute phase of stroke.

Evidence   The sensitivity and specificity of MRA to detect substantial intracranial stenosis when compared with digital subtraction angiography (DSA) has been reported to range from 80 to 100 percent.[66-68] The accuracy of MRA in detecting and grading cervical internal carotid artery stenosis versus a catheter angiographic gold standard has been found to range from 85 to 96 percent.[64,65,69,70] These angiographic comparison studies, however, have generally been performed in the subacute or chronic phase, and MRA's ability to detect vascular abnormalities in the acute setting has not been fully explored. One small salient series is that of Ohue and colleagues, who reported on six patients who underwent intra-arterial thrombolysis for acute ischemic stroke.[71] Preprocedural MRA identified the acute vascular occlusion in all patients, confirmed at subsequent digital subtraction angiography, and postprocedural MRA proved accurate in monitoring recanalization and reocclusion. The impact of MRA on early diagnosis was explored in the study of Lee and colleagues, who obtained both cervical and intracranial MRAs in 46 acute ischemic stroke patients within an average of 32 h of stroke onset.[72] Large vessel occlusion or stenosis was noted in 28 percent of patients. MRA results altered the etiologic diagnosis in 59 percent of cases, yielding diagnoses that correlated more closely with the final diagnosis.

Recommendations   MRA is a useful adjunct to conventional brain imaging in acute ischemic stroke, providing information regarding presence and site of large vessel occlusion not available by examining vessel flow voids on conventional MRI. MRA findings correlate strongly, but not perfectly, with catheter angiography. An efficient imaging strategy is to obtain acute MRA concomitantly with acute MRI to aid in determining stroke etiology in the first hours after onset. In select cases when MRA findings are unexpected or suggest a treatment intervention of some risk, findings may need to be confirmed with additional vascular studies.

Diffusion-Weighted Magnetic Resonance Imaging

Background   Diffusion-weighted magnetic resonance imaging (DWI) signals reflect the mobility of water molecules within tissues. In ischemic tissues, energy failure and impairment of membrane function result in movement of water into the cell (cytotoxic edema). Intracellular water restricts diffusion and produces high signal on DWI images. The major potential advantage of DWI in imaging acute ischemic stroke is the rapid appearance of abnormal signal soon after onset of blood flow impairment. In animal models, affected cerebral tissues exhibit high signal on DWI within <10 min of vessel occlusion.[73,74] DWI sequences can be obtained in 30 to 60 s of scanner time on MR units equipped with echo planar hardware.

Evidence   DWI has been shown to be exquisitely sensitive to ischemic change within the first 6 h of stroke onset (Fig. 2-1). Warach and colleagues found that among nine scans obtained within 6 h of symptom onset, DWI was abnormal in 100 percent, whereas T2-weighted images were abnormal in 0 percent.[75] Tong and colleagues reported that in ten patients imaged

within 6.5 h of stroke onset, DWI was abnormal in 90 percent, whereas T2-weighted images were abnormal in 10 percent.[76] Lee and colleagues found that in 46 patients imaged an average of 32 h after onset, DWI was abnormal in 98 percent, and T2-weighted images were abnormal in 73 percent.[72] DWI imaging offers a number of additional advantageous features. The volume of DWI abnormality correlates closely with the severity of neurologic deficit at the time of imaging and predicts long-term clinical outcome with a high degree of accuracy.[76–78] In patients with a history of multiple prior infarcts, abnormal DWI signal discriminates acute lesions responsible for the current deficit from old lesions not presently symptomatic.[79] In patients with an exacerbation of an old neurologic deficit, abnormal DWI signal adjacent to old infarction allows recognition of progression of ischemic injury, whereas absent DWI signal suggests systemic metabolic or infectious insult or other cause of decompensation of prior recovery other than new ischemia.[79] Information provided by acute DWI frequently modifies the clinician's judgement of ischemia location, size, and mechanism. In the study of Lee and colleagues, DWI images improved the localization diagnosis from 67 percent of patients using CT and physical exam to 100 percent of patients using DWI. The etiologic diagnosis was correctly determined using DWI in 78 percent of patients, improving correlation with final diagnosis.[72]

DWI signal alterations are reversible in animal models if reperfusion is rapidly established. In humans, reversal of DWI change with early reperfusion has been observed (Fig. 2-2), but in general by 3 to 6 h after onset, DWI abnormalities are not rapidly reversible.[79b]

Recommendations   Diffusion-weighted MR imaging is effective in establishing the presence, the site, and the extent of cerebral ischemia within 6 h of symptom onset. In facilities where DWI is available, and when patients are stable for MRI scanning, DWI imaging is a useful adjunct to conventional imaging strategies.

Magnetic Resonance Perfusion Imaging

Background   Magnetic resonance (MR) perfusion imaging is performed with the bolus injection of a paramagnetic contrast agent or bolus noninvasive magnetic labeling of arterial blood, tracking the first pass of contrast through brain tissues to derive a concentration-time curve.[80] Different parameters, including bolus ar-

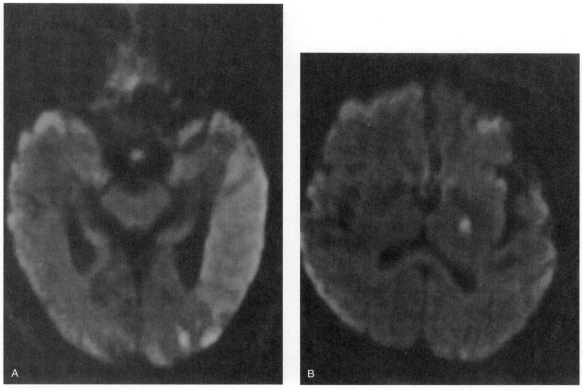

Figure 2-1.
A *DWI hyperintensity involving left middle cerebral artery territory.* B *DWI hyperintensity involving left internal capsule.*

rival time, relative mean transit time, and relative cerebral blood volume, may be calculated and displayed as perfusion maps. Perfusion MR techniques provide a relative measure of regional blood flow, rather than an absolute quantitative measure. In this respect, perfusion MR is similar to single-photon emission computerized tomography (SPECT) scanning. Perfusion data can be obtained in 5 min of scanning time but often require 10 to 40 min of additional postprocessing time before final images are generated.

It has been suggested that perfusion MR can be combined with diffusion MR to define distinct physiologic tissue states. The simplest version of this hypothesis suggests that regions with both diffusion and perfusion abnormality are suffering both ongoing bioenergetic compromise and ongoing hypoperfusion and likely are already irreversibly infarcted or shortly will be. Regions with perfusion but no diffusion abnormality

constitute a salvageable penumbra, experiencing hypoperfusion, but not yet advanced bioenergetic failure. Regions with diffusion but no perfusion abnormality are areas that have already been reperfused, and their current bioenergetic compromise may well spontaneously improve.

Evidence Recent studies in the 1 to 10-h epoch have shown perfusion deficits can be detected before an area of abnormality is seen on conventional MRI.[59,76–78,81] Moreover, acute perfusion lesion volumes correlate even more closely with current clinical deficit and long-term stroke outcome than diffusion-weighted MR lesion volumes.[76,77] Hypotheses regarding the ability of combined DWI/PWI imaging to define the physiologic state of ischemic tissues have not yet been adequately tested in humans. Several studies have suggested that when perfusion lesion volumes exceed diffusion lesion vol-

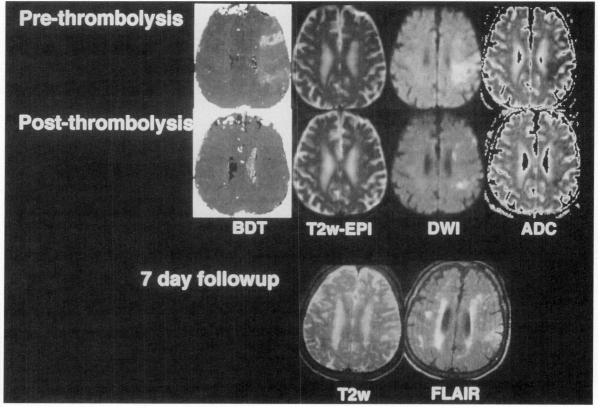

Figure 2-2.
Top. Prethrombolysis images including bolus delay time (BDT) with delayed flow shown as hyperintensity, T2-weighted image, diffusion-weighted image (DWI), and apparent diffusion coefficient (ACD). Middle. 3 hours post-thrombolysis images depicting decreased lesion volume on DWI and BDT without evidence of ischemia on T2-weighted images. Bottom. 7-day follow up depicting decreased final lesion volume on T2-weighted and fluid-attenuated inversion recovery (FLAIR) images.

umes on the initial scan, the DWI lesion will tend to expand into the remainder of the hypoperfused field on follow-up imaging.[76–78,81]

Recommendations Perfusion MR is a promising but not yet thoroughly validated technique for acutely measuring regional cerebral perfusion. It should continue to be evaluated in research settings but is not ready for adoption as a standard acute imaging technique.

Computerized Tomography Angiography

Background Computerized tomography angiography (CTA) employs helical scan acquisition tech-

niques to rapidly map vessel caliber and anatomy during the bolus passage of iodinated contrast material. Images may be reconstructed and rotated in three dimensions (Fig. 2-3). A substantial amount of contrast, generally about 150 to 170cc, is required, making the procedure unsuitable for patients with renal impairment and contrast allergies. Compared with MRA, CTA has advantages of allowing scanning of patients who are critically ill, claustrophobic, and have metallic implants. In addition, CT technology is more widely available in the acute setting than MRI and ultrasound, and CTA can be performed immediately following the screening brain CT that is obtained in most ischemic stroke patients.

Evidence   CTA in the first few hours after stroke onset has been examined in several small to moderate size series. In a study of 21 patients, CTA performed within 6 h of stroke onset accurately identified vessel occlusions confirmed by subsequent digital subtraction.[82] In addition, CTA was able to characterize the length of the occluded arterial segment. The degree of collateral circulation to the ischemic field was also felt to be well characterized by assessing the amount of contrast enhancement in arterial branches beyond the occlusion and the extent of diminished parenchymal enhancement. In another study, in five patients studied within 3 h of ictus, CTA documented vascular occlusions that correlated with clinical deficits and perfusion impairments.[83] In a series of 40 patients studied within 6 h of ictus, CTA showed vascular occlusions in 85 percent.[84] Subsequent digital subtraction angiography confirmed vessel occlusion in six of seven patients studied. Among 20 patients in this series treated with thrombolysis, CTA measures of leptomeningeal collateral flow correlated with eventual clinical outcome.

Recommendations   CTA shows promise as an acute large vessel imaging technique but has not yet been thoroughly validated. Drawbacks of CTA in the acute setting at present include prolonged postprocessing times to yield final images and exposure to iodinated contrast. Further investigations are needed to clarify the utility of this new technology in the acute stroke setting.

Xenon-Computerized Tomography

Background   Xenon is an inert gas that is radiopaque. When inhaled and absorbed in the blood stream, its rate of appearance in a cerebral region is directly proportional to the amount of blood flow received. Serial CT images allow derivation of a time-concentration curve that can be processed to provide a map of regional perfusion (Fig. 2-4 and color insert 1). An advantage of xenon-CT (XCT) over other measures of regional cerebral perfusion like SPECT and perfusion MR is that xenon-CT provides an absolute, quantitative measure of blood flow, not a relative measure. However, xenon itself is a vasodilator that increases cerebral blood flow, thereby disturbing resting physiology, and the spatial resolution of xenon-CT is less precise than O15 positron emission tomography. Xenon-CT images can be acquired in 8 min of scan time and require 10 to 25 min of postprocessing. Some amount of patient cooperation is required for correct mask placement during xenon uptake. A drawback of xenon methods is that xenon can produce a transient acute confusional state.

Evidence   In a series of 53 patients with acute hemispheric stroke symptoms studied within 8 h of onset, XCT frequently identified regions of hypoperfusion before lesions were evident on conventional CT. Patients destined to evolve permanent deficits could be differentiated from those who would experience transient symptoms by degree of perfusion impairment (mean CBF 17.3 mL/100 g/min in permanent deficit patients, 35.4 mL/100 g/min in transient deficit patients).[85] In a subgroup of 20 patients with middle cerebral artery infarcts studied under 6 h, xenon CT was abnormal in 100 percent, whereas conventional CT was felt to be abnormal in only 55 percent.[86] The utility of xenon-CT as a guide to thrombolytic therapy has been explored. In 26 patients, many treated with intra-arterial thrombolysis, pretreatment XCT seemed to distinguish irreversibly infarcted tissue (profound perfusion impairment <10 mL/100 g/min) and threatened but salvageable tissue (moderate perfusion impairment between 10 and 30 mL/100 g/min).[87]

Recommendations   Xenon-CT is a potentially useful acute adjunct to conventional CT, providing regional perfusion imaging. However, it awaits validation in diverse acute stroke cohorts, and its requirement for mask inhalation and occasional transient effect on mental state poses practical challenges to acute implementation. Its use in acute ischemic stroke imaging remains exploratory.

Single-Photon Emission Computerized Tomography

Background   SPECT uses intravenous injection of an isotope to evaluate cerebral blood flow. Most commonly employed in acute stroke studies in 99m Tc-hexamethylpropylene amine oxime (HMPAO), which readily crosses the blood-brain barrier and rapidly localizes in brain in proportion to blood flow. SPECT measures relative, not absolute, regional cerebral perfusion. After injection, the tracer is taken up by brain tissues within 2 min. Imaging obtained anytime within the next 4 h will reflect the physiologic state at the time of the initial injection. Accordingly, tracer may be injected in the emergency department, procedure suite, or other site to capture initial physiology and scans acquired after a delay. A drawback to hyperacute SPECT scanning is the preparation time of HMPAO, which takes 20 to 30

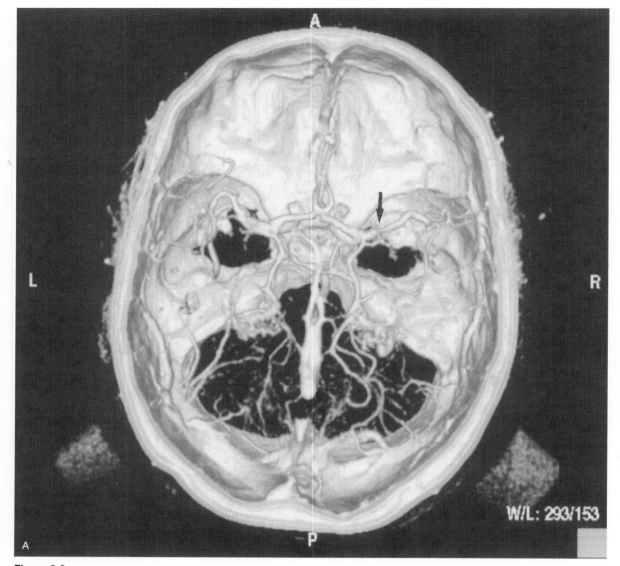

Figure 2-3.
A *CTA of right middle cerebral artery stenosis.*

min. Also, in contrast to the competing perfusion imaging modalities of xenon CT and magnetic resonance perfusion imaging that may be obtained on the same scanner as obligatory structural imaging in acute ischemic stroke, SPECT requires patient transport to a second imaging facility.

Evidence Several studies have demonstrated that SPECT can visualize perfusion abnormalities in the acute period before structural change appears on conventional CT images.[88–90] SPECT has the potential to differentiate areas that are markedly hypoperfused from areas only mildly hypoperfused. A study examin-

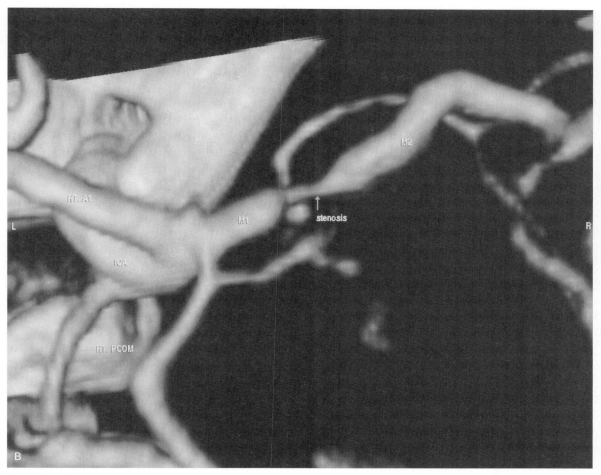

Figure 2-3 (*Continued*).
B *CTA magnified view of right middle cerebral artery stenosis. A1, anterior cerebral artery A1 segment; ICA, internal carotid artery; PCOM, posterior communicating artery; M1, middle cerebral artery M1 segment; M2, middle cerebral artery M2 segment.*

ing patients within 6 h of stroke onset delineated areas of moderate hypoperfusion surrounding areas of more profound hypoperfusion. This peri-infarction area was found to have a 40 percent reduction of blood flow in comparison with the corresponding contralateral normal parenchyma and proposed to represent the ischemic penumbra.[89] SPECT has been employed to demonstrate reperfusion after thrombolytic therapy.[90] Because of the limited spatial resolution of SPECT, lacunar infarcts are not reliably detected.[90]

Recommendations SPECT is able to demonstrate perfusion defects in advance of the appearance of structural lesions in acute ischemic stroke. Further investigation is needed to determine whether SPECT has the ability to distinguish viable parenchyma from irreversibly damaged parenchyma. Difficulties in operating SPECT facilities around the clock and the need for transport to a second imaging suite will limit the widespread adoption of SPECT in acute stroke imaging.

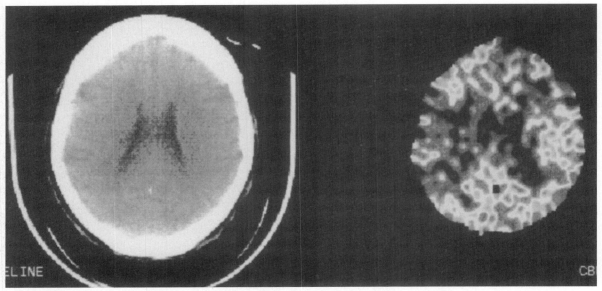

Figure 2-4.
Simultaneous CT and xenon CT. Left. CT scan without evidence of ischemia. Right. Xenon CT with significantly decreased blood flow in right middle cerebral artery territory shown in blue (range 27–38 mL/100g/min). Normal blood flow in homologous area in left middle cerebral artery territory shown as yellow-orange (range 45–72 mL/100 g/min). (See also color insert 1.)

Ultrasound Procedures

Background Ultrasound studies of the carotid bifurcation are a well-established noninvasive test in the diagnosis of stroke but have not been extensively studied in the acute period. A full carotid ultrasonography battery includes continuous wave Doppler measurement of blood velocity, B-mode imaging of vessel anatomy, and color-flow imaging of flow direction and lumen caliber (see Chap. 33). Carotid ultrasound visualizes only the proximal cervical carotid arteries and very limited segments of the cervical vertebral arteries. Transcranial Doppler (TCD) ultrasound employs a low frequency probe to penetrate the skull and interrogate the major basal intracranial arteries.[91] Ultrasound procedures have the advantage of being performed at the bedside in a timely fashion. The costs are minimal, and patient cooperation is not essential. Disadvantages of ultrasound include being highly operator dependent and having difficulty distinguishing high-grade stenosis from complete occlusion.

Evidence Continuous wave and color-flow Doppler have widespread acceptance for the evaluation of carotid disease and demonstrate a 90 to 95 percent sensitivity and specificity for high-grade carotid stenosis in experienced laboratories.[69,92] Studies employing carotid ultrasound in the acute setting, however, are few. Two series employing combined carotid and transcranial ultrasound in the acute phase reported multimodal ultrasound was helpful in identifying patterns of extracranial, intracranial, and combined vascular occlusions and stenoses but did not systematically employ confirmatory angiography.[93,94] The utility of acute TCD sonography has been somewhat more extensively explored. Several groups have demonstrated that TCD assessment of MCA patency, impaired flow or preserved flow in the first 6 h after ictus can predict subsequent clinical course.[95–97] For example, in the series of Toni and colleagues, 93 MCA stroke patients underwent TCD 6 h after ischemic stroke onset.[95] Abnormal TCD findings of absence MCA signal or MCA asymmetry were present in 29 percent of patients who demonstrated early improvement, 65 percent of patients who maintained a stable neurologic deficit, and 85 percent of patients with early deterioration. TCD abnormality was an independent predictor of early worsening, increasing the odds of deterioration fivefold. Serial TCD examinations have been employed to monitor the occurrence of spontaneous and thrombolytic-induced MCA recanalization.[95,98]

Preliminary studies employing TCD to detect asymptomatic microemboli have demonstrated that recurrent artery-to-artery and cardiogenic embolic signals appear most frequently in the first 6 h after stroke onset and decline thereafter.[99,100] There is suggestive evidence that TCD embolus detection can measure the impact of acute anticoagulation in reducing asymptomatic microemboli. For example, in a study of 100 acute stroke patients, microembolic signals were detected on admission in 46 percent of patients without anticoagulation vs. 32 percent of patients on anticoagulation.[99] However, a relation between suppression of microembolic signals and prevention of symptomatic macroembolism has not yet been conclusively established.

Recommendations Carotid duplex ultrasound and TCD ultrasound are of established value in identifying stenoses and occlusions of cervicocephalic vessels and establishing collateral patterns of flow. When available in the acute setting, they can aid in identifying the site and mechanism of arterial insult. Preliminary data suggest that TCD can provide additional prognostic information not available from clinical exam and CT scan alone. Serial TCD examinations to monitor recanalization or progression to occlusion and TCD embolus detection are emerging strategies of promise in the acute phase but are not yet validated outside of facilities with extensive experience in TCD research.

Catheter Angiography

Background Conventional angiography is the gold standard for evaluating cerebrovascular abnormalities. With the development of reliable noninvasive methods for large vessel imaging, such as MRA, CTA, and multimodal ultrasound, the use of catheter angiography in acute ischemic stroke is becoming more selective. Advantages include better visualization of medium and small vessels than with noninvasive techniques and the ability to proceed directly to an endovascular intervention after diagnostic imaging. Catheter angiography can detect arterial dissection with sensitivity and can define the route and to some degree the adequacy of collateral circulation. Disadvantages include periprocedural risks of stroke, exposure to iodinated contrast with nephrotoxicity and potential for allergic re-

sponse, and lack of around the clock availability outside of large medical centers.

Evidence Systematic angiographic studies performed within the first few hours of stroke onset are sparse. In 139 patients studied within 8 h of onset of moderate focal ischemia, angiography demonstrated occlusions of cervical or cephalic large or medium-sized arteries in 81 percent.[101] The site of angiographic occlusion has been demonstrated to predict outcome in conservatively treated patients and to predict likelihood of recanalization and of hemorrhagic transformation in patients treated with thrombolytic therapy.[101,102] In a randomized trial of intra-arterial thrombolysis performed within 6 h of symptom onset, among patients with clinical evidence of large vessel middle cerebral artery syndromes, initial angiography demonstrated acute vascular occlusions in 73 percent.[103]

The risks of angiography in the hyperacute ischemic stroke setting have not been well-defined. An overview of eight prospective and seven retrospective studies of angiographic complications in patients with mild, generally subacute, or chronic cerebrovascular disease found a permanent neurologic complication rate of about 1 percent, a risk of any neurologic complication of about 4 percent, and a mortality rate less than 0.1 percent.[104]

Recommendations Although less utilized than in the past, angiography still plays a role in acute stroke evaluation and remains the definitive method for evaluating the cerebral vasculature.[53] It remains the only way to confidently make a diagnosis of diseases affecting small caliber vessels such as vasculitis. It is also often of help in the rapidly deteriorating patient, the patient with conflicting or unrevealing noninvasive vascular imaging, the patient with suspected dissection, and the young stroke patient.

EARLY SUPPORTIVE THERAPY

Respiratory Management

Background Systemic oxygen desaturation will exacerbate and extend brain injury originating from focal cerebral hypoxia. Acute stroke patients are at risk for respiratory compromise owing to aspiration, hypoventilation, upper airway obstruction, atelectasis, or rarely a reduction in the ventilatory drive or neurogenic pulmonary edema.

Evidence   One-third of acute ischemic stroke patients exhibit overt or silent aspiration.[105] Pneumonia complicates acute stroke in 5 to 12 percent of cases.[103,106,107] In recent large series, intubation has been pursued in between 6 and 8 percent of acute ischemic stroke patients, frequently on Emergency Department arrival or within the first 6 h of onset.[108,109] Although as a group patients requiring intubation generally have much worse prognoses than those who do not, good clinical outcomes in individual cases are obtainable.[109]

Recommendations   All acute stroke patients should be monitored for hypoxia with a goal of maintaining serum oxygen saturation levels of greater than 95 percent. If this cannot be achieved on room air, supplemental oxygen should be used. No evidence supports the routine use of supplemental oxygen for patients with adequate blood oxygen saturation when breathing room air.[19] If ventilatory assistance is required to achieve adequate oxygenation, or if the upper airway is threatened because of obtundation or laryngeal dysfunction, endotracheal intubation and mechanical ventilation should proceed with dispatch. Intubation and the use of hypnotics may elevate intracranial pressure. To reduce this risk, short-acting sedatives with minimal cardiac side effects should be used, such as thiopental, etomidate, and propofol.[110] Benzodiazepines and opioids are useful in maintaining anesthesia during mechanical ventilation because they lower intracranial pressure, which potentially improves cerebral blood flow.[110,111]

Blood Pressure Management

The treatment of hypertension in the acute stroke patient has long been the subject of debate.[112,113] Although it is well known that chronic hypertension is an independent risk factor for the occurrence of ischemic stroke, lowering elevated blood pressure during an episode of cerebral ischemia has the potential to extend the area of ischemia.

Elevated blood pressures occur naturally in the first few hours of ischemic stroke for a variety of reasons, including response to stress, full bladder, pain, underlying hypertension, physiologic compensation for hypoxia, and increased intracranial pressure. Untreated, pressures will usually spontaneously decline substantially within 24 h of onset and return to the patient's likely baseline by 4 to 7 days.[114,115] This observation underlies the adage passed down by neurologists that the most effective treatment to lower hypertension in the stroke patient is to wait 5 min and recheck it.

In the normal brain, to ensure adequate oxygenation, cerebral blood flow is maintained at a constant level over a wide range of systemic perfusion pressures through cerebrovascular autoregulation. When systemic blood pressure rises, cerebral arterioles constrict, increasing vascular resistance, and net cerebral blood flow remains unchanged. In contrast, a drop in blood pressure results in dilatation of cerebral arterioles to reduce resistance and avoid a fall in blood flow. Patients who have a background history of hypertension will have chronically shifted their autoregulatory range upward so that cerebral blood flow declines at a higher mean arterial pressure than in normotensives.[116]

Autoregulation is impaired in the ischemic field of patients with acute ischemic stroke. The cerebrovascular endothelium in these regions is itself experiencing ischemia and loses the ability to respond fully to autoregulatory signals. As a consequence, in the ischemic field cerebral blood flow varies directly with systemic blood pressure.[117,118] Reducing the systemic blood pressure may diminish blood flow to the ischemic penumbra and promote extension of the infarct. On the other hand, although it makes sense to prevent precipitous drops in blood pressure in stroke patients, it is also possible that markedly elevated blood pressures could cause further damage by promoting edema formation, increasing the risk of hemorrhagic transformation, and exacerbating vascular damage.

Evidence   Against this theoretical background largely based on observations in animal models, data on the efficacy of alternative blood pressure management strategies in acute human ischemic stroke are sparse. In one small randomized clinical trial of 16 patients, both the placebo group and the antihypertensive-treated group experienced equal drops in blood pressure over the first 72 h of therapy and did not differ in clinical outcome.[119] Suggestive data against active lowering of blood pressure have come from large observational series.[8,120,121] For example, 868 consecutive acute ischemic stroke patients were observed to determine correlates of stroke progression. Two groups were identified, those with early progression (within 36 h of stroke onset) and those with late progression (within 1 week of stroke onset). In patients with early stroke progression, two variables were independently associated with progression: admission blood pressure and history of diabetes.[121] In patients with early progression, for every 20-mmHg drop in systolic blood pressure, the relative risk of worsening within 36 h of stroke onset increased by a factor of 0.66.

Conversely, the strategy of actively raising the blood pressure in all patients with ischemic stroke has also not directly been tested in major clinical trials. Indirect observations from randomized clinical trials of hemodilution (sometimes associated with volume expansion and blood pressure elevation) suggest that many elderly stroke patients with coexisting cardiac morbidities do not tolerate induced hypertension well, and congestive heart failure, myocardial infarction, and other complications of therapy negate possible gains in cerebral perfusion.[122] In select patients carefully managed in the intensive care unit, induced hypertension with phenylephrine has been shown to improve cerebral perfusion and possibly favorably influence the clinical course.[123]

Recommendations Antihypertensive therapy should be withheld in the first few hours after ischemic stroke onset, unless blood pressure is in hypertensive encephalopathy range on two consecutive measurements at least 5 min apart, with systolic blood pressure above 220 mmHg or mean arterial pressure greater than 130 mmHg.[13,19,20,23] This recommendation is modified if a patient has a concurrent condition that independently requires moderation of blood pressure, including acute myocardial infarction, aortic dissection, acute renal failure owing to accelerated hypertension, or early hemorrhagic transformation of cerebral infarct. In these circumstances, a compromise must be struck between the need to maintain systemic blood pressure to maximize cerebral perfusion and the need to lower blood pressure to avoid extension of visceral injury. Another exceptional case is in the first 24 h after tissue plasminogen activator administration, when, to minimize the risk of cerebral hemorrhagic transformation, the systolic blood pressure should be maintained at less than 180 mmHg and diastolic blood pressure less than 105 mmHg.

The choice of antihypertensive medications must take into account the effect of drugs on the cerebrovascular as well as the systemic circulation.[117] Nitroglycerin, sodium nitroprusside, calcium channel blockers, and hydralazine are cerebral venodilators that increase cerebral blood volume and may thereby increase intracerebral pressure and impair autoregulation. In contrast, alpha- and beta-adrenergic blockers, ganglion blockers, and angiotensin-converting enzyme inhibitors have little effect on cerebral blood volume. Parenteral agents that allow rapid, controlled titration to target pressures are often useful in the hyperacute setting and include enalapril, labetalol, and nitroprusside. Regimens for management of blood pressure in both thrombolytic and non-thrombolytic patients adapted from the NINDS-TPA trialists approach are shown in Table 2-5.[124]

Hypotension is uncommon in ischemic stroke, but when present, vigorous treatment is warranted. First, a treatable cause such as decreased volume status (e.g., dehydration or hemorrhage), pump failure (e.g., arrhythmia, myocardial infarction, or congestive heart failure), or decreased peripheral vascular resistance (e.g., sepsis) should be sought and corrected if identified. If the pressure falls below 90/60 mmHg, or if blood pressure is in low normal range and collateral insufficiency seems to be producing stroke progression, colloid solutions, hypervolemic therapy, and vasopressor agents should be employed. Often in these circumstances, central venous or Swan-Ganz monitoring should be employed because coexisting cardiac disease is common in the elderly ischemic stroke population. Raising blood pressure to the patient's baseline level is a reasonable initial target.

Fluid Management

Background The majority of strokes occur in the elderly, who are liable to fluid and electrolyte disturbance. Decades ago, it was common to restrict fluid intake in acute ischemic stroke patients because of concern about cerebral edema. However, diminished fluid input decreases intravascular volume, promoting collateral failure, and increases blood viscosity, promoting recurrent arterial and venous thrombosis.

Evidence Patients with ischemic stroke are often dehydrated upon hospital arrival.[125] Large cohort studies have demonstrated that only 10 to 20 percent of ischemic stroke patients develop edema that produces clinical deterioration.[126–128] Edema generally peaks 3 to 5 days after stroke onset and is essentially never a concern in the first few hours post-ictus.

Recommendations Careful management of fluids is mandatory in patients with acute cerebral ischemia. Because of the frequency of aspiration, oral feedings should be avoided or minimized in the first few hours. All acute stroke patients require an intravenous access line. Although cerebral edema is rarely a concern in the acute setting, hypotonic intravenous fluids are best avoided. Most patients should receive normal saline at full maintenance volume, with infusion rates of 75 to 125 mL/h to maintain intravascular volume and optimize brain perfusion.[13,19,20,23]

Table 2-5.
Blood pressure management algorithms for patients with acute ischemic stroke

For patients not treated with thrombolysis
Monitor BP q 15 min for 1 h after ER arrival
    Then q 1 h × 3 for 3 h
    Then q 2 h × 2 for 4 h
    Then q 4 h × 4 for 16 h
For SBP > 220 mmHg or DBP 120–140 mmHg on 2 readings 5–10 min apart
    Give labetolol 10 mg IV over 1–2 min
    May repeat or double every 10–20 min, up to 150 mg
    If response not satisfactory, use nitroprusside 0.5–10 μg/kg/min
    Monitor BP at least every 15 min
    Observe for hypotension
For DBP > 140 mmHg
    Nitroprusside 0.5–10 μg/kg/min
    Monitor BP at least every 15 min
    Observe for hypotension

For patients treated with thrombolytics
Monitor BP q 15 min for 2 h after initiation of TPA
    Then q 30 min × 12 for 6 h
    Then q 60 min × 16 for 16 h
For SBP > 230 mmHg or DBP 121–140 mmHg on 2 readings 5–10 min apart
    Give labetolol 10 mg IV over 1–2 min
    May repeat or double every 10–20 min, up to 150 mg
    If response not satisfactory, use nitroprusside 0.5–10 μg/kg/min
    Monitor BP at least every 15 min
    Observe for hypotension
For SBP 180–230 mmHg and/or DBP 105–120 mmHg
    Give labetolol 10 mg IV over 1–2 min
    May repeat or double every 10–20 min, up to 150 mg
For DBP > 140 mmHg
    Nitroprusside 0.5–10 μg/kg/min
    Monitor BP at least every 15 min
    Observe for hypotension

Glucose Management

Background Hyperglycemia is the most common metabolic derangement in acute ischemic stroke. Many patients have a background history of diabetes that predisposed to their stroke. Even in nondiabetic patients, the physiologic stress of stroke frequently evokes a systemic sympathetic nervous system response that elevates blood sugar acutely.

    Studies in animal models of focal and global ischemia have suggested that acute hyperglycemia may increase infarct size.[129] Deprivation of oxygen forces ischemic neuronal tissues to convert from aerobic to anaerobic metabolism. In ischemic regions, serum glucose is metabolized to lactate by anaerobic glycolysis. The greater the glucose level in the blood entering an ischemic neuronal field, the greater the resulting lactic acidosis. Consequently, avoidance of hyperglycemia in the acute stage might improve stroke outcome. However, overaggressive lowering of serum glucose levels to produce symptomatic hypoglycemia may also adversely affect patient course.

Evidence Several large observational studies have demonstrated that elevated blood glucose at admission in acute ischemic stroke correlates with poor outcome.[41,130–132] However, it has not been demonstrated whether this association reflects a primary adverse effect of hyperglycemia on outcome or an epiphenomenon of severe initial brain injury producing a secondary rise in blood sugar. The benefits of insulin or combined glucose-insulin infusions to rapidly reduce blood sugar acutely will not be fully clarified until the results of the Normoglycemia in Cerebral Events (NICE) trial become available. In patients undergoing intravenous thrombolysis, acute hyperglycemia is an independent risk factor for hemorrhagic transformation.[125]

Recommendations Although definitive studies are pending, current basic science and clinical observations suggest that hyperglycemia should be treated promptly in acute stroke. Employing sliding insulin scale to maintain a glucose level of <200 mg/dL is a reasonable strategy.[19,20] In patients with profound hyperglycemia, glucose reduction should be limited to 75 to 100 mg/dL per hour to reduce the risk of osmotic injury to the brain.[129] Dextrose containing intravenous solutions in general should be avoided in the first several hours after stroke onset, except in symptomatic hypoglycemia.

Temperature Management

Background Hyperthermia markedly worsens ischemic and traumatic brain injury in animal models.[133,134] Several mechanisms have been proposed to explain the deleterious effects of hyperthermia. Enhanced release of neurotransmitters, increased numbers of potentially damaging ischemic depolarizations in the focal ischemic penumbra, impaired recovery of energy metabolism, enhanced inhibition of protein kinases, and worsening of cytoskeletal proteolysis have all been implicated.[133]

Evidence A few large acute ischemic stroke cohort studies have found hyperthermia on admission to be an independent risk factor for poor outcome from acute ischemic stroke.[135,136] In the series of Reith and colleagues,[135] 390 consecutive acute ischemic stroke patients had body temperature measured within 6 h of stroke onset (median 2.4 h postonset). For every 1-degree Centigrade increase in body temperature, the relative risk of death or severe final deficit increased by 2.2. These observations are intriguing, but they cannot exclude the possibility that early hyperthermia is a consequence of severe stroke rather than a promoter of increased injury. Induced hypothermia has shown bene-

fit in randomized clinical trials in traumatic brain injury[137] and is actively being investigated in human stroke.[138] Conventional hypothermic therapy, however, requires intubation and paralysis of musculature to prevent shivering, steps which may pose risk to patients, especially those with milder strokes. Large-scale interventional trials are needed to determine whether systemic or selective cerebral hypothermic treatment can improve stroke outcome.

Recommendations Acute stroke patients with fever should be investigated for a source of infection and treated. In addition, the fever should be reduced promptly with antipyretics and cooling blankets if necessary. Induced hypothermia is a promising treatment intervention but remains investigational at present.

THROMBOLYTIC THERAPY

Intravenous

Background Thrombolytic agents activate plasminogen to form plasmin, which actively digests fibrin strands. The thrombolytic agents that have been most extensively investigated in ischemic stroke are recombinant tissue plasminogen activator (TPA) and streptokinase. TPA is a serine protease endogenously released in human tissues from vascular endothelium. Unlike urokinase and streptokinase, TPA preferentially activates plasminogen that is bound to fibrin. It has been proposed that this specificity results in fibrinolysis somewhat confined to localized thrombus, minimizing systemic fibrinolytic activation. Streptokinase is a protein synthesized by streptococci that complexes with and activates both circulating plasminogen and bound plasminogen.

By promoting early recanalization of occluded vessels and early reperfusion of ischemic fields, pharmacologic thrombolysis has the potential to salvage penumbral neuronal tissue. However, by exposing injured brain to lytic agents, thrombolytic therapy also increases the risk of hemorrhagic transformation of infarct with worsening of clinical deficit. Only large-scale clinical trials can determine whether, and when, intravenous thrombolytic therapy confers overall benefit (or harm) in acute ischemic stroke (Table 2-6).

Evidence Eight large-scale clinical trials of intravenous thrombolytic therapy have been completed. We

Table 2-6.

Clinical trials of intravenous thrombolytics in acute ischemic stroke

Trial	Agent	Dose (% of MI dose)	Time window (mean time)	Ischemic stroke type	Sample size	Hematoma/ symptomatic hemorrhage (%)		Good outcome*	
						Drug	Placebo	Drug	Placebo
NINDS Trial 1	TPA	75	<3 h (~2.2 h)	All	291	6	0	47	27
NINDS Trial 2	TPA	75	<3 h (~2.2 h)	All	333	7	1	39	26
ECASS I	TPA	85		Mod-Sev MCA	620	20	7	36	29
ECASS II	TPA	75		Mod-Sev MCA	800	8.8	3.4	40	37
MAST-E	SK	100	<6 h (4.4 h)	Mod-Sev MCA	310	21	3	20	18
MAST-I	SK	100	<6 h (NA)	All	622	8	1	37	35
ASK	SK	100	<6 h (4.6 h)	All	340	13	2	34	35
			<6 h (NA)						
			<4 h (3.5 h)						

ASK, Australian Streptokinase Trial; ECASS, European Cooperative Acute Stroke Study; MAST-E, Multicenter Acute Stroke Trial-Europe; MAST-I, Multicenter Acute Stroke Trial-Italy; MCA, middle cerebral artery; MI, myocardial infarction; NA, not available; NINDS, National Institute of Neurologic Diseases and Stroke; TPA, tissue plasminogen activator; SK, streptokinase.

*Good outcome measures: NINDS Trials 1 and 2, Rankin disability score <2; ECASS I and II, MAST-E, and MAST-I, Rankin <3; ASK, Barthel Index 95–100.

will briefly delineate the chief features and results of the individual trials and then analyze their collective import. Trial features and results are summarized in Table 2-7.

The European Cooperative Acute Stroke Study I assigned 620 patients to either placebo or 1.1 mg/kg of intravenous TPA.[139] Inclusion criteria included symptom onset within 6 h and a stable moderate to severe hemispheric stroke. Patients were excluded if examination revealed a complete hemispheric syndrome, rapidly improving symptoms, CT evidence of hemorrhage, or early CT signs of major infarction involving one-third or greater of the MCA territory. The primary outcome measures included the Barthel Index activities of daily living and a modified Rankin scale disability score at 90 days.

One-hundred nine patients (17 percent) were inadvertently enrolled in the study even though they had major protocol violations. A majority of the violations were because of incorrect CT scan interpretations. The study design had anticipated difficulty in rapid judgement of CT and other enrollment criteria and specified both an intention to treat analysis of the entire study population and a "targeted patient" analysis confined to patients fully meeting formal enrollment criteria. In the intention to treat analysis, no statistically significant differences in the primary endpoints were noted. Mild

trends in favor of the treatment group were noted on secondary analyses. For example, 36 percent of TPA patients vs. 29 percent of placebo patients had Rankin disability scores >2 at 90 days. In the targeted patient subgroup, statistically significant differences in some outcome measures were noted in favor of the treatment group. Safety analyses showed that in the intention to treat groups, parenchymal hematomas were more frequent in the TPA group than with placebo, 20 percent vs. 7 percent. However, overall mortality did not differ between the two groups. Subjects inappropriately enrolled in the trial, including those with early signs of infarction, experienced an increased risk of mortality at day 30 as well as a significant increase in parenchymal hemorrhage.

The findings of the two NINDS-TPA trials provided the foundation for FDA approval of ischemic stroke as an added indication for TPA. They differed from the ECASS trial in several important respects. Patients were enrolled within 3 h of stroke onset (half within 90 min of onset), and the total dose administered was 0.9 mg/kg.[140] The only CT exclusion criterion was hemorrhage; enrollment of patients with early signs of infarction was permitted.

In trial 1, the primary endpoint was a measure of early drug effect, the percent of patients who improved by 4 points or more on a neurologic deficit scale, the

Table 2-7.
Algorithm for thrombolytic therapy

Inclusion criteria
1. Ischemic stroke with a defined onset of <3 h from time TPA is to be started
   Ascertain last time patient known to be awake and deficit-free
2. Measurable deficit on NIH Stroke Scale
   Neurologic deficit > minimal weakness, isolated ataxia, isolated sensory, or isolated dysarthria
3. CT scan shows no evidence of intracranial hemorrhage
   If early signs of new major hemisphere infarct are present (e.g., edema, mass effect, sulcal effacement) reassess time of onset; the presence of these CT findings may be associated with an increased risk of hemorrhage

Exclusion criteria
History
 1. Stroke or serious head trauma within past 3 months
 2. Major surgery or serious trauma within past 14 days
 3. History of intracranial hemorrhage, AVM, or aneurysm
 4. GI or urinary tract hemorrhage within previous 21 days
 5. Arterial puncture at a noncompressible site OR lumbar puncture within previous 7 days

Clinical
 6. Rapidly improving neurologic signs or minor symptoms
 7. Systolic blood pressure > 185 mmHg OR diastolic blood pressure > 110 mmHg OR aggressive (IV) treatment required to reduce patient's blood pressure to specified limits
 8. Seizure at onset
 9. Symptoms suggestive of subarachnoid hemorrhage
10. Recent myocardial infarction-induced pericarditis

Laboratory
11. Patient taking anticoagulants OR prothrombin time >15 s (international normalized ratio >1.7)
12. Patient received heparin within 48 h preceding stroke onset AND has an elevated partial-thromboplasatin time
13. Platelet count <100,000 per mm^3
14. Glucose concentration <50 mg/dL (2.7 mmol/L) OR >400 mg/dL (22.2 mmol/L)
15. Women with a positive pregnancy test

Discuss the risks and benefits of thrombolytic therapy with the patient and family (if possible) and document the discussion in the medical record.

Before administering TPA
Review checklist to confirm inclusion and exclusion criteria
Confirm patient is not spontaneously improving

Treatment and management
 1. TPA 0.9 mg/kg total or maximum 90 mg
 2. Administer 10% of TPA dose as a bolus
 3. Administer remaining 90% of TPA as a constant infusion over 1 h
 4. DO NOT give anticoagulants for 24 h from start of TPA administration
 5. DO NOT give antiplatelet agents for 24 h from start of TPA administration
 6. Admit to intensive care unit OR acute stroke unit
 7. Maintain systolic blood pressure UNDER 180 mmHg and diastolic blood pressure UNDER 115 mmHg
 8. Restrict central venous line placement OR arterial puncture for 24 h
 9. DO NOT insert indwelling bladder catheter for >30 min after TPA administration
10. AVOID insertion of nasogastric tube for 24 h after TPA administration

---

NIH Stroke Scale. Trial 1 enrolled 291 patients. In the TPA group, 47 percent of patients improved by the 4-point threshold vs. 39 percent of the placebo group, a difference that did not reach statistical significance ($p = .21$). Other measures of early activity were positive, including, for example, the average NIHSS score decline from admission to 24 h. Both the control and the TPA groups had an NIHSS score of 14 upon admission. At 24 h, the TPA group scored 8 vs. 12 in the placebo group, a statistically significant group difference ($p < .02$).[141] Also, 3-month secondary endpoints were positive, including statistically significant differences in Barthel, Rankin, and NIHSS scores. These differences were taken as hypothesis-generating observations, requiring a second trial for confirmation.

Trial 2 was alike in all design and dose regimen respects to trial 1, differing only in the prespecified primary endpoint. This consisted of a global statistic combining 3-month scores on the Barthel, Rankin, and NIHSS scales and the Glasgow Outcome Scale. A total of 333 patients were enrolled. The primary endpoint and each of its component outcome measures were significantly favorable for the TPA arm. For example, no or minimal disability on the Barthel Index was present in 50 percent of the TPA group vs. 38 percent of the placebo group. No or minimal residual neurologic deficits measured on the NIHSS were present in 31 percent of the TPA group vs. 20 percent of the placebo group. The absolute risk difference of 12 percent in the Barthel outcome translates into a number needed to treat of 8.3. For every 8.3 patients treated with IV TPA, one more patient will have no or minimal disability at 3 months. Patients at all degrees of initial stroke severity and with large vessel atherothrombotic, small vessel lacunar, and cardioembolic stroke subtypes seemed to benefit in subgroup analysis. Safety data in the NINDS-TPA trials demonstrated a tenfold-increased incidence of symptomatic intracerebral hemorrhage with TPA, 6.4 percent vs. 0.6 percent. However, no difference was noted in overall 3-month mortality, 17 percent in the TPA group vs. 21 percent with placebo.

In multifactorial analysis, two variables independently predicted the development of symptomatic hemorrhage with TPA therapy in the combined NINDS-TPA trials. Early signs of mass effect, hypodensity, and edema on the pretreatment CT increased the risk of symptomatic hemorrhage 7.8-fold, and severe neurologic deficit at baseline with NIHSS >20 increased the risk 1.8-fold.[51] For this reason, some authorities have recommended caution or avoidance of TPA in patients with these features. However, both patients with early

hypodensity on CT and patients with baseline NIHSS >20 tended to fare better if assigned to thrombolytic therapy.[141] The overall prognosis is guarded for both sets of patients, who have evidence of severe ischemia at time of therapeutic decision making. For example, of those patients with an NIHSS >20, 10 percent of the TPA group had a favorable outcome compared with 4 percent of the control group. An analysis of the combined trial populations, analyzing 26 patient variables with 90 percent power to detect an influence on treatment response, found no single variable or combination of variables that identified nonresponders to therapy, suggesting a generalized efficacy of TPA for patients who met trial inclusion and exclusion criteria.[142]

Three randomized placebo-controlled trials of intravenous streptokinase were conducted in the mid 1990s.[143–145] The Multicentre Acute Stroke Trial-Italy (MAST-I) and the Multicentre Acute Stroke Trial-Europe (MAST-E) had a 6-h time window, and a dose of 1.5 million units of streptokinase was administered intravenously. The Australian Streptokinase Trial (ASK) employed the same dose of streptokinase but in a time window of 4 h. The MAST-E and ASK trials were terminated because of a disproportionate number of deaths and symptomatic intracranial hemorrhage in patients who received streptokinase. Similarly, the MAST-I trial was halted because of an increased 10-day fatality rate in patients treated with streptokinase.

The disparate findings of these first six fully reported clinical trials of intravenous thrombolysis occasioned a great deal of controversy.[141,146,147] The uniquely positive findings of the two NINDS-TPA trials, however, can be fully explained by several distinctive, biologically salient aspects of their conduct (Table 2-7). Perhaps most crucially, the time window for entry and the median time poststroke at treatment were markedly shorter in the NINDS trials than in the remaining studies. Also, based on preliminary dose-escalation safety trials, the NINDS investigators employed a thrombolytic dose approximately 75 percent of the standard myocardial infarction dose vs. 85 percent in ECASS I and 100 percent in the streptokinase studies. Also, management of blood pressure and other supportive care may have been more uniform and intensive in the smaller number of centers participating in the NINDS studies than in the geographically more diverse comparator trials. The combination of shorter time to treatment, lower dose, agent type, and intensive supportive care is fully adequate to account for differences in trial results.

Extending the time window of the 0.9 mg/kg dose of TPA beyond 3 h was the focus of two more recent clinical trials. ECASS II enrolled 800 patients within 0 to 6 h of symptom onset, randomized to 0.9 mg/kg of TPA or placebo. In contrast to the NINDS-TPA trial, a substantial majority (80 percent) of the patients enrolled in ECASS II were treated during the 3 to 6-h time window.[148] The primary endpoint of a favorable outcome as determined by the modified Rankin scale at 90 days was achieved by 40.3 percent of TPA patients vs. 36.6 percent of placebo patients. This 3.7 percent difference was not significant. A post-hoc analysis using a different cutoff on the modified Rankin scale found a significant difference between the groups if outcome was classified according to independence (Rankin 0-2 vs. 3-5). This analysis revealed an absolute difference of 8.3 percent in favor of the TPA group in reaching independence. The ATLANTIS trial randomized patients who were 3 to 5 h post-stroke onset to 0.9 mg/ kg TPA or placebo. The study was stopped early when an interim analysis showed no major difference in the primary endpoint between treatment arms, and futility analysis suggested little chance of an important difference emerging. These data suggest that 3 h post-onset is a critical time point for intravenous TPA therapy. Under 3 h, therapy confers substantial benefit on average, whereas beyond 3 h, TPA offers little overall gain.

Important additional information regarding the use of intravenous TPA comes from observations in a large cohort of patients treated in actual clinical practice after marketing.[149] Among 960 patients treated according to the NINDS trial/FDA-approved criteria, symptomatic hemorrhages occurred in only 6 percent.[149] However, in 57 patients in whom treatment deviated from NINDS trial/FDA-approved criteria, symptomatic hemorrhages occurred in 10.7 percent.[150] These data suggest that strict adherence to FDA-approved criteria is required to maximize the safety of therapy.

Recommendations Substantial clinical trial evidence supports the use of intravenous TPA in patients who meet the inclusion and exclusion criteria of the NINDS-TPA trials. Patients are candidates for thrombolysis if they have an acute neurologic deficit thought to be caused by cerebral ischemia that is potentially disabling, their CT scan shows no hemorrhage, and therapy can be started within 3 h of symptom onset. (A detailed checklist for determining eligibility is provided in Table 2-7.) As with any potentially harmful treatment, the risks and benefits of thrombolytic therapy must be discussed with the patient and/or the patient's representative. TPA is administered at a dose of 0.9 mg/kg with a maximum dose of 90 mg. Ten percent of the total

dose is given as a bolus over 1 min, and the remainder is infused over 1 h. Anticoagulants and antiplatelet agents are not to be administered within the first 24 h following thrombolytic treatment.

After infusion, close monitoring of blood pressure and neurologic status is mandatory and is best carried out in a neurologic intensive care unit or stroke unit (Table 2-5). Neurologic deterioration, new onset headache, acute hypertension, nausea, or vomiting may be signs of intracranial hemorrhage and must be investigated immediately. An acute rise in blood pressure may be the first indication of intracerebral hemorrhage. If the patient is still receiving TPA, the infusion should be discontinued and a CT obtained immediately. A stat prothrombin time (PT), partial thromboplastin time (PTT), platelet count, and fibrinogen level should be sent. If the CT shows hemorrhage, then the laboratory results should be evaluated for abnormalities and corrected with fibrinogen, cryoprecipitate, and/or platelets. A neurosurgical consultation may be warranted for hematoma evacuation or intervention to relieve increased intracranial pressure. If the guidelines for intravenous TPA are rigorously adhered to, this therapy is effective in treating patients with acute ischemic stroke.

Intra-arterial and Combined Intravenous and Intra-arterial Thrombolysis

Background In superselective, intra-arterial thrombolysis, a catheter is positioned in an occluded cerebral vessel, and thrombolytic agent is infused directly into the clot. Often, the catheter is passed several times back and forth through the clot to mechanically disrupt the thrombus and promote widespread access of thrombolytic agent to target fibrin strands. Since the pioneering study of Zeumer and colleagues in 1983, continuous improvements in catheter technology have further advanced this technique.[151]

Intra-arterial thrombolysis possesses several theoretical advantages over intravenous thrombolysis. Higher concentrations of thrombolytic agent are delivered to the clot, increasing the likelihood of recanalization. Conversely, lower concentrations of thrombolytic agent escape into the systemic circulation, potentially decreasing the risk of systemic hemorrhagic complications. Gentle mechanical disruption may be employed to potentiate the pharmacologic thrombolytic intervention. The diagnostic angiogram that immediately precedes intervention provides precise information regarding stroke pathophysiology not available from noninvasive testing. The time at which recanalization is achieved is known with certainty and supportive therapy, such as fluid and blood pressure management can immediately be adjusted for a reopened rather than occluded vessel.

These benefits must be weighted against several theoretical disadvantages of intra-arterial thrombolysis vs. intravenous thrombolysis. Start of thrombolytic therapy is substantially delayed by the need to move the patient to an angiography suite, prep the patient for the procedure, mobilize the interventional team, and catheterize the involved vessel. In controlled trials, the time delay from completion of CT scan to catheter on clot and start of thrombolysis has generally ranged from 70 to 120 min. Intra-arterial therapy requires manipulation of a catheter in the ischemic bed and injured vessels, possibly increasing the risk of cerebral hemorrhage. Intra-arterial treatment is both labor and capital intensive and requires highly experienced interventional neuroradiologists to perform the angiogram and infuse the thrombolytic agent. Consequently, if it is found to be beneficial, it is likely to remain an intervention confined to tertiary stroke critical care centers.

Combined intravenous and intra-arterial thrombolysis strategies have evolved as an attempt to combine the advantage of rapid start of treatment of intravenous therapy and the eventual more definitive recanalization of intra-arterial therapy. Intravenous thrombolysis is begun immediately upon completing the CT scan. Simultaneously, the patient is transported to the angiography suite and catheterization begins. When the catheter arrives on clot, intravenous infusion is ended (or it has ended earlier after reaching a prespecified maximal dose), and intra-arterial infusion begins.

Evidence   Although numerous case series report the effectiveness of intra-arterial thrombolysis, only a limited number of prospective randomized trials within the first 6 h of stroke onset have been conducted. In a study by Mori et al, 31 patients were enrolled with a carotid artery territory stroke and randomized to receive TPA (20 or 30 mega-international units (MIU)) or placebo. Postinfusion angiogram showed only 17 percent reperfusion in the placebo group in comparison with 50 percent in the 30-MIU TPA arm and 44 percent in the 20-MIU arm. In follow-up, patients treated with 30 MIU had a significantly earlier and better clinical improvement than those who received placebo.[152]

The safety and recanalization efficacy of intra-arterial pro-urokinase was investigated by the PROACT investigators.[103] Forty-six patients treated within 6 h of stroke onset who had angiographic evidence of complete occlusion or minimal perfusion involving the M1 or M2 middle cerebral artery were randomized 2:1 to intra-arterial pro-urokinase plus systemic heparin or intra-arterial placebo plus systemic heparin. Median time to treatment was 5.5 h. Early recanalization occurred significantly more often with pro-urokinase. Recanalization rates were 82 percent in the pro-urokinase plus high dose heparin group, 40 percent in the pro-urokinase plus low dose heparin group, and 14 percent in the combined placebo group. Though associated with excellent recanalization rates, the high intra-arterial pro-urokinase plus high dose heparin group had an unacceptable high incidence of symptomatic hemorrhagic transformation (27 percent). Based on the encouraging findings of this phase 2 study, a larger phase 3 trial was conducted, and preliminary results suggest a substantial clinical benefit of intra-arterial pro-urokinase up to 6 h after symptom onset.

The feasibility and safety of combined intravenous/intra-arterial TPA therapy was investigated in the Emergency Management of Stroke (EMS) Bridging Trial. The investigators randomized 35 patients within 3 h of stroke onset to receive intravenous TPA plus intra-arterial TPA or intravenous placebo plus intra-arterial TPA.[153] The intravenous TPA dose was two-thirds of the standard intravenous dose, infused rapidly (0.6 mg/kg, 10% bolused IV over 1 to 2 min, and the remaining infused IV over 30 min). The intra-arterial TPA dose was up to 20 mg over 2 h. Clot was visualized at angiography in 22 of 34 patients. Complete recanalization was achieved more often in the combination intravenous/intra-arterial group (55 percent) than the intra-arterial group alone (10 percent). However, there was no difference in functional outcome at 7 to 10-day and 3-month follow-up. Two patients in the combined treatment arm experienced fatal bleed complications not clearly related to treatment assignment. There was no difference between the groups with regard to symptomatic intracerebral hemorrhage or other moderate to severe bleeding complications. This pilot study demonstrates the feasibility of combined intravenous and intra-arterial thrombolytic therapy.

Recommendations   Intra-arterial and combined intravenous/intra-arterial thrombolysis have the potential to become powerful tools to reverse ischemia in the acute setting. These techniques have not yet been fully proven to be effective and continue to be evaluated in research settings. Until safety and efficacy are definitely demonstrated, these treatment modalities should not be used outside a research or compassionate care protocol.

ANTIPLATELET THERAPY

Background

Antiplatelet agents are of potential benefit in acute ischemic stroke by reducing the formation of "white
thrombi," platelet and fibrin aggregates that form in
fast-moving arterial streams on damaged endothelial
surfaces. Antiplatelet therapy may discourage propagation of the initial thrombus to block additional vessels
and recurrent embolization. However, antiplatelet therapy may also increase the risk of hemorrhagic transformation of infarct.

Current antiplatelet agents modulate platelet
function via four different pathways. Aspirin irreversibly inhibits platelet cyclo-oxygenase, preventing generation of the pro-aggregrant metabolite, thromboxane.
The thienopyridines, ticlopidine and clopidogrel, block
ADP-induced platelet aggregation. Dipyridamole inhibits phosphodiesterase, which leads to increased cyclic
AMP levels and subsequent impaired platelet adhesion.
G2P3 blocker agents block the platelet membrane glycoprotein receptor that mediates platelet aggregation.

An extensive body of clinical trial data demonstrates the effectiveness of long-term antiplatelet therapy in the secondary prevention of serious vascular
events such as stroke, myocardial infarction, or vascular
death.[154] Only a few studies, however, have examined
the use of antiplatelet therapy in the setting of acute ischemic stroke.

Evidence

Two megatrials have examined the efficacy of aspirin
therapy within 48 h of ischemic stroke onset. The Chinese Acute Stroke Trial (CAST) enrolled 21,106 patients within 48 h of stroke onset and randomized patients to 160 mg of aspirin a day or placebo.[155] Treatment
was administered daily for 4 weeks. Ninety-seven percent of the patients completed the 4 weeks of medication, whether they remained hospitalized for 4 weeks
or discharged before that time. The primary endpoint
for the study was death from any cause during the first
4 weeks following stroke and death or dependence at
discharge. Secondary endpoints included fatal or nonfatal recurrent stroke and death or nonfatal stroke within
4 weeks. Study results for the primary endpoint demonstrated a significant reduction in death at 4 weeks from
3.9 percent in the control group to 3.3 percent in the
aspirin group. Secondary analyses demonstrated modest
but statistically significant reductions with aspirin in

recurrent ischemic strokes at 4 weeks and 4-week
mortality.

The International Stroke Trial (IST) employed a
3×2 factorial design to investigate whether aspirin,
low-dose heparin, high-dose heparin, or a combination
of aspirin and heparin are safe and efficacious in the
treatment of ischemic stroke.[156] There were 19,435 patients enrolled within 48 h of symptom onset with an
average time to randomization of 19 h. Sixteen percent
of patients were enrolled within 6 h of symptom onset.
Subjects were randomized to one of the six following
groups: heparin 5000 IU SQ bid, heparin 12,500 IU SQ
bid, aspirin 300 mg qd, aspirin 300 mg qd + heparin
5000 IU SQ bid, aspirin 300 mg qd + 12,500 IU SQ bid,
or avoid aspirin and heparin. Subjects were treated for
14 days or until time of discharge. The average duration
of treatment was 11 days, with the main reason for early
discontinuation being hospital discharge. The primary
outcomes for the study were death within 14 days and
death or dependency at 6 months.

Aspirin-treated patients had significantly fewer
recurrent ischemic strokes with no significant increase
in hemorrhagic strokes within 14 days. The recurrent
ischemic stroke rate declined from 3.9 percent to 2.8
percent with aspirin therapy. A nonsignificant decrease
in mortality within 14 days was observed. At 6 months,
there was a nonsignificant trend toward a smaller percentage of the aspirin group being dead or dependent
(62.2 percent vs. 63.5 percent).

One much smaller trial specifically investigated
the initiation of aspirin within the very first few hours
of ischemic stroke onset. MAST-I employed a 2×2
factorial design to test aspirin, streptokinase, both, or
neither in patients enrolled within 6 h of stroke onset.[143]
The aspirin regimen was 300 mg daily vs. avoid aspirin
for the first 10 days after onset. One-hundred fifty-three
patients were randomized to the aspirin alone sub-arm
and 156 to the neither aspirin nor streptokinase sub-arm.
No statistically significant differences in early recurrent
stroke, symptomatic cerebral hemorrhage, or death or
disability at 6 months were noted.

A meta-analysis combining the results of 40,397
randomized subjects from the IST, CAST, and MAST-
I demonstrates the following statistically significant effects of aspirin: early recurrent ischemic stroke is reduced from 3.2 percent to 2.4 percent, symptomatic
hemorrhagic transformation is increased from 0.8 percent to 1.0 percent and overall death or nonfatal stroke
at 6 months is reduced from 9.1 percent to 8.2 percent.
These findings suggest a statistically significant, but biologically quite small, benefit of aspirin. Use of aspirin
in the first weeks after onset yields a reduction of 9

deaths or recurrent strokes per 1000 patients treated. The number needed to treat with aspirin to prevent one death or disability at 6 months is 111. It is unclear from these trials to what, if any, degree this small treatment effect of aspirin reflects beneficial actions in the first hours after stroke onset, rather than usefulness in preventing secondary strokes in the subsequent 14 to 28 days.

Other antiplatelet agents have not been systematically investigated in the acute stroke setting. Ticlopidine takes 4 to 5 days and clopidogrel 2 to 4 days to reach maximal effectiveness at standard dosing, limiting their theoretical utility in the first few hours, although loading doses of clopidogrel might allow a more rapid onset of action. Phase II dose-escalation trials of G2P3 platelet antagonists in acute ischemic stroke are under way.

Recommendations

Clinical trial evidence supports the use of aspirin in the first 2 weeks after ischemic stroke onset and provides some support for the use of aspirin at a dose of 160 to 325 mg in the first few hours. All patients not receiving thrombolytic or anticoagulant therapy should be treated with aspirin, unless there is a history of hypersensitivity to aspirin, active peptic ulcer disease, recent gastrointestinal bleeding, or other contraindication. To promote rapid therapeutic effect, patients able to take pills orally should be instructed to chew the aspirin tablet prior to swallowing. Patients unable to swallow safely should receive therapy either by nasogastric tube or rectal suppository.

ANTICOAGULATION THERAPY

Administering anticoagulation therapy in acute stroke is a time-honored, but until recently essentially untested, therapeutic practice. Theoretically, anticoagulation is most effective on red thrombi, which tend to form in areas of low flow or stagnation. It has been hypothesized that anticoagulation may prevent recurrent embolization, clot propagation, and thrombotic occlusion of a stenotic lesion. Conversely, acute anticoagulation may increase the risk of hemorrhagic transformation.

Heparin

Background Unfractionated heparin has been employed in acute ischemic stroke for over 40 years. Unfractionated heparin is a mixture of glycosaminoglycans isolated from porcine intestinal mucosa. Heparin binds to endothelial cell surfaces and works by binding and accelerating one thousandfold the actions of antithrombin III. Antithrombin III forms stable complexes with and inhibits several clotting factor proteases. Heparin catalyzes this reaction without being consumed. Once an antithrombin-protease complex is formed, heparin is released intact for binding to another antithrombin molecule.

Evidence Unfractionated heparin was initially tested in several small, clinical trials, some in the pre-CT era when some enrolled patients may have had hemorrhage present on entry. A meta-analysis of all trials of acute anticoagulation (chiefly with unfractionated heparin) reported through 1993 identified 10 trials enrolling a total of only 1047 patients.[157] Across all studies of ischemic stroke, acute anticoagulation showed a nonsignificant trend toward reduction in the odds of death.

The subsequent IST examined the effects of aspirin, subcutaneous heparin, and a combination of these two drugs in ischemic stroke patients who presented within 48 h of stroke onset.[156] As noted above, subjects were randomized to six treatment arms in a 3 × 2 factorial design: low-dose heparin alone (5000 IU SQ bid), high-dose heparin alone (12,500 IU SQ bid), aspirin 300 mg alone, aspirin 300 mg + low-dose heparin, aspirin 300 mg + high-dose heparin, and avoid aspirin and heparin. Treatment was continued for 14 days or until time of discharge, and the average duration of treatment was 11 days.

Patients treated with heparin had significantly fewer recurrent ischemic strokes within 14 days (2.9 percent vs. 3.8 percent), but this benefit was offset by a similar increase in hemorrhagic strokes (1.2 percent vs. 0.4 percent). Treatment groups showed no difference in the incidence of death and disability at 6 months. No net benefit of acute anticoagulation was seen when analysis was confined to the subgroup of 3169 patients who had atrial fibrillation and likely cardioembolic stroke. Considering each of the six treatment group subarms across the entire trial population, there was a trend to best outcome in patients assigned to aspirin plus low-dose heparin daily.

The results of the International Stroke Trial argue against a policy of fixed, high-dose, subcutaneously administered heparin for all comers with acute ischemic stroke. Whether these findings are generalizable to the more common U.S. practice of adjusted-dose, intravenous heparin for selected patients is uncertain. Avoiding acute treatment of patients with risk factors for hemorrhagic transformation might improve the benefit-risk ratio. Large series have suggested that large infarct size, severely elevated blood pressures, and older age increase the risk of hemorrhage.[107,158–160]

Recommendations Clinical trial data do not suggest major net benefit or harm of unfractionated intravenous dose heparin in acute ischemic stroke. Therefore, no firm recommendation can be given, and use of unfractionated high-dose heparin remains at the discretion of the treating physician. Our own algorithm for the use of antiplatelet and anticoagulant therapy is provided in Table 2-8. The use of low-dose subcutaneous heparin is recommended in patients with hemiparesis or otherwise rendered immobile by stroke for prophylaxis against deep venous thrombosis and pulmonary embolism. Using high-dose heparin in patients with severe hypertension should generally be avoided because of increased risk of hemorrhage.[107,158,159] We recommend gently lowering blood pressure to a MAP of 130 mmHg before administering heparin.

Low Molecular Weight Heparins and Heparinoids

Background Heparin can be fractionated by either chemical or enzymatic depolymerization to yield fragments about one-third the size of the average molecular component of unfractionated heparin. Purified, low molecular weight heparins (LMWH) also work by binding to antithrombin III. LMWHs differ in several important respects, however, from unfractionated heparin. They exert relatively less effect on clotting factor IIa, which has been associated with hemorrhagic complications in animal models, but equal effect on factor Xa, associated with beneficial antithrombotic activity.[161] They are much less likely than unfractionated heparin to provoke an antibody response and the syndrome of heparin-induced thrombocytopenia with in vivo thrombosis. They have high bioavailability and a more prolonged half-life, yielding a more predictable anticoagulant response, and consequently can be administered at arterial disease treatment levels with once or twice daily subcutaneous

---

Table 2-8.
Algorithm for antithrombotic therapy in acute ischemic stroke

---

Initial IV heparin with a bolus, aim PTT 50–60 for:
  Suspected critical, symptomatic carotid artery stenosis, when exam suggests infarct size is small to moderate (<5 cm)
  Suspected basilar artery thrombosis
  Suspected dissection of extracranial vessels, when exam suggests infarct size is small to moderate (<5 cm)
  Dissection of intracranial vessels without subarachnoid hemorrhage, when exam suggests infarct size is small to moderate (<5 cm)
Initial IV heparin without bolus or SQ low molecular weight heparin* at arterial disease dose for:
  Cardioembolic stroke, when exam suggests infarction size is small to moderate (<5 cm)
Initial aspirin 325 mg, crush and chew, for all others
Initial subcutaneous heparin, 5,000 units bid, for all nonambulatory patients not on full-dose anticoagulation

Subsequent IV heparin with a bolus, aim PTT 50–60, for:
  Large vessel atherothrombotic stroke in progression despite aspirin, when the physician believes the progression may be due to clot propagation or recurrent embolism
  Lacunar stroke in progression despite aspirin, when the physician believes the progression may be due to clot propagation
Subsequent IV heparin without bolus or SQ low molecular weight heparin* at arterial disease dose for:
  Cardioembolic stroke when infarct size is large (>5 cm), after 5–7-days delay and repeat CT shows no hemorrhagic transformation

---

*e.g., Enoxaparin 1 mg/kg SQ bid or dalteparin 100 anti-Xa units/kg SQ bid.

injections without requiring laboratory monitoring and dose adjustment.

Heparinoids are mixtures of LMWH, dermatan sulphate, and chondroitin sulphate. Their mode of action and relative advantages compared with unfractionated heparin are comparable with LMWHs, although their half-lives are considerably longer.[162]

Evidence Two double-blinded placebo-controlled trials of a LMWH, nadroparine, in acute ischemic stroke have been performed. The first compared two dosages of LMWH with placebo in the treatment of 306 patients with acute ischemic stroke.[163] Patients who presented within 48 h of stroke onset received high-dose LMWH, low-dose LMWH, or placebo for 10 days. The average time to treatment was 27 h. There was a significant dose-dependent reduction in the risk of death and dependency for activities of daily living at 6 months for patients treated with LMWH. In the high-dose arm, 45 percent of patients were dead or dependent at 6 months vs. 65 percent in the placebo arm. In contrast to studies involving heparin, there was no significant difference in the rates of hemorrhagic transformation or systemic bleeding in patients receiving LMWH or placebo.

These promising results, however, were not replicated in a second larger confirmatory trial.[164] In this study, 767 patients were randomized within 24 h of stroke onset to high-dose LMWH, low-dose LMWH, or placebo for 10 days. There was no difference between the three treatment groups in the primary endpoint of death or disability at 6 months. Pulmonary embolism occurred less frequently in the LMWH groups than the placebo group. Hemorrhagic transformation occurred more frequently in the high-dose LMWH group than the other treatment arms.

The first multicenter trial of a heparinoid in acute ischemic stroke was carried out in the Trial of Org 10172 in Acute Stroke Treatment (TOAST).[165] This randomized double-blind trial compared danaparoid with placebo for 7 days in 1281 patients enrolled within 24 h of stroke onset. Danaparoid was administered by continuous intravenous infusion, dose-adjusted by laboratory monitoring of factor Xa. On the primary outcome measure of favorable Barthel activities of daily living score at 3 months, no difference between the treatment groups was observed. Subgroup analysis did suggest a beneficial effect in patients with large vessel (primarily carotid) atherothrombotic stroke mechanisms, with very favorable 3-month outcomes in 43.3 percent of the danaparoid groups vs. 29.1 percent of the placebo group. No benefit at all was detected in patients with cardioembolic and lacunar stroke mechanisms.

It is instructive to consider event rates observed in the control arms in recent trials of anticoagulant therapy. In the TOAST trial, progression/recurrence of infarct was observed in only 1.3 percent of placebo patients over the first 7 days, despite the absence of aspirin, heparin, or heparinoid. In the cardioembolic TOAST placebo subgroup, recurrent infarct occurred in only 1.6 percent of patients not receiving anticoagulant therapy. Similarly, in atrial fibrillation patients enrolled in the International Stroke Trial and assigned to the avoid aspirin and avoid heparin arm, recurrent infarct occurred in only 1.1 percent of patients over 14 days. These observations suggest that with modern fluid management and general supportive care, progression or recurrence of infarct occurs very infrequently in acute ischemic stroke patients even in the absence of antithrombotic therapy. As a result, opportunities for anticoagulation therapy to be beneficial are circumscribed.

Recommendations Clinical trial data provide no firm evidence of net benefit or net harm of LMWHs or heparinoids in acute ischemic stroke. Therefore, no firm recommendation can be given, and their use remains at the discretion of the treating physician. The TOAST trial suggests that patients with large vessel atherothrombotic stroke may benefit from heparinoid treatment, but this subgroup analysis requires prospective confirmation in a new trial. The risk-benefit ratio of these agents may be improved by avoiding their use in the first 5 to 7 days in patients with large cerebral infarcts (e.g., those involving greater than 5 cm of tissue in longest dimension). Our current approach to antithrombotic therapy is illustrated in Table 2-8.

Ancrod

Background Ancrod is an enzyme that is derived from the venom of the Malaysian pit viper and cleaves circulating fibrinogen into soluble fibrin fragments. The conversion of fibrinogen to fibrin results in inhibition of thrombus formation, and lowering fibrinogen levels will reduce the tendency to clot formation. Because fibrinogen is a major contributor to plasma viscosity, its cleavage by ancrod results in a lowered blood viscosity. Theoretically, this allows for increased perfusion, especially in the microcirculation. In addition to these properties, ancrod has also been found to induce the release of endogenous plasminogen activator from the vessel wall. This combination of properties makes ancrod an attractive candidate agent for treating acute stroke patients.

Evidence Two international, randomized, placebo-controlled trials of ancrod has been conducted. The first 132 acute ischemic stroke patients enrolled within 6 h of stroke onset.[166] Patients randomized to ancrod received 0.5 units/kg over 6 h and then daily infusions with a target fibrinogen level of 0.7 to 1.0 g/L for a total of 7 days. The average fibrinogen level after the 6-h infusion was 1.3 g/L, and only 23 percent of patients achieved the target level of < 1.0 g/L. The study failed to show a difference in outcome at 3 months between the two groups. No increase in major systemic bleeding or hemorrhagic transformation was observed. Because the target fibrinogen level was not achieved in most patients during the initial 6-h infusion, a follow-up, higher dose study was performed to determine whether ancrod is effective in acute ischemic stroke. The Stroke Treatment with Ancrod Trial (STAT) was an international randomized double-blind placebo-controlled trial investigating the efficacy of ancrod within 3 h of ischemic stroke onset. Although the results of this study have not been published, interim analysis showed that 90 percent of ancrod recipients achieved a target 12-h post-treatment fibrinogen level of <0.7 g/L.

Recommendations Until the results of the STAT trial are published, ancrod cannot be recommended for treatment of the acute ischemic stroke patient.

CONCLUSIONS

Our concepts of the pathophysiology and treatment of stroke have changed dramatically over the past 10 years. Basic science and clinical studies have emphasized the importance of rapid intervention to restore blood flow and prevent permanent ischemic damage. With the recent development of effective thrombolytic acute stroke therapy, the era of therapeutic nihilism is at an end. Now, stroke is recognized as an eminently treatable medical emergency, and every minute counts when caring for an acute stroke patient. Care according to the consensus principles outlined in this chapter will help to reduce the personal, familial, and societal burden of this devastating disease.

REFERENCES

1. Brott, TG, Haley EC, Jr, Levy DE, et al: Urgent therapy for stroke: Part I. Pilot study of tissue plasminogen activator administered within 90 minutes. *Stroke* 23:632, 1992.
2. The National Institute of Neurological Disorders and Stroke (NINDS) rt-PA Stroke Study Group: A systems approach to immediate evaluation and management of hyperacute stroke: Experience at eight centers and implications for community practice and patient care. *Stroke* 28:1530, 1997.
3. A Working Group on Emergency Brain Resuscitation: Emergency brain resuscitation: A Working group on emergency brain resuscitation. *Ann Intern Med* 122: 622, 1995.
4. Hossmann K: Viability thresholds and the penumbra of focal ischemia. *Ann Neurol* 36:557, 1994.
5. Heiss WD, Fink GR, Pietrzyk U, Huber M, Herholz K: Do PET Data Support a Therapeutic Window in Ischemic Stroke?, in O.-S.H. Krieglstein J (ed): *Pharmacology of Cerebral Ischemia.* Wisenschaftliche Verlagsgesellschaft, Stuttgart, 1992, pp 529–536.
6. Heiss W, Graf R: The ischemic penumbra. *Curr Opin Neurol* 7:11, 1994.
7. Zivin J: Factors determining the therapeutic window for stroke. *Neurology* 50:599, 1998.
8. Bratina P, Greenberg L, Pasteur W, Grotta JC: Current emergency department management of stroke in Houston, Texas. *Stroke* 26:409, 1995.
9. Gomez CR, Malkoff MD, Sauer CM, Tulyapronchote R, Burch CM, Banet GA: Code stroke: An attempt to shorten inhospital therapeutic delays. *Stroke* 25:1920, 1994.
10. Wentworth DA, Atkinson R: Implementation of an acute stroke program decreases hospitalization costs and length of stay. *Stroke* 27:1040, 1996.
11. Zweifler RM, Brody ML, Graves GC, et al: Intravenous t-PA for acute ischemic stroke: Therapeutic yield of a stroke code system. *Neurology* 50:501, 1998.
12. Rapp K, Bratina P, Barch C, et al: Code stroke: Rapid transport, triage and treatment using rt-PA therapy. *J Neurosci Nurs* 29:361, 1997.
13. The European Ad Hoc Consensus Group: Optimizing intensive care in stroke: A European perspective. *Cerebrovasc Dis* 7:113, 1997.
14. Kasner S, Grotta J: Emergency identification and treatment of acute ischemic stroke. *Ann Emerg Med* 30:642, 1997.
15. American College of Emergency: Guidelines for trauma care systems. *Ann Emerg Med* 22:1079, 1993.
16. National Heart Attack Alert Program Coordinating Committee, M.t.T.W.G: Emergency department: Rapid identification and treatment of patients. *Ann Emerg Med* 23: 311, 1994.
17. Kidwell CS, Saver J, Schubert GB, Eckstein M, Starkman

S: Design and retrospective analysis of the Los Angeles Prehospital Stroke. *Prehosp Emerg Care* 2:267, 1998.

18. Broderick J: Logistics in acute stroke management. *Drugs* 3:109, 1997.

19. Adams HP Jr, Brott TG, Crowell RM, et al: Guidelines for thrombolytic therapy for acute stroke: A supplement to the guidelines for the management of patients with acute ischemic stroke. *Stroke* 25:1901, 1994.

20. Saver JL, Starkman S: State of the art medical management of acute ischemic stroke. *J Stroke Cerebrovasc Dis* 6:189, 1997.

21. American Heart Association: Acute stroke, in *Textbook of Advanced Cardiac Life Support.* Dallas, American Heart Association, 1997, pp 10-1 to 10–21.

22. Azzimondi G, Bassein L, Fiorani L, et al: Variables associated with hospital arrival time after stroke: Effect of delay on the clinical efficiency of early treatment. *Stroke* 28: 537, 1997.

23. National Stroke Association Consensus Panel: Stroke: The first hours. *Stroke Clinical Updates* 1, 1997.

24. Mohr JP, Caplan LR, Melski JW, et al: The Harvard Cooperative Stroke Registry: A prospective registry. *Neurology* 28:754, 1978.

25. Foulkes MA, Wolf PA, Price TR, Mohr JP, Hier DB: The Stroke Data Bank: design, methods, and baseline characteristics. *Stroke* 19:547, 1988.

26. Caplan L, Hier D, Cruz ID: Cerebral embolism in the Michael Reese Stroke Registry. *Stroke* 14:530, 1983.

27. Bogousslavsky J, Van Melle G, Regli F: The Lausanne Stroke Registry: Analysis of 1,000 consecutive patients with first stroke. *Stroke* 19:1083, 1988.

28. Caplan L: *Stroke: A Clinical Approach.* Newton, Butterworth-Heinemann, 1993, p 562.

29. Moossy J: Pathology of cerebral atherosclerosis: Influence of age, race, and gender. *Stroke* 24(Suppl 12):122-3; 131-2, 1993.

30. Feldmann E, Daneault N, Kwan E, et al: Chinese-white differences in the distribution of occlusive cerebrovascular disease. *Neurology* 40:1541, 1990.

30a. Singh R, Cohen SN, Krup R, Abedi AG: Racial differences in ischemic cerebrovascular disease. *J Stroke and Cerebrovasc Dis* 7:352, 1998.

31. Bamford J: Clinical examination in diagnosis and subclassification of stroke. *Lancet* 339:400, 1992.

32. Bogousslavsky J, Castillo V: What is the place of clinical assessment in acute stroke management, in B. J (ed): *Acute Stroke Treatment.* St. Louis, Mosby, 1997, pp 15–32.

33. Bamford J, Sandercock P, Dennis M, et al: A prospective study of acute cerebrovascular disease in the community: The Oxfordshire Community Stroke Project 1981-86. 1. Methodology, demography and incident cases of first-ever stroke. *J Neurol Neurosurg Psychiatry* 51:1373, 1988.

34. Brott T, Tilley B, Welch KM, et al: Improved reliability of the NIH Stroke Scale using video training. *Stroke* 25:2220, 1994.

35. Adams HP, Jr, Brott TG, Furlan AJ, et al: Guidelines

for thrombolytic therapy for acute stroke: A supplement to the guidelines for the management of patients with acute ischemic stroke. *Stroke* 27:1711, 1996.

36. Quality Standards Subcommittee of the American Academy of Neurology: *Practice advisory: Thrombolytic therapy for acute ischemic stroke. Neurology* 47:835, 1996.

37. Kaarisalo MM, Immonen-Raiha P, Marttila RJ, et al: Atrial fibrillation and stroke: Mortality and causes of death after the first acute ischemic stroke. *Stroke* 28: 311, 1997.

38. Oppenheimer S, Hachinski V: The cardiac consequences of stroke. *Neurol Clin* 10:167, 1992.

39. Oppenheimer S: The anatomy and physiology of cortical mechanisms of cardiac control. *Stroke* 24(12 Suppl):I3, 1993.

40. DiPasquale G, Urbinettis S, Pinelli GC: Cardiac arrhythmias following acute brain injuries, in P.G. DiPasquale (ed): Heart-Brain Interactions. Berlin, Springer-Verlag, 1992, pp 19–30.

41. Weir CJ, Murray GD, Dyker AG, Lees KR: Is hyperglycaemia an independent predictor of poor outcome after acute stroke? Results of a long-term follow up study. *Br Med J* 314:1303, 1997.

42. Myllyla V, Sotaniemi K, Pyhtinen J: Significance of cerebral CT in neurological practice. *Acta Neurol Scand* 78:228, 1988.

43. Morgenstern L, Luna-Gonzales H, Huber JC, Jr, Wong SS, Uthman M, Gurian JH: Worst headache and subarachnoid hemorrhage: Prospective, modern computed tomography and spinal fluid analysis. *Ann Emerg Med* 32:297, 1998.

44. Tarr RW, Hecht ST, Horton JA: Nontraumatic intracranial hemorrhage, in LRE (ed): *Magnetic Resonance and Computerized Tomography Imaging of the Head, Neck, and Spine,* St. Louis, Mosby, 1991, pp 267–299.

45. Moulin T, Cattin F, Crepin-LeBlond T, et al: Early CT signs in acute middle cerebral artery infarction: Predictive value for subsequent infarct locations and outcome. *Neurology* 47:366, 1996.

46. von Kummer R, Nolte PN, Schnittger H, Thron A, Ringelstein EB: Detectability of cerebral hemisphere ischaemic infarcts by CT within 6 hours. *Neuroradiology* 38:31, 1996.

47. Truwit CL, Barkovich AJ, Gean-Marton A, Hibri N, Norman D: Loss of the insular ribbon: Another early CT sign of acute middle cerebral artery infarction. *Radiology* 176:801, 1990.

48. Tomura N, Uemura K, Inugami A, Fujita H, Higano S, Shishido F: Early CT finding in cerebral infarction: Obscuration of the lentiform nucleus. *Radiology* 168:463, 1988.

49. Gacs G, Fox A, Barnett HJ, Vinuela F: CT visualization of intracranial arterial thromboembolism. *Stroke* 14: 756, 1983.

50. Bates, VE, Vereczkey-Porter K, Bakshi R, Empey HS, Kamran S, Wright P: Staging acute stroke using cranial

computerized tomography findings and neurological deficit. *Neurology* 50:A195, 1998.

51. The NINDS t-PA Stroke Study Group: Intracerebral hemorrhage after intravenous t-PA therapy for ischemic stroke. *Stroke* 28:2109, 1997.

52. Schriger D, Kalafut M, Starkman S, Krueger M, Saver JL: Cranial computed tomography interpretation in acute stroke: Physician accuracy in determining eligibility for thrombolytic therapy. *JAMA* 279:1293, 1998.

53. Johnston K, Haley EC: Emergency imaging of the acute stroke patient. *J Neuroimaging* 7:111, 1997.

54. Bryan RN, Levy LM, Whitlow WD, Killian JM, Preziosi TJ, Rosario JA: Diagnosis of acute cerebral infarction: Comparison of CT and MR imaging. *Am J Neuroradiol* 12:611, 1991.

55. Shuaib A, Lee D, Pelz D, Fox A, Hachinski VC: The impact of magnetic resonance imaging on the management of acute ischemic stroke. *Neurology* 42:816, 1992.

56. Yuh WT, Crain MR, Loes DJ, Greene GM, Ryals TJ, Sato Y: MR imaging of cerebral ischemia: Findings in the first 24 hours. *Am J Neuroradiol* 12:621, 1991.

57. Mohr J, Biller J, Hilal SK, et al: Magnetic resonance versus computed tomographic imaging in acute stroke. *Stroke* 26:807, 1995.

58. Hommel M, Besson G, Le Bas JF, et al: Prospective study of lacunar infarction using magnetic resonance imaging. *Stroke* 21:546, 1990.

59. Rother J, Guckel F, Neff W, Schwartz A, Hennerici M: Assessment of regional cerebral blood volume in acute human stroke by use of single-slice dynamic susceptibility contrast-enhanced magnetic resonance imaging. *Stroke* 27:1088, 1996.

60. Kates R, Atkinson D, Brant-Zawadzki M: Fluid-attenuated inversion recovery (FLAIR): Clinical prospectus of current and future applications. *Top Magn Reson Imaging* 8:389, 1996.

61. Patel M, Edelman R, Warach S: Detection of hyperacute primary intraparenchymal hemorrhage by magnetic resonance imaging. *Stroke* 27:2321, 1996.

62. Singer MB, Atlas S, Drayer BP: Subarachnoid space disease: Diagnosis with fluid-attenuated inversion-recovery MR imaging and comparison with gadolinium-enhanced spin-echo MR imaging-blinded reader study. *Radiology,* 208:417, 1998.

63. Campbell BG, Zimmerman R: Emergency magnetic resonance of the brain. *Top Magn Reson Imaging* 9:208, 1998.

64. Willig DS, Turski P, Frayne R, Graves VB, et al: Contrast-enhanced 3D MR DSA of the carotid artery bifurcation. *Radiology,* 208:447, 1998.

65. Remonda L, Heid O, Schroth G: Carotid artery stenosis, occlusion, and pseudo-occlusion: First-pass, gadolinium-enhanced, three-dimensional MR angiography— preliminary study. *Radiology* 209:95, 1998.

66. Stock K, Radue E, Jacob AL, et al: Intracranial arteries: Prospective blinded comparative study of MR angiography and DSA in 50 patients. *Radiology* 195:451, 1995.

67. Korogi Y, Takahshi M, Nakagawa T, et al: Intracranial vascular stenosis and occlusion: MR angiographic findings. *Am J Neuroradiol* 18:135, 1997.

68. Qureshi AI, Isa A, Cinnamon J, et al: Magnetic resonance angiography in patients with brain infarction. *J Neuroimaging* 8:65, 1998.

69. Jackson MR, Chang AS, Robles HA, et al: Determination of 60% or greater carotid stenosis: A prospective comparison of magnetic resonance angiography and duplex ultrasound with conventional angiography. *Ann Vasc Surg* 12:236, 1998.

70. Magarelli N, Scarabino T, Simeone AL, et al: Carotid stenosis: A comparison between MR and spiral CT angiography. *Neuroradiology* 40:367, 1998.

71. Ohue S, Kohno K, Kusunoki K, et al: Magnetic resonance angiography in patients with acute stroke treated by local thrombolysis. *Neuroradiology* 40:536, 1998.

72. Lee LJ, Krowell C, Alger J, Starkman S, Saver J: Impact upon stroke subtype diagnosis of early diffusion-weighted MR and MRA imaging. *Neurology* 50:A298, 1998.

73. Moseley ME, Cohen Y, Mintorovitch J, Chileuitt L, et al: Early detection of regional cerebral ischemia in cats: Comparison of diffusion- and T2-weighted MRI and spectroscopy. *Magn Reson Med* 14:330, 1990.

74. Pierpaoli C, Alger J, Righini A, Mattiello J, et al: High temporal resolution diffusion MRI of global cerebral ischemia and reperfusion. *J Cereb Blood Flow Metab* 16:892, 1996.

75. Warach S, Gaa J, Siewert B, Wielopolski P, Edelman RR: Acute human stroke studied by whole brain echo planar diffusion—weighted magnetic resonance imaging. *Ann Neurol* 37:231, 1995.

76. Tong DC, Yenari M, Albers GW, O'Brien M, Marks MP, Moseley ME: Correlation of perfusion- and diffusion-weighted MRI with NIHSS score. *Neurology* 50:864, 1998.

77. Barber PA, Darby DG, Desmond PM et al: Prediction of stroke outcome with echoplanar perfusion- and diffusion-weighted MRI. *Neurology* 51:418, 1998.

78. Warach S, Dashe J, Edelman R: Clinical outcome in ischemic stroke predicted by early diffusion-weighted and perfusion magnetic resonance imaging: A preliminary analysis. *J Cereb Blood Flow Metab* 16:53, 1996.

79. Lutsep H, Albers GW, DeCrespigny A, et al: Clinical utility of diffusion-weighted magnetic resonance imaging in the assessment of ischemic stroke. *Ann Neurol* 41:574, 1997.

79a. Kidwell CS, Saver JL, Mattiello J, et al: Thrombolytic reversal of acute human cerebral ischemic injury demonstrated by diffusion/perfusion magnetic resonance imaging. *Neurology* 52(Suppl 2):A536, 1999.

80. Siewert B, Schlaug G, Edelman RR, Warach S: Comparison of EPISTAR and T2*-weighted gadolinium-enhanced perfusion imaging in patients with acute cerebral ischemia. *Neurology* 48:673, 1997.

81. Rordorf GKW, Copen WA, Cramer SC, et al: Regional ischemia and ischemic injury in patients with acute middle

cerebral artery stroke as defined by early diffusion-weighted and perfusion-weighted MRI. *Stroke* 29:939, 1998.

82. Knauth M, von Kummer R, Jansen O, Hahnel S, Dorfler A, Sartor K: Potential of CT angiography in acute ischemic stroke. *Am J Neuroradiol* 18:1001, 1997.

83. Hunter GJ, Hamburg L, Ponzo JA, et al: Assessment of cerebral perfusion and arterial anatomy in hyperacute stroke with three-dimensional functional CT: Early clinical results. *Am J Neuroradiol* 19:29, 1998.

84. Wildermuth S, Knauth M, Brandt T, Winter R, Sartor K, Hacke W: Role of CT angiography in patient selection for thrombolytic therapy in acute hemispheric stroke. *Stroke* 29:935, 1998.

85. Firlik AD, Rubin G, Yonas H, Wechsler LR: Relation between cerebral blood flow and neurologic deficit resolution. *Neurology* 51:17, 1998.

86. Firlik AD, Kauffman A, Wechsler LR, Firlik KS, Fukui MB, Yonas H: Quantitative cerebral blood flow determinations in acute ischemic. *Stroke* 28:2208, 1997.

87. Kaufmann AM, Firlik A, Yonas H, Wechsler L, et al: Emergent stroke therapy and quantitative cerebral blood flow. *Stroke* 28:253, 1997.

88. Limburg M, van Royen EA, Hijdra A, Verbeeten B, Jr: rCBF-SPECT in brain infarction: When does it predict outcome? *J Nucl Med* 32:382, 1991.

89. Shimosegawa E, Hatazawa J, Inugami A, et al: Cerebral infarction within six hours of onset: Prediction of completed infarction with technetium-99m-HMPAO SPECT. *J Nucl Med* 35:1097, 1994.

90. Baird AE, Donnan GA, Austin MC, Fitt GJ, Davis SM, McKay WJ: Reperfusion after thrombolytic therapy in ischemic stroke measured by single-photon emission computed tomography. *Stroke* 25:79, 1994.

91. Saver JL, Feldman E: Basic transcranial doppler examination: Technique and anatomy, in Babikian VL (ed): *Transcranial Doppler Ultrasonography.* St. Louis, Mosby, 1993, pp 11–28.

92. Schmidt P, Sliwka U, Simon SG, Noth J: High-grade stenosis of the internal carotid artery assessed by color and power Doppler imaging. *J Clin Ultrasound* 26:85, 1998.

93. Martin PJ, Pye IF, Abbott RJ, Naylor AR: Color-coded ultrasound diagnosis of vascular occlusion in acute stroke. *J Neuroimaging* 5:152, 1995.

94. Camerlingo M, Casto L, Censori B, Servalli MC, Ferraro B, Mamoli A: Prognostic use of ultrasonography in acute non-hemorrhagic carotid stroke. *Ital J Neurol Sci* 17:215, 1996.

95. Toni D, Fiorelli M, Zanette EM, et al: Early spontaneous improvement and deterioration of ischemic stroke. *Stroke* 29:1144, 1998.

96. Goertler M, Kross R, Baeumer M, et al: Diagnostic impact and prognostic relevance of early contrast-enhanced transcranial color-coded duplex sonography in acute stroke. *Stroke* 29:955, 1998.

97. Alexandrov AV, Black S, Ehrlich LE, Caldwell CB, Nor-ris JW: Predictors of hemorrhagic transformation occurring spontaneously and on anticoagulants in patients with acute ischemic stroke. *Stroke* 28:1198, 1997.

98. Zanette EM, Roberti C, Mancini G, Pozzilli C, Bragoni M, Toni D: Spontaneous middle cerebral artery reperfusion in ischemic stroke: A follow-up study with transcranial Doppler. *Stroke* 26:430, 1995.

99. Sliwka U, Lingnau A, Stohlmann WD, et al: Prevalence and time course of microembolic signals in patients with acute stroke: A prospective study. *Stroke* 28:358, 1997.

100. Tong D, Albers G: Transcranial Doppler-detected microemboli in patients with acute stroke. *Stroke* 26:1588, 1995.

101. del Zoppo GJ, Poeck K, Pessin MS, et al: Recombinant tissue plasminogen activator in acute thrombotic and embolic stroke. *Ann Neurol* 32:78, 1992.

102. Yokogami K, Nakano S, Ohta H, Goya T, Wakisaka S: Prediction of hemorrhagic complications after thrombolytic therapy for middle cerebral artery occlusion: Value of pre- and post-therapeutic computed tomographic findings and angiographic occlusive site. *Neurosurgery* 39:1102, 1996.

103. del Zoppo G, Higashida R, Furlan A, et al: PROACT: A phase II randomized trial of recombinant prourokinase by direct arterial delivery in acute middle cerebral artery stroke. *Stroke* 29:4, 1998.

104. Hankey GJ, Warlow C, Sellar RJ: Cerebral angiographic risk in mild cerebrovascular disease. *Stroke* 21:209, 1990.

105. Daniels SK, Brailey K, Priestly DH, Herrington LR, Weisberg LA, Foundas AL: Aspiration in patients with acute stroke. *Arch Phys Med Rehabil* 79:14, 1998.

106. Johnston KC, Li JY, Lyden PD, et al: Medical and neurological complications of ischemic stroke: Experience from the RANTTAS trial. *Stroke* 29:447, 1998.

107. Cerebral Embolism Study Group: Immediate anticoagulation of embolic stroke: A randomized trial. *Stroke* 14:668, 1983.

108. Gujjar AR, Diebert E, Manno EM, Duff S, Diringer MN: Mechanical ventilation for ischemic stroke and intracerebral hemorrhage: Indications, timing, and outcome. *Neurology* 51:447, 1998.

109. Grotta J, Pasteur W, Khwaja G, Hamel T, Fisher M, Ramirez A: Elective intubation for neurologic deterioration after stroke. *Neurology* 45:640, 1995.

110. Mirski MA, Muffelman B, Ulatowski JA, Hanley DF: Sedation for the critically ill neurologic patient. *Crit Care Med* 23:2038, 1995.

111. Hartmann A, Stingele R, Schnitzer M: General treatment strategies for elevated intracranial pressure, in HW. (ed): *Neuro Critical Care.* Berlin, Springer Verlag, 1994. pp 101–116.

112. Yatsu FM, Zivin J: Hypertension in acute ischemic strokes: Not to treat. *Arch Neurol* 42:999, 1985.

113. Spence J, Del Maestro R: Hypertension in acute ischemic strokes. Treat. *Arch Neurol* 42:1000, 1985.

114. Broderick J, Brott T, Barsan W, et al: Blood pressure

during the first minutes of focal cerebral ischemia. *Ann Emerg Med* 22:1438, 1993.

115. Carlsberg B, Asplun DK, Hagg E: Course of blood pressure in different subsets of patients after acute stroke. *Cerebrovasc Dis* 1:281, 1991.

116. Strandgaard S: Autoregulation of cerebral blood flow in hypertensive patients: The modifying influence of prolonged antihypertensive treatment on the tolerance to acute, drug-induced hypotension. *Circulation* 53:720, 1976.

117. Powers W: Acute hypertension after stroke: The scientific basis for treatment. *Neurology* 43:461, 1993.

118. Meyer JS, Shimazu K, Fukuuchi Y, Ouchi T, Okamoto S, Koto AA: Impaired neurogenic cerebrovascular control and dysautoregulation after stroke. *Stroke* 4:169, 1973.

119. Lisk DR, Grotta J: Lamki LM, Tran HD, Taylor JW, Molony DA, Barron BJ: Should hypertension be treated after acute stroke? A randomized controlled trial using single photon emission computed tomography. *Arch Neurol* 50:855, 1993.

120. Kimura K, Yasaka M, Yamaguchi T: Antihypertensive drugs in acute stage of atherothrombotic infarction. *Rinsho Shinkeigaku* 34:114, 1994.

121. Jorgensen HS, Nakayama H, Raaschou HO, Olsen TS: Effect of blood pressure and diabetes on stroke in progression. *Lancet* 344:156, 1994.

122. Ledingham J: Management of hypertensive crises. *Hypertension* 5:III114, 1983.

123. Rordorf G, Cramer S, Efird JT, Schwamm LH, Buonanno F, Koroshetz WJ: Pharmacological elevation of blood pressure in acute stroke: Clinical effects and safety. *Stroke* 28:2133, 1997.

124. Brott T, Lu M, Kothari R, et al: Hypertension and its treatment in the NINDS rt-PA stroke trial. *Stroke* 29:1504, 1998.

125. Malkoff MD, Gomez C, Tulyapronchote R, Clark WR, Woolson RF, Adams HP, and the TOAST Investigators: Incidence and significance of dehydration in patients with ischemic stroke. *Stroke* 25:246, 1994.

126. Toni D, Fiorelli M, Gentile M, et al: Progressing neurological deficit secondary to acute ischemic stroke: A study on predictability, pathogenesis, and prognosis. *Arch Neurol* 52:670, 1995.

127. Plum F: Brain swelling and edema in cerebral vascular disease. *Res Publ Assoc Res Nerv Ment Dis* 41:318, 1966.

128. White OB, Norris JW, Hachinski VC, Lewis A: Death in early stroke, causes and mechanisms. *Stroke* 10:743, 1979.

129. Wass C, Lanier W: Glucose modulation of ischemic brain injury: Review and clinical recommendations. *Mayo Clin Proc* 71:801, 1996.

130. Candelise L, Landi G, Orazio EN, et al: Prognostic significance of hyperglycemia in acute stroke. *Arch Neurol* 42:661, 1985.

131. Mankovsky BN, Patrick J, Metzger BE, Saver JL: The size of subcortical ischemic infarction in patients with and without diabetes mellitus. *Clin Neurol Neurosurg* 98:137, 1996.

132. Pulsinelli WA, Levy DE, Sigsbee B, Scherer P, Plum F: Increased damage after ischemic stroke in patients with hyperglycemia. *Am J Med* 74:540, 1983.

133. Ginsberg M, Busto R: Combating hyperthermia in acute stroke: A significant clinical concern. *Stroke* 29:529, 1998.

134. Maher J, Hachinski V: Hypothermia as a potential treatment for cerebral ischemia. *Cerebrovasc Brain Metab Rev* 5:277, 1993.

135. Reith J, Jorgensen HS, Pedersen PM, et al: Body temperature in acute stroke: Relation to stroke severity, infarct size, mortality, and outcome. *Lancet* 347:422, 1996.

136. Azzimondi G, Bassein L, Nonino F, Fiorani L, Vignatelli L, Re GD, Alessandro R: Fever in acute stroke worsens prognosis: A prospective study. *Stroke* 26:2040, 1995.

137. Marion DW, Penrod L, Kelsey SF, et al: Treatment of traumatic brain injury with moderate hypothermia. *N Engl J Med* 336:540, 1997.

138. Schwab S, Schwarz S, Aschoff A, Keller E, Hacke W: Moderate hypothermia and brain temperature in patients with severe middle cerebral artery infarction. *Acta Neurochir Suppl* 71:131, 1998.

139. Hacke W, Kaste M, Fieschi C, et al: Intravenous thrombolysis with recombinant tissue plasminogen activator for acute hemispheric stroke. *JAMA* 274:1017, 1995.

140. The National Institute of Neurological Disorders and Stroke rt-PA Stroke Study Group: Tissue plasminogen activator for acute ischemic stroke. *N Engl J Med* 333:1581, 1995.

141. Haley EC, Jr, Lewandowski C, Tilley BC: Myths regarding the NINDS rt-PA Stroke Trial: Setting the record straight. *Ann Emerg Med* 30:676, 1997.

142. The NINDS t-PA Stroke Study Group: Generalized efficacy of t-PA for acute stroke: Subgroup analysis of the NINDS t-PA Stroke Trial. *Stroke* 28:2119, 1997.

143. Multicentre Acute Stroke Trial-Italy (MAST-I) Group: Randomised controlled trial of streptokinase, aspirin, and combination of both in treatment of acute ischaemic stroke. *Lancet* 346:1509, 1995.

144. The Multicenter Acute Stroke Trial-Europe Study Group: Thrombolytic therapy with streptokinase in acute ischemic stroke. *N Engl J Med* 335:145, 1996.

145. Donnan GA, Davis SM, Chambers BR, et al: Streptokinase for acute ischemic stroke with relationship to time of administration. *JAMA* 276:961, 1996.

146. Hoffman J: Thrombolytic therapy of strokes: Part II. *Emerg Med Acute Care Essays* 20:1, 1986.

147. Wardlaw J, Warlow C, Counsell C: Systematic review of evidence on thrombolytic therapy for acute ischemic stroke. *Lancet* 350:607, 1997.

148. Hacke W, Kaste M, Fieschi C, et al: Randomised double-blind placebo-controlled trial of thrombolytic therapy with intravenous alteplase in acute ischaemic stroke. *Lancet* 352:1245, 1998.

149. Tanne D: A large multinational investigation to predict t-PA related symptomatic ICH in patients with acute ischemic stroke. *Stroke* 30, 1999.

150. Tanne D, Mansbach H, Verro P, Binder JR, Karanjia PN, Dayno J, Dulli D, Book D, Levine SR, and the rt-PA in Clinical Practice Stroke Survey Group: Intravenous rt-PA therapy for stroke in clinical practice: A multicenter evaluation of outcome. *Stroke* 29:288, 1998.

151. Zeumer H, Hacke W, Ringelstein EB: Local intraarterial thrombolysis in vertebrobasilar thromboembolic disease. *Am J Neuroradiol* 4:401, 1983.

152. Mori E, Yoneda Y, Tabuchi M, et al: Intravenous recombinant tissue plasminogen activator in acute carotid artery territory stroke. *Neurology* 42:976, 1992.

153. The EMS Bridging Trial Investigators: Combined intravenous/intra-arterial thrombolytic therapy: Safety, time-to-treatment, and frequency of clot. *Stroke* 27:165, 1996.

154. Antiplatelet Trialists' Collaboration: Collaborative overview of randomised trials of antiplatelet therapy—I: Prevention of death, myocardial infarction, and stroke by prolonged antiplatelet therapy in various categories of patients. *Br Med J* 308:81, 1994.

155. Chinese Acute Stroke Trial Collaborative Group: CAST: Randomised placebo-controlled trial of early aspirin use in 20,000 patients with acute ischaemic stroke. *Lancet* 349:1641, 1997.

156. International Stroke Trial Collaborative Group: The International Stroke Trial (IST): A randomised trial of aspirin, subcutaneous heparin, both, or neither among 19,435 patients with acute ischaemic stroke. *Lancet* 349:1569, 1997.

157. Sandercock PA, van den Belt AG, Lindley RI, Slattery J: Antithrombotic therapy in acute ischaemic stroke: An overview of the completed randomised trials. *J Neurol Neurosurg Psychiatry* 56:17, 1993.

158. Shields RW Jr, Laureno R, Lachman T, Victor M: Anticoagulant-related hemorrhage in acute cerebral embolism. *Stroke* 15:426, 1984.

159. Cerebral Embolism Study Group: Cardioembolic stroke, early anticoagulation, and brain hemorrhage. *Arch Intern Med* 147:636, 1987.

160. Chamorro A, Vila N, Saiz A, Alday M, Tolosa E: Early anticoagulation after large cerebral embolic infarction: A safety study. *Neurology* 45:861, 1995.

161. Hirsh J, Levine M: Low molecular weight heparin. *Blood* 79:1, 1992.

162. Nurmohamed M, ten Cate H, ten Cate J: Low molecular weight heparin(oid)s: Clinical investigations and practical recommendations. *Drugs* 53:736, 1997.

163. Kay R, Wong KS, Yu YL, et al: Low-molecular-weight heparin for the treatment of acute ischemic stroke. *N Engl J Med* 333:1588, 1995.

164. Hommel M: Fraxiparine in ischemic stroke study. *Cerebrovasc Dis* 8:(Suppl 4):19A, 1998.

165. TOAST Investigators: Usefulness of a low molecular weight heparinoid in improving outcomes at 7 days and 3 months after stroke. *Stroke* 29:286, 1998.

166. The Ancrod Stroke Study Investigators: Ancrod for the treatment of acute ischemic brain infarction. *Stroke* 25:1755, 1994.

Chapter 3

THE SUBACUTE STROKE PATIENT: HOURS 6 TO 72 AFTER STROKE ONSET

Askiel Bruno
Darryl L. Kaelin
Engin Y. Yilmaz

INTRODUCTION

The time period from 6 to 72 h after onset of ischemic stroke can be considered subacute, because the time to administer thrombolytic therapy with proven efficacy and safety has expired. The possible exception to this may be thrombosis in the vertebrobasilar circulation,[1] but this remains to be proven. There are promising cytoprotective therapies for acute stroke, and it is possible that some of them will prove beneficial beyond the first 6 h (see Chap. 13). Management during the subacute period is focused on preventing and managing stroke complications, identifying the most likely stroke mechanism, prophylaxis against stroke recurrence, stroke education, and initiating rehabilitation.

Where to Admit

Background The increasing complexity of optimal medical care for acute stroke victims is making the advantages of acute stroke units more apparent. An acute stroke unit can be defined as an area in a hospital, staffed by a Stroke Team, where all acute and subacute stroke victims are admitted. As most stroke victims do not need to be admitted to an intensive care unit, acute stroke units located on general hospital wards will accommodate most stroke victims.

Special monitoring should include neurologic checks, which would detect a decrease in the level of consciousness and an increase in paresis in addition to other neurologic signs. Continuous heart rhythm and oxygen saturation monitoring during subacute stroke is also useful.

A Stroke Team should consist of designated physicians, nurses, and other health care personnel with experience and interest in the special care of acute and subacute stroke victims. For those stroke victims who need to be admitted to or transferred to an intensive care unit, a specialized neurointensive unit is preferred. A neurointensive unit is an intensive care unit where acute and subacute stroke victims are cared for by a Stroke Team. Such arrangements are likely to optimize multiple aspects of patient evaluation and treatment, reduce length of hospital stay, and probably minimize cost.

Evidence Strand and colleagues,[2] in a prospective, nonrandomized study, compared the outcomes of 110 stroke patients admitted to a stroke unit to 183 similar patients admitted to general medical wards. Patients with stroke symptoms for up to 7 days were included and were admitted either to the stroke unit or a general ward, based on availability of beds in the stroke unit. Mortality rate 3 months after stroke was the same in the two groups (34 percent). Survivors were significantly more independent 1 year after stroke in the stroke unit group than in the general wards group with respect to personal hygiene ($p < .05$) and dressing ($p < .01$).

Inderdavik and colleagues,[3] in a prospective, randomized study, compared the outcomes of 110 stroke patients admitted to a stroke unit to 110 similar patients admitted to a general medical ward. Patients with stroke symptoms for up to 7 days were included. Mortality rate 6 weeks after stroke was 7 percent in the stroke unit group and 17 percent in the general ward group ($p = .03$). Mortality rate at 1 year remained lower in the stroke unit group than the general ward group (25 percent vs. 33 percent, respectively) but was no longer statistically significant. Patients assigned to the stroke unit were more likely to be living at home 6 weeks after stroke than patients assigned to the general ward (56 percent vs. 33 percent, respectively, $p < .001$). Functional outcomes 1 year after stroke were significantly better in the stroke unit group than the general ward group, according to the Barthel Index ($p = .001$) and a neurologic score ($p = .004$).

Jorgensen and colleagues,[4] in a prospective, non-randomized study, compared the outcomes of 936 stroke patients admitted to a stroke unit to 305 similar patients admitted to general medical or neurologic wards. The patients in these two groups were consecutive admissions to the stroke unit or a general medical ward, which were located in different hospitals in neighboring communities. Ninety-five percent of patients were admitted within 7 days of stroke onset. In-hospital mortality was significantly lower in the stroke unit group than the general wards group (23 percent vs. 29 percent, respectively, $p = .02$). Mortality rate at 6 months was also significantly lower in the stroke unit group than the general wards group (28 percent vs. 35 percent, respectively, $p = .01$). Length of hospital stay was significantly shorter for the stroke unit patients than the general wards patients (mean 39 days vs. 55 days, respectively, $p < .001$). Patients treated in the stroke unit were more likely to be discharged home than patients treated on the general wards (65 percent vs. 56 percent, respectively, $p = .02$).

Recommendations   We recommend admission or transfer of all acute stroke patients to a specialized stroke unit if possible. For patients at high risk for complications, such as large strokes or severe dysphagia, and for patients with medical complications, such as unstable angina, we recommend initial admission to a neurointensive unit for a duration that depends on the condition of the patient. Although patients with acute stroke usually receive intravenous fluids, there have been no clinical trials testing the efficacy of various hydration protocols. Because dehydration may enhance thrombosis and decrease perfusion of the ischemic brain region, and overhydration may augment stroke-associ-ated cerebral edema, euvolemia seems optimal. Isotonic solutions, such as 0.9% NaCl (*normal saline*), are preferred.

MANAGING STABLE SUBACUTE STROKE

Many stroke patients remain stable or begin to improve during the subacute period. These patients usually have relatively small strokes and, because of the small amount of brain injury, usually do not have the complications discussed later in this chapter. The most important issue in treating stable subacute stroke patients is optimal prophylaxis against stroke recurrence and complications.

Treatments to Limit Stroke Size and Prevent Early Recurrence

Background   Many treatments for subacute stroke have been tested. In this section, we will discuss only those treatments that have been tested in randomized clinical trials. These treatments include anticoagulation, hypervolemic hemodilution, cytoprotective drugs, and aspirin. Anticoagulation with intravenous heparin is probably the most popular treatment for acute ischemic stroke[5] despite lack of evidence for its efficacy in randomized clinical trials. Intravenous tissue plasminogen activator has been proven effective in the treatment of acute ischemic stroke in selected patients within 3 h from stroke onset.[6] However, it does not seem to be beneficial beyond the first 3 h, and clinical trials testing other thrombolytic agents have been negative.

Evidence   There have been only two randomized clinical trials of intravenous heparin treatment in acute ischemic stroke. In one trial, 225 patients with stable ischemic stroke were randomized to anticoagulation with intravenous heparin or indistinguishable placebo for 7 days, starting within 48 h of stroke onset.[7] Patients with suspected embolism or uncontrolled hypertension were excluded from this study. Partial thromboplastin time (PTT) was maintained at 50 to 70 s. Patients were followed for up to 1 year, and no significant difference was detected in neurologic status between the two treatment groups. Mortality at 1 year was significantly higher in the heparin than placebo group (15 percent vs. 7 percent, respectively, $p < .01$). Most deaths occurred 3 to 12 months after the stroke and seemed to be unrelated to the acute stroke treatment.

****

The other randomized intravenous heparin treatment trial for acute stroke patients was not blinded and was designed to compare the short-term stroke recurrence rates between anticoagulated and not anticoagulated patients with cardioembolic stroke.[8] In this study, 45 patients within 48 h of stroke onset were randomized to immediate anticoagulation or no anticoagulation and no antiplatelet therapy for the initial 10 days following stroke. Mean PTT during the study period was 1.5 to 2.5 times control in 23 of the 24 anticoagulated patients. There were no major bleeding complications in either group. Thromboembolic complications occurred in 3 (14 percent) patients during the 14-day study period: recurrent cerebral embolism in 2 and deep vein thrombosis in 1, all in the nonanticoagulated group. Although this difference did not reach statistical significance ($p = .09$), this study was terminated based on this trend and the apparent safety of immediate anticoagulation.

One study of subcutaneous low molecular weight heparin (nadroparin) treatment, given within 48 h of stroke onset,[9] suggests that it may be beneficial. In this study, 312 patients were randomized to three groups: high-dose (4100 antifactor Xa IU twice daily), low-dose (4100 IU once daily), or indistinguishable placebo treatment for 10 days. There was a statistically significant dose-dependent effect in favor of nadroparin after 6, but not 3 months of follow-up ($p = .005$). Functional independence was reached by 35 percent of patients in the placebo group, 48 percent in the low-dose group, and 55 percent in the high-dose group. Recurrent ischemic stroke during the 10-day treatment period occurred in 1 to 2 percent of patients in all three groups. Serious bleeding complications during the 10-day treatment period occurred in 2 patients, 1 gastrointestinal and 1 symptomatic hemorrhagic transformation of an infarct, both in the placebo group.

A larger study of a low molecular weight heparinoid (danaparoid, a heparin analog), given within 24 h of stroke onset, showed no significant benefit at 3 months.[10] In this study, 1281 patients were randomized to intravenous danaparoid or indistinguishable placebo treatment for 7 days. Favorable outcome at 3 months was achieved by 74 percent of patients in the placebo group and 75 percent in the danaparoid group. Recurrent ischemic stroke during the 7-day treatment period occurred in 1.1 percent of patients in each group. Among patients with cardioembolic stroke, recurrent ischemic stroke occurred in 2 of 123 (1.6 percent) placebo-treated patients and none of 143 danaparoid-treated patients. Serious bleeding complications, both extra- and intracranial, during the 7-day treatment period occurred in 7 of 628 (1.1 percent) placebo-treated patients and 25 of 638 (3.9 percent) danaparoid-treated patients ($p < .005$).

Three multicenter, randomized trials tested the efficacy of hemodilution in subacute ischemic stroke to augment cerebral perfusion of the ischemic region and improve patient outcome. In the nonblinded Scandinavian Stroke Study,[11] 373 patients with ischemic stroke and hematocrits 38 to 50 percent were randomized to hemodilution ($n = 183$) or no hemodilution ($n = 190$) treatment within 48 h of stroke onset. Hemodilution was accomplished by removal of 250 to 1000 mL of blood during the first 2 days and infusion of dextran 40, 500 mL daily for 5 days. In the hemodilution group, mean hematocrit was reduced from 44 to 37 percent. There were no statistically significant differences in complications between the two treatment groups. After 3 months of follow-up, there were no statistically significant differences in mortality (16 percent with hemodilution and 12 percent without hemodilution) or neurologic outcome between the two treatment groups.

In the nonblinded Hemodilution in Stroke Study,[12] 88 patients were randomized to hypervolemic hemodilution ($n = 45$) or no hemodilution ($n = 43$) within 24 h of stroke onset. Hemodilution was accomplished with pentastarch while monitoring the pulmonary wedge pressure. The target hematocrit was 30 to 33 percent. At the end of the 3-day treatment period, average hematocrit decreased in the hemodilution group by 7 percent and in the nonhemodilution group by 2 percent. During follow-up for 3 months, no statistically significant differences in mortality (20 percent with hemodilution and 7 percent without hemodilution) or neurologic outcome were found. However, because of the higher mortality rate in the hemodilution group, this study was terminated by the safety monitoring committee.

The efficacy of mild hypervolemic hemodilution was tested more recently in the Austrian Hemodilution Stroke Trial.[13] In this multicenter, double-blind trial 200 patients with ischemic stroke in the middle cerebral artery territory were randomized to hypervolemic hemodilution ($n = 98$) or placebo hydration ($n = 102$) within 6 h of stroke onset. Hemodilution was accomplished with 10% hydroxyethyl starch and the placebo hydration with Ringer's lactate given over 5 days. At the end of the 5-day treatment period, hematocrit decreased in the hemodilution group by 3.7 percent and in the placebo group by 1.9 percent. During a 3-month follow-up, there were no statistically significant differences in mortality (13 percent with hemodilution and 17 percent with placebo) or neurologic outcome between the two treatment groups.

There are several acute stroke treatment trials of the calcium channel blocker nimodipine. One relatively small study suggests that treatment with nimodipine starting within 24 h of ischemic stroke onset may be somewhat beneficial.[14] In this study, 186 patients were randomized to nimodipine 30 mg orally every 6 h for 28 days or to an indistinguishable placebo treatment. In the nimodipine group, there were significantly less deaths during the 28-day treatment period (8.6 percent vs. 20.4 percent with placebo, $p < .05$) and significantly more favorable neurologic outcomes ($f < .03$). However, a subsequent larger study of nimodipine treatment in ischemic stroke started within 48 h of onset showed no benefit from this drug.[15] In this study, 1215 patients were randomized to nimodipine 40 mg orally 3 times daily for 21 days or indistinguishable placebo treatment. At 6 months, functional independence was present in 55 percent of patients in the nimodipine group and 58 percent in the placebo group, and there were no significant differences in mortality between these two groups.

In another large nimodipine trial,[16] 1064 patients with acute ischemic stroke were randomized within 48 h of stroke onset to nimodipine 60 mg, 120 mg, or 240 mg orally daily or an indistinguishable placebo treatment for 21 days. Primary analysis showed no significant differences in death or neurologic outcome among the four treatment groups. However, secondary analysis showed that patients in the 120-mg nimodipine group, treated within 18 h of stroke onset, had a significantly better outcome ($p = .005$) than placebo-treated patients.

A trial of intravenous nimodipine treatment, given within 24 h of ischemic stroke onset, was terminated because of unacceptable safety issues.[17] In this study, 295 patients were randomized to three groups: 1 or 2 mg/h intravenous nimodipine for 5 days followed by nimodipine 120 mg orally daily for a total period of 21 days, or to indistinguishable placebo treatment. Patients in the placebo group had significantly better outcomes at 21 days and 24 weeks. There were no significant differences in mortality among the three groups. However, there were significant reductions in blood pressure in the nimodipine groups, mainly on day 2, which were thought to be responsible for the worse outcome in these patients compared with the placebo-treated patients. Thus, whether nimodipine is truly beneficial in acute stroke, and at what dose, remains to be proven.

In the International Stroke Trial,[18] 19,435 patients with ischemic stroke were randomized to unblinded treatment with subcutaneous heparin alone (5000 or 12,500 IU twice daily), aspirin alone (300 mg daily),

aspirin with the low-dose and the high-dose heparin, or placebo. Treatment started within 48 h of stroke onset and continued for up to 14 days. Heparin was associated with a lower rate of recurrent ischemic stroke (2.9 percent with heparin and 3.8 percent without heparin, $p < .01$) but a higher rate of intracerebral hemorrhage (1.2 percent with heparin and 0.4 percent without heparin, $p < .001$) during the 14-day treatment period. Heparin was not associated with a significantly different mortality at 14 days (9 percent with and without heparin) or likelihood of poor outcome at 6 months (63 percent in both groups). Aspirin was associated with a somewhat lower rate of recurrent ischemic stroke during the 14-day treatment period (2.8 percent with aspirin and 3.9 percent without aspirin, $p < .001$), a trend toward less poor outcomes at 6 months (62 percent with aspirin and 64 percent without aspirin, $p = .07$), but not with intracerebral hemorrhage (0.9 percent with aspirin and 0.8 percent without aspirin) or mortality at 14 days (9 percent in both groups).

In the Chinese Acute Stroke Trial,[19] 21,106 patients with ischemic stroke were randomized to blinded treatment with aspirin 160 mg/day or placebo. Treatment started within 48 h of stroke onset and continued for up to 4 weeks. Aspirin was associated with significantly fewer deaths (3 percent with aspirin and 4 percent without aspirin, $p = .04$) and significantly fewer recurrent ischemic strokes (1.6 percent with aspirin and 2.1 percent without aspirin, $p = .01$) at 4 weeks. Rates of intracerebral hemorrhage were not significantly different between the two treatment groups (1.1 percent with aspirin and 0.9 percent without aspirin).

Several other cytoprotective drugs have been found somewhat effective in the treatment of subacute ischemic clinical stroke. However, subsequent larger trials have not confirmed the initial results, are currently in progress, or are being planned. Some cytoprotective drugs work by inhibiting the effects of excitotoxic amino acids, some by inhibiting calcium accumulation in ischemic cells, and some like nimodipine by protecting cell membranes against oxidative damage. It is possible that one or more of them will prove useful in the treatment of ischemic stroke in the near future (see Chap. 13).

Recommendations   As aspirin has been shown to have a short-term small beneficial effect when started during the subacute stroke period, and it is usually the initial treatment of choice for secondary stroke prevention, we recommend starting aspirin, 325 mg daily, for those patients who are not already taking aspirin regularly and who are not being treated with anticoagulation.

There are no other proven effective treatments for ischemic stroke beyond the first 3 h. In certain situations discussed later in this chapter, anticoagulation therapy seems appropriate.

Dysphagia

Background   Dysphagia has been demonstrated in 22 to 54 percent of patients with recent stroke by bedside and videofluoroscopic testing.[20–22] Dysphagia predisposes to aspiration pneumonia, which increases morbidity and mortality. In a prospective study of 121 patients with stroke evaluated with bedside tests and videofluoroscopy, dysphagia was associated with increased risk of pneumonia ($p = .05$), poor nutritional state ($p = .001$), higher mortality ($p = .001$), longer hospital stay ($p < .001$), and institutional care ($p < .05$).[23]

Proper swallowing involves the integrated function of several oropharyngeal muscles and the brainstem nuclei that regulate the swallowing mechanism. The swallowing process is modified by the cerebral cortex through corticobulbar pathways. The neuroanatomic correlates of dysphagia are not well understood. The swallowing mechanism is cortically represented in both cerebral hemispheres.[24] Additionally, there seems to be cerebral hemispheric dominance for swallowing independent of handedness.[25] Robins and Levine, in their controlled and prospective study, showed that left-sided cortical strokes are more likely to cause impairment in the oral phase and right-sided cortical strokes in the pharyngeal phase of swallowing.[26] However, other studies report that lesions in either cerebral hemisphere may cause dysphagia.[27,28] The exact role of each cortical lobe in dysphagia is not well understood, but the anterior insula seems to play an important role.[29] Despite recent advances in understanding dysphagia, correlation between cortical location of stroke and dysphagia remains weak.

Evidence   In a study of 37 consecutive stroke patients who had videofluoroscopic barium swallow examination within 1 month of stroke, 54 percent had aspiration, and aspiration was associated with an impaired cough reflex.[22] Among patients with impaired cough reflex, aspiration was seen in 91 percent and among those with intact cough reflex in 38 percent ($p < .01$). Furthermore, an impaired cough reflex has been associated with dysphonia, dysarthria, abnormal gag reflex, impaired volitional cough, cough after swallowing, and voice change after swallowing.[29,30] In another study to determine the frequency and clinical predictors of aspiration, 55 consecutive stroke patients were evaluated with oromotor examination and videofluoroscopic swallow study within 5 days of stroke onset.[31] Aspiration on videofluoroscopy was seen in 21 (38 percent) patients, and 14 of them (67 percent) had an impaired cough reflex. Abnormal volitional cough and cough on swallowing, when present together, were significantly associated with aspiration ($p < .001$) and predicted aspiration with 78 percent accuracy.

The gag reflex is often used in the assessment of swallowing. However, in a study of 140 healthy subjects, gag reflex was absent bilaterally in 29 (43 percent) of elderly subjects and in 18 (26 percent) of young subjects ($p = .046$).[32] By contrast, pharyngeal sensation was absent in only 1 patient and therefore, this may be more indicative of a pathologic finding than an absent gag reflex.

Screening for dysphagia by practical bedside swallowing evaluation has been recommended by different authors. DePippo and colleagues, in a study of 44 consecutive patients, detected 80 percent of aspirating patients with a 3-oz. water swallow test, confirmed with videofluoroscopy.[33] Other tests reported to predict aspiration include the Burke Dysphagia Screening Test and Repetitive Oral Suction Swallow (ROSS) Test.[30,34]

In a prospective study of 122 consecutive subacute stroke patients using a special dysphagia screening test, 30 (25 percent) patients were identified as being at high risk for aspiration.[35] Of these, 45 percent remained dysphagic, 34 percent required alternate feeding methods, 10 percent had significant weight loss, and 10 percent were admitted with pneumonia during a 60-day follow-up. Prevalence of atrial fibrillation, coronary artery disease, or smoking was significantly higher ($p < .05$) in patients at high risk for aspiration. Severe and left-sided infarcts were associated with dysphagia. In another, retrospective study of 70 stroke patients who had videofluoroscopic swallow study, stroke location, patient age, unilateral vs. bilateral neurologic signs, or dysphonia did not correlate with aspiration.[36]

Specific dietary recommendations for dysphagic patients are based on observational reports of swallowing problems associated with different types of food in patients with various severities of dysphagia.[37] In a prospective 3-year study of 115 patients with stroke, to investigate the effect of diet, patients were randomized to three dysphagia treatment groups.[38] Each group represented graded levels of diet and reinforcement of compensatory swallowing techniques. In group A, patients selected a diet, and compensatory swallowing techniques were taught. In group B, a therapist prescribed the diet based on the modified barium swallow test, and compensatory swallowing techniques were taught. In group C, a therapist prescribed a customized diet based on the modified barium swallow test, and compensatory swallowing techniques were taught and emphasized daily. The main outcome measures in the study were the occurrence of pneumonia, dehydration, calorie-nitrogen deficit, recurrent upper airway obstruction, and death. Results showed no significant difference between the three treatment groups for any of the endpoints.

Recommendations Early identification of stroke patients with dysphagia and specific interventions are believed to decrease the risk of aspiration (Table 3-1). A swallowing assessment should always precede initiation of feeding during subacute stroke and can be done at bedside with a simple swallowing test, such as the 3-oz. water swallow test.[33] This test consists of observing a patient drink 3 oz. of water from a cup without interruption. The test is abnormal if there is drooling, coughing, or change in voice for up to 1 min after drinking the water. Videofluoroscopy using modified barium swallow may help to define the nature and extent of dysphagia.

Speech and dietary evaluation, followed by a customized feeding recommendation, is believed to improve nutritional state and decrease length of hospital stay. A four-level dysphagia diet plan has been proposed, based on the American Dietetic Association recommendations.[37] Diet considerations include food temperature and texture. For example, foods that form a bolus in the mouth are easier to swallow than liquids.

The prescribed diet is as nutritious as possible and relatively safe to swallow, based on the severity of dysphagia. For mildly dysphagic patients, a soft diet with liquids as tolerated is suggested. For severely dysphagic patients, pureed diets with no thin liquids is suggested. For severely dysphagic patients, tube feedings may be needed to maintain daily calorie requirements and to sufficiently reduce the risk of aspiration. If tube feeding is anticipated beyond 2 weeks, we recommend early percutaneous gastric tube placement.

Intraluminal Arterial Thrombus

Background An intraluminal thrombus in a large cerebral artery is occasionally found on arteriography upstream from the region of ischemia.[39–44] The concern is that this thrombus will break loose and occlude a major cerebral artery with devastating consequences. Usually, such thrombi develop because an atherosclerotic plaque becomes ulcerated, exposing the thrombogenic subendothelium.

Evidence Some reports recommend initial medical treatment with anticoagulation. Biller and colleagues[42] reported 9 patients with intraluminal clot in the internal carotid artery among 2250 (0.4 percent) patients who had an arteriogram because of cerebral ischemia. Six patients had urgent carotid endarterectomy, and two of them developed new neurologic deficits perioperatively.

Table 3-1.
Conditions thought or known to predispose to stroke-associated pneumonia and corresponding management suggestions

Condition	Management
Decreased consciousness	Optimal treatment of underlying cause
Seizures	Anticonvulsants
Decreased upper airway reflexes	Swallowing therapy
Decreased cough reflex	Swallowing therapy
Feeding tubes	Discontinue as soon as possible or place PEG[a]
Gastric distension	Avoid overfeeding
Vomiting	Antiemetics and treat underlying cause
Decreased mobility	Early mobilization
Decreased chest movements on the side contralateral to brain injury	Incentive spirometry, chest therapy

[a]Percutaneous endoscopic gastrostomy

The remaining three patients were managed medically (two with anticoagulation and one with antiplatelet therapy) and had no neurologic deterioration. Buchan and colleagues[43] report 30 patients with intraluminal clot in the internal carotid artery identified during a 10-year period. Of these, 16 had urgent carotid endarterectomy, with perioperative neurologic complications in 4. The remaining 14 patients were initially treated medically (11 with anticoagulation and 3 with antiplatelet therapy) without complications. Repeat arteriograms in 8 of the medically treated patients showed resolution of the clot in 7. Delayed carotid endarterectomy in 6 patients was associated with a perioperative stroke in 1.

Some reports suggest that urgent surgical removal of the clot may be the optimal treatment of this problem. Donnan and Blandin[40] report three patients with long intraluminal clots, two in the carotid artery and one in the vertebral artery, treated successfully by early surgical embolectomy. Other reports indicate that good outcomes can result from either approach. Caplan and colleagues[41] report nine patients with intraluminal clot in the internal carotid artery. Six had early carotid endarterectomy with clot removal and three were treated medically, and none had recurrent cerebral ischemia. Yarnell and colleagues[39] reported three patients with intraluminal clot in the internal carotid artery. Two were treated with anticoagulation and one with early endarterectomy, and all did well.

Recommendations Optimal management of intraluminal arterial thrombus is unproven and thus remains controversial. There are no randomized treatment trials of this problem to guide medical decision making. We suggest rapid anticoagulation with intravenous heparin or subcutaneous enoxaparin plus concomitant warfarin (see "Starting Anticoagulation Therapy"). When the international normalized ratio (INR) reaches 2.0, the heparin or enoxaparin is discontinued. We recommend a target INR of 2.5 for approximately 4 weeks. However, when deciding on the intensity and duration of anticoagulation therapy, the physician must consider the associated bleeding risks (see "Starting Anticoagulation Therapy"). After that, a repeat arteriogram is done to reevaluate the thrombus. If the clot has resolved, warfarin is stopped and antiplatelet therapy is begun. If the clot has resolved and severe extracranial carotid stenosis is present, carotid endarterectomy is considered. In the unlikely event of clot persistence, warfarin is continued for an additional 4 weeks and arteriogram repeated again.

Severe (Preocclusive) Arterial Stenosis

Background Severe (preocclusive, usually >95 percent diameter reduction) arterial stenosis is occasionally identified on arteriography during stroke evaluation. This situation is associated with angiographically visible slow poststenotic blood flow, which fails to opacify the entire poststenotic vascular bed. This definition is based on that used for coronary artery perfusion in the thrombolysis in myocardial infarction (TIMI) studies and corresponds to grade 1 perfusion (grade 0 is no perfusion due to occlusion, with no visible antegrade flow). As a result of this oligemia, it is postulated that the risk of local thrombosis is increased. There is concern that if thrombotic occlusion develops, a stroke might result and subsequent endarterectomy would be very difficult, risky, or impossible.

Evidence There are no controlled trials to suggest that during the subacute stroke period one form of antithrombotic treatment is better than another in patients with symptomatic preocclusive arterial stenosis. Ringelstein and colleagues[46] described nine patients with severe preocclusive stenosis of the extracranial carotid artery. Six were treated with emergency endarterectomy and had no complications or recurrent stroke during several months of follow-up. In one patient with unspecified medical treatment, the carotid artery became occluded within 3 h of diagnosis without neurologic worsening. In another patient who refused surgery, the medical treatment was not stated, and the carotid artery was found to be occluded 4 weeks later without symptoms. One patient died during cerebral aneurysm surgery, before planned carotid endarterectomy.

O'Leary and colleagues[47] reported 34 patients with preocclusive extracranial internal carotid artery stenosis documented with arteriography, 9 of whom were treated medically without anticoagulation. Two of these nine patients had a stroke during arteriography, three had a stroke ipsilateral to the severely stenosed carotid artery within 11 months (1 week, 3 months, and 11 months), and the remaining four had no recurrence of cerebral ischemic events during follow-up for an unspecified period. However, follow up noninvasive studies showed occlusion of the severely stenosed carotid artery in all nine nonanticoagulated medically treated patients.

Recommendations Based on visualization of severely reduced arterial flow and the concern that this might soon lead to an occlusion with tragic consequences, we recommend consideration of immediate anticoagulation of TIMI grade 1 cerebrovascular arterial stenosis, with serious consideration given to the associated bleeding risks (see "Starting Anticoagulation Therapy"). If an endarterectomy is planned, anticoagulation should continue until surgery. If anticoagulation beyond 2 weeks is anticipated, we recommend anticoagulation with warfarin to a target INR of 2.5.

Sometimes, the stenosis regresses as the thrombus dissolves and becomes fibrotic. Therefore, it is worthwhile to repeat the arteriogram approximately 4 weeks after the start of anticoagulation therapy to reevaluate the degree of stenosis and poststenotic flow. MRA or CT arteriogram do not demonstrate filling of vascular beds sufficiently to adequately grade the stenosis according to TIMI criteria. If the stenosis remains TIMI grade 1, we recommend indefinite anticoagulation. If the stenosis decreases to TIMI grade 2 (the entire poststenotic vascular bed is opacified although local blood flow may be reduced), we usually recommend switching to antiplatelet therapy unless there is another specific indication for continued anticoagulation.

Asymptomatic Hemorrhagic Transformation of an Infarct

Background   A small amount of bleeding into the infarct is sometimes seen on repeat cerebral CT even in patients not treated with thrombolysis or anticoagulation. This occurs because the damaged blood vessels are leaky. Because the amount of extravasated blood is small, there is no clinical deterioration, and there may even be continuous improvement. In the NINDS tissue plasminogen activator (TPA) in acute stroke study,[6] asymptomatic hemorrhagic transformation of an infarct within 36 h of treatment occurred in 3 percent of placebo and 4 percent of TPA-treated patients. In the TOAST study,[10] asymptomatic hemorrhagic transformation of an infarct within 10 days occurred in 8 percent of placebo and 8 percent of low molecular weight heparinoid-treated patients. The usual question is: when can anticoagulation be started after an asymptomatic hemorrhagic transformation of an infarct?

Evidence   There are no clinical studies to guide the antithrombotic treatment of patients with asymptomatic hemorrhagic transformation of an infarct.

Recommendations   Based on the available information, there is no reason to withhold antiplatelet therapy

in patients with asymptomatic hemorrhagic transformation of an infarct. If for some reason anticoagulation is recommended, we decide when to start it based on the size and density of the blood within the infarct visible on CT. If the bleeding is petechial and confined to a small (<50 percent) portion of the infarcted region, we recommend no delay in anticoagulation. If, however, the bleeding is more dense (hyperdensity is more homogeneous or more confluent than petechial), we recommend waiting 4 to 7 days and repeating the CT. The CT is repeated until the hemorrhagic lesion is petechial and occupies < 50 percent of the infarct. At that time, we feel that starting anticoagulation is reasonably safe.

Starting Anticoagulation Therapy

Background   Anticoagulation therapy is sometimes recommended for patients with suspected or documented hypercoagulability, recurrent thromboembolism, a serious source of emboli, or progressing thrombosis (Table 3-2). For immediate anticoagulation, intravenous heparin is usually used. However, fixed doses

Table 3-2.
Abnormalities in subacute stroke patients for which temporary or indefinite anticoagulation therapy is often recommended

Unstable stroke deficits
Serious source of emboli[a]
  Prosthetic heart valve
  Chronic or intermittent atrial fibrillation, atrial flutter,
    or sick sinus syndrome
  Akinetic or aneurysmal myocardial wall
  Severely decreased myocardial contractility (ejection
    fraction <25%)
  Mural thrombus
  Rheumatic heart disease
  Atrial septal defect
  Large patent foramen ovale
  Intraluminal arterial thrombus
  Arterial dissection
Severe (preocclusive) arterial stenosis (TIMI grade 1[b])
Hypercoagulable disorders
  Antiphospholipid antibody syndrome
  Activated protein C resistance (factor V Leiden mutation)
  Disseminated intravascular coagulation
  Deficiency of protein C, protein S, or antithrombin III

[a]Adapted from Ref. 115.

[b]See "Severe (Preocclusive) Arterial Stenosis."

of low molecular weight heparin (LMWH) compounds produce rapid and more predictable anticoagulation than unfractionated heparin, they can be given subcutaneously instead of intravenously, and they do not require monitoring of the coagulation system. In addition, LMWH compounds are less likely to cause thrombocytopenia and perhaps bleeding than unfractionated heparin.

Long-term anticoagulation is started with warfarin. Because warfarin does not exert its full anticoagulant effect until 3 to 6 days after start of treatment, temporary anticoagulation with heparin or a LMWH during the first few days of warfarin therapy is often recommended. In addition, there is concern that the concentration of the anticoagulant proteins C and S will decrease before the concentration of the procoagulant factors II, IX, and X, resulting in a transient hypercoagulable state.[49] However, it has not been demonstrated that immediate anticoagulation is better than starting warfarin alone and waiting a few days for the desired anticoagulation to occur. Thus, immediate anticoagulation may not be necessary, and intravenous heparin may not be superior to subcutaneous heparin or a LMWH. In this section, we will discuss the methods of anticoagulation. The possible reasons for anticoagulation therapy during subacute stroke are discussed in other sections in this chapter.

Evidence   When considering anticoagulation therapy in a patient with subacute stroke, the risk of hemorrhage into the infarct must always be kept in mind in addition to extracerebral bleeding. In one retrospective study, 19 patients with cardioembolic infarcts complicated by symptomatic hemorrhagic transformations while being treated with intravenous heparin anticoagulation were compared with 24 similar patients without hemorrhagic complications.[50] Large infarcts (involving the entire middle cerebral artery territory) were associated with hemorrhagic transformation, but patient age, embolic source, and intensity of anticoagulation were not. Large infarcts were present in 57 percent of patients with symptomatic hemorrhagic transformation but in 21 percent of patients without hemorrhagic transformation.

One prospective, nonblinded, uncontrolled study analyzed 45 patients with carotid territory nonlacunar infarcts treated with intravenous heparin within 5 h of stroke onset for 4 days.[51] The PTT ratio was 2.0 to 2.5. Symptomatic cerebral hemorrhage occurred in 2 (4.4 percent) patients, nonserious extracranial bleeding in 6 (13 percent), and serious extracranial bleeding in none.

Possibly because of the low frequency of cerebral hemorrhagic complications in this small study, none of the clinical features analyzed were associated with an increased risk of cerebral hemorrhage.

In an attempt to achieve a therapeutic effect as soon as possible, it is common practice to start oral warfarin with 10 mg on the first 1 or 2 days and then continue with 5 mg/day. However, this approach does not seem to be better than starting and continuing with 5 mg/day mainly because the likelihood of excessive anticoagulation is increased. In a trial comparing 5 mg vs. 10 mg of warfarin on the first day of anticoagulation, followed by 5 mg/day, 49 patients were randomized.[52] After 3.5 days, INR of 2.0 to 3.0 was achieved by 79 percent of patients in the 5-mg group and 63 percent in the 10-mg group. Excessive elevation of INR occurred in 4 patients in the 10-mg group and 1 patient in the 5-mg group.

There are no published studies of LMWH compounds as bridging therapy for stroke patients being started on warfarin, but treatment of deep vein thrombosis with subcutaneous enoxaparin 1 mg/kg, twice daily, given concomitantly with warfarin until the INR reaches 2.0, seems safe and effective. In one study,[53] 55 patients with deep vein thrombosis were treated with subcutaneous enoxaparin until the INR reached 2.0 from concomitant warfarin treatment. There were no ischemic or hemorrhagic complications, the average duration of enoxaparin treatment was 5.6 days, and 294 hospital days were avoided.

Recommendations   There is no universally accepted protocol for initiating anticoagulation with heparin. Absence of intracranial hemmorrhage should be confirmed with a CT scan or an MRI of the brain within 24 h prior to starting anticoagulation. Our protocol for starting anticoagulation with intravenous heparin is based on published suggestions.[8] Some experts recommend a heparin bolus and some do not. Those who recommend a bolus, suggest 5000 to 10,000 U. The usual recommendation is to adjust the constant heparin infusion rate to achieve a PTT of 1.5 to 2.5 times control. We usually start intravenous heparin anticoagulation with a bolus of 5000 U followed by an infusion rate of 1000 U/h. Then, the PTT is checked every 4 h, and the heparin infusion rate adjusted if needed to keep the PTT between 75 and 85 s (2.0 to 2.5 times control). After two consecutive PTT values show little change, the interval between the PTT tests is increased to twice daily and sometimes once daily.

Our protocol for starting anticoagulation with warfarin is also based on published suggestions.[49] We start anticoagulation with subcutaneous enoxaparin, 1 mg/kg twice daily together with oral warfarin 4.0 mg daily. We check the INR daily after the first 3 days and stop the enoxaparin when the INR reaches 2.0. The warfarin dose may need to be adjusted. This method allows for patients to be discharged from an acute care hospital before the INR is 2.0, if they are otherwise stable.

MANAGING UNSTABLE SUBACUTE STROKE

Neurologic deterioration during subacute stroke occurs in 22 to 43 percent of patients.[54,55] It can result from multiple neurologic and non-neurologic problems. Some problems increase the extent of brain injury, whereas other problems further impair ischemic brain function until the problem is corrected. Effective treatment requires rapid identification of the cause of deterioration and appropriate intervention.

Symptomatic Hemorrhagic Transformation of an Infarct

Background   Hemorrhagic transformation of a cerebral infarct is usually the initial concern when an anticoagulated patient has neurologic deterioration. Because the infarcted tissue contains damaged blood vessels that receive some blood flow, extravasation of blood from these leaky vessels on a microscopic level is common. This complication is of practical significance primarily in medium-to-large strokes, because as infarct size increases, the number and extent of leaky vessels increases. A small amount of blood within an infarct can be seen on MRI and histologically in most large cerebral infarcts, but a larger amount of blood is needed to be visible on CT. If the hemorrhagic transformation of an infarct involves a relatively small amount of blood within the already damaged tissue, the patient will most likely remain stable and may even improve. However, when the amount of extravasated blood is sufficiently large to cause damage to previously unaffected tissue or to produce a mass effect, clinical worsening occurs. A hemorrhagic transformation may be diagnosed as symptomatic when a neurologic deficit progresses and the CT shows dense blood in the ischemic region.

Hemorrhagic transformation of cerebral infarcts occurs in patients treated with placebo or antiplatelet therapy, but it occurs at a significantly higher rate in patients treated with anticoagulation or thrombolytic drugs.[6,10,18] In the International Stroke Trial,[18] 19,435 patients with subacute ischemic stroke were randomized to unblinded treatment with subcutaneous heparin alone (5000 or 12,500 IU twice daily), aspirin alone (300 mg daily), aspirin with the low-dose and the high-dose heparin, or placebo. During the 14-day treatment period, symptomatic hemorrhagic stroke, including hemorrhagic transformation of the infarct, occurred at a rate of 0.3 percent in the placebo group, 0.5 percent in the aspirin group, approximately 0.5 percent in the low-dose heparin group, and approximately 1.6 percent in the high-dose heparin group. The difference between the low- and high-dose heparin groups is relatively small, but statistically significant ($p < .00001$). In addition to the cerebral hemorrhages, the rate of serious extracerebral hemorrhages during the treatment period was also significantly higher in the heparin vs. aspirin-treated groups (1.3 percent vs. 0.4 percent, respectively, $p < .00001$).

In a trial of a low molecular weight heparinoid (danaparoid) vs. placebo in acute ischemic stroke,[10] serious cerebral bleeding during treatment occurred in 3 of 628 (0.5 percent) of patients on placebo and 10 of 638 (1.6 percent) of anticoagulated patients (statistically not significantly different). In the NINDS TPA in acute stroke trial,[6] symptomatic intracerebral hemorrhage within 36 h of treatment occurred at a rate of 0.6 percent in the placebo group and 6.4 percent in the TPA group ($p < .001$).

Evidence   There are no clinical studies on the treatment of hemorrhagic complications during subacute stroke. In the NINDS TPA in acute stroke trial,[6] 13 patients with symptomatic intracerebral hemorrhage received blood products (fresh frozen plasma, cryoprecipitate, or platelets) to limit the bleeding, and 12 of them died within 90 days. The American Heart Association guidelines recommend to correct the fibrinolytic state before any surgery is undertaken.[56]

The surgical management of hemorrhagic transformation of an infarct is based on that of spontaneous intracerebral hemorrhage. Management is guided by (1) the size of the hematoma, (2) the location of the hematoma, and (3) the likelihood of neurologic worsening or death. A review of the four randomized trials of surgical vs. nonsurgical management of supratentorial intracerebral hematomas[57] indicates that the role of craniotomy and stereotactic surgery has not been adequately studied and that the efficacy of endoscopic evacuation seems promising. Superficial brain hematomas are easier to remove with less damage to neighboring structures than are deep hematomas. Cerebellar hematomas are more likely to be resected than supratentorial hematomas because of the concern that swelling will compress the nearby brainstem or the cerebral aqueduct with tragic consequences. This concern is based on the reported natural history of cerebellar hematomas.[58,59] Zieger and colleagues[58] reported 32 patients with cerebellar hematoma. Patients with hematomas measuring 25 cm^3 (approximately 3.7 cm in diameter) had a relatively stable clinical course and were likely to survive with either conservative or surgical treatment (6 of 7 with conservative only and 7 of 8 with surgical). However, patients with hematomas measuring 47 cm^3 (approximately 4.5 cm in diameter) had a progressing clinical course and were more likely to survive with surgical treatment (0 of 6 with conservative only and 6 of 11 with surgical).

In addition to cerebellar hematoma size, CT evidence of compression of the quadrigeminal cistern seems to be an additional useful indicator of prognosis. Taneda and colleagues[59] report 75 patients with cerebellar hematomas. Among patients without cistern compression 38 of 43 (88 percent) recovered well regardless of the type of treatment given. However, among patients with cistern compression without obliteration, 11 of 16 (69 percent) recovered well. In this group, good outcome was dependent on hematoma evacuation within 48 h of onset. Among patients with cistern obliteration, 0 of 16 recovered well despite hematoma evacuation within 48 h in eight of them. There are no data from randomized clinical treatment trials on this topic.

Recommendations   As soon as symptomatic hemorrhagic transformation of an infarct is suspected or diagnosed, thrombolytic or anticoagulation therapy should be stopped immediately. In the case of heparin or low molecular weight heparin compounds, pharmacologic reversal of anticoagulation is not recommended. However, fibrinogen can be used to reverse the effects of TPA. Cryoprecipitate contains approximately 250 mg of fibrinogen per unit and raises the fibrinogen level approximately 8 mg/dL per unit. If the hematoma is large or located in the cerebellum, a consultation with a neurosurgeon is warranted. In most situations, supportive therapy is recommended, but occasionally neurosurgical decompression of the hematoma, cerebrospinal fluid drainage, or both are indicated. Anticoagulation may later be resumed, when the hematoma has resolved, the infarct has healed, and there are no contra-

indications. Usually, we recommend to wait 4 weeks before resuming anticoagulation, but there is no clinical evidence that this is the optimal time.

Cerebral Edema

Background   Cerebral edema is by far the most common fatal complication of ischemic stroke within the first week (78 percent), and it is most likely to occur 3 to 4 days after stroke onset.[60] Redistribution of water in the extracellular and intracellular spaces occurs in every acute cerebral infarct. This process results in the visible hypodensity on CT or hyperintensity on T2-weighted MRI, which represents the ischemic region. Therefore, every cerebral infarct is associated with edema within the infarct, but only large infarcts are at risk of severe swelling with potentially life-threatening mass effect.[60] It is important to limit cerebral edema and mass effect to prevent the damage from extending beyond the initial infarct.

Swelling of large hemispheric infarcts can produce subfalcine (under the falx cerebri), transtentorial (under the tentorium cerebelli), or downward (through the foramen magnum) brain herniation. Subfalcine herniation can compress the contralateral cerebral hemisphere and result in bilateral cerebral dysfunction, plus occlude one or both anterior cerebral arteries, which run along the falx cerebri, and cause additional cerebral ischemia. In transtentorial herniation, the medial temporal lobe pushes medially under the tentorium cerebelli to compress the midbrain, plus it is likely to occlude the posterior cerebral artery, which runs along the tentorium cerebelli, and cause additional cerebral ischemia. In downward brain herniation, the medulla oblongata is compressed as it is pushed down through the limited opening of the foramen magnum. Swelling of large cerebellar infarcts produces compression of the adjacent brainstem against the clivus. This usually leads to rapid development of coma and is seldom reversible. In addition to compressing adjacent brain tissue and cerebral vessels, cerebral edema decreases cerebral blood flow by raising the intracranial pressure and thus lowering the cerebral perfusion pressure (cerebral perfusion pressure = mean arterial pressure − intracranial pressure).

Evidence   It is important to know which patients are at higher than average risk of cerebral swelling and herniation so that preventive or therapeutic steps can be taken. Toni and colleagues[54] analyzed the predictors of neurologic deterioration in 152 consecutive acute stroke patients. They found that 39 (26 percent) patients deteriorated during the initial 4 days after stroke onset. Independent predictors of deterioration were elevated blood glucose level on admission and ischemic hypodensity seen on CT within 5 h of stroke onset. Also, patients who deteriorated had significantly larger infarcts than those who did not deteriorate ($p < .001$). Only 10 percent of the patients who deteriorated achieved a favorable outcome compared with 53 percent of those who did not deteriorate ($p < .001$). In our experience, a useful rule is that a cerebral infarct larger than one-half of the middle cerebral artery territory or a cerebellar infarct larger than one-half of a cerebellar hemisphere has a higher than average risk of swelling with mass effect.

Recommendations Several therapies are recommended to limit cerebral swelling and mass effect. We recommend that patients with an increased risk of stroke-related cerebral swelling and mass effect (large cerebral or cerebellar infarct) be monitored for signs of deterioration closer than more stable patients. Ideally, they should be admitted to a specialized stroke unit. Avoidance of hypoosmolar intravenous solutions, such as 5% dextrose in water, and avoidance of overhydration are recommended.

Seizures

Background Because stroke produces a cerebral lesion, it increases the likelihood of seizure. In addition to the usual dangers of seizures, such as aspiration and injury, seizure at the onset of stroke can make the stroke seem more severe than it is, and seizures during the subacute stroke period can mimic deterioration from other causes. A seizure may not be witnessed, and the patient may be amnestic for the event and have postictal hemiparesis. If there are no recurrent seizures, postictal hemiparesis usually resolves within several hours.

Evidence Seizures after ischemic stroke have been recorded in 2.0 to 6.0 percent of patients within the first 15 days after the stroke.[61–64] Risk of early seizure after stroke was associated with cortical lesion, carotid territory lesion, and large infarcts. Most seizures were partial and readily controlled with antiepileptic medications.

Kilpatrick and colleagues[61] prospectively studied 601 consecutive patients with acute ischemic stroke and found that 24 (4.0 percent) of them had a seizure within 14 days of stroke onset. All the seizures were in patients with cortical infarcts in the carotid territory. Mechanism of cerebral infarction did not predict occurrence of seizure. Most seizures were partial and easily controlled with antiepileptic medications. Seizures were not associated with worse clinical outcome during mean follow-up of 7 months.

Giroud and colleagues[62] prospectively studied 1202 consecutive patients with acute ischemic stroke and found that 60 (5.0 percent) of them had a seizure within 15 days of stroke onset. Seizures were more common in patients with cortical infarcts 57 of 929 (6.1 percent) than with lacunar infarcts 3 of 273 (1.1 percent). Most seizures were partial and occurred only once during the first 15 days after stroke onset.

So and colleagues[63] studied 535 consecutive patients with acute ischemic stroke in a community and found that 33 (6.2 percent) of them had a seizure within 7 days of stroke onset. Of these seizures, 78 percent were within 24 h of stroke onset. In multivariate analysis, the only predictor of early seizure was location of the infarct in the carotid territory (odds ratio 4.0, 95 percent confidence interval 1.2 to 13.7).

Arboix and colleagues[64] studied 793 consecutive patients with acute ischemic stroke and found that 16 (2.0 percent) of them had a seizure within 48 h of stroke onset. Most seizures (63 percent) were generalized, without an apparent focal onset. Analysis included additional patients with hemorrhagic stroke and transient ischemic attack and showed that early seizures were associated with advanced age, confusion, hemorrhagic stroke, large stroke, involvement of the parietal and temporal lobes, concurrent medical complications, and in-hospital mortality (33.3 percent with seizures and 14.2 percent without seizures, $p = .02$).

Recommendations Although some clinical features have been associated with early poststroke seizures, the likelihood of this complication is relatively low, and we do not recommend prophylactic treatment with antiepileptic medications. If a seizure occurs after stroke, we recommend treatment with antiepileptic medication, because in the presence of an underlying lesion the risk of recurrence is increased, and this is a standard of practice. Early poststroke seizures seem to be readily controlled with antiepileptic medications. As always, pharmacologic monotherapy is preferable to polytherapy.

Wide Blood Pressure Fluctuations

Background Fluctuations in blood pressure within certain limits are normally tolerated by the brain because the cerebrovascular resistance adjusts to maintain constant cerebral blood flow. This response, called cerebrovascular autoregulation, is impaired in ischemic brain regions. Consequently, a decrease in blood pressure is accompanied by a decrease in cerebral perfusion, possibly resulting in increased brain injury.[65] Blood pressure is elevated in 69 to 84 percent of patients with subacute stroke.[66,67] This elevation occurs in both previously hypertensive and nonhypertensive patients and spontaneously decreases over the subsequent several days. This is most likely a physiologic response to brain ischemia and stress in general, and seems to have some beneficial effects.

Evidence Physiologic studies show that ischemic brain regions have impaired vascular autoregulation, and as a result cerebral perfusion in the ischemic regions fluctuates with blood pressure changes.[68] Evidence for such a physiologic reaction comes from animal experiments,[69] anecdotal case reports,[70] a prospective observational study,[72] and clinical acute stroke trials.[17,73]

Lisk and colleagues[73] prospectively randomized 16 hypertensive patients within 72 h of ischemic stroke onset to placebo ($n = 6$) or antihypertensive treatment ($n = 10$). Baseline mean arterial blood pressure was 120 to 140 mmHg, and the aim was to lower the blood pressure 10 to 15 percent from the baseline value. Cerebral blood flow (CBF) was measured at baseline and on day 3 with single photon emission computed tomography. Blood pressure decreased on days 1 through 3 by a similar amount in both groups. However, blood pressure decreased significantly more in patients treated with nicardipine ($n = 5$) as compared with captopril or clonidine combined ($n = 5$). The greater was the blood pressure reduction, the less was the CBF increase between baseline and day 3 ($p < .05$). In patients treated with nicardipine, there was no increase in CBF on day 3, whereas in patients treated with captopril or clonidine there was a significant 16 percent increase ($p = .03$). There was no significant difference in clinical outcome between the two treatment groups. This could be because this study was too small to detect such a difference.

The Intravenous Nimodipine West European Stroke Trial[17] was prematurely terminated because treatment with nimodipine was associated with significant blood pressure reductions and with worse clinical outcome. In this study, 100 patients with acute ischemic stroke were randomly assigned to placebo treatment and 195 patients to a low (1 mg/h) or a high (2 mg/h) dose of nimodipine treatment within 24 h of stroke onset. Outcome was significantly better ($P < .001$) and blood pressure significantly higher on day 2 ($P < .001$) in the placebo group than the high-dose nimodipine group. There was a strong correlation between the extent of blood pressure reduction and unfavorable neurologic outcome ($P < .001$).

However, a recent retrospective study showed that a decrease in mean arterial pressure between the first and third day after admission for ischemic stroke is associated with improved outcome.[74] In this study, 481 patients were studied within 48 h of onset of stroke (mean 21 h). Of these, 235 (49 percent) were treated with oral antihypertensive agents during transport to the hospital or while in the emergency room. Two days after stroke, the mean arterial pressure dropped significantly more in the treated patients (14 mmHg vs. 10 mmHg, $p < .05$). Full recovery at day 7 was seen in 252 (52 percent) patients and was 2.9 times more common among patients with a 20 to 30 percent drop in mean arterial pressure. This retrospective study must be interpreted with caution. Most likely, patients who were destined to full recovery had spontaneous blood pressure reductions, and had a largely intact cerebrovascular autoregulation. It would be incorrect and dangerous to interpret this study as showing that reduction of blood pressure during subacute stroke contributed to full recovery.

Recommendations Lowering the blood pressure during the subacute ischemic stroke period should be avoided, unless a strong indication is present, such as severe blood pressure elevation (>230 systolic or >120 diastolic), arterial dissection, or end organ damage. If the blood pressure needs to be lowered during the subacute ischemic stroke period, this should be done slowly with an intravenous agent, such as labetalol, and only down to an intermediate level. The risk of lowering blood pressure during subacute ischemic stroke should be weighed against its benefits.

If thrombolytic therapy is administered within the first few hours after stroke onset, elevated blood pressure increases the risk of hemorrhagic transformation of an infarct. Therefore, in that special situation, the blood pressure should be maintained below 180 systolic and below 105 diastolic.[56] Ideally, to compromise between the risk of hemorrhagic transformation and the risk of infarct extension, the blood pressure should probably be 170 to 179 systolic and 95 to 104 diastolic. Unless the patient is in shock, raising the blood pressure to these levels is not recommended. For mild to moderate blood pressure elevations (180 to 230 mmHg systolic or 105 to 120 mmHg diastolic) after thrombolytic therapy, intravenous labetalol is recommended. Recommended dose is 10 mg over 1 to 2 min, repeated or doubled if needed every 10 to 20 min, up to a total dose of 150 mg. For severe blood pressure elevations (>230 mmHg systolic or 121 to 140 mmHg diastolic), initial treatment with intravenous labetalol is recommended followed by sodium nitroprusside, starting with 0.5 to 1.0 (μg/kg per min, if blood pressure remains elevated >180/105 mmHg.

Metabolic and Toxic Complications

Background Although metabolic and toxic complications have systemic effects, they can exacerbate focal neurologic deficits when there is an underlying brain lesion, such as stroke. In this section, we will discuss selected metabolic and toxic complications that are most likely to be encountered during subacute stroke.

Hyperglycemia is often present during subacute stroke, usually in diabetic patients. Central nervous system effects of hyperglycemia are usually seen when the blood glucose level is >600 mg/dL. Some studies suggest that there may be a direct relationship between blood glucose level during subacute stroke and extent of ischemic brain injury. Of the 279 placebo-treated acute ischemic stroke patients in the Randomized Trial of Tirilazad Mesylate in Patients with Acute Stroke (RANTTAS) study,[75] 30 (11 percent) had hyperglycemia, nonserious in all of them. The impact of different degrees of hyperglycemia during subacute ischemic stroke and in different stroke subtypes remains unresolved. For further discussion of this topic, see Chap. 5.

Infections are a well recognized cause of impaired mentation, which is likely to make the neurologic deficits seem worse than before the infection. Infections are the most common toxic complications during subacute stroke. Of the 279 placebo-treated acute ischemic stroke patients in the RANTTAS study,[75] at least 65 (23 percent) developed an infection within 10 days of stroke onset. These infections were urinary in 30 (11 percent) patients, pneumonia in 27 (10 percent), cellulitis in 5 (2 percent), and sepsis in 3 (1 percent). Additional infections with a frequency of <1 percent included wound infection, bronchitis, and septic joint. Unselected stroke patients are likely to be sicker and thus have more infectious complications than those eligible to participate in a clinical treatment trial such as RANTTAS.

In a hospital study of 607 consecutive patients, Davenport and colleagues[76] found that infection occurred in 212 (35 percent) patients within 37 days of the stroke. Urinary tract infection occurred in 98 (16 percent) patients, chest infections in 70 (12 percent), and other infections in 44 (7 percent). Most chest infections (approximately 60 percent) occurred in the first 10 days, whereas urinary tract infections occurred at a constant rate throughout the study.

Hypoxia is also a well-known cause of impaired mentation. There are many reasons for patients with subacute stroke to develop hypoxia, such as lung infections, pulmonary edema, and atelectasis. Of the 279 placebo-treated acute ischemic stroke patients in the RANTTAS study,[75] 8 (3 percent) had hypoxia within 10 days of stroke onset. Of these, two (1 percent) were categorized as serious.

Sedating medications are sometimes given to patients with subacute stroke. By virtue of their known action, sedating medications can impair a patient's mentation and make the neurologic deficits seem worse than before sedation.

Evidence There are no clinical studies on the treatment of metabolic complications in subacute stroke patients in particular. Our recommendations are based on the logical assumption that if a metabolic or toxic derangement known to adversely affect the central nervous system is identified, correction of this derangement will improve neurologic function.

Recommendations Metabolic derangements should be corrected as soon as they are identified to prevent them from getting bigger and to optimize neurologic function as soon as possible. The exact treatment to correct a metabolic or toxic derangement depends on the underlying cause, but until proven otherwise, should be the same as in other situations. Toxic medications should be discontinued or replaced with less toxic alternatives if possible (see "Delirium").

Hyperthermia

Background An increase in body temperature is another possible cause for neurologic deterioration during subacute stroke. The extent of ischemic brain injury seems to be directly related to body temperature. The explanations for this observation are: (1) hyperthermia increases cellular metabolic demand which cannot be met because of ischemia, (2) toxic substances, such as excitatory amino acids and free radicals, accumulate to a greater extent than in normothermia, and (3) the activity of lytic enzymes increases with the temperature. Consequently, the rate of cell damage is accelerated at higher temperatures. The mechanisms responsible for augmentation of ischemic brain injury at elevated temperatures have recently been reviewed.[77] The lower the temperature, the lower is the metabolic rate and the more stable are the cellular components. As the metabolism slows, so does the process of cell death. This can explain cold weather hibernation by some animals, possibility of good recovery from ice-water drowning compared with warm-water drowning, preservation of myocardium during open heart surgery employing cold cardioplegia, and prolonged stability of biologic products at reduced temperatures. Normal human body temperature is 37.0°C (98.6°F), and it can be thought of as a point on a line representing the relationship between temperature and rate of ischemic cell damage. The lower the temperature, the slower the damage.

Evidence Results from animal experiments consistently show that as brain temperature decreases or increases, so does the extent of ischemic brain injury. Clinical studies in acute stroke show that elevated body temperature is associated with worse outcome.[78–80] Azzimondi and colleagues[78] analyzed the relationship between body temperature during the first 7 days of stroke and the 30-day survival in 183 prospective randomly selected patients. Fever (axillary $T > 37.2°C$) during the first 7 days after stroke onset occurred in 78 (43 percent) patients; in 15 percent it developed on day 1 and in 49 percent on day 2. The overall 30-day mortality was 29 percent (53 patients), and fever was an independent predictor of death (odds ratio 3.4, $p = .006$).

Reith and colleagues[79] analyzed the relationship between body temperature within 6 h of ischemic stroke onset and clinical outcome in 390 consecutive patients. On admission, hypothermia (tympanic $T \leq 36.5°C$) was present in 11 percent of patients, normothermia (tympanic T 36.6 to 37.5°C) in 64 percent and hyperthermia (tympanic $T > 37.5°C$) in 25 percent. Elevated body temperature was independently associated with greater stroke severity ($p < .009$), larger infarcts ($p < .001$), greater mortality ($p < .02$), and worse outcome in survivors ($p < .003$). For each 1°C increase in body tempera-

ture, the relative risk of poor outcome (death or severe disability) rose by a factor of 2.2 ($p < .002$).

Castillo and colleagues[80] measured body temperature every 2 h for 72 h in 260 patients with ischemic stroke, starting <24 h from onset. Hyperthermia (axillary $T > 37.5°C$) was measured in 158 (61 percent) patients, and in 91 (58 percent) of them an infectious cause was found. Hyperthermia during the first 24 h after stroke onset, but not later, was independently associated with larger stroke ($p < .001$), worse neurologic deficit ($p < .001$), and dependency ($p = .002$) at 3 months. Mortality at 3 months was 1 percent in the normothermic and 16 percent in the hyperthermic patients ($p < .001$).

It remains to be proven whether strokes cause hyperthermia, hyperthermia augments ischemic brain injury, or both, and whether lowering body temperature during acute stroke will improve the clinical outcome. Ginsberg and Busto[77] recently reviewed the evidence in support of aggressive treatment of hyperthermia during subacute stroke.

Recommendations Hypothermia therapy has not been sufficiently studied in the treatment of acute ischemic stroke, and it is technically difficult and risky. However, because there is good evidence that hyperthermia is detrimental during acute ischemic stroke and it can be treated relatively easily, we recommend that elevated body temperature during the subacute stroke period be reduced promptly. Hyperthermia may be treated with antipyretic drugs, reduced ambient temperature, and cooling blankets.

Recurrent Ischemic Stroke

Background A recurrent ischemic stroke is a new arterial occlusion that causes another ischemic stroke. This usually results in new symptoms and signs, as opposed to the other causes of progressing stroke mentioned above, which result in worsening of the preexisting deficits. Recurrent ischemic stroke during the subacute period is serious. It results in additional brain damage, increased likelihood of complications, decreased likelihood of a favorable outcome, and indicates that the prescribed treatment was not effective in preventing the recurrent stroke. Recurrent ischemic stroke during the subacute stroke period is relatively rare. If patients at greatest risk for recurrent ischemic stroke could be reliably identified, they might benefit from a more aggressive stroke prevention treatment than patients with a lower risk of stroke recurrence.

Evidence In the Stroke Data Bank,[81] recurrent ischemic stroke occurred in <1 percent of 1273 patients within 7 days of hospitalization for acute ischemic stroke. Recurrent stroke was associated with longer hospitalization (27 vs. 14 days) and higher 30-day fatality (20 percent vs. 7 percent). In multivariate analysis, coexisting arterial hypertension ($p = .01$) and blood glucose > 140 mg/dL ($p = .001$) were good predictors of recurrent stroke.

In the International Stroke Trial,[18] 19,435 patients with acute ischemic stroke were studied (see "Treatments to Limit Stroke Size and Prevent Early Recurrence"). Recurrent ischemic stroke within 14 days occurred in 283 (2.9 percent) patients treated with heparin (half of them also received aspirin) and 370 (3.8 percent) patients not treated with heparin (half of them also received aspirin) ($p < .01$). However, the apparent benefit from heparin was offset by an increased rate of intracerebral hemorrhage (1.2 percent with heparin and 0.4 percent without heparin, $p < .001$). Recurrent ischemic stroke within 14 days occurred in 275 (2.8 percent) patients treated with aspirin (half of them also received heparin) and 378 (3.9 percent) patients not treated with aspirin (half of them also received heparin) ($p < .001$). Aspirin use was not associated with increased rate of intracerebral hemorrhage (0.9 percent with aspirin and 0.8 percent without aspirin).

In the study of intravenous low molecular weight heparinoid (danaparoid) vs. placebo (see "Treatments to Limit Stroke Size and Prevent Early Recurrence"),[10] recurrent ischemic stroke during the 7-day treatment period occurred in 7 of 638 (1 percent) patients in the danaparoid group and 7 of 628 (1 percent) patients in the placebo group. Among patients with cardioembolic stroke, typically thought to have the highest stroke recurrence rate, recurrent stroke occurred in 2 of 123 (1.6 percent) patients in the placebo group and none of 143 patients in the active drug group.

Among patients with cardioembolic stroke in the Cerebral Embolism Study,[8] recurrent stroke during the 14-day treatment period occurred in 2 of 21 (10 percent) non-anticoagulated patients and none of 24 anticoagulated patients. The nonanticoagulated patients did not receive antiplatelet therapy.

Recommendations Although patients with hypertension and hyperglycemia during subacute ischemic stroke seem to have an increased risk of early recurrence, it is premature to recommend prophylactic aggressive treatment for this subgroup of patients. Because early recurrent ischemic stroke during the subacute period is rare (<2 percent), a large proportion of patients would most likely be treated aggressively unnecessarily. However, we do recommend immediate anticoagulation for patients who have early recurrent ischemic stroke, if it is reasonably safe to do so (see "Starting Anticoagulation Therapy"). As always, the possible benefits of anticoagulation therapy must be weighed against the associated risks. Duration of anticoagulation therapy depends on the underlying cause. Antiplatelet agents are usually discontinued during anticoagulation.

Delirium

Background Delirium is a form of acute confusion. The fundamental abnormality in all confusional states is the inability to maintain normal attention. Delirium (agitated confusion) is distinguished from other forms of acute confusion by the behavior of the patient, which includes hyperactivity, agitation, hallucinations, delusions, possible violence, and autonomic instability. The autonomic instability may result in flushing, diaphoresis, tachycardia, and fluctuating arterial hypertension. The list of possible causes of confusional state, including delirium, is long and includes a large variety of toxic and metabolic derangements, deficiency states, and withdrawal from sedatives. In addition, delirium can complicate stroke. During the subacute stroke period, delirium may alternate with nonagitated confusion. The distinction between delirium and nonagitated confusion is clinically important, because the symptoms of delirium usually need to be treated together with the underlying cause. As the pharmacologic treatment for the symptoms of delirium may inhibit recovery from stroke, it must be done with caution.

It is difficult to estimate the prevalence of delirium during subacute stroke because definitions between studies differ widely, and delirium is often tabulated together with nonagitated confusion. Of the 279 placebo-treated stroke patients in the RANTTAS study,[75] 22 (8 percent) had agitation during the first 10 days after stroke.

The brain lesions associated with acute delirium can be in either the right or left cerebral hemisphere, or both.[82] It has been postulated that the lesions responsible for acute delirium affect posterior hemispheric structures, sparing the reticular activating system and disinhibiting the limbic system. This can explain the agitation as opposed to lethargy and the abnormal behavior.

Evidence Animal studies suggest that some drugs may enhance whereas others may inhibit the complex process of recovery from stroke.[83] Amphetamines and acetylcholine have been reported to enhance recovery from stroke, mainly in laboratory animals. Neuroleptics, benzodiazepines, phenytoin, and certain antihypertensives have been reported to inhibit recovery from stroke, also mainly in experimental animals.

In an interesting retrospective clinical study, Goldstein and colleagues[84] compared stroke recovery between 24 patients treated during the recovery period with at least one of the drugs implicated to inhibit recovery (neuroleptics, benzodiazepines, phenytoin, clonidine, or prazosin) and 34 patients not treated with these drugs. The two groups were similar with respect to important baseline characteristics that might effect the results. Recovery was measured prospectively by examiners blinded to the drugs that the patients were receiving. At 30 days after stroke onset, sensorimotor function recovered significantly slower ($p = .004$), and the likelihood of being independent was significantly lower ($p = .02$) among patients treated with the "deleterious drugs" than patients not treated with these drugs. Multivariate analysis showed that the drug group predicted recovery ($p = .03$) independent of other important predictors.

Recommendations Although it is premature to recommend drugs such as catecholamines to enhance the recovery from stroke, we recommend to avoid, if possible, those drugs that seem to inhibit recovery from stroke, such as neuroleptics, benzodiazepines, phenytoin, clonidine, and prazosin. For the treatment of arterial hypertension and seizures, many good alternative drugs are available. For the treatment of the symptoms of delirium, nonpharmacologic measures should be optimized first. Some patients may respond favorably to frequent reassurances from sympathetic hospital staff, relatives, or friends. Keeping the room adequately lit at all times is believed to help as well. When pharmacologic treatment with an antipsychotic or a sedative medication is needed, the potency and frequency of administration of such drugs should be minimized.

Neurologic Worsening for No Apparent Reason

Background When none of the above specific problems are identified in a patient with progressing subacute stroke deficits, a propagating thrombus is often implicated. Consequently, anticoagulation therapy is usually recommended. However, propagation of a thrombus in a stroke patient is difficult to document and seldom is. An alternative explanation for progressing subacute stroke is offered by Fisher and Garcia.[55] They suggest that, as a result of the many biochemical alterations induced by ischemia, the full extent of brain injury becomes manifest over the first 2 days of ischemic stroke. This includes the deleterious effects of excitatory amino acids, free radicals, and lytic enzymes. This is the natural course of ischemic brain damage, without any of the specific complications discussed above. In this situation, antithrombotic therapy is not expected to be beneficial. This may account for the negative results of anticoagulation therapy trials in progressing ischemic stroke. However, some form of cytoprotective therapy could possibly provide protection from ischemia until perfusion is improved.

Evidence Despite the common use of heparin anticoagulation in progressing ischemic stroke, the evidence from recent clinical trials suggests that this treatment may not be beneficial for a large proportion of patients and is associated with hemorrhagic complications. Haley and colleagues,[85,86] in a study of 36 consecutive patients with progressing ischemic stroke, found that 18 (50 percent) patients continued to deteriorate neurologically, despite anticoagulation with intravenous heparin. One of these deteriorations was related to hemorrhagic transformation of an infarct, and bleeding complications occurred in 5 (14 percent) patients. In all 5 patients with bleeding complications, the PTT was in the therapeutic range.

Slivka and Levy[86] studied 69 consecutive patients treated with intravenous heparin anticoagulation for progressing ischemic stroke. They found that 27 (39 percent) patients continued to deteriorate neurologically while anticoagulated. Two of these deteriorations were related to hemorrhagic transformation of the infarcts, and overall, bleeding complications occurred in 10 (14 percent) patients. Deterioration did not correlate with the PTT. Because these studies were not controlled, it remains unknown whether the anticoagulation treatments were beneficial. It is possible that the outcome of the patients in these studies would have been worse if they were not anticoagulated.

Toni and colleagues[54] studied factors associated with neurologic deterioration in 152 consecutive patients with first-ever ischemic stroke. The conditions of 39 (26 percent) patients deteriorated during the initial 4 days of the stroke. Independent risk factors for deterioration were elevated serum glucose level at admission, hypodensity on cerebral CT within 5 h of stroke onset, and carotid siphon occlusion. The authors suggest that cerebral edema is probably the most common cause of subacute stroke deterioration.

Recommendations   When faced with a patient with progressing ischemic stroke without an apparent etiology, other than possible thrombus extension or recurrent thromboembolism, we recommend immediate anticoagulation with intravenous heparin for at least 3 days (see "Starting Anticoagulation Therapy"). Subsequently, treatment depends on the neurologic stability of the patient and findings on evaluation. If the patient continues to have recurrent thromboembolic events, has a hypercoagulable disorder, or has a serious source of emboli, we recommend anticoagulation with warfarin for at least 3 months (no evidence) and periodic reassessment of the need for anticoagulation.

MANAGING MEDICAL COMPLICATIONS OF SUBACUTE STROKE

There are many possible medical complications during the subacute stroke period. Keeping them all in mind and taking steps to prevent them are essential for optimal patient management. The ability to do this effectively by specialized stroke teams, in acute stroke units as compared with general hospital wards, is probably the reason why better stroke outcomes have been measured for patients treated in the acute stroke units.

Venous Thromboembolism

Background   Deep vein thrombosis (DVT) of the lower extremities is a common and serious complication of stroke. Without prophylaxis, DVT can be demonstrated in approximately one-half of patients with paresis within 10 days of stroke.[87] The most serious complication of DVT is pulmonary embolism (PE). If DVT is not treated, the likelihood of developing PE is 30 percent during the subsequent 2 years.[87] Risk of PE is greater with clots in the thigh veins than with clots in the calf veins.[88] The mortality rate from PE is difficult to determine because many small emboli are asymptomatic and remain undetected.

Approximately one-half of patients with DVT are asymptomatic.[87] Typical symptoms and signs are pain, warmth, swelling, and erythema of the affected leg and a low-grade fever. Differential diagnosis includes celluli-

tis, muscle injury, superficial thrombophlebitis, Achilles tendonitis, and long bone fracture. Duplex ultrasound and impedance plethysmography are very useful diagnostic tests for DVT. If performed and interpreted by experienced personnel, both have a sensitivity and specificity greater than 90 percent.[89]

The most common symptoms and signs of PE are dyspnea, pleuritic chest pain, cough, and tachypnea. Additional symptoms and signs of PE may include tachycardia, right heart failure, hemoptysis, pulmonary rales, pulmonary consolidation, pleural effusion, hypoxia, hypotension, and rapid death. Ventilation/perfusion nuclear lung scan has a greater than 90 percent sensitivity in diagnosing PE. Pulmonary arteriogram is the most definitive test.

Evidence   The main risk factor for DVT in stroke patients is immobility.[88,89] In one study,[90] DVT developed in <1 percent of ambulatory patients and in 25 percent of similarly treated nonambulatory patients ($p < .001$). Presumably, decreased muscular contractions in the paretic leg decrease venous blood flow, resulting in blood stasis, which enhances thrombosis. Another potential risk factor for DVT during the subacute stroke period is blood hypercoagulability, which is present in some patients, mainly those with nonlacunar-type stroke, and persists for up to 4 weeks.[91] This may be why in some stroke patients, DVT develops in the unaffected leg.

Several studies indicate that the rate of DVT in stroke patients can be reduced with antithrombotic prophylaxis, such as subcutaneous heparin, LMWH, LMWH analogs (heparinoids), and with intermittent pneumatic compression (IPC) devices.[92–99] Table 3-3 summarizes the randomized clinical trials of DVT prophylaxis after stroke.

Three nonblinded trials compared prophylaxis with subcutaneous heparin to no prophylaxis.[92,94,95] All showed that prophylaxis with heparin, 5000 units TID (two studies) or BID (one study) significantly reduces the rate of DVT. The two studies using 500 units TID had an objective endpoint (^{125}I-fibrinogen leg scan), but the study using 5000 units BID had only a subjective clinical endpoint (clinical signs of DVT).

Three blinded trials compared prophylaxis with LMWH to placebo.[92–98] Prophylaxis with LMWH was significantly more effective than placebo in one of these studies,[96] borderline in another,[97] and not effective in the third study.[98] The study that showed a benefit used Danaparoid (a LMWH analog), 750 units BID.

Table 3-3.

Randomized clinical trials of deep vein thrombosis prophylaxis after ischemic stroke

Author, year, study type	Treatment #1 (# patients)	Treatment #2 (# patients)	Endpoint	Result
McCarthy, 1977, nonblinded	Heparin SQ 5000 U TID for 14 days (*n* = 16)	No prophylaxis (*n* = 16)	^{125}I-Fibrinogen leg scan	DVT in 13% patients in heparin group and 75% in no prophylaxis group (*p* < .01)
Turpie, 1977, nonblinded	IPC for 5 days (*n* = 65)	No prophylaxis (*n* = 63)	^{125}I-Fibrinogen leg scan	DVT in 2% patients in IPC group and 19% in no prophylaxis group (*p* < .001)
Gelmers, 1980, nonblinded	Heparin SQ 5000 U BID until mobilized (*n* = 42)	No prophylaxis (*n* = 40)	Clinical signs of DVT	DVT in 2% patients in heparin group and 23% in no prophylaxis group (*p* < .001)
McCarthy, 1986, nonblinded	Heparin SQ 5000 U TID for 14 days (*n* = 144)	No prophylaxis (*n* = 161)	^{125}I-Fibrinogen leg scan	DVT in 22% patients in heparin group and 73% in no prophylaxis group (*p* < .001)
Turpie, 1987, blinded	LMWH[a] SQ 750 U BID for 14 days (*n* = 50)	Placebo (*n* = 25)	^{125}I-Fibrinogen leg scan and plethysmography	DVT in 4% patients in LMWH group and 28% in placebo group (*p* = .005)
Prins, 1989, blinded	LMWH[b] 2500 U SQ BID for 14 days (*n* = 27)	Placebo (*n* = 30)	^{125}I-Fibrinogen leg scan	DTV in 22% patients in LMWH group and 50% in placebo group (*p* = .05)
Sandset, 1990, blinded	LMWH[b] 3000–5500 U/day for 14 days (*n* = 42)	Placebo (*n* = 50)	Venography	DVT in 36% patients in LMWH group and 34% in placebo group (NS)
Turpie, 1992, blinded	LMWH[a] SQ 750 U BID for 14 days (*n* = 45)	Heparin SQ 5000 U BID for 14 days (*n* = 42)	^{125}I-Fibrinogen leg scan and plethysmography	DVT in 9% patients in LMWH group and 31% in heparin group (*p* = .01)

Abbreviations: LMWH, low molecular weight heparin compound; TID, three times daily; BID, twice daily; SQ, subcutaneously; DVT, deep vein thrombosis; IPC, intermittent pneumatic compression; NS, not statistically significant.

[a]Danaparoid (a low molecular weight heparinoid).

[b]Fragmin (a low molecular weight heparin).

The study with borderline benefit and the one with no benefit, both used Fragmin 3000–5500 units per day.

One blinded study compared two effective DVT prophylaxis treatments, an LMWH analog, Danaparoid, and subcutaneous heparin.[99] The Danaparoid dose was 750 units BID, and the heparin dose was the lower dose previously shown to be effective, 5000 units BID. Danaparoid was significantly better than heparin. However, it has not been definitively proven which form of antithrombotic prophylaxis and at what dose has the best efficacy to complications ratio.

IPC is an alternative to anticoagulation for DVT prophylaxis in stroke patients. This is accomplished with devices that fit around the legs and periodically alternately compress them, simulating muscle move-

ments. One randomized, nonblinded clinical trial compared IPC with no prophylaxis and found that IPC significantly reduced the DVT rate in patients with various intracranial diseases, including stroke.[93] More recently, a nonrandomized study of consecutive stroke patients found that IPC in addition to subcutaneous heparin 5000 units BID and antithrombotic stockings was more effective than the heparin and antithrombotic stockings only.[90] In this study, 432 patients had IPC and 249 did not. Confirmed DVT occurred in <1 percent of patients who had IPC and 9 percent of patients who did not (*p* < .001). This difference was even greater in nonambulating patients, <1 percent with IPC and 25 percent without IPC (*p* < .001). Elastic compression stockings help prevent superficial thrombophlebitis but do not seem to be effective in DVT prophylaxis.[88]

Recommendations   Every effort should be made to achieve ambulation as soon after stroke as possible. DVT prophylaxis should be used in all nonambulating patients. There is no universally accepted protocol for DVT prophylaxis in subacute stroke patients. We recommend subcutaneous heparin 5000 units TID and IPC. For patients with active extracranial bleeding, we initially recommend IPC only.

Both DVT and PE need to be treated with full-dose anticoagulation to inhibit thrombus extension and embolism. Intravenous heparin and oral warfarin should be started as soon as the diagnosis is made (see "Starting Anticoagulation Therapy"). Target INR for maintenance anticoagulation is 2.0 to 3.0. Optimal duration of anticoagulation therapy has not been established by an ideally designed clinical trial, and it is best to individualize treatment based on each patient's risk factors. Usually, at least 3 months of anticoagulation therapy is recommended for both DVT and PE.[100,101]

The most dreaded complication of long-term oral anticoagulation therapy is bleeding. The likelihood of bleeding during warfarin anticoagulation increases with increasing intensity of anticoagulation, with the presence of certain underlying disorders, such as renal insufficiency or anemia, and with concomitant use of aspirin.[49] If anticoagulation for DVT or PE is contraindicated, such as in a patient with active bleeding, an inferior vena cava filter can be placed to stop the emboli from reaching the lungs. Intravenous thrombolytic therapy, with streptokinase, urokinase, or tissue plasminogen activator, is sometimes considered for patients with acute PE, but probably should not be used in patients with a subacute ischemic stroke because of the possibility of hemorrhagic transformation of the infarct.

Pneumonia

Background   Pneumonia occurs in 2 to 5 percent of patients with recent stroke. In one study of 441 stroke patients, 2.7 percent developed pneumonia while in the hospital.[102] Of the 279 placebo-treated stroke patients in the RANTTAS trial,[75] 14 (5 percent) developed pneumonia within 30 days of stroke onset. Pneumonia was the most common serious medical complication, and aspiration pneumonia accounted for 60 percent of the serious pneumonias.

Aspiration pneumonia develops because of dysphagia and the associated endotrachial aspiration of oropharyngeal or gastric secretions. Several clinical conditions, such as depressed level of consciousness, seizures, and impaired upper airway reflexes, predispose stroke patients to aspiration (see Table 3-1). Nasogastric and other feeding tubes, gastroesophageal reflux, gastric distention, and vomiting have been cited as predisposing factors for aspiration.[103] Reduced chest movements ipsilateral to hemiparesis, inefficient cough reflex, and decreased inspiratory volume predispose to atelectasis and result in impaired clearance of pulmonary secretions. This, in turn, predisposes to pneumonia. In addition, decreased mobility, being in an intensive care unit, or being on a respirator increases the risk of developing pneumonia. The likelihood of ventilator-associated pneumonia can be decreased with prophylactic cefuroxime treatment.[104]

Aspiration pneumonia affects dependent lung regions. Infiltration is usually multilobar and bilateral. The location of pneumonia varies according to patient's position at the time of aspiration. In the supine position, superior segments of the lower lobes, posterior segment of the right upper lobe, and posterior subsegment of the left upper lobe are usually involved.

Aspiration pneumonia is caused by mixed anaerobic and aerobic infection, with up to 80 percent of cases caused by multiple organisms. Aerobic bacteria associated with community-acquired aspiration pneumonias are mostly streptococci, whereas nosocomial infections are usually caused by Gram-negative organisms, particularly *Klebsiella* and *Escherichia coli*. The major anaerobic organisms include *Fusobacterium nucleatum, Peptostreptococcus, Bacteroides melaninogenicus,* and *Bacteroides intermedius.* Sputum Gram stain and culture have limited diagnostic usefulness because of low sensitivities and specificities. Complications of aspiration pneumonia include necrotizing pneumonitis and lung abscess.

Evidence   The recommendations for prevention of pneumonia listed in Table 3-1 are based on our current understanding of the pathophysiology of stroke-related pneumonia. There are no clinical studies on the treatment of stroke-associated pneumonia in particular.

Recommendations   The steps recommended to prevent the development of pneumonia during the subacute stroke period are listed in Table 3-1. When stroke-associated pneumonia is diagnosed or suspected, until proven otherwise, treatment should be similar to that for nosocomial or aspiration pneumonia associated with other disorders.

Cardiac Complications

Background Electrocardiographic changes during subacute stroke include various arrhythmias, ST segment depression, QT segment prolongation, and abnormal U waves. Such complications could result in angina, myocardial infarction, congestive heart failure, and cerebral hypoperfusion. These cardiac complications are most common in patients with subarachnoid hemorrhage, less common with intracerebral hemorrhage, and least common with cerebral infarction. Cardiac ischemic events during subacute stroke are partly related to premorbid heart disease and partly to the acute stroke itself.

Of the 279 placebo-treated stroke patients in the RANTTAS trial,[75] 16 (6 percent) had ischemic cardiac events within 3 months of stroke. In addition, congestive heart failure developed in 30 (11 percent) patients and cardiac arrest in 5 (2 percent). Most episodes of congestive heart failure (23 of 30, 77 percent) and cardiac ischemia (12 of 16, 75 percent) were classified as not serious.

In a study of cardiac enzymes during subacute stroke, Norris and colleagues[105] measured creatine phosphokinase (CK), lactate dehydrogenase (LDH), and serum glutamic oxalo-acetic transaminase (SGOT) for 4 days after admission in 224 patients with acute stroke and in 64 hospitalized controls with various disorders. They also measured CK isoenzymes in another group of 230 patients with acute stroke and 53 non-stroke controls. At least two of the three cardiac enzymes were elevated in 13 of 162 (8 percent) patients with ischemic stroke, 4 of 23 (17 percent) patients with intracranial hemorrhage, 1 of 39 (3 percent) patients with transient ischemic attack (TIA), and 8 of 64 (13 percent) controls. Compared with the controls, enzyme levels were highest in patients with intracranial hemorrhage ($p < .001$), somewhat elevated in patients with ischemic stroke (borderline statistically significant, $p = .05$), and not significantly different in patients with TIA. Cardiac enzymes rose progressively during the 4 days of study.

In the second group of patients studied by Norris and colleagues, elevated cardiac muscle CK (CK-MB) was found in 19 of 168 (11 percent) patients with ischemic stroke, 4 of 32 (13 percent) patients with intracranial hemorrhage, 2 of 30 (7 percent) patients with TIA, and 3 of 53 (6 percent) controls. Elevated CK-MB was

significantly associated with new cardiac arrhythmias (92 percent vs. 50 percent, $p < .001$) and ECG changes of ST segment depression and T-wave inversion (68 percent vs. 40 percent, $p < .05$). Supraventricular or ventricular ectopic beats accounted for >90 percent of the arrhythmias.

In a study of 33 patients with acute ischemic stroke and 17 patients with recent TIA monitored continuously for 48 h, McDermott and colleagues[106] found ST segment depression in 29 percent and ventricular arrhythmias in 35 percent of patients. The ST segment depression was associated with increasing age and left cerebral ischemia.

The pathologic substrate for the cardiac ischemic events during subacute stroke has been identified as myocytolysis.[107] This is characterized as scattered foci of swollen myocytes, surrounded by monocytes, interstitial hemorrhages, and myofibrillary degeneration. These changes surround intracardiac nerves and are usually not seen beyond 2 weeks after stroke, largely based on animal experiments. This complication has been attributed to sympathetic nervous system hyperactivity and lesions involving the insular cortex.

Evidence There is no clinical evidence that cardiac abnormalities during subacute stroke should be treated differently than the same abnormalities not associated with stroke, except that anticoagulation and thrombolysis are more risky as discussed in previous sections.

Recommendations Until proven otherwise, treatment of cardiac arrhythmias during subacute stroke should be the same as in other situations. Many arrhythmias are ectopic beats not associated with hemodynamic complications or symptoms and usually do not need to be treated. Treatment of cardiac ischemia should also be similar to that in other situations, except that thrombolytic therapy is contraindicated and anticoagulation is more risky, owing to an increased risk of hemorrhagic transformation of the infarct.

Urinary Incontinence

Background Urinary incontinence is defined as inability to control the outflow of urine. Urinary incontinence predisposes to skin breakdown and is a very bothersome problem. Urinary continence requires adequate mobility, mentation, motivation, dexterity, and the integrated control of bladder function. Consequently, there are multiple potential causes of incontinence. The prevalence of incontinence increases with age.[108] Major urinary incontinence has been measured at 6.1 percent (5.3 percent in men and 6.5 percent in women), among persons older than 74 years living at home in England,[109] and at 9.6 percent among community residents in Texas.[110] Therefore, urinary incontinence in some stroke patients precedes the stroke.

Stroke can cause or add to pre-existing urinary incontinence in three ways[111]: one, the brain lesion can interrupt the inhibitory input to the reflex arc between the bladder and the spinal cord, resulting in bladder overactivity; two, the bladder function may be normal, but the patient may not be able to get to the toilet, use the toilet, or communicate the need to void; and three, certain medications may produce or exacerbate urinary incontinence, such as diuretics, anticholinergics, and (α adrenergic blockers. In addition, hyperglycemia and urinary tract infection (UTI) can augment incontinence. Urinary incontinence has been associated with stroke in the frontal, parietal, and temporal lobes, but not the occipital lobe.[108]

In one study,[112] 151 consecutive patients with subacute stroke were followed to determine the prevalence and outcome of urinary incontinence. Premorbid urinary incontinence was present in 26 (17 percent) patients. The prevalence of urinary incontinence decreased over time from 60 percent at the end of the first week to 42 percent after 4 weeks, and 29 percent after 12 weeks. Of the 279 placebo-treated stroke patients in the RANTTAS trial,[75] 14 (5 percent) had urinary incontinence within 10 days of stroke. In the Copenhagen Stroke Study,[113] 935 patients admitted with acute stroke were studied and urinary incontinence was present on admission in 47 percent of patients and at 6 months in 19 percent. Independent predictors of urinary incontinence on admission were older patient age, larger stroke, presence of diabetes mellitus, hypertension, other disabling diseases, and worse neurologic deficits.

In a study of 607 consecutive hospitalized acute stroke patients, Davenport and colleagues[76] found UTI in 98 (16 percent) patients during a mean observation of 37 days. UTI developed at a constant rate during the initial 30 days after stroke. Of the 279 vehicle-treated stroke patients in the RANTTAS trial,[75] 30 (11 percent) developed UTI within 30 days of stroke. In 3 (1 percent) of these patients, the UTI was considered serious.

Evidence   There are no data on the optimal management of urinary incontinence or UTI in subacute stroke patients in particular. Chronic indwelling urinary catheters, like other chronic catheters, are well known to predispose to infections. However, there is no evidence that using an indwelling urinary catheter during the subacute stroke period only, significantly increases the risk of developing UTI.

Recommendations   Because the risk of developing UTI during the first 3 days of placement of an indwelling bladder catheter seems to be low, such catheters may be used for all incontinent patients. However, indwelling urinary catheters should be removed as soon as they are no longer required, preferably by day 4. For patients without urinary outflow obstruction, external catheters could be used for men and diapers for women. Alternatively, patients with outflow obstruction could be treated with intermittent catheterization. This issue is more important beyond the subacute period.

Antibiotic treatment for prophylaxis against UTI or for asymptomatic bacteruria is not recommended because this may result in infection with resistant bacteria. If UTI develops, initial antibiotic treatment is empirical with a broad spectrum of coverage, given parenterally for at least 3 days. Inadequate therapy may result in kidney infection, loss of renal function, and sepsis. Nosocomial UTI usually involves more virulent bacteria than out-of-hospital-acquired UTI.

DIAGNOSTIC TESTING DURING SUBACUTE STROKE

The history and physical examination form an indispensable foundation of accurate diagnosis, which is essential for optimal management. Without a confident understanding of the nature of the patient's symptoms, and the localization of neurologic dysfunction that produces these symptoms, a physician is vulnerable to being misled by results of various diagnostic tests. For example, brain MRI often demonstrates nonspecific white matter lesions, and vascular ultrasonography sometimes shows vascular lesions, both of which require clinical correlation.

Stroke workup should be tailored to the individual patient with the goal of determining the mechanism of the stroke. Based on the history, a decision should be made whether a stroke or another process, such as a brain tumor or subdural hematoma, is causing the symptoms. With the history and neurologic examination, the location of the stroke should be defined as precisely as possible. Neuroimaging should be done to confirm the location, size, and ischemic vs. hemorrhagic nature of the stroke. Additional workup includes determination of the degree of stenosis in the responsible artery, search for sources of emboli, and in selected cases search for unusual causes, such as a hypercoagulable condition or drug abuse (Table 3-4).

During evaluation, it is important to distinguish between cerebral infarcts in the carotid and vertebrobasilar territories because proven stroke prevention treatment in the former includes endarterectomy, whereas in the latter it does not. This can usually be reliably determined on history and physical examination by an experienced physician. Neuroimaging helps confirm the localization.

A special situation exists with strokes in the distribution of the posterior cerebral artery. This artery usually receives blood flow from the basilar artery, but in approximately 15 percent of people the flow has an embryonic pattern from the carotid artery. Thus, it seems reasonable to investigate the carotid artery in

Table 3-4.

Diagnostic tests during subacute ischemic stroke

Test	Ischemia in carotid territory	Ischemia in vertebrobasilar territory
Initial CT or MRI	Always	Always
CBC, RPR or VDRL, ESR, PT, PTT, blood glucose, electrolytes	Always	Always
Electrocardiogram	Always	Always
Chest x-ray	Always	Always
Urine for illicit drugs	Always in young patients and if suspected in older patients	Always in young patients and if suspected in older patients
Carotid duplex	If carotid endarterectomy is an option	No
Transthoracic echocardiogram	If lacunar stroke with evidence of heart disease or nonlacunar stroke with probable etiology found prior to echocardiogram	If lacunar stroke with evidence of heart disease or nonlacunar stroke with probable etiology found prior to echocardiogram
Transesophageal echocardiogram	All nonlacunar strokes without probable etiology found prior to echocardiogram	All nonlacunar strokes without probable etiology found prior to echocardiogram
Special tests for hypercoagulability	If suspected, usually in young patients	If suspected, usually in young patients
Repeat CT or MRI	If infarct not well seen on initial scan, or anticoagulation or carotid endarterectomy planned	If infarct not well seen on initial scan or anticoagulation planned
Diffusion MRI	If new infarct needs to be distinguished from old infarct(s)	If new infarct needs to be distinguished from old infarct(s)
MRA	If severe carotid stenosis or occlusion on duplex, to look for intracranial stenosis and vascular malformation, and to screen young patients	If severe basilar artery stenosis suspected, to look for vascular malformations, and to screen young patients
Lumbar puncture	If infectious or autoimmune vasculitis suspected	If infectious or autoimmune vasculitis suspected
Catheter arteriogram	If noninvasive carotid studies are inconclusive or vasculitis suspected and LP is not diagnostic	If noninvasive studies are inconclusive or vasculitis suspected and LP is not diagnostic
Meningeal and brain biopsy	If vasculitis suspected on arteriogram and LP is not diagnostic	If vasculitis suspected on arteriogram and LP is not diagnostic

Abbreviations: CT, computed tomography; MRI, magnetic resonance imaging; CBC, complete blood count; RPR, rapid plasma reagin test; VDRL, venereal disease research laboratory test; ESR, erythrocyte sedimentation rate; PT, prothrombin time; PTT, partial thromboplastin time; MRA, magnetic resonance arteriogram.

patients with an infarct in the posterior cerebral artery territory.

Initial Neuroimaging

Background Initial neuroimaging of stroke is essential to distinguish between ischemic and hemorrhagic stroke as well as other intracranial lesions.[114] Because of the ability to easily and reliably rule out cerebral hemorrhage and widespread availability, cranial CT is usually the first neuroimaging test done in acute stroke or when a hemorrhagic transformation is suspected.

MRI is also able to reliably distinguish between ischemic and hemorrhagic stroke. Because MRI is more sensitive than CT in demonstrating any brain pathology, more care needs to be taken to distinguish clinically relevant from irrelevant findings. Also, MRI technology is more complex than CT technology and thus requires much more knowledge to perform and interpret the test. MRI is able to provide more information about the acute stroke and will undoubtedly soon be the initial test of choice in acute stroke evaluation in those medical centers where it is available.

Evidence As the evaluation and management of patients with ischemic stroke is considerably different than patients with hemorrhagic stroke, initial neuroimaging to confirm one or the other is obviously necessary. For detailed discussion on the usefulness of cerebral CT and MRI in stroke, please see Chaps. 34 and 35.

Recommendations We recommend cerebral CT as the initial test in subacute stroke, if not done during the acute period. Cerebral CT for stroke evaluation should be done with thin (approximately 5.0 mm) slice thickness, as thicker slices result in decreased visibility of small strokes, particularly in the posterior fossa. If readily available, MRI could be done instead.

Repeat Neuroimaging

Background Because ischemic strokes are usually not fully seen on acute imaging and because of cerebral complications that occasionally develop after the initial imaging, repeat neuroimaging is often indicated.

Evidence Repeat neuroimaging is most useful in determining hemorrhagic transformation of an infarct and confirming the location and size of an infarct. Although

not proven, anticoagulation therapy in the presence of asymptomatic hemorrhagic transformation of an infarct may produce a serious symptomatic hematoma. Also, larger strokes seem to be at greater risk for hemorrhagic transformation than smaller strokes[50] (see "Starting Anticoagulation Therapy"). In addition, although not supported by rigorous scientific data, the delay between stroke and carotid endarterectomy is often based on the size of the stroke.

Recommendations We recommend repeating neuroimaging within several days after stroke when (1) there is neurologic deterioration, (2) the initial scan does not fully demonstrate the acute infarct and the patient is expected to survive with a reasonable quality of life, (3) anticoagulation is to be started, or (4) carotid endarterectomy is planned. In our experience, visualization of the infarct helps confirm the vascular territory involved and extent of injury. In case of stroke recurrence, this could serve as a comparison. Although not supported by clinical studies, if a hemorrhagic transformation is seen on repeat cerebral CT, we wait and repeat cerebral CT until the hemorrhage has nearly completely resolved before recommending anticoagulation. We estimate the time between the serial CTs based on the density of the hematoma. We consider CT a better test for following hemorrhagic transformation of an infarct than MRI, because MRI is so sensitive that it often demonstrates small amounts of residual blood within an infarct, over a much longer period than CT.

We usually prefer to repeat neuroimaging with MRI than CT because of the following advantages: (1) better visualization of small strokes, particularly in the posterior fossa, (2) ability to predict low-flow regions based on flow-void images in large cerebral arteries and veins, (3) ability to visualize arterial dissection on cross-sectional images, and (4) the possibility of performing magnetic resonance arteriography (MRA), magnetic resonance venography (MRV), or diffusion-weighted MRI during the same session using little addition time (see Chap. 35).

Vascular Evaluation

Background Vascular evaluation of stroke is usually completed during the subacute period. This includes evaluation of the relevant cerebral vessels for the presence of stenosis, quantification of stenosis, and determination of the cause of stenosis. Multiple noninvasive and invasive tests are available for vascular evaluation. They confirm each other as well as offer additional information. Optimal treatment often depends on the vascular findings.

Evidence   For discussion of vascular ultrasonography, CT angiography, MRA, and catheter arteriography in cerebrovascular disease, see Chaps. 33 to 36.

Recommendations   For patients with carotid territory ischemia who are potential candidates for carotid endarterectomy, we recommend initial testing of the cervical carotid arteries with duplex ultrasound. It is essential that this test be performed by a properly trained and certified technologist and that the vascular laboratory be validated by comparing the ultrasound results to the gold standard catheter arteriography. When the carotid duplex is negative (normal or mild stenosis of the symptomatic artery, <50 percent), additional vascular testing is usually not necessary. When the carotid duplex shows moderate stenosis (50 to 79 percent) of the symptomatic artery, we recommend a catheter arteriogram to precisely measure the stenosis. When the carotid duplex shows severe stenosis (80 to 99 percent) of the symptomatic artery, we recommend MRA to confirm severe stenosis. If the MRA confirms severe stenosis, a catheter arteriogram does not seem necessary. Some experts argue that prior to carotid endarterectomy, all patients should have a catheter arteriogram to visualize the intracranial vessels in detail, which may provide useful information to the surgeon. MRA is able to provide this information, but in less detail than catheter arteriogram. This issue remains unresolved. When the carotid duplex shows occlusion, we recommend a catheter arteriogram to rule out a preocclusive lesion with very little blood flow, which may be treatable with endarterectomy. However, MRA seems to be sufficiently sensitive for this purpose. Whenever carotid duplex and MRA are conflicting, a catheter arteriogram is needed to clarify the situation.

The confirmation of carotid disease with catheter arteriography is helpful because (1) the decision to recommend carotid endarterectomy is usually based on finding (≥70 percent internal carotid artery stenosis, which usually cannot be confidently determined with duplex ultrasound or MRA, (2) ultrasound findings consistent with occlusion, which usually cannot be treated with endarterectomy, are sometimes associated with severe preocclusive stenosis, which can be treated with endarterectomy, (3) MRA often overestimates the degree of arterial stenosis, and (4) certain lesions, such as intraluminal thrombi, are better defined by catheter arteriography than by the noninvasive tests.

For patients with vertebrobasilar territory, ischemia vascular evaluation helps determine the mechanism of stroke, but may not be necessary. Surgical procedures, such as vertebral artery endarterectomy or anastomosis, have not been proven beneficial. Although not proven beneficial, symptomatic severe basilar artery stenosis is often treated with anticoagulation therapy because of the concern that a brainstem stroke with tragic consequences may develop in the near future.

In some patients, the clinical presentation and course, and the initial diagnostic studies, lead to a suspicion of an unusual condition, such as cerebral vasculitis or moyamoya disease. MRA can sometimes be used as a screening test, but for definitive diagnosis such patients should have a detailed vascular evaluation with a catheter arteriogram. Also, young stroke victims, without a good explanation for their stroke based on other tests, should have an arteriogram. A high quality MRA may be adequate for this purpose. If it is normal, we do not recommend a catheter arteriogram. If the MRA is abnormal and the abnormality is of uncertain nature and severity, we usually recommend a catheter arteriogram. Catheter arteriography is safer in younger patients than older patients.

Echocardiography

Background   Because emboli from the heart can travel to any cerebral artery, every ischemic stroke may be considered as possibly cardioembolic. However, certain clinical features have been associated with cardiac sources of emboli and are thus considered consistent with cardioembolic stroke. The features associated with a cardiac source of emboli can be divided into clinical features and neuroimaging findings. The clinical features linked to cardioembolic stroke are abrupt onset of symptoms, presence of systemic emboli, decreased consciousness, aphasia, visual field defect, and hemineglect.[115,116] On the other hand, patients with a lacunar stroke syndrome, such as pure motor hemiparesis for example, most likely have intrinsic small vessel disease as the cause of their stroke. These patients are less likely to have a serious source of cardiac emboli. The neuroimaging findings associated with probable cardioembolic stroke are large infarct and bilateral infarcts.[117]

Virtually any intracardiac abnormality carries a risk of thrombosis and embolism, but the risk varies greatly depending on the specific abnormality. Table 3-2 lists the abnormalities considered to be serious sources of emboli. With the introduction of transesophageal echocardiography (TEE), various intracardiac lesions are being identified more frequently than with transthoracic echocardiography (TTE), but the clinical significance of many of the mild abnormalities remains to be determined.

In addition, the finding of other abnormalities that could account for the stroke, such as severe carotid artery disease, increases the challenge of patient management. Usually, there is no definitive way to determine which mechanism was responsible for a given stroke, and the best approach seems to be to treat all relevant abnormalities.

Evidence   In an analysis of the NINDS Stroke Data Bank,[115] there were 1290 patients, divided into high ($n = 250$), medium ($n = 167$), and low ($n = 873$) risk of cardiac embolic findings based on echocardiograms. Increasing risk of cardioembolic stroke was significantly associated with abrupt onset of stroke symptoms, decreased consciousness at onset of symptoms, and evidence of systemic embolism. Abrupt onset of symptoms occurred in 47 percent of patients in the high-risk group, 39 percent in the medium-risk group, and 38 percent in the low-risk group ($p = .008$). Decreased consciousness was present in 29 percent of patients in the high-risk group, 18 percent in the medium-risk group, and 11 percent in the low-risk group ($p < .001$). Evidence of systemic embolism was present in 5 percent of patients in the high-risk group, 2 percent in the medium-risk group, and 2 percent in the low-risk group ($p = .005$).

In another analysis of the NINDS Stroke Data Bank,[116] increasing risk of cardioembolic stroke was significantly associated with decreased consciousness on examination, aphasia, visual field defect, and hemineglect. Decreased consciousness was found in 36 percent of patients in the high-risk group, 23 percent in the medium-risk group, and 17 percent in the low-risk group ($p < .001$). Aphasia was found in 33 percent of patients in the high-risk group, and 23 percent in the medium-risk group, and 23 percent in the low-risk group ($p = .006$). Visual field defect was found in 30 percent of patients in the high-risk group, 28 percent in the medium-risk group, and 15 percent in the low-risk group ($p < .001$). Hemineglect was found in 21 percent of

patients in the high-risk group, 14 percent in the medium-risk group, and 9 percent in the low-risk group ($p < .001$). On the other hand, patients with pure motor hemiparesis or sensorimotor lacunar strokes had significantly less serious sources of cardiac emboli than patients with other stroke types. Pure motor hemiparesis was found in 13 percent of patients in the high-risk group, 21 percent in the medium-risk group, and 30 percent in the low-risk group ($p < .001$). Sensorimotor lacunar syndrome was found in 8 percent of patients in the high-risk group, 13 percent in the medium-risk group, and 14 percent in the low-risk group ($p = .017$).

In further analysis of the NINDS Stroke Data Bank,[117] 1267 patients who had cerebral CT were divided into high ($n = 244$), medium ($n = 165$), and low ($n = 858$) risk of cardiac embolic findings based on echocardiograms. Increasing risk of cardioembolic stroke was significantly associated with a large infarct (one-half a lobe or greater) and mass effect on the initial CT. Prevalence of large infarcts was 28 percent in the high-risk group, 16 percent in the medium group, and 13 percent in the low-risk group ($p < .001$). Prevalence of mass effect was 9 percent in the high-risk group, 5 percent in the medium-risk group, and 3 percent in the low-risk group ($p < .001$). In addition, based on the last CT done during hospitalization, increasing risk of cardioembolic stroke was significantly associated with bilateral infarcts. Prevalence of bilateral carotid territory infarcts was 9 percent in the high-risk group, and 4 percent in the medium- and low-risk groups ($p = .003$).

Although some experts suggest that the prevalence of hemorrhagic conversion of an infarct is more likely in cardioembolic stroke, the large and prospective NINDS Stroke Data Bank does not fully support this suspicion. The prevalence of hemorrhagic conversion of an infarct as detected on repeat CT was 6 percent in the high cardioembolic risk group, 1 percent in the medium-risk group, and 3 percent in the low-risk group ($p = .09$).

Recommendations   For patients who present with a lacunar stroke (subcortical or brainstem infarct ≤2.0 cm in diameter) and have no evidence of heart disease on examination, ECG, or chest x-ray, an echocardiogram does not seem necessary. We recommend TTE as a screening test for two categories of stroke patients: (1) those with a lacunar stroke and evidence of heart disease and (2) those with a nonlacunar stroke and a probable etiology for the stroke found prior to an echocardiogram. If a TTE shows a possible source of emboli, TEE is often needed to define the abnormality in more detail.

We recommend TEE for all nonlacunar stroke patients with no probable etiology found prior to an echocardiogram. When our suspicion that a given stroke is cardioembolic is high, based on the clinical and neuroimaging features described above, we recommend TEE with contrast to look for a right-to-left intracardiac shunt. For additional discussion on TEE, see Chap. 37. A right-to-left intracardiac shunt can also be detected with a transcranial Doppler after intravenous saline contrast injection by identifying the saline bubbles in a cerebral artery Doppler signal.

Other Tests

Background When the standard tests discussed above do not indicate a probable cause of the stroke, additional tests are often recommended to achieve this goal. These tests are tailored to the individual patient depending mainly on the medical history and the age of the patient. In addition, some tests, such as diffusion-weighted MRI, are currently being evaluated for their ability to contribute further information, which might improve patient management.

Evidence For discussion of hypercoagulable conditions and the appropriate tests, see Chap. 15. For discussion of cerebral perfusion studies using CT and MRI, see Chaps. 34 and 35.

Recommendations We routinely recommend complete blood count (CBC) including platelets, partial thromboplastin time (PTT), prothrombin time, blood glucose, and electrolytes. Severe thrombocytosis may be uncovered by the CBC and be responsible for the stroke, or a prolonged PTT may indicate the presence of an antiphospholipid antibody. Occasionally, a metabolic derangement is responsible for neurologic deficits. We recommend special blood tests for hypercoagulability in selected stroke patients. These are unusually young stroke patients (<55 years old) without another clear cause for their stroke identified after the preliminary workup as described above.

We also recommend urine testing for illicit drug use in all young patients with stroke. Some stroke patients may be unaware that they were given a dangerous drug to consume at a party, for example. Sympathomimetic drugs, such as cocaine or amphetamines, have been linked to stroke through vasoconstriction and acute arterial hypertension. Intravenous drug abuse may cause a stroke through endocarditis and paradoxical embolism of foreign material, such as talc.

We recommend lumbar puncture (LP) as part of a stroke workup for patients with suspected vasculitis. If the vasculitis is infectious, such as that associated with fungal meningitis or neurosyphilis, the LP may be diagnostic. Unfortunately, the LP is often nonspecific, and additional testing is needed. It is important to remember that a normal cerebrospinal fluid does not rule out cerebral vasculitis.

There are currently several tests of cerebral perfusion that could be done during the subacute stroke period, such as single photon emission computed tomography (SPECT), stable xenon CT, perfusion-weighted MRI, and positron emission tomography (PET). PET is least practical and most expensive. Stable xenon CT is quantitative and combined with the existing standard CT imaging. Initial clinical studies suggest that stable xenon CT may be useful by predicting the extent of irreversible and reversible cerebral tissue within an ischemic region. However, further studies of perfusion during acute and subacute ischemic stroke are needed to establish a clear clinical application for these tests. Perfusion studies are presently not considered essential for the optimal management of acute or subacute stroke patients.

We occasionally recommend superficial brain and meningeal biopsy to confirm the diagnosis of primary cerebral vasculitis and to rule out other conditions, such as intravascular carcinomatosis or infectious vasculitis. These patients usually have recurrent ischemic strokes within a short period of time and no definite cause based on other tests. Definitive diagnosis is important before recommending specific therapy, because different therapies are indicated for the different diagnoses, and there are side effects from each therapy.

REHABILITATION

When a stroke patient is medically and neurologically stable, it is appropriate to begin rehabilitation. Basic principals of rehabilitation including proper positioning, range of motion, and education can start immediately. The role of rehabilitation is to reduce chronic disability and prevent stroke-related complications to improve functional outcome. Rehabilitation aims to exert a direct effect on neurologic recovery and to teach compensation strategies and the use of assistive devices. An interdisciplinary approach to the management of functional deficits after stroke, where each health provider works together toward commonly understood goals, is ideal. Although team members focus on their area of expertise, they also incorporate the treatment plans and philosophies of other rehabilitation team members (Table 3-5).

Physical Therapy

Background   Physical therapy (PT) during the first 72 h involves initiation of treatment to correct abnormal muscle tone (usually flaccid) and to promote active movement through sensorimotor re-education. Such therapies include stretching, neuromuscular facilitation, and both passive and active assisted range of motion exercises.

Evidence   Although general consensus favors early rehabilitation interventions, there has been little research on the impact of physical therapy in the first 72 h on outcome. A retrospective study comparing similar groups of stroke patients treated with standard PT within 72 h vs. those treated after the first 4 days showed that early PT may shorten acute hospitalization (24 vs. 39 days) and improve ambulation and self-care skills ($p < .05$).[118] The early therapy group was more likely

to be discharged home than the delayed therapy group (33 percent vs. 13 percent). In another randomized study of 63 subacute stroke patients, early mobilization reduced the occurrence of orthostatic hypotension.[119] The optimal type of PT during subacute stroke remains to be proven.

Recommendations   We recommend consulting PT to evaluate and treat any stroke patient who is medically stable and suffers residual weakness, abnormal muscle tone, or loss of balance. Those whose functional decline preceded their stroke may also benefit from a conditioning program to regain endurance and tolerance to activity. For patients with minor residual deficits who return home alone at discharge, PT evaluation for possible home safety concerns and equipment needs is recommended.

Occupational Therapy

Background   The methods of treatment used by occupational therapists are similar to those described previously for physical therapists. Occupational therapy

Table 3-5.
Rehabilitation services for stroke patients

Physical therapy	Occupational therapy
Positioning	Positioning
Range of motion exercises	Visual perceptual skills
Mobilization	Activities of daily living
Strength and endurance exercises	Equipment
Gait training	Upper extremity splinting
Equipment	Psychological and social support
Lower extremity splinting	General psychological support
Speech and language pathology	Patient and family education
Speech evaluation	Neuropsychological testing
Swallowing evaluation	Community resources
Nutritional support	Discharge planning
Nursing	Physiatrist
Positioning	Nutrition/hydration
Skin checks	Sleep assessment
Neurologic checks	Medication assessment
Breathing/coughing exercises	DVT[a] prophylaxis
Safety evaluation	Bladder and bowel programs
Bladder and bowel programs	Patient and family education
Patient and family education	Social support
Patient and family goals	Patient and family goals
	Supervision of rehabilitation

[a]DVT, deep vein thrombosis.

(OT), however, focuses on activities of daily living, such as feeding, grooming, dressing, and toileting. OT teaches the use of assistive devices and compensation strategies to promote better use, primarily of the upper extremities. OT is also involved in treating acquired visual-spatial deficits that limit self-care skills. Such problems as ocular dysmotility, visual field deficit, and hemineglect syndrome can be quantified and early retraining or compensation strategies developed. In addition, shoulder pain is an important complication of upper extremity paralysis after stroke.[120] It has been reported in 70 to 84 percent of patients with a paralyzed upper extremity.

Evidence   No study has investigated the impact of starting OT within 72 h of stroke onset compared with starting it later.

Recommendations   Despite the lack of evidence, we see no reason to delay starting OT beyond the first 72 h of stroke onset, if the patient is medically ready for OT. It is the strong consensus of the Agency for Healthcare Policy and Research that patients with functional deficits and some voluntary movement be encouraged to use the affected limb and to perform functional tasks directed at improving strength, motor control, relearning sensorimotor relationships, and improving functional performance.[121] Although rarely needed within the first 72 h, OT usually customizes and acquires a wheelchair and a seating system.

We recommend that patients with a flaccid upper extremity, predisposed to inferior subluxation at the glenohumeral joint and possible painful shoulder syndrome, be evaluated by OT to set guidelines for shoulder support during transfers and ambulation. Preventative measures include supporting the shoulder in a position that maintains normal scapulohumeral orientation. Range of motion exercises should not carry the shoulder beyond 90 degrees of flexion or abduction unless there is upward rotation of the scapula and external rotation of the humeral head.

Speech and Language Therapy

Background   A speech and language pathologist's role in the first 72 h after stroke is mainly to identify and classify aphasia and dysphagia. Patients with different types of aphasia have different communication problems and need different therapies and communication

strategies. Identification, classification, and quantification of dysphagia is important to implement optimal strategies for aspiration prophylaxis and nutrition (see "Dysphagia").

Evidence   No study has investigated the impact of starting speech therapy within 72 h of stroke onset compared with starting it later.

Recommendations   Despite the lack of evidence, we see no reason to delay starting speech and language evaluation and therapy beyond the first 72 h of stroke onset, if the patient is medically ready for therapy. We recommend evaluation by a speech and language pathologist to (1) classify a patient's aphasia and start therapy to help the patient, the family, and the hospital staff to communicate better and (2) identify, classify, and help manage dysphagia. Depending on the type of dysphagia, different swallowing techniques can be taught to decrease the likelihood of aspiration. Depending mainly on the severity of dysphagia, foods with different consistency (degree to which food remains as a bolus in the mouth) are recommended to decrease the likelihood of aspiration, keeping in mind the need for adequate nutrition (see "Dysphagia").

Psychological and Social Support

Background   Strokes often lead to sudden and dramatic changes in function and social roles. A psychologist can be helpful in assessing the impact of these changes on patients and their families. By providing needed support and education, the psychologist can facilitate appropriate decision making and coping mechanisms. Identification of present and possible future problems is likely to result in earlier intervention. Anxiety and depression can be reduced with psychological support. Because depression is felt to be a determining factor in functional outcome after stroke, counseling could possibly lead to better long-term quality of life. Similarly, a licensed social worker is responsible for evaluating family and community resources, securing needed community services, and facilitating discharge planning. Social workers can also provide counseling and education where appropriate.

Evidence   No study has investigated the impact of starting psychological and social services within 72 h of stroke onset compared with starting them later.

Recommendations   Despite the lack of evidence, we see no reason to delay starting psychological and social services beyond the first 72 h of stroke onset. It is the strong consensus of the Agency for Healthcare Policy and Research that discharge planning begin at the time of admission and that patients and families be thoroughly instructed on the effects and prognosis of the stroke, potential complications, and needs and rationales for treatment.[121]

Nursing Care

Background   Along with the usual nursing interventions during the subacute stroke period, nurses can help implement rehabilitation plans and treatments. Some of the important patient care issues involving considerable nursing input include decubitus ulcers, incontinence, and falls. Decubitus ulcers result from compromise of circulation to the skin as a consequence of prolonged compression of a specific region, such as the heal or hip. Decubitus ulcers have been documented in 14.5 percent of stroke patients and are associated with coma, paralysis, spasticity, obesity, and incontinence.[122]

Bowel incontinence has been documented in 40 percent of stroke patients on admission and 9 percent at 6 months.[113] Falls are the most common cause of injury in hospitalized stroke patients and are associated with sensorimotor deficits, confusion, visual-perceptual impairment, and aphasia.

Evidence   There are no studies comparing different nursing care protocols within 72 h of stroke onset.

Recommendations   Nursing care orders for stroke patients should include consideration of each organ system and should be aimed at reducing comorbidities and improving outcomes. Examples include proper positioning, periodic repositioning, skin checks, neurologic checks, and deep breathing and coughing exercises to reduce pulmonary complications. Constant pressure applied to the skin, as little as 70 mmHg, for 2 h or more has been shown to produce irreversible tissue damage. Therefore, patients with decreased mobility should be placed in positions that minimize skin pressure and should be repositioned periodically. Proper positioning in bed includes anatomic alignment of the head, trunk, and extremities to prevent pathologic reflexes and contractures. Also, heels should be elevated and hips slightly flexed to reduce heel and sacral pressure. While sitting, the hips, knees, and elbows should be supported at a 90-degree angle, and a molded head rest can be used to prevent head turning in patients with hemineglect or gaze preference. Patients with sensory, motor, or cognitive limitations may not be able to shift weight to redistribute pressure and prevent skin breakdown. Repositioning is recommended at least every 2 h.

Minimum neurologic check should include level of alertness (alert, drowsy, stuporous, or comatose), pupillary size and reaction, and a simple test of the affected function tailored to each patient. The frequency of neurologic checks should be tailored to the severity of the stroke. For severe strokes, during the first 72 h we recommend neurologic checks every 2 h. For moderately severe strokes, a lower frequency of neurologic checks is appropriate.

Clearance of pulmonary secretions is essential to reduce the work of breathing and to limit infections and atelectasis. For patients with a decreased cough reflex or hypoventilation, techniques for clearing secretions include postural drainage, chest percussion and vibration, incentive spirometry, and controlled coughing with compression of the abdomen. These techniques can be applied by a nurse with assistance from a respiratory therapist.

The Foley catheter should be removed as soon as possible and a bladder program with frequent scheduled voiding and measurement of postvoid residuals begun. Incontinence can be caused by decreased alertness, decreased sensation of bladder fullness, physical inability to get to a toilet or use a urinal, or lack of voluntary inhibition of the micturition reflex due to the stroke. Scheduled toileting every 2 to 4 h reduces urgency and heightens awareness of the need to void. Checking postvoid residuals helps distinguish between an uninhibited and a hypotonic bladder. We recommend catheterization if a patient is unable to void within 8 to 10 h, bladder volume is >300 mL, or postvoid residuals are >150 mL. Constipation is not uncommon after stroke and can be prevented with early mobilization, monitoring intake and output, and use of bowel medications as needed.

The nurse should assess the patient's safety needs and institute fall protocols when indicated (Table 3-6). A physician should be notified when a patient's safety is compromised. Finally, nurses should be directed to begin patient and family education early after stroke to reduce the fear and anxiety that often accompany such a significant change in health.

Table 3-6.
Suggested fall precautions during subacute stroke

Bed rails up at all times

Bed at lowest reasonable height when unattended

Patient room as close to nurses station as reasonably possible

Nonslip footwear worn when out of bed

Assist or observe patient when out of bed as much as reasonably possible and notify physician of any hazard

Physiatrist Role

Background   Physiatrists are physicians trained in Physical Medicine and Rehabilitation. This specialty includes the diagnosis, treatment, and rehabilitation for patients with various neurologic and musculoskeletal impairments. In addition to standard medical treatments, physiatry employs physical agents, assistive devices, and therapeutic exercises.

Evidence   There are no studies on the impact of physiatrists' contribution to coordinated patient care within 72 h of stroke onset.

Recommendations   Consultation with a physiatrist is appropriate for all stroke patients with a residual deficit. A physiatrist can help by: (1) suggesting means to lower the likelihood of complications related to stroke, (2) supervising rehabilitation by different types of therapists, which should coincide with the patient's and family's needs, (3) participating in patient and family education about stroke, and (4) suggesting an optimal discharge plan and subsequent rehabilitation setting (see "Rehabilitation Programs"). The optimal type of rehabilitation setting is largely dependent on the extent of brain injury.

Rehabilitation Programs

Comprehensive Inpatient Rehabilitation Units   Such units may be directly connected to an acute care hospital or free-standing. They generally provide an interdisciplinary approach, including PT, OT, speech and language therapy, recreational therapy, social work assistance, and psychological evaluation. Patients in such facilities are usually more medically complex and need 3 to 4 h of multiple types of physical therapy daily.

Discharge goals are usually to home, either alone or with assistance.

Subacute Rehabilitation Units   In recent years, there has been an emergence of less intense rehabilitation units that are classified as Skilled Nursing Facilities. These are subacute rehabilitation units that are usually connected to an acute care hospital or an extended care facility. They, too, provide multiple types of rehabilitation therapies but for less than 3 h per day. Patients need less intensive rehabilitation to reach their disposition goals or are so impaired that they cannot tolerate a more rigorous rehabilitation program.

Day Rehabilitation Programs   Many stroke victims continue to benefit from a comprehensive rehabilitation program after they have been discharged home. These programs provide similar levels of rehabilitation to that in inpatient rehabilitation units but allow the patient to live at home. Most day rehabilitation programs set goals of more independent living. Many such programs provide transportation to and from the rehabilitation center.

Outpatient Rehabilitation Therapy.   Individual therapy services can be obtained through hospitals or independent therapy facilities. The experience among therapists in treating neurologically impaired patients may be limited compared with the above-mentioned rehabilitation units. Patients may visit multiple types of therapists two to three times per week, but the efforts of the therapists are not as well coordinated as in a rehabilitation unit. Transportation to and from therapy is usually not provided.

Home Health Rehabilitation Therapy   When a patient's community access is limited for medical or functional reasons, in-home rehabilitation therapies can be arranged. This allows the therapist to adapt the treatment plan to the patient's environment and make recommendations to increase safety, such as build a ramp, remove area carpets, or widen bathroom doors. The down side of in-home rehabilitation therapy is that most therapy equipment is not transportable to the homes.

REFERENCES

1. Brandt T, von Kummer R, Müller-Küppers M, Hacke W: Thrombolytic therapy of acute basilar artery occlusion:

Variables affecting recanalization and outcome. *Neurology* 27:875, 1996.

2. Strand T, Asplund K, Eriksson S, et al: A non-intensive stroke unit reduces functional disability and the need for long-term hospitalization. *Stroke* 16:29, 1985.

3. Indredavik B, Bakke F, Solberg R, et al: Benefit of a stroke unit: A randomized controlled trial. *Stroke* 22:1026, 1991.

4. Jorgensen HS, Nakayama H, Raaschou HO, et al: The effect of a stroke unit: Reductions in mortality, discharge rate to nursing home, length of hospital stay, and cost. A community-based study. *Stroke* 26:1178, 1995.

5. Marsh EE III, Adams HP Jr, Biller J, et al: Use of antithrombotic drugs in the treatment of acute ischemic stroke: A survey of neurologists in practice in the United States. *Neurology* 39:1631, 1989.

6. The National Institute of Neurological Disorders and Stroke rt-PA Stroke Study Group: Tissue plasminogen activator for acute ischemic stroke. *N Engl J Med* 333: 1581, 1995.

7. Duke RJ, Bloch RF, Turpie AG, Trebilcock R, Bayer N: Intravenous heparin for the prevention of stroke progression in acute partial stable stroke. *Ann Intern Med* 105:825, 1986.

8. Cerebral Embolism Study Group: Immediate anticoagulation of embolic stroke: A randomized trial. *Stroke* 14:668, 1983.

9. Kay R, Wong KS, Yu YL, et al: Low-molecular-weight heparin for the treatment of acute ischemic stroke. *N Engl J Med* 333:1588, 1995.

10. The Publications Committee for the Trial of ORG 10172 in Acute Stroke Treatment (TOAST) Investigators: Low molecular weight heparinoid, ORG 10172 (danaparoid), and outcome after acute ischemic stroke. *JAMA* 279: 1265, 1998.

11. Scandinavian Stroke Study Group: Multicenter trial of hemodilution in acute ischemic stroke: I. Results in the total patient population. *Stroke* 18:691, 1987.

12. The Hemodilution in Stroke Study Group: Hypervolemic hemodilution treatment of acute stroke: Results of a randomized multicenter trial using pentastarch. *Stroke* 20: 317, 1989.

13. Aichner FT, Fazekas F, Brainin M, et al: Hypervolemic hemodilution in acute ischemic stroke: The Multicenter Austrian Hemodilution Stroke Trial (MAHST). *Stroke* 29:743, 1998.

14. Gelmers HJ, Gorter K, de Weerdt CJ, Wiezer HJ: A controlled trial of nimodipine in acute ischemic stroke. *N Engl J Med* 318:203, 1988.

15. Trust Study Group: Randomised, double-blind, placebo-controlled trial of nimodipine in acute stroke. *Lancet* 336:1205, 1990.

16. The American Nimodopine Study Group: Clinical trial of nimodipine in acute ischemic stroke. *Stroke* 23:3, 1992.

17. Wahlgren N, MacMahon D, De Keyser J, Indredavik B, Ryman T, for the INWEST Study Group: Intravenous Nimodipine West European Stroke Trial (INWEST) of nimodipine in the treatment of acute ischaemic stroke. *Cerebrovasc Dis* 4:204, 1994.

18. International Stroke Trial Collaborative Group: The international stroke trial (IST): A randomized trial of aspirin, subcutaneous heparin, both, or neither among 19,435 patients with acute ischaemic stroke. *Lancet* 349:1569, 1997.

19. CAST (Chinese Acute Stroke Trial) Collaborative Group: CAST: Randomized placebo-controlled trial of early aspirin use in 20,000 patients with acute ischaemic stroke. *Lancet* 349:1641, 1997.

20. Horner J, Buoyer FG, Alberts MJ, Helms MJ: Dysphagia following brain-stem stroke: Clinical correlates and outcome. *Arch Neurol* 48:1170, 1991.

21. Smithard DG, O'Neill PA, England RE, et al: The natural history of dysphagia following a stroke. *Dysphagia* 12:188, 1997.

22. Yilmaz EY, Gupta SR, Mlcoch AG, Moritz T: Aspiration following stroke. *J Neuro Rehab* 12:61, 1998.

23. Smithard DG, O'Neill PA, Parks C, Morris J: Complications and outcome after acute stroke: Does dysphagia matter? *Stroke* 27:1200, 1996. Erratum. 29:1480, 1998.

24. Hamdy S, Aziz Q, Rothwell JC, et al: The cortical topography of human swallowing musculature in health and disease. *Nat Med* 2:1217, 1996.

25. Hamdy S, Aziz Q, Rothwell JC, et al: Explaining oropharyngeal dysphagia after unilateral hemispheric stroke. *Lancet* 350:686, 1997.

26. Robbins J, Levine RL, Maser A, Rosenbek JC, Kempster GB: Swallowing after unilateral stroke of the cerebral cortex. *Arch Phys Med Rehabil* 74:1295, 1993.

27. Horner J, Massey EW: Silent aspiration following stroke. *Neurology* 38:317, 1988.

28. Horner J, Massey EW, Riski JE, Lathrop DL, Chase KN: Aspiration following stroke: clinical correlates and outcome. *Neurology* 38:1359, 1988.

29. Daniels SK, Foundas AL: The role of the insular cortex in dysphagia. *Dysphagia* 12:146, 1997.

30. Nilsson H, Ekberg O, Olsson R, Hindfelt B: Dysphagia in stroke: A prospective study of quantitative aspects of swallowing in dysphagic patients. *Dysphagia* 13:32, 1998.

31. Daniels SK, Brailey K, Priestly DH, et al: Aspiration in patients with acute stroke. *Arch Phys Med Rehabil* 79:14, 1998.

32. Davies AE, Kidd D, Stone SP, MacMahon J: Pharyngeal sensation and gag reflex in healthy subjects. *Lancet* 345:487, 1995.

33. DePippo KL, Holas MA, Reding MJ: Validation of the 3-oz water swallow test for aspiration following stroke. *Arch Neurol* 49:1259, 1992.

34. DePippo KL, Holas MA, Reding MJ: The Burke dysphagia screening test: Validation of its use in patients with stroke. *Arch Phys Med Rehabil* 75:1284, 1994.

35. Gupta SR, Yilmaz EY, Micoch AM, Day J, Belanger L: Poststroke dysphagia: Identification of high-risk patients. *Ann Neurol* 44:519, 1998.

36. Horner J, Massey EW, Brazer SR: Aspiration in bilateral stroke patients. *Neurology* 40:1686, 1990.

37. Martin AW: Dietary management of swallowing disorders. *Dysphagia* 6:129, 1991.

38. DePippo KL, Holas MA, Reding MJ, Mandel FS, Lesser ML: Dysphagia therapy following stroke: A controlled trial. *Neurology* 44:1655, 1994.

39. Yarnell P, Earnest M, Kelly G, Sanders B: Disappearing carotid defects. *Stroke* 9:258, 1978.

40. Donnan G, Blandin P: The stroke syndrome of long intraluminal clot with incomplete vessel obstruction. *Clin Exp Neurol* 16:41, 1979.

41. Caplan L, Stein R, Patel D, et al: Intraluminal clot of the carotid artery detected radiographically. *Neurology* 34:1175, 1984.

42. Biller J, Adams HP, Jr, Boarini D, et al: Intraluminal clot of the carotid artery: A clinical angiographic correlation of nine patients and literature review. *Surg Neurol* 25:467, 1986.

43. Buchan A, Gates P, Pelz D, Barnett HT: Intraluminal thrombus in the cerebral circulation: Implications for surgical management. *Stroke* 19:681, 1988.

44. Levine SR, Quint DJ, Pessin MS, Boulos RS, Welch KMA: Intraluminal clot in the vertebrobasilar circulation: Clinical and radiologic features. *Neurology* 39:515, 1989.

45. The TIMI Study Group: The Thrombolysis in Myocardial Infarction (TIMI) trial: Phase I findings. *N Engl J Med* 312:932, 1985.

46. Ringelstein EE, Berg-Dammer E, Zeumer H: The so-called atheromatous pseudoocclusion of the internal carotid artery. *Neuroradiology* 25:147, 1983.

47. O'Leary DH, Mattle H, Potter JE: Atheromatous pseudoocclusion of the internal carotid artery. *Stroke* 20:1168, 1989.

48. Weitz JI: Low-molecular-weight heparins *N Engl J Med* 337:688, 1997. Erratum. 337:1567, 1997.

49. Hirsh J: Oral anticoagulant drugs. *N Engl J Med* 324:1865, 1991.

50. Cerebral Embolism Study Group: Cardioembolic stroke, early anticoagulation, and brain hemorrhage. *Arch Intern Med* 147:636, 1987.

51. Camerlingo M, Cast L, Censori B, et al: Immediate anticoagulation with heparin for first-ever ischemic stroke in the carotid artery territories observed within 5 hours of onset. *Arch Neurol* 51:462, 1994.

52. Harrison L, Johnston M, Massicotte MP, et al: Comparison of 5-mg and 10-mg loading doses in initiation of warfarin therapy. *Ann Intern Med* 126:133, 1997.

53. Dedden P, Chang B, Nagel D: Pharmacy-managed program for home treatment of deep vein thrombosis with enoxaparin. *Am J Health Syst Pharm* 54:1968, 1997.

54. Toni D, Fiorelli M, Gentile M, et al: Progressing neurological deficit secondary to acute ischemic stroke. *Arch Neurol* 52:670, 1995.

55. Fisher M, Garcia JH: Evolving stroke and the ischemic penumbra. *Neurology* 47:884, 1996.

56. Adams HP Jr, Brott TG, Furlan AJ, et al: Guidelines for thrombolytic therapy for acute stroke: A supplement to the guidelines for the management of patients with acute ischemic stroke. *Stroke* 27:1711, 1996.

57. Prasad K, Browman G, Srivastava A, Menon G: Surgery in primary supratentorial intracerebral hematoma: A meta-analysis of randomized trials. *Acta Neurol Scand* 95:103, 1997.

58. Zieger A, Vonofakos D, Steudel WI, Dusterbehn G: Non-traumatic intracerebellar hematomas: Prognostic value of volumetric evaluation by computed tomography. *Surg Neurol* 22:491, 1984.

59. Taneda M, Hayakawa T, Mogami H: Primary cerebellar hemorrhage: Quadrigeminal cistern obliteration on CT scans as a predictor of outcome. *J Neurosurg* 67:545, 1987.

60. Oppenheimer S, Hachinski V: Complications of acute stroke. *Lancet* 339:721, 1992.

61. Kilpatrick CJ, Davis SM, Tress BM, et al: Epileptic seizures in acute stroke. *Arch Neurol* 47:157, 1990.

62. Giroud M, Gras P, Fayolle H, et al: Early seizures after acute stroke: A study of 1,640 cases. *Epilepsia* 35:959, 1994.

63. So EL, Annegers JF, Hauser WA, O'Brien PC, Whisnant JP: Population-based study of seizure disorders after cerebral infarction. *Neurology* 46:350, 1996.

64. Arboix A, Comes E, Massons J, García L, Oliveres M: Relevance of early seizures for in-hospital mortality in acute cerebrovascular disease. *Neurology* 47:1429, 1996.

65. Strandgaard S, Paulson OB: Cerebral autoregulation. *Stroke* 15:413, 1984.

66. Wallace JD, Levy LL: Blood pressure after stroke. *JAMA* 246:2177, 1981.

67. Britton M, Carlsson A, De Faire U: Blood pressure course in patients with acute stroke and matched controls. *Stroke* 17:861, 1986.

68. Powers WJ: Acute hypertension after stroke: The scientific basis for treatment decisions. *Neurology* 43:461, 1993.

69. Waltz AG: Effect of blood pressure on blood flow in ischemic and nonischemic cerebral cortex. *Neurology* 18:613, 1968.

70. Graham DI: Ischaemic brain damage of cerebral perfusion failure type after treatment of severe hypertension. *Br Med J* 4:739, 1975.

71. Lavin P: Management of hypertension in patients with acute stroke. *Arch Intern Med* 146:66, 1986.

72. Jorgensen HS, Nakayama H, Raaschou HO, Olsen TS: Effect of blood pressure and diabetes on stroke in progression. *Lancet* 344:156, 1994.

73. Lisk DR, Grotta JC, Lamki LM, et al: Should hypertension be treated after acute stroke? A randomized controlled trial using single photon emission computed tomography. *Arch Neurol* 50:855, 1993.

74. Chamorro A, Vila N, Ascaso C, et al: Blood pressure and functional recovery in acute ischemic stroke. *Stroke* 29:1850, 1998.

75. Johnston KC, Li JY, Lyden PD, et al: Medical and neuro-

logical complications of ischemic stroke: Experience from the RANTTAS trial. *Stroke* 29:447, 1998.

76. Davenport RJ, Dennis MS, Wellwood I, Warlow CP: Complications after acute stroke. *Stroke* 27:415, 1996.

77. Ginsberg MD, Busto R: Combating hyperthermia in acute stroke: A significant clinical concern. *Stroke* 29:529, 1998.

78. Azzimondi G, Bassein L, Nonino F, et al: Fever in acute stroke worsens prognosis: A prospective study. *Stroke* 26:2040, 1995.

79. Reith J, Jorgensen HS, Pedersen PM, et al: Body temperature in acute stroke: Relation to stroke severity, infarct size, mortality, and outcome. *Lancet* 347:422, 1996.

80. Castillo J, Davalos A, Marrugat J, Noya M: Timing for fever-related brain damage in acute ischemic stroke. *Stroke* 29:2455, 1998.

81. Sacco RL, Foulkes MA, Mohr JP, et al: Determinants of early recurrence of cerebral infarction: The Stroke Data Bank. *Stroke* 20:983, 1989.

82. Brust JC. Agitation and delirium, in Bogousslavsky J, Caplan L, (eds.): *Stroke Syndromes.* New York, Cambridge University Press, 1995; p 134–9.

83. Goldstein LB: Basic and clinical studies of pharmacologic effects on recovery from brain injury. *J Neur Transplant Plast* 4:175, 1993.

84. Goldstein LB, Matchar DB, Morgenlander JC, Davis JN: Influence of drugs on the recovery of sensorimotor function after stroke. *J Neuro Rehab* 4:137, 1990.

85. Haley EC, Jr, Kassell NF, Torner JC: Failure of heparin to prevent progression in progressing ischemic infarction. *Stroke* 19:10, 1988.

86. Slivka A, Levy D: Natural history of progressive ischemic stroke in a population treated with heparin. *Stroke* 21:1657, 1990.

87. Warlow C, Ogston D, Douglas AS: Deep venous thrombosis of the legs after strokes: Part I. Incidence and predisposing factors. Part II. Natural history. *Br Med J* 1:1178, 1976.

88. Brandstater ME, Roth EJ, Siebens HC: Venous thromboembolism in stroke: Literature review and implications for clinical practice. *Arch Phys Med Rehabil* 73:S-379, 1992.

89. Verstraete M: The diagnosis and treatment of deep-vein thrombosis. *N Engl J Med* 329:1418, 1993.

90. Kamran SI, Downey D, Ruff RL: Pneumatic sequential compression reduces the risk of deep vein thrombosis in stroke patients. *Neurology* 50:1683, 1998.

91. Feinberg WM, Bruck DC, Jeter MA, Corrigan JJ Jr: Fibrinolysis after acute ischemic stroke. *Thromb Res* 64:117, 1991.

92. McCarthy ST, Turner JJ, Robertson D, Hawkey CJ: Low-dose heparin as a prophylaxis against deep-vein thrombosis after acute stroke. *Lancet* ii:800, 1977.

93. Turpie AGG, Gallus AS, Beattie WS, Hirsh J: Prevention of venous thrombosis in patients with intracranial disease by intermittent pneumatic compression of the calf. *Neurology* 27:435, 1977.

94. Gelmers HJ: Effects of low-dose subcutaneous heparin on the occurrence of deep vein thrombosis in patients with ischemic stroke. *Acta Neurol Scandinav* 61:313, 1980.

95. McCarthy ST, Turner J: Low-dose subcutaneous heparin in the prevention of deep-vein thrombosis and pulmonary emboli following acute stroke. *Age Ageing* 15:84, 1986.

96. Turpie AGG, Levine MN, Hirsh J, et al: Double-blind randomised trial of ORG 10172 low-molecular-weight heparinoid in prevention of deep-vein thrombosis in thrombotic stroke. *Lancet* i:523, 1987.

97. Prins MH, Gelsema R, Sing AK, van Heerde LR, den Ottolander GJH: Prophylaxis of deep venous thrombosis with a low-molecular-weight heparin (Kabi 2165/Fragmin®) in stroke patients. *Haemostasis* 19:245, 1989.

98. Sandset PM, Dahl T, Stiris M, et al: A double-blind and randomized placebo-controlled trial of low molecular weight heparin once daily to prevent deep-vein thrombosis in acute ischemic stroke. *Sem Thromb Hemost* 16:25, 1990.

99. Turpie AGG, Gent M, Côte, R, et al: A low-molecular-weight heparinoid compared with unfractionated heparin in the prevention of deep vein thrombosis in patients with acute ischemic stroke: A randomized, double-blind study. *Ann Intern Med* 117:353, 1992.

100. Tierney LM, Jr, Messina LM: Blood vessels and lymphatics, in Tierney LM, Jr, McPhee SJ, Papadakis MA, (eds): *Current Medical Diagnosis and Treatment,* 36th ed. London, Appleton and Lange, 1997, pp 452–454.

101. Stauffer JL: Lung, in Tierney LM, Jr, McPhee SJ, Papadakis MA, (eds): *Current Medical Diagnosis and Treatment,* 36th ed. London, Appleton and Lange, 1997, pp 290–297.

102. Teasell RW, McRae M, Marchuk Y, Finestone HM: Pneumonia associated with aspiration following stroke. *Arch Phys Med Rehabil* 77:707, 1996.

103. Stollerman GH: Infectious diseases: Medical disorders, in Cassel CK, Cohen HJ, Larson EB, Meier DE, Resnick NM, Rubenstein LZ, Sorenson LB (eds): *Geriatric Medicine.* 3rd ed. New York, Springer-Verlag, 1997, pp 615–619.

104. Sirvent JM, Torres A, El-Ebiary M, et al: Protective effect of intravenously administered cefuroxime against nosocomial pneumonia in patients with structural coma. *Am J Respir Crit Care Med* 155:1729, 1997.

105. Norris JW, Hachinski VC, Myers MG, et al: Serum cardiac enzymes in stroke. *Stroke* 10:548, 1979.

106. McDermott MM, Lefevre F, Arron M, Martin GJ, Biller J: ST segment depression detected by continuous electrocardiography in patients with acute ischemic stroke or transient ischemic attack. *Stroke* 25:1820, 1994.

107. Oppenheimer SM, Hachinski VC: The cardiac consequences of stroke. *Neurol Clin* 10:167, 1992.

108. Brittain KR, Peet SM, Castleden CM: Stroke and incontinence. *Stroke* 29:524, 1998.

109. McGrother C, Castleden CM, Duffin H, Clarke M: A profile of disordered micturition in the elderly at home. *Age Ageing* 16:105, 1987.

110. Teasdale TA, Taffet GE, Luchi RJ, Adam E: Urinary incontinence in a community-residing elderly population. *J Am Geriatr Soc* 36:600, 1988.
111. van der Worp HB, Kappelle LJ: Complications of acute ischaemic stroke. *Cerebrovasc Dis* 8:124, 1998.
112. Borrie MJ, Campbell AJ, Caradoc-Davies TH, Spears GFS: Urinary incontinence after stroke: A prospective study. *Age Ageing* 15:177, 1986.
113. Nakayama H, Jorgensen HS, Pedersen PM, Raaschou HO, Olsen TS: Prevalence and risk factors of incontinence after stroke: The Copenhagen Stroke Study. *Stroke* 28:58, 1997.
114. Libman RB, Wirkowski E, Alvir J, Rao TH: Conditions that mimic stroke in the emergency department. *Arch Neurol* 52:1119, 1995.
115. Kittner SJ, Sharkness CM, Price TR, et al: Infarcts with a cardiac source of embolism in the NINDS Stroke Data Bank: Historical features. *Neurology* 40:281, 1990.
116. Kittner SJ, Sharkness CM, Sloan MA, et al: Infarcts with a cardiac source of embolism in the NINDS Stroke Data Bank: Neurologic examination. *Neurology* 42:299, 1992.
117. Kittner SJ, Sharkness CM, Sloan MA, et al: Features on initial computed tomography scan of infarcts with a cardiac source of embolism in the NINDS Stroke Data Bank. *Stroke* 23:1748, 1992.
118. Hayes SH, Carroll SR: Early intervention care in the acute stroke patient. *Arch Phys Med Rehabil* 67:319, 1986.
119. Asberg KH: Orthostatic tolerance training of stroke patients in general medical wards: An experimental study. *Scand J Rehabil Med* 21:179, 1989.
120. Gowland C: Management of hemiplegic upper limb, in Brandstater ME, Basmhajian JV, (eds): *Stroke Rehabilitation,* Baltimore, Williams & Wilkins, 1987, pp 237–241.
121. Gresham GE, Duncan PW, Stason WV, et al: Post-stroke rehabilitation. Clinical practice guideline. Rockville, MD: U.S. Department of Health and Human Services. Public Health Service, Agency for Health Care Policy and Research. May 1995. Report No. 16.
122. Walker AE, Robins M, Weinfeld FD: The National Survey of Stroke: Clinical findings. *Stroke* 12:113, 1981.

Chapter 4

THE SUBACUTE STROKE PATIENT: PREVENTING RECURRENT STROKE

Stanley N. Cohen

INTRODUCTION

Once the issues of the acute and subacute management and diagnostic workup have been resolved and the patient is stable, the next focus must be on decreasing the risk of recurrent stroke and death. The diagnostic workup described in the prior chapters will enable the treating physician to segregate out those patients with nonatherosclerotic etiologies who require specific disease-oriented interventions (e.g., hypercoagulable states, cerebral vasculitis, etc.). Atherosclerosis involving large and small arteries supplying the brain is the most common cause of ischemic stroke in the United States. The patients with stroke due to atherosclerosis and those with "cryptogenic" stroke will require medical management, consideration of surgical intervention, and risk reduction. The mainstay of medical management for stroke prevention in patients with underlying atherosclerosis is antiplatelet therapy. The mainstay of surgical intervention is carotid endarterectomy (CEA). Risk reduction for the major risk factors, hypertension, diabetes, and hypercholesterolemia, are discussed in separate chapters in this volume. This chapter will focus on choosing an antiplatelet agent, selecting patients who may benefit from CEA, managing secondary risk factors, and selecting patients for cardiac workup.

USE OF PLATELET ANTAGONISTS

Background

The most common underlying cause of ischemic stroke in adults is atherosclerosis.[1] Fatty streaks, one of the earliest forms of atherosclerosis, can be found as early as the first and second decades of life.[2] Atherosclerotic plaques develop over the course of years. Although the pathogenesis of atherosclerosis is multifactorial, it is thought that disruption of the endothelial lining over the plaques plays an important role in causing the formation of intra-arterial thrombi.[3] Studies have shown that stenoses of $\geq$50 percent can be associated with endothelial damage and thrombus formation.[4] Platelets are an integral part of these thrombi. The platelet-rich arterial thrombi differ from venous thrombi, which are composed primarily of red cells in a fibrin mesh. Venous thrombi have been shown to be responsive to anticoagulants such as heparin and warfarin rather than antiplatelet agents.

The normal undamaged endothelium promotes blood flow by producing locally acting antiplatelet and anticoagulant agents. When platelets are exposed to damaged endothelium, thrombogenic subendothelium containing collagen, or other types of pathologic and physiologic stimuli, platelet activation occurs leading to adhesion and aggregation. Platelets adhere by using pseudopods and form a thin layer over the damaged endothelium. They also release potent vasoconstrictive agents, thromboxane A_2 and serotonin, and other agents that stimulate excitatory reactions leading to platelet aggregation such as adenosine diphosphate, β-thromboglobulin, platelet factor 4, von Willebrand factor, and fibrinogen.[5] The platelets provide a surface for activation of soluble coagulation factors. With platelet aggregation, thrombi are formed composed primarily of platelets and fibrin. Platelet aggregation is mediated by the glycoprotein IIb/IIIa (GP IIb/IIIa) complex receptor, found only on platelets and megakaryocytes.[6]

Therapeutic approaches for preventing athero-sclerotic ischemic stroke have focused on reducing intra-arterial thrombus formation by inhibiting platelet function. There are four agents available in the United States for stroke prevention whose action is primarily through antagonism of platelet function (Fig. 4-1). Aspirin (ASA) inhibits platelet function by irreversibly acetylating platelet cyclooxygenase. Ticlopidine and clopidogrel act by inhibiting the binding of adenosine diphosphate (ADP) to its platelet receptors and thereby inhibiting ADP-induced platelet aggregation. Dipyridamole (DP) inhibits platelet adhesion, but the mechanism of action is not fully known. Because these agents inhibit platelet function, they should be able to reduce the formation of intra-arterial thrombi and therefore reduce cerebral ischemic events.[7]

Aspirin inhibits thrombogenesis by irreversibly inactivating cyclooxygenase, which results in inhibition of thromboxane A_2, a potent stimulator of platelet activation. This inhibition is reversible. Aspirin also promotes thrombogenesis by blocking production of prostacyclin in the vascular endothelium. Platelets circulate for 7 to 10 days. Inhibition of platelet function by ASA lasts for the lifespan of the platelet.[8] This inhibition impairs platelet aggregation but not adhesion. Aspirin, in doses commonly used in stroke prevention, will inhibit thrombus formation but not stop the progression of atherosclerosis.[9] The onset of action for ASA is rapid,

with maximal effect taking place within 15 to 30 min of ingestion.[1] A single dose of ASA will prolong bleeding time for 24 to 48 h. Restoration of bleeding time is probably due to the production of unexposed platelets with normal aggregation.

Ticlopidine is a thienopyridine derivative. It is inactive in vitro and requires breakdown in the liver to metabolites, still unidentified, for in vivo activity.[2] Like ASA, it inhibits platelet aggregation. However, it does not interfere with prostaglandin synthetase. It inhibits platelet aggregation primarily by irreversibly inhibiting ADP-induced aggregation by inhibiting the ADP receptor on the platelet. Ticlopidine platelet inhibition is seen within 24 to 48 h of administration, peaks at 4 to 10 days, and lasts for the lifespan of the platelet. Bleeding time is prolonged twofold and remains prolonged for 4 to 10 days after the last dose.[2,3]

Clopidogrel is also a thienopyridine derivative. It is also inactive in vitro and is thought to work in vivo through an active metabolite. Like ticlopidine, it inhibits platelet function by irreversibly binding the ADP receptor on the platelet, preventing subsequent ADP-mediated activation of the GP IIb/IIIa complex.[4] Clopidogrel has a dose-related inhibition of platelet aggregation and prolongation of bleeding time, with 75 mg being roughly equivalent to 500 mg of ticlopidine.[5] The onset of action is faster than ticlopidine at about 2 h. Maximal platelet inhibition occurs between 3 and 7 days. Like ticlopidine,

Figure 4-1.

Schematic representation of the proposed mechanisms of action of aspirin, dipyridamole, ticlopidine, and clopidogrel in platelet inhibition. ADP, adenosine diphosphate; TXA_2, thromboxane A_2; COX, cyclooxygenase. Adapted from Bousser et al.[4]

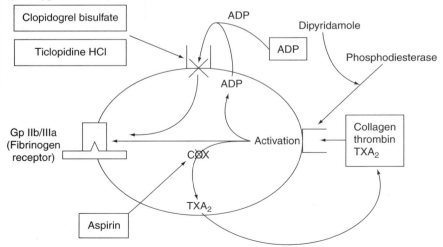

bleeding time remains prolonged for 4 to 10 days after the last dose.

Dipyridamole is an inhibitor of platelet adhesion.[6] The mechanism of action is uncertain. It may act by stimulating prostacyclin synthesis, inhibiting phosphodiesterase to raise platelet cyclic AMP levels, or blocking the uptake of adenosine into vascular and blood cells, causing accumulation of a platelet-inhibitory and vasodilatory compound in the thrombotic microenvironment.[1] The average time to peak concentration is about 75 min. It is metabolized in the liver. Dipyridamole is highly protein bound.

Fibrinogen binding to the platelet is the final step in the platelet aggregation pathway. The GP IIb/IIIa complex is the binding site for fibrinogen on the surface of the activated platelet. The binding of fibrinogen and von Willebrand factor to the platelet is mediated by the tripeptide amino acid sequence, arginine-glycine-aspartic acid (RGD). Two methods of inhibiting the GP IIb/IIIa complex that are being tested in stroke include monoclonal antibodies to GP IIb/IIIa and RGD analogs that compete with ligand binding to GP IIb/IIIa complex.[7] Inhibiting the GP IIb/IIIa complex has the potential for reducing the growth of a thrombus and causing its deaggregation.[8] GP IIb/IIIa inhibitors have shown potential in the treatment of myocardial infarction and unstable angina.[9,10]

Evidence

Aspirin Since the late 1970's, there have been many prospective randomized trials testing the efficacy of platelet antagonists in patients at high risk for ischemic stroke. The first large multicenter trial reported on 178 patients with hemispheric TIAs who were not referred for carotid endarterectomy (the selection of patients for surgical or medical treatment was not done on a randomized basis).[11] Patients were treated with 650 mg ASA twice daily or placebo. They found that the number of unfavorable outcomes was significantly reduced at 6 months in the ASA-treated group. However, no difference was found in the endpoints of death or cerebral or retinal infarction. The Canadian Cooperative Study was the second large randomized trial of platelet antagonists in stroke prevention.[12] Five-hundred eighty-five patients were randomized to ASA, sulfinpyrazone, ASA plus sulfinpyrazone, or placebo. During an average 26-month follow-up, 14 percent of the men on ASA alone suffered a stroke, whereas 16 percent on placebo had a stroke. When comparing all patients taking ASA with

those not taking ASA (independent of sulfinpyrazone), the men taking ASA had a significantly decreased risk of the combined endpoints of continuing TIA, stroke, or death. The study was not designed to show, and did not show, that ASA decreases the risk of stroke. Over the next decade, many studies further examined the potential benefit of ASA in patients at high risk for stroke. Of all of the studies comparing ASA with placebo, only the French Accidents, Ischemiques Cerebraux Lies a l'Atherosclerose (AICLA) study and the European Stroke Prevention Study 2, demonstrated a significant benefit for ASA in risk reduction for stroke[13,14] (see Table 4-1). Each of the others failed to show a statistically significant reduced stroke risk, but most showed a significantly reduced unfavorable vascular outcome for ASA.[11,12,15–19]

Conflicting results of individual studies produced controversy as to the efficacy of ASA in stroke or vascular death prevention. It was thought that a modest risk reduction might be missed because the number of subjects in the individual trials may be too small to reach statistical significance. Therefore, several meta-analyses of pooled data have been reported. The Antiplatelet Trialists' Collaboration analyzed the results of 25 trials that used antiplatelet medications (ASA, DP, sulfinpyrazone, and ticlopidine) in 29,000 patients with TIA, ischemic stroke, unstable angina, or myocardial infarction.[20] They found that antiplatelet treatment reduced the risk of vascular mortality by 15 percent, nonfatal MI or stroke by 30 percent, and unfavorable vascular events by 25 percent. In the 13 cerebrovascular trials, the risk of nonfatal stroke was reduced by 22 percent. Sze and co-workers performed a meta-analysis of randomized trials that compared antiplatelet drugs with placebo in 1928 patients with TIA or minor stroke.[21] For ASA compared with placebo, they found a non-significant 15 percent reduction in stroke risk. For ASA combined with DP or sulfinpyrazone, there was a significant reduction of 39 percent in stroke risk ($p < .05$). However, ASA combinations also had a 350 percent higher risk of serious gastrointestinal side effects ($p < .05$), whereas ASA alone was not significantly different than placebo. There was no significant reduction in mortality for either ASA alone or ASA combinations.

In a meta-analysis of trials that compared ASA with placebo (nine trials) or ASA plus DP to placebo (three trials) or ASA to ASA plus DP (three trials) in 9256 patients with a history of TIA or minor stroke, Gelmers and Tijssen reported that for ASA vs. placebo, there was a small but significant 15 percent risk reduction in favor of ASA for all vascular events and for

Table 4-1.
Prospective randomized trials comparing ASA to placebo

Study	No. patients	Mean follow-up in months	ASA dose in mg/day	No. strokes in ASA (%)	No. strokes in placebo (%)	No. strokes & death ASA (%)	No. strokes & death placebo (%)
SALT[19]	1360	32	75	93 (14)	112 (16)[a]	138 (20)	171 (25)
Danish[17]	301	21	50–100	9 (6)	11 (7)[a]	21 (14)	17 (11)
UK-TIA[18]	2435	48	300 or 1200	201 (12)	238 (15)[a]	346 (21)	205 (25)
AICLA[13]	402	36	1000	17 (9)	31 (15)[b]	27 (14)	38 (19)
Danish[15]	203	25	1000	17 (17)	11 (11)[a]	21 (21)	17 (17)
Canadian[12]	283	26	1300	22 (15)	20 (14)[a]	26 (18)	30 (22)
AITIA[11]	178	6	1300	5 (6)	10 (11)[a]	7 (8)	14 (16)
Swedish[16]	505	24	1500	32 (13)	32 (13)[a]	65 (26)	65 (26)
ESPS 2[14]	6602	24	50	206 (12.2)	250 (15.2)[b]	330	378

[a]Indicates difference in stroke between drug and placebo groups is not significant.

[b]Indicates difference in stroke between drug and placebo groups $p < .05$.

ASA, aspirin.

Adapted from Cohen.[12]

stroke (95 percent CI 0.75 to 0.97).[22] Tijssen updated the meta-analysis, including the results of the ESPS 2 trial.[23] In the 10 trials comparing ASA with placebo, there was a 19.7 percent rate of vascular events in the ASA group compared with 22.2 percent in the placebo group. This is a relative risk reduction of 13 percent ($p = .0011$). There was no difference in the relative risk reduction for high-, medium-, or low-dose ASA.

The Antiplatelet Trialists' Collaboration analyzed data from 145 trials comparing antiplatelet therapy with control in about 70,000 high-risk patients and 30,000 low-risk patients.[24] This included 11,707 patients in 18 studies entered with stroke or TIA. They found reduction in vascular events of about 25 percent in each of four main high-risk categories of patients (prior MI, acute MI, stroke/transient ischemic attack, other high risk). Subgroup analyses showed that the reductions were statistically significant in middle age and old age, in men and women, in hypertensive and normotensive patients, and in diabetic and nondiabetic patients. In patients presenting with stroke or TIA, there was a significant 23 percent risk reduction in subsequent nonfatal stroke. There was no significant reduction in the risk of fatal stroke. In patients with stroke or TIA, the authors concluded that prolonged antiplatelet therapy reduced both vascular mortality and all causes of mortal-

ity. In low-risk patients, there was no benefit in stroke prevention and a small, marginally significant increase in the risk for hemorrhagic stroke.

The results of each meta-analysis must be viewed with some caution. These analyses pool a heterogeneous group of clinical trials (transient ischemic attack, stroke, surgical trials, myocardial infarction, unstable angina), a heterogeneous group of endpoints (nonfatal stroke, nonfatal myocardial infarction, vascular death, and death from all causes), and various antiplatelet medications at various doses.[25]

The optimal dose of ASA remains controversial.[25–27] The prospective trials used doses ranging from 75 to 1500 mg per day.[11–13,15–19] Of these, only the UK-TIA trial compared placebo, low-dose ASA (325 mg/day), and high-dose ASA (1300 mg/day).[18] No difference was found between the two ASA doses in terms of stroke prevention. Given the study power, differences of up to 25 percent could have failed to have been detected. The low-dose ASA group did have significantly fewer gastrointestinal side effects. The Dutch Trial compared low-dose ASA (283 mg/day) with very low-dose ASA (30 mg/day).[28] They found no difference between the two doses in vascular death, nonfatal stroke, or myocardial infarction. The very low-dose group had fewer adverse effects. In the VA Cooperative

Asymptomatic Carotid Artery Stenosis Study, all patients were started on regular (nonenteric coated) ASA 650 mg twice a day.[29] Only 25 percent had no adverse effects and were still on that dose of regular ASA at study end.[30] There were 837 adverse reactions to ASA during the 4954 follow-up visits, with 45 percent of patients having gastrointestinal side effects. The authors concluded that high-dose ASA therapy is poorly tolerated and that adverse reactions to even low-dose enteric-coated ASA are common. The antithrombotic effect of ASA combined with the dose-related erosive effect on the gastric mucosa may explain the increased risk of major gastrointestinal bleeding with higher doses of ASA.[27]

The North American Symptomatic Carotid Endarterectomy Trial (NASCET) investigators, in a post hoc, retrospective analysis, found that patients on high-dose ASA (650 to 1300 mg/day) had significantly fewer postoperative strokes than did patients on low-dose ASA (81 to 350 mg/day).[31] Based on these data, the NASCET investigators studied ASA dosing in the perioperative period in a prospective randomized trial. They found that patients on low-dose ASA (81 to 350 mg/day) had significantly fewer unfavorable outcomes than those assigned to high dose.[32] Perhaps the most important take-home message from this trial is to interpret post hoc retrospective analyses with caution, even when they are generated from well-done large prospective trials. The data from the ACE trial suggest that low-dose ASA is better than high-dose ASA in the perioperative period. Because of the short duration of follow-up, it does not address the issue of the optimal ASA dose for long-term stroke prophylaxis.

ASA is attractive for long-term prophylaxis because of its low cost and its perceived low side-effect profile. However, the gastrointestinal hemorrhage rate for ASA in a stroke population is not negligible. In a meta-analysis of ASA trials, Roderick and colleagues reported a 2.48 percent GI hemorrhage rate with 1.7 percent requiring hospitalization.[33] In stroke trials with ASA dosing from 30 to 1300 mg per day reporting serious GI hemorrhages, there was a 2 to 3 percent hemorrhage rate.[18,19,28,34,35]

Ticlopidine   There have been two large prospective randomized trials using ticlopidine as the platelet antagonist in at-risk patients.[36,37] The Ticlopidine Aspirin Stroke Study (TASS) randomized 3069 patients with TIA or mild ischemic stroke within 3 months of the event and followed them for a mean of 3.4 years. The authors reported that ticlopidine significantly reduced the risk of stroke (RR 21 percent, $p = .024$) and the risk of stroke and death (RR 12 percent, $p = .048$) as compared with ASA in the intent-to-treat analysis. In the efficacy analysis, in which only the patients remaining on the assigned treatment at the time of the endpoint or at the end of the trial were considered for analysis, the risk reduction for stroke rose to 27 percent ($p = .011$) in favor of ticlopidine. In this analysis, at the end of the first year after entry, ticlopidine reduced the risk of stroke compared with ASA by 48 percent (3.4 vs. 6.4 percent, respectively, $p = .0004$).[38] The Canadian American Ticlopidine Study (CATS) compared ticlopidine with placebo in 1053 patients with completed ischemic stroke in the last 1 month and followed for a mean of 2.0 years. In the intent-to-treat analysis, ticlopidine reduced the endpoint of stroke, MI, or vascular death (RR 23 percent, $p = .02$) but did not show a benefit for reducing the risk of stroke alone.[36] However, the efficacy analysis did show a significant risk reduction for stroke or stroke death (RR 34 percent, $p = .008$) in favor of ticlopidine. In both TASS and CATS, the ticlopidine-treated group had a 1 percent incidence of severe neutropenia requiring discontinuation of the drug. Each case of severe neutropenia occurred in the first 3 months after initiating therapy and reversed with cessation of the drug. Compared with ASA, the ticlopidine patients had significantly more diarrhea and rash but significantly less gastritis, ulcer, or gastrointestinal bleeding. The patients assigned to ticlopidine had a mean rise in cholesterol of 9 percent. However, this increase did not result in an increase in fatal or nonfatal MI, and the cholesterol level was not a predictor of MI.[39] There have been reports of thrombotic thrombocytopenic purpura (TTP) associated with ticlopidine use.[40] Of 60 cases reviewed by Bennett and colleagues, 12 developed TTP within 3 weeks of starting the drug. Only one developed TTP outside of the first 12 weeks on the drug. In a post hoc retrospective analysis of data from TASS, Grotta et al reported ticlopidine to be significantly more effective than ASA in preventing subsequent strokes in patients whose angiograms did not show associated high-grade stenosis (10 percent vs. 19 percent).[41] Other subgroup analyses from TASS have reported benefit from ticlopidine in women, blacks, patients with minor stroke, and diabetics.[41-43] As noted in discussing the post hoc analysis of NASCET, caution must be used when interpreting post hoc subgroup analyses.[44] There is a 5 percent chance of a type 1 error (in 100 subgroup analyses, 5 significant results can be expected by chance alone).

Clopidogrel   There has been only one large prospective randomized trial assessing the safety and efficacy of clopidogrel, the Clopidogrel versus ASA in Patients at Risk of Ischemic Events (CAPRIE).[35] This trial included 19,185 patients, including 6431 entering with ischemic stroke. Forty percent of the stroke patients had lacunar infarctions. Patients were entered up to 6 months after the qualifying event. The study also included patients with MI and peripheral arterial disease (PAD). In the intent-to-treat analysis, clopidogrel showed a reduction in recurrent stroke, MI, or vascular death compared with ASA (5.32 percent per year vs. 5.83 percent per year). This represents an absolute risk reduction of 0.5 percent per year with a relative risk reduction of 8.7 percent ($p = .043$). In the on-treatment analysis, the relative risk reduction improved to 9.4 percent. For the subgroup entering with stroke, the unfavorable outcome rate was 7.15 percent with clopidogrel and 7.71 percent with ASA. This is an absolute risk reduction of 0.6 percent per year and a relative risk reduction of 7.3 percent ($p = .26$). In the patients entering with stroke, the recurrent stroke rate was 5.2 percent per year for the clopidogrel group and 5.7 percent per year for ASA. The difference is not significant. There was a differential response in the three subgroups entering the study, with only the PAD subgroup showing an improvement on clopidogrel compared with ASA. It must be remembered that the study was designed with the power to find a difference in total atherosclerotic complications from all groups but not in each of the three subgroups. The side-effect profile was roughly equivalent to ASA, with no difference in neutropenia and no reports of TTP. The clopidogrel group had more rashes and diarrhea, whereas the ASA group had more gastric irritation and gastrointestinal hemorrhage.

Dipyridamole   There have been five large prospective trials comparing DP and ASA, alone or in combination, in the treatment of TIA and stroke patients.[13,14,45–47] The earlier placebo-controlled trials (AICLA and the Toulouse TIA Trial) showed a benefit in favor of ASA plus dipyridamole (DP) vs. placebo for decreasing stroke risk.[13,47] However, both AICLA and the American-Canadian Co-Operative Study failed to show a benefit from ASA plus DP when compared with ASA alone in preventing stroke or death.[13,45] Over 40 percent of patients taking high-dose ASA withdrew from treatment in each of these studies.[48] It is possible that the failure to find a difference was due to the failure of the studies to be powered to find a difference with the small number of endpoints.

The European Stroke Prevention Study (ESPS) compared ASA 330 mg plus DP 75 mg TID with placebo in 2500 patients with a 2-year follow-up.[46] They found a 33.5 percent reduction in the primary endpoint of stroke and death from any cause ($p < .001$) and a 38.1 percent reduction in stroke ($p < .001$). They reported no gender difference, with both men and women having significantly reduced endpoints ($p < .001$ each). The reduction in the rate of stroke was 40.1 percent for men ($p < .001$) and 37.8 percent for women ($p = .018$).[49] Although the risk reduction seemed much better than prior reports using ASA alone, because there was no ASA only group in this study, no conclusion could be drawn regarding the benefit of combination therapy vs. ASA alone.

In Gelmers and Tijssen's meta-analysis of trials comparing ASA and ASA plus dipyridamole with placebo, for stroke prevention, there was a significant 39 percent relative risk reduction with a combination of DP and ASA vs. placebo (95 percent CI 0.50 to 0.75).[22] In analyzing studies that compared ASA alone with ASA plus DP, the addition of DP had no benefit in reducing risk of mortality or stroke. The authors felt that further study is needed before the combination of ASA plus DP is discarded from the therapeutic armamentarium.

In the European Stroke Prevention Study 2 (ESPS 2), 6602 patients were randomized to ASA alone (50 mg/day), DP alone (400 mg/day), a combination of ASA plus DP, or placebo with a 2-year follow-up.[14] The risk of stroke was reduced by 18 percent for ASA alone ($p = .013$), 16 percent for DP alone ($p = .039$), and 37 percent for the combination ($p < .001$). There was a relative risk reduction for stroke of 23 percent favoring the combination compared with ASA alone ($p = .006$). The ASA-treated groups had an 8.5 percent risk of bleeding from any site, significantly higher than placebo ($p < .001$), with severe or fatal hemorrhage occurring in 1.5 percent. Controversy surrounded the report of these data due to ethical questions regarding a placebo arm in a stroke prevention trial and to allegations of fraud at one of the centers in the study.[50] The data from this center were excluded prior to trial unblinding.

In the updated meta-analysis that included the ESPS 2 trial results, Tijssen reported a 14.6 percent vascular event rate for the dipyridamole plus ASA group ($n = 2,473$) and a 17.2 percent rate for those in the ASA group ($n = 2436$).[23] This is a 15 percent relative risk reduction for the combination therapy compared with ASA alone ($p = .012$). Comparing the combination of ASA plus dipyridamole with placebo, the combination therapy had an event rate of 14.2 percent (n = 3239) vs. placebo at 20.1 percent (n = 3259). This is a relative risk reduction of 30 percent ($p < .00001$). The author concluded that the addition of dipyridamole to ASA in high-risk patients would reduce the vascular event rate by an additional 15 percent compared with ASA alone. Others have opined that the reason for the benefit of combination therapy vs. monotherapy was the choice of very low-dose ASA, which may have been suboptimal in effectiveness.[26]

Treatment Recommendations

Platelet antagonists are widely accepted in secondary stroke prevention. The choice of which drug to use as a first choice and, in the case of ASA, the optimal dose, is controversial. In a survey of "stroke experts," about half of the European neurologists who use ASA used low dose (30 to 175 mg/day) and half used medium dose (200 to 400 mg/day).[51] The North Americans surveyed split with about 60 percent using medium dose and about 40 percent using high dose (500 to 1300 mg/day). The choice of treatment in the case of ASA failure becomes even more controversial. There are four platelet antagonists to chose from, each with advantages and disadvantages shown in controlled trials.

Aspirin has the advantages of being very inexpensive, available without a prescription, convenient once a day dosing, and an acceptable level of serious side effects. The major disadvantages are that it is only a weak protector against recurrent stroke (about 15 to 20 percent better than placebo) and the risk of serious GI bleeding (about 1 to 2 percent), with the risk of hemorrhage continuing for the duration of the use of the drug. The frequent "minor" side effects that will interfere with compliance include GI irritation.

Ticlopidine has the advantage of being about 20 percent better than ASA in preventing a recurrent stroke in patients at high risk for stroke and less frequent GI pain, GI hemorrhage, and peptic ulcers than ASA. It has the disadvantages of expense, inconvenient twice a day dosing, inconvenient frequent blood testing, and the high frequency of "minor" side effects. The risk of severe neutropenia is about 1 percent. This requires monitoring of the CBC every 2 weeks for the first 3 months after initiating therapy. Unlike the bleeding risk with ASA, the risk of severe neutropenia seems to be significant only in the first 3 months, and monitoring is not needed after that. The frequency of TTP occurring with ticlopidine use is unknown. Although the majority of reported cases occurred in the first 3 months of ther-

apy, there are reports of cases occurring outside that time window. The most frequent "minor" side effects are diarrhea and rash, each occurring about twice as often with ticlopidine than with ASA. The frequency with which diarrhea occurs can be reduced by initiating therapy at 250 mg/day after meals for the first week.

Clopidogrel has the advantage of being slightly more effective than ASA in preventing vascular endpoints in patients with atherosclerosis, convenient once a day dosing, significantly less GI hemorrhage, indigestion, nausea and vomiting, and a very low "minor" side-effect profile. Its disadvantage is expense. The minor side effects include increased rash and diarrhea when compared with ASA. Although the relative risk reduction for all endpoints in the CAPRIE study was significant, the absolute risk reduction was very small. Considering all outcomes, there was a 0.5 percent/year reduction for all patients. The absolute risk reduction of 0.6 percent/year for those entering the study with stroke was not statistically or clinically significant.

Slow-release dipyridamole has the advantage of being about as effective as ASA in preventing vascular endpoints and stroke in patients with prior stroke or TIA. It also has a decreased risk of bleeding. The expense is uncertain because the formulation used in ESPS 2 is not yet available in the United States but almost certainly will be more expensive than ASA. It has the disadvantage of inconvenient twice a day dosing and increased risk of headache, diarrhea, and vomiting compared with ASA.

The combination of ASA plus DP has the advantage of being more effective than ASA in preventing stroke in high-risk patients. It has the disadvantages of twice a day dosing and side-effect profile that combines the side effects of ASA and DP. The relative risk reduction for stroke as an endpoint was 23.1 percent ($p = .006$), with an absolute risk reduction of 1.4 percent/year.

Which is the appropriate first choice for secondary stroke prevention? ASA has been the gold standard for many years. In view of its low cost, ease of use, and accepted efficacy of about 20 percent better than placebo, it remains an appropriate choice in many patients. Ticlopidine carries a higher risk profile, expense, and considerable inconvenience especially in regard to frequent blood draws. Because of this, ticlopidine is not often chosen as a first drug of choice despite its favorable efficacy. It should be considered in patients who are unable to tolerate ASA or have a history of ulcers or gastritis. Clopidogrel does not carry the inconvenience or risk of ticlopidine, but the small benefit relative to

ASA in stroke patients combined with the increased expense does not justify choosing clopidogrel over ASA as a first drug of choice. Clopidogrel should be considered a first drug of choice in patients who cannot take ASA and are not reliable enough to take ticlopidine. Dipyridamole as a single agent has no advantage in efficacy or expense over ASA and is more inconvenient to use because of frequency of dosing and frequency of nausea, vomiting, and diarrhea. The combination of delayed release DP plus ASA is attractive. There is a statistically and clinically significant decrease in the frequency of stroke with an acceptable increase in side-effect profile (Fig. 4-2).

What is the best approach in the patient who presents with ischemic stroke while on ASA? Obviously, the patient should be evaluated to ensure that there is no superimposed etiology requiring more specific therapy

(see Chap. 3). Once it has been determined that platelet antagonism is still the treatment of choice, therapeutic options include:

1. Continue on the same dose of ASA.

For the patient presenting with a new ischemic event while on ASA, continuing on ASA without changing dose initially seems counterintuitive. However, if the patient has been without ischemic symptoms for a period of time while on ASA, the new symptoms may not necessarily be viewed as a treatment failure but rather a "breakthrough event." This can be viewed in the same way as a stable epilepsy patient having a single seizure. It is considered a breakthrough seizure rather than a treatment failure. It may not warrant changing therapy. Although this approach is not "wrong," considering that there are reasonable alter-

Figure 4-2.
Dipyridamole, ticlopidine, and clopidogrel compared with aspirin in cerebrovascular disease. Results are shown of three large trials. Data derived from Refs. 14, 35, and 37. Adapted from Albers et al.[120]

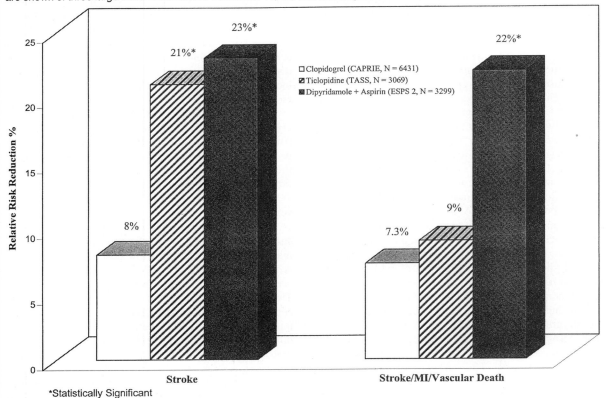

native strategies, this nihilistic approach should not be first choice.

2. Continue on ASA, only change the dose.

There is a widely held belief that argues that high-dose ASA may be better than low dose. Patients on low-dose ASA coming in with a new event can be switched to high-dose ASA. Although this is a strategy that is frequently chosen, the absence of good data to support this position makes this a less desirable option.

3. Change to ticlopidine or clopidogrel.

Ticlopidine is more effective than ASA in preventing stroke in patients who present with stroke or TIA. This is a reasonable justification for switching the "ASA failure" to ticlopidine so long as the patient will be able to comply with the blood monitoring required of ticlopidine. If the patient is noncompliant or has difficulty tolerating ticlopidine, clopidogrel is a reasonable second choice. Although not proven to be better than ASA in this setting, the mechanism of action is different than ASA, and the side-effect profile is better.

4. Change to a combination of ASA plus dipyridamole.

The combination of ASA plus dipyridamole has been shown to be more effective in preventing recurrent strokes than ASA in this population. Although the side-effect profile of the two drugs combined is additive, so is the benefit. This is a very attractive strategy.

5. Change to a combination of ASA plus ticlopidine or clopidogrel.

ASA has a different mechanism of action than the thienopyridine derivative drugs in inhibiting platelet aggregation. In theory, the combining of two types of drugs should be complementary. The combination has been used successfully after cardiac stent placement. There have been no trials of this combination in stroke prophylaxis. No evidence-based recommendation can be made for this approach.

6. Change to oral anticoagulants.

Although there is a wealth of good clinical data on the role of oral anticoagulants in stroke prevention in atrial fibrillation, there is a dearth when it comes to anticoagulation for prophylaxis in atherothrombotic stroke. Retrospective, observational data support the use of warfarin in patients with symptomatic intracranial stenosis.[52] In the only major prospective randomized trial comparing antiplatelet agents with warfarin for non-cardioembolic stroke, the study was stopped after only 14 months of average follow-up.[53] Warfarin was inferior to aspirin due to bleeding side effects. However, this trial used warfarin with a target INR of 3.0 to 4.5. The authors calculated that two-thirds of the hemorrhages would be avoided with an INR of 2.0 to 3.0.

Despite the absence of data supporting the use of warfarin in patients without atrial fibrillation, when patients "fail" platelet antagonists, and they are deemed to be good candidates for anticoagulation, some experts will choose to anticoagulate, keeping the INR below 3.0.

ROLE OF CAROTID ENDARTERECTOMY

Background

Carotid stenosis was first clearly recognized as a potential cause of stroke in the 1950's. Since that time, physicians have been trying to refine a mechanical solution, carotid endarterectomy (CEA), for a potentially mechanical problem. The purpose of CEA is to remove an atherothrombotic lesion from the region of the carotid bifurcation. The surgery involves exposing the carotid bifurcation in the neck, clamping the common, internal, and external carotid arteries, performing an arterotomy on the carotid artery, and removing the plaque.[54] During the late 1970's and early 1980's, despite the lack of any large, prospective randomized trials proving the safety and efficacy of CEA for any indication, the number of procedures performed per year grew.[55] In 1970, about 12,000 CEAs were performed annually in the United States. By 1980, that number had grown to over 50,000; by 1985, this number had passed 100,000. Associated with some negative publicity, the number dropped to below 75,000 in 1990. Since the publication of the CEA trials in the early 1990's, the number has again dramatically grown.[56]

Evidence

The role of CEA in patients with symptomatic stenosis remained controversial until the early 1990's. The first large randomized clinical trial presented equivocal results.[57] In a study assessing the use of CEA in five California Veterans Affairs Medical Centers, based on indications developed by a consensus of experts, only 55 percent of CEAs performed were considered clearly appropriate.[58] To help resolve the controversy, three clinical trials were started to compare medical management plus CEA vs. medical management alone: the European Carotid Surgery Trial (ECST), the VA Cooperative Trial, and the North American Symptomatic Carotid Endarterectomy Trial (NASCET).

ECST entered 2518 patients in three groups: mild stenosis (<30 percent), moderate stenosis (30 to 69 percent), and severe stenosis (70 to 99 percent).[59] Stenosis was calculated by comparing the narrowest residual carotid lumen with the estimated diameter of the normal carotid bulb. All patients had nondisabling strokes, TIA, or retinal infarction in the territory of the stenosed carotid artery within the previous 6 months. After a prerandomization angiogram, a neurologist and a surgeon evaluated the patient. If they were reasonably certain, for any reason, that surgery was either indicated or not indicated, the patient was declared ineligible. Only if the doctors were substantially uncertain whether CEA was indicated was the patient entered. There were no standard criteria for what constituted reasonable certainty or reasonable uncertainty. The study was terminated prematurely for the mild stenosis and severe stenosis groups. The 30-day surgical stroke or death rate was 4.6 percent for patients with mild stenosis and 7.5 percent for those with severe stenosis. For the 374 patients with mild stenosis, the risk of ipsilateral stroke at 3 years was so small that any 3-year benefit of surgery would be outweighed by the early risk of surgery. For the 778 patients with severe stenosis, at 3 years, the risk of surgical death or stroke, or any stroke, was 12.3 percent for the surgical group and 21.9 percent for the control group. The 3-year risk of disabling or fatal stroke was 6.0 percent for surgery and 11.0 percent for controls. These differences are statistically significant in favor of surgery ($2p < .01$ and $2p < .05$, respectively).

In 1998, the ECST reported the final results of the study.[60] There was a total of 3024 patients randomized, 60 percent to surgery, 40 percent control. The perioperative major stroke or death rate was 7.0 percent (major stroke defined as a stroke with symptoms lasting more than 7 days). In the control group, the risk of recurrent stroke was related to the severity of stenosis only in the first 2 to 3 years after randomization. Comparing outcomes for those having successful surgery (not counting surgical strokes or deaths) with control, there is clear benefit to surgery with stenosis at ≥80 percent. At 3 years, for 80 to 99 percent stenosis, the absolute risk reduction in major stroke and death was 11.6 percent with the number needed to treat to prevent a major stroke at 3 years equal to nine. Subgroup analysis showed a higher surgical risk for women with less overall benefit. Men derived benefit from surgery with stenosis ≥80 percent, whereas women got benefit only with stenosis ≥90 percent.

NASCET was more rigorously designed.[61] To participate, a surgeon had to have performed at least 50 endarterectomies in the prior 24 months with <6 percent stroke or death rate. Patients had to have ischemic symptoms in the prior 120 days ipsilateral to a stenosis of 30 to 99 percent. In NASCET, percent stenosis was calculated with the formula $(1 - [MRL/DL]) \times 100$. Minimum residual lumen (MRL) was the narrowest diameter at the site of the stenosis. Distal lumen (DL) was measured distal to the stenosis beyond the carotid bulb at a point where the artery walls were parallel and disease free. (See Chap. 36, Fig. 36-5.) In severe disease, where the decreased pressure due to the stenosis caused collapse and narrowing of the distal carotid, DL was estimated using the diameter of the external carotid artery or the contralateral internal carotid. This method gave very different results than the ECST method. A 50 percent stenosis by ECST was equal to a 16 percent stenosis in NASCET.[62] An ECST stenosis of 70 percent was equal to a 50 percent in NASCET, and an ECST stenosis of 80 percent was roughly equal to 70 percent in NASCET. All patients received aspirin and optimal medical management and were randomized to CEA or medical therapy alone.

In 1991, the NINDS monitoring committee stopped the trial for the 70 to 99 percent stenosis group. In 659 patients with severe stenosis, Kaplan-Meier estimates indicated that the risk of ipsilateral stroke at 2 years was 9 percent for the surgical group and 26 percent for the medical group ($p < .001$).[34] For major ipsilateral or fatal stroke, the risks were 2.5 percent vs. 13.1 percent for the surgical and medical groups, respectively. Statistically significant risk reduction was found in favor of surgery for the endpoints of any stroke, any stroke or death, any major or fatal stroke, and any major stroke or death.

Subgroup analysis was performed to help identify patients with increased risk of recurrent stroke. Within the medical group, risk of ipsilateral stroke was stratified based on the number of risk factors present. Those with 0 to 5 risk factors had a 17 percent risk of ipsilateral stroke in 2 years, those with 6 risk factors had a 23 percent risk, and those with ≥7 risk factors had a 39 percent risk.

In the medical group, if there were no recurrent symptoms by 3 years after the qualifying event, the yearly rate of ipsilateral stroke was comparable with the surgical group.[31] This indicates there is little to be gained by performing a CEA 3 years after an event.

The presence of an angiographically defined ulcer was an independent risk for stroke.[63] The risk of ipsilateral stroke at 2 years in the medical group with ulcerated plaques increased from 26.3 to 73.2 percent as the degree of stenosis increased from 75 to 95 percent. For patients with no ulcer, the risk of stroke remained constant at 21.3 percent for all degrees of stenosis.

The 2-year risk of stroke in patients presenting with hemispheric TIA was significantly higher than for those presenting with transient monocular blindness (43.5 percent vs. 16.6 percent).[64] Surgically treated patients with carotid occlusion contralateral to the severe symptomatic stenosis had a 14 percent risk of operative stroke or death.[65] However, medically treated patients in this subgroup had a 69 percent 2-year risk of stroke compared with 22 percent for the surgically treated patients, more than offsetting the higher operative risk.

Of 58 medically treated patients with near occlusion of the symptomatic carotid, only one suffered a stroke in the 32-day postrandomization period, no different than the rate of patients entered with lesser degrees of stenosis.[66] This suggests that symptomatic near occlusion does not require emergency CEA and can be managed in the same fashion as surgical candidates with lesser degrees of stenosis. Of the 48 near-occlusion patients treated surgically, the postoperative complication rate was no different than for those with lesser degrees of stenosis. This implies that there is no added danger in operating on near occlusion compared with lesser degrees of stenosis.

In 1998, NASCET investigators reported the results for the 2226 patients in the moderate stenosis group.[31] For patients with 50 to 69 percent stenosis, the surgical group had a 15.7 percent 5-year ipsilateral stroke rate compared with 22.2 percent for the medical group ($p = .045$). This is a relative risk reduction of 29 percent with an absolute risk reduction of 6.5 percent. For those with a stenosis less than 50 percent, no significant difference was found between surgical and medical groups. Post hoc analysis suggested that within the 50 to 69 percent group, the largest benefit is in patients who are male, have hemispheric events, do not have diabetes, and are taking high-dose ASA. The 30-day surgical stroke or death rate was 6.7 percent. By way of comparison, the medical group had a 32-day postrandomization stroke or death rate of 2.4 percent. The primary results from the NASCET trial are summarized in Table 4-2.

The VA Cooperative Trial (VACT) randomized 189 men with angiographically proven symptomatic carotid stenosis of $\geq$50 percent.[67] Stenosis was calculated by the same method used in NASCET. After a mean follow-up of 11.9 months, the study was stopped because of the positive results published by NASCET and ECST. The number of ipsilateral strokes was too small to show a difference between treatment groups. When endpoints of stroke and crescendo TIA were combined, a difference in favor of surgery was found.

Goldstein and colleagues, in a meta-analysis of these three trials, found that there were no significant differences in outcome event rates among the trials, and the outcome event rates were similar for men and women.[68]

The benefit of CEA is dependent on maintaining a low postoperative complication rate. Half of the formula for maintaining low complication rates is proper patient selection. In 1975, Sundt and colleagues analyzed risk factors for postoperative stroke or death in patients undergoing CEA.[69] In neurologically stable patients with no medical or angiographic risks, the complication rate was 1 percent. Patients with angiographic risks but no medical or neurologic risks had a 2 percent rate. Those with medical risks but no neurologic risks had a 7 percent rate. Those with neurologic risks, independent

Table 4-2.

K-M Estimate of ipsilateral stroke by stenosis stratification in NASCET

	Patients		Failure rate (%)		Absolute RR (%)	RRR (%)	NNT	p value
Stenosis	Med	Surg	Med	Surg				
70–99%	331	328	26.1[a]	12.9	13.2	51	8	0.000051
50–69%	428	430	22.2[b]	15.7	6.5	29	15	0.045
<50%	690	678	18.7[b]	14.9	3.8	20	26	0.16

[a]2-year estimate.

[b]5-year estimate.

Adapted from Barnett HJM; personal communication with permission.

of the medical or angiographic risks, had a 10 percent complication rate. Goldstein and colleagues reviewed 697 CEAs performed for symptomatic stenosis at 12 academic medical centers.[70] The postoperative stroke, MI, and death rate was 8.5 percent. They found that patients over 75 years had a higher risk of MI postoperatively. Contralateral carotid occlusion, ipsilateral intraluminal thrombus, and ipsilateral siphon stenosis had higher rates of complication, though only occlusion was significant. Patients with none of these four risk factors had a significantly lower complication rate compared with those with one or more. In NASCET, risk for postoperative stroke or death was associated with contralateral carotid occlusion, left-sided carotid disease, taking less than 650 mg of ASA, absence of history of MI or angina, lesion on brain imaging ipsilateral to the CEA, history of diabetes, and diastolic blood pressure >90 mmHg. In reviewing results of CEA for Medicare beneficiaries in 1996, Hsia and colleagues reported that patients age 85 and older had twice the average perioperative mortality.[71] In a retrospective review of 291 CEAs, Wong and colleagues found risks for increased perioperative stroke, death, or cardiac complications included history of angina, history of congestive heart failure, lack of preoperative antiplatelet agent, and age >75 years.[72]

The other half of the formula for low postoperative complication rates is proper selection of surgeons. Ruby and colleagues studied surgical volume as a risk for postoperative stroke and death in 3997 CEAs.[73] They found that surgeons with an annual volume of ≤1 CEA were 2.5 times more likely to have a complication than those performing ≥10 CEAs per year. Postoperative mortality for CEA was found to be higher with low-volume surgeons (≤1 CEA per year) operating in low-volume hospitals (≤100 CEAs per year) than high-volume surgeons operating in high-volume hospitals.[74]

After a stroke, the timing of a CEA has been controversial. The Joint Study of Extracranial Arterial Occlusion reported in 1969 that surgical mortality was 42 percent for those operated in under 2 weeks compared with 5 percent when the surgery was delayed at least 2 weeks.[75] This, combined with numerous anecdotal reports, led to the recommendation that surgery be delayed 5 to 6 weeks following an acute stroke.[76] Piotrowski and colleagues reported a series of 129 CEAs, examining outcome in relation to timing of surgery.[77] They found no difference between patients operated 2, 4, 6, or >6 weeks after acute stroke. NASCET investigators examined the results of surgery done from 3 to 30 days (mean of 16 days) after nondisabling stroke compared with more than 30 days after stroke.[78] There was no difference in the postoperative stroke rates between early and late groups.

Treatment Recommendations

Based on the three large prospective trials, CEA can be recommended as the treatment of choice in symptomatic patients below the age of 80 with nondisabling strokes or TIAs associated with ipsilateral angiographically measured extracranial carotid stenosis of 70 to 99 percent. The patients must be good surgical candidates, and the surgeons must be able to perform the surgery with less than a 6 percent stroke or death rate. For symptomatic patients with 50 to 69 percent, the benefit is marginal, and patient selection must be even more vigilant. Most patients with less than 50 percent stenosis get no benefit from surgery.

There are no good data on patients with both atrial fibrillation (AF) and severe carotid stenosis ipsilateral to an ischemic stroke. Absent the data, it is reasonable to recommend in patients that, with ≥70 percent stenosis ipsilateral to stroke who have AF and who are otherwise good surgical candidates, endarterectomy should be done followed by chronic anticoagulation.[79]

The proper imaging method for selecting patients for CEA is controversial.[80] Advocates of replacing angiography with duplex scanning stress the increase in safety and the decrease in cost compared with angiography.[81] Angiography carries between 0.5 and 1 percent complication rate in cerebrovascular patients. The monetary cost of the angiogram is between $3000 and $6000. Advocates of maintaining angiography as the "gold standard" stress the better accuracy, the ability to differentiate between a near occlusion and a complete occlusion, the ability to identify intraluminal thrombus, and the ability to assess the intracranial vessels.[82] Magnetic resonance angiography has potential for becoming the imaging study of choice, but because of the tendency to overestimate degree of stenosis, it is not ready to replace angiography. To use duplex as a replacement for angiography for selecting patients for CEA, the duplex lab must be validated against angiography. We currently require a peak systolic velocity cut point that has been shown to give a 99 percent specificity for a ≥70 percent stenosis. If an MRA confirms the stenosis and fails to reveal a vascular lesion that might preclude CEA (such as distal intracranial aneurysm or large artery occlusion), the patient can proceed to CEA without an angiogram. If the ultrasound indicates stenosis but fails to hit parameters indicative of a ≥70 percent stenosis with a 99 percent specificity, or the MRA does not confirm the lesion or is unclear regarding the intracranial vessels, we recommend proceeding to contrast angiography.

Regarding timing of the CEA after an acute stroke, there are no large prospective randomized trials to guide who would be a good candidate for early surgery or even define what is "early" surgery. One of the fears of early surgery is opening a tight stenosis and exposing a cerebrovascular tree that has been protected from a high-pressure head by the stenosis to increased pressures in the face of impaired autoregulation. This could result in intracranial hemorrhage. One of the fears of delayed surgery is recurrent stroke or progression of a tight stenosis to a complete occlusion occurring prior to the operation. After reviewing the literature on the subject, Pritz stratified patients with acute stroke based on CT scan hypodensity, shift, level of consciousness, and vascular territory of the infarct.[83] It seems reasonable that patients with a small lesion, on both clinical grounds and imaging, who are clinically stable and have a normal level of consciousness, can undergo CEA by 1 week after the event. For patients with larger lesions, it is prudent to wait longer, individualizing based on the size of the lesion and the clinical condition of the patient.

Selecting a surgeon with a complication rate below 7 percent for symptomatic patients is critical. The studies showing benefit of surgery set minimal standards for all participating surgeons. NASCET required that surgeons demonstrate <6 percent perioperative stroke or death rate in 50 cases in the prior 24 months.[61] The VA Cooperative Study required participating hospitals to demonstrate 25 or more CEAs annually for 3 years with a perioperative complication rate below 6 percent with individual surgeons performing at least 10 operations annually for 3 years.[67] Unfortunately, most physicians do not have access to volume of surgeries done by the doctors to whom they refer, let alone the complication rates.[84] We recommend that doctors referring patients for CEA demand that their surgeons maintain an ongoing audit CEA volume and complication rate. If this information is not available, consideration should be given to referring to a center where the data are known.

For the patient with symptomatic stenosis ≥70 percent who has increased surgical risk making carotid endarterectomy untenable, consideration may be given to carotid angioplasty (see Chap. 11). Although angioplasty and stent placement are well established in treating cardiac disease, the risks and durability of this procedure in the cerebrovascular tree are still uncertain. Carotid angioplasty should only be considered at centers with expertise in invasive radiology and experience in cerebrovascular angioplasty.

RISK FACTOR MANAGEMENT

Introduction

When caring for a stroke victim, there is a tendency to focus on disease-specific interventions such as those dealt with in the prior two sections. However, stroke prophylaxis requires attempting to decrease all potentially modifiable risk factors. Even after risk factors are identified, treatment of the risk factors often meets with limited success.[85]

Certain risk factors have been identified that cannot be modified including age, gender, race, ethnicity, and heredity (Table 4-3).[86] Of the modifiable risk factors, hypertension, diabetes, hyperlipidemia, cardiac disease including atrial fibrillation, recreational drug use, oral contraceptive use, migraine, and the hypercoagulable states are dealt with in separate chapters later in this volume. This section will review some of the other important modifiable risk factors.

Asymptomatic Carotid Stenosis

Background Patients with stroke may be found to have carotid stenosis remote from their symptomatic brain lesion. Prior to 1990, there were no rigorous scientific trials on the role of CEA for asymptomatic stenosis. The literature was filled with conflicting observational series and anecdotal reports. In 1978, Thompson and coworkers reported a retrospective review of 270 patients who had been evaluated by them for carotid stenosis.[87] One-hundred thirty-two had CEA, whereas 138 did not receive an operation. With follow-up up to 192 months, the authors reported that 91 percent of the operated patients remained asymptomatic, whereas only 56 percent of the nonoperated patients were asymptomatic. Other reports indicated that the natural history of symptomatic stenosis may be benign and surgery may not be warranted.[88] Though these were not prospective randomized trials, many papers suggested that CEA may benefit some patients with asymptomatic carotid stenosis.

Many series reported on the risks of CEA in asymptomatic patients with very variable results. Thompson and colleagues reported a 0 percent surgical stroke or death rate in patients with asymptomatic

Table 4-3.
Risk factors for first ischemic stroke

Well-documented risk factors
  Modifiable, value established
    Hypertension
    Cardiac disease
    Atrial fibrillation
    Infective endocarditis
    Mitral stenosis
    Recent large myocardial infarction
    Cigarette smoking
    Sickle cell disease
    Transient ischemic attacks
    Asymptomatic carotid stenosis
  Potentially modifiable
    Diabetes mellitus
    Hyperhomocysteinemia
    Left ventricular hypertrophy
  Nonmodifiable
    Age
    Gender
    Hereditary/familial factors
    Race/ethnicity
    Geographic location
Less well-documented risk factors
  Potentially modifiable
    Elevated blood cholesterol and lipids
    Cardiac disease
      Cardiomyopathy
      Segmental wall motion abnormalities
      Nonbacterial endocarditis
      Mitral annular calcification
      Mitral valve prolapse
      Valve strands
      Spontaneous echocardiographic contrast
      Aortic stenosis
      Patent foramen ovale
      Atrial septal aneurysm
    Use of oral contraceptives
    Consumption of alcohol
    Use of illicit drugs
    Physical inactivity
    Obesity
    Elevated hematocrit
    Dietary factors
    Hyperinsulinemia and insulin resistance
    Acute triggers (stress)
    Migraine
    Hypercoagulability and inflammation
      Fibrin formation and fibrinolysis
      Fibrinogen
      Anticardiolipin antibodies
      Genetic and acquired causes
      Subclinical diseases
      Intimal-medial thickness
      Aortic atheroma
      Ankle-brachial blood pressure ratio
      Infarct-like lesions on MRI
    Socioeconomic features
  Nonmodifiable
    Season and climate

From Sacco et al.[86]

bruit.[89] Fode and colleagues reported a retrospective analysis of 396 patients undergoing CEA at multiple centers for asymptomatic stenosis.[90] The surgical stroke or death rate was 5.1 percent. Brott and Thalinger reported on CEA results in Cincinnati in a 1-year period.[91] They analyzed 67 operations for asymptomatic bruit and 63 operations for asymptomatic stenosis. There was a 7.7 percent postoperative stroke rate with a 3.1 percent death rate. Easton and Sherman reported the CEA complication rate in 228 consecutive patients operated in two 600-bed community hospitals in Illinois.[92] In the asymptomatic patients, the surgical stroke or death rate was 18.2 percent. Many other series through 1985 reported CEA complication rates for asymptomatic patients between 0 and 20 percent.

Evidence By the mid-1980's, four major randomized studies were organized to examine the role of CEA in asymptomatic carotid stenosis. Investigators at the Mayo Clinic performed a randomized controlled trial comparing CEA with medical management using low-dose ASA in patients with asymptomatic carotid stenosis ≥50 percent.[93] The medical patients were treated with 80 mg ASA per day, whereas for those randomized to surgery, ASA was discouraged except if there were known cardiac indications. Both groups had established vascular risk factors aggressively managed. In 30 months, 71 patients were randomized, 35 surgical, 36 medical. With a mean follow-up of 24 months, the medical group had four TIAs, no strokes, and no MIs, whereas the surgical group had no TIAs, three strokes, and eight MIs. The difference in MIs between groups was highly significant ($p = .004$). The study was stopped because of the excessive number of MIs in the surgical group. It was felt that the absence of ASA in the surgical arm might have been responsible for the high rate of MI in the follow-up period. When the study was stopped, the number of patients entered, the duration of follow-up, and the total number of endpoints were small. The study was not powered to draw a conclusion about the benefit or lack of benefit from CEA in this setting.

The Carotid Artery Stenosis with Asymptomatic Narrowing: Operation vs. Aspirin (CASANOVA) Study Group examined a somewhat different population.[94] They followed 410 patients with 50 to 90 percent stenosis for 3 years. They divided the patients in two groups. Group A had unilateral surgery for unilateral stenosis or bilateral surgery for bilateral stenosis. Group B had no surgery for unilateral stenosis or unilateral surgery for bilateral stenosis. Patients who progressed to >90 percent stenosis developed bilateral stenosis of

>50 percent, developed a carotid stenosis >50 percent contralateral to the operated side, developed restenosis >50 percent, or had a TIA with >50 percent stenosis were crossed over to surgery. During follow-up, an additional 26 percent of group B patients underwent CEA. All patients received ASA 330 mg plus dipyridamole 75 mg TID. The endpoints were perioperative stroke or death or stroke during follow-up. Surgical complications included 0.3 percent "minor" stroke, 2.7 percent stroke, and 1.2 percent death. Including pulmonary embolism, MI, and permanent cranial nerve damage, the rate of major surgical complications was 6.9 percent. During follow-up, the rate of primary endpoints for group A was 10.7 percent and for group B 11.3 percent. The study failed to find a statistically significant difference between treatments. Three design problems may have impaired the study's ability to find a difference. First, patients with high-grade stenosis (>90 percent) were excluded. Second, the study called for intentional crossovers to surgery with asymptomatic progression of the stenosis. Third, the study may not have been powered to detect a small difference between groups. Because of these design problems, the absence of a significant difference between groups must be interpreted with caution.

The VA Cooperative Study entered 444 men with angiographically proven ≥50 percent asymptomatic carotid stenosis.[29] The study compared optimal medical treatment including antiplatelet medication (aspirin) plus carotid endarterectomy (n = 211) with optimal medical treatment alone (n = 233). All patients were given 1300 mg aspirin per day (although the dose was reduced if dose-related intolerance developed). All patients had an angiogram prior to entry. The angiographic complication rate was 0.5 percent. The surgical stroke or death rate was 4.3 percent. One of the big surprises in the study was that over 30 percent of the patients died during the 4-year follow-up, half from cardiac causes.[95,96] The primary endpoint was the combined incidence of ipsilateral TIA (including amaurosis fugax) or stroke. The incidence of all ipsilateral neurologic events was 8.0 percent in the surgical group and 20.6 percent in the medical group (p < .001), giving a relative risk for the surgical group vs. the medical group of 0.38 (95 percent confidence interval [CI], 0.22 to 0.67). The authors concluded that carotid endarterectomy, combined with optional medical management, can reduce the incidence of ipsilateral neurologic events in high-risk men with arteriographically confirmed asymptomatic carotid stenosis. The study showed no difference between groups when ipsilateral stroke was examined as the only end-

point. However, the study was not powered to find a difference in stroke as the only endpoint. Also, the high mortality rate may have lowered the stroke rate, potentially obscuring a difference between groups.

Each center in the Asymptomatic Carotid Atherosclerosis Study (ACAS) had to prove that it would be able to contribute 50 cases per year for 2 years, be able and willing to follow patients for 5 years, and have an angiographic morbidity <1 percent and angiographic mortality <0.1 percent.[97,98] Surgeons had to show evidence of a minimum of 12 endarterectomies per year with a combined neurologic morbidity and mortality rate no greater that 3 percent for asymptomatic patients and 5 percent for symptomatic patients.[99] Patients were considered eligible if they had at least one of the following: (1) angiogram within 60 days indicating ≥60 percent stenosis, (2) Doppler ultrasound within 60 days showing a frequency or velocity greater than the instrument-specific 95 percent positive predictive value for >60 percent stenosis, or (3) Doppler ultrasound within 60 days showing a frequency or velocity greater than the instrument-specific 90 percent positive predictive value for >60 percent stenosis confirmed by ocular pneumoplethysmography (OPG-Gee). Patients were excluded for one of the following: (1) clinical evidence of prior symptomatic cerebrovascular events in the study artery or in the vertebrobasilar circulation, (2) symptoms referable to the contralateral side in the prior 45 days, (3) contraindication to ASA therapy, (4) medical disorder that could complicate surgery, or be (5) medical condition that would prevent follow-up or be likely to produce death or disability within 5 years. Patients randomized to surgery based on noninvasive testing had postrandomization presurgery angiography. Surgery was canceled if the angiogram showed a stenosis measured <60 percent, a distal AVM, an aneurysm, or a siphon stenosis greater than proximal randomized stenosis. Of the 825 patients randomized to surgery, 104 did not undergo the operation. The reasons for not having the surgery included refusal to have surgery despite prior consent (45), angiogram showing <60 percent stenosis or significant intracranial stenosis (33), cardiac contraindications (12), and stroke prior to CEA (6). The patients randomized to the surgical group but not undergoing surgery were retained in the surgical arm for the analysis. In total, 1659 patients were entered. Initially, the study's main endpoints were ipsilateral TIA or stroke or perioperative TIA, stroke, or death. In March 1993, after the report of the VA Cooperative Study, the primary endpoints were changed to ipsilateral stroke or perioperative stroke or death. The study was stopped after an average follow-up of 2.7 years because a benefit from surgical management was demonstrated. Using the Kaplan-Meier estimation, it was projected that after 5 years, the surgical group would have a 5.1 percent risk of reaching an endpoint, whereas the medical group would have an 11 percent risk. This is an aggregate risk reduction of 53 percent (95 percent CI 22, 72). The benefit of surgery was apparent by 10 months and significant by 3 years. There was a gender difference with men having an absolute risk reduction of 8 percent and relative risk reduction of 66 percent compared with women with an absolute risk reduction of 1.4 percent and relative risk reduction of 17 percent. This difference was not significant (the study was not powered to find gender differences).

A common misconception about ACAS is that the study is flawed because there was only a median follow-up of 2.7 years rather than the originally planned 5 years.[100] It must be remembered that the study was terminated by the Data Safety and Monitoring Committee 7 years after it began because of the power of the results at that point in time (probability of error <0.05). The Kaplan-Meier method does not extrapolate or guess what will happen with patients in the future. Rather, each patient contributes data only for those intervals for which the patient was observed. ACAS followed 50 percent of patients for 2.7 years, 44 percent of patients for greater than 3 years, 26 percent for greater than 4 years, and 9 percent for the full 5 years.[101] This method of handling data from clinical trials is standard.[102] Another concern about the ACAS conclusions stems from the fact that approximately 30 percent of patients were not truly asymptomatic because they had a prior contralateral TIA, stroke, or CEA.[103] However, 70 percent were truly asymptomatic, and the relative risk reduction in this subgroup is nearly the same as in the entire group (46 percent vs. 53 percent).

Therapeutic Recommendations   Three of the four large prospective trials examining CEA in asymptomatic patients failed to show a significant benefit for surgery in the prevention of stroke. Each of these studies had serious design flaws that may have prevented showing a difference between treatments. ACAS did find a significant difference between treatments. The 53 percent relative risk reduction is impressive. However, this translates to a 1 percent per year absolute risk reduction in ipsilateral strokes. This means that 19 CEAs are needed to prevent one stroke of any severity. An important factor in achieving the positive results in this trial is the surgical stroke or death rate of less than 2 percent,

less than half that of the VA Coop trial and the CASA-NOVA trial. If the ACAS surgeons had a surgical stroke or death rate of 4.5 percent, benefit of surgery would not have been apparent until nearly 3 years, and significant reduction of risk would not have been achieved by 5 years.

The physician evaluating a patient with an asymptomatic stenosis needs to consider the surgical risk vs. stroke risk without surgery. In the VA study, patients with a history of coronary artery disease (CAD) had a significantly higher rate of neurologic complications from CEA than did those with no CAD history.[104] A history of peripheral vascular disease or angina significantly predicted serious complication from CEA in the asymptomatic patient (11 vs. 2 percent and 13 vs. 4 percent, respectively). In ACAS, history of diabetes (3.9 percent vs. 1.4 percent), contralateral siphon stenosis (15.4 vs. 1.4 percent), and never drinking (2.9 vs. 0.4 percent) were associated with significantly higher risk of perioperative stroke.[99] History of stroke (5.7 vs. 3.4 percent), contralateral stenosis of >60 percent (5.5 vs. 2.2 percent), contralateral siphon stenosis (15.4 vs. 3.1 percent), and never drinking (4.7 vs. 1.5 percent) predicted a significantly higher risk of any perioperative complication. Neither study found age to be a significant risk factor for CEA complication. Because of the rigorous selection criteria for patients entering these studies and because of the relatively small number of complications in each study, it is difficult to generalize from these findings. It may be wise to be more cautious in recommending surgery for a patient with several of these risk factors as compared with the patient with none.

Before recommending CEA, the treating physician should also evaluate the radiologist, the surgeon, and the operative team. If the asymptomatic patient is to have potential benefit from surgery, a cerebrovascular team must be selected who can perform vascular imaging, CEA, and perioperative care with <3 percent stroke or mortality.

Based on the ACAS results, if a patient has an acceptable surgical risk (<3 percent), is likely to survive long enough to get benefit from the surgery (>3 years), and the radiological/surgical team can perform the procedure at a proven low risk, CEA is considered proven appropriate for asymptomatic patients with angiographically measured stenosis at ≥60 percent.[105] The surgery is neither urgent nor mandatory. The patient should be informed that the benefit of the surgery, although statistically significant, is small in absolute terms (1 percent per year). Aggressive management of medical risk factors is mandatory, whether or not the patient proceeds with surgical intervention.[95]

Cigarette Smoking

Early studies on the association between cigarette smoking and stroke reported variable results. The Framingham Study, in a multivariate analysis, found that when hypertension and age were taken into account, smoking is a significant risk factor.[106] It is a more important risk factor at younger ages.[107,108] Howard and colleagues reported an ordered association of smoking with silent cerebral infarction, with nonsmokers < nonsmokers exposed to environmental smoke < former smokers < current smokers.[109] In a prospective study of 7735 men, Wannamethee and colleagues found benefit to stopping smoking, with light smokers dropping to the level of nonsmokers and heavy smokers dropping to about a twofold risk of nonsmokers in 5 years.[110] The benefit was greatest in hypertensive patients.

With the data now available, it is clear that cigarette smoking is a well-documented modifiable risk factor for ischemic infarction. Patients at risk for stroke should be given assistance in smoking cessation.

Alcohol Use and Abuse

The relationship between alcohol consumption and stroke risk is complex, with risk associated with heavy use differing from light use. There may be racial differences in regard to alcohol risk and stroke.

Palomaki and colleagues found a protective effect of light alcohol use, with ≤50 g per week reducing the risk of ischemic stroke.[111] Haapaniemi and colleagues found that heavy drinking was more common in patients under the age of 60 years with infarction than in controls. Light to moderate drinking before the illness did not increase the risk, whereas heavy (>120 g/day ethanol) drinking did (RR 7.57, 95 percent CI 1.97, 29.10).[112] You and colleagues also found heavy alcohol use to be a significant risk but did not find that heavy ingestion the day before the stroke a risk.[113] Although the data are not completely clear, it is reasonable to recommend avoiding heavy alcohol consumption as a measure of stroke risk reduction.

Physical Activity

Regular exercise is known to be beneficial for general health and has been shown to reduce the risk of cardiovascular disease. Exercise has the potential for decreasing blood pressure, reducing obesity, and improving glucose homeostasis, each of which should help reduce stroke risk. Studies looking for an association between exercise and reduced stroke risk have produced mixed results. Sacco and colleagues studied the leisure activities of 369 patients with first stroke and 678 case-control subjects.[114] Controlling for other risk factors, they found a significant protective effect of physical activity in younger and older patients, men and women, and in each ethnic group studied. In the older patients, even light to moderate exercise was protective. The Harvard Alumni Health Study prospectively followed 11,130 alumni over an 11-year period.[115] They found that energy expenditure up to 3000 kcal/week was associated with reduced stroke risk in men. Other studies have failed to find a benefit in reducing the ischemic stroke risk.

The results of case-control studies and prospective trials have given mixed results. An evidence-based recommendation cannot be made. However, in view of the low cost and low risk of the intervention, instituting a program of progressive physical activity as part of a risk reduction program after stroke is a reasonable recommendation.

Homocysteine

Homocysteine is a sulfur-containing amino acid formed during the metabolism of methionine.[116] Hyperhomocysteinemia has been associated with increased risk of atherosclerosis, heart attack, and stroke. The Physicians' Health Study measured homocysteine levels and prospectively followed subjects for 5 years. Elevated homocysteine levels were associated with increased risk of MI during follow-up.[117] Using carotid stenosis of ≥25 percent as a marker, Selhub and colleagues reported high plasma homocysteine levels and low concentrations of folate and vitamin B_6 associated with carotid disease.[118] In a meta-analysis of case-control studies and population studies, Boushey and colleagues found that elevated homocysteine levels are associated with increased risk of heart disease and stroke and act independently of other risk factors.[119] Folate, vitamin B_6, and vitamin B_{12} supplementation can lower homocysteine levels. It is not known if this type of supplementation will lower vascular outcomes. Until the results of clinical trials are available, no evidence-based recommendations can be made. However, considering the benign nature of vitamin supplementation, it is reasonable to recommend supplemental vitamins in stroke patients with elevated homocysteine levels.

REFERENCES

1. Schafer AI: Antiplatelet therapy. *Am J Med* 101:199, 1996.
2. Sharis PJ, Cannon CP, Loscalzo J: The antiplatelet effects of ticlopidine and clopidogrel. *Ann Intern Med* 129:394, 1998.
3. Ponzillo J, Chow M: Focus on ticlopidine: A platelet aggregation inhibitor for stroke prophylaxis. *Hosp Formul* 25:517, 1990.
4. Bousser MG, Roberts RS, Gent M: Ticlopidine and clopidogrel in secondary stroke prevention. *Cerebrovasc Dis* 7(Suppl 6):17, 1997.
5. Boneu B, Destelle G: Platelet anti-aggregating activity and tolerance of clopidogrel in atherosclerotic patients. *Thromb Haemost* 76:939, 1996.
6. Arky R: *Physicians' Desk Reference.* Montvale, Medical Economics Company 1999, 3477.
7. Schafer AI: Antiplatelet therapy with glycoprotein IIb/IIIa receptor inhibitors and other novel agents. *Txa Heart Inst J* 24:90, 1997.
8. Chesebro JH, Badimon JJ: Platelet glycoprotein IIb/IIIa receptor blockade in unstable coronary disease. *N Engl J Med* 338:1439, 1998.
9. The platelet receptor inhibition in ischemic syndrome management study investigators: A comparison of aspirin plus tirofiban with aspirin plus heparin for unstable angina. *N Engl J Med* 338:1498, 1998.
10. The platelet receptor inhibition in ischemic syndrome management in patients limited by unstable signs and symptoms study investigators: Inhibition of the platelet glycoprotein IIb/IIIa receptor with tirofiban in unstable angina and non-Q-wave myocardial infarction. *N Engl J Med* 338:1488, 1998.
11. Fields WS, Lemak NA, Frankowski RF, Hardy RJ: Controlled trial of aspirin in cerebral ischemia. *Stroke* 8:301, 1977.
12. Canadian Cooperative Study Group: A randomized trial of aspirin and sulfinpyrazone in threatened stroke. *N Engl J Med* 299:53, 1978.
13. Bousser MG, Eschwege E, Hagenah M, et al: "AICLA" controlled trial of aspirin and dipyridamole in the secondary prevention of athero-thrombotic cerebral ischemia. *Stroke* 14:5, 1983.
14. Diener H, Cunha L, Forbes C, et al: European Stroke Prevention Study: 2. Dipyridamole and acetylsalicylic acid in the secondary prevention of stroke (see Comments). *J Neurol Sci* 143:1, 1996.
15. Sorensen PS, Pedersen H, Marquardsen J, et al: Acetylsalicylic acid in the prevention of stroke in patients with reversible cerebral ischemic attacks. *Stroke* 14:15, 1983.
16. Swedish Cooperative Study: High-dose acetylsalicylic acid after cerebral infarction. *Stroke* 18:325, 1987.
17. Boysen G, Sorensen S, Juhler M, et al: Danish very-low-dose aspirin after carotid endarterectomy trial. *Stroke* 19:1211, 1988.
18. UK-TIA Study Group: United Kingdom transient ischaemic attack (UK-TIA) aspirin trial: Interim results. *Br Med J* 296:316, 1988.
19. SALT Collaborative Group: Swedish Aspirin Low-Dose Trial (SALT) of 75 mg aspirin as secondary prophylaxis after cerebrovascular ischaemic events (see Comments). *Lancet* 338:1345, 1991.
20. Antiplatelet Trialists' Collaboration: Secondary prevention of vascular disease by prolonged antiplatelet treatment. *Br Med J* 296:320, 1988.
21. Sze PC, Reitman D, Pincus MM, et al: Antiplatelet agents in the secondary prevention of stroke: Meta-analysis of the randonized control trials. *Stroke* 19:436, 1988.
22. Gelmers H, Tijssen J: Platelet antiaggregants in secondary prevention after stroke: Does dipyridamole add to the effect of aspirin? J Stroke Cerebrovasc Dis 3:115, 1993.
23. Tijssen JG: Low-dose and high-dose acetylsalicylic acid, with and without dipyridamole: A review of clinical trial results. *Neurology* 51(Suppl 3):S15, 1998.
24. Antiplatelet Trialists' Collaboration: Collaborative overview of randomised trials of antiplatelet therapy 3: I. Prevention of death, myocardial infarction, and stroke by prolonged antiplatelet therapy in various categories of patients. *Br Med J* 308:81, 1994.
25. Dyken ML, Barnett HJM, Baston JD, et al: Low-dose aspirin and stroke. *Stroke* 23:1395, 1992.
26. Barnett HJM, Kaste M, Meldrum H, Elisasziw M: Aspirin dose in stroke prevention: Beautiful hypothesis slain by ugly facts. *Stroke* 27:588, 1996.
27. Hart RG, Rohack JJ, Solomon DH, Feinberg WM: What's new in stroke? *Tx Med* 91:46, 1995.
28. Dutch TIA Trial Study Group: A comparison of two doses of aspirin (30 mg vs. 283 mg a day) in patients after a transient ischemic attack or minor ischemic stroke (see Comments). *N Engl J Med* 325:1261, 1991.
29. Hobson RW, Weiss DG, Fields WS, et al: Efficacy of carotid endarterectomy for asymptomatic carotid stenosis: The Veterans Affairs Cooperative Study Group. *N Engl J Med* 328:221, 1993.
30. Krupski WC, Weiss DG, Rapp JH, et al: Adverse effects of aspirin in the treatment of asymptomatic carotid artery stenosis: The VA Cooperative Asymptomatic Carotid Artery Stenosis Study Group. *J Vasc Surg* 16:588, 1992. Discussion, 597.
31. Barnett HJ, Taylor DW, Eliasziw M, et al: Benefit of carotid endarterectomy in patients with symptomatic moderate or severe stenosis: North American Symptomatic Carotid Endarterectomy Trial Collaborators (see Comments). *N Engl J Med* 339:1415, 1998.
32. Taylor DW, Barnett HJM, Haynes RB, et al: Low-dose and high-dose acetyl salicylic acid for patients undergoing carotid endarterectomy. A randomized controlled trial. *Lancet* 353:2179, 1999.
33. Roderick J, Wilkes HC, Meade TW: The gastrointestinal toxicity of aspirin: An overview of randomized controlled trials. *J Clin Pharmacol* 35:219, 1993.

34. North American Symptomatic Carotid Endarterectomy Trial Collaborators: Beneficial effect of carotid endarterectomy in symptomatic patients with high grade stenosis. *N Engl J Med* 325:445, 1991.

35. CAPRIE Steering Committee: A randomized blinded trial of clopidogrel versus aspirin in patients at risk of ischaemic events (CAPRIE). *Lancet* 348:1329, 1996.

36. Gent M, Blakely JA, Easton, JD, et al: The Canadian American ticlopidine strudy (CATS) in thromboembolic stroke. *Lancet* 1:1215, 1989.

37. Hass WK, Easton JD, Adams HP, et al: A randomized trial comparing ticlopidine hydrochloride with aspirin for the prevention of stroke in high-risk patients. *N Engl J Med* 321:501, 1989.

38. Ticlopidine Aspirin Study Group: Ticlopidine versus aspirin for stroke prevention: On-treatment results from the ticlopidine aspirin stroke study. *J Stroke Cerebrovasc Dis* 3:168, 1993.

39. Hass WK, Molony, BA, Anderson S, Kamm B: Comparison of ticlopidine and aspirin for the prevention of stroke (Letter). *N Engl J Med* 322:405, 1990.

40. Bennett CL, Weinberg PD, Rozenberg-Ben-Dror K, et al: Thrombotic thrombocytopenic purpura associated with ticlopidine. *Ann Intern Med* 128:541, 1998.

41. Grotta JC, Norris JW, Kamm B: Prevention of stroke with ticlopidine: Who benefits most? TASS Baseline and Angiographic Data Subgroup. *Neurology* 42:111, 1992.

42. Harbison J, Ticlopidine Aspirin Study Group: Ticlopidine versus aspirin for the prevention of recurrent stroke. *Stroke* 23:1723, 1992.

43. Weisberg L, Ticlopidine Aspirin Study Group: The efficacy and safety of ticlopidine and aspirin in non-whites: Analysis of a patient subgroup from the Ticlopidine Aspirin Stroke Study. *Neurology* 43:27, 1993.

44. van Gijn J, Algra A: Ticlopidine, trials, and torture (Editorial: Comment). *Stroke* 25:1097, 1994.

45. American-Canadian Co-Operative Study Group: Persantine aspirin trial in cerebral ischemia: Part II. Endpoint results. *Stroke* 16:406, 1985.

46. European Stroke Prevention Study Group: European stroke prevention study. *Stroke* 21:1122, 1990.

47. Guiraud-Chaumeil B, Rascol A, David J, et al: Prevention des recidives des accidents vasculaires cerebraux ischemiques par les anti-agregants plaquettaires. *Rev Neurol (Paris)* 138:367, 1982.

48. Diener HC: Dipyridamole trials in stroke prevention. *Neurology* 51 (Suppl 3):S17, 1998.

49. Sivenius J, Laakso M, Penttila IM, et al: The European Stroke Prevention Study: Results according to sex. *Neurology* 41:1189, 1991.

50. Enserink M: Fraud and ethics charges hit stroke drug trial (news) (see Comments). *Science* 274:2004, 1996.

51. Mashur F, Bursch M, Einhaupl KM: Differences in medical and surgical therapy for stroke prevention between leading experts in North America and Western Europe. *Stroke* 29:339, 1998.

52. Chimowitz MI, Kokkinos J, Strong J, et al: The Warfarin-Aspirin Symptomatic Intracranial Disease Study. *Neurology* 45:1488, 1995.

53. The Stroke Prevention in Reversible Ischemia Trial Study Group: A randomized trial of anticoagulants versus aspirin after cerebral ischemia of presumed arterial origin. *Ann Neurol* 42:857, 1997.

54. Moore W: Technique of carotid endarterectomy, in Moore W (ed): *Surgery for Cerebrovascular Disease,* New York, Churchill Livingstone, 1987, pp 491–502.

55. Dyken M, Pokras R: The performance of endarterectomy for disease of the extracranial arteries of the head. *Stroke* 13:948, 1984.

56. Tu JV, Hannan EL, Anderson GM, et al: The fall and rise of carotid endarterectomy in the United States and Canada (see Comments). *N Engl J Med* 339:1441, 1998.

57. Fields WS, Maslenikov V, Meyer JS, et al: Joint study of extracranial arterial occlusion: V. Progress report of prognosis following surgery or nonsurgical treatment for transient cerebral ischemic attacks and cervical carotid artery lesions. *JAMA* 211:1993, 1970.

58. Merrick NJ, Brook RH, Fink A, Solomon DH: Use of carotid endarterectomy in five California Veterans Administration medical centers. *JAMA* 256:2531, 1986.

59. European Carotid Surgery Trialists Group: MRC European Carotid Surgery Trial: Interim results for symptomatic patients with severe (70–99%) or with mild (0–29%) carotid stenosis. *Lancet* 337:1235, 1991.

60. European Carotid Surgery Trialists Collaborative Group: Randomised trial of endarterectomy for recently symptomatic carotid stenosis: Final results of the MRC European Carotid Surgery Trial (ECST). *Lancet* 351:1379, 1998.

61. North American Symptomatic Carotid Endarterectomy Trial Steering Committee: North American Symptomatic Carotid Endarterectomy Trial. *Stroke* 22:711, 1991.

62. European Carotid Surgery Trialists Collaborative Group: Endarterectomy for moderate symptomatic carotid stenosis: Interim results from the MRC European Carotid Surgery Trial. *Lancet* 347:1591, 1996.

63. Eliasziw M, Streifler JY, Fox AJ, et al: Significance of plaque ulceration in symptomatic patients with high-grade carotid stenosis: North American Symptomatic Carotid Endarterectomy Trial. *Stroke* 25:304, 1994.

64. Streifler JY, Eliasziw M, Benavente OR, et al: The risk of stroke in patients with first-ever retinal vs hemispheric transient ischemic attacks and high-grade carotid stenosis: North American Symptomatic Carotid Endarterectomy Trial. *Arch Neurol* 52:246, 1995.

65. Gasecki AP, Eliasziw M, Ferguson GG, et al: Long term prognosis and effect of endarterectomy in patients with symptomatic severe carotid stenosis and contralateral carotid stenosis or occlusion: Results from NASCET. *J Neurosurg* 83:778, 1995.

66. Morgenstern LB, Fox AJ, Sharpe BL, et al: The risks and benefits of carotid endarterectomy in patients with near

occlusion of the carotid artery: North American Symptomatic Carotid Endarterectomy Trial (NASCET) Group. *Neurology* 48:911, 1997.

67. Mayberg MR, Wilson SE, Yatsu F, et al: Carotid endarterectomy and prevention of cerebral ischemia in symptomatic carotid stenosis. *JAMA* 266:3289, 1991.

68. Goldstein LB, Hasselblad V, Matchar DB, McCrory DC: Comparison and meta-analysis of randomized trials of endarterectomy for symptomatic carotid artery stenosis. *Neurology* 45:1965, 1995.

69. Sundt TM, Sandock BA, Whisnan JP: Carotid endarterectomy: Complications and preoperative assessment of risk. *Mayo Clin Proc* 50:301, 1975.

70. Goldstein LB, McCrory DC, Landsman PB, et al: Multicenter review of preoperative risk factors for carotid endarterectomy in patients with ipsilateral symptoms. *Stroke* 25:1116, 1994.

71. Hsia DC, Moscoe LM, Krushat WM: Epidemiology of carotid endarterectomy among Medicare beneficiaries: 1985-1996 update. *Stroke* 29:346, 1998.

72. Wong JH, Findlay JM, Suarez-Almazor ME: Regional performance of carotid endarterectomy: Appropriateness, outcomes, and risk factors for complications. *Stroke* 28:891, 1997.

73. Ruby ST, Robinson RN, Lynch JT, Mark H: Outcome analysis of carotid endarterectomy in Connecticut: The impact of volume and specialty. *Ann Vasc Surg* 10:22, 1996.

74. Hannan EL, Popp AJ, Tranmer B, et al: Relationship between provider volume and mortality for carotid endarterectomies in New York state. *Stroke* 29:2292, 1998.

75. Blaisdell WF, Clauss RH, Galbraith JG, et al: Joint Study of Extracranial Arterial Occlusion: IV. A review of surgical considerations. *JAMA* 209:1889, 1969.

76. Caplan LR, Skillman J, Ojemann R, Fields WS: Intracerebral hemorrhage following carotid endarterectomy: A hypertensive complication? *Stroke* 9:457, 1978.

77. Piotrowski JJ, Bernhard VM, Rubin JR, et al: Timing of carotid endarterectomy after acute stroke. *J Vasc Surg* 11:45, 1990.

78. Gasecki AP, Ferguson GG, Eliasziw M, et al: Early endarterectomy for severe carotid artery stenosis after a nondisabling stroke: Results from the North American Symptomatic Carotid Endarterectomy Trial. *J Vasc Surg* 20:288, 1994.

79. Hart RG, Sherman DG, Easton JD, Cairns JA: Prevention of stroke in patients with nonvalvular atrial fibrillation. *Neurology* 51:674, 1998.

80. Hachniski V: The issue is standards, not techniques. *Arch Neurol* 52:834, 1995.

81. Strandness DE: Angiography before carotid endarterectomy: No. *Arch Neurol* 52:832, 1995.

82. Barnett HJM, Eliaziw M, Meldrum HE: The identification by imaging methods of patients who might benefit from carotid endarterectomy. *Arch Neurol* 52:827, 1995.

83. Pritz MB: Timing of carotid endarterectomy after stroke. *Stroke* 28:2563, 1997.

84. Goldstein LB, Moore WS, Robertson JT, Chaturvedi S: Complication rates for carotid endarterectomy: A call to action (Editorial). *Stroke* 28:889, 1997.

85. Joseph LN, Babikian VL, Allen NC, Winter MR: Risk factor modification in stroke prevention. *Stroke* 30:16, 1999.

86. Sacco RL, Benjamin EJ, Broderick JP, et al: Risk factors. *Stroke* 28:1507, 1997.

87. Thompson JE, Patman RD, Talkington CM: Asymptomatic carotid bruit: Long term outcome of patients having endarterectomy compared with unoperated controls. *Ann Surg* 188:308, 1978.

88. Humphreys DM: Antiplatelet therapy in ischaemic events (Letter; Comment). *Lancet* 349:1914, 1997.

89. Thompson J, Austin D, Patman R: Carotid endarterectomy for cerebrovascular insufficiency: Long term results in 592 patients followed up at thirteen years. *Surg Clin North Am* 66:233, 1986.

90. Fode NC, Sundt TM, Robertson JT, et al: Multicenter retrospective review of results and complications of carotid endarterectomy in 1981. *Stroke* 17:370, 1986.

91. Brott T, Thalinger K: The practice of carotid endarterectomy in a large metropolitan area. *Stroke* 15:950, 1984.

92. Easton J, Sherman D: Stroke and mortality rate in carotid endarterectomy: 228 consecutive operations. *Stroke* 8:565, 1977.

93. Mayo Asymptomatic Carotid Endarterectomy Study Group: Results of a randomized controlled trial of carotid endarterectomy for asymptomatic carotid stenosis: Mayo Asymptomatic Carotid Endarterectomy Study Group. *Mayo Clin Proc* 67:513, 1992.

94. CASANOVA Study Group: Carotid surgery versus medical therapy in asymptomatic carotid stenosis. *Stroke* 22:1229, 1991.

95. Chimowitz MI, Weiss DG, Cohen SN, et al:, Cardiac prognosis of patients with carotid stenosis and no history of coronary artery disease: Veterans Affairs Cooperative Study Group 167. *Stroke* 25:759, 1994.

96. Cohen SN, Hobson RW, Weiss DG, Chimowitz M: Death associated with asymptomatic carotid artery stenosis: Long-term clinical evaluation. VA Cooperative Study 167 Group. *J Vasc Surg* 18:1002, 1993. Discussion, 1009.

97. Executive Committee for the Asymptomatic Carotid Atherosclerosis Study: Endarterectomy for asymptomatic carotid artery stenosis. *JAMA* 273:1421, 1995.

98. Asymptomatic Carotid Atherosclerosis Study Group: Study design for randomized prospective trial of carotid endarterectomy for asymptomatic atherosclerosis. *Stroke* 20:844, 1989.

99. Young B, Moore WS, Robertson JT, et al: An analysis of perioperative surgical mortality and morbidity in the asymptomatic carotid atherosclerosis study. *Stroke* 27:2216, 1996.

100. Foster D: Endarterectomy for asymptomatic carotid artery stenosis (Letter). *JAMA* 274:1505, 1995.

101. Toole J, ACAS Executive Committee: Endarterectomy for asymptomatic carotid stenosis (Letter). *JAMA* 274: 1506, 1995.

102. Kalbleisch J, Prentice R: *The Statistical Analysis of Failure Time Data.* New York, John Wiley & Sons, Inc., 1980.

103. Hennerici M, Daffertshofer M, Meairs S: Concerns about generalisation of premature ACAS recommendations for carotid endarterectomy. *Lancet* 346:1041, 1995.

104. Cohen SN, Weiss DG, Chimowitz MI, et al: Preoperative prediction of complication in carotid endarterectomy (CEA). *Neurology* 44:A128, 1994.

105. Biller J, Feinberg MW, Castaldo JE, et al: Guidelines for carotid endarterectomy: A statement for healthcare professionals from a Special Writing Group of the Stroke Council, American Heart Association. *Circulation* 97:501, 1998.

106. Wolf PA, D'Agostino RB, Kannel WB, et al: Cigarette smoking as a risk factor for stroke. *JAMA* 259:1025, 1988.

107. Love BB, Biller J, Jones MP, et al: Cigarette smoking: A risk factor for cerebral infarction in young adults. *Arch Neurol* 47:693, 1990.

108. Shinton R, Beevers G: Meta-analysis of relation between cigarette smoking and stroke. *Br Med J* 298:789, 1989.

109. Howard G, Wagenknecht LE, Cai J, et al: Cigarette smoking and other risk factors for silent cerebral infarction in the general population. *Stroke* 29:913, 1998.

110. Wannamethee SG, Shaper AG, Whincup PH, et al: Smoking cessation and the risk of stroke in middle-aged men. *JAMA* 274:155, 1995.

111. Palomaki H, Kaste M, Raininko R, et al: Risk factors for cervical atherosclerosis in patients with transient ischemic attack or minor ischemic stroke. *Stroke* 24:970, 1993.

112. Haapaniemi H, Hillbom M, Juvela S: Lifestyle-associated risk factors for acute brain infarction among persons of working age. *Stroke* 28:26, 1997.

113. You RX, McNeill JJ, O'Malley HM, et al: Risk factors for stroke due to cerebral infarction in young adults. *Stroke* 28:1913, 1997.

114. Sacco RL, Gan R, Boden-Albala B, et al: Leisure-time physical activity and ischemic stroke risk. *Stroke* 29:380, 1998.

115. Lee I, Paffenbarger RS: Physical activity and stroke incidence: The Harvard Alumni Health Study. *Stroke* 29:2049, 1998.

116. Welch GN, Loscalzo J: Homocysteine and atherosclerosis. *N Engl J Med* 338:1042, 1998.

117. Stampfer MJ, Malinow MR, Willett WC: A prospective study of plasma homocyst(e)ine and risk of myocardial infarction in US physicians. *JAMA* 268:877, 1992.

118. Selhub J, Jacques PF, Boston AG, et al: Association between plasma homocysteine concentrations and extracranial carotid artery stenosis. *N Engl J Med* 332:286, 1995.

119. Boushey CJ, Beresford AA, Omenn GS, Motulsky, AG: A quantitative assessment of plasma homocysteine as a risk factor for vascular disease. *JAMA* 274:1049, 1995.

120. Albers GW, Easton JD, Sacco AL, Teal P, et al: Antithrombotic and thrombolytic therapy for ischemic stroke. *Chest* 114:683S, 1998.

121. Cohen SN: Antiplatelet drugs in patients with carotid bifurcation disease. *Semin Vasc Surg* 8:2, 1995.

Chapter 5

THE SUBACUTE STROKE PATIENT: GLUCOSE MANAGEMENT

Sangeeta Rao Kashyap
Seymour R. Levin

BACKGROUND

Introduction

Hyperglycemia is observed in at least 30 percent of patients with acute cerebral infarction.[1] The hyperglycemic reaction in acute stroke may be attributed to several etiologies. These include: a nonspecific reaction to acute stress and tissue injury, uncovering of underlying diabetes by the acute stroke, previously known diabetes, and iatrogenic causes such as the administration of steroids and dextrose infusion at the onset of acute stroke. The prevalence of previously unrecognized diabetes diagnosed by elevated glycosylated hemoglobin level during stroke is high and varies widely from 6 to 42 percent.[2] Melamed reported a higher incidence of "stress hyperglycemia" in patients with brainstem infarction and hemorrhagic stroke as compared with ischemic hemispheric infarction.[3]

The effect of hyperglycemia on the outcome of stroke is believed by some to be detrimental. However, the data are not consistent, and this is a topic of debate. Additionally, very little is known about postischemic hyperglycemia on the outcome of stroke. Hypoglycemia in the setting of acute stroke may exacerbate neuronal injury,[4] although there are some animal data that suggest it may improve neurologic outcome during cerebral ischemia.[5]

This chapter will provide management strategies for hyperglycemia of various causes in the setting of acute and chronic stroke. However, we will first discuss the significance of hyperglycemia in the setting of acute stroke followed by the pathophysiology of cerebral ischemia under hyperglycemic conditions. There will also be a brief discussion of hypoglycemia in the setting of stroke.

Epidemiology and Prognosis

Epidemiologic and postmortem studies show that diabetic patients have a higher incidence of ischemic stroke than nondiabetic patients. In the Framingham Study, the incidence of thrombotic stroke was 2.5 times higher in diabetic men and 3.6 times higher in diabetic women than in those without diabetes.[6] Palumbo and colleagues reported that the frequencies of transient ischemic attacks and stroke in patients with diabetes were 3.0 and 1.7 times greater, respectively, than those in nondiabetic patients.[7] In addition to the diabetic population, patients with impaired glucose tolerance also have a higher prevalence of stroke. In the prospective Honolulu Heart Study, patients with serum glucose >120 mg/dL after a 50-g glucose load had an increased prevalence of thromboembolic stroke.[8]

Once patients with diabetes experience a stroke, they have a worse outcome than do nondiabetics. Several studies have shown an increase in short- and long-term mortality in the diabetic patient who has had a cerebral ischemic event. The increased morbidity seems to be related not only to the predisposing metabolic status but also on the initial glucose level.[9] In most studies, the cut-off point is a serum glucose of 120 mg/dL. A study from England showed that only in those patients with a presenting blood glucose of <120 mg/dL did complete recovery of the hemiparesis occur within

4 weeks, and none of those with a presenting serum glucose >120 mg/dL had complete recovery of the hemiparesis within that time.[10] Pulsinelli and colleagues showed, in diabetic patients <65 years of age, a higher percentage of those with a random serum glucose <120 mg/dL returned to work when compared with those with a glucose >120 mg/dL.[11]

Pathophysiology of Cerebral Ischemia in Hyperglycemic Conditions

A number of pathophysiologic events occur in an area of cerebral ischemia. Cerebral ischemia leads to energy depletion, decrease of adenosine triphosphate (ATP) levels, and loss of ion homeostasis with intracellular accumulation of calcium, sodium, chloride, and osmotically obligated water.[25] There are three possible explanations for the worsening of stroke damage in the presence of hyperglycemia. The first is that under hypoxic conditions caused by a stroke, glucose is metabolized by anaerobic glycolysis that produces lactic acid. Lactic acid accumulates and results in damage to neuronal, glial, and vascular tissue. It is probable that the production of lactic acid in the ischemic area is augmented by changes in the blood-brain barrier or at the cell membranes of neurons and glial cells that allow an increase in glucose delivery to the cell.

The second potential explanation is that during conditions of hyperglycemic ischemia, the extracellular concentration of the neurotransmitters glutamate and aspartate is increased, which activates neurons and increases injury.[25] The increase in these neurotransmitters is due to excessive release combined with a failure of energy-dependent reuptake.

The third theory is that with hyperglycemic ischemia and neuronal hyperstimulation, an increase occurs in intracellular calcium, which may cause neuronal damage. Additionally, severe hyperglycemia may cause depletion of water and electrolytes, leading to cardiac arrhythmias and infarction, which in turn may exacerbate cerebral ischemia.

A number of possible changes may occur in the area of cerebral ischemia in hyperglycemic compared with normoglycemic conditions: (1) elevation of cerebral lactate levels, (2) decreased local glucose metabolism, (3) ion metabolic disturbance, and (4) changes of blood-brain barrier function. The relative importance of each of these remains speculative because there are few human studies of brain biochemical changes after acute stroke.

EVIDENCE

Laboratory Studies

Animal models of cerebral infarction suggest that glucose is an important modulator of brain injury during ischemia. In these models, induced hyperglycemia augments ischemic damage as evidenced by clinical signs and neuropathologic changes and is associated with impaired postischemic cerebral perfusion. Campbell first demonstrated that if rats were fed a diet of low carbohydrates, they survived hypoxia longer than rats fed a normal diet.[12] Craven et al reported similar protection against hypoxia in fasted rats and concluded that weight loss and carbohydrate depletion were responsible for the better neurologic outcome.[13] Myers and Yamaguchi demonstrated that animals made hyperglycemic before cerebral ischemia suffered greater neurologic deficits, more severe morphologic brain damage, and had poor recovery of glucose metabolism than normoglycemic controls.[14] Pulsinelli et al demonstrated that glucose given before onset of ischemia was followed by severe brain injury, with necrosis of the majority of neocortical neurons and glia, substantial neuronal damage through the remainder of forebrain, and severe brain edema as compared with rats given saline before induction of ischemia.[15] Despite numerous reports from animal data of worse neurologic outcome with hyperglycemia, this finding has not been consistent. Models of end-artery infarction suggest that glucose may diminish stroke severity.[16]

Clinical Studies

Clinical studies also indicate an adverse effect on outcome when cerebral ischemia occurs in the setting of hyperglycemia. Davalos demonstrated that peri-ischemic hyperglycemia in either diabetic or nondiabetic patients was associated with a significant increase in mortality in comparison with normoglycemia.[17] Longsteth and colleagues performed a retrospective analysis of 389 consecutive patients who were successfully resuscitated after out-of-hospital cardiac arrest.[18] In this patient population, hyperglycemia (defined as a blood glucose concentration of 300 mg/dL or higher) at the time of hospital admission correlated with a low probability of awakening. In a subsequent study, Longsteth and Inui retrospectively evaluated neurologic outcome of 430 consecutive patients who were resuscitated after out-of-hospital cardiac arrest.[19] All received infusions of 5% glucose before hospital admission. At admission, mean blood glucose values from patients who did not awaken after cardiac arrest were significantly higher than those in patients who did awaken. Of patients who awakened, those with persistent neurologic deficits had a significantly greater mean blood concentration at admission than did patients without deficits. The problem with the above studies is that due to the retrospective analysis of the studies, they do not determine a direct causal link between hyperglycemia and neurologic outcome. They also did not account for other contributing factors that may have led to poor outcome.

Some studies compared mortality rates in three groups of patients: (1) those with previously known or newly diagnosed diabetes, (2) those with transitory hyperglycemia without diabetes, and (3) those with normoglycemia. Candelise et al found mortality was higher in hyperglycemic patients with no history of diabetes mellitus (78 percent) than in diabetic (45 percent) or in normoglycemic nondiabetic patients (29 percent) who sufffered acute hemispheric stroke.[20] Reactive hyperglycemia, due to a major stress response, accounts for the worse prognosis. Kiers et al found that among patients who suffered an acute stroke, transient hyperglycemia was more often present in patients who suffered a hemorrhagic stroke than an ischemic stroke.[21] Woo et al showed that a high fasting glucose level was associated with an increased mortality, but this was observed only among patients with intracerebral hemorrhage as opposed to ischemic infarction. He concluded from his study, as did the above two authors, that the association between glucose concentration and stroke outcome is a reflection of stress relating to stroke severity rather than a direct harmful effect of glucose on damaged neurons.[22]

The above studies suggest that hyperglycemia may not be independently correlated to stroke outcome but may be a marker of stroke severity and tissue injury and, in this way, indicates a poor prognosis. Thus, although some experimental and clinical studies have found a relationship between the level of glycemia and outcome of stroke, the relationship may not be a causal one. Matchar et al, in a prospective, multicenter cohort study, found no association between level of glycemia and outcome from acute stroke.[23] In the past, it was recommended to keep surgical patients at high risk for perioperative ischemia euglycemic (blood glucose less than 120 mg/dL). However, largely due to this study and the previous studies discussed above, this is no longer the current teaching. Furthermore, there are no clinical studies on the additional risk of hypoglycemia on cerebral ischemia. Some animal data suggest that hypoglycemia induced with insulin may lessen the severity of stroke[24]; however, it is unclear whether this is due to the direct effects of insulin on ischemic tissue or hypoglycemia.

THERAPEUTIC RECOMMENDATIONS

Glucose Management in Acute Stroke

Because there are no prospective randomized trials on glucose control in the poststroke period, our recommendations are Grade C, based on Level V evidence and based on principles to avoid extreme hyperglycemia and hypoglycemia (Fig. 5-1). During the acute and subacute stroke periods (i.e., the first 24 to 48 h after the onset of neurologic deficits), it is not necessary to keep patients euglycemic because, as discussed above, the data regarding the effect of hyperglycemia on stroke outcome are still unclear. Early identification of glucose levels in patients who have a stroke is critical. Care should be taken to identify and, if possible, avoid unwanted sources of hyperglycemia, including physiologic stress and indiscriminate use of corticosteroid drugs. For the patient with known diabetes on either oral agents or insulin, we consider the ideal blood glucose concentration to be 100 to 250 mg/dL. Patients with serial blood glucose levels greater than 300 mg/dL and with ischemic neurologic deficits should be placed in an intensive care setting for frequent blood glucose monitoring every 1 to 2 h. It should be determined whether diabetic ketoacidosis exists by measuring serum ketones and serum pH levels. Patients with serum glucose levels usually greater than 300 mg/dL should be started on an insulin drip at an initial rate of 1 unit/h. The infusion should be titrated 1 to 1.5 units/h with the goal of reducing glucose at a rate of about 60 to 90 mg/dL/h. Care must be taken to reduce the insulin infusion by 50 percent and starting IV dextrose when the serum glucose level reaches 150 mg/dL to avoid hypoglycemia. Excessively rapid correction of blood glucose may induce cerebral edema and induce osmotic injury to the brain.[26] In addition to reducing glucose levels, the fluid and electrolytic status of the patient needs to be determined and deficiencies replaced as deemed appropriate.

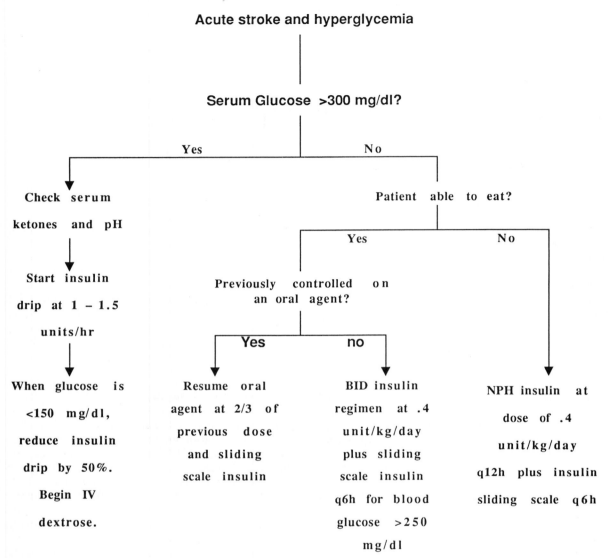

Figure 5-1.
Management of hyperglycemia in acute stroke.

Once this period after the stroke has passed (i.e., after 24 to 48 h), it is necessary to assess if the patient is able to eat. Once the patient is able to safely swallow and begin eating, a regimen of NPH combined with twice daily regular insulin should be started. Insulin can be dosed as 0.4 unit/kg/day with two-thirds in the morning and one-third before dinner (Fig. 5-2). Serum glucose levels should be monitored every 6 h. A conservative sliding scale of regular insulin should then be used to treat serum glucose over 250 mg/dL (Table 5-1). Increases in NPH and regular insulin from the original regimen may be required as the patient begins to take food in required caloric amounts. A sliding scale of regular insulin alone should not be used to avoid the potential "peaks and valleys" of this type of regimen.[27] For the diabetic patient whose glycemia was previously controlled on oral agents and has become hemodynamically stable, these agents may be restarted to maintain

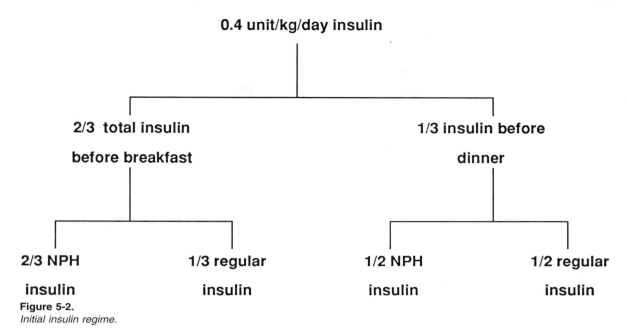

Figure 5-2.
Initial insulin regime.

a blood glucose level in the 100 to 250 mg/dL range. Generally, many ill patients who are hospitalized eat only one-half to two-thirds of what they normally eat at home. Thus, their oral agent dose or their insulin dose may also be reduced by this amount to avoid hypoglycemia (blood glucose less than 60 mg/dL).

For the diabetic patient who is unable to eat or drink due to dysphagia, insulin would be the agent of choice to control blood glucose levels. If the patient is being fed with a constant drip via a nasogastric tube, NPH insulin can be given every 12 h at a starting dose of .4 unit/kg/day, increasing the dose by 2 unit amounts every 12 h to attain desired glucose levels. For patients receiving total parenteral nutrition, 25 units of regular insulin may be added to each liter bag. Usually, this is sufficient to maintain glycemia in the suggested ranges. If these levels are not achieved, additional insulin added to each liter or additional NPH or "sliding scale" regular insulin can be added.

For the patient with no prior history of diabetes, hyperglycemia presenting at the onset of acute stroke may represent predisposition to this disorder or "stress hyperglycemia." Again, we recommend maintaining the blood glucose level in the 100 to 250 mg/dL range. A hemoglobinA1c will help to determine if the patient had abnormal glucose metabolism in the 6 to 8 weeks prior to the acute stroke. A patient with no known

history of diabetes may present with hyperosmolar coma as the first presentation of diabetes under the physiologic stress of having a stroke. Replacement of fluids and administration of an insulin drip as described above in an intensive care setting is critical. Profound hypovolemia associated with this condition, owing to osmotic diuresis, may exacerbate ischemic injury to the brain. Once the patient is neurologically stable, the hyperglycemia may represent new onset diabetes or previously undiagnosed diabetes. Under these circumstances physicians must initiate ongoing appropriate diet, exercise, educational, and pharmacologic therapy. Consultation with an endocrinologist is advised.

Glucose Management in Chronic Stroke

Glucose management in the weeks or months after a stroke requires a multidisciplinary team effort. This includes a physician, nurse, diabetes educator, dietitian, physiotherapist, and family members. The person with diabetes who has had a stroke is subject to numerous cognitive, perceptual, communicative, and motor disturbances depending on the location and extent of the brain damage. Many of these impairments have a significant impact on the ability of the person to carry out activities of daily living including aspects of a diabetes regimen. Exercise and diet regimens should be individualized.

Table 5-1.
Sliding scale regular insulin in patients with stroke

Serum glucose (mg/dL)	Regular insulin (units)
250–300	2
301–350	4
351–400	6
>400	8
	Re-evaluate insulin regimen. Evaluate for ketoacidosis

"Sliding scale insulin is used as a supplement to IV insulin drip or intermediate acting insulin (NPH or Lente) regimen. As serum blood glucose rises above 300 mg/dL osmotic diuresis will occur, resulting in water and electrolyte losses. Presence of ketoacidosis should be determined with plasma ketones and pH when serum glucose is over 300 mg/dL. Re-evaluation of the insulin regimen is necessary when serum glucose levels are greater than 300 mg/dL.

Self-glucose monitoring should be done regularly and can be done daily for the patient on oral agents or two to four times daily for the patient on insulin. Monitoring may need to be done by a family member or a nurse if the patient is unable to monitor himself. Glycemic goals, in our opinion, should be somewhat lower than during the acute stroke period. Pre-meal levels at 100 to 160 mg/dL seem reasonable. The dose of insulin or oral agent should be monitored frequently and changed when needed as the patient's physical exercise and diet changes. Patients in the chronic phase of a stroke may be undergoing rigorous physical rehabilitation. Extremes of physical activity may precipitate hypoglycemia. Advising the patient to eat regularly and check blood glucose levels before going to physical therapy can prevent hypoglycemia. Blood glucose levels below 100 mg/dL should be treated with glucose containing food or liquid before proceeding with physical therapy.

CONCLUSION

Glucose management in the setting of acute and chronic stroke should be designed to avoid extremes of glycemia. The prognostic significance of initial hyperglycemia on stroke outcome remains unclear. In the absence of randomized clinical trials in the setting of acute stroke, it seems reasonable to aim treatment toward avoiding extremes of hyperglycemia and hypoglycemia. Further

clinical studies need to be performed to evaluate the relationship between glycemia and neurologic outcome in stroke. For the chronic stroke patient with diabetes, careful adjustments in hypoglycemic agents need to be made as exercise and diet changes with neurologic recovery.

REFERENCES

1. Gray CS, Taylor R, French JM, et al: The prognostic value of stress hyperglycemia and previously unrecognized diabetes in acute stroke. *Diabet Med* 4:237, 1987.
2. Makovsky B, Metzger B, Molitch M, et al: Cerebrovascular disorders in patients with diabetes mellitus. *J Diabetes Complications* 10:228, 1996.
3. Melamed E: Reactive hyperglycemia in patients with acute stroke. *J Neurol Sci* 29:267, 1976.
4. Ibayashi S, Fujishima M, Sadoshima S, et al: Cerebral blood flow and tissue metabolism in experimental cerebral ischemia of spontaneously hypertensive rats with hyper, normo, and hypoglycemia. *Stroke* 17:261, 1986.
5. Sappey-Marinier D, Chileuitt L, Weiner M, et al: Hypoglycemia prevents increase in lactic acidosis during reperfusion after temporary cerebral ischemia in rats. *NMR Biomed* 8:171, 1995.
6. Kannel WB, Mcgee DL: Diabetes and cardiovascular disease: The Framingham study. *JAMA* 241:2035, 1979.
7. Palumbo PJ, Elveback LR, Whisnant JP, et al: Neurologic complications of diabetes mellitus: Transient ischemic attacks, stroke and peripheral neuropathy. *Adv Neurol* 19:593, 1978.
8. Abbott RD, Donahue RP, MacMahon SW, et al: Diabetes and the risk of stroke. The Honolulu Heart Program. *JAMA* 257:949, 1987.
9. Lehto S, Ronnemaa T, Pyorala K, et al: Predictors of stroke in middle-aged patients with non-insulin-dependent diabetes. *Stroke* 27:63, 1996.
10. Gray CS, Taylor R, French JM, et al: The prognostic value of stress hyperglycemia and previously unrecognized diabetes in acute stroke. *Diabet Med* 4:237, 1987.
11. Pulsinelli WA, Levy DE, Sigsbee B, et al: Increased damage after ischemic stroke in patients with hyperglycemia with or without established diabetes mellitus. *Am J Med* 74:540, 1983.
12. Cambell JA: Increase of resistance to oxygen want in animals on certain diets. *Q J Exp Physiol* 28:231, 1983.
13. Craven C, Chinn H, MacVicar R: Effect of carrot diet and restricted feeding on the resistance of the rat to hypoxia. *J Aviation Med* 21:256, 1950.
14. Myers RE, Yamaguchi S: Nervous system effects of cardiac arrest in monkeys. *Arch Neurol* 34:65, 1977.
15. Pulsinelli WA, Waldman S, Sigsbee B, et al: Experimental hyperglycemia and diabetes mellitus worsen stroke outcome. *Trans Am Neurol Assoc* 105:21, 1980.

16. Ginsberg MD, Prado R, Dietrich WD, et al: Hyperglycemia reduces the extent of cerebral infarction in rats. *Stroke* 18:570, 1987.

17. Davalos A, Cendra E, Ternel J, et al: Deteriorating ischemic stroke: Risk factors and prognosis. *Neurology* 40: 1865, 1990.

18. Longstreth WT, Jr, Diehr P, Inui TS: Prediction of awakening after out-of-hospital cardiac arrest. *N Engl J Med* 308:1378, 1983.

19. Longstreth WT, Jr, Inue TS: High blood glucose level on hospital admission and poor neurological recovery after cardiac arrest. *Ann Neurol* 15:59, 1984.

20. Candelise L, Landi G, Orazio EN, Boccardi E: Prognostic significance of hyperglycemia in acute stroke. *Arch Neurol* 42:661, 1985.

21. Kiers L, Davis SM, Larkins R, et al: Stroke topography and outcome in relation to hyperglycemia and diabetes. *J Neurol Neurosurg Psychiatry* 55:263, 1992.

22. Woo J, Lam CW, Kay R, et al: The influence of hyperglycemia and diabetes mellitus on immediate and 3-month morbidity and mortality after acute stroke. *Arch Neurol* 47:1174, 1990.

23. Matchar D, Divine G, Heyman A, et al: The influence of hyperglycemia on outcome of cerebral infarction. *Ann Intern Med* 177:449, 1992.

24. Tyson R, Peeling J, Sutherland G: Metabolic changes associated with altering blood glucose levels in short duration forebrain ischemia. *Brain Res* 608:288, 1993.

25. Bell D: Stroke in the diabetic patient. *Diabetes Care* 17:213, 1994.

26. McGarry JD: The metabolic derangements and treatment of diabetic ketoacidosis. *N Engl J Med* 309:159, 1983.

27. Queale WS, Seidler AJ, Brancati FL: Glycemic control and sliding scale insulin use in medical inpatients with diabetes mellitus. *Arch Intern Med* 157:545, 1997.

Chapter 6

THE SUBACUTE STROKE PATIENT: LIPID MANAGEMENT

Daniel A. Streja

BACKGROUND

In 1993, the National Cholesterol Education Program (NCEP) published guidelines in the form of the second report of the expert panel for detection, evaluation, and treatment of high cholesterol in adults (Adult Treatment Panel II).[1] The purpose of the guidelines was to "make a significant contribution in reducing the toll from coronary heart disease." The report of the expert panel states:

> Substantial carotid atherosclerosis is documented by cerebral symptoms (transient ischemic attacks or stroke) accompanied by the demonstration of significant atherosclerosis on sonogram or angiogram. For patients with established coronary heart disease or other clinical atherosclerotic disease that puts them at equivalent risk, it is reasonable to set a lower target value for LDL cholesterol lowering than is recommended for primary prevention.

The panel recommended initiation of diet therapy in all patients with cerebrovascular disease and an LDL cholesterol of over 3.4 mM (130 mg/dL). Drug therapy with lipid-lowering drugs was recommended for patients with LDL cholesterol over 3.4 mM after a maximum 3 months of diet intervention. In patients with an LDL cholesterol between 2.6 and 3.4 mM (100–130 mg/dL), the panel recommended careful evaluation and optional drug therapy depending on physician's estimate of the balance of cost and risk of therapy vs. potential benefit.

This chapter will review the evidence currently available to support the 1993 NCEP guidelines for treatment of hyperlipidemia in stroke patients. On reviewing the guidelines, four pertinent questions come to mind:

1. Do patients with cerebrovascular disease have the same risk of a coronary event as patients with coronary artery disease?

2. What is the evidence that lipid intervention will reduce coronary events and risk of death in patients with cerebrovascular disease?

3. Is cholesterol lowering expected to have an effect on recurrent stroke rates?

4. How is treatment of hyperlipidemia initiated and monitored in patients with cerebrovascular disease?

RISK OF CORONARY EVENTS IN CEREBROVASCULAR DISEASE PATIENTS

Early autopsy studies have documented the association between the extent of atherosclerosis in carotid and coronary arteries. Subsequent clinical and epidemiologic studies have shown similar rates of fatal and nonfatal coronary events in patients with cerebrovascular and coronary artery disease. Cohorts of patients with cerebrovascular disease include patients free of coronary artery disease with lower risk of coronary events, but these cohorts are usually 10 to 15 years older than cohorts of patients with coronary artery disease. The older age increases coronary risk in patients with cerebrovascular disease, offsetting the decrease in risk related to the improved survival of patients free of coronary artery disease.

Coronary Events after Stroke

Stroke increases markedly the risk of recurrent cerebrovascular events, and, traditionally, prevention of recurrent strokes has been one of the main concerns in poststroke management. Multiple studies have attempted to find strategies for prevention of recurrent cerebrovascular events. Prevention of cardiac events in patients with cerebrovascular disease has received less attention despite the fact that the risk of fatal acute myocardial infarction (MI) or sudden cardiac death is higher in these patients than the risk of fatal stroke.[2] In cohorts of elderly patients, there is a high prevalence of concurrent, clinically significant, cerebrovascular, coronary, and peripheral vascular disease. The occurrence of a stroke increases the long-term mortality of acute MI survivors, and, similarly, pre-existing coronary artery disease increases the risk of death in stroke patients. Up to 86 percent of the stroke victims will eventually die of a vascular cause, mostly coronary or cerebrovascular disease.[3] The ratio between the risk of death from a coronary and a cerebrovascular cause is low after the initial event and increases progressively in the first 6 months, subsequently reaching levels of between 2 and 7. The risk of cardiovascular death in stroke patients is related to the level of risk factors for coronary artery disease. Male gender, diabetes, and hypertension significantly increase mortality of patients with stroke. Stroke patients have an increased risk of nonfatal coronary events. The 5-year incidence of documented MI in stroke survivors is estimated at 19 percent or approximately 4 percent per year, equivalent with the rate reported in survivors of acute MI.[4] Pre-existing coronary artery disease and diabetes increase the risk of nonfatal coronary events in stroke patients.

Coronary Events in Patients with Transient Ischemia and/or Postendarterectomy

Stroke-free patients with cerebrovascular disease have an increased rate of coronary events. Patients with carotid stenosis, whether treated with endarterectomy and antiplatelet agents or with antiplatelet agents alone, have a high risk of cardiovascular death.[5] The same high cardiovascular mortality rate has been documented in cohorts of patients with asymptomatic carotid bruits, followed up prospectively. Patients with transient ischemic attacks treated with medical therapy have a 25 to 70 percent increased risk of cardiovascular death, depending on the length of follow-up. This is at least twice the risk of death through a cerebrovascular event. Patients undergoing endarterectomy have a decreased risk of ipsilateral neurologic events but the same high rate of fatal coronary events.[6] There is a high risk of perioperative death in patients with coronary artery disease undergoing endarterectomy. In long-term follow-up of endarterectomy patients, the risk of coronary events is two to four times higher than the risk of stroke. Approximately one-third to one-half of the patients with cerebrovascular disease have symptomatic coronary artery disease, which accounts for a large proportion of excess cardiovascular risk in these patients.

Asymptomatic Coronary Artery Disease in Patients with Cerebrovascular Disease

NCEP guidelines recommend aggressive cholesterol lowering in all patients with cerebrovascular disease. The implication is that patients with cerebrovascular disease who are free of clinical coronary or peripheral vascular disease are also at high cardiovascular risk. In the Veteran Administration Study of Endarterectomy for Asymptomatic Carotid Stenosis, 102 of 444 patients (23 percent) fit this description.[7] These patients had a 25 percent event risk at 4 years' median follow-up, in the range reported for patients with documented coronary artery disease. Other studies document the high prevalence of undiagnosed coronary disease in cerebrovascular disease patients. Among patients undergoing elective carotid endarterectomy with no history of MI, 29 percent had severe coronary artery disease, documented by angiogram.[8] One-fourth to one-third of patients with cerebrovascular disease and no symptoms or history of coronary artery disease had an abnormal coronary perfusion, documented by thallium-201 scintigraphic testing.[9,10] Asymptomatic coronary artery disease documented by these imaging studies did not seem to affect perioperative mortality but strongly influenced long-term prognosis.[11]

Carotid Ultrasound Detected Abnormalities and Coronary Artery Disease

Carotid artery disease documented by carotid ultrasound is associated with the levels of standard risk factors for coronary events and may substitute for them as a risk predictor. Carotid intima/media thickness (IMT) has become the most reported index of carotid atherosclerosis, and it predicts both coronary and cerebrovascular events.[12] In many studies, carotid IMT has been associated with the severity of coronary artery disease documented by quantitative angiogram. This confirms that atherosclerosis should be viewed as a generalized disease process.

Summary

Patients with cerebrovascular disease, symptomatic or asymptomatic, have a risk of fatal or nonfatal coronary events similar to that of younger patients with coronary artery disease.

TREATMENT OF HYPERLIPIDEMIA AND CORONARY ARTERY DISEASE

LDL cholesterol is the main form of transport of cholesterol in human serum. Hyperlipidemia in patients with documented atherosclerosis is defined as the presence of an LDL cholesterol over 2.6 mM (100 mg/dL). This is different than the broader definition of hyperlipidemia, which includes abnormalities of other lipoprotein fractions. The reason for this narrow definition is that, although other lipoproteins are predictors of cardiovascular risk, only LDL cholesterol lowering has been documented to be effective in preventing coronary events. Prior to 1993, numerous studies have attempted to reduce cardiovascular events through cholesterol lowering. The pharmacologic intervention in these studies used:

• bile acid binding resins acting through a reduction of bile acid pool, resulting in a compensatory increased uptake of circulating LDL cholesterol by the liver;

• niacin, an inhibitor of synthesis of lipoproteins; and

• fibrates, acting mostly by modifying the metabolism of triglyceride-containing particles, very low density lipoproteins, and chylomicron remnants.

The advent of hepatic hydroxymethylglutaryl coenzyme A (HMG CoA) reductase inhibitors (statins), acting by inhibiting cholesterol synthesis and increasing the uptake of low-density cholesterol particles, has resulted in a simplified, evidence-based therapy plan for treatment of hyperlipidemia in secondary prevention.

Successful Non-Statin Trials of Secondary Prevention

The Newcastle Study enrolled 497 patients (20 percent women), over 65 years of age, with a history of

MI and/or angina.[13] They were randomized between clofibrate 1.5 g/day and corn oil-placebo for a duration of 5 years. A difference of 15 to 20 percent in total cholesterol between the groups was maintained throughout the study. There was a 43 percent decrease in total mortality ($p = .02$) and a 35 percent decrease in first nonfatal MI, significant only in patients who were not being treated with anticoagulants ($p = .032$).

The Oslo Diet-Heart Study included 412 male MI survivors, 30 to 64 years of age, randomized to a diet-treated group or a control group.[14] The diet was low in saturated fat and cholesterol and high in polyunsaturated fat and resulted in a 15 percent difference in total cholesterol between the groups. At 5 years' follow-up, there was a 25 percent reduction in fatal and nonfatal MI ($p = .05$). At 11 years' follow-up, there was a 44 percent decrease in fatal MI ($p = .004$). Of note is the fact that most of the reduction in fatal MI occurred in patients aged over 60 years.

The UPJOHN Colestipol Study enrolled 2278 patients, men and women, with cholesterol over 6.5 mM (250 mg/dL), for a duration of 3 years.[15] The average age was 51 years for men and 57 years for women. An average difference of 10 percent in total cholesterol between the treated and control group was maintained throughout the study. In a subgroup of 337 men with coronary artery disease, there were 15 coronary artery disease (CHD) deaths in the placebo group and 5 deaths in the control group ($p = .01$). There was no significant difference in CHD mortality in women.

The Coronary Drug Project enrolled 8341 men, 30 to 64 years of age, with documented previous MI, in six treatment arms: conjugated estrogens 2.5 mg/day (1101), conjugated estrogens 5.0 mg/day (1119), dextrothyroxine sodium (1103), clofibrate 1.8 g/day (1110), niacin 3.0 g/day (1119), and placebo (2789).[16,17] The only successful arm was the niacin arm. Patients had at baseline an average cholesterol of 6.5 mM (250 mg/dL), which, on niacin, was maintained at an average 10 percent lower throughout the study. There was a significant (27 percent) decrease in the rate of nonfatal MI at 5 years' follow-up, which was maintained at 7 years. There was also a threefold decrease in the rate of revascularization procedures at 5 years. At 15 years' follow-up, there was a 9 percent improved survival ($p = 0.0012$), attributable to a decrease in CHD mortality in patients treated with niacin during the study. The study identified a time lag of 2 to 3 years before the occurrence of a beneficial trend in nonfatal MI and a 6- to 8-year lag for the occurrence of a beneficial trend in total mortality. There was also a high rate of discontinuation and a very high side effect profile in the niacin-treated group.

The Stockholm Ischemic Heart Disease Secondary Prevention Study enrolled 555 survivors of acute MI, 20 percent women, and less than 70 years of age.[18] Only 13 percent patients were considered hypercholesterolemic (total cholesterol over 90th percentile of Stockholm population). Insulin-requiring diabetics were excluded. Patients were randomized for duration of 5 years between clofibrate 2 g/day plus niacin 3 g/day and placebo. The average difference in total cholesterol between the groups was 13 percent. The study reported a 26 percent decrease ($p = .05$) in total mortality in all treated patients and a 28 percent decrease ($p = .05$) in total mortality in treated patients over 60 years of age. There was a 36 percent decrease ($p = .01$) in CHD mortality in the treated group. The authors reported that the benefits of the drug regimen used were obtained mostly in hypertriglyceridemic patients and were dependent on a significant triglyceride lowering.

The Program of Surgical Control of Hyperlipidemia (POSCH) Study enrolled 838 patients, MI survivors, 90 percent men, and 30 to 64 years of age.[19] They were nondiabetic and had a total cholesterol of over 5.7 mM (220 mg/dL) after at least 6 weeks of compliance with a step II American Heart Association diet. In the treatment group, a partial ileal bypass was performed in all patients. This resulted in a 23 percent decrease in total cholesterol and a 38 percent decrease in LDL cholesterol. At a median 9.7 years' follow-up, the treatment group had a 35 percent decrease in combined coronary artery disease death and nonfatal MI ($p < .001$) and a 62 percent reduction in revascularization procedures ($p = .0001$). Total mortality was affected only in patients with a normal ejection fraction (36 percent decrease; $p = .012$). Semiquantitative angiograms were performed serially in most of the patients. There was a highly significant difference in disease progression between treated and control groups at 3, 5, 7, and 10 years' follow-up ($p = .001$). This was statistically significant in women ($p = .013$), showing for the first time benefit of cholesterol lowering in both genders.

The VA-HIT trial enrolled 2531 men, age <73 years, with documented coronary artery disease.[69] They had HDL cholesterol <1.1 mM, LDL cholesterol < 3.6 mM, and triglycerides <2.7 mM. Twenty-five percent of the patients had diabetes, and over 505 had fasting hyperinsulinemia and at least one feature of "dysmetabolic syndrome." Patients were randomized to double-blind treatment with gemfibrozil 600 mg BID or placebo. After a mean follow-up of 5.1 years, there was a 22 per-cent decrease in coronary heart disease death and myocardial infarction ($p = .006$) and a 22 percent decrease in nonfatal myocardial infarction ($p = .027$). There was a 29 percent decrease in the risk of stroke as defined by the investigators ($p < .04$). After panel adjudication of stroke cases, the difference became borderline significant (<5 percent, $p = .10$). There was a 59 percent decrease in risk of TIA ($p < .001$) and a 65 percent decrease in risk of carotid endarterectomy ($p < .01$).

Summary The non-statin studies of treatment of hyperlipidemia have documented that coronary events and revascularization procedures can be decreased by effective therapy in middle-age men with coronary disease. Only suggestive evidence using surrogate outcomes was documented in women. Studies using niacin reported a decrease in total mortality, attributable to a decrease in coronary death. There was no significant decrease in the rate of recurrent nonfatal MI. The benefits could not be demonstrated in patients with decreased ejection fraction. No information was obtained concerning coronary prevention in diabetics. There was a substantial lag in the occurrence of clinical benefit.

Statin Trials of Secondary Prevention

The Scandinavian Simvastatin Survival (4S) Study enrolled 4444 patients with angina pectoris or previous MI and total cholesterol 5.5 to 8.0 mM (212 to 308 mg/dL) after diet instructions.[20–22] There were 827 women in the study. Forty-three percent of the patients were over 65 years of age, and 202 patients had diabetes mellitus. Patients were randomized to double-blind treatment with simvastatin (average daily dose = 26 mg) or placebo. Over the 5.4 years of follow-up, total cholesterol was decreased by 15 percent and LDL cholesterol by 35 percent. There was a 30 percent decrease in total mortality in the treatment group, which occurred with a lag of 1 to 2 years. Coronary death was decreased by 42 percent and all cardiovascular death by 35 percent. All of these benefits were at the $p = .00001$ level. There were no significant side effects and no increase in noncardiovascular mortality. There was a significant increase in the proportion of survivors free of either coronary events or all atherosclerosis-related events. There was a 37 percent decrease in revascularizations. Consequently, there was a significant decrease in hospitalization rates. Women enrolled in the study had a 35 percent decrease in major coronary event rate ($p = .01$). Patients over 65 years of age had a 34 percent decrease in total mortality ($p = .01$), a 43 percent decrease in cardiovascular mortality, and a 34 percent decrease in major coronary event rate (p = .001). There was an impressive 55 percent decrease in the rate of coronary events in diabetics (p = .002). The benefits of cholesterol reduction were independent of baseline LDL cholesterol level in this cohort of hypercholesterolemic patients. The investigators reported higher benefits at higher levels of LDL cholesterol reduction.

The Cholesterol and Recurrent Events (CARE) Study enrolled 4159 MI survivors (3583 men and 576 women) with a total cholesterol less than 6.2 mM (240 mg/dL).[23] They were randomized between pravastatin 40 mg/day and placebo and followed for 5 years. A 28 percent difference in LDL cholesterol between the arms was maintained throughout the study. Half of the patients were over 60 years of age, and 15 percent of the patients had diabetes. The study reported a 24 percent decrease in CHD death and nonfatal MI (p = .003). Nonfatal MI was reduced 23 percent (p = .02). There was a 26 percent reduction in coronary bypass surgery (p = .005), a 23 percent decrease in coronary angioplasty rates (p = .01), and a 27 percent decrease in all revascularization procedures (p = .001). The reduction in major coronary events was 20 percent in men (p = .001) and 46 percent in women (p = .001). Patients over 60 years had a 27 percent reduction in major coronary events (p = .001) compared with a 20 percent reduction in younger patients (p = .02). The reduction in event rates was significant in diabetics (25 percent; p = .05), hypertensive patients (23 percent; p = .005), and current smokers (33 percent; p = .006). Patients with previous revascularization procedures had a decrease of 22 percent in the rate of major coronary events (p = .006). The study reported a 28 percent decrease in major coronary events in patients with a left ventricular ejection fraction of less than 40 percent (p = .02). The reduction in major coronary events in patients with total cholesterol 5.5 to 6.2 mM (212 to 240 mg/dL) was in the same range as reported in the Scandinavian Simvastatin Study. In patients with lower baseline LDL cholesterol, the benefit was diminished, and no benefit could be demonstrated in patients with an LDL cholesterol of less than 3.2 mM (125 mg/dL). The study reported that, after a small reduction in LDL cholesterol was achieved, there was no demonstrable relationship between the magnitude of LDL cholesterol reduction and clinical benefit.

The Lipid Intervention in Prevention of Ischemic Disease (LIPID) Study enrolled 9014 patients with angina pectoris or previous MI and total cholesterol 4 to 7 mM (155 to 270 mg/dL) after diet instructions.[24] There were 1516 women in the study. Fifteen percent of the patients were over 70 years of age, and 9 percent of the patients had diabetes mellitus. Patients were randomized to double-blind treatment with pravastatin 40 mg/day or placebo. Over the 6 years' follow-up, LDL cholesterol was decreased by 25 percent. There was a 23 percent decrease in total mortality in the treatment group. Coronary death and cardiovascular death were decreased by 24 percent each. All of these benefits were at the p < .001 level, and the lag in the occurrence of clinical benefit was approximately 1 year. There were no significant side effects and no increase in noncardiovascular mortality. There was a significant increase in the proportion of survivors free of either coronary events or all atherosclerosis-related events. There was a 24 percent decrease in revascularizations. Women, patients over 70 years of age, and diabetics had benefits similar to the rest of the group. Preliminary data show no LDL cholesterol threshold for benefit in these patients. Four percent of patients had a history of stroke, and 3 to 4 percent had a history of TIA. At the time of the preparation of this chapter, a subgroup analysis in these patients was not available.

Summary The statin studies of treatment of hyperlipidemia have confirmed that coronary events and revascularization procedures can be decreased by effective therapy in middle-age men with coronary artery disease. Significant therapeutic benefit was documented also in women and patients over 60 years of age. A significant decrease in total mortality and the rate of recurrent nonfatal MI was reported in two of three studies. The benefits were demonstrated in patients with decreased ejection fraction. Diabetics with hypercholesterolemia had a very impressive therapeutic benefit. The lag in the occurrence of clinical benefit was much shorter than the lag of non-statin trials. The drugs were well tolerated with no significant side effects.

Statin Studies in Patients with Abnormal Carotid Ultrasound

None of the studies listed specifically enrolled patients with cerebrovascular disease. In four smaller studies, patients were randomized between statin therapy and placebo. Progression of carotid atherosclerosis as assessed by carotid ultrasound was the main outcome. Follow-up was for 2 to 4 years. Clinical events were also recorded.

The Asymptomatic Carotid Artery Progression (ACAPS) Study enrolled 919 asymptomatic patients 40 to 79 years of age with an IMT of 1.5 to 3.5 mm at least in

1 of 12 sites measured.[25] The patients were randomized between lovastatin 20 to 40 mg/day and placebo. Half of the patients in each group received warfarin 1 mg/day. Half of the patients were women, and more than half were over 60 years. Lovastatin therapy resulted in a 28 percent reduction in LDL cholesterol. At 3 years' follow-up, the changes in maximum IMT were significantly different ($p = .001$) independent of age gender and baseline LDL cholesterol. There were 14 major cardiovascular events in the placebo group and 5 in the treatment group ($p = .04$). Nine patients died during the study, eight in the placebo group, and one in the treatment group ($p = .02$).

The Pravastatin, Lipids, and Atherosclerosis in the Carotids (PLAC II) Study enrolled 151 men with documented coronary artery disease and carotid IMT of more than 1.3 mm at least in one site.[26,27] Patients were randomized between pravastatin 40 mg/day and placebo. A 28 percent difference in LDL cholesterol between groups was maintained throughout the study. Active treatment at 3 years' follow-up resulted in decrease of the rate of progression of atherosclerosis in the common carotid. The authors reported a 35 percent reduction in the mean annualized progression rate of intima/media thickness after adjustment for cardiovascular risk factors, baseline thickness, and reader effects. There were 13 deaths or coronary events in the placebo group and 5 in the treatment group ($p = .04$).

The Kuopio Atherosclerosis Prevention (KAPS) Study enrolled 447 asymptomatic men 44 to 65 years of age with a LDL cholesterol over 4.0 mM (155 mg/dL).[28] They were randomized between pravastatin 40 mg/day and placebo with a 28 percent difference in LDL cholesterol maintained throughout the study. The mean baseline IMT in the common carotid was 1.35 mm. There was a threefold decrease in the rate of progression of atherosclerosis in the common carotid in the treated group. The treatment effect was larger in the subjects with higher IMT baseline values. There were 15 cardiovascular events in the placebo group and 11 in the treatment group.

The Carotid Atherosclerosis Italian Ultrasound (CAIUS) Study enrolled 305 asymptomatic patients (47 percent women) with at least one lesion with IMT 1.3 to 3.5 mm.[29] They were randomized between pravastatin 40 mg/day and placebo, with a 23 percent difference in LDL cholesterol being maintained throughout the study. The mean maximum IMT decreased in the treatment group and increased in the placebo group, and this difference was significant ($p = .0007$). There were six events in each treatment arm.

Summary   There are no studies documenting the benefit of cholesterol lowering after a cerebrovascular event. The best information available to date is from the studies where patients were selected to have anatomic abnormalities of the extracranial carotid arteries. In these studies, statin therapy uniformly decreased the progression of atherosclerosis as documented by ultrasound. A trend toward a decreased number of cardiovascular events was noted in most studies.

CHOLESTEROL LOWERING AND RECURRENT STROKE

The risk of a cerebrovascular event increases tenfold in patients with ischemic stroke or transient ischemia. The risk of stroke varies with the age group. A meta-analysis of 45 cohorts reports a crude annual stroke rate of 0.22 percent in patients age 45 to 64 years and a rate of 1.22 percent in patients over age 65 years.[30] In large randomized stroke prevention trials in patients with transient ischemia, the annual risk of stroke in the placebo group is 4 to 12 percent. Cholesterol lowering is viewed as an intervention for prevention or treatment of atherosclerosis, but no direct information is available to date concerning its effect on stroke recurrence. Some inference could be drawn from data concerning the effect of cholesterol lowering on primary prevention of stroke in patients with coronary artery disease.

Cholesterol Concentration and Risk of Death and Stroke

There is overwhelming evidence that cholesterol level predicts the risk of cardiovascular events and cardiovascular death. The relationship seems to be exponential as there is no threshold, and hypercholesterolemic patients have progressively larger increases in risk with each increment of cholesterol concentration. A U-shaped relationship between cholesterol and total mortality has been reported in most studies.[31] This is because of an increase in noncardiovascular death rate at very low cholesterol concentration. The relationship has been extensively analyzed because of initial concerns of detrimental effects of cholesterol lowering. Most authors have attributed the U-shaped curve to low cholesterol concentrations being a marker for chronic illnesses and poor nutritional status. In some cohorts studied prospectively, the relationship was no longer apparent after a few years during which patients with terminal illnesses died. The risk of stroke of all subtypes is unrelated to cholesterol concentration. This apparent lack of relationship between cholesterol and cerebrovascular disease conceals a positive association with ischemic stroke and a negative association with hemorrhagic stroke.[30] In larger studies, when these two types of events are reported separately, the risk of ischemic stroke increases slightly but significantly with cholesterol concentration, whereas the risk of hemorrhagic stroke is increased at low cholesterol levels due to a small subgroup with low cholesterol and uncontrolled diastolic hypertension.[32] In addition, in most studies, subtypes of strokes are not identified and, although ischemic stroke is an atherosclerotic event, risk factors for atherosclerosis would not be expected to be associated with cardioembolic strokes. Smaller studies found that only patients with very high cholesterol levels are at increased risk of ischemic stroke, which is in keeping with an exponential relationship.[33] A recent study has reported an increase in long-term mortality after stroke in patients with low cholesterol and has requested a moratorium on cholesterol reduction after stroke.[34] Such data can also be attributed to an increased mortality in patients with poor nutrition and low cholesterol. A placebo-controlled trial of prevention of stroke recurrence with cholesterol-lowering agents could clarify this problem but would be unethical in the age range in which the benefit of secondary prevention of coronary events has already been documented.

Cholesterol Lowering and Risk of Stroke

In the early 1970's, two small studies attempted to reduce the incidence of recurrent stroke by cholesterol reduction with clofibrate.[35,36] No recent studies have attempted to decrease the incidence of stroke in patients with cerebrovascular disease by lowering cholesterol. Some studies of cholesterol lowering for prevention of recurrent coronary events have reported the incidence of strokes, and some, more recent, have included stroke as an outcome. Stroke prevention through cholesterol lowering seems to be related to the method used for lipid intervention.[37-42] The data of the main studies are shown in Table 6-1.

The results of this analysis show a striking difference between studies using statins and studies using other methods of cholesterol lowering. Old fibrate studies seem to show a trend toward increased risk, and one of the meta-analyses mentioned showed a significantly increased risk of fatal stroke.[37] In contrast, the VA-HIT trial showed a striking benefit.[70] Other non-statin studies did not report any benefit with the exception of the

study of Dayton et al.[43] In the CDP, a total follow-up endpoint analysis showed a 24 percent decrease in the risk of fatal and nonfatal cerebrovascular events ($z_N = -2.46$). Statin studies of secondary prevention have shown a consistently significant decrease in the risk of stroke and transient ischemic events. The reason for the spectacular effect of statins is not clear. It could be the result of a more effective cholesterol lowering or because of mechanisms of action other than cholesterol lowering.

Other Lipoprotein-Related Risk Factors for Ischemic Stroke

In addition to total and LDL cholesterol, other lipoprotein factors have been associated with an increased stroke rate or documented cerebrovascular disease.

Fasting Triglycerides   The association of triglyceride concentration with ischemic stroke has been addressed in a few studies.[54,55] In some, no relationship was found; in others, a strong relationship was present. Fasting triglycerides have been positively associated with atherosclerosis of large arteries of the Willis circle on autopsy, the severity of angiographic cerebrovascular lesions, and the progression of carotid IMT. Intermediate density lipoproteins, the atherogenic product of metabolism of triglyceride-containing lipoprotein particles, have been associated with ischemic stroke. Triglycerides and apolipoproteins C-III and E, mostly carried in triglyceride-containing particles, have been associated with the rate of progression of carotid IMT.

Triglycerides have been associated with the presence of "echo-lucent carotid lesions," presumably the ultrasound equivalent of unstable plaques. Hypertriglyceridemia is considered a marker of insulin resistance, and insulin levels have been positively associated with IMT in Asians, Hispanics, and non-Hispanic whites.

HDL Cholesterol   High density lipoprotein (HDL) cholesterol levels are the single best biochemical predictors of coronary artery disease.[56] Subjects with low HDL cholesterol or low levels of apolipoprotein A1 (the main apolipoprotein in HDL) are at increased risk of stroke.[57] Low HDL cholesterol levels are associated with the severity of carotid atherosclerosis, carotid IMT, and progression of carotid IMT. Patients with low HDL cholesterol are more likely to have early recurrent stenosis after endarterectomy caused by intimal hyperplasia. HDL cholesterol and fasting triglyceride concentrations

Table 6-1.
Cerebrovascular outcomes in randomized studies of cholesterol lowering

Study	Size (#)	Cerebrovascular events: number (%) Treatment	Control	Risk ratio (95% CI)
Dietary studies				
Dayton VA Study[43]	846	13 (3.06)	25 (5.92)	0.53 (0.28–1.01)
Minnesota Diet Study[44]	4,393	13 (0.59)	11 (0.50)	1.04 (0.58–1.88)
Multiple intervention studies				
Hjerman—Oslo Study[45]	1,232	9 (0.48)	3 (0.48)	1.04 (0.24–4.56)
MRFIT[46]	12,866	49 (0.76)	41 (0.64)	1.19 (0.79–1.80)
Miettinen et al.[47]	1,222	0 (0)	8 (1.31)	0.06 (0–1.01)
Fibrate studies				
Stockholm HS (clofibrate + niacin)[13]	555	6 (2.15)	5 (1.81)	1.17 (0.38–3.60)
CDP—clofibrate arm[16]	3,892	136 (12.3)	311 (11.2)	1.05 (0.73–1.52)
WHO—clofibrate[48]	10,627	26 (0.48)	20 (0.38)	1.32 (0.78–2.22)
Helsinki Heart Study (gemfibrozil)[49]	4,081	20 (0.98)	18 (0.89)	1.43 (0.43–4.75)
Other interventions				
CDP—niacin arm[16]	3,908	95 (8.49)	311 (11.2)	0.86 (0.57–1.26)
UPJOHN—colestipol study[15]	2,278	0 (0)	1 (0.09)	0.33 (0–8.03)
LRC Study (cholestyramine)[50]	3,806	19 (0.98)	16 (0.84)	1.18 (0.61–2.26)
POSCH (ileal bypass)[19]	838	14 (3.32)	15 (3.50)	1.65 (0.22–12.4)
VA-HIT (gemfibrozil)[69–70]	2,531	88 (6.9)	64 (5.1)	0.71
Statin studies				
Pravastatin Multinational Study[51]	1,062	0 (0)	5 (0.94)	0.14 (0–2.77)
Scandinavian Simvastatin Study[20–22]	4,444	75 (3.38)	102 (4.59)	0.72 (0.52–0.96)
CARE (pravastatin)[23]	4,159	54 (2.63)	78 (3.75)	0.69 (0.49–0.97)
LIPID (pravastatin)[24]	9,014	169 (3.75)	204	0.81 (0.04–0.99)
PAIP (pravastatin)[24,52]	1,891	5 (5.26)	13 (1.37)	0.38 (0.01–1.09)
WESCOPS (pravastatin)[53]	6,595	46 (1.39)	51 (1.55)	0.90 (0.61–1.33)

are the main determinants of removal of postprandial triglycerides. Impaired clearance of postprandial triglycerides has been associated with carotid atherosclerosis.

Lipoprotein (a) The association of lipoprotein (a) (Lp (a)) with coronary artery disease has been a subject of debate in the medical literature and was not completely resolved at the time of the submission of this manuscript. A few studies have attempted to establish the relationship between Lp (a) and cerebrovascular disease. In case control studies, the concentration of Lp (a) was

reported to be twice as high in stroke patients.[58] There is a twofold increase in stroke risk in patients with Lp (a) >30 mg/dL. In prospective studies, however, Lp (a) is not a predictor of stroke.[59] High levels of Lp (a) have been associated with increased IMT in type 2 diabetics.

Apo E Polymorphism Apolipoprotein E4 allele has been associated with an increased risk of coronary artery disease and Alzheimer disease. In case control studies, a twofold increase in the frequency of this allele was reported in stroke patients.[60] There is also an increased frequency of E4 allele in patients with restenosis after endarterectomy. E4 allele is associated with increased IMT at all sites independent of other cardiovascular risk factors.

Dietary Fat   Intake of total dietary fat and saturated fat has been associated with coronary artery disease independent of cholesterol level. The risk of stroke seems to have a much more complex relationship with dietary fat.[61,62]

The relationship of saturated fat intake with stroke risk is equivocal. Some studies have reported a decreased risk with the intake of saturated fat. Other studies show an association of stroke risk and meat intake, which usually parallels saturated fat intake.

Monounsaturated fat intake is associated with a decreased stroke risk in all prospective studies. Phospholipids of red blood cell membranes in patients with stroke have a decreased content of oleate, indicating a decreased intake of monounsaturated fat.

Total polyunsaturated fat intake does not seem to be associated with stroke risk. Alpha linolenic acid is decreased in patients with stroke. This is in agreement with the studies showing benefit for coronary prevention from its addition to diet of patients at high risk. Fish intake, presumably through its content in omega 3 fatty acids, has been associated with a decreased recurrent MI risk and stroke risk.

Dietary Antioxidants   The intake of fresh fruits has been associated with a decreased risk of stroke, presumably through its content in antioxidants.[63] Associations of different antioxidants with risk of stroke have been reported in some studies:

There is a significant decrease in the risk of stroke in the upper quartile of flavonoid intake compared with the lower quartile.

A low beta-carotene intake has been associated with a doubling of the risk of stroke.

Vitamin C intake is negatively associated with IMT. Vitamin E intake is negatively associated with IMT only in women.

Antibodies to oxidized LDL have been reported to be increased in stroke patients.

Caloric Intake   Abdominal obesity has a positive association with all strokes.[64,65] In ischemic stroke, the relationship has been documented to be independent of

traditional risk factors. In women, weight gain is an independent risk factor for stroke.

TREATMENT PLAN

Based on the evidence presented, pharmacologic intervention has become the first line therapy for secondary prevention. Statins are the drugs of choice because of better outcomes, side effect and safety profile, and compliance. In most practices, diet and other lipid-lowering drugs have become an adjuvant therapy in the treatment of hyperlipidemia in high-risk patients.

Diagnosis and Plan of Management of Hyperlipidemia after a Cerebrovascular Event

NCEP guidelines recommend treatment with lipid-lowering drugs in patients with atherosclerosis and an LDL over 3.4 mM (130 mg/dL) after a short diet trial. These patients represent 70 to 80 percent of all patients with documented atherosclerosis. Some experts recommend treatment with statins in all patients immediately after a coronary event. In this alternative, initial evaluation of hyperlipidemia is not necessary. The wisdom of this policy in stroke patients, where some concerns exist about unnecessarily low cholesterol levels, is questionable. An accurate determination of lipoprotein concentrations can be obtained in the first 48 h after a stroke.[66] Subsequently, the concentrations of lipoproteins no longer reflect the prestroke levels until 3 months after the event. After the initiation of therapy, the levels should be monitored at intervals of a minimum of 3 months. According to the NCEP, the goal of treatment should be a reduction of LDL cholesterol below 2.6 mM (100 mg/dL). There is agreement that a minimum 20 to 25 percent decrease in LDL cholesterol and an LDL cholesterol under 3.4 mM is necessary to achieve benefit, but there is disagreement over the need, the risks, and the cost effectiveness of achieving the NCEP goals in all patients. Consequently, the minimum goal is a reduction in LDL cholesterol concentration under 3.4 mM.

Diet Therapy

The current practice is to request a consult from a registered dietician prior to the discharge of the patient from the specialized stroke care proram. Diet recommendations should be made available to all stroke patients. In patients with 2.6 to 3.4 mM LDL cholesterol, diet therapy is sufficient for control of lipoprotein concentrations. The diet should consist of caloric reduction for overweight patients, limitation of fat content to 30 percent calories, and isocaloric substitution of simple carbohydrates with complex carbohydrates and of saturated fat with monounsaturated fat. The diet should be enriched in fresh fruits and vegetables. The so-called "Mediterranean diet" will best fit the needs of stroke patients.[67,68] They could also be allowed a moderate alcohol intake (no more than two drinks per day), with the exception of patients with hypertriglyceridemia, which will be exacerbated by alcohol intake.

Drug Therapy

Because diet therapy has at best only moderate effects on LDL cholesterol, patients should be started on drug therapy as soon as the diagnosis of hyperlipidemia is established. The drugs of choice are statins.

Statins   Currently, there are six statins on the U.S. market:

Lovastatin: dosage 20 to 80 mg; LDL cholesterol lowering up to 39 percent.

Pravastatin: dosage 10 to 40 mg; LDL cholesterol lowering up to 34 percent.

Simvastatin: dosage 10 to 80 mg; LDL cholesterol lowering up to 54 percent.

Fluvastatin: dosage 20 to 80 mg; LDL cholesterol lowering up to 35 percent.

Atorvastatin: dosage 10 to 80 mg; LDL cholesterol lowering up to 60 percent

Cerivastatin: dosage 0.2 to 0.4 mg; LDL cholesterol lowering up to 37 percent.

The treatment is usually initiated with the statin of choice with an average dose, expected to result in a 25 percent reduction in LDL cholesterol. Subsequently, the management is adjusted until the pre-established target level is reached. The dose of statin is usually changed by multiples of two. Each doubling of the statin dose will result in an additional 6 percent LDL cholesterol lowering. The choice of statin depends on the physicians' perception of the relative value of drug-specific clinical evidence, LDL cholesterol lowering, and cost.[69]

Fibrates   In patients with LDL cholesterol under 3.4 mM or triglycerides over 7 mM, a viable alternative is the use of a fibrate as a first line drug. There are two fibrates on the U.S. market: gemfibrozil (dosage 600 mg BID) and fenofibrate (dosage 200 mg QD).[70] Fibrates could also be added to statin therapy, but clinical monitoring is necessary because of increased risk of myositis. The combination fibrate-statin should not be used in patients with renal failure.

Niacin   Niacin could be used as monotherapy in patients with cerebrovascular disease, but the expected benefit, safety, and side effect profile does not match that of statins. Niacin can be used in addition to statins to increase the LDL lowering, to reduce hypertriglyceridemia, or to increase HDL cholesterol. Myositis has been reported occasionally in patients taking combinations of statin and niacin. Some patients with premature atherosclerosis have high levels of Lp (a) as the only risk factor. These patients are usually treated with niacin, the only lipid-lowering drug effective in decreasing Lp (a) levels. Initiation of cristaline niacin therapy should include a gradual increase in dose because of the severe flushing experienced by most patients. The usual starting dose is 100 mg TID with weekly 100-mg increments in each dose. Recently, niacin has been made available as a prescription drug (Niaspan; KOS Pharmaceuticals). This preparation is easier to administer, better tolerated, and safe in doses up to 2 g. Monitoring of blood glucose, uric acid, and transaminase levels is recommended in all niacin-treated patients.

Bile Acid Binding Resins   Bile acid binding resins have been used mostly in combination with statins or niacin to increase the effectiveness of LDL lowering. In elderly patients, bile acid binding resins are usually poorly tolerated because of their gastrointestinal side effects.

COMPLIANCE ISSUES

Despite overwhelming evidence of benefit, hyperlipidemic patients with documented atherosclerosis are grossly undertreated. Only a fraction of the patients are being started on drug therapy, and half of these patients discontinue their medication within a year after the initiation of therapy. Physician compliance problems, patient compliance problems, miscommunication, and administrative errors account for this suboptimal health care delivery. Computerized monitoring of treatment in high-risk patients seems to be an acceptable solution in types of practices where this is feasible. It increases the physician compliance with guidelines without unduly increasing physician-patient contact time.

REFERENCES

1. National Cholesterol Education Program: Summary of the second report of the National Cholesterol Education Program (NCEP) Expert Panel on Detection, Evaluation, and Treatment of High Blood Cholesterol in Adults. *JAMA* 269:3015, 1993.
2. Dennis MS, Burn JP, Sandercock PA, et al: Long-term survival after first-ever stroke: The Oxfordshire Community Stroke Project. *Stroke* 24:796, 1993.
3. von Arbin M, Britton M, de Faire U: Mortality and recurrences during eight years following stroke. *J Intern Med* 231:43, 1992.
4. Viitanen M, Eriksson S, Asplund K: Risk of recurrent stroke, myocardial infarction and epilepsy during long-term follow-up after stroke. *Eur Neurol* 28:227, 1988.
5. Cohen SN, Hobson RW II, Weiss DG, et al: Death associated with asymptomatic carotid artery stenosis: Long-term clinical evaluation. VA Cooperative Study 167 Group. *J Vasc Surg* 18:1002, 1993.
6. Hertzer NR, Arison R: Cumulative stroke and survival ten years after carotid endarterectomy. *J Vasc Surg* 2:661, 1985.
7. Chimowitz MI, Weiss DG, Cohen SL, et al: Cardiac prognosis of patients with carotid stenosis and no history of coronary artery disease. Veterans Affairs Cooperative Study Group 167. *Stroke* 25:759, 1994.
8. Hertzer NR, Young JR, Beven EG, et al: Coronary angiography in 506 patients with extracranial cerebrovascular disease. *Arch Intern Med* 145:849, 1985.
9. Di Pasquale G, Andreoli A, Pinelli G, et al: Cerebral ischemia and asymptomatic coronary artery disease: A prospective study of 83 patients. *Stroke* 17:1098, 1986.
10. Love BB, Grover-McKay M, Biller J, et al: Coronary artery disease and cardiac events with asymptomatic and symptomatic cerebrovascular disease. *Stroke* 23:939, 1992.
11. Urbinati S, Di Pasquale G, Andreoli A, et al: Frequency and prognostic significance of silent coronary artery disease in patients with cerebral ischemia undergoing carotid endarterectomy. *Am J Cardiol* 69:1166, 1992.
12. Bots ML, Hoes AW, Koudstaal PJ, et al: Common carotid intima-media thickness and risk of stroke and myocardial infarction: The Rotterdam Study. *Circulation* 96:1432, 1997.
13. Trial of clofibrate in the treatment of ischaemic heart disease. Five-year study by a group of physicians of the Newcastle upon Tyne region. *Br Med J* 4:767, 1971.
14. Leren P: The Oslo diet-heart study: Eleven-year report. *Circulation* 42:935, 1970.
15. Dorr AE, Gundersen K, Schneider JC Jr, et al: Colestipol hydrochloride in hypercholesterolemic patients: Effect on serum cholesterol and mortality. *J Chronic Dis.* 31:5, 1978.
16. Coronary Drug Project report on clofibrate and niacin. *Atherosclerosis* 30:239, 1978.
17. Canner PL, Berge KG, Wenger NK, et al: Fifteen year mortality in Coronary Drug Project patients: Long-term benefit with niacin. *J Am Coll Cardiol.* 8:1245, 1986.
18. Carlson LA, Rosenhamer G: Reduction of mortality in the Stockholm Ischaemic Heart Disease Secondary Prevention Study by combined treatment with clofibrate and nicotinic acid. *Acta Med Scand* 223:405, 1988.
19. Buchwald H, Varco RL, Matts JP, et al: Effect of partial ileal bypass surgery on mortality and morbidity from coronary heart disease in patients with hypercholesterolemia: Report of the Program on the Surgical Control of the Hyperlipidemias (POSCH). *N Engl J Med* 323:946, 1990.
20. Scandinavian Simvastatin Survival Study Group: Randomised trial of cholesterol lowering in 4444 patients with coronary heart disease: The Scandinavian Simvastatin Survival Study (4S). *Lancet* 344:1383, 1994.
21. Miettinen TA, Pyorala K, Olsson AG, et al: Cholesterol-lowering therapy in women and elderly patients with myocardial infarction or angina pectoris: Findings from the Scandinavian Simvastatin Survival Study (4S). *Circulation* 96:4211, 1997.
22. Pedersen TR, Kjekshus J, Pyorala K, et al: Effect of simvastatin on ischemic signs and symptoms in the Scandinavian simvastatin survival study (4S). *Am J Cardiol* 81:333, 1998.
23. Sacks FM, Pfeffer MA, Moye LA, et al: The effect of pravastatin on coronary events after myocardial infarction in patients with average cholesterol levels. *N Engl J Med* 335:1001, 1996.
24. The Long-Term Intervention with Pravastatin in Ischemic Disease (Lipid) Study Group: Prevention of cardiovascular events and death with presentation in patients with coronary heart disease and a broad range of initial cholesterol levels. *N Engl J Med* 339:1349, 1998.
25. Furberg CD, Adams HP Jr, Applegate WB, et al: Effect of lovastatin on early carotid atherosclerosis and cardiovascular events: Asymptomatic Carotid Artery Progression Study (ACAPS) Research Group. *Circulation* 90:1679, 1994.
26. Crouse JR III, Byington RP, Bond MG, et al: Pravastatin, lipids, and atherosclerosis in the carotid arteries (PLAC-II). *Am J Cardiol* 75:455, 1995.
27. Furberg CD, Pitt B, Byington RP, Park JS, McGovern ME: Reduction in coronary events during treatment with pravastatin: PLAC I and PLAC II investigators. Pravastatin limitation of atherosclerosis in the coronary arteries. *Am J Cardiol* 76:60C, 1995.
28. Salonen R, Nyyssonen K, Porkkala E, et al: Kuopio Atherosclerosis Prevention Study (KAPS): A population-based primary preventive trial of the effect of LDL lowering on atherosclerotic progression in carotid and femoral arteries. *Circulation* 92:1758, 1995.
29. Mercuri M, Bond MG, Sirtori CR, et al: Pravastatin reduces carotid intima-media thickness progression in an asymptomatic hypercholesterolemic mediterranean population:

The Carotid Atherosclerosis Italian Ultrasound Study. *Am J Med* 101:627, 1996.

30. Cholesterol, diastolic blood pressure, and stroke: 13,000 strokes in 450,000 people in 45 prospective cohorts. Prospective studies collaboration. *Lancet* 346:1647, 1995.

31. Jacobs D, Blackburn H, Higgins M, et al: Report of the conference on low blood cholesterol: Mortality associations. *Circulation* 86:1046, 1992.

32. Iso H, Jacobs DR Jr, Wentworth D, et al: Serum cholesterol levels and six-year mortality from stroke in 350,977 men screened for the multiple risk factor intervention trial. *N Engl J Med* 320:904, 1989.

33. Lindenstrom E, Boysen G, Nyboe J: Influence of total cholesterol, high density lipoprotein cholesterol, and triglycerides on risk of cerebrovascular disease: The Copenhagen City Heart Study. *Br Med J* 309:11, 1994.

34. Dyker AG, Weir CJ, Lees KR: Influence of cholesterol on survival after stroke: Retrospective study. *Br Med J* 314:1584, 1997.

35. Acheson J, Hutchinson EC: Controlled trial of clofibrate in cerebral vascular disease. *Atherosclerosis* 15:177, 1972.

36. The treatment of cerebrovascular disease with clofibrate: Final report of the Veterans Administration Cooperative Study of Atherosclerosis, Neurology Section. *Stroke* 4:684, 1973.

37. Atkins D, Psaty BM, Koepsell TD, et al: Cholesterol reduction and the risk for stroke in men: A meta-analysis of randomized, controlled trials. *Ann Intern Med* 119:136, 1993.

38. Hebert PR, Gaziano JM, Hennekens CH: An overview of trials of cholesterol lowering and risk of stroke. *Arch Intern Med* 155:50, 1995.

39. Hebert PR, Gaziano JM, Chan KS, et al: Cholesterol lowering with statin drugs, risk of stroke, and total mortality: An overview of randomized trials. *JAMA* 278:313, 1997.

40. Blauw GJ, Lagaay AM, Smelt AH, et al: Stroke, statins, and cholesterol: A meta-analysis of randomized, placebo-controlled, double-blind trials with HMG-CoA reductase inhibitors. *Stroke* 28:946, 1997.

41. Delanty N, Vaughan CJ: Vascular effects of statins in stroke. *Stroke* 28:2315, 1997.

42. Bucher HC, Griffith LE, Guyatt GH: Effect of HMGcoA reductase inhibitors on stroke: A meta-analysis of randomized, controlled trials. *Ann Intern Med* 128:89, 1998.

43. Dayton S, Pearce ML, Hashimoto S: A controlled clinical trial of a diet high in unsaturated fat preventing complications of atherosclerosis. *Circulation* 40 (Suppl II):1, 1969.

44. Frantz ID Jr, Dawson EA, Ashman PL, et al: Test of effect of lipid lowering by diet on cardiovascular risk: The Minnesota Coronary Survey. *Arteriosclerosis* 9:129, 1989.

45. Hjermann I, Velve Byre K, Holme I: Effect of diet and smoking intervention on the incidence of coronary heart disease: Report from the Oslo Study Group of a randomised trial in healthy men. *Lancet* 2:1303, 1981.

46. Multiple risk factor intervention trial: Risk factor changes and mortality results: Multiple Risk Factor Intervention Trial Research Group. *JAMA* 248:1465, 1982.

47. Miettinen TA, Huttunen JK, Naukkarinen V, et al: Multifactorial primary prevention of cardiovascular diseases in middle-aged men: Risk factor changes, incidence, and mortality. *JAMA* 254:2097, 1985.

48. A co-operative trial in the primary prevention of ischaemic heart disease using clofibrate: Report from the Committee of Principal Investigators. *Br Heart J* 40:1069, 1978.

49. Frick MH, Elo O, Haapa K, et al: Helsinki Heart Study: Primary-prevention trial with gemfibrozil in middle-aged men with dyslipidemia: Safety of treatment, changes in risk factors, and incidence of coronary heart disease. *N Engl J Med* 317:1237, 1987.

50. The Lipid Research Clinics Coronary Primary Prevention Trial results: I. Reduction in incidence of coronary heart disease. *JAMA* 251:351, 1984.

51. The Pravastatin Multinational Study Group for Cardiac Risk Patients: Effects of pravastatin in patients with serum total cholesterol levels from 5.2 to 7.8 mmol/liter (200 to 300 mg/dL) plus two additional atherosclerotic risk factors. *Am J Cardiol* 72:1031, 1993.

52. Byington RP, Jukema JW, Salonen JT, et al: Reduction in cardiovascular events during pravastatin therapy: Pooled analysis of clinical events of the Pravastatin Atherosclerosis Intervention Program. *Circulation* 92:2419, 1995.

53. Shepherd J, Cobbe SM, Ford I, et al: Prevention of coronary heart disease with pravastatin in men with hypercholesterolemia: West of Scotland Coronary Prevention Study Group. *N Engl J Med* 333:1301, 1995.

54. Lehto S, Ronnemaa T, Pyorala K, and Laakso M: Predictors of stroke in middle-aged patients with non-insulin-dependent diabetes. *Stroke* 27:63, 1996.

55. Njolstad I, Arnesen E, Lund-Larsen PG: Body height, cardiovascular risk factors, and risk of stroke in middle-aged men and women: A 14-year follow-up of the Finnmark Study. *Circulation* 94:2877, 1996.

56. Wilson PW: High-density lipoprotein, low-density lipoprotein and coronary artery disease. *Am J Cardiol* 66 (Suppl 6):7A, 1990.

57. Woo J, Lau E, Lam CW, Kay R, et al: Hypertension, lipoprotein(a), and apolipoprotein A-I as risk factors for stroke in the Chinese. *Stroke* 22:203, 1991.

58. Pedro-Botet J, Senti M, Nogues X, et al: Lipoprotein and apolipoprotein profile in men with ischemic stroke: Role of lipoprotein(a), triglyceride-rich lipoproteins, and apolipoprotein E polymorphism. *Stroke* 23:1556, 1992.

59. Ridker PM, Stampfer MJ, Hennekens CH: Plasma concentration of lipoprotein(a) and the risk of future stroke (see Comments). *JAMA* 273:1269, 1995.

60. Margaglione M, Seripa D, Gravina C, et al: Prevalence of apoliprotein E alleles in healthy subjects and survivors of ischemic stroke: An Italian Case-Control Study. *Stroke* 29:399, 1998.

61. McGee D, Reed D, Stemmerman G, et al: The relationship

of dietary fat and cholesterol to mortality in 10 years: The Honolulu Heart Program. *Int J Epidemiol* 14:97, 1985.

62. Gillman MW, Cupples LA, Millen BE, et al: Inverse association of dietary fat with development of ischemic stroke in men. *JAMA* 278:2145, 1997.

63. Keli SO, Hertog MG, Feskens EJ, et al: Dietary flavonoids, antioxidant vitamins, and incidence of stroke: The Zutphen study. *Arch Intern Med* 156:637, 1996.

64. Shinton R, Sagar G, Beevers G: Body fat and stroke: Unmasking the hazards of overweight and obesity. *J Epidemiol Community Health* 49:259, 1995.

65. Walker SP, Rimm EB, Ascherio A, et al: Body size and fat distribution as predictors of stroke among US men. *Am J Epidemiol* 144:1143, 1996.

66. Woo J, Lam CW, Kay R, Wong HY, Teoh R, Nicholls MG: Acute and long-term changes in serum lipids after acute stroke. *Stroke* 21:1407, 1990.

67. De Lorgeril M, Salen P, Martin JL, et al: Effect of a mediterranean type of diet on the rate of cardiovascular complications in patients with coronary artery disease: Insights into the cardioprotective effect of certain nutriments. *J Am Coll Cardiol* 28:1103, 1996.

68. Assmann G, de Backer G, Bagnara S, et al: International consensus statement on olive oil and the Mediterranean diet: Implications for health in Europe. The Olive Oil and the Mediterranean Diet Panel. *Eur J Cancer Prev* 6:418, 1997.

69. Bloomfield-Rubins H, Robins S, Iwane M, et al: Rationale and Design of the Department of Veteran Affairs High Density Lipoprotein Intervention Trial for Secondary Prevention of Coronary Artery Disease in men with low high density lipoprotein cholesterol and desirable low density lipoprotein cholesterol. *Am J Cardiol* 71:45, 1993.

70. Bloomfield-Rubins H, Robins SJ, Collins, et al: Gemifibrozil for the secondary prevention of coronary heart disease in men with low levels of high-density lipoprotein cholesterol. *N Engl J Med* 341:410, 1999.

Chapter 7

THE SUBACUTE STROKE PATIENT: BLOOD PRESSURE MANAGEMENT

Peter A. Glassman
Marion Ho

BACKGROUND

Hypertension is defined as a persistent systolic blood pressure (SBP) greater than or equal to 140 mmHg and/or diastolic blood pressure (DBP) greater than or equal to 90 mmHg. Isolated systolic hypertension (ISH) is defined as a systolic blood pressure 140 mmHg or greater but a diastolic blood pressure below 90 mmHg.[1]

Although these definitions conveniently divide normal from elevated blood pressure, the risk of stroke is linearly related to differences in blood pressure throughout the range of measurement. For example, persons with a blood pressure of 120/80 have an estimated fourfold *reduction* in risk compared with persons with a blood pressure of about 150/90. Persons with a blood pressure of 170/105 have an approximately fourfold *elevation* in risk compared with persons with a blood pressure of 150/90.[2]

Patients who are hypertensive and already have had a stroke are at high risk for another cerebrovascular event.[3] In fact, the Joint National Committee in their Sixth Report (JNC VI) on Prevention, Detection, Evaluation, and Treatment of High Blood Pressure, issued in 1997, classifies them as the highest risk.[1] As such, these patients should receive appropriate intervention even when their blood pressure is nominally elevated (i.e., 140/90 mmHg or higher).

The main issue, though, is deciding which patients have the diagnosis of hypertension after an ischemic infarction.[4] Blood pressure is frequently elevated during the acute and post-acute stages of stroke. Only about one-third of patients with high blood pressure after an acute stroke have high blood pressure 10 days later.[5] Thus, the desire to intervene on seemingly hypertensive patients in the early postacute stages of stroke must be balanced by the knowledge that many such patients will turn out to be normotensive in the coming weeks. Whether stroke patients whose blood pressures fall within the normal range require further blood pressure reduction is unknown.

Once the decision is made to initiate therapy, patients should be started on medication(s) and educated on adjunctive lifestyle recommendations. The goal of therapy is to gradually reduce blood pressure to below 140/90 and, if tolerated, toward 120/80 mmHg without causing orthostatic hypotension. The choice of medications should be prioritized in terms of which drugs have the strongest evidence in reducing vascular events <u>and</u> overall mortality. Lifestyle recommendations should be oriented toward helping control blood pressure and toward improving overall health and well being.

EVIDENCE

Antihypertensive Treatment and Primary Prevention of Stroke

The evidence from prospective observational studies and from drug trials has been extensively documented and analyzed at length elsewhere but in toto indicates that elevated blood pressure increases the risk for stroke, cardiac events, and mortality.[6,7] With specific regard to stroke, data from seven of nine prospective observational studies (418,343 lives for all studies) suggest that the risk of stroke is "directly and continuously" associated with blood pressure measurements, with a persistent 5 mmHg difference in diastolic blood pressure, altering stroke risk by about one third.[2] This is illustrated in Fig. 7-1.[2]

Randomized clinical trials on antihypertensive therapy support the data from observational studies regarding primary prevention of stroke. A 1994 overview of 4 large and 13 small unconfounded randomized trials (approximately 48,000 individuals) found that antihypertensive therapy decreased stroke risk by about 38 percent (95 percent confidence interval, 31 to 45 percent).[2] As noted in observational studies, a decrease in diastolic blood pressure by 5 to 6 mmHg was required to achieve that degree of risk reduction.[2] Figure 7-2, from JNC VI, summarizes the findings for the major primary prevention trials.[1]

Overwhelming evidence from randomized controlled trials indicates that controlling systolic and/or diastolic blood pressure with a diuretic and/or beta

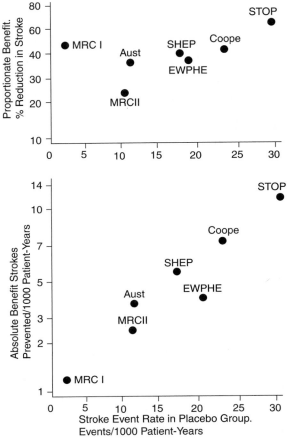

Figure 7-2.
Comparison of proportionate (relative) and absolute benefit from reduction in the incidence of stroke in six trials under review and in one other with a similar design but in which the absolute risk for stroke was much lower.

Figure 7-1.
Relative risks of stroke and of coronary heart disease, estimated from combined results. (From MacMahon S, Peto R, Cutler J, et al: Epidemiology: Blood pressure, stroke, and coronary heart disease—Part 1. Lancet 335:765, 1990.)

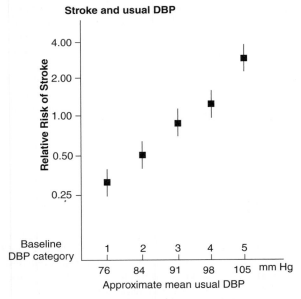

blocker-based regimen reduces the risk for stroke, cardiac event, and mortality.[1,2] One question that continues to perplex researchers and clinicians alike is whether the clinical effects of one antihypertensive agent can be assumed to be the clinical effects of another. In other words, do newer agents achieve the same benefit as regimens based on beta blockers and diuretics?

Unfortunately, apart from one recent study (discussed below), there are little data in this regard, and the answer remains elusive. However, unless a newer agent confers some additional advantageous mechanism of action, such as does angiotensin-converting enzyme inhibitors (ACEI) for diabetics with diabetic nephropathy, there is little likelihood that it will provide substantially greater clinical benefit than that seen with diuretic and beta blocker-based interventions.[2,8]

One recent study looked at isolated systolic hypertension in patients 60 years and older and evaluated a therapeutic intervention primarily based on nitrendipine, an intermediate-acting dihydropyridine calcium channel blocker not currently available in the United States. The study found that compared with placebo, nitrendipine alone or in combination with enalapril and/or hydrocholorthiazide reduced relative risk for stroke (nonfatal and fatal) by 42 percent.[9] Mortality between the two groups was not statistically different (−14 percent in favor of intervention group, $p = .22$). Little information was available for the group on nitrendipine alone, making assessment of this drug (vs. placebo) difficult.

Putting this study into context, it is important to note that the results on vascular events fall into the range noted in earlier trials.[2] However, as opposed to earlier trials, overall mortality did not improve compared with placebo. Moreover, there is legitimate concern that dihydropyridine calcium channel blockers may not have the clinical effectiveness of other antihypertensives and may, in fact, be harmful to certain types of patients such as those with diabetes.[10,11] In particular, dihydropyridine calcium channel blockers may increase the rate of untoward vascular events relative to ACE inhibitors and diuretics.[10,11] Taken as a whole, the evidence raises concerns concerning long-term safety, especially when compared with other agents.

Antihypertensive Treatment and Secondary Prevention of Stroke

These issues above may all be moot because those studies were focused on preventing a first stroke (i.e., primary prevention) and not on what should be done about high blood pressure after a stroke (i.e., secondary prevention). Unfortunately, there is a paucity of clinically relevant evidence in this regard.[2] It is not clear that results from primary prevention trials can be extrapolated to poststroke survivors, especially because persons with one stroke have a far higher risk of another stroke than patients enrolled in primary prevention trials.[12] In fact, an actuarial study from Rochester, Minnesota looking at patients who had a stroke between 1950 and 1979 found that "neither blood pressure before the first stroke nor management of hypertension after the stroke had any apparent effect on stroke recurrence."[13] This result, although interesting, was based on a retrospective

unadjusted cohort analysis, making any firm conclusion on secondary prevention (or lack thereof) difficult.

Other data on secondary prevention do support evidence from primary prevention studies.[14] A recent meta-analysis found that stroke recurrence, fatal and nonfatal, was reduced by 38 percent in patients treated with antihypertensive therapy.[15] This finding is similar to a prior but much smaller study that found that managing hypertension reduced relative risk of subsequent stroke by about 40 percent.[16] The risk reduction appeared even larger (e.g., 50% to 75 percent) for patients whose hypertension was well controlled.[3,16,17]

There is some evidence that elevated diastolic pressure, rather than systolic pressure, is more closely associated with risk of stroke recurrence,[3] but the relevance of this result remains unclear given the dramatic reduction in stroke risk for elderly patients with isolated systolic hypertension in primary prevention studies.[18,19] Overall, the evidence can be summarized by the following: (1) patients with stroke and hypertension are at high risk for recurrent stroke, (2) managing blood pressure after a stroke reduces the risk of recurrent stroke, and (3) well-controlled blood pressure reduces the risk for recurrent stroke greater than poorly controlled blood pressure.

Yet, although few would now argue against treating hypertension in ischemic stroke survivors, it is unknown what constitutes the optimal intervention for and degree of blood pressure control for these patients. Current consensus suggests that stroke patients should receive intervention for blood pressure control if it is persistently 140/90 mmHg or above[1] and that optimal risk reduction for cardiovascular events is at a blood pressure of 120/80 mmHg.[1]

A point of contention, though, is whether a diastolic pressure of 80 mmHg is truly optimal. One study on recurrent stroke supports the diastolic recommendation of 80 to 84 mmHg,[20] whereas another suggests that diastolic blood pressures below 85 mmHg may be associated with an increased risk of cardiac events.[21] The principal results of the Hypertension Optimal Treatment (HOT) trial found that the lowest risk of stroke occurred at diastolic blood pressures below 80 mmHg; the lowest risk of cardiovascular mortality occurred at 86.5 mmHg, although further reduction was found to be safe.[22] These results, however, may not pertain to stroke survivors.

It is also unknown when the optimal time is for initiating (or restarting) antihypertensive therapy in the poststroke period. This is in large part because of the difficulty in determining the diagnosis of hypertension shortly after an acute cerebrovascular event. Several studies have found that most patients (70 to 85 percent) have high blood pressure after an acute stroke.[5,23] However, blood pressure tends to fall dramatically as patients become clinically stable,[24,25] with only about 30 percent having high blood pressure 1 to 2 weeks later.[4,5] Whether the blood pressure stays low is controversial, though, with one study indicating that two-thirds of patients have substantial blood pressure increases over the course of a month.[26] Thus, patients should be followed regularly after a stroke to monitor blood pressure, regardless of the initial therapeutic decision.

There is no evidence that early intervention for elevated blood pressure, when not associated with an emergent situation (e.g., coronary ischemia), reduces mortality after stroke. In fact, such intervention may cause further harm by precipitating cerebral hypoperfusion and should be avoided, if possible.[25,27,28]

Owing to the paucity of evidence, the basis for and type of blood pressure intervention after a stroke must rely heavily on information derived from clinical trials on primary prevention and from expert opinion. This combination has been well used by the Joint National Committee on Prevention, Detection, Evaluation, and Treatment of High Blood Pressure in their periodic updates on diagnosis and management of hypertension. Our recommendations generally follow the current recommendations found in JNC VI.[1] The basic management plan is summarized in Table 7-1.

THERAPEUTIC RECOMMENDATIONS

Initiation of Therapy

When to initiate therapy after a stroke must remain in the domain of clinical judgment, given that a variety of physiological and psychological factors can prompt elevated blood pressure readings in patients who have recently suffered a cerebrovascular event. As a general rule, unless the patient requires emergent treatment for high blood pressure, it is prudent to hold off altering pre-existing hypotensive therapy until the patient is clinically stable and without the dramatic blood pressure changes that are so often seen shortly after a stroke.[5,23,24] In most instances, therapy can wait until the patient is in the ambulatory setting, 7 to 14 days after a stroke.[4,29]

To properly diagnose high blood pressure, the following technique is recommended.[1] Patients should be in a sitting position with their backs supported and arms bared. The arm should be at heart level. Measure-

Table 7-1.

Managing high blood pressure in the poststroke period

1. Patients with a cerebrovascular event (stroke or TIA) and hypertension are in the highest risk category and should be treated with medication if blood pressure is persistently ≥140/90. Lifestyle modification should be used as adjunctive therapy.
2. Blood pressure should be reduced gradually, after the patient is clinically stable, to <140/90. A further gradual reduction may be warranted, as tolerated, toward 120/80. This is considered the "optimal" level for reducing cardiovascular risk.[1]
3. Choose, whenever possible, a regimen including beta blockers and/or thiazide diuretics as these are safe, effective, and cost-effective and have been shown to reduce the risk of stroke, coronary heart disease, and mortality associated with hypertension.
4. Reasonable alternatives, when patients cannot tolerate either of the above medications, include a number of hypotensive drugs from other pharmaceutical classes. Clinicians should consider patient preferences and comorbidities and the cost of pharmacologic treatment.

ments should be made after at least 5 min of resting. The patient should not have consumed caffeinated drinks or used tobacco within 30 min of measurement.

The inflatable portion of cuff should comfortably encircle at least 80 percent of the arm because an inappropriately small cuff may yield a spuriously elevated reading. Clinicians should use the first appearance of sound (phase 1) as the systolic blood pressure and disappearance of the last sound (phase 5) as the diastolic reading. Initial blood pressure measurements should be taken in both arms, and the higher reading should be used as the patient's baseline level. The same arm should be used for monitoring blood pressure control. Initial blood pressure assessment should also include measurements in a sitting and standing position to help detect any baseline postural changes. Two or more readings separated at least by 2 min should be averaged. If the first two readings differ by more than 5 mmHg, additional readings should be obtained and averaged.[1]

For patients without a previously known history of hypertension, a history and physical exam should assess several areas. First, it should focus on any possible reversible or secondary causes of hypertension. Clinical findings that may suggest a secondary cause include an enlarged thyroid gland, cushingoid features, abdominal bruits, aortic pulsation, diminished femoral pulses or absent lower extremity pulses, or abdominal or flank masses. Low serum potassium in a patient not on diuretics may indicate primary hyperaldosteronism.

Second, a clinical evaluation should assess the presence of longstanding target organ damage. Clinicians should ask whether the patient has (or has had) angina or claudication, myocardial infarction, coronary revascularization, heart failure, or peripheral vascular disease. A focused examination should look for retinopathy (i.e., arteriolar narrowing, arteriovenous changes, hemorrhages, and exudates), left ventricular hypertrophy (e.g., a third or fourth heart sound, increased size, precordial heave), and vascular bruits and abnormalities (e.g., abdominal aortic bruits/aneurysm, diminished peripheral pulses). Laboratory evidence that suggests chronic organ damage includes a raised serum creatinine, proteinuria, cardiomegaly on chest radiograph, or electrocardiographic changes (i.e., left ventricular hypertrophy, nonspecific ST changes, or old infarction).

Third, other risk factors for cardiovascular diseases such as diabetes, dyslipidemia, renal diseases, and coronary artherosclerotic disease should be identified for subsequent intervention. Clinicians should also inquire about consumption of alcohol, sodium, and tobacco products. The patient's basic dietary habits should be explored. Serum chemistries and lipid studies can assist in establishing the presence of some cardiovascular risks. Many of these issues are dealt with elsewhere in this book.

Before starting medications, clinicians should ensure that the appropriate laboratory tests have been completed.[1] These include a urinalysis, complete blood count, serum chemistries (serum creatinine, fasting blood glucose, potassium), and lipid analysis. A recent 12-lead electrocardiogram is also needed. Other tests that may be considered include a uric acid and thyroid-stimulating hormone and, especially for diabetics, calcium and magnesium. Creatinine clearance and 24-h urine are usually not needed unless initial laboratory testing detects a relevant abnormality. Further cardiovascular evaluation (e.g., echocardiography, ambulatory blood pressure monitoring, ankle-brachial blood pressures) are only helpful in selected patients and are not used routinely.

Lifestyle Changes

There are two basic components of therapy: pharmacologic and nonpharmacologic. No matter what medication is eventually used, patients, and those that help care for

them, should receive education on lifestyle changes (Table 7-2).[1] Some recommendations will be more difficult for patients whose mobility and/or cognitive function are impaired. Nevertheless, the recommendations should be viewed as overall goals to move toward over time.

Aerobic exercise, particularly low impact activities such as walking, swimming, or stationary cycling, should be increased gradually to between 30 and 45 min a day. If the patient cannot walk, there are exercise machines available that promote aerobic exercises through arm activity. Similarly, weight loss, if needed, should be done gradually and with reasonable goals. Even losing 5 to 10 pounds can assist in blood pressure control. Clinicians will need to tailor weight loss and exercise programs to the capabilities and preferences of the individual patient.

In terms of specific diets, the Dietary Approaches to Stop Hypertension (DASH) diet is "heart" healthy and lowers blood pressure. The DASH diet combines low total fat and low saturated fat (e.g., low-fat dairy products) with fruits, vegetables, and nuts and legumes.[30] The basic components of the DASH diet are given in Table 7-3. As with exercise and weight loss, patients

Table 7-2.
Lifestyle changes

Recommended lifestyle changes
1. Lose weight, if needed (e.g., 5 to 10 lb. over 2 to 3 months)
2. Reduce alcohol intake to no more than 1 ounce per day of any type of alcohol (e.g., 24 ounces of beer, 10 ounces of wine, 2 ounces of 100 proof whiskey). Lightweight persons and women should have no more than half that amount.
3. Increase aerobic activity to 30 to 45 min a day (gradually, as tolerated).
4. Sodium intake should be <100 mmol/day (2.4 g of sodium or 6 g of sodium chloride) (e.g., avoid store-bought salty foods and do not add salt to home-cooked or restaurant foods).
5. Consume foods that provide adequate potassium, calcium, and magnesium (e.g., emphasize low-fat dairy products, fresh fruits and juices, and vegetables and nuts)
6. Stop smoking and reduce overall dietary fats, saturated fats, and cholesterol.

From the Sixth Report of the Joint National Committee on Prevention, Detection, Evaluation, and Treatment of High Blood Pressure. *Arch Intern Med* 157:2422, 1997.

Table 7-3.

The DASH diet[a]

Food group	Daily serving	Serving sizes	Examples and notes
Grain and grain products	7–8	1 slice bread ½ c (0.12 L) dry cereal ½ c (0.12 L) cooked rice, pasta, or cereal	Whole wheat bread, English muffin, pita bread, bagel, cereals, grits, oatmeal
Vegetables	4–5	1 c (0.24 L) raw leafy vegetables ½ c (0.12 L) cooked vegetables 6 oz (180 mL) vegetable juice	Tomatoes, potatoes, peas, carrots, squash, broccoli, turnip greens, collards, kale, spinach, artichokes, beans, sweet potatoes
Fruits	4–5	6 oz (180 mL) fruit juice 1 medium fruit ½ c (0.06 L) dried fruit ¼ c (0.12 L) fresh, frozen, or canned fruit	Apricots, bananas, dates, grapes, oranges, orange juice, grapefruit, grapefruit juice, mangos, melons, peaches, pineapples, prunes, raisins, strawberries, tangerines
Low-fat or nonfat dairy foods	2–3	8 oz (240 mL) milk 1 c (0.24 L) yogurt 1.5 oz (45 g) cheese	Skim or 1% milk, skim or low-fat buttermilk, nonfat or low-fat yogurt, part-skim mozzarella cheese, nonfat cheese
Meats, poultry, and fish	≤2	3 oz (84 g) cooked meats, poultry, or fish	Select only lean meats; trim away visible fats; broil, roast, or boil instead of frying; remove skin from poultry
Nuts, seeds, and legumes	(4–5/wk)	1.5 oz (42 g) or ⅓ c (0.08 L) nuts; 0.5 oz (14 g) or 2 tbsp (3 mL) seeds; ½ c (0.12 L) cooked legumes	Almonds, filberts, mixed nuts, peanuts, walnuts, sunflower seeds, kidney beans, lentils

[a]Modified from the Sixth Report of the Joint National Committee on Prevention, Detection, Evaluation, and Treatment of High Blood Pressure. *Arch Intern Med* 157:2421, 1997. Based on the Dietary Approaches to Stop Hypertension (DASH) study.[30] Diet plan based on 2000 calories a day (400 J/d). Depending on energy needs, the number of daily servings in a food group may vary from those listed.

and/or their caregivers should attempt to integrate changes gradually, as tolerated, to maximize long-term adherence. Discussion with a dietitian about practical use of this diet plan may be helpful for patients and family members.

Pharmacologic Management

The general algorithm for managing hypertension after stroke (Fig. 7-3) modified from JNC VI,[1] is given below. Patients with high blood pressure (≥140/90) and clinical evidence suggesting a prior history of hypertension can

be started on antihypertensive therapy and lifestyle modifications when clinically stable. For those with high blood pressure but no evidence of previous hypertension, it would seem prudent to reassess blood pressure at about 7 to 14 days poststroke before making the decision to begin antihypertensive medication. If doubt still exists at that time (i.e., the trend in blood pressure continues downward) or the patient is not yet clinically stable, clinicians can delay their decision. The goal of therapy is to reduce blood pressure gradually, without causing orthostatic hypotension, and without interfering with the patient's quality of life.

Figure 7-3.
Algorithm for Managing Hypertension in Post-Stroke Period. (Modified from the Sixth Joint report of the National Committee on Prevention, Detection, Evaluation, and Treatment of High Blood Pressure. Arch Intern Med *157:2430, 1997.)*

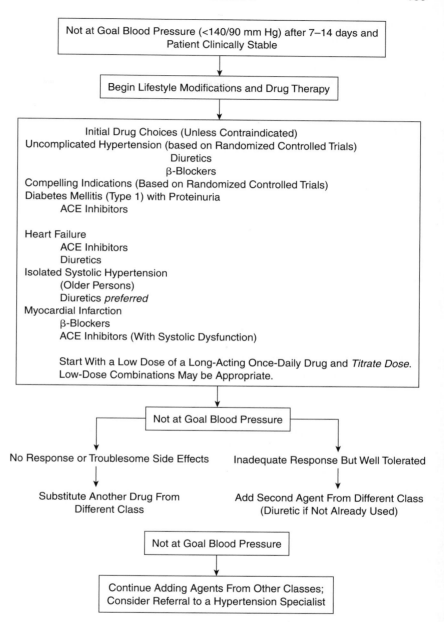

When deciding on which drug(s) to prescribe, clinicians should plan on using as few medications as possible. Longer-acting preparations are preferred to make adherence easier for the patient, although there is not a lot of evidence to indicate that patients are more or less adherent with once daily vs. twice daily therapy.

Clinicians should keep in mind drug costs and monetary outlays required of patients, particularly those paying for part or all of their medications. It is a good idea to discreetly inquire how patients will be paying for their drugs and whether these payments create a hardship. If so, effort should be made to choose the least expensive medications and/or to assist the patient through pharmaceutical programs aimed at getting medications to those in need.

JNC VI suggests that drug therapy be tailored to the patients' comorbidities when possible.[1] Such an approach adds to convenience and reduces the potential for polypharmacy. Tailoring is helpful if the patient is already on a medication, or is to be started on a medication, that can be dosed to reduce blood pressure (e.g., an alpha blocker for prostatism or a beta blocker for coronary heart disease).

On the other hand, newer evidence on low-dose diuretics and on beta blockers supports older evidence for using thiazide diuretics and beta blockers as primary agents in treating hypertension.[31–33] Thus, tailoring medications should usually take a secondary role except if the patient has a compelling reason to use a specific drug (Table 7-4, below). In fact, the evidence is so overwhelmingly in favor of diuretics and beta blockers that, as a general rule of thumb, clinicians should seriously consider using one or both before using other antihypertensive drugs.

A reasonable alternative to these is an ACE inhibitor, as this class of medication has been shown to reduce morbidity and mortality for selected cardiac patients and has beneficial effects on left ventricular hypertrophy.[34] Appendix 7-1 gives several approaches to controlling blood pressure using these classes of medications. In practical terms, physicians should become comfortable with one or two medications from each class of pharmaceutical they routinely use. We include a selected list of all classes of medications in Appendix 7-2.

Secondary alternatives to beta blockers and thiazide diuretics and ACE inhibitors include drugs with little or no data on hypertensive or vascular morbidity and mortality. These include angiotensin II receptor antagonists and nondihydropyridine calcium channel blockers. Other drugs such as alpha blockers and centrally acting agents can be used, at clinicians' discretion, with the understanding that these medications can have adverse effects in elderly patients.

The issues concerning potential benefits and harms of dihydropyridine calcium channel blockers are complex. As discussed earlier, one study supports use of dihydropyridines for preventing stroke in patients with isolated systolic hypertension.[19] Other studies have found that dihydropyridines caused an unwanted increase in vascular events.[8,10,11] It is important to remember that none of these studies focused on poststroke patients. It may be that the risk-benefit profile improves for secondary stroke prevention. It is equally possible that the risk-benefit profile becomes worse. Given the controversy on long-term safety issues, we recommend that dihydropyridine calcium channel blockers be reserved for patients whose blood pressure is not controlled on or who cannot tolerate diuretics, beta blockers, and/or ACE inhibitors.

Medications

Thiazide diuretics may be used as monotherapy, in combination therapy, or as part of multiple drug regimens.[36] Diuretics should preferentially be relatively low dose such as hydrochlorothiazide (HCTZ) 12.5 or 25 mg daily (or equivalent), as higher doses may be associated with more adverse effects.[37] Low-dose diuretics have few contraindications (or side effects), but clinicians should be cautious with patients who may be volume depleted or who have gout, symptomatic prostatism, or poorly controlled diabetes. Potassium-sparing diuretics are not

Table 7-4.
Compelling indications to use specific medications

Diabetes mellitus (type 1) with proteinuria[a]	ACE inhibitors
Heart failure (systolic)	ACE inhibitors, diuretics
Isolated systolic hypertension (older patients)	Diuretics preferred
Myocardial infarction	Beta blocker (non-ISA) + ACE inhibitor (with systolic dysfunction)

[a]Some may argue that type II diabetics with proteinuria should receive ACE inhibitors.[35]
+ refers to beta blockers without intrinsic sympathomimetic activity.
Adapted from the Sixth Report of the Joint National Commission.[1]

usually used alone for antihypertensive therapy but are helpful in combination products (e.g., HCTZ and triamterene), especially when higher doses of thiazide diuretics are used or when a patient is also taking digoxin.[36] Clinicians should be aware that even with combined drugs, hypokalemia may still occur, particularly when the combined product uses higher doses of hydrochlorothiazide (or equivalent).

Beta blockers may be used as monotherapy, in combination with diuretics, or as part of multiple drug regimens. Beta blockers come with various attributes such as those with intrinsic sympathomimetic activity (e.g., acebutolol, carteolol, pindolol). These have fewer effects on lipids than beta blockers without intrinsic sympathomimetic activity. However, what relevance lipid alterations (or lack of) have for beta blockers is unclear, given that the cardioselective agents (e.g., metoprolol, propanolol) have been shown to benefit cardiac events and mortality.[1] As such, beta blockers without intrinsic sympathomimetic activity should be used in patients with a history of myocardial infarction.[1] Beta blockers should be used with caution in patients with a history of bronchospasm, systolic heart failure, diabetes, and heart block or in patients who are already taking an opthalmic beta blocker for glaucoma. Note that diabetics with coronary heart disease benefit from beta blockers and should not be denied these potentially beneficial drugs, when appropriate.[32]

Although ACE inhibitors do not have clinical outcome data regarding hypertensive morbidity and mortality, they have proven benefits for selected cardiac patients, particularly those with systolic heart failure or systolic dysfunction (i.e., low ejection fraction) and patients who have recently suffered a myocardial infarction.[34] They have good efficacy in reducing blood pressure and work well alone or when combined with diuretics. The most common adverse effect of ACE inhibitor is chronic cough, occurring in a small number of patients (2 to 10 percent). ACE inhibitors should be used very cautiously with potassium-sparing diuretics, as this combination may result in hyperkalemia. Bilateral renal artery stenosis is a contraindication to using ACE inhibitors. Patients on ACE inhibitors should have serum potassium, creatinine, and blood urea nitrogen checked shortly after starting the medication.

Angiotensin II receptor antagonists have a similar mechanism of action to ACE inhibitors but lack the cumulative evidence on morbidity and mortality for selected cardiac patients. They are reasonable alternatives to ACE inhibitors, especially when an ACE inhibitor is indicated but cannot be tolerated.

Calcium channel blockers have good efficacy in reducing blood pressure and, in the case of longer-acting preparations, have the benefit of being easy to prescribe and being convenient for many patients. However, as discussed above, some data on longer-acting dihydropyridines are concerning. Clinicians may wish to use these agents in patients who have not reached their blood pressure goal with beta blockers, diuretics, or ACE inhibitors. Dihydropyridines should be avoided in diabetic patients, if possible.[10] When a dihydropyridine is used, it is prudent to use longer-acting (e.g., once daily) preparations. Immediate-release nifedipine should no longer be used in the management of hypertension owing to serious questions about short-term and long-term safety.[8,38] Dihydropyridines can cause peripheral edema, often occurring shortly after starting the medication or after a dose increase. Diuretics will not necessarily resolve the edema, and the medication usually needs to be stopped.

When a longer-acting calcium channel blocker is warranted, clinicians can also consider any among the once-daily verapamil or diltiazem preparations. It should be understood that these have little evidence of benefit or harm in patients with cardiac ischemia[39] and that there are no data to suggest that these agents reduce the risk of stroke. However, these agents are generally well tolerated and are efficacious in reducing blood pressure. Diltiazem, in particular, may assist in reducing blood pressure in black men.[40] Both diltiazem and verapamil should be avoided in patients with heart block or decreased systolic function. Verapamil may cause constipation.

Other medications that are available include alpha blockers (prazosin, doxazosin, and terazosin), centrally acting drugs (clonidine and methyldopa), combined alpha and beta blockers (labetalol, carvedilol), direct vasodilators (hydralazine and minoxidil), and peripheral adrenergic inhibitors (e.g., reserpine). Although the use of these drugs should not be downplayed, they play a secondary role in managing stroke patients because of potential adverse effects on the central nervous and/or vascular systems.[1]

Many of the above medications are available as combined products (see Appendix 7-2). For some patients and clinicians, these products represent extra convenience. They may also represent extra expense, and use may need to be constrained because of financial considerations. Clinicians should be wary of products that together might increase the risk of orthostatic hypotension. Moreover, if an adverse event is noted by the patient, it is often difficult to know which agent is the offending drug, and both may have to be discontinued.

Although no drug or drug combination is guaranteed to reduce blood pressure, clinicians should reconsider their management plan if a patient has no or little response to antihypertensive medications. Common problems include nonadherence to therapy (including forgetfulness or taking the wrong pills), improper dosing or combination of medications, volume overload from too much salt or from lack of a diuretic in the drug regimen, high alcohol intake, and chronic pain.[1] Drug interactions can also interfere with good blood pressure control, including interactions with nasal decongestants, adrenal steroids, antidepressants, and nonsteroidal anti-inflammatory drugs.[1] Appendix 7-3 lists some of the more common drug interactions.

Some patients' blood pressure will be difficult to control even on multiple drug regimens. Patients who do not meet their basic blood pressure goal (<140/90 mmHg) on three properly dosed medications (one of which should be a diuretic) may have resistant hypertension.[1] Whenever possible, the above factors should be addressed and corrected. Lifestyle modifications should be reinforced. If the blood pressure is still not controlled, clinicians should seek advice from someone with expertise in managing hypertension.

Finally, in the office setting clinicians will occasionally see poststroke patients who have very high blood pressures (e.g., SBP ≥200 or DBP ≥110). Without acute organ damage, such as ongoing ischemia, cerebral encephalopathy, or progressive renal deterioration, asymptomatic patients should have their blood pressure lowered over hours and days, rather than emergently. Oral or sublingual nifedipine should not be used because of its rapid and unpredictable action on blood pressure.[38] Rather, prudent measures of blood pressure reduction include raising the dose of an existing medication or beginning a new medication (or class of medication) that can be continued for subsequent care. Examples include a short-acting ACE inhibitor such as captopril or a short-acting beta blocker such as metoprolol. After an initial monitoring in the office, patients can be followed closely to assure a gradual decline in blood pressure by titrating or adding medications, as needed.

REFERENCES

1. The sixth report of the Joint National Committee on Prevention, Detection, Evaluation, and Treatment of High Blood Pressure. *Arch Intern Med* 157:2413, 1997.

2. Collins R, MacMahon S: Blood pressure, antihypertensive drug treatment and the risks of stroke and of heart disease. *Br Med Bull* 50:272, 1994.

3. Alter M, Friday G, Lai SM, O'Connell J, Sobel E: Hypertension and risk of stroke recurrence. *Stroke* 25:1605, 1994.

4. O'Connell JE, Gray CS: Treating hypertension after stroke. *Lancet* 344:519, 1994.

5. Wallace JD, Levy LL: Blood pressure after stroke. *JAMA* 246:2177, 1981.

6. MacMahon S, Peto R, Cutler J, et al: Blood pressure, stroke, and coronary heart disease. Part 1. Prolonged differences in blood pressure: Prospective observational studies corrected for dilution bias. *Lancet* 335:765, 1990.

7. Collins R, Peto R, MacMahon S: Blood pressure, stroke, and coronary heart disease. Part 2. Short-term reductions in blood pressure: Overview of randomized drug trials in their epidemiological context. *Lancet* 335:827, 1990.

8. Psaty BM, Heckbert SR, Koepsell TD, et al: The risk of myocardial infarction associated with antihypertensive therapies. *JAMA* 274:620, 1995.

9. Staessen JA, Fagard R, Thijs L, et al: Randomized double-blind comparison of placebo and active treatment for older patients with isolated systolic hypertension. *Lancet* 350:757, 1997.

10. Estacio RO, Jeffers BW, Hiatt WR, Biggerstaff SL, Gifford N, Schrier RW: The effect of nisoldipine as compared with enalapril on cardiovascular outcomes in patients with non-insulin dependent diabetes and hypertension. *N Engl J Med* 338:645, 1998.

11. Borhani NO, Mercuri M, Borhani PA, et al: Final outcome results of the Multicenter *Isradipine Diuretic* Atherosclerosis Study (MIDAS): A randomized controlled trial. *JAMA* 276:785, 1996.

12. Burn J, Dennis M, Bamford J, Sandercock P, Wade D, Warlow C: Long-term risk of recurrent stroke after a first-ever stroke. The Oxfordshire Community Stroke Project. *Stroke* 25:333, 1994.

13. Meissner I, Whisnant JP, Garraway M: Hypertension management and stroke recurrence in a community (Rochester, Minnesota, 1950–1979). *Stroke* 19:459, 1988.

14. MacMahon S, Rodgers A: Primary and secondary prevention of stroke. *Clin Exp Hypertens* 18:537, 1996.

15. Gueyffier F, Boissel J, Boutie F, et al: Effect of antihypertensive treatment in patients having already suffered from stroke: Gathering the evidence. *Stroke* 28:2557, 1997.

16. Carter AB: Hypotensive therapy in stroke survivors. *Lancet* 1:485, 1970.

17. Beevers DG, Hamilton M, Faiman MJ, Harpur JE: Antihypertensive treatment and the course of established cerebral vascular disease. *Lancet* 1:1407, 1973.

18. SHEP Cooperative Research Group: Prevention of stroke by anti-hypertensive drug treatment on older persons with isolated systolic hypertension. Final Results of the Systolic Hypertension in the Elderly Program (SHEP). *JAMA* 265:3255, 1991.

19. Insua JT, Sacks HS, Lau T-S, et al: Drug Treatment of hypertension in the elderly. *Ann Intern Med* 121:355, 1994.
20. Irie K, Yamguchi T, Minematsu K, Omae T: The J-curve phenomenon in stroke recurrence. *Stroke* 24:1844, 1993.
21. Farnett L, Mulrow C, Linn WD, Lucey CR, Tuley MR: The J-curve phenomenon and the treatment of hypertension: Is there a point beyond which pressure reduction is dangerous? *JAMA* 265:489, 1991.
22. Hansson L, Zancheti A, Carruthers SG, et al: Effects of intensive blood-pressure lowering and low-dose aspirin in patients with hypertension: Principal results of the Hypertension Optimal Treatment (HOT) randomised trial. *Lancet* 351:1755, 1998.
23. Harper G, Castleden CM, Potter JF: Factors affecting changes in blood pressure after acute stroke. *Stroke* 25:1726, 1994.
24. Britton M, Carlsson A, de Faire U: Blood pressure course in patients with acute stroke and matched controls. *Stroke* 17:861, 1986.
25. Durodami RL, Grotta JC, Lamki LM, et al: Should hypertension be treated after acute stroke? A randomized controlled trial using single photon emission computed tomography. *Arch Neurol* 50:855, 1993.
26. Carlsson A, Britton M: Blood pressure after stroke. A one-year follow-up study. *Stroke* 24:195, 1993.
27. Lavin P: Management of hypertension in patients with acute stroke. *Arch Intern Med* 146:66, 1986.
28. Strandgaard S: Hypertension and stroke. *J Hypertens* 14(Suppl 3):S23, 1996.
29. O'Connell JE, Gray CS: Treatment of post-stroke hypertension. *Drugs Aging* 6:408, 1996.
30. Appell LJ, Moore TJ, Obarzanek E, et al., for the DASH Collaborative Research Group: A clinical trial of the effects of dietary patterns on blood pressure. *N Engl J Med* 336:1117, 1997.
31. Philipp T, Anlauf M, Distler A, Holzgreve H, Michaelis J, Weleck S: Randomised, double blind, multicentre comparison of hydrochlorothiazide, atenolol, nitrendipine and enalapril in antihypertensive treatment: Results of the HANE study. *Br Med J* 315:154, 1997.
32. Shorr RI, Ray WA, Daugherty JR, Griffin MR: Antihypertensives and the risk of serious hypoglycemia in older persons using insulin or sulphonureas. *JAMA* 278:40, 1997.
33. Curb JD, Pressel SL, Cutler JA, Savage PJ, et al: Effect of diuretic-based antihypertensive treatment on cardiovascular disease risk in older diabetic patients with isolated systolic hypertension. *JAMA* 276:1886, 1996.
34. Latini R, Maggioni AP, Flather M, Sleight P, Tognoni G: ACE inhibitor use in patients with myocardial infarction: Summary of evidence from clinical trials. *Circulation* 92:3132, 1995.
35. Ravid M, Lang R, Rachmani R: Long-term renoprotective effect of angiotensin-converting enzyme inhibition in non-insulin-dependent diabetes mellitus: A 7-year follow-up study. *Arch Intern Med* 156:286, 1996.
36. Ogilvie RI, Burgess ED, Cusson JR, Feldman RD, Leiter LA, Myers MG: Report of the Canadian Hypertension Society Consensus Conference. 3. Pharmacologic treatment of essential hypertension. *Can Med Assoc J* 149:575, 1993.
37. Fries ED: The efficacy and safety of diuretics in treating hypertension. *Ann Intern Med* 122:223, 1995.
38. Grossman E, Messerli FH, Grodzicki T, Kowey P: Should a moratorium be placed on sublingual nifedipine capsules given for hypertensive emergencies and pseudoemergencies? *JAMA* 276:1328, 1996.
39. Yusuf S, Held P, Furberg C: Update of effects of calcium antagonists in myocardial infarction or angina in light of the second Danish Verapamil Infarction Trial (DAVIT-II) and other recent studies. *Am J Cardiol* 67:1295, 1996.
40. Materson BJ, Reda DJ, Cushman WC, et al: Single-drug therapy for hypertension in men: A comparison of six antihypertensive agents with placebo. *N Engl J Med* 328:914, 1993.

Appendix 7-1.

The authors' preferred regimens for controlling blood pressure

Regimen	Diuretic	ACEI or beta blocker
Initiate	Begin HCTZ 12.5 or 25 mgs daily (or equivalent) Begin lifestyle education	Begin once-daily ACE inhibitor or Beta blocker Begin lifestyle education
Follow-up	See 1 to 2 weeks If BP does not meet goal, raise HCTZ to 25 mgs (if not already done) or Add ACE inhibitor or Beta blocker	See 1 to 2 weeks Titrate gradually to standard maintenance dosing or until BP reaches goal
Further follow-up	Titrate ACE inhibitor or beta blocker to standard maintenance dosing or until BP meets goal If goal not reached, add third agent and titrate upward, as before Reinforce lifestyle education, as needed	If BP does not meet goal, add HCTZ 12.5 mg daily and titrate to 25 mg, if needed If goal not reached, add third agent and titrate upward, as before Reinforce lifestyle education, as needed
Laboratory tests	Repeat serum chemistries and creatinine/blood urea nitrogen shortly after starting ACE inhibitor or diuretic	Repeat serum chemistries and creatinine/ blood urea nitrogen shortly after starting ACE inhibitor or diuretic
Clinical monitoring	Once stable, see every 3 to 6 months to assess compliance, BP control, and adherence to lifestyle changes	Once stable, see every 3 to 6 months to assess compliance, BP control, and adherence to lifestyle changes

Appendix 7-2.

Selected list

Drug	Trade name	Usual dose range, total mg/day[a] (frequency per day)	Selected side effects and comments[a]
1. Diuretics (partial list)			Short-term: increases cholesterol and glucose levels; biochemical abnormalities: decreases potassium, sodium, and magnesium levels, increases uric acid and calcium levels; rare: blood dyscrasias, photosensitivity, pancreatitis, hyponatremia
a. *Thiazides*			
Chlorothalidone (G)[b]	Hygroton	12.5–50 (1)	
Hydrochlorothiazide (G)	Hydrodiuril, Micro-zide, Esidrix	12.5–50 (1)	
Indapamide	Lozol	1.25–5 (1)	Less or no hypercholesterolemia

(continues)

Appendix 7-2.
Selected list (Continued)

Drug	Trade name	Usual dose range, total mg/day[a] (frequency per day)	Selected side effects and comments[a]
b. *Loop diuretics*			Not routinely used alone for hypertension
Ethacrynic acid	Edecrin	25–100 (2–3)	Only nonsulfonamide diuretic, ototoxicity
Furosemide (G)	Lasix	40–240 (2–3)	Short duration of action, no hypercalcemia
c. *Potassium sparing agents*			Not routinely used alone for hypertension
Amiloride hydrochloride (G)	Midamor	5–10 (1)	
Spironolactone (G)	Aldactone	25–100 (1)	Gynecomastia
Triamterene (G)	Dyrenium	25–100 (1)	
Diuretic Combinations			
Triamterene, 37.5, 50 or 75 mg/ hydrochlorothiazide, 25 or 50 mg	Dyazide, Maxide		
Spironolactone, 25 or 50 mg/ hydrochlorothiazide, 25 or 50 mg	Aldactazide		
Amiloride hydrochloride, 5 mg/ hydrochlorothiazide, 50 mg	Moduretic		
2. Beta blockers			Bronchospasm, bradycardia, heart failure, may mask insulin-induced hypoglycemia; less serious: impaired peripheral circulation, insomnia, fatigue, decreased exercise tolerance, hypertriglyceridemia (except agents with intrinsic sympathomimetic activity)
Acebutolol[b,c]	Sectral	200–800 (1)	
Atenolol (G)[b]	Tenormin	25–100 (1–2)	
Betaxolol[b]	Kerlone	5–20 (1)	
Bisoprolol fumarate[b]	Zebeta	2.5–10 (1)	
Carteolol hydrochloride[c]	Cartrol	2.5–10 (1)	
Metoprolol tartrate (G)[b]	Lopressor	50–300 (2)	
Metoprolol succinate[b]	Toprol-XL	50–300 (1)	
Nadolol (G)	Corgard	40–320 (1)	
Penbutolol sulfate[c]	Levatol	10–20 (1)	
Pindolol (G)[c]	Visken	10–60 (2)	
Propranolol hydrochloride (G)	Inderal	40–480 (3)	
	Inderal LA	40–480 (1)	
Timolol maleate (G)	Blocadren	20–60 (2)	

(continues)

Appendix 7-2.
*Selected list (**Continued**)*

Drug	Trade name	Usual dose range, total mg/day[a] (frequency per day)	Selected side effects and comments[a]
Beta-adrenergic blockers and diuretics			
Atenolol, 50 or 100 mg/ chlorthalidone, 25 mg	Tenoretic		
Bisoprolol fumarate, 2.5, 5, or 10 mg/hydrochlorothi- azide, 6.25 mg	Ziac[a]		
Metoprolol tartrate, 50 or 100 mg/hydrochlorothiazide, 25 or 50 mg	Lopressor HCT		
Nadolol, 40 or 80 mg/ben- droflumethiazide, 5 mg	Corzide		
Propranolol hydrochloride, 40 or 80 mg/hydrochlorothiazide, 25 mg	Inderide		
Propranolol hydrochloride (ex- tended release), 80, 120, or 160 mg/hydrochlorothiazide, 50 mg	Inderide LA		
Timolol maleate, 10 mg/hydro- chlorothiazide, 25 mg	Timolide		
3. ACE inhibitors			
Benazepril hydrochloride	Lotensin	5–40 (1–2)	Common: cough; rare: angioedema, hyperkalemia, rash, loss of taste, leukopenia
Captopril (G)	Capoten	25–150 (2–3)	
Enalapril maleate	Vasotec	5–40 (1–2)	
Fosinopril sodium	Monopril	10–40 (1–2)	
Lisinopril	Prinivil, Zestril	5–40 (1)	
Moexipril	Univasc	7.5–15 (2)	
Quinapril hydrochloride	Accupril	5–80 (1–2)	
Ramipril	Altace	1.25–20 (1–2)	
Trandolapril	Mavik	1–4 (1)	
ACE inhibitors and diuretics			
Benazepril hydrochloride, 5, 10, or 20 mg/hydrochlorothiazide, 6.25, 12.5, or 25 mg	Lotensin HCT		
Captopril, 25 or 50 mg/hydro- chlorothiazide, 15 or 25 mg	Capozide[a]		
Enalapril maleate, 5 or 10 mg/ hydrochlorothiazide, 12.5 or 25 mg	Vaseretic		

(continues)

Appendix 7-2.
*Selected list (**Continued**)*

Drug	Trade name	Usual dose range, total mg/day[a] (frequency per day)	Selected side effects and comments[a]
Lisinopril, 10 or 20 mg/hydro-chlorothiazide, 12.5 or 25 mg	Prinzide, Zestoretic		
4. Angiotensin II receptor blockers			Angioedema (very rare), hyperkalemia
Losartan potassium	Cozaar	25–100 (1–2)	
Valsartan	Diovan	80–320 (1)	
Irbesartan	Avapro	150–300 (1)	
Candesartan	Atacand	8–32 (1–2)	
Telmisartan	Micardis	40–80 (1)	
Angiotensin II receptor antagonists and diuretics			
Losartan potassium, 50 mg/ hydrochlorothiazide, 12.5 mg	Hyzaar		
5. Calcium antagonists			
Nondihydropyridines			Conduction defects, worsening of systolic dysfunction, gingival hyperplasia
Diltiazem hydrochloride	Cardizem SR	120–360 (2)	Nausea, headache
	Cardizem CD	120–360 (1)	
	Dilacor XR, Tiazac		
Verapamil hydrochloride	Isoptin SR, Calan SR,	90–480 (2)	Constipation
	Verelan, Covera HS	120–480 (1)	
Dihydropyridines			Edema of the ankle, flushing, headache, gingival hypertrophy
Amlodipine besylate	Norvasc	2.5–10 (1)	
Felodipine	Plendil	2.5–20 (1)	
Isradipine	DynaCirc	5–20 (2)	
	DynaCirc CR	5–20 (1)	
Nicardipine	Cardene SR	60–90 (2)	
Nifedipine	Procardia XL, Adalat CC	30–120 (1)	
Nisoldipine	Sular	20–60 (1)	

(continues)

Appendix 7-2.
*Selected list (**Continued**)*

Drug	Trade name	Usual dose range, total mg/day[a] (frequency per day)	Selected side effects and comments[a]
Calcium antagonists and ACE inhibitors			
Amlodipine besylate, 2.5 or 5 mg/benazepril hydrochloride, 10 or 20 mg	Lotrel		
Diltiazem hydrochloride, 180 mg/enalapril maleate, 5 mg	Teczem		
Verapamil hydrochloride (extended release), 180 or 240 mg/trandolapril, 1, 2, or 4 mg	Tarka		
Felodipine, 5 mg/enalapril maleate, 5 mg	Lexxel		
6. Alpha blockers			
Doxazosin mesylate	Cardura	1–16 (1)	
Prazosin hydrochloride (G)	Minipress	2–30 (2–3)	
Terazosin hydrochloride	Hytrin	1–20 (1)	
7. Central alpha agonists			Can use tablet or patch
Clonidine hydrochloride (G)	Catapres	0.2–1.2 (2–3)	
8. Combined alpha and beta blockers			Postural hypotension, bronchospasm; should be used cautiously due to potential orthostasis
Carvedilol	Coreg	12.5–50 (2)	
Labetalol hydrochloride (G)	Normodyne, Trandate	200–1,200 (2)	
9. Direct vasodilators			Headaches, fluid retention, tachycardia
Hydralazine hydrochloride (G)	Apresoline	50–300 (2)	
Minoxidil (G)	Loniten	5–100 (1)	Lupus syndrome Hirsutism

From the Sixth Report of the Joint National Committee on Prevention, Detection, Evaluation, and Treatment of High Blood Pressure. *Arch Intern Med* 157:2425–2426, 1997.
[a]Approved for initial therapy.
[b]Cardioselective.
[c]Has intrinsic sympathomimetic activity.

Appendix 7-3.
Selected drug interactions

Drug class	May increase hypotensive effect	May decrease hypotensive effect	Other effects
Diuretics	Diuretics that act at different sites in the nephron (e.g., furosemide + thiazides)	Resin-binding agents NSAIDs Steroids	Diuretics raise serum lithium levels Potassium-sparing agents + ACE inhibitors may cause hyperkalemia
β blockers	Cimetidine + quinidine may increase effect of hepatically metabolized β blockers	NSAIDs Withdrawal of clonidine Agents that induce hepatic enzymes including rifampin and phenobarbital	Propranolol hydrochloride can induce hepatic enzymes β blockers may worsen effects of hypoglycemia Heart block may occur with β blockers verapamil or diltiazem May worsen cocaine effects on coronary arteries
ACE inhibitors	Chlorpromazine or clozapine	NSAIDs Antacids Food decreases absorption (moexipril)	ACE inhibitors may raise serum lithium levels ACE inhibitors with potassium-sparing diuretics may cause hyperkalemia
Calcium antagonists	Grapefruit juice (some dihydropyridines) Climetidine or ranitidine (hepatically metabolized calcium antagonists)	Agents that induce hepatic enzymes including rifampin and phenobarbital	Some calcium channel blockers (CCBs) alter cyclosporine levels Verapamil and diltiazem may increase digoxin, quinidine, sulfonylureas, and theophylline levels Verapamil hydrochloride may lower serum lithium levels
α blockers			Prazosin hydrochloride may decrease verapamil hydrochloride clearance
Central α_2-agonists and peripheral neuronal blockers		Tricyclic antidepressants (and probably phenothiazines) Monoamine oxidase inhibitors Iron salts may reduce methyldopa absorption	Methyldopa may increase serum lithium levels Severity of clonidine hydrochloride withdrawal may be increased by β blockers Some anesthetic agents are potentiated by clonidine hydrochloride

Modified from the Sixth Report of the Joint National Committee on Prevention, Detection, Evaluation, and Treatment of High Blood Pressure. *Arch Intern Med* 157:2431, 1997.

Chapter 8

THE SUBACUTE STROKE PATIENT: NEUROREHABILITATION FOR STROKE PATIENTS

Bruce H. Dobkin

OVERVIEW OF NEUROREHABILITATION

For the recently and chronically disabled stroke survivor, neurorehabilitation aims to increase functional independence, lessen the burden of care provided by significant others, reintegrate the patient back into the family and community, and improve quality of life. Efforts begin with the prevention of medical complications that accompany immobility and physical and cognitive impairments. They proceed with the evaluation and treatment of impairments and disabilities in an inpatient or outpatient setting. The long-term goal is to lessen disability and handicap.

Impairments include sensorimotor and other neurologic, physical, and cognitive deficits, such as a new left hemiparesis and left hemianopsia with hemi-inattention to the surrounds. A chronic hip contracture is another type of impairment. Neurologic impairments are often measured using the physical examination, the National Institutes of Health Stroke Scale, the Scandinavian Stroke Scale, or the Fugl-Meyer Scale. *Disabilities* are the functional restrictions induced by impairments, such as not being able to walk across a room without assistance because of the hemiparesis. The Barthel Index and the Functional Independence Measure are examples of ordinal scales for quantification of level of independence in activities of daily living (ADLs). *Handicaps* arise from impairments and disabilities. These include the disadvantages that limit or prevent the fulfillment of a usual role, such as no longer being able to visit a friend because the left hemiparesis prevents stair climbing. They can be measured, in part, by the Frenchay Activities Index.[1] Health-related quality of life, which includes a patient's perception of his or her physical functioning and mental, psychosocial, and emotional state, has been measured with the Sickness Index Profile and the SF-36.[2] Many other scales have been used in neurorehabilitation studies.[3,4]

Just as rehabilitation differs from the usual practices of neuromedicine that focus on disease mechanisms and their treatment, the practice of rehabilitation differs in that it includes a wide range of participants. Important roles are played not only by physicians and nurses but by physical, occupational, recreational, and speech-language therapists, social workers, neuropsychologists, orthotists, dietitians, and sometimes engineers. They work as a team to optimize the physical, cognitive, behavioral, psychosocial, and vocational potential of people who are disabled by their neurologic impairments.

Successful interventions depend on understanding potential mechanisms of recovery, the natural history of gains over time, and specific outcomes that arise with present therapeutic strategies. Because stroke rehabilitation includes many forms of intervention for a wide range of impairments, disabilities, and handicaps carried out in a multidisciplinary fashion, space only allows for a look into some of the more common evidence-based practices. More detailed critiques and additional approaches can be found in dedicated texts.[4,5]

Rationale For Gains

Table 8-1 outlines some of the potential mechanisms that might contribute to changes in impairments and

Table 8-1.
Mechanisms that might support recovery of function

Network plasticity

1. Recovery of neuronal excitability
   Resolution of cellular toxic-metabolic dysfunction
   Resolution of edema; resorption of blood products
   Resolution of diaschisis

2. Activity in neurons adjacent to injured ones and in partially spared pathways

3. Alternative behavioral strategies

4. Representational adaptations in neuronal assemblies
   Expansion of representational maps
   Recruitment of cells not ordinarily involved in an activity

5. Recruitment of parallel and subcomponent pathways
   Altered activity of the distributed functions of cortical and subcortical neural networks
   Activation of pattern generators (e.g., for stepping)
   Recruitment of networks not ordinarily involved in an activity
   Dependence on task-related stimulation

Neuronal plasticity

1. Altered efficacy of synaptic activity
   Activity-dependent unmasking of previously ineffective synapses
   Learning tied to activity-dependent changes (e.g., long-term potentiation, long-term depression) in synaptic strength in
      peri-injury and remote regions
   Increased neuronal responsiveness from denervation hypersensitivity
   Decline in number of neurons, as in apoptosis
   Change in number of a variety of receptors
   Change in neurotransmitter release and uptake

2. Regeneration and sprouting of axons and dendrites
   Signaling gene expression for cell viability, growth, and remodeling proteins
   Modulation by neurotrophic factors
   Actions of chemoattractants and inhibitors in the milieu

3. Remyelination

4. Trans-synaptic degeneration

5. Ion channel changes on fibers for impulse conduction

6. Actions of neurotransmitters and neuromodulators

Adapted from Ref. 4.

disabilities. These mechanisms overlap. Some will depend on each other over time. In addition, biologic therapeutic approaches such as tissue implants may enhance these mechanisms when applied to human studies of recovery in the near future. Although care must be taken in extrapolating from animal studies of recovery to their implications for human interventions,[6] at least a few of these potential mechanisms suggest strategies that can be used by the rehabilitation team to improve outcomes.

Many lines of animal and human research suggest that partial recovery after a stroke can be due to a functional shift to neighboring neurons. For example,

Nudo and colleagues induced a less than 1-mm injury to the motor arm area of primates. The perilesional neuronal representations for movements of the digits decreased if the monkey did not practice using the hand to scoop pellets out of a narrow well,[7] but neighboring representations for the digits and wrist and forearm increased with practice.[8] Thus, cortical representational changes are especially likely to arise during training paradigms that involve learning and the acquisition of specific skills. The neurons of the ischemic penumbra of an acute cerebral infarction may play an important role in functional gains, as this region has a large potential for the learning mechanism of long-term potentiation. In rat studies, however, sensorimotor cortex lesions that were followed by very early contralateral forelimb overuse of perilesional neurons caused greater injury.[9,10] This plasticity probably arises when previously silent synapses from thalamocortical and intracortical circuits are unmasked.[11] In some instances, it might arise from sprouting of dendrites over short distances.[12]

The combination of partially spared pathways after a stroke, flexible neuronal assemblies that represent movements and sensation, and multiple representational maps for movements in a parallel, distributed system offers a rich vein for exploration by rehabilitationists. Behaviorally relevant tasks that are shaped with an optimal schedule of practice and feedback might increase human recovery, as it has enhanced upper extremity and locomotor functions in animal studies. The optimal duration and intensity of training is uncertain for human rehabilitation strategies, but more intensive practice seems to enhance subsequent performance.[13] Unfortunately, most patients get only a few months of formal inpatient and outpatient retraining at a modest level of intensity, spread across many tasks.

Overview of Practices

Background Rehabilitation efforts in the first few days after a stroke usually include a physical and occupa-tional therapy evaluation and an assessment of swallowing and language when needed. With shortened inpatient hospitalizations, a decision is then made to send patients for inpatient rehabilitation, to home perhaps with visits by therapists and a nurse who will initiate rehabilitation, to an outpatient setting, or to a skilled nursing facility for ongoing care that can include up to several hours of physical, occupational, swallowing, and language therapy a day. Patients who are at a supervised or minimal assisted level of self-care usually return home. By the end of the first week after a stroke, from 12 to 20 percent of patients are appropriated for inpatient rehabilitation.

Medicare guidelines allow for inpatient care for patients who need ongoing supervision by physicians and nurses, have enough stamina to participate in rehabilitation therapies for at least 3 h a day, and have adequate psychosocial supports to permit a discharge to home or to a board and care. Motivation and cognition must be adequate for learning compensatory strategies. In weekly conferences, the team reassesses progress toward reasonable functional goals that will allow the patient to return home. Family training and support are essential. The majority of these patients will have a moderate level of disability on admission in ADLs with a Barthel Index (BI) score of 40 to 60 or a Functional Independence Measure (FIM) score of 40 to 80. These disability scales are shown in Tables 8-2 and 8-3. Average lengths of stay range from 18 to 30 days, in part depending upon the amount of

Table 8-2.

The Barthel Index

	Help	Independent
1. Feeding (If food needs to be cut up = help)	5	10
2. Moving from wheelchair to bed and return (includes sitting up in bed)	5–10	15
3. Personal toilet (wash face, comb hair, shave, clean teeth)	0	5
4. Getting on and off toilet (handling clothes, wipe, flush)	5	10
5. Bathing self	0	5
6. Walking on level surface (or, if unable to walk, propel wheelchair)	10	15
	0[a]	5[a]
7. Ascend and descend stairs	5	10
8. Dressing (include tying shoes, fastening fasteners)	5	10
9. Controlling bowels	5	10
10. Controlling bladder	5	10

[a]Score only if unable to walk.

Table 8-3.

Functional independence measure (FIM) items

Bladder management
Bowel management
Social interaction
Problem solving
Memory
Comprehension
Bed-to-chair and wheelchair-to-chair transfer
Toilet transfer
Tub and shower transfer
Locomotion (walking or wheelchair)
Climbing stairs
Eating
Grooming
Bathing
Dressing (upper body)
Dressing (lower body)
Toileting
Burden of care
  7. Complete independence (timely, safely)
  6. Modified independence (device)
  5. Supervision
  4. Minimal assistance (subject does at least 75 percent of task)
  3. Moderate assistance (50 percent)
  2. Maximal assistance (25 percent)
  1. Total assistance (<25 percent)

help available to the patient upon leaving inpatient care and the level of third-party payor support. Table 8-4 shows the range of FIM admission and discharge scores from patients entered into the Uniform Data System for Medical Rehabilitation (UDS$_{MR}^{SM}$) of the University of Buffalo Foundation Activities, Inc.

Across a range of retrospective and prospective observational studies, unfavorable prognosticators for recovery and a home discharge include advanced age and neurologic impairments such as profound paresis, loss of proprioception, visuospatial hemineglect, and bowel and bladder incontinence at the time of transfer to a rehabilitation unit. Also, the higher the admission score on the BI or FIM, the higher the discharge score and the greater the likelihood that the patient will return to living at home. An epidemiologic report from the Framingham Study is one of the very few studies that has compared functional disabilities in survivors of stroke with a control group matched for age and sex from the same cohort.[14] About 80 percent of cases were over age 65. Of the 148 cases who had survived for 6

months after their stroke, testing on the BI revealed that 20 percent were dependent in ambulation, one-third were dependent in ADLs, and over two-thirds socialized much less than they had prior to the stroke. In the stroke-free controls, 28 percent showed decreased socialization inside and outside the home, 20 percent were limited in household tasks, 9 percent were dependent in self-care activities, and 6 percent were dependent in mobility. When Gresham and colleagues removed the disabilities attributed to comorbid conditions, the percent who were disabled primarily from their stroke fell by as much as 50 percent.[15] Thus, premorbid functional disabilities may commonly account for limitations in recovery when superimposed upon stroke-induced impairments.

The discharge plan from inpatient or outpatient rehabilitation should be done with adequate warning and family preparation. Patients should have appropriate durable medical equipment and follow-up medical and disability-oriented community care.

Evidence   Do focused programs of stroke rehabilitation improve important outcomes beyond the natural history of recovery?[16,17] This controversy has been ad-

Table 8-4.

UDS$_{MR}^{SM}$ first admissions for stroke rehabilitation in 1995 (57,486 patients)[a]

Mean subscore	Admission	Discharge
Self-care	3.5	4.9
Sphincter control	3.9	5.2
Transfers	2.8	4.5
Locomotion	1.9	3.8
Communication	4.6	5.3
Social cognition	4.2	5.0
Mean FIM total	62.7 (SD 21)	86.4 (SD 24)
Median FIM	64	91
Mean onset (days)	15	
Length of stay	23 (SD 17)	
FIM gain/week	7.2	
Discharge (%)		
Community	76	
Long-term care	17	
Acute care	5	
Mean age (yrs)	70 (SD 12)	

[a]Adapted from Ref. 127.

dressed in a variety of retrospective and prospective studies that look at where and how a program of therapy is provided or examine the value of particular interventions for patients. Questions addressed include: Is the rehabilitation of disabilities caused by stroke effective? Is a particular therapeutic approach better than another? Is rehabilitation delivered on a specialized unit more effective than care on a general medical ward? What is the most efficient setting that provides a particular level of care for a patient with a given level of disability?

In this day of strategies to lower health-care costs, the issue of locus of treatment takes on special significance. At least 20 trials have compared outcomes in patients managed on specialized stroke rehabilitation units vs. standard medical ward care.[18] In general, these patients were not too low or too high-level for inpatient rehabilitation as practiced in the United States today. The mean age for each trial was 65 to 75 years, and subjects were randomized within a few days to 2 to 4 weeks after the stroke. These trials suggest that the milieu and the usually greater frequency of rehabilitation therapies on a dedicated unit lead to better outcomes in moderately impaired patients, at least for the first 3 to 6 months after the stroke. The specialized unit also returns more patients home who are more independent. Even with the same type and intensity of physical and occupational therapy services provided by people with the same level of experience, functional recovery on BI tasks was greater and more rapid on the dedicated unit that directed therapy toward adapting the patients' residual abilities to their future needs in their homes.[19] Indeed, patients in one British trial who reached the median BI score associated with discharge had significantly shorter lengths of stay after having reached that level of function when managed on the stroke unit compared with those who were just as functional on a medical unit.[20] This suggests a better organization for assessment and goal-oriented services on a dedicated unit. The stroke unit with its rehabilitation team also seems to lower death rates, especially for causes related to immobility. Significantly greater survival extended for up to 18 months in one study[21] and increased long-term survival and functional independence at 5 years in another.[22]

On the other hand, the results of several European community studies of all stroke survivors suggested that patients who received therapy in the hospital or with an organized outpatient approach performed as well as those who received little or no remedial treatment.[23,24] This finding is likely to vary with the severity

of stroke and availability of home supports; patients with BI scores of less than 40 may not benefit from very intensive therapy over a short time and those with scores over 80 might do well as long as psychosocial supports are available. A study of Medicare patients has reopened the controversy about inpatient vs. skilled nursing facility stroke rehabilitation programs. The latter are favored by many health maintenance organizations for their lower initial cost. This prospective study showed that stroke patients who were admitted to a rehabilitation hospital were significantly more likely to return to the community and recover ADLs than patients sent to subacute or traditional nursing facilities for therapy and management.[25]

Do neurorehabilitation practices, overall, lessen disability or impairment? After reviewing 124 investigations drawn from a literature search of studies done from 1960 to 1990, Ottenbacher carried out a meta-analysis on 36. These met the criteria of including hemiparetic patients with stroke who were given a rehabilitation service in a design that compared at least two groups or conditions for change in a functional measure that could be quantified.[26] Outcomes included gait, hand function, ADLs, response times, and visuoperception. From 173 statistical evaluations recorded on the 3717 acute and chronic patients in the 36 trials, the analysis showed that the average patient who received a program of focused stroke rehabilitation or a particular procedure performed better than about 65 percent of the patients in the comparison group. Larger treatment effect sizes were associated with an earlier intervention and younger patients. No association was found with the duration of a program. The authors point out that this synthesis of data is imperfect. The review could not assess the intensity of the interventions and how well they were carried out, detect systematic biases, or account for missing data.

Medical Complications

Medical complications often interfere with a patient's ability to participate in therapy.[27,28] During inpatient rehabilitation, about one-third of patients will have a urinary tract infection, urinary retention, musculoskeletal pain, or depression. About 20 percent develop a rash or need continuous management of blood pressure (see Chap. 7), hydration, nutrition, and glucose levels (see Chap. 5). About 10 percent will develop a transient toxic-metabolic encephalopathy, pneumonia, cardiac arrhythmias, or thrombophlebitis. Up to 5 percent may develop serious skin ulcers, a pulmonary embolus, seizures, gastrointestinal bleeding, obstructive sleep apnea, and other medical complications. Prophylactic measures for these potential problems, where feasible, are essential.

Bladder Dysfunction

Background Urinary incontinence occurs in up to 60 percent of patients in the first week after a stroke but tends to improve without a specific medical treatment. Urinary dribbling and involuntary emptying affect 30 percent of healthy, noninstitutionalized people over the age of 65. Across studies, about 18 percent of those who were incontinent at 6 weeks poststroke are still so at 1 year. By the end of outpatient rehabilitation, the incidence is about 10 percent in patients with a motor-only stroke and about 70 percent with large hemispheric strokes.[29] Urinary tract infections develop in about 40 percent of patients during their acute stroke and rehabilitation care.

Treatment In patients with retention of urine volumes greater than 300 cc, intermittent bladder catheterization with a clean technique probably lessens the risk of a UTI in men and women, though the specific evidence from small trials is slim. Perineal cleanliness should lessen the risk of infection by contamination. The procedure may not work for the male with prostatic enlargement. If retention persists, an indwelling catheter is best for the short run. Medications may reduce the outlet obstruction, or prostatic surgery may be indicated

once the patient is a stable outpatient. The use of medications is usually on a trial-and-error basis, though the yield is best when urodynamic testing points to a specific abnormality of urine filling and storage, bladder emptying, or a combination of both.

Most patients with incontinence after a hemispheric stroke have a small-volume bladder and are unable to suppress the micturition reflex or become aware of filling too late to void in a urinal, commode, or toilet. Scheduled voiding is one good approach. An anticholinergic agent such as 5 mg of oxybutynin just at night or up to TID may allow greater filling. Persistent bladder dyscontrol is often secondary to an unstable detrusor and detrusor-sphincter dyssynergia.[30] Table 8-5 lists the potential benefits of specific drug interventions.

Musculoskeletal and Central Pain

Background Pain is common after a stroke and can limit the participation of people in therapy.[31] Central pain can become a major source of disability. It is most common after a thalamoparietal stroke and affects fewer than 5 percent of all patients with stroke. Some patients only need assurance that the pain does not represent a serious complication or a warning signal of another stroke. Others will need to help the physician set goals about moderating the severity, frequency, duration, and time of day of the pain. Musculoskeletal pain is far more common. Shoulder pain at the hemiparetic arm develops in from 5 percent to 50 percent of patients.[32] Nociception can exacerbate hypertonicity and trigger flexor and ex-

Table 8-5.
Pharmacologic manipulation of bladder dysfunction

Medication	Indication	Mechanism of action
Bethanechol 25 mg bid-50 mg qid	Facilitate emptying	Increase detrusor contraction
Prazosin 1 mg BID-2 mg tid	Decrease outlet obstruction Prostatic hypertrophy	Alpha blockade of external sphincter to decrease tone
Tamsulosin 0.4 mg qd		
Hyoscyamine 0.125 mg hs-0.25 mg tid	Urge incontinence Frequency	Relax detrusor; increase internal sphincter tone
Oxybutinin 2.5 mg hs-5 mg qid Tolterodine-2 mg BID		
Imipramine 25 mg-100 mg hs	Urge incontinence Enuresis	Increase internal sphincter tone; decrease detrusor contractions

tensor spasms and dystonic postures. A painful shoulder can cause the hemiplegic arm to flex at the elbow and wrist. The shoulder-hand syndrome with reflex-sympathetic dystrophy[33] has been described in over 25 percent of patients in prospective studies.[34] Even more common, most patients during their rehabilitation will suffer with cervical, lumbar, hip, knee, or ankle pain secondary to musculoligamentous injuries, overuse, overstretching, and poor resting postures.

Evidence Nonsteroidal anti-inflammatory medications and passive and active joint range of motion can reduce shoulder pain.[35] Functional electrical stimulation to reduce subluxation may also prevent pain.[36]

Treatment Physical modalities, analgesics, anti-inflammatory agents, and local anesthetics or steroids can benefit most sources of musculoligamentous pain. Examples of prevention of further injury include using an orthotic for a shoulder subluxation and controlling hyperextension-induced pain with an ankle-foot orthosis. Tricyclic and selective serotonin reuptake inhibitor antidepressants, carbamazepine, clonidine, gabapentin, benzodiazepines, and baclofen are among the drugs that may diminish dysesthetic or lancinating pain in some patients.

Depression

Background Depression is very common after a stroke. The community-based Framingham Study diagnosed depression in 47 percent of 6-month stroke survivors with no difference found in the incidence between those with left- and right-sided lesions.[37] The investigators used the Center for Epidemiologic Studies-Depression Scale, which also revealed depression in 25 percent of age- and sex-matched controls. In a population-based cohort of Swedish stroke patients whose mean age was 73 years, the prevalence of major depression was 25 percent at hospital discharge, 30 percent at 3 months' poststroke, 16 percent at 1 year, 19 percent at 2 years, and 29 percent at 3 years.[38] A left anterior infarct, dysphasia, and living alone have been shown in many studies to predict depression upon discharge. At 3 months, greater dependence in ADLs and social isolation have been associated with depression.

Evidence Early treatment of depression with tricyclic or serotonin-specific reuptake inhibitor antidepressants or methylphenidate can alleviate the mood disorder and improve rehabilitation outcomes.[39,40]

Treatment Counseling and positive reinforcement for any progress during rehabilitation seems to help lessen the concerns that patients have about becoming a burden on others. The social worker's help is critical during the inpatient stay in providing a feasible discharge plan that the patient finds agreeable. Counseling about emotional incontinence, visits by patients who have had a recent stroke and now live at home, and outpatient support groups for patients and caregivers can also improve a person's outlook. Especially in the elderly, drug therapy must start at a low dose. The specific medication used will depend upon medical risk factors (anticholinergic side effects might cause cardiac arrhythmias, drowsiness, confusion, or urinary retention), the presence of anxiety (some SSRI and tricyclic medications seem to be more useful here), insomnia (a tricyclic might aid sleep), and speed of onset (methylphenidate can act within a few days, though effects may wane over the next 4 weeks).

Dysphagia

Background Swallowing disorders can lead to malnutrition, dehydration, or to aspiration. The stroke and an associated metabolic encephalopathy can cause lethargy, inattention, poor judgement, and impaired control or sensitivity of the tongue or cheek, all of which might impair the oral stage of swallowing. Patients may take too much food or liquid, which then enters the airway before the swallow reflex is triggered. They may not form a bolus and many pocket solids in the cheek. Slow oral intake or a cough or wet voice after swallowing points to the potential for aspiration and pneumonia.

Evidence A videofluoroscopic modified barium swallow (MBS) study revealed a much greater risk for pneumonia in aspirators compared with nonaspirators in stroke patients during their inpatient rehabilitation.[41] Nasogastric feeding tubes and gastrostomies do not seem to appreciably lessen the risk of aspiration, probably due to gastric reflux, aspiration of oral secretions, and errors in tube placement.

Treatment Adequate hydration and nutrition are important during rehabilitation to prevent muscle breakdown, renal insufficiency and an encephalopathy, and other toxic-metabolic sequelae. An MBS with less than a teaspoonful of thin and thickened barium and a barium-coated piece of cookie will document problems at the oral, pharyngeal, and esophageal stages. The therapist can assess the effect of changes in head and neck position on deglutition.

Therapy is indicated when aspiration occurs with any of these tasks. Most commonly with hemispheric strokes, the swallowing reflex is delayed, the bolus slides over the base of the tongue and collects in the valleculae and hypopharynx, and sometimes the pharyngeal constrictor malfunctions. Therapies include compensatory head repositioning such as flexing or turning to one side, tongue and sucking exercises, double swallowing, and supraglottic and dry coughing. In most cases, the feeding of pureed foods and thickened liquids allows the dysphagic person to get adequate nutrition. Nasogastric feedings can supplement oral intake. They should be given after each meal so they do not blunt the patient's appetite and only when caloric and fluid intake by mouth is less than the daily need. A dietitian can help determine optimal caloric intake for each patient. If dysphagia persists toward the time of discharge from inpatient rehabilitation, a gastrostomy or gastrojejunostomy tube is a comfortable portal for nutrition.

Skin Ulcers

Background Education in skin management during rehabilitation provides an important opportunity for preventing later morbidity and mortality. Ischemia of the skin and underlying tissues occurs particularly in weight-bearing areas adjacent to bony prominences. Model Systems data for patients admitted within 24 h of traumatic SCI showed that 4 percent subsequently developed pressure sores and 13 percent of these were graded as severe.[42] They occurred over the sacrum, heel, scapula, foot, and trochanter. Raising the head of the bed by only a few inches especially increases shearing forces over the sacrum. Sores related to sitting are most frequently associated with the ischial tuberosities, where tissue pressure can exceed 300 mmHg on an unpadded seat. A 2-inch-thick foam pad may only decrease that local pressure to 150 mmHg. Even with the use of cushions designed to distribute weight-bearing skin surfaces, pressures in the sitting position are far above the 11 to 33-mmHg pressures in the capillaries and venules.

Evidence A standard four-stage classification for degrees of integument breakdown, prophylactic measures, and wound care is available from the Agency for Health Care Policy and Research.[43] No particular intervention for a pressure sore, other than antibiotics

and debridement for stage 3 to 4 ulcers, seems to be better than another.

Treatment Rubor, induration, and blistering are signs that precede a break in the skin. Pressure relief is the best approach provided every 2 to 3 h in patients with intact sensation after a hemiplegic stroke. Patients must develop a skin care program based on their general health, nutrition, continence, the toughness of their skin, the most used positions, type of wheelchair seat, presence of old skin scars, and other factors. Lubricants can minimize friction, and pillows and wedges protect bony areas. Gas-permeable films can protect a stage 1 ulcer, hydrocolloids and hydrogels may help a stage 2 or 3 ulcer heal, and debridement is essential for a large, infected wound. Topical antibiotics can impair healing.

Seizures

Background Across prospective studies, seizures occur in about 5 percent of patients within 2 weeks of a stroke. The great majority occurs within 72 h of onset. In the Copenhagen Stroke Study, a cortical injury, an intracerebral hemorrhage, and greater severity of stroke by the Scandinavian Stroke Scale were associated with a greater frequency of partial or generalized seizures.[44] However, a seizure in that prospective study within 2 weeks of onset did not increase mortality or lead to greater neurologic impairment. Some studies have suggested greater mortality, perhaps related to a greater size of the stroke. A seizure focus might arise from the ischemic penumbra; if this area were preserved, a better outcome might be anticipated, despite the early seizure.[45–47] After a subarachnoid hemorrhage (SAH) that produces a rather large basal cistern collection of blood, seizure frequency in the first days postbleed is greater than when less blood is evident by CT scan.

Evidence No clinical trials have been designed to assess the use of prophylactic anticonvulsants in subjects who suffer an acute ischemic or intracerebral hemorrhagic stroke, particularly not those who are at higher risk for a seizure. However, no efficacy has been found for prophylaxis beyond the first week after a traumatic brain injury or neurosurgical procedure on the brain.

Treatment Anticonvulsant therapy is indicated following a first seizure and perhaps following an SAH. Discontinuation depends upon the early course; if no seizures recur within 3 months, a trial off medication should be considered. Some studies suggest that the major anticonvulsants can impede recovery, so serum levels of phenytoin, carbamazepine, or valproate should be kept at the lower end of a therapeutic range, if possible.[48]

Sexual Dysfunction

Background After stroke, sexual desire persists, but many men and women who had been active will experience dysfunction.[49] Premorbid problems from diabetes, medications, vascular disease, and psychogenic causes can be exacerbated by new neural dysfunction, decreased mobility, pain, and new medications that complicate the stroke.

Evidence Little research in the form of clinical trials has been attempted for stroke-related sexual dysfunction. However, counseling and medication approaches and prostheses for men are perhaps as likely to work after stroke as with other people who are impotent for medical and psychological causes.

Treatment Counseling and exploration of different sexual techniques may help those who lose self-esteem or fear rejection because the partner is now, to some degree, a caretaker. New systemic and genital agents that promote an erection may be appropriate for men. The "Viagra revolution" has aided men with erectile dysfunction, though use is limited to those who do not have ischemic heart disease.

Sleep Disorders

Background During rehabilitation, insomnia, sleep apnea, and excessive daytime sleepiness can interfere with attention and learning. Medications, pain, anxiety, depression, and chronically poor sleep habits contribute. Reversed sleep-wake cycles seem most common in patients with cognitive dysfunction. Up to one-third of stroke inpatients may have a sleep disorder. Central and obstructive sleep apnea have been associated with a higher risk for stroke.[50] Pharyngeal muscle weakness and impaired neural control during sleep of the nasopharyngeal and pharyngolaryngeal muscles due to a stroke contribute to the risk for obstructive apnea. Polysomnography is indicated when the rehabilitation team observes a hypersomnolent, confused, and snoring or apneic patient.

Evidence One study found an average of 52 sleep-disordered breathing events per hour in selected subjects within 1 year of stroke.[51] The number of oxygen desaturation events and the oximetry measures during sleep-disordered breathing correlated with poorer functional recovery scores at 1 and 12 months after stroke.[52,53]

Treatment Insomnia during the first week or two of rehabilitation can be managed with short-acting hypnotics (chloral hydrate can be especially useful), nighttime non-narcotic analgesics, and careful positioning in bed. Nocturia more than two times that awakens the patient can be diminished by holding liquid intake after dinner and using medications that lessen detrusor activation (see above). Melatonin may help correct a reversed day-night sleep cycle. A nasal or oral positive-pressure breathing apparatus can prevent the consequences of obstructive sleep apnea.

Spasticity

Background A number of still ill-defined mechanisms alter membrane properties and morphologically and physiologically reorganize spinal circuits, leading to hypertonicity.[54] Spasticity can lead to dystonic postures and, in some instances, limit function. However, the paresis, slowness, and fatigability that accompany an upper motor neuron syndrome are usually more serious contributors to impairment and disability.

Evidence No studies offer convincing data on the benefits of systemic antispasticity medications following a stroke. A few trials suggest some value of local botulinum injections to reduce flexor or extensor tone and abnormal muscle activation during movement.[55]

Treatment Pathologically increased tone in patients with hemiplegia can usually be managed by aiming to maintain normal length of the muscle and soft tissue across a joint and helping patients avoid abnormal flexor and extensor patterns at rest and during movement. Spasticity should be treated more aggressively when it interferes with nursing care and perineal hygiene or contributes to contractures and pressure sores.

Dantrolene, baclofen, a benzodiazepine such as clonazepam, and tizanidine can reduce hypertonicity-related flexor or extensor postures and, occasionally, improve the pattern of ambulation. A clear effect should be evident, and attempts should be made after further physical therapy to eliminate the drug. Each can cause more difficulty with weight bearing and can produce sedation, confusion, and other central and systemic side effects (Table 8-6).

Chemical agents such as phenol have been injected into a nerve, motor point, or muscle to lessen inappropriate muscle co-contraction, spasms, and dystonic postures. As motor point blocks can partially spare voluntary movement and could reduce reciprocal inhibition when given to an antagonist muscle, they could improve some aspects of motor control. Intramuscular injections of ethanol or botulinum-A toxin will reduce local features of spasticity for about 3 months.[55-57] Botulinum injections have seemed most efficacious for the wrist and finger flexors and plantar flexors.

Although rarely used after a stroke, a variety of surgical procedures, including tendon lengthening, tenotomy, and tendon transfer, can correct deformities induced by spasticity and improve function. A gait analysis with EMG helps determine which procedure might aid mobility. Tendon lengthening of the hamstrings, Achilles, and toe or finger and wrist flexors is occasionally considered. Physical therapy must follow surgery.

Cognitive Dysfunction and Dementia

Background A range of cognitive impairments arise following stroke. Careful neuropsychologic testing often reveals executive, visuoperceptual, and disconnection syndromes. Memory loss and hemi-inattention or neglect are among those that especially interfere with rehabilitation.

The incidence and risk factors for memory loss and dementia caused by one or more strokes has become increasingly appreciated.[58-60] In a population study, dementia was nine times greater in the first year after a stroke compared with the expected incidence in an age-controlled group and twice the risk for the stroke population each subsequent year.[61] In other community-based studies, the incidence ranged from 20 percent at 3 months after a stroke to 30 percent of all stroke survivors.[62-64] The frequency of dementia rises with increasing age and varies with the definition that is used to designate dementia. Even a mild aphasia may affect verbal memory and can interfere with verbal learning during rehabilitation.[65] The rehabilitation team depends upon teaching that can be encoded and retrieved. Memory disturbances can have a profoundly negative influence on the compensation and new learning that underlies much of the rehabilitation process.

Visual neglect was found in 38 percent of 150 consecutive patients with moderate disability after a new stroke.[66] The neglect was modestly associated with poorer ADL scores and slower recovery, though severe neglect was rare beyond 6 months. The NINDS Stroke Data Bank also looked at the effect of hemineglect on the ADL scores at 7 to 10 days and 1 year after onset of a first stroke.[67] Patients who had anosognosia, visual neglect, tactile extinction, motor impersistence, or auditory neglect had the lowest BI scores at 1 year, even after adjusting the data for initial ADL scores and for poststroke rehabilitation.

Recovery across reports has been most rapid within the first 2 weeks, regardless of the side of stroke, and has plateaued at 3 months, when most patients have little visual neglect. Many patients have more subtle and lingering impairments that depend upon what test is used to detect them. Severe visual neglect and anosognosia in the first week predict some level of persistent impairment at 6 months.

Table 8-6.
Dosages of medications for symptomatic spasticity

First line use
  Dantrolene–25 mg BID to 50 mg QID
  Baclofen–5 mg BID to 40 mg QID
  Clonidine–0.05 mg QD to 0.2 mg TID
  Tizanidine–2 mg BID to 8 mg QID
  Clonazepam–0.5 to 2 mg BID to TID

Occasionally useful additions
  Gabapentin–400 mg TID to 600 mg QID
  Intrathecal baclofen–50-μg trial dose
  Phenytoin–serum concentration 10 to 20 mg%
  Cyproheptadine–4 mg BID to 8 mg QID

Evidence No specific form of cognitive therapy has proven to be useful for memory loss and dementia, though trials of anticholinesterases are ongoing for multi-infarct dementia. In normal subjects, constant feedback enhances immediate performance, but an intermittent schedule of reinforcement improves long-term retention. The optimal way to enhance learning in people with a focal brain injury is less certain, and probably much more variable, depending upon what type of memory, attention, or other cognitive process has been affected. Amnestic subjects and those with impaired episodic memory have been shown to do worse with trial-and-error training. More frequent feedback and errorless learning were shown to improve retention.[68]

Well-described behavioral interventions have been employed to improve attention to the left.[69,70] The techniques include an anchoring stimulus on the left and the use and gradual withdrawal of left-sided cues to draw visual attention there, work on sensory awareness to physical stimuli, and tasks to aid spatial organization. No studies have clearly shown that this approach works better than any other, but it is a reasonable starting point.

Treatment An approach that uses cognitive remediation for amnestic disorders trains patients to use the postulated subcomponent processes that underlie declarative and nondeclarative memory. Procedural memory tends to be better preserved and can be used to regain or learn motor skills. Therapists also employ a restorative or compensatory approach to affect particular memory skills for functionally important activities. A common compensatory intervention is to limit subjects to one task at a time, block out interruptions during learning tasks and in daily activities, rehearsal, and keeping lists in a calendar book of what needs to be done.

Table 8-7 lists some of the traditional and rather ingenious ways rehabilitationists have tried to clinically manage hemi-inattention. None has produced robust results. Noradrenergic and dopaminergic stimulants including methylphenidate and bromocriptine are especially worth trying.

Table 8-7.
Interventions for hemi-inattention[a]

Multisensory visual and sensory cues, then fading cues[70]
Verbal elaboration of visual analysis[71]
Visual imagery[72]
Environmental adaptations[73]
Video feedback[74]
Monocular and binocular patches and prisms[75–78]
Left limb movement in left hemispace[79]
Head and trunk midline adjustments[80–84]
Vestibular stimulation[85–87]
Reduce hemianopic defects[88]
Pharmacotherapy[89]
Computer training[90,91]

[a]Adapted from Ref. 4.

General Approaches

Physical Therapies and Mobility Training

Background In the Copenhagen Study, 51 percent of patients initially were unable to walk, 12 percent walked with assistance, and 37 percent were independent.[92] At discharge, 22 percent could not walk, 14 percent walked with assistance, and 64 percent of survivors walked independently. About 80 percent of those who were initially nonwalkers reached their best walking function within 6 weeks and 95 percent within 11 weeks. In patients who walked with assistance, 80 percent reached best function within 3 weeks and 95 percent within 5 weeks. Independent walking was achieved by 34 percent of the survivors who had been dependent and 60 percent of those who initially required assistance. Recovery of ambulation correlated directly with residual leg strength. In general, walking can be achieved readily if a patient can flex the hip and extend the hemiparetic knee against gravity.

More detailed information about outcomes in relationship to impairment and disability was reported in a prospective study of 95 consecutive inpatients admitted to a rehabilitation center after a hemispheric stroke.[93] Patients were followed until they reached a plateau of recovery. Life table analyses of the probability of recovering BI functions were made for patients who were divided into three categories of impairment and examined at 2-week intervals. Over 90 percent of patients with a pure motor (M) deficit became independent in walking 150 feet by week 14, but only 35 percent of those with motor and proprioceptive (SM) loss by week 24, and 3 percent of those with motor, sensory, and hemianoptic deficits (SMH) by week 30. The probability of walking over 150 feet with assistance increased to 100 percent with M impairment by week 14 (80 percent by week 8) and to over 90 percent in those with SM loss by week 26 and with SMH deficits by 28 weeks after the stroke. About 65 percent achieved a BI score of over 95 by 15 weeks if they had only M deficits and by 26 weeks with SM loss, but only 10 percent scored that high with SMH deficits after 18 to 30 weeks. However, 100 percent achieved a score of >60 by 14 weeks with M loss only, 75 percent by 23 weeks with SM deficits, and 60 percent by 29 weeks with SMH loss.

Evidence The sensorimotor impairments caused by stroke can be managed by at least four general approaches: exercise, facilitation and neurodevelopmental techniques, compensatory training, and drawing upon theories of motor control and motor learning. When compared with each other, no differences have been found among the traditional schools of facilitative therapy; a mild benefit seems apparent with strengthening exercises.[94,95] Motor control approaches stress task-oriented practice and optimal schedules of practice and reinforcement.[96] Few clinical trials have been reported, but the results look promising as part of a physical and occupational therapy strategy.[97-101] Treadmill walking is a potential task-oriented therapy for ambulation.[102] In patients with stroke, single case studies and small clinical trials have suggested that body weight-supported treadmill training (BWSTT) increased the likelihood of achieving more independent ambulation and at greater speeds than by conventional locomotor therapy.[103-105] Gait symmetry clearly improves during treadmill step training.[106,107] A Canadian trial randomized about 100 patients to BWSTT or treadmill training without BWS during inpatient rehabilitation for stroke and showed significant increases in overground speed in those managed with BWS.[108]

BWSTT, in theory, allows the spinal cord and supraspinal locomotor regions to experience sensory inputs that are more like ordinary stepping compared with the atypical locomotor inputs created by compensatory gait deviations and difficulty with loading a paretic limb.[109] More normal input may improve the timing and increase the activation of residual descending locomotor outputs on the motor pools. Sensory inputs related to the level of loading and to treadmill speed have been shown to modulate the EMG output during BWSTT, even when the legs are fully assisted during the step cycle.[110,111]

A great variety of trials have employed electromyographic, visual, and auditory biofeedback to increase muscle contraction or lessen cocontractions, improve the pattern of arm or leg movements, and improve balance.[112,113] Although some results show promise, no technique has come into common usage. Gains during biofeedback sessions often do not carry over to movements made during walking.

Treatment   Range of motion in the paretic arm and leg is maintained with positioning, splints, and slow rhythmic rotation and stretch of all joints several times a day, along with weight bearing as soon as possible. Patient and family are taught to assist. This activity can also reduce unwanted hypertonicity. The dominant synergistic movement in the leg is the extensor pattern at the hip and knee with adduction of the hip and plantar flexion at the ankle. At the onset of therapy, the physical

therapist might stimulate this pattern just enough to allow weight bearing on the leg. At the same time, flexion at the hip, knee, and ankle would be encouraged by such mat exercises as rolling onto the side and bringing the knee to the chest with whatever sensory stimulation and physical assistance is needed. The patient is trained to increase the amount of weight bearing and the amount of time spent on the paretic leg and works on truncal control and balance. Once the patient has adequate endurance and stability to stand in the parallel bars or at a hemibar with the therapist's help to control the paretic leg, gait training begins. The therapist may concentrate on the most prominent deviations from normal during the gait cycle such as circumduction of the hip, pelvic drop, hyperextension or flexor give-way of the knee, inadequate dorsiflexion of the ankle, and toe clawing. The physical therapist also encourages more weight bearing on the paretic leg, and a longer reciprocal step length.

Hemiparetic patients who recover little ankle movement, whose foot tends to turn over during gait, or who lack enough knee control to prevent it from snapping back usually can be managed with a polypropylene ankle-foot orthosis that is fitted to the patient's needs. Bracing can improve the gait pattern.[114] In those with profound sensorimotor impairment, a double upright metal brace is occasionally indicated. As inpatient therapy for gait progresses away from the parallel bars to increasing distances walked with a quadcane, then to stair climbing and outdoor ambulation on uneven surfaces, therapy can continue in the outpatient setting, where mobility in the home and community is stressed.

Occupational Therapies and Self-Care Skills

Background   The occupational therapist brings to the rehabilitation team expertise with assistive devices for ADLs and often works with the neuropsychologist in addressing visuospatial inattention, memory loss, apraxia, dysphagia, and difficulties in problem solving. Tables 8-2 and 8-3 provide an overview of the kinds of self-care tasks that the therapist addresses. Outcomes across prospective and retrospective studies in patients undergoing rehabilitation or in the general acute stroke population suggest that about 60 to 70 percent of patients recover the ability to manage basic self-care skills, although the majority do not return to their premorbid level of socialization.

The Copenhagen Stroke Study was a community-based population study that prospectively followed about 1200 patients admitted acutely and nearly all of the 800 survivors.[115] Using the BI and Scandinavian Stroke Scale, the study graded recovery before and after acute and rehabilitative inpatient stays and at 6 months. Within the same facility, all who needed rehabilitation received services for an average total stay of 35 days (S.D. 41). By then, 11 percent had severe impairments, 11 percent had moderate, and 78 percent had mild or no deficits. At the same time, 20 percent had severe disability, 8 percent moderate, 26 percent mild, and 46 percent had no disability. ADLs plateaued by 9 weeks in those with initially mild strokes, within 13 weeks in the moderate, within 17 weeks in the severe, and within 20 weeks for the most severe stroke patients.[116] Best upper extremity function was assessed with the BI feeding and grooming score for the affected arm.[117] Within 9 weeks, 95 percent of patients achieved their best function. With mild paresis, this was accomplished by 6 weeks after onset. With severe paresis, best function was achieved by 11 weeks. Many studies suggest that no more than about 10 percent of patients who have no movement of the hand by several weeks after onset will recover independent feeding and dressing with that hand. Patients who do have some finger flexion and extension can continue to improve their hand coordination for tasks for 6 to 12 months if they practice those tasks.

Evidence The studies cited in the physical therapy section hold for occupational therapies. No general approach has been shown to be better than another. Forced use of the affected upper extremity and gradual shaping of a variety of functional movements to overcome what is theorized as learned nonuse of the paretic limb has been accomplished with some success.[118] Failed early attempts to use the affected limb can lead to behavioral suppression. The primary intervention uses a variety of techniques that prevent the use of the unaffected arm by placing it in a sling or glove. The patient practices skills and ADLs exclusively with the affected arm. In chronic stroke patients who could dorsiflex the wrist at least 10 degrees and extend and fingers of the paretic hand, much of the improvement in daily use was evident within days of restraint of the unaffected arm plus therapy, which suggests that a latent capability had succumbed to learned nonuse.[119]

Treatment At first, emphasis is often placed on visually or manually patterning the patient through parts of a task, then through the entire task, with frequent positive feedback. Techniques that conserve energy and promote independence in dressing, grooming, bathing, and toileting involve relearning how to carry out the task and much practice. The therapist also provides a wheelchair with proper seating, a clear plastic lap board or arm trough to rest the paretic limb where it can be seen by the patient, an arm sling if shoulder subluxation or pain arises, a compression glove to reduce hand edema if elevation and massage fail, and static and dynamic splints to maintain wrist and finger position. A visit to the home of a patient who is less than fully independent is the best way to establish the need for assistive devices such as grab bars, rails, ramps, and environmental controls, architectural changes such as widening a doorway to allow wheelchair access, and for an emergency remote control calling system.

Speech and Language Therapies

Background In the Copenhagen Study, 38 percent of 881 patients were aphasic on admission, with 20 percent of the admissions rated as severe on the Scandinavian Stroke Scale.[120] Nearly one-half of the severe aphasics died early after onset, and one-half of the mild aphasics recovered by 1 week. Only 18 percent of community survivors were still aphasic at the time of their acute and rehabilitation hospital discharge. Up to 28 percent received early speech therapy as needed. Patients were retested for 6 months. Ninety-five percent with a mild aphasia reached their best level of recovery at 2 weeks, with a moderate aphasia at 6 weeks, and with severe aphasia within 10 weeks. Only 8 percent of the severe aphasics fully recovered on the scoring system used by 6 months. Mild language deficits might not be ascertained by the scale. The best predictor of recovery was a lesser severity of aphasia close to the time of the stroke.

Evidence A meta-analysis was performed on 55 interventional trials of speech/language therapy in aphasic patients after stroke.[121] Significant effects were found for treated over untreated patients at all stages of recovery, with the greatest effect found when therapy was started early after stroke. Treatments in excess of 2 h per week gave greater gains than lesser amounts of therapy. Severe aphasics showed large gains when treated by a speech-language pathologist. Only one defined intervention, multimodal stimulation, was tested in enough cases to show its greater average effect. An inadequate number of studies were found to allow the analysis to demonstrate any differential effects of treatments for differing types of aphasia. A large variety of approaches for particular language and linguistic impairments have been described.[122–124] Melodic intonation therapy for nonfluent aphasics who have good comprehension has been found to have value for increasing expression.[125]

Treatment For the aphasic patient, speech therapists attempt to find ways to circumvent, deblock, or compensate for impairments in the comprehension and expression of language. Visual and verbal cueing techniques include picture matching and sentence completion tasks. Frequent repetition and positive reinforcement are used as the patient approaches the desired responses.

CONCLUSIONS

The amount of disability is reduced during the time of stroke rehabilitation, particularly when an organized program of care is offered. On average, both the amount of impairment and disability lessens during the period of inpatient and outpatient therapy. Although a skeptic might suggest that neurologic recovery alone could account for functional gains, more than one study has demonstrated a likely independent role for stroke rehabilitation in reducing disability.[126–128] Beyond spontaneous recovery, methods that emphasize problem solving, adaptation, the learning and practice of compensatory skills, and motor learning in the face of sensorimotor impairments should lead to improvements in ADLs and more sophisticated activities.

Stroke rehabilitation requires a team approach to optimize outcomes. An organized therapeutic mileu during inpatient rehabilitation helps to account for better functional outcomes and discharge placements, particularly for patients with moderate initial disability. However, few studies have shown the benefit of one approach over another. Only small trials have offered well-defined strategies for the treatment of particular impairments and disabilities, such as walking, ataxia, grasping, aphasia syndromes, hemineglect, and other cognitive impairments. Much energy is spent on the difficult economics of providing an ideal amount of therapy services. More effort is needed on the part of therapists and clinical and basic neuroscientists to draw upon concepts of neuroplasticity and motor learning to devise better theory-based interventions.

REFERENCES

1. Pedersen P, Jorgensen H, Nakayama H, et al: Comprehensive assessment of activities of daily living in stroke: The Copenhagen Stroke Study. *Arch Phys Med Rehabil* 78:161, 1997.
2. Garratt A, Rutta D, Abdulla M, et al: The SF36 health survey questionnaire: An outcome measure suitable for routine use within the NHS? *Br Med J* 306:1440, 1993.
3. Wade D: *Measurement in Neurological Rehabilitation.* New York, Oxford University Press, 1992, p 388.
4. Dobkin B: Neurologic rehabilitation, in Gilman S (ed): *Contemporary Neurology Series,* vol. 47. Philadelphia, F A Davis, 1996.
5. Gresham C, Duncan P, Stason W, et al: *Post-Stroke Rehabilitation: Assessment, Referral, and Patient Management.* Clinical Practice Guideline No. 16: U.S. Public Health Service, Agency for Health Care Policy and Research, 1995.
6. Dobkin B: Experimental brain injury and repair. *Curr Opin Neurol* 10:493, 1997.
7. Nudo R, Milliken G: Reorganization of movement representations in primary motor cortex following focal ischemic infarcts in adult squirrel monkeys. *J Neurophysiol* 75:2144, 1996.
8. Nudo R, Wise B, SiFuentes F, Milliken G: Neural substrates for the effects of rehabilitative training on motor recovery after ischemic infarct. *Science* 272:1791, 1996.
9. Kozlowski D, von Stuck S, Lee S, Hovda D, Becker D: Behaviorally-induced contusions following traumatic brain injury: Use-dependent secondary insults. *Abstracts of the 26th meeting of the Society for Neuroscience* 22:1905, 1996.
10. Kozlowski D, James D, Schallert T: Use-dependent exaggeration of neuronal injury after unilateral sensorimotor cortex lesions. *J Neurosci* 16:4776, 1996.
11. Donoghue J: Limits of reorganization in cortical circuits. *Cereb Cortex* 7:97, 1997.
12. Jones T, Kleim J, Greenough W: Synaptogenesis and dendritic growth in the cortex opposite unilateral sensorimotor cortex damage in adult rats: A quantitative electron microscopic examination. *Brain Res* 733:142, 1996.
13. Kwakkel G, Wagenaar R, Koelman T: Effects of intensity of rehabilitation after stroke. *Stroke* 28:1550, 1997.
14. Gresham GE, Phillips TF, Wolf PA: Epidemiologic profile of long-term stroke disability: The Framingham Study. *Arch Phys Med Rehabil* 60:487, 1979.
15. Gresham GE, Granger CV: Overview: Patient evaluation and treatment program, in Brandstater ME, Basmajian JV (eds): *Stroke Rehabilitation.* Baltimore, Williams & Wilkins, 1987, pp 399–405.
16. Dobkin BH: Controversies in neurology: Focused stroke rehabilitation programs do not affect outcome. *Arch Neurol* 46:701, 1989.
17. Reding M, McDowell F: Focused stroke rehabilitation programs improve outcome. *Arch Neurol* 46:700, 1989.
18. Collaboration SUT: How do stroke units improve patient outcomes? A collaborative systematic review of the randomized trials. *Stroke* 28:2139, 1997.

19. Kalra L, Dale P, Crome P: Improving stroke rehabilitation: A controlled trial. *Stroke* 24:1462, 1993.
20. Kalra L: The influence of stroke unit rehabilitation on functional recovery from stroke. *Stroke* 25:821, 1994.
21. Ronning O, Guldvog B: Stroke units versus general medical wards: I. Twelve- and eighteen-month survival. *Stroke* 29:58, 1998.
22. Indredavik B, Slordahl S, Bakke F: Stroke unit treatment. *Stroke* 28:1861, 1997.
23. Davies P, Bamford J, Warlow C: Remedial therapy and functional recovery in a total population of first-stroke patients. *Int Disabil Studies* 11:40, 1989.
24. Wade D, Skilbeck C, Bainton D: Controlled trial of a home-care service for acute stroke patients. *Lancet* 1985:323, 1985.
25. Kramer A, Steiner J, Schlenker R, et al: Outcomes and costs after hip fracture and stroke: A comparison of rehabilitation settings. *JAMA* 277:396, 1997.
26. Ottenbacher K, Jannell S: The results of clinical trials in stroke rehabilitation research. *Arch Neurol* 50:37, 1993.
27. Kalra L, Yu G, Wilson K, Roots P: Medical complications during stroke rehabilitation. *Stroke* 26:990, 1995.
28. Dromerick A, Reding M: Medical and neurological complications during inpatient stroke rehabilitation. *Stroke* 25:358, 1994.
29. Reding M, Winter S, Thompson M: Urinary incontinence after unilateral hemispheric stroke. *J Neurol Rehab* 1:25, 1987.
30. Gelber D, Jozefczyk P, Good D, et al: Urinary retention following acute stroke. *J Neurol Rehab* 8:69, 1994.
31. Teasell R: Pain following stroke. *Crit Rev Phys Med Rehabil* 3:205, 1992.
32. Sunderland A, Tinson D, Bradley E: Enhanced physical therapy improves recovery of function after stroke: A randomised controlled trial. *J Neurol Neurosurg Psychiatry* 55:530, 1992.
33. Rowbotham MC: Complex regional pain syndrome type I (reflex sympathetic dystrophy). *Neurology* 51:4, 1998.
34. Werner R, Priebe M, Davidoff G: Reflex sympathetic dystrophy syndrome associated with hemiplegia. *Neuro Rehabil* 2:16, 1992.
35. Poduri K: Shoulder pain in stroke patients and its effects on rehabilitation. *J Stroke Cerebrovasc Dis* 3:261, 1993.
36. Faghri P, Rodgers M, Glaser R: The effects of functional electrical stimulation on shoulder subluxation, arm function recovery, and shoulder pain in hemiplegic stroke patients. *Arch Phys Med Rehabil* 75:73, 1994.
37. Wolf P, Bachman D, Kelly-Hayes M: Stroke and depression in the community: The Framingham Study. *Neurology* 40 (Suppl 1):416, 1990.
38. Astrom M, Adolfsson R, Asplund K: Major depression in stroke patients: A 3-year longitudinal study. *Stroke* 24:976, 1993.
39. Reding M, Orto L, Winter S, McDowell F: Antidepressant therapy after stroke. *Arch Neurol* 43:763, 1986.
40. Andersen G, Vsetergaard K, Lauritzen L: Effective treatment of poststroke depression with the selective serotonin reuptake inhibitor citalopram. *Stroke* 25:1099, 1994.
41. DePippo K, Holas M, Reding M: Dysphagia therapy following stroke: A controlled trial. *Neurology* 44:1655, 1994.
42. Stover S: *Spinal Cord Injury: The Facts and Figures.* Birmingham, AL, University of Alabama, 1986.
43. Agency for Health Care Policy and Research: *Pressure Ulcers in Adults: Prediction and Prevention.* U.S. Department of Health and Human Services, 1992.
44. Reith J, Jorgensen H, Nakayama H, Olsen T: Seizures in acute stroke: Predictors and prognostic significance. The Copenhagen Stroke Study. *Stroke* 28:1585, 1997.
45. Furlan M, Marchal G, Viader F, Derlon J-M, Baron J-C: Spontaneous neurological recovery after stroke and the fate of the ischemic penumbra. *Ann Neurol* 40:216, 1996.
46. Dobkin B: Activity-dependent learning contributes to motor recovery. *Ann Neurol* 44:158, 1998.
47. Marchal G, Beaudouin V, Rioux P: Prolonged persistence of substantial volumes of potentially viable brain tissue after stroke: A correlative PET-CT study with voxel-based data analysis. *Stroke* 27:599, 1996.
48. Goldstein L: Influence of common drugs and related factors on stroke outcome. *Curr Opin Neurol* 10:52, 1997.
49. Boldrini P, Basaglia N, Calanca M: Sexual changes in hemiparetic patients. *Arch Phys Med Rehabil* 72:202, 1991.
50. Partinen M, Palomaki H: Snoring and cerebral infarction. *Lancet* 1:1325, 1985.
51. Mohsenin V, Valor R: Sleep apnea in patients with hemispheric stroke. *Arch Phys Med Rehabil* 76:71, 1995.
52. Bassetti C, Aldrich M, Quint D: Sleep-disordered breathing in patients with acute supra- and infratentorial strokes: A prospective study of 39 patients. *Stroke* 28:1765, 1997.
53. Good D, Henkle J, Gelber D, Welsh J, Verhulst S: Sleep-disordered breathing and poor functional outcome after stroke. *Stroke* 27:252, 1996.
54. Young R, Emre M, Nance P: Current issues in spasticity management. *Neurologist* 3:261, 1997.
55. Hesse S, Krajnik J, Luecke D, Jahnke M, Gregoric M, Mauritz K: Ankle muscle activity before and after botulinum toxin therapy for lower limb extensor spasticity in chronic hemiparetic patients. *Stroke* 27:455, 1996.
56. Simpson D, Alexander D, O'Brien C, et al: Botulinum toxin type A in the treatment of upper extremity spasticity: A randomized, double-blind, placebo-controlled trial. *Neurology* 46:1306, 1996.
57. Chutorian A, Root L: Management of spasticity in children with botulinum-A toxin. *Int Pediatr* 9:35, 1994.
58. Moroney J, Bagiella E, Desmond D, Paik M, YS, Tatemichi T: Risk factors for incident dementia after stroke. *Stroke* 27:1283, 1996.
59. Gorelick P: Status of risk factors for dementia associated with stroke. *Stroke* 28:459, 1997.
60. Tatemichi T, Desmond D, Mayeux R: Dementia after stroke. *Neurology* 42:1185, 1992.
61. Kokmen E, Whisnant J, O'Fallon W, Beard C: Dementia

after ischemic stroke: A population based study in Rochester, Minn. *Neurology* 46:154, 1996.

62. Pohjasvaara T, Erkinjuntti T, Vataja R, Kaste M: Dementia three months after stroke: Baseline frequency and effect of different definitions of dementia in the Helsinki Stroke Aging Memory Study (SAM) Cohort. *Stroke* 28:785, 1997.

63. Henon H, Pasquier F, Durieu I: Preexisting dementia in stroke patients. *Stroke* 28:2429, 1997.

64. Desmond D, Moroney J, Sano M, Stern Y: Recovery of cognitive function after stroke. *Stroke* 27:1798, 1996.

65. Ween J, Verfaellie M, Alexander M: Verbal memory function in mild aphasia. *Neurology* 47:795, 1996.

66. Kalra L, Perez I, Gupta S, Wittink M: The influence of visual neglect on stroke rehabilitation. *Stroke* 28:1386, 1997.

67. Marshall R, Sacco R, Lee S, Mohr J: Hemineglect predicts functional outcome after stroke (Abstract). *Ann Neurol* 36:298, 1994.

68. Wilson B, Baddeley A, Evans J, Shiel A: Errorless learning in the rehabilitation of memory impaired people. *Neuropsychol Rehabil* 4:307, 1994.

69. Gordon W, Diller L, Lieberman A, et al: Perceptual remediation in patients with right brain damage: A comprehensive program. *Arch Phys Med Rehabil* 66:353, 1985.

70. Ben-Yishay Y, Diller L: Cognitive remediation in traumatic brain injury: Update and issues. *Arch Phys Med Rehabil* 74:204, 1993.

71. Hanlon R, Dobkin B: Effects of cognitive rehabilitation following a right thalamic infarct. *J Clin Exp Neuropsychol* 14:433, 1992.

72. Smania N, Bazoli F, Piva D, Guidetti G: Visuomotor imagery and rehabilitation of neglect. *Arch Phys Med Rehabil* 78:430, 1997.

73. Loverro J, Reding M: Bed orientation and rehabilitation outcome for patients with stroke and hemianopsia or visual neglect. *J Neurol Rehabil* 2:147, 1988.

74. Tham K, Tegner R: Video feedback in the rehabilitation of patients with unilateral neglect. *Arch Phys Med Rehabil* 78:410, 1997.

75. Rossi P, Kheyfets S, Reding M: Fresnel prisms improve visual perception in stroke patients with homonymous hemianopia or unilateral visual neglect. *Neurology* 40:1597, 1990.

76. Butter C, Kirsch N: Combined and separate effects of eye patching and visual stimulation on unilateral neglect following stroke. *Arch Phys Med Rehabil* 73:1133, 1992.

77. Serfaty C, Soroker N, Glicksohn J, Sepkuti J, Myslobodsky M: Does monocular viewing improve target detection in hemispatial neglect? *Restor Neurol Neurosci* 9:7, 1995.

78. Arai T, Ohi H, Sasaki H, et al: Hemispatial sunglasses: Effect on unilateral spatial neglect. *Arch Phys Med Rehabil* 78:230, 1997.

79. Robertson I, North N: Spatio-motor cueing in unilateral neglect: The role of hemispace, hand and motor activation. *Neuropsychologia* 30:553, 1992.

80. Karnath H, Schenkel P, Fischer B: Trunk orientation as the determining factor of the contralateral deficit in the neglect syndrome and as the physical anchor of the internal representation of body orientation in space. *Brain* 114:1997, 1991.

81. Taylor D, Ashburn A, Ward C: Asymmetrical trunk posture, unilateral neglect and motor performance following stroke. *Clin Rehabil* 8:48, 1994.

82. Mennemeier M, Chatterjee A, Heilman K: A comparison of the influences of body and environment centered reference frames on neglect. *Brain* 117:1013, 1994.

83. Simon E, Hegarty A, Mehler M: Hemispatial and directional performance biases in motor neglect. *Neurology* 45:525, 1995.

84. Wiart L, Bon Saint Come A, Debelleix X, et al: Unilateral neglect syndrome rehabilitation by trunk rotation and scanning training. *Arch Phys Med Rehabil* 78:424, 1997.

85. Rode G, Charles N, Perenin M-T: Partial remission of hemiplegia and somatoparaphrenia through vestibular stimulation in a case of unilateral neglect. *Cortex* 28:203, 1992.

86. Rubens A: Caloric stimulation and unilateral visual neglect. *Neurology* 35:1019, 1985.

87. Vallar G, Sterzi R, Bottini G: Temporary remission of left hemianesthesia after vestibular stimulation: A sensory neglect phenomenon. *Cortex* 26:123, 1990.

88. Kerkhoff G, MunBinger U, Meier E: Neurovisual rehabilitation in cerebral blindness. *Arch Neurol* 51:474, 1994.

89. Fleet W, Valenstein E, Watson R, Heilman K: Dopamine agonist therapy for neglect in humans. *Neurology* 37:1765, 1987.

90. Robertson I, Gray J, Pentland B, Waite L: Microcomputer-based rehabilitation for unilateral left visual neglect: A randomized controlled trial. *Arch Phys Med Rehabil* 71:663, 1990.

91. Gray J, Robertson I, Pentland B, Anderson S: Microcomputer-based attentional retraining after brain damage: A randomised group controlled trial. *Neuropsychol Rehabil* 2:97, 1992.

92. Jorgensen H, Nakayama H, Raaschou H, Olsen T: Recovery of walking function in stroke patients: The Copenhagen Stroke Study. *Arch Phys Med Rehabil* 76:27, 1995.

93. Reding M, Potes E: Rehabilitation outcome following initial unilateral hemispheric stroke: Life table analysis approach. *Stroke* 19:1354, 1988.

94. Ashburn A, Partridge C, De Souza L: Physiotherapy in the rehabilitation of stroke: A review. *Clin Rehabil* 7:337, 1993.

95. Giuliani C: Strength training for patients with neurological disorders. *Neurol Report* 19:29, 1995.

96. Lister M: *Contemporary Management of Motor Control Problems: Proceedings of the II Step Conference.* Alexandria, VA, Foundation for Physical Therapy, 1991, p 278.

97. Schmidt R: Motor learning principles for physical therapy, in Lister M (ed): *Contemporary Management of Motor*

Control Problems. Alexandria, VA, Foundation for Physical Therapy, 1991, pp 49–63.

98. Poole J: Application of motor learning principles in occupational therapy. *Am J Occup Ther* 45:531, 1991.

99. Winstein C, Merians AS, Sullivan, KJ: Motor learning after unilateral brain damage: *Neuropsychologia* 37:975, 1999.

100. Hanlon R: Motor learning following unilateral stroke. *Arch Phys Med Rehabil* 77:811, 1996.

101. Dean C, Shepherd R: Task-related training improves performance of seated reaching tasks after stroke. *Stroke* 28:722, 1997.

102. Richards C, Malouin F, Wood-Dauphinee S, et al: Task-specific physical therapy for optimization of gait recovery in acute stroke patients. *Arch Phys Med Rehabil* 74:612, 1993.

103. Dobkin B, Fowler E, Gregor R: A strategy to train locomotion in patients with chronic hemiplegic stroke. *Ann Neurol* 30:278, 1991.

104. Hesse S, Bertelt C, Schaffrin A, et al: Restoration of gait in nonambulatory hemiparetic patients by treadmill training with partial body-weight support. *Arch Phys Med Rehabil* 75:1087, 1994.

105. Hesse S, Jahnke M, Bertelt C: Gait outcome in ambulatory hemiparetic patients after a 4-week comprehensive rehabilitation program and prognostic factors. *Stroke* 25:1999, 1994.

106. Hesse S, Helm B, Krajnik J, Gregoric M, Mavritz KHM: Treadmill training with partial body weight support: Influence of body weight release on the gait of hemiparetic patients. *J Neurol Rehabil* 11:15, 1997.

107. Hassid E, Rose D, Dobkin B, et al: Improved gait symmetry in hemiparetic patients during body weight-supported treadmill stepping. *J Neurol Rehabil* 11:21, 1997.

108. Visintin M, Korner-Bitensky N, Barbeau H, Mayo N: *A New Approach to Retraining Gait Following Stroke Through Body Weight Support and Treadmill Stimulation*. World Confederation for Physical Therapy Congress, Washington, D.C., June 25, 1995.

109. Dobkin B: Recovery of locomotor control. *Neurologist* 2:239, 1996.

110. Dobkin B, Harkema S, Requejo P, Edgerton V: Modulation of locomotor-like EMG activity in subjects with complete and incomplete chronic spinal cord injury. *J Neurol Rehabil* 9:183, 1995.

111. Harkema S, Dobkin B, Edgerton V: *Activity-Dependent Plasticity after Complete Human Spinal Cord Injury*. Seventh International Symposium on Neural Regeneration, Asilomar Conference, Pacific Grove, CA, 1997.

112. Glanz M, Klawansky S, Stason W, et al: Biofeedback therapy in poststroke rehabilitation: A meta-analysis of the randomized controlled trials. *Arch Phys Med Rehabil* 76:508, 1995.

113. Moreland J, Thomson M, Fuoco A: Electromyographic biofeedback to improve lower extremity function after stroke: A meta-analysis. *Arch Phys Med Rehabil* 79:134, 1998.

114. Lehmann J, Condon S, Price R, de Lateur B: Gait abnormalities in hemiplegia: Their correction by ankle-foot orthoses. *Arch Phys Med Rehabil* 68:763, 1987.

115. Jorgensen H, Nakayama H, Raaschou H, et al: Outcome and time course of recovery in stroke: Part I. Outcome. The Copenhagen Stroke Study. *Arch Phys Med Rehabil* 76:399, 1995.

116. Jorgensen H, Nakayama H, Raaschou H, et al: Outcome and time course of recovery in stroke: Part II. Time course. The Copenhagen Stroke Study. *Arch Phys Med Rehabil* 76:406, 1995.

117. Nakayama H, Jorgensen H, Raaschou H, Olsen T: Recovery of upper extremity function in stroke patients: The Copenhagen Stroke Study. *Arch Phys Med Rehabil* 75:394, 1994.

118. Taub E, Wolf S: Constraint induced movement techniques to facilitate upper extremity use in stroke patients. *Top Stroke Rehabil* 3:38, 1997.

119. Taub E, Miller N, Novack T: Technique to improve chronic motor deficit after stroke. *Arch Phys Med Rehabil* 74:347, 1993.

120. Pedersen P, Jorgensen H, Nakayama H, Raaschou H, Olsen T: Aphasia in acute stroke: Incidence, determinants, and recovery. *Ann Neurol* 38:659, 1995.

121. Robey R: A meta-analysis of clinical outcomes in the treatment of aphasia. *J Speech Lang Hear Res* 41:172, 1998.

122. LaPointe L: *Aphasia and Related Neurogenic Language Disorders*. New York, Thieme Medical Publishers, 1990, p 238.

123. Helm-Estabrooks N, Albert M: *Manual of Aphasia Therapy*. Austin, TX, Pro-Ed, 1991.

124. Caplan D: Toward a psycholinguistic approach to acquired neurogenic language disorders. *Am J Speech Lang Pathol* 12:59, 1993.

125. Neurology Assessment (a committee report): Melodic intonation therapy. *Neurology* 44:566, 1994.

126. Roth E, Heinemann A, Lovell L, et al: Impairment and disability: Their relation during stroke rehabilitation. *Arch Phys Med Rehabil* 79:329, 1998.

127. Fiedler R, Granger C: Uniform data system For medical rehabilitation: Report of first admissions for 1995. *Am J Phys Med Rehabil* 76:76, 1997.

128. Kwakkel G, Wagenaar RC, Twisk JWR, et al: Intensity of leg and arm training after primary middle-cerebral-artery stroke: A randomised trial: *Lancet* 354:191, 1999.

Chapter 9

THE CHRONIC STROKE PATIENT: MANAGEMENT OF COMMON MEDICAL PROBLEMS

Freddi Segal-Gidan
Helena C. Chui

INTRODUCTION

The gradual, continuous decline in stroke mortality over the past several decades has resulted in increasing numbers of stroke survivors. Many of these stroke survivors have physical and mental impairments, as well as varying degrees of disability. Survivors of stroke frequently experience one or more ongoing medical problems after their acute stroke rehabilitation is complete. These problems, often referred to as long-term complications, may affect function and quality of life. Guidelines for the prevention and treatment of complictions during poststroke rehabilitation have been developed based largely on expert opinion because research-based evidence is not available for most of the problems to be discussed here.[1]

Despite good neurologic recovery, the quality of life for most stroke survivors is diminished compared with their self-reported quality of life before stroke.[2] In addition, global life satisfaction is decreased in 42 to 61 percent of stroke survivors 4 to 6 years poststroke, depending on which factors are included in the measure.[3] Among the more frequently encountered poststroke problems are spasticity and contractures, depression, urinary dysfunction, pain/neuralgia, skin breakdown/decubitus ulcers, and sexual dysfunction. This chapter will provide background on the prevalence of each of these problems and the impact each problem

has on poststroke function. The evidence-based literature is then reviewed to elucidate what is known about effective treatment. Lastly, recommendations are outlined for the rational management of each problem.

WEAKNESS, SPASTICITY, AND CONTRACTURE

Background

Free passive and active mobility is critical to normal function. Hemiplegia following a stroke, however, commonly limits mobility by three mechanisms. These are weakness, spasticity, and contracture. The prevalence of spasticity and/or contracture of one or more joints in long-term stroke survivors is not known.

The interruption of cortical motor control pathways following stroke causes muscle weakness. The effect is incomplete muscle activation. Impaired selective control leads to the emergence of primitive flexor and extensor patterns.[4] As a result, the quality of the individual's available voluntary muscle action is compromised. Inability to move the limb against gravity will allow the tissues to stiffen. Motor recovery from the initial flaccid state begins with a flexor synergy of the hip, knee, and ankle muscles. This is soon accompanied by a similar extensor synergy, which then progresses to normal rapidity and dexterity of motion if recovery is complete. For many stroke survivors, however, recovery terminates at the primitive synergy. In the lower extremity, this can provide a simplistic form of stepping and stance, but the upper extremity requires more versatility even for basic function.

Spasticity is the hallmark of an upper motor neuron disorder and among the most frequent motor complications found in stroke survivors. It is common, but not universal, among stroke survivors. The consensus definition is that spasticity is a motor disorder characterized by a velocity-dependent increase in tonic stretch reflexes (motor tone).[5–7] In simpler language, this is an excessive reaction to hyperexcitable quick stretch reflex. The signs are increased muscle tone and exaggerated tendon jerks. The current understanding is that spasticity occurs when there is an imbalance of inhibition and excitation at the motor neuron level of the spinal cord. During an activity such as walking, spasticity impedes joint motion by creating an antagonistic force.

Contractures represent stiffening of the fibrous connective tissues within the muscles, tendons, ligaments, and joint capsules. The cause is immobility usually because of weakness, spasticity, or pain.[8] Contractures may exacerbate pain, spasticity, and loss of function. In a study of 100 hemiplegic patients, one-quarter were found to have painful contracture of the shoulder.[9]

Although collagen provides the main supporting forces of connective tissue, the component most susceptible to the absence of motion is the proteoglycan gel, which lubricates and separates the collagen fibers. Proteoglycan is metabolically very active. Experimental immobilization for 9 weeks is associated with early and progressive proteoglycan deterioration in the joint capsule without changes in total collagen.[10] By 9 weeks, complete extension was lost, and mobility in the available range was three times stiffer compared with controls. However, the histologic sequence of change associated with the development of contracture suggests potential reversibility if motion is reinstituted sufficiently early. Increased resistance to passive motion at the ankle and fingers may begin within 3 days of stroke onset, preceding any evidence of spasticity,[11] hence the rationale for the initiation of early motion. In hemiplegia, the muscles may be a greater source of passive resistance than the joint capsule. Spasticity also isolates fibrous connective tissue from stretch. Clinically, the muscles also seem to be the greater barrier, as significant motion can be recovered in a paralytic deformity by surgical tendon release without touching the joint capsule.

Evidence

Primary treatment of poststroke spasticity relies on physical therapy. Early mobilization prevents contractures, which in turn makes the tissue more pliable so spasticity is diminished. Manual stretch has been shown to be effective in improving finger control with selected patients.[12] Range of motion in an immobilized joint has been found to decrease in as little as 3 days.[13] Limb positioning and bracing are used to reduce mild to moderate spasticity, as well as to control associated pain and enhance function. Splints, casts, and static orthoses are used to maintain proper joint position between mobilization sessions. Lying prone for as little as 2 h a day, even while asleep, can prevent hip flexion contractures. Upper extremity splints can be employed to maintain a spastic hand in maximal extension. In the hemiplegic lower leg with foot drop due to spastic equinovarus, a short leg orthotic device (ankle foot orthosis [AFO]) has been shown useful to control the ankle and to improve stability of the knee for ambulation.[14,15] Serial casting is also used to reduce spasticity and to treat an established contracture. In a rigid contracture, serial casting is ineffective. Dense but semielastic contractures will respond. The use of these techniques is based largely on clinical experience and early studies that compared a single intervention with no treatment. There are no longitudinal studies reported in the medical or rehabilitation literature on the long-term efficacy of any of these interventions, on comparisons of various regimens, or on the ability of patients or their caregivers to routinely and persistently carry out programs over months or years.

Pharmacotherapy of spasticity in the stroke patient is controversial and lacks sound scientific evidence. Medications are used primarily to decrease pain associated with the spasticity and secondarily to improve function. The most commonly used oral medications in patients with persistent spasticity of central origin are baclofen, dantrolene, and benzodiazepines.[16] Baclofen and benzodiazepines appear clinically to act at the level of the spinal cord, whereas dantrolene exerts its action peripherally on muscle fibers.[17] Theoretically, these drugs can be used concurrently, but there have been no clinical trials to support this approach. The FDA approved tizanidine for spasticity associated with multiple sclerosis. Studies in the acute poststroke period have shown little to no effect of these drugs on spasticity,[18] but no radomized clinical control studies have been done in stroke survivors with spasticity beyond several months. There has been a case report of decreased spasticity secondary to a brainstem stroke with the use of clonidine.[19] Several other case reports note improvement in spasticity associated with other neurologic conditions using a variety of different agents.[20–22] Intrathecal baclofen has been shown to be effective in reducing spasticity, increasing range of motion, and improving function in patients with spinal cord injury[23,24] and with spasticity of central origin because of cerebral palsy,[25] but no studies on its efficacy in stroke patients have been done.

Local injection of phenol near nerve motor points has been shown to be effective in patients with severe upper extremity spasticity.[26] Improvement with phenol injection usually lasts for 6 to 8 weeks. Intramuscular injection of botulinum toxin has been shown to be safe and effective in reducing spasticity and subsequent disability in stroke patients with severe spasticity of the upper or lower limb.[27,28] One double-blind, placebo-controlled study using botulinum toxin injections demonstrated significant reductions in chronic poststroke spasticity with the use of botulinum toxin injections without adverse effects.[29] Reduced spasticity was seen within several days to a week and lasted from between 1 and 11 months. Another study has shown botulinum toxin injections to be an effective treatment of dystonia associated with spastic equinovarus deformity.[30]

Permanent correction of an obstructive spasticity or contracture by surgical intervention may be considered after spontaneous recovery has plateaued (between 6 and 12 months) and when the patient is medically and neurologically stable, usually 9 to 12 months after the stroke. Such procedures generally involve the release of the appropriate tendons, by selected neurectomies, or by transferring tendons to produce antagonistic action.[31] Long-term improvement in function is the ultimate goal, but no studies demonstrating efficacy of surgical releases beyond several months have been done.

Therapeutic Recommendations

A rational integrated treatment plan that employs a variety of tools, nonpharmacologic, pharmacologic, and procedural, is needed to successfully manage poststroke weakness, spasticity, and contracture. Although spasticity cannot be prevented, it should be aggressively

managed when it interferes with function. Contractures can be prevented.

The current standard of clinical practice includes early range of motion exercises a minimum of twice a day and positioning to maintain normal joint alignment. This regimen is designed to minimize spasticity and prevent contracture formation. Passive range of motion for as little as 30 min a day has been reported by clinical experience to be sufficient to prevent contracture formation.[32] A goal of early rehabilitation programs should be the development of a daily plan of therapeutic exercises that the patient can engage in independently or with the aid of a caregiver to prevent contracture formation. Health-care providers should (1) routinely question the patient and/or caregiver about their daily exercise program and (2) monitor affected limbs to identify increased spasticity, loss of range of motion, and early contracture formation. Providers need to offer ongoing encouragement to both patients and caregivers to persist in the daily range of motion program. If negative changes are noted, referral to outpatient or home physical or occupational therapy should be considered.

Pharmacotherapy is recommended for spasticity when it negatively impacts function or is associated with pain (see below). The choice of oral medication for chronic spasticity is usually guided by the patient's other medical conditions and should be reserved for those with multiple areas of spasticity. Table 9-1 summarizes currently available medications for the treatment of spasticity. Side effects and concurrent medical conditions often dictate the choice of medication. Both baclofen and dantrolene are eliminated in the urine

Table 9-1.

Medications used for the treatment of spasticity

Site of action	Drug
Opioid receptor	Opioid analgesics
$GABA_B$ receptor	Baclofen
Benzodiazepine receptor	Clonazepam
$GABA_A$ receptor	??
α_2-adrenergic receptor	Clonidine
Intra- and extrafusal fiber	Dantrolene
Nerve	Phenol
Neuromuscular junction	Botulinum toxicity
NMDA receptor	??

and should be used with caution in the presence of renal disease. Dantrolene is metabolized by the liver and is known to be hepatotoxic in about 1 percent of people. Benzodiazepines and baclofen act centrally and cross the blood-brain barrier, which may cause sedation and confusion at doses sufficient to affect spasticity. These problems may be more apparent among the elderly, who are prone to adverse drug effects and in those stroke patients with significant cognitive impairment. Whether one selects a short- or long-acting benzodiazepine depends on the patient's specific needs. In either case, the dosage is generally titrated upward slowly until spasticity is controlled or adverse effects occur. Baclofen is usually started at 5 mg two to three times a day and the dose increased every 3 to 5 days to a maximum of 80 mg/day, depending on patient response. The starting dose of dantolene is usually 25 mg once or twice daily, and the dose is increased by 25-mg increments to a maximum of 100 mg four times/day.

For the treatment of localized areas of spasticity, where improvement in range of motion, function, or reduction in pain is desired, the use of botulinum toxin injections is preferred over phenol injections. Phenol chemodenervation with motor point blocks requires clinical and technical proficiency using electromyographic motor stimulation. Caution must be exercised to select pure motor nerves, as causalgia may occur if the myelin sheath of a sensory nerve or a mixed sensory and motor nerve is injured. Electromyography is also required for the identification of overactive muscles appropriate for botulinum toxin injection. Current recommendations are that injections should be given in doses below 250 to 300 units and no more frequently than every 12 weeks.[33] Phenol injections are preferred by some clinicians because they last longer and are less expensive.

Activity is another means of preventing late development of contractures. Muscle strengthening and functional training should be part of the rehabilitation program and should be continued following discharge.

Splints and orthotic devices to maintain positioning should be examined regularly, at least every 3 to 4 months, for appropriate fit and use. It is important to examine the underlying skin to be certain that pressure points and skin breakdown (see below) are not occurring. When a patient stops using a device, the reason should be ascertained. Over time, daily use causes wear and tear. Splints may break, attachments can become loose and break off, and changes in the patient's habitus or function may cause a device that once fit to become too loose or tight and to no longer be appropriate or useful.

Referral to orthopedic surgery should be considered only after an adequate trial of physical therapy, occupational therapy, and pharmacologic management strategies. Surgery may be warranted when (1) spasticity causes pain that is resistant to pharmacologic therapy and other interventions, or (2) when contracture or unbalanced muscle control (primitive pattern) interferes with function or impairs adequate hygiene, placing the patient at risk for skin breakdown and other problems.[34]

DEPRESSION

Background

Depression is considered the most common psychiatric condition following stroke. This is not surprising as depressive symptoms commonly occur with physical illness, especially among older people.[35] In a study of depression among community-dwelling older people, a strong link was found between depression and functional decline[36] as well as between depressed mood and having had a stroke. However, the presence and severity of depression among stroke survivors does not seem to be strongly related to the severity of physical or cognitive impairment, including aphasia.[37,38] Although depression is known to be common among the nursing home population, there are no studies that specifically address the prevalence of depression among the poststroke institutionalized population.

Estimates of the prevalence of clinically significant depression among community-dwelling stroke survivors vary greatly from 18 to 63 percent.[39-41] Approximately one-fifth of persons with stroke have been reported to have depressive symptoms at 3 months, with a similar proportion reporting symptoms at 1 year after the stroke.[42] One study found that some cases of depression in the first several months after stroke resolve spontaneously, but about one-third of stroke patients not initially depressed become depressed during the first year.[40] Another study found that over the course of the first year after a stroke the number of individuals with depressive symptoms declined, and persistent depressive symptoms were present in a small number of individuals, primarily those with pre-existing psychiatric disorders.[43] Thus, the prevalence of depression 1 year after stroke has been reported to increase, remain the same, or to decrease compared with 3 months after stroke.

The high-risk period for poststroke depression may last for up to 2 years.[44] One-third of patients who did not have a depression in the acute poststroke period later developed depression between three months and 2 years following their stroke.[45]

The overall prevalence of poststroke depression does not seem to increase further after the first 1 to 2 years. It has been reported that depression is more likely to develop among survivors during the first 2 years following a stroke than from 3 to 10 years after the stroke.[46] The prevalence of symptoms of major depression at 3 years poststroke has been reported between 18 and 29 percent.[47,48] Responses among 36 percent of stroke survivors 4 to 5 years after their stroke suggested they were depressed.[49]

The association between poststroke depression and mortality is unclear. Major depressive disorders are associated with increased mortality, usually secondary to accidents and suicide.[50] There are no comparable data demonstrating a relationship between poststroke depression and increased mortality.

There has been a considerable body of research devoted to studying the association of depression and lesion location in stroke patients. This association is now believed to be complex and multifactorial. Depression was initially thought to be associated with left-sided lesions. Further studies demonstrated poststroke depression also associated with right-sided lesions, particularly those involving the right parietal lobe.[51,52] The relationship between depression, physical impairment, recovery, and daily function is complex, and it is difficult to sort out cause and effect. Though one might think that depression would be correlated with the severity of neurologic impairment, this has not been demonstrated in any studies to date. In one study, physical impairment has been shown to account for no more than 10 percent of the variance in scores on depression rating instruments.[53] In the early poststroke period, the presence of depressive symptoms has been shown to negatively influence physical recovery.[54,55] Depression has also been shown to be a major factor impeding participation and progress in rehabilitation.[56,57]

Depression has been shown to be associated with impaired functioning in individuals with and without chronic medical conditions.[58–60] It would therefore seem likely that depression in stroke survivors would have a negative impact on function and well-being. However, there are few studies that document the effect of chronic poststroke depression on function. Poststroke patients who were initially depressed have been shown to be more impaired when followed at 1 and 2 years than nondepressed patients.[61,62] Thus, depression does not seem to be strongly associated with the initial severity of neurologic impairment but seems to have a small, significant negative effect on functional improvement in the rehabilitation setting, but not beyond.[63]

Evidence

The effectiveness of treating poststroke depression is believed to be as good as that for primary depression alone. Most of the clinically available antidepressants have been used in the treatment of poststroke depression. The tricyclic antidepressants (TCA) have been shown to be an effective treatment for poststroke depression. A retrospective chart review of poststroke patients with psychiatric evaluations revealed improvement within 6 weeks among a subgroup of those treated with one of several "cyclic" antidepressants.[64] In a double-blind, placebo-controlled study, depressed stroke patients treated with nortriptyline had significantly improved depression rating scores.[65] A trend toward greater improvement in both depression and activities of daily living has also been reported with the use of trazodone in poststroke patients with depression.[66] However, between 20 and 40 percent of antidepressant-treated patients dropped out of these studies because of the development of central nervous system (CNS), cardiac, and other anticholinergic side effects. In a comparison trial, methylphenidate was shown to be as effective as the tricyclic antidepressant nortriptyline in treating poststroke depression, but with a shorter peak response time.[67] The selective serotonergic reuptake inhibitors (SSRIs) have also been shown effective in the treatment of poststroke depression.[68] Table 9-2 summarizes the limited studies published on the treatment of poststroke depression. No studies comparing the efficacy of the different classes of antidepressants in the treatment of depression in long-term stroke survivors have been reported.

There is limited information about nonpharmacologic treatments for poststroke depression. Electroconvulsive therapy remains a viable option for poststroke depression that is refractory to antidepressants when there is a high suicide risk or psychotic symptoms. It has been shown to be safe and effective in this population[69] but is usually not used within 3 months of the stroke. Psychological treatments, including group and behavioral therapy, have been shown effective in treating depression in the acute poststroke phase, but their role in depression among poststroke survivors after acute rehabilitation has not been well-researched. A

Table 9-2.
Published studies on the treatment of depression in stroke patients

Author/year	Type of study	Treatment	Outcome/result
Oradei & Waite 1974[130]	Case report	Group psychotherapy knowledge	Enhanced socialization Improved coping
Watziawick & Coyne 1980[131]	Case report	Problem-focused family therapy	Change in behavior
Feibel & Springer 1982[132]	ECT	Retrospective chart review	Improved mood
Lipsey et al 1984[65]	Randomized double-blind	Nortriptyline Placebo-control	Improved depression scale No functional improvement
Reding et al 1986[66]	Double-blind placebo-control	Trazodone	Improved ADL score
Murray et al 1986[69]	Retrospective study	ECT	Clinical improvement
Finkelstein et al 1987[64]	Retrospective study	TCAs	Improved severity rating in subgroup
Thompson et al 1989[133]	Case report	Cognitive & family therapy	Clinical improvement
Andersen et al 1994[68]	Double-blind placebo-control	Citalopram	Improved depression scale
Lauritzen et al 1994[134]	Controlled clinical trial	Imipramine, desipramine, mianserin	Improved depression scale
Dam et al 1996[135]	Randomized, 3-group assignment	Fluoxetine or maprotiline	Improved functional recovery

randomized trial of a social support intervention to stroke survivors who were not being treated for depression found no significant differences between the treated and nontreated groups on measures of social support or psychosocial outcomes.[70]

Therapeutic Recommendations

Early identification of poststroke depression is the key to early treatment and prevention of further disability as a result of depression. Given what is known about the prevalence of depression among stroke survivors, a high index of suspicion must be maintained by the clinician working with this population. In our experience, an early and often overlooked indicator of underlying depression is failure to progress in rehabilitation. Identification of depression is often complicated by the presence of aphasia and/or cognitive impairment. Published guidelines for the identification and treatment of depression seem to be equally applicable to the long-term stroke population, as any other group.[71,72] Depression scales (e.g., Hamilton Depression Questionnaire, Yesavage Depression Questionnaire, Zung Self-Rating Depression Scale, Beck Depression Inventory) may be

useful but have not been validated in the stroke population.

There is no simple algorithm to guide the clinician in the diagnosis of depression or the choice of therapeutic intervention. The choice of antidepressant medication should be guided by the patient's other medical conditions and the agent's side-effect profile (Table 9-3), along with cost and the ability to monitor therapy. The use of TCAs in stroke survivors is limited by their anticholinergic, antihistaminergic, and alpha-receptor blockade. The potential for orthostatic hypotension and anticholinergic delirium is especially high with the use of amitriptyline in patients with brain injury, including stroke. When a TCA is appropriate, nortriptyline is the preferred drug, usually starting with a low dose (10 to 20 mg) before bedtime and increasing at weekly intervals. Trazodone, a non-TCA, has fewer side effects and in our experience is better tolerated. The usual starting dose is 50 mg once or twice daily, increasing by 25 to 50 mg every 3 to 4 days. The SSRI agents have fewer side effects and are often thought of as more activating, or energizing, than the older agents. This may be advantageous in some stroke patients but may not be ideal when anxiety is a major component.

Table 9-3.

Common side effects of antidepressant medications

Drug	Dose range	Side effects
Amitriptyline	75–300 mg/d	Anticholinergic, drowsiness, hypotension, weight gain, cardiac
Nortriptyline	40–150 mg/d	Hypotension, cardiac
Imipramine	75–300 mg/d	Anticholinergic, drowsiness, hypotension, weight gain, cardiac
Desipramine	75–300 mg/d	Hypotension, cardiac
Doxepin	75–400 mg/d	Anticholinergic, drowsiness, hypotension, weight gain, cardiac
Trazodone	50–60 mg/d	Drowsiness, hypotension, cardiac
Amoxapine	75–600 mg/d	Anticholinergic, drowsiness, insomnia, hypotension, cardiac
Fluoxetine	10–80 mg/d	Insomnia
Sertraline	25–200 mg/d	Insomnia, wt gain
Paroxetine	10–60 mg/d	Drowsiness, insomnia, weight gain
Bupropion	150–450 mg/d	Insomnia, cardiac

Regardless of the pharmacologic agent chosen, it is important to monitor the patient closely for side effects as well as clinical improvement. Ideally, there should be contact with the patient at least weekly. The drug dosage should be adjusted until symptoms have begun to improve or side effects require a reduction in the dose. It usually requires 3 to 6 weeks to see symptomatic improvement (longer with TCAs than with SSRIs) and at least 6 months of continuous medication therapy to adequately treat the depression. If the patient's depression is refractory to treatment with one antidepressant medication, after maximum dosage or 6 to 8 weeks of therapy, this agent should be discontinued and a second drug initiated. Depression that is nonresponsive to a trial of two separate antidepressant medication regimens probably warrants referral to a psychiatrist for consideration of alternative therapy, including combined drug therapy or ECT. Antidepressant therapy should be continued for a minimum of 6 months, and even up to a year, before gradually decreasing the dose until the medication can be stopped, or depressive symptoms reappear.

URINARY INCONTINENCE

Background

The most common form of urinary dysfunction among stroke survivors is urinary incontinence. Approximately half (51 percent) of stroke survivors acknowledge experiencing urinary incontinence sometime during the first year after stroke.[73] At 12 weeks poststroke, urinary incontinence was found among 29 percent of survivors.[74] The reported prevalence declines to 12 to 19 percent at several months to 1 year poststroke.[73,75,76] A small percentage of subjects have persistent urinary incontinence beyond several months. However, these numbers do not distinguish pre-existing from incident poststroke urinary incontinence. In one study, 2.5 percent of poststroke patients with urinary incontinence were incontinent prior to their stroke.[73]

Urinary incontinence is a well-known marker for stroke severity in the acute phase,[77] but its value as a predictor of functional outcome past several months is poorly documented. In the first few weeks poststroke, urinary incontinence is the best single predictor of severe or moderate disability at 3 months and is associated with a poor prognosis for acute rehabilitation.[73] Initial urinary incontinence is also the single best predictor of disability at 12 months poststroke.[78] The long-term association between initial continence and functional outcome beyond 12 months has not been specifically researched.

The pathophysiology of persistent urinary incontinence in poststroke survivors is also not well studied. In general, urinary incontinence in poststroke patients may be related to one of three underlying problems: primary bladder dysfunction, cognitive impairment, or physical impairment.[79] Detrusor instability, also known as uninhibited neurogenic bladder, is the most common form of primary bladder dysfunction in poststroke incontinence.[80] Both detrusor hyperreflexia and areflexia have been demonstrated in poststroke patients with incontinence.[81] How much each of these contributes to persistent urinary incontinence is not known. Incomplete bladder emptying has been demonstrated in about one-third of poststroke patients admitted for rehabilitation.[82] The combined presence of moderate to severe cognitive impairment and urinary incontinence is a major predictor for institutionalization. However, the impact of impaired cognition or physical impairment on urinary incontinence over the long term is not well understood.

Evidence

The treatment of urinary incontinence in the poststroke patient has not been systematically studied. The potential benefits of treating incontinence in stroke survivors are suggested by recent reports in the Japanese literature.[83] Thus, the same principles that guide treatment of urinary incontinence in the general population should be followed for the poststroke patient with persistent incontinence.

A number of randomized controlled trials have shown that bladder training is effective in reducing urinary incontinence because of detrusor instability.[84] These studies employed various forms of habit training using a timed voiding schedule and fluid intake management in patients with incontinence owing to detrusor hyperactivity. Use of low-dose anticholinergic agents can help detrusor hyperactivity and assist in regaining continence. However, there are no controlled trials that specifically focus on the use of anticholinergic agents in the stroke population. In the poststroke patient, such a regimen may be complicated by the presence of cognitive impairment. In such cases, prompted voiding, a variation of habit training where a caregiver checks for wetness at scheduled intervals and prompts the patient to void, has proven to be successful. Timed voiding alone has been shown effective in managing urinary incontinence in poststroke patients with a normally functioning bladder and dementia, aphasia, or severe functional impairment.[85]

Outflow obstruction in men is usually caused or exacerbated by prostatic enlargement. Pharmacologic treatment with terazosin or doxazosin may be beneficial when there is mild obstruction.[86] Surgery is the treatment of choice when there is moderate to severe obstruction because of prostatic enlargement. The sur-

gical risk in the weeks to months after a stroke must be weighed against the benefits. Transurethral prostatectomy for the treatment of prostatic enlargement (prostatism) in male poststroke patients has been shown to be most effective when done more than 1 year poststroke.[87]

The management of urinary incontinence may require considerable effort by the patient and/or caregiver. Urinary incontinence is a well-known source of caregiver stress.[88] The presence of urinary incontinence has frequently been cited by caregivers as one of the primary reasons for institutionalization of stroke survivors.[89,90]

Therapeutic Recommendations

Treatment of urinary incontinence begins with appropriate identification of the underlying etiology. A history of the frequency and amount of urine loss during the day and at night should be obtained from the patient or caregiver. It is important to ask about continence and urination habits prior to the stroke to ascertain what impact, if any, the stroke has had on continence. The development of new urinary incontinence several weeks or months after a stroke usually signals an underlying problem not directly related to the stroke. In such a case, the most common causes are an underlying infection or medication side effects.

A comprehensive physical examination including complete neurologic, rectal, and, in women, pelvic examination is essential. A urinalysis is important to rule out infection as a cause or contributing factor in all cases of chronic or recurring urinary incontinence. Next, a post-void residual test should be performed. The patient is asked to void and then a bladder scan is done or a catheter is inserted through the urethra to determine the quantity of urine remaining in the bladder. If the patient has an indwelling catheter, this should be removed. A post-void residual test should be done after voiding, or intermittent catheterization should be performed every 4 to 6 h if no voiding has occurred. If the post-void residual volume is high (>100 cc), then intermittent catheterization, or an indwelling catheter, is needed to reduce the risk of hydronephrosis.

A trial of a timed voiding or prompted voiding schedule is usually worthwhile for several days. We generally recommend the patient be taken to the toilet, or if confined to bed provided a urinal or bedpan, every 2 h initially. The time period between voidings is then gradually lengthened by 30 to 60-min intervals, depending on the patient's ability to remain dry. If the patient becomes incontinent within the 2-h time frame, the schedule should be shortened to every 1 to $1\frac{1}{2}$ h. If a patient fails to void during a 4 to 6-h period, then intermittent catheterization is performed.

Male patients with urinary incontinence, an enlarged prostate, and normal prostate-specific antigen (PSA) can be placed on an empirical trial of terazosin. This is especially useful when the patient is also hypertensive but requires frequent monitoring for hypotension, particularly orthostatic changes.

Urge incontinence due to detrusor hyperactivity is best approached with behavioral therapy supplemented by an anticholinergic pharmacologic agent. Because of their side effects, these agents should be used at the lowest dose possible to achieve decreased episodes of incontinence, if not total continence, without interfering side effects. Propantheline is inexpensive, but its effectiveness is often limited by side effects. Oxybutynin has been shown in several short-term controlled trials (1 to 4 weeks) to be superior to placebo in both reducing incontinence frequency and in producing continence.[91-93] The recommended dose is 2.5 to 5 mg orally three to four times/day.

When incontinence is secondary to overflow and an areflexic bladder, clean intermittent self-catheterization every 4 h is the treatment of choice. The ability of the poststroke patient to manage such a regimen is often complicated by lack of sufficient motor control and cognitive ability. The use of an indwelling Foley catheter to control continence is a readily available and inexpensive solution that is employed too frequently without regard to its potential serious adverse consequences. Recurrent urinary tract infections, often leading to urosepsis, are common in individuals with long-term indwelling urinary catheters.[94] The use of external collection devices (condom catheters), adult diapers, or other continence undergarments is preferable to the long-term placement of an indwelling catheter, although this can be an expensive and labor-intensive solution.

POSTSTROKE PAIN/NEURALGIA

Background

Pain is not uncommon in stroke patients, but its incidence and prevalence after the acute rehabilitation phase is not known. Central poststroke pain, originally called "thalamic pain" or "thalamic pain syndrome," was first described by Dejerine and Roussy in 1906.[95] In this condition, patients experience persistent pain without stimulation of peripheral nociceptors. The pain is believed to be of neurogenic origin, caused by a brain lesion (most commonly an intracranial infarct or hemorrhage) affecting central pain pathways. Decades later, it has become apparent that many, if not the majority, of the patients with this condition have strokes in regions other than the thalamus.[96-98]

The physical exam findings may be unique in the stroke patient with central poststroke pain. The presence of allodynia—elicitation of pain by a nonpainful stimulus—is pathognomonic of neurogenic pain and has been reported in about 60 percent of patients with central poststroke pain.[94] Hypersthesia or hyperesthesia associated with pinprick or thermal sensation may be seen. Parasthesias in the absence of stimulation may also be present.

Only a small number, between 2 and 6 percent, of stroke patients experience central pain. Pain may begin at the time of the stroke or up to several months poststroke. The median time to onset of pain has been reported as 3 months; 95 percent of patients report onset of pain between 3 and 9 months.[99]

The impact of central poststroke pain on function and quality of life has not been studied in a systematic manner. Pain may interfere with the sleep-wake cycle, the ability to carry out activities of daily living, and participation in a therapeutic exercise program.[100] However, pain problems in stroke survivors have not been found to be indicators of poor stroke recovery.[101]

Evidence

Treatment of central poststroke pain syndrome has proven to be very difficult. In most cases, response to treatment is either minimal or incomplete. The literature primarily includes case reports with few randomized controlled clinical trials. Conventional analgesics, including opioids, and destructive neurosurgery have been tried over the years without success.[102] Naloxone has been tried, but in a double-blind crossover trial no therapeutic effect was demonstrated.[103]

Current treatment for neurogenic pain, including central poststroke pain, centers on the use of antidepressants. A positive response was initially demonstrated in 10 of 15 patients in a double-blind crossover trial with amitriptyline.[104] Several studies of other neurogenic pain syndromes have demonstrated the superior effect of adrenergically active over the purely serotonergically active antidepressants.[105,106] There are no published studies comparing the different adrenergic antidepressants or different doses of an individual antidepressant for the treatment of poststroke neurogenic pain.

Other classes of pharmaceutical agents have been tried without much success in treating patients with poststroke pain. Anticonvulsants have been proven effective for the treatment of several different neurologic pain syndromes[107] but ineffective as monotherapy for poststroke pain. The newer anticonvulsants, such as gabapentin, show promise in treating some types of neurologic pain but have not been studied in poststroke pain patients. GABA agonists (e.g., baclofen) have been shown beneficial in postherpetic neuralgia with allodynia and therefore may also be effective for poststroke central pain, especially in the presence of allodynia.[108] It has been suggested that combined anticonvulsant and antidepressant therapy may be beneficial, but there is no evidence to indicate the improved efficacy of such a regimen. Anti-arrhythmics and calcium channel blocker have also been suggested as possible therapeutic agents for neurogenic pain, but there have been no case reports or controlled studies of their use in poststroke central pain.

What proportion of individuals with central poststroke pain are successfully treated pharmacologically, or how many of these patients eventually become pain free without medication is not known. Anecdotally, it has been reported that about half of the patients obtain pain relief from antidepressants or antidepressant plus anticonvulsant therapy.

Various other therapeutic techniques have been tried with patients with poststroke central pain refractory to pharmacologic therapy. Transcutaneous electrical nerve stimulation (TENS) has been shown to significantly reduce, but not eliminate, pain in some patients with central poststroke pain.[109] Chronic electrical stimulation of the gasserian ganglion has been reported especially effective for the treatment of chronic medically intractable facial pain when the pain is of central origin.[110] Sympathetic blockade by stellate ganglion injection or intravenous fusion of guanethidine into the affected limb has been shown to temporarily relieve pain.[111] Subthreshold stimulation of the motor cortex has shown promise in recent years.[112]

Treatment Recommendations

Clinically, the general approach has been to begin antidepressant therapy at the first appearance of pain, to select the agent with the highest adrenergic activity, and to gradually increase to the highest dose that can be tolerated without side effects. Pain relief, when it does occur, is not immediate, but usually begins after the patient has been on a maximally tolerated dose for several weeks. The optimal length of treatment has not been formally studied. When the pain has been successfully abolished or significantly reduced, dosage is usually maintained for 6 months. After this period of time, current clinical practice is to slowly reduce the dosage in a stepwise manner, allowing several weeks between dosage reduction. It is important to emphasize that these drugs are being used for neurogenic pain relief, which is believed to be unrelated to their mood-elevating effects.

The use of anticonvulsants for neurogenic pain is commonly employed clinically but, as noted above, is not supported by solid data. When antidepressants are ineffective or not tolerated by the patient because of side effects, and other modalities have been exhausted, then it is reasonable to consider a trial of an anticonvulsant. Carbamazepine is currently the most often employed pharmacologic agent in this class. Gabapentin is also being used off label for neurogenic pain and seems clinically to work as well as carbamazepine but requires less laboratory monitoring and may be better tolerated.

SKIN BREAKDOWN/PRESSURE SORES

Background

Impaired mobility, such as that found among some long-term stroke survivors, is a well-known risk factor for pressure sore formation. When there is associated sensory impairment, incontinence (urinary or fecal), and cognitive impairment, the risk for skin breakdown is further increased. Pressure sores are known to contribute to functional disability. The true incidence and prevalence of pressure sores in long-term stroke survivors is not known. Pressure sore formation has been estimated to occur in 3 to 5 percent of institutionalized patients with immobility due to underlying neurologic impairment, many of whom have had a stroke.[113,114]

A pressure sore can develop over any bony prominence where there is unrelieved pressure for a prolonged period of time. Besides pressure, sliding and sheering forces on the skin and the underlying tissues contribute to skin breakdown. The majority of pressure sores occur on the lower half of the body. Over 90 percent involve the sacrum, ischium, trochanter, iliac crest, medial or lateral malleolus, and calcaneus. A classification system based on the depth of tissue damage has been established by the National Pressure Ulcer Advisory Panel (Table 9-4).[115]

Evidence

The management of pressure sores should follow the same principles regardless of the patient's underlying medical condition. Standards of care that emphasize identification of risk factors (Table 9-5), prevention, early recognition, and aggressive therapy have been established to guide care in all settings.[116,117] Cost effectiveness of a specialized air bed has been shown for both the treatment and prevention of pressure ulcers in a few studies.[118,119] Combined use of a pressure ulcer risk assessment scale with a labor-intensive low-technology program has been shown to reduce the incidence of pressure ulcer development, to lengthen the time to ulcer development, and to be cost effective.[120] This program involved the use of simple preventive measures based on each patient's risk for skin breakdown, in a setting where no measures were previously in use: pressure-reducing mattresses, chair cushions, frequent repositioning with a turning schedule, and moon boots to protect heels. Patients were either at-risk for skin breakdown or had early small pressure ulcers (stage 1 or 2), with no large or deep ulcers (stage 3 or 4). Cost savings may not reflect

Table 9-4.
Pressure ulcer staging

Stage I	Nonblanching erythema of intact skin
Stage II	Partial-thickness tissue injury involving the epidermis and dermis, which presents as an abrasion or blister
Stage III[a]	Full-thickness tissue loss involving the subcutaneous tissue, which may extend down to, but not through, the fascial layer
Stage IV[a]	Full-thickness tissue damage to the level of bone, muscle, tendon, joint, or other supporting structures

[a]Both stage III and IV ulcers may present with varying amounts of necrotic tissue, undermining, or sinus tracts. Ulcers that are covered with eschar cannot be definitively staged until debridement has been performed.

Source: The National Pressure Ulcer Advisory Panel.

Table 9-5.
Risk factors for the development of pressure ulcer formation

Immobility
Vascular disease
Diabetes mellitus
Immune deficiency
Malignancy
Malnutrition
Psychosis
Depression

what would occur in facilities that already have in place some aspects of pressure ulcer prevention but not a comprehensive preventive program.

Treatment Recommendations

Prevention is the cornerstone of a pressure sore management program. Measures to avoid prolonged unrelieved pressure should begin during the acute and rehabilitation phases of stroke management.[121] Stroke survivors and their families must be taught early about pressure relief measures. These include frequent turning of the patient who cannot roll over in bed and positioning of immobile extremities to avoid prolonged pressure on bony prominences.

Health care providers must be vigilant in performing frequent skin examinations of the stroke patient who is bed bound or immobile to identify early signs of excess pressure and skin breakdown. This requires routinely undressing the patient, especially from the waist down, including the removal of stockings and shoes, and visual inspection of the areas known to be prone to skin breakdown. Particular attention must be paid to any extremity that is immobile or has impaired sensation. Available tools to help reduce pressure and position immobile limbs include special beds, heel protectors, special mattresses, and special wheel chair cushions. When these devices are employed, it is imperative that they be inspected regularly for wear and tear or soiling and their continued use be routinely re-evaluated for appropriateness to the patient's current physical and functional status.

When a stage II or greater pressure sore develops, wound dressing techniques and frequent dressing changes every day should be instituted to aid healing. A shallow stage II or small stage III lesion can be successfully treated with wound cleansing with normal saline and mechanical debridement with wet-to-dry saline-soaked gauze dressings. A larger stage III or stage IV ulcer requires more aggressive debridement. If eschar or necrotic tissue is present, this must be removed before wound healing can take place. This often requires surgical debridement in the office, at the bedside, or if the lesion is very large or there are several lesions, in the operating room. Such wounds should be treated locally by cleansing thoroughly with normal saline and then dressing with local antibacterial cream, such as silver sulphadiazine (Silvadene). This is done to reduce the amount of bacterial colonization, prevent sepsis, and promote granulation tissue formation in the wound. It is important to provide the patient with adequate pain relief medication before undertaking such a procedure. Debridement with enzymatic or autolytic agents may be used once the majority of necrotic tissue has been removed. There has been a proliferation of such agents: tapes, gels, foams, and beads. We recommend that the provider become familiar with one or two in each class to use as needed.

SEXUAL DYSFUNCTION

Background

Studies have shown that stroke has a profound effect on all aspects of a survivor's life, including sexuality and sexual function. A marked decline in various aspects of sexual function in the poststroke patient has been reported. However, most of the published studies are over a decade old, report the responses of small groups of stroke survivors at one period of time, and do not provide longitudinal data on changes in sexual function over time.

Stroke may affect both physical and psychological aspects of sexuality. Sexual interest and desire are reported to remain the same, but function is often impaired among stroke survivors.[122] There are conflicting data regarding frequency of sexual activity among stroke survivors. One study reported no significant change in the amount of time spent in foreplay and the resumption of intercourse in a majority of patients within 3 months of their stroke.[123] An earlier study found that two-thirds of stroke patients with hemiplegia and a regular sex partner reported major changes in their sexual life 1 and 6 years poststroke.[124] Only 36 percent of individuals with regular life partners who were sexually active prior to their stroke had continued sexual activity

at the same frequency poststroke. Diminished libido and frequency of intercourse have been reported to occur in both younger[125] and older[126] stroke survivors 1 year after stroke. Reduced foreplay activity, including decreased frequency of caressing and touching, has been reported.[127] Hypersexuality has been reported to be a rare occurrence, associated with a history of poststroke seizures and temporal lobe lesions.[128]

Sexual function is impaired in many, but not all, stroke survivors of both genders. Male poststroke patients report a significant decrease in the ability to achieve an erection and to ejaculate.[124,126] Males have been reported to experience a greater decrease in frequency of sexual intercourse poststroke compared with prestroke activity levels.[126] Female stroke survivors report fewer changes in frequency of intercourse and less sexual dissatisfaction than males.[127] Both males and females cited fatigue as a major reason for both decreased sexual frequency and pleasure poststroke. Use of antihypertensive medication was thought to be a contributing factor to decreased sexual function in the poststroke patient, but this has been shown not to be the case.[129]

Little is known about the interaction between sexual dysfunction and overall function and quality of life among stroke survivors. One study of quality of life among long-term stroke survivors did use sexual satisfaction as one aspect of quality of life.[3]

Evidence

There are no published studies that specifically focus on therapeutic interventions for the treatment of sexual dysfunction among stroke survivors. Several studies of the treatment of sexual dysfunction in people with chronic diseases have included stroke survivors, but whether the problems and needs of this specific subgroup differ from those with other chronic diseases remains unknown.

Treatment Recommendations

Clinicians must be aware of the prevalence of sexual dysfunction among stroke survivors and its impact on quality of life. Clinicians must also be willing to broach the subject with patients and their partners. The key to being able to recommend possibly effective therapeutic interventions for sexual dysfunction is the willingness and openness of clinical providers to broach the sensitive, and often taboo, subject of sexuality with their patients. In general, patients with sexual functioning problems are reluctant to approach a health-care pro-

Table 9-6.

Antihypertensive medications with impotence as a reported potential adverse reaction

Chemical name	Manufacturer name
Ace inhibitors	
Ramipril hydrochloride	Altace
Benazepril hydrochloride	Lotensin
Enalapril maleate	Vasotec
Lisinopril	Zestril, Prinivil
α_1 *antagonists*	
Abetolol hydrochloride	Normodyne, Trandate
Doxazosin mesylate	Cardura
Terazosin hydrochloride	Hytrin
Prazosin hydrochloride	Prazosin
β *blockers*	
Betaxolol hydrochloride	Kerlone
Timolol maleate	Blocarden
Propranolol hydrochloride	Inderal
Penbutolol sulfate	Levatolol
Ca channel blockers	
Diltiazem hydrochloride	Dilacor
Felodipine	Plendil
Nifedipine	Procardia, Adalat
Other	
Methyldopa	Aldomet
Clonidine	Catapres
Guinfacine hydrochloride	Tenex
Guanabenze acetate	Wytensin
Guanadrel sulfate	Hylorel
Valsartan	Diovan

vider for assistance. By asking the patient who is several months poststroke whether s/he has resumed sexual activity, the clinician signals to the patient a willingness to discuss the subject and assist the patient.

The clinician caring for a stroke survivor must acknowledge whether s/he has the skills, knowledge, time, and interest to evaluate and treat sexual dysfunction. Often, referral to a gynecologist for a female or urologist for a male stroke survivor is necessary to ascertain whether there is any organic etiology underlying the dysfunction. A review of medications is important to ascertain whether sexual dysfunction could be a side effect, such as from some of the commonly prescribed antihypertensive agents (Table 9-6).

The recent approval of sildenafil provides a welcome pharmacologic solution for the male patient with erectile dysfunction. However, the clinical drug trials did not specifically include (or exclude) stroke patients, so there are no data on its use in this particular population. Its use is contraindicated in patients using an organic nitrite, and the Federal Drug Agency, the American Heart Association, and American College of Cardiology all advise caution when prescribing it for individuals with other cardiovascular conditions, including stroke and hypertension. Its use by stroke survivors should be considered on a case-by-case basis with particular attention to medical history, contributing factors, and medications.

CONCLUSION

Research on the chronic medical problems of stroke survivors beyond the acute rehabilitation phase (3 months) is very limited. There are a few studies of small groups of stroke survivors 1 to 2 years poststroke. However, there are no longitudinal studies beyond the first few years of the types of problems encountered and how they impact function or quality of life. As the number of stroke survivors continues to increase, it is imperative that greater attention be paid to understanding, not just the epidemiology of medical problems encountered by these patients but also what can be done to diminish their occurrence and to improve their outcome.

ACKNOWLEDGMENTS

We wish to thank Jacqueline Perry, MD, for her critical review and invaluable additions to the section of the manuscript on weakness, spasticity and contracture. We would also like to acknowledge Bryan Kemp, PhD, Salah Rubayi, MD, and Karen Pires, RN, for their willingness to share their expertise in specific topic areas in a review of an earlier draft of this manuscript.

Work on this chapter was indirectly supported by NIH/NIA Grant # PO 1AG12435 and NIH/NIA Grant #AG00093-16

REFERENCES

1. United States Department of Health and Human Services, Agency for Health Care Policy and Research. *Post Stroke Rehabilitation*. Clinical Practice Guideline No. 16. 1995.
2. Niemi M-L, Laaksonen R, Kotila M, et al: Quality of life 4 years after stroke. *Stroke* 19:1101, 1988.

3. Viitanen, M, Fugl-Meyer KS, Bemspang B, et al: Life satisfaction in long-term survivors after stroke. *Scan J Rehabil Med* 20:17, 1988.

4. Perry J: Determinants of muscle function in the spastic lower extremity. *Clin Orthop* 288:10, 1993.

5. Lance JW: Symposium synopsis, in Feldman RG, Young RR, Koella WP (eds): *Spasticity, Disordered Motor Control.* Year Book Medical, 1980.

6. Bodine-Fowler SC, Bottee MJ: Muscle spasticity, in Nicket VL, BotteMJ (eds): *Orthopaedic Rehabiliation,* 2nd ed. New York, Churchill Livingstone, 1992.

7. Young RR, Wegner AW: Spasticity, *Clin Orthop* 219:50, 1987.

8. Akeson WH, Woo SL-Y, Amiel D, et al: The connective tissue response to immobility: Biochemical changes in periarticular connective tissue of the immobilized rabbit knee. *Clin Orthop* 93:356, 1973.

9. Caldwell CB, Wilson DJ, Braun RH: Evaluation and treatment of the upper extremity in the hemiplegic stroke patient. *Clin Orthop* 63:69, 1969.

10. Woo SL-Y, Akeson MW, et al: Connective tissue response to immobility. *Arthritis Rheum* 18:257, 1975.

11. Twitchell TE: The restoration of motor function following hemiplegia in man. *Brain* 74:443, 1951.

12. Carey JR: Manual stretch: Effect on finger movement control and force in stroke subjects with spastic extrinsic finger flexor muscles. *Arch Phys Med Rehabil* 71:888, 1990.

13. Sharpless JW: *Mossman's a Problem Oriented Approach to Stroke Rehabilitation.* Springfield, Charles C Thomas, 1982.

14. Perry J: Lower extremity bracing in hemiplegia. *Clin Orthop* 63:32, 1969.

15. Perry J, Montgomery J: Gait of the stroke patient and orthotic indications, in Brandstater ME, Basmajian JV (eds): *Stroke Rehabilitation.* Baltimore, William & Wilkins, 1987.

16. Katz RT: Management of spasticity. *Am J Phys Med Rehabil* 67:108, 1988.

17. Davidoff RA: Antispasticity drugs: Mechanisms of action. *Ann Neurol* 17:107, 1985.

18. Katrak PH, Cole AMD, Poulos CJ, et al: Objective assessment of spasticity, strength and function with early exhibition of dantolene sodium after cerebrovascular acident: A randomized double-blind study. *Arch Phys Med Rehabil* 73:4, 1992.

19. Sandford PR, Spengler SE, Sawasky KB: Clonidine in the treatment of brainstem spasticity. *Am J Phys Med Rehabil* 71:301, 1992.

20. Zachariah SB, Borges EF, Varghese R, et al: Positive response to oral divalproex sodium (Depakote) in patients with spasticity and pain. *Am J Med Sci* 308:38, 1994.

21. Jimi T, Wakayama Y: Mexiletine for treatment of spasticity due to neurological disorders (Letter). *Muscle Nerve* 16:885, 1993.

22. Jaeken J, DeCock P, Casaaer P: Vigabatrin as a spasmolytic drug (Letter). *Lancet* 338:1603, 1991.

23. Penn RD, Savoy SM, Corcos D, et al: Intrathecal baclofen for severe spinal spasticity. *N Engl J Med* 320:1517, 1989.

24. Acland RH: Intrathecal baclofen for the management of severe spasticity. *N Z Med J* 106:129, 1993.

25. Albright AL, Barron WB, Fasick P, et al: Continuous intrathecal baclofen infusion for spasticity of cerebral origin. *JAMA* 270:2475, 1993.

26. Keenan MAE, Eufrocina ST, Stone L, et al: Percutaneous block of the musculocutaneous nerve to control elbow flexor spasticity. *J Hand Surg* 15A:340, 1990.

27. Bhakata BB, Cozens JA, Bamform JM, et al: Use of botulism toxim in stroke patients with severe upper limb spasticity. *J Neurol Neurosurg Psychiatry* 61:30, 1996.

28. Hesse S, Leucke D, Malezic M, et al: Botulism toxin treatment for lower limb extensor spasticity in chronic hemiparetic patients. *J Neurol Neurosurg Psychiatry* 57:1321, 1994.

29. Simpson DM, Alexander DN, O'Brien CF, et al: Botulinum toxin type A in the treatment of upper extremity spasticty: A randomized, double-blind, placebo-controlled trial. *Neurology* 46:1306, 1996.

30. Dengler R, Neyer U, Wohlfarth K. et al: Local botulinum toxin in the treatment of spastic footdrop. *J Neurol* 239:375, 1992.

31. Botte MJ, Waters RL, Keenan MAE, et al: Orthopaedic management of the stroke patient: Part II. Treating deformities of the upper and lower extremities. *Ortho Rev* 17:891, 1988.

32. Roper, BA. The orthopedic management of the stroke patient. *Clin Ortho Rel Res* 219:78, 1987.

33. O'Brien FC, Seeberger LC, Smith DB: Spasticity after stroke: Epidemiology and optimal treatment. *Drugs Aging* 9:332, 1996.

34. Waters RL: Upper extremity surgery in stroke patients. *Clin Ortho Related Res* 131:31, 1978.

35. Hermann N: Clinical features and pathogenesis of depression in old age, in Shulman KI, Tohen M, Kucher SP (eds): *Mood Disorders Across the Life Span.* New York, Wiley-Liss, Inc., 1996, pp. 341–360.

36. Penninx B, Guralnik J, Ferrucci I, et al: Depressive symptoms and physical decline in community-dwelling older persons. *JAMA* 279:1720, 1998.

37. Morris PLP, Robinson RG, Raphael B: The prevalence and course of post-stroke depression in the hospitalized patient. *Int J Psychiatry Med* 20:349, 1990.

38. Starkstein SE, Robinson RG: Aphasia and depression. *Aphasiology* 2:1, 1988.

39. Kelly-Hayes M, Aige C: Assessment and psychologic factors in stroke rehabilitation. *Neurology* S29, 1995.

40. Stern RA, Bachman DL: Depressive symptoms following stroke. *Am J Psychiatry* 148:351, 1992.

41. House A: Mood disorders after stroke: A review of the evidence. *Int J Geriatr Psychiatry* 2:211, 1987.

42. Hermann N, Black SE, Lawrence J, et al: The Sunnybrook

Stroke Study: A prospective study of depressive symptoms and functional outcome. *Stroke* 29:618, 1998.

43. House A, Dennis M, Mogridge L, et al: Mood disorders in the year after first stroke. *Br J Psychiatry* 158:83, 1991.

44. Robinson RG, Boduc PL, Price TR: Two-year longitudinal study of post-stroke mood disorders: Diagnosis and outcome at one and two years. *Stroke* 18:837, 1987.

45. Robinson RG, Pisey JR, Rao K, et al: A two-year longitudinal study of post-stroke mood disorders: A comparison of acute onset with delayed-onset depression. *Am J Psychiatry* 143:1238, 1986.

46. Robinson RG, Price TR: Poststroke depressive disorders: A follow-up study of 103 patients. *Stroke* 13:635, 1982.

47. Astrom M, Adolfsson R, Asplund K: Major depression in stroke patients: A 3-year longitudinal study. *Stroke* 24:976, 1993.

48. Schwartz JA, Speed NM, Brunberg JA, et al: Depression in stroke rehabilitation. *Biol Psychiatry* 33:694, 1993.

49. Wilkinson PR, Wolfe CDA, Warburton FG, et al: A long-term follow-up of stroke patients. *Stroke* 28:507, 1997.

50. Wells KB: *Depression as a Tracer Condition for the National Study of Medical Care Outcomes: Background Review.* Santa Monica, RAND, 1985.

51. Finset A: Depressed mood and reduced emotionality after right hemisphere brain damage, in Kinsbourne M, (ed): *Cerebral Hemisphere Function in Depression.* Washington, DC, American Psychiatric Press, 1990.

52. Starkstein SE, Robinson RG, Honig MA, et al: Mood changes after right-hemisphere lesions. *Br J Psychiatry* 155:79, 1989.

53. Robinson RG, Kubos KL, Starr LB, et al: Mood disorders in stroke patients: Importance of location of lesion. *Brain* 107:81, 1984.

54. Sinyor D, Amato P, Kaloupek P: Post-stroke depression: Relationship to functional impairment, coping strategies, and rehabilitation outcome. *Stroke* 17:112, 1986.

55. Kottila M, Waltimo O, Niemi ML, et al: The profile of recovery from stroke and factors influencing outcome. *Stroke* 15:1039, 1984.

56. Robinson RG, Starr LB, Kubos KL, et al: Two-year longitudinal study of post-stroke mood disorders: Findings during initial evaluation. *Stroke* 14:736, 1983.

57. Robinson RG, Starr LB, Lipsey JR, et al: Two-year longitudinal study of post-stroke mood disorders: Dynamic changes in associated variables over first six months of follow-up. *Stroke* 15:510, 1984.

58. Omel J, Kempen GI, Deeg DJ, et al: Functioning, well-being and health perception in late middle-aged and older people: Comparing the effects of depressive symptoms and chronic medical conditions. *J Am Geriatr Soc* 46:39, 1998.

59. Wells KB, Steward A, Hays RD, et al: The functioning and well-being of depressed patients: Results from the Medical Outcome Study. *JAMA* 262:914, 1989.

60. Von Korff M, Ormel J, Katon W, Lin EHB. Disability and depression among high utilizers of health care: A longitudinal analysis. *Arch Gen Psychiatry* 49:91, 1992.

61. Parikh RM, Robinson RG, Lipsey JR, et al: The impact of poststroke depression on recovery in activities of daily living over a 2-year follow-up. *Arch Neurol* 47:785, 1990.

62. Morris PL, Raphael B, Robinson RG: Clinical depression is associated with impaired recovery from stroke. *Med J Aust* 157:239, 1992.

63. Eastwood MR, Rifat SL, Nobbs H, et al: Mood disorder following cerebrovascular accident. *Br J Psychiatry* 154:195, 1989.

64. Finklestein SP, Weintraub RJ, Karmouz N, et al: Antidepressant drug treatment for poststroke depression: Retrospective study. *Arch Phys Med Rehabil* 68:772, 1987.

65. Lipsey JR, Robinson RG, Pearlson GD, et al: Nortriptyline treatment for poststroke depression: A double-blind study. *Lancet* 1:287, 1964.

66. Reding MJ, Orto LA, Winer SW, et al: Antidepressant therapy after stroke: Double-blind trial. *Arch Neurol* 43:763, 1986.

67. Lazarus LW, Moberg PJ, Langsley PR, Lingam VR: Methylphenidate and nortriptyline in the treatment of poststroke depression: A retrospective comparison. *Arch Phys Med Rehabil* 75:403, 1994.

68. Andersen G, Vestergaard K, Lauritzen L: Effective treatment of poststroke depression with the selective serotonin reuptake inhibitor citalopram. *Stroke* 25:1099, 1994.

69. Murray GB, Shea V, Conn DK: Electroconvulsive therapy for post-stroke depression. *J Clin Psychiatry* 47:258, 1986.

70. Friedland J, McCall MA: Social support intervention after support: Results of a randomized trial. *Arch Phys Med Rehabil* 73:573, 1992.

71. American Psychiatric Association: *Diagnostic and Statistical Manual of Mental Disorders,* 4th ed. Washington, DC, American Psychiatric Association, 1994.

72. U.S. Dept. of Health and Human Services, Agency for Health Care Policy and Research: *Depression in Primary Care, Vol 2. Treatment of Major Depression* (AHCPR Pub. No. 39-0551). Washington, DC, Government Printing Office, 1993.

73. Brocklehurst JC, Andrews SK, Richards BR, et al: Incidence and correlates of incontinence in stroke patients. *J Am Geriatr Soc* 33:540, 1985.

74. Borrie MJ, Campbell AJ, Spears GF: Urinary incontinence after stroke: A prospective study. *Age Aging* 15:177, 1988.

75. Barer DH: Continence after stroke: Useful predictor or goal of therapy? *Age Aging* 18:183, 1989.

76. Nakayama H, Jogensen HS, Pedersen PM, et al: Prevalence and risk factors of incontinence after stroke: The Copenhagen stroke study. *Stroke* 28:58, 1997.

77. Wade DT, Hewer RL: Outlook after an acute stroke: Urinary incontinence and loss of consciousness compared in 532 patients. *Q J Med* 56:601, 1985.

78. Taub NA, Wolfe CDA, Richardson E, Burney PGJ: Predicting the disability of first-time stroke sufferers at one

year: 12-month follow-up of a population-based cohort in southeast England. *Stroke* 25:352, 1994.

79. Arunabh MB. Badlani G: Urologic problems in cerebrovascular accidents. *Probl Urol* 7:41, 1993.

80. Khan Z, Stazer P, Yong WC, et al: Analysis of voiding disorders in patients with cerebrovascular accidents. *Urology* 35:265, 1990.

81. Badlani GH, Vohra S, Motola JA: Detrusor behavior in patients with dominant hemisphere strokes. Neurourol *Urodynamics* 10:119, 1991.

82. Garrett VE, Scott JA, Costich J, et al: Bladder emptying assessment of stroke patients. *Arch Phys Med Rehabil* 70:41, 1989.

83. Brittain KR, Peet SM, Castleden CM: Stroke and incontinence. *Stroke* 29:524, 1998.

84. Fantl JA, Newman DK, Colling J, et al: *Urinary Incontinence in Adults: Acute and Chronic Management.* Clinical Practice Guideline No. 2, 1996 Update. Rockville, MD, Agency for Health Care Policy and Research, AHCPR Publication No. 96-0682.

85. Gelber DA, Good DC, Laven LJ, et al: Causes of urinary incontinence after acute hemispheric stroke. *Stroke* 24:378, 1993.

86. Hu T: Impact of urinary incontinence on health care cost. *J Am Geriatr Soc* 38:292, 1990.

87. Lum SK, Marshall VR: Results of prostatectomy in patients following a cerebrovascular accident. *Br J Med* 54:186, 1982.

88. Flaherty IH, Miller DK, Coe RM: Impact on caregivers of supporting urinary function in noninstitutionalized chronically ill seniors. *Gerontologist* 32:541, 1992.

89. Ouslander JG: Urinary incontinence in the elderly. *West J Med* 135:482, 1981.

90. Ouslander JG, Kane RL, Abrass B: Urinary incontinence in elderly nursing home patients. *JAMA* 248:1134, 1992.

91. Tapp AJ, Cardozo LD, Versi E, et al: The treatment of detrusor instability in post-menopausal women with oxybutynin chloride: A double-blind placebo controlled study. *Br J Obstet Gynaecol* 97:521, 1990.

92. Zeegers AGM, Kiesswetter H, Kramer AEJL, et al: Conservative therapy of frequency, urgency and urge incontinence: A double-blind clinical trial of flavoxate hydrochloride, oxybutynin chloride, emepronium bromide and placebo. *World J Urol* 5:57, 1989.

93. Holmes DM, Montz FJ, Stanton SL: Oxybutynin versus propantheline in the management of detrusor instability: A patient-regulated variable dose trial. *Br J Obstet Gynaecol* 96:607, 1989.

94. Ouslander JG, Greengold B, Ches S: Complications of chronic indwelling urinary catheters among male nursing home patients: A prospective study. *J Urol* 138:1191, 1987.

95. Dejerine J, Roussy J: Le syndrome thalamique. *Rev Neurol* 14:521, 1906.

96. Agnew DC, Shetter AG, Segall HD, et al: Thalamic pain. *Adv Pain Res Ther* 5:941, 1983.

97. Bowsher D, Lahuerta J, Brock LG: Twelve cases of cen-

tral pain, only three with thalamic lesions. *Pain* 2 (Suppl):83, 1984.

98. Bowsher D, Smith T, Lewis-Jones H, et al: Magnetic resonance pathology of central post-stroke pain (CPSP). *Proc XIth Int Congr Neuropathol* 384, 1990.

99. Bowsher D: Pain syndromes and their treatment. *Curr Opini Neurol Neurosurg* 6:257, 1993.

100. Roth EJ: Natural history of recovery and influence of comorbid conditions on stroke outcome, in Gorelick P (ed): *Atlas of Cerebrovascular Disease.* Philadelphia, Current Medicine, 1996.

101. Jongbloed L: Prediction of function after stroke: A critical review. *Stroke* 17:765, 1986.

102. Bowsher D: Neurogenic pain syndromes and their management. *Br Med Bull* 47:644, 1991.

103. Bainton T, Fox M, Bowsher D, et al: A double-blind trial of naloxone in central post-stroke pain. *Pain* 48:159, 1992.

104. Leijon G, Boivie J: Central post-stroke pain: A controlled trial of amitriptyline and carbamazepine. *Pain* 36:27, 1989.

105. Lynch S, Max MB, Muir J, et al: Efficacy of antidepressants in relieving diabetic neuropathy pain: Amitriptyline vs desipramine, and fluoxitene vs placebo. *Neurology* 40 (Suppl 1):437, 1990.

106. Max MB, Schafer SC, Culnane M, et al: Amitriptyline, but not lorazepam, relieves postherpetic neuralgia. *Neurology* 38:1427, 1988.

107. McQuay H, Carroll D, Jadad AR, et al: Anticonvulsant drugs for management of pain: A systematic review. *Br Med J* 311:1047, 1995.

108. Nurmikko T, Wells C, Bowsher D: Pain and allodynia in postherpetic neuralgia: Role of somatic and sympathetic systems. *Acta Neurol Scand* 84:146, 1991.

109. Leijon G, Boivie J: Central post-stroke pain: The effect of high and low frequency TENS. *Pain* 38:187, 1989.

110. Taub E, Munz M, Tasker RR: Chronic electrical stimulation of the gasserian ganglion for the relief of pain in a series of 34 patients. *J Neurosurg* 86:197, 1997.

111. Loh I, Nathat PW, Scott GD: Pain due to lesions of central nervous system removed by sympathetic block. *Br Med J* 282:1026, 1981.

112. Tsubokawa T, Katayama Y, Ymamoto T, et al: Chronic motor cortex stimulation in patients with thalamic pain. *J Neurosurg* 78:393, 1993.

113. Moolten SE: Bed sores in the chronically ill patient. *Arch Phys Med Rehabil* 53:450, 1972.

114. Guralnik M, Hans TB, White LR, et al: Occurrence and predictors of pressure sores in the National Health Examination Survey Follow-up. *J Am Geriatr Soc* 36:807, 1988.

115. National Pressure Ulcer Advisory Panel. Pressure ulcer prevalence, cost and risk assessment: Consensus development conference statement. *Decubitus* 24, 1989.

116. U.S. Department of Health & Human Services, Agency for Health Care Policy and Research: *Pressure Ulcers in Adults: Prediction and Prevention.* Clinical Practice Guidelines No 3, Washington, DC, 1994.

117. U.S. Department of Health & Human Services, Agency

for Health Care Policy and Research: *Treatment of Pressure Ulcers.* Clinical Practice Guidelines No. 15, Washington, DC, 1994.

118. Ferrell Bam Jeeker E, Siu AL, et al: Cost-effectiveness of low-air-loss beds for treatment of pressure ulcers. *J Gerontol A Biol Sci Med Sci* 50A:M141, 1995.

119. Inman KJ, Sibbald WJ, Rutledge FS, et al: Clinical utility and cost-effectiveness of an air suspension bed in the prevention of pressure ulcers. *JAMA* 269:1139, 1993.

120. Xakellis GC, Framtz RA, Lewis A, Harvey P: Cost-effectiveness of an intensive pressure ulcer prevention protocol in long term care. *Adv Wound Care* 11:22, 1998.

121. Mackelbust J, Sieggreen M: *Pressure Ulcers: Guidelines for Prevention and Nursing Management.* West Dundee, IL, S-N Publications, 1991.

122. Bray GP, DeFrank RS, Wolfe TL: Sexual functioning in stroke survivors. *Arch Phys Med Rehabil* 62:286, 1981.

123. Boldrini P, Basaglia N, Calanca MC: Sexual changes in hemiparetic patients. *Arch Phys Med Rehabil* 72:202, 1991.

124. Fugl-Meyer AR, Jaasko L: Post-stroke hemiplegia and sexual intercourse. *Scan J Rehabil Med* 7:158, 1980.

125. Kalliomaki JL, Markkanen TK, Mustonen VA: Sexual behavior after cerebral vascular accident: Study on patients below age 60 years. *Fertil Steril* 12:156, 1961.

126. Monga TN, Lawson JS, Inglis J: Sexual dysfunction in stroke patients. *Arch Phys Med Rehabil* 67:19, 1986.

127. Sjogren K: Sexuality after stroke with hemiplegia: II. With special regard to partnership adjustment and to fulfillment. *Scan J Rehabil Med* 15:63, 1983.

128. Monga TN, Monga M, Raina MS, et al: Hypersexuality in stroke. *Arch Phys Med Rehabil* 67:415, 1986.

129. Sjogren K, Damber J-E, Liliequist B: Sexuality after stroke with hemiplegia: I. Aspects of sexual function. *Scand J Rehabil Med* 15:55, 1983.

130. Oradei DM, Waite NS: Group psychotherapy with stroke patients during immediate recovery phase. *Am J Orthopsychiatry* 44:386, 1974.

131. Watziawick P, Coyne JC: Depression following stroke: Brief, problem-focused family therapy. *Family Treatment* 19:13, 1980.

132. Feibel JH, Springer CJ: Depression and failure to resume social activities after stroke. *Arch Phys Med Rehabil* 63:276, 1982.

133. Thompson SC, Sobolew-Shobin A, Graham MA, Jenigion AS: Psychosocial adjustment following stroke. *Soc Sci Med* 28:139, 1981.

134. Laurtzen L, Bjerg Bendseb B, Vilmar T, et al: Post-stroke depression: Combined treatment with imipramine or desipramine and mianserin: A controlled clinical study. *Psychopharmacology* 114:119, 1994.

135. Dam M, Tonin P, De Boni A, et al: Effects of fluoxetine and maprotiline on functional recovery in poststroke hemiplegic patients undergoing rehabilitation therapy. *Stroke* 27:1211, 1996.

Chapter 10

THE CHRONIC STROKE PATIENT: MANAGEMENT OF COGNITIVE IMPAIRMENT

Helena C. Chui

INTRODUCTION

Cognitive impairment is commonly experienced after stroke, but the pattern and severity of cognitive impairment are highly variable. Depending upon the arterial distribution and location of vascular brain injury, a wide range of cognitive functions may be affected. These include attention, memory, language, motor planning, visual-spatial perception, reasoning, and executive function. Characteristic cognitive syndromes associated with major artery (e.g., aphasia and neglect) and minor artery syndromes (e.g., executive dysfunction following lacunar infarcts in the basal ganglia and thalamus) have been amply described in the literature.[1] Dementia, a multifaceted decline in memory and cognitive impairment sufficiently severe to interfere with an individual's usual level of social and occupational function,[2] may result from multiple strokes or single strokes in locations that are strategically important for cognition.

In this chapter, we first review the magnitude, impact, and outlook for the problem, namely, cognitive impairment following stroke. Then, we undertake a critical review of the evidence regarding (1) methods of evaluation, (2) treatment using rehabilitative and pharmacologic interventions, (3) prevention of secondary complications, and (4) supportive care. Each section concludes with a summary of recommendations for management and treatment. If available, we cite the 1995 clinical guidelines for poststroke rehabilitation published by the Agency for Health Care Policy and Research (AHCPR).[3] Finally, we offer our own recommendations for treatment, management, and future research.

Magnitude of the Problem: Prevalence within the First 3 Months of Stroke

Memory Impairment Impairments in immediate verbal and visual memory were noted in 29 percent and 39 percent of 138 patients drawn from the Frenchay Stroke registry and examined 3 to 6 months poststroke.[4] Impairment in verbal recall and delayed verbal and visual recognition memory was found in 21 to 26 percent of 227 patients 3 months poststroke.[5]

Aphasia Speech or language disorders occur in approximately 30 to 40 percent of patients with stroke[6–8] and are associated with injury to the left or dominant hemisphere. In a study of 192 patients with acute aphasia, the distribution of aphasic subtypes was as follows: anomic 53, global 38, Broca 34, Wernicke 23, conduction 18, sensory 16, motor 7, and isolation 3.[6]

Visual Neglect Acutely, unilateral neglect is noted in 32 to 55 percent of patients with right hemisphere stroke and 25 to 42 percent of those with left hemisphere injury.[9–11] Three months after stroke, the prevalence of unilateral neglect was reported to be 33 percent with right hemisphere and 0 percent with left hemisphere lesions.[10] Thus, right hemisphere stroke seems to produce more frequent and long-lasting neglect.

Dementia One-quarter to one-third of stroke survivors meet DSM (Diagnostic and Statistical Manual)[2] criteria for dementia when examined 3 months following hospitalization for acute stroke.[12,13] Demographic risk factors for dementia include greater age and fewer years of education.[6] If the incidence of stroke in the United States is 500,000 per year, then the incidence of stroke-related dementia would be an estimated 150,000 per year. In the United States, these patients tend to be followed in stroke rather than dementia clinics. Thus, despite the substantial number of subjects who meet DSM criteria, relatively few first-time stroke survivors receive a formal diagnosis of dementia.

The pattern of cognitive deficits observed in stroke-related dementia is heterogeneous. Memory may not be the most prominent or defining feature, as it is in Alzheimer disease. Cortical infarcts resulting from large-artery disease may produce a combination of focal cognitive deficits, such as aphasia, neglect, etc. Subcortical infarcts resulting from small-artery disease are more likely to cause apathy, slowing, and dysexecutive function. Dementia syndromes associated with small-artery disease have been reviewed elsewhere.[14–16]

Impact of the Problem: Predictors of Functional Outcome

Poststroke cognitive impairment has an adverse effect on level of autonomy, mobility, and quality of life.[17,18] Hemineglect has been most consistently associated with poor outcome at the time of discharge from acute rehabilitation therapy.[9,19–21] In one study, the presence of visual neglect was associated with lower Barthel Index Scores, longer duration of rehabilitation, and greater numbers of therapy hours but similar rates of discharge home.[11] In a prospective study of 273 stroke patients admitted for rehabilitation, severity of stroke and cognitive impairment (including neglect) predicted less favorable outcome at discharge.[21] Risks for poor autonomy and impaired mobility were significantly increased in the presence of hemineglect (relative risk [RR] = 7.30; confidence interval [CI] 4.04 to 13.18; RR = 9.25 [CI 4.63 to 18.45]) or global aphasia (RR = 4.51 [CI 2.74 to 7.41]; RR = 4.71 [CI 2.79 to 7.97]). Similarly, cognitive impairment increased the risk for discharge to dependent living (either home with an attendant or to a nursing home) (odds ratio [OR] = 2.4 [CI 1.3 to 4.4]), even after adjusting for age and physical disability.[22] The adverse impact of cognitive compromise on functional outcome has been confirmed by multiple investigators.

Lincoln et al.[8] reported the growing importance of cognitive impairment as a predictor of function after longer times following stroke. At the time of discharge, performance on Raven Coloured Progressive Matrices predicted 6 percent of the variance in activities of daily living (ADL). By 9 months poststroke, recognition memory for faces predicted 33 percent of variance in ADL; reading and writing predicted a significant proportion of variance for extended ADL (15 percent for kitchen activities and 34 percent for leisure activities). Thus, severity of cognitive impairment may assume increasing importance as a predictor of longer-term functional outcome and quality of life.

Outlook for the Problem: Natural History More Than 6 Months after Stroke

With time, patients and caregivers inquire increasingly more often about the psychologic sequelae of stroke (e.g., concentration and memory impairment).[23] Yet, compared with the outlook for motor function, far less is known about the recovery of cognitive ability. Three longitudinal neuropsychologic studies extending beyond 6 months poststroke were identified by this review. In these studies, no attempt has been made to subgroup patients by type and location of stroke, despite recognized differences in the degree of early functional recovery between major vs. minor stroke.[24–26]

Based on clinical observation, the greatest improvement in cognitive function seems to occur during the first 3 months following stroke.[7,27] Based on comparisons of prevalence at different time points, improvement may continue through the first year. For example, the frequencies of neuropsychologic deficits decreased when assessed at 3 to 12 months: visuoperceptual from 60 percent to 41 percent, memory from 55 percent to 31 percent, and aphasia 33 percent to 30 percent.[7] Thus, like motor function, the greatest improvements in cognition occur during the first 3 months but may continue through the first year.

A prospective longitudinal study of 151 patients hospitalized for stroke sheds important insights.[28] Improvement in neuropsychologic testing was observed in 12.6 percent of patients at 12 compared with 3 months poststroke. Improvement was noted for memory, orientation, visual spatial function, and attention but not for language or abstract reasoning. The investigators noted that the likelihood of improvement was greater for left hemisphere vs. brainstem/cerebellar stroke (OR 5.57; CI 1.96 to 29.25). However, this particular finding should be interpreted with caution because patients with severe aphasia were excluded, possibly leading to an over-representation of milder left hemisphere strokes. Fourteen of the 19 patients who had shown improvement at 1 year were re-evaluated at subsequent annual intervals, but none showed additional improvement. Diabetes mellitus was a predictor of poor cognitive outcome (OR 0.12; CI 0.02 to 0.63). The reason for this is not known but may be related to diffuse microangiopathy, impaired autoregulation, reduced cerebral blood flow, or silent brain infarcts associated with chronic hyperglycemia.

Increased risk for subsequent deterioration in cognitive function has also been observed in this cohort. In the absence of further symptomatic strokes, the relative risk of developing dementia 1 year following stroke was increased 5.5-fold compared with a nonstroke comparison group; the risk was particularly high among elderly persons.[6] Reasons for the delayed development of dementia are unknown but may include recurrent silent strokes, subclinical hypoxic ischemic brain injury, or concomitant Alzheimer disease, which becomes increasingly more common after age 65 years. An association between dementia risk with seizures, cardiac arrhythmias, and pneumonia provides some support for the hypothesis that dementia may be mediated via adverse effects of hypoxia or ischemia.[29] In summary, the outlook for cognition following stroke seems to be highly variable, encompassing a longer time frame for recovery, as well as the risk of subsequent decline.

METHODS FOR EVALUATING COGNITIVE IMPAIRMENT

Background

Because cognitive deficits affect length of stay, rate of recovery, and short- and long-term functional outcome, cognitive assessment is essential for prognosis and treatment. Cognitive deficits vary independently of physical mobility and ability to care for self;[30] they must be assessed specifically. This can be performed first with brief screening tools and then, if indicated, by using longer neuropsychologic tests or test batteries. A comprehensive compendium of neuropsychologic tests is available.[31] Thus, the following section is not meant to be exhaustive. Conceptual issues are highlighted, but only a few of the available neuropsychologic tests are mentioned.

Assessment of cognition in stroke patients may be complicated by the presence of significant deficits in motor, perceptual, or language function, depressed mood, as well as by level of education and cultural background. For example, patients with weakness of the dominant hand may have difficulty performing cognitive tests that require fine motor coordination. Patients with visual neglect may not respond to objects presented in one visual field; stimuli should be presented in their good field.[20] Patients with severe aphasia may also perform poorly on tests of verbal memory and reasoning; mem-

ory should be tested with nonverbal stimuli (e.g., the hidden objects test). Depression is commonly experienced by stroke survivors (see Chap. 9) and may worsen cognitive performance, particularly on tests that tax attention and concentration. Educational and cultural differences often influence performance on cognitive tests.[32] Thus, for stroke patients, the selection of appropriate tests and the interpretation of test results must be individualized.

A number of screening tests have been used in the stroke literature. These tests include the Mini-Mental State Exam (MMSE), Neurobehavior Cognitive Status Examination (NCSE), and the Cognitive Capacity Screening Examination (CCSE). The Folstein MMSE[33] is one of the most popular mental status screening tests, as it takes but 8 to 10 min to administer. Notably, 29 of its 30 points depend upon verbal abilities; hence, the MMSE score may be lowered disproportionately among aphasic stroke patients. In addition, the MMSE is not sensitive for detecting deficits in reasoning or executive function. The modified Mini-Mental State (3MS) has been expanded[34] to broaden the spectrum of cognitive domains but so far has not been commonly used among stroke patients. The CCSE is similar to the MMSE.[35] The NCSE provides a profile of functioning for several cognitive domains (i.e., orientation, attention, language, repetition, naming, construction, memory, calculations, reasoning judgment) rather than a single summative score.[36] Thus, the level of information provided falls between a brief screening tool and more detailed neuropsychologic testing.

Individual neuropsychologic tests or test batteries are commonly used for in-depth assessment. The reader is referred elsewhere[31] for more information regarding the statistical structure, reliability, and validity for the following tests.

Attention Digit span of the WAIS and Mental Control of the WMS-R provide measures of verbal attention, whereas the visual span of the Memory Assessment Scales (MAS)[37] assesses visual attention.

Memory The Wechsler Memory Scale-Revised (WMS-R)[38] and the Benton Visual Retention Test (BVRT)[39] are commonly used to assess memory.

Language The Boston Diagnostic Aphasia Examination (BDAE),[40] Western Aphasia Battery (WAB),[41] Multilingual Aphasia Examination (MAE),[42] and the Porch Index of Communicative Ability (PICA)[43] are commonly chosen to assess aphasia.

Visual-Spatial Abilities   Performance subtests of the Wechsler Adult Intelligence Scale-R (WAIS-R)[44] (e.g., block design, picture arrangement, picture completion) are used to evaluate visual perception and visual-spatial reasoning. The Rivermead Perceptual Assessment Battery (RPAB) was developed specifically to assess perceptual abilities in hemiparetic stroke patients, regardless of speech deficits.[45] The RPAB comprises 16 perception tests, ranging from simple tasks such as picture, object, and color matching to more complex tasks such as cancellation, figure-ground, sequencing, body image, and copying shapes, words, and three-dimensional figures.

Concept Formation and Executive Function   Individual tests are usually selected to assess concept formation and reasoning (e.g., similarities test from the WAIS-R, Raven's Progressive Matrices,[46] Wisconsin Card Sorting Test,[47] and Modified Stroop Test.)[48]

Motor Speed   The finger tapping test may be used to assess motor speed.[49]

Evidence

There is limited information comparing the reliability or validity of test instruments among patients with strokes or stroke subtypes. Simple screening tools for severity of dementia (e.g., MMSE, CCSE, Hasegawa Dementia Rating Scale) have been correlated with reductions in mean cortical gray-matter cerebral blood flow, severity, location, and number of cerebral infarcts.[50–52] Most of the tests described in the background section have been used to characterize the neuropsychologic profile of patients with vascular brain injury.[31,53] But there is no evidence in the literature identifying any one superior method of neuropsychologic assessment for patients with stroke or stroke-related dementia.

Recommendations

Based on expert consensus, the AHCPR guideline[3] states that "a clinical psychological examination should be performed in patients who show evidence of cognitive or emotional problems on clinical examination or a mental status screening test. Complete neuropsychological testing is required when more precise understanding of deficits will facilitate treatment."

In selecting appropriate tests, the examiner should consider cultural and motivational factors, as well as perceptual, linguistic, or motor deficits that might influence the interpretation of test results. Because the pattern and severity of cognitive impairment evolves rapidly during the first 3 months, follow-up evaluation (e.g., at 3 or 12 months) is often advisable for long-term planning. Future research might be directed toward developing algorithms for reliable and cost-effective screening and evaluation.

TREATMENT I: COGNITIVE REHABILITATION

Background

Language and perceptual impairments (i.e., major hemispheral syndrome) have been most frequently targeted for rehabilitation. Strategies have been directed toward remediation or compensation by the patient and toward adaptation and compensation by the family/caregiver.

Techniques used by speech pathologists to treat aphasia include traditional stimulus-response modality-specific drills, compensatory strategies designed to circumvent language deficits, and alternative and augmentative communication systems. A variety of interventions have been used to decrease neglect. Some investigators have used the caloric stimulation of the semicircular canal[54] or opticokinetic stimulation[55] to force gaze transiently toward the neglected side.[54] Others have attempted to augment the level of sensory stimulation on the neglected side (e.g., by applying vibratory stimuli to the neglected side of the neck[56] or extra visual stimulation in the neglected field.[57] Fresnel prisms have been used to shift portions of what would normally fall in the neglected into the nonneglected field of view.[58] Finally, the eye on the neglected side has been patched.[59]

Evidence

Evidence regarding the effectiveness of speech therapy for aphasia is mixed. To examine the effectiveness of speech therapy vs. no therapy, two randomized[60,61] and one "partially" randomized controlled trial[62] were reviewed. The sample size, intensity, and duration of therapy differed. Significant differences between treatment and nontreatment groups were reported by two of three studies. Wertz et al.[61] randomized 121 subjects to three crossover groups; the treatment phase comprised 8 to 10 h of treatment per week for 12 weeks. At 12 weeks, the treatment group was significantly better than the non-treatment group; the home treatment group was intermediate but not significantly different. Shewan and Kertesz[62] randomized 100 subjects among three types of treatment vs. control (note the control group was self-selected). Treatment consisted of 3 h of therapy per week for 1 year. Analysis of covariance, controlling for score at entry, showed a significant favorable effect for the three treatment groups combined vs. the untreated controls. On the other hand, no significant treatment effect was found by Lincoln et al,[60] who randomized 191 subjects among two groups, with the treatment group receiving 2 h of therapy for 24 weeks. The results of these few randomized controlled studies are consistent with the hypothesis that low-intensity speech therapy may not be significantly better than no therapy, but high-intensity therapy might be.

Few studies specifically address the subtype of aphasia, timing of intervention, or type or intensity of intervention. Greater improvement has been observed incidentally for Broca's aphasia compared with other subtypes of aphasia.[62] One study[61] reported no significant differences in outcome when speech therapy was delayed 12 weeks. Wertz et al.[63] reported slightly better outcome among patients receiving individual vs. group treatment. Small but non-significant differences have been noted between intensive outpatient speech therapy vs. in-home volunteer support.[61] No significant differences were observed between 2 h per week of speech therapy vs. supportive counseling.[64] Questions regarding which types of patients are most likely to benefit, the optimal time for intervention, the ideal intensity, and type of intervention remain unanswered.

Seven randomized and two "quasi" randomized controlled trials for perceptual deficits have been reviewed.[3] Acute benefits were found in seven of the nine studies,[65,66] but these were limited to short-term effects on outcome measures sharing stimulus characteristics with the intervention.[58] After 4 weeks, patients fitted with Fresnel prisms were reported to show better performance on perceptual tests but not in activities of daily living.[58] A randomized trial among 50 stroke patients with visual neglect showed a trend toward higher Barthel scores at 12 weeks and a significant reduction in median length of hospital stay among the group receiving spatiomotor cueing and early emphasis on functional rehabilitation.[11] In an earlier quasi-randomized study, Gordon et al[66] also reported greater improvement in a treatment group at the time of discharge, but these differences had disappeared by 4 months postdischarge. Thus far, the data supporting effectiveness of cognitive rehabilitation for visual neglect beyond the time of discharge are extremely limited.

Recommendations

Based on several randomized controlled trials, "patients with aphasia should be offered treatment targeted at the identified language retrieval or comprehension deficits and aimed at improving functional communication."[3] Although several randomized trials support the efficacy of speech therapy, the optimal type, timing intensity, and duration of therapy are still unknown. Expert opinion and a single RCT support the recommendation that "cognitive and perceptual problems not severe enough to preclude rehabilitation require goal-directed treatment plans.[67] Clearly, more randomized controlled trials are needed, not only during acute rehabilitation but in the months to year following stroke.

TREATMENT II: PHARMACOLOGIC TREATMENT OF VASCULAR DEMENTIA

Background

To date, most randomized controlled pharmacologic trials relevant to cognitive impairment associated with stroke can be indexed via the term "multi-infarct dementia (MID)." In the past, MID has been defined operationally by Hachinski Ischemia Score >7[68] or by a modified Hachinski Ischemia Score >4.[69] During the past decade, a number of new criteria have been promulgated to broaden the conceptualization of vascular dementia and to incorporate neuroimaging findings. These include Erkinjutti criteria,[70] DSM IV,[2] ICD-10,[71] California ADDTC,[72] and NINDS-AIREN.[73] These criteria are not interchangeable,[74,75] but absent clinicopathologic validation, none has emerged as better than the other.[76] The traditional Hachinski Ischemia Score seems to have higher inter-rater reliability than the newer criteria,[77] but does not identify certain subtypes of vascular dementia such as Binswanger-type vascular dementia or mixed Alzheimer-vascular dementia.[29] Most frequently, recent pharmacologic trials have adapted the NINDS-AIREN criteria,[73] which behave relatively conservatively in identifying cases of vascular dementia (VaD) cases.[74]

The choice of pharmacologic agent is often borrowed from Alzheimer studies, where the rationale is presumably different. Treatment duration has usually traditionally been short (e.g., 12 weeks) although getting substantially longer (6 to 12 months). Patients with MID VaD and primary degenerative dementia (PDD)/AD are often combined. A rationale for treating patients with vascular dementia may be proposed, but patients are not selected based upon the relevant pathophysiology. Rarely is attention paid to the subtype of vascular dementia (e.g., large-vessel thrombosis, cardioembolism, small-artery thrombosis, or stenosis). Therapeutic effects are generally small, and post hoc analyses show similar effects for patients with diagnoses of Alzheimer disease (AD)/PPD or VaD/MID.

Evidence

A few randomized, double-blind, placebo-controlled trials have been conducted for a wide variety of compounds in patients with MID. Experience with these drugs has been recently reviewed.[78,79] Results of several double-blind placebo-controlled (DBPC) studies during the past 10 years are also summarized below.

Alkaloid derivatives, such as hydergine or nicergoline, have been used because of their vasoactive and metabolic-activating effects.[80,81] Hydergine is a mixture of derivatives from three ergot alkaloids with weak vasodilator and dopaminergic effects. In a meta-analysis of 49 placebo-controlled comparisons ($n = 2576$), hydergine was consistently more effective than placebo on the Sandoz Clinical Assessment Geriatric Scale (SCAGS), clinical global ratings, and overall neuropsychologic measures. Effect sizes were greater in vascular dementia ($d = 0.35$, $p < .0001$) than AD ($d = 0.24$, $p = .0004$).[82] Among 315 patients with mild to moderate dementia (subtype not specified), Battaglia et al[81] reported favorable differences in SCAGS scores at 3 and 6 months in the treatment compared with the placebo group.

Pentoxifylline (Trental) is a xanthine derivative and phosphodiesterase inhibitor that increases red cell deformability, decreases blood viscosity, inhibits platelet aggregation and thrombus formation, and suppresses leukocyte adhesion.[83–85] In a DBPC trial of pentoxifylline among 64 patients with MID, there was a nonsignificant trend showing less deterioration on the Alzheimer Disease Assessment Scale (ADAS) in the treatment group.[83] Propentofylline has similar hemorrheologic properties but also some neuroprotective effects including inhibiting of excessive glutamate release, calcium accumulation, and free radical formation.[78] In a 3-month, phase II clinical trial[86] and both 6- and 12-month phase III DBPC trials,[87] a beneficial effect of propentofylline was observed for dementia attributed to either AD or VaD.

Similarly, piracetam and its analogs (antiracetam, etiracetam, oxiracetam, and pramiracetam) seem to enhance cerebral metabolism and modulate neurotransmitter functions.[88–90] Several DBPC trials in patients with vascular dementia showed improvement in subjective complaints ($n = 40$),[91] social isolation, overall dysfunction, and sleep disturbance ($n = 60$),[92] MMSE and SCAGS ($n = 11$),[93] and the ADAS ($n = 64$).[83] In a 12-week DBPC study of 272 patients with primary dementia (primary degenerative dementia = 77, MID = 107), the treatment group (regardless of diagnosis) did significantly better on the Blessed Dementia Scale, Newcastle Memory Information Concentration Test, and an inventory of psychic and somatic complaints.[94] In a 90-day DBPC trial of oxiracetam in 60 patients with either AD or MID, the treatment group was significantly better for MMSE, Rey auditory learning, world fluency, Luria alternating series, and instrumental activities of daily living.[95] In a DBPC trial among 73 patients with either MID or PDD, oxiracetam was associated with better word fluency in both types of patients but with improvement in the Relatives Assessment of Global Symptomatology in the PDD group only.[96]

Calcium channel antagonists (e.g., nimodipine) exert a neuroprotective effect in acute experimental ischemia.[79] In a 12-week DBPC trial among 178 subjects with cognitive decline, nimodipine was associated with significantly better global impression of cognitive improvement and scores on the Wechsler Memory Scale, MMSE, and SCAGS.[97]

A number of other compounds have been studied including glycosaminoglycan,[98] xantinolnicotinate,[99] and ateroid.[100] Vinca alkaloids (e.g., vincamine, vinburine, vinpocetine) increase cerebral blood flow, activate cerebral metabolism, and modulate neurotransmitter release.[101,102] Multicenter trials of memantidine, a reversible GABA antagonist, and donepezil, an acetylcholinesterase inhibitor (already approved by the Federal Drug Administration for the treatment of AD) are now under way.

In summary, many of the compounds studied so far have shown only modest benefit (i.e., often statistically, but not clinically significant). The effects of these compounds are usually of similar magnitude in patients with Alzheimer disease and vascular dementia, suggesting that their mode of action may be common to both types of dementia or a non-specific form of tertiary amelioration.

Recommendations

Because of lack of evidence, we cannot make recommendations at this time for the pharmacologic treatment of cognitive impairment associated with cerebrovascular disease. Treatment recommendations for depression, a common associated symptom complex, can be found in Chap. 9. Hopefully, novel compounds will be developed in the future to target basic pathophysiologic mechanisms of ischemia or to enhance neuroplasticity. We suggest that future trials of vascular dementia should identify the targeted pathophysiologic mechanism, then use a corresponding pathophysiologic measure to select and characterize subjects. This would either complement or replace the current practice of enrolling subjects using combinations of already broad clinical diagnoses.

PREVENTION I: AVOIDING EXCESS DISABILITY

Background

For several reasons, patients with cognitive impairment are at increased risk for excess disability. First, the threshold for superimposed confusional state or delirium is lowered. Second, the patient may be less aware or able to report symptoms of comorbid illness (e.g., depression, pneumonia, urinary tract infection). Thus, the burden of increased vigilance falls upon the primary care physician and caregiver. Certain classes of medications are more likely to cause adverse cognitive side effects, particularly those with strong anticholinergic or sedating properties.

Evidence

In a study of elderly persons with global cognitive impairment (not necessarily related to stroke), the following medications were most commonly associated with confusion: sedatives, hypnotics, antihypertensives, and major tranquilizers.[103] Specifically, diazepam, cimetidine, digoxin, propranolol, phenytoin, phenobarbital, levodopa, amantadine, prednisone, indomethacin, and amitriptyline have been commonly implicated.[104]

In the Oxfordshire Community Stroke Project, the following coexisting pathologic conditions were found among 675 patients with first-ever stroke: previous angina (16 percent), previous myocardial infarction (17 percent), intermittent claudication (17 percent), previous dependency (15 percent), previous malignancy (11 percent), diabetes mellitus (9 percent), cardiac failure (8 percent), and previous epileptic seizures (3 percent) (note: no data were available on respiratory or musculoskeletal problems).[105] Diagnosis of new or recurrent

problems related to these medical conditions might be delayed in persons who are cognitively impaired and less aware or able to communicate their symptoms.

A model to predict the development of delirium was derived from 196 elderly hospitalized persons and validated in 312 comparable patients.[106] These data are instructive, even though they were not derived from patients with stroke. Five independent precipitating factors were identified: use of physical restraints, malnutrition, more than three medications added, use of a bladder catheter, and any iatrogenic event. Note that four of these five risk factors can be considered iatrogenic.

Recommendations

Physicians should recognize medications that are more likely to cause confusion in elderly persons, particularly those who are cognitively impaired. These medications should be used judiciously, if at all. As a general practice, medication lists should be reviewed periodically, and unnecessary medications should be discontinued. Physicians and caregivers should be alert to the possible presence of medical comorbidity, even if the patient does not or is unable to complain of the usual symptoms. Sudden declines in cognitive function should prompt an evaluation for recurrent ischemic events or for comorbid conditions. In addition, risk data in elderly hospitalized subjects suggest that the use of physical restraints and Foley catheters should be minimized, with special attention given to nutritional status.

PREVENTION II: MANAGEMENT OF VASCULAR RISK FACTORS

Background

Patients and caregivers commonly express fear of stroke recurrence[23] and seek information about how to reduce risk. Although experimental drugs are being investigated for their beneficial effects on cognition (see "Treatment II" above), the simple effectiveness of managing vascular risk factors has been relatively neglected.

Evidence

Several studies underscore the importance of continued management of vascular risk factors to prevent stroke recurrence. A meta-analysis of nine randomized controlled clinical trials showed that active treatment with blood pressure-lowering drugs reduces the risk of recurrent stroke by 28 percent (RR = 0.72; CI 0.61 to 0.85, $p < .0001$).[107,108] The evidence supporting treatment of vascular risk factors is discussed in further detail in Chaps. 4, 5, 6, and 7 of this text.

Evidence regarding the effectiveness of controlling vascular risk factors for cognitive outcome is meager, with virtually all data originating from a single laboratory. In a prospective observational study of 29 hypertensive patients with MID, maintenance of systolic BP between 135 and 150 was associated with stabilization of cognition, whereas lowering of systolic BP below 135 was associated with decline.[109] To our knowledge, no randomized trials of BP control have been conducted in patients with MID. Meyer et al.[110] reported a randomized, nonplacebo-controlled trial of 325 mg/day aspirin vs. no aspirin among 70 patients with MID. After a mean follow-up of 15 months, the aspirin-treated group showed significantly higher scores on the CCSE, as well as higher CBF, than the untreated group. Diabetes mellitus has been recently identified as a marker for failure to recover,[28] but the effect of glucose control on cognitive outcome is unstudied.

Recommendations

According to the AHCPR Guidelines,[3] "high priority should be given to the prevention of stroke recurrence and stroke complications and to health promotion more generally, after the stroke survivor returns to the community." Management of vascular risk factors is clearly important to prevent stroke recurrence; the benefits for cognitive function directly merit further study.

SUPPORTIVE CARE IN THE COMMUNITY SETTING

Background

The main provider of long-term supportive care to stroke survivors is the non-professional caregiver, usually the patient's spouse or other family member. For many stroke survivors, the presence of a committed caregiver is required for successful discharge to the community.[26] In a long-term follow-up study (average 4.9 years poststroke), no one with a moderate or severe disability was living at home without a caregiver.[111] However, the toll exacted from the caregiver can be high. Over half of persons caring for stroke survivors report significant emotional distress.[112] Caregiver burden, such as depression, increases with severity of the patient's

dependency, emotional distress,[112,113] and severity of cognitive impairment.[114] Interventions to reduce caregiver burden and stress are likely to benefit the quality of life for both the patient and caregiver.

Other sources of community support to the patient and caregiver include home health workers, home chore workers, day care, and support groups. Home health workers assist with medical care. Home chore workers provide the patient with companionship and assistance with activities of daily living while providing relief to the primary caregiver. Day care provides a rich source of mental, social, and physical activities and therapy for the patient, as well as respite to caregivers. Educational information and emotional support are shared at peer-support groups. These options are available to stroke survivors living in the community, with and without significant cognitive impairment.

Evidence

Randomized controlled studies of interventions for caregivers of stroke survivors are limited. Forster and Young[115] report a randomized controlled study of home visits for 240 patient-caregiver dyads. For the treatment group, a nurse specialist provided information, advice, and support for a minimum of six visits during the first 6 months. No significant improvement was found in caregivers' perceived health, social activities, or stress at 3, 6, or 12 months.[115] Although several observational studies have noted increased risk of caregiver depression with restricted activity[113] or lack of availability of community activity programs,[116] randomized trials of caregiver activity were not identified.

A few studies were located regarding the impact of home health care among stroke survivors, but not specifically related to those cognitively impaired. In a randomized controlled trial of 240 stroke patients, home visits by a nurse specialist resulted in a small improvement in social activities for a subgroup of mildly disabled patients.[115] In a retrospective study of 755 Medicare beneficiaries 6 weeks after hospital discharge following acute stroke (or other medical conditions), use of home health care hours did not have significant effect on the patient's functional status.[117] In a randomized controlled trial among 417 stroke patients, Dennis et al[112] found that the addition of a family care worker improved patient and caregiver satisfaction but not the patient's physical well-being. These studies suggest that supportive home health interventions may improve consumer satisfaction, increase socialization for the mildly disabled, keep patients at home, and compensate for functional limitations but do not seem to promote restoration of physical function. Randomized controlled trials of home health care specifically upon cognitive outcome could not be identified.

Case series and anecdotal experience suggest that other support modalities, such as home chore workers, day care, and support groups, improve quality of life for both patients and caregivers. However, few randomized studies have been performed.

Recommendations

Presence of a caregiver is often the major factor determining whether a patient will live at home. The AHCPR guidelines[3] state: "Clinicians need to be sensitive to potential adverse effects of caregiving on family functioning and the health of the caregiver. They should work with the patient and caregivers to avoid negative effects, promote problem solving, and facilitate reintegration of the patient into valued family and social roles." At the present time, there is no clearly proven method to reduce caregiver burden; randomized controlled trials of enhanced physical activity may be considered. The effectiveness of other types of supportive care, including day care and support groups, should also be studied.

CONCLUSION

The best treatment for stroke-related cognitive impairment is prevention: (1) prevention of the stroke in the first place, (2) prevention of a repeated stroke, and (3) prevention of secondary comorbidity and excess disability. Evidence supporting the effectiveness of rehabilitation or medications to improve cognition is limited, and effect sizes have been small. Thus, the burden of supportive treatment continues to fall upon the caregiver. We suggest the following research priorities related to the treatment and management of persons with stroke-related cognitive impairment:

Effective support for caregivers

Cognitive rehabilitation in community settings

Effectiveness of controlling vascular risk factors

Pharmacologic treatment to minimize ischemic brain injury and to enhance neuroplasticity.

ACKNOWLEDGMENT

Supported by NIH/NIA Grant #P01 AG12435.

REFERENCES

1. Adams RD, Victor M, Ropper AH: *Principles of Neurology.* New York, McGraw-Hill, 1997.
2. American Psychiatric Association: *Diagnostic and Statistical Manual of Mental Disorders.* 4th Ed. Washington DC, American Psychiatric Association, 1994.
3. Gresham GE, Duncan PW, Stason WB, Adams HP, Adelman AM, et al: Post-stroke rehabilitation. Clinical Practice Guideline, Number 16 (No. 95-0662). Rockville: Agency for Health Care Policy and Research, U.S. Department of Health and Human Services, 1995.
4. Wade DT, Parker V, Langton-Hewer R: Memory disturbance after stroke: Frequency and associated losses. *Int Rehabil Med* 8:60, 1986.
5. Tatemichi TK, Desmond DW, Stern Y, Paik M, Sano M, Bagiella E: Cognitive impairment after stroke: Frequency, patterns, and relationship to functional abilities. *J Neurosurg, Psychiatry* 57:202, 1994a.
6. Kertesz A, Sheppard A: The epidemiology of aphasic and cognitive impairment in stroke: Age, sex, aphasia type and laterality differences. *Brain* 104:117, 1981.
7. Kotila M, Waltimo O, Niemi ML, Laaksonen R, Lempinen M: The profile of recovery from stroke and factors influencing outcome. *Stroke* 15:1039, 1984.
8. Lincoln NB, Balckburn M, Ellis S, Jackson J, Edmaus JA, Nouri FM Walrer MF, Haworth H: An investigation of factors influencing progress of patients on a stroke unit. *J Neurol Neurosurg Psychiatry* 52:493, 1989.
9. Fullerton KJ, McSherry D, Stout RW: Albert's test: A neglect test of perceptual neglect. *Lancet* 1:430, 1986.
10. Stone SP, Wilson B, Wroot A, Halligan PW, Lange LS, Marshall JC, Greenwood RJ: The assessment of visuospatial neglect after acute stroke. *J Neurol Neurosurg Psychiatry* 54:345, 1991.
11. Kalra L, Perez I, Gupta S, Wittink M: The influence of visual neglect on stroke rehabilitation. *Stroke* 28:1386, 1997.
12. Tatemichi TK, Desmond DW, Mayeux R, et al: Dementia after stroke: Baseline frequency, risks, and clinical features in a hospitalized cohort. *Neurology* 42:1185, 1992.
13. Pohjasvaara T, Erkinjuntti T, Ylikoski R, Hietanen M, Vataja R, Kaste M: Clinical determinants of poststroke dementia. *Stroke* 29:75, 1998.
14. Cummings JL: Frontal-subcortical circuits and human behavior. *Arch Neurol* 50:873, 1993.
15. Chui HC: Rethinking vascular dementia: moving from myth to mechanism, in Growdon JH, Rossor M (eds): *The Dementias: Blue Books of Practical Neurology.* Newton, Butterworth-Heinemann, 1998, pp 377–402.
16. Chui HC, Willis L: Vascular diseases of the frontal lobes, in Cummings JC, Miller B (eds): *The Frontal Lobes.* Guilford Press, 1999, pp 370–401.
17. Galski T, Bruno RL, Zorowitz R, Walker J: Predicting length of stay, functional outcome, and aftercare in the

rehabilitation of stroke patients: The dominant role of higher-order cognition. *Stroke* 24:1794, 1993.

18. Sisson RA: Cognitive status as a predictor of right hemisphere stroke outcomes. *J Neurosc Nurs* 27:152, 1995.

19. Jongbloed L: Prediction of function after stroke: A critical review. *Stroke* 17:765, 1986.

20. Denes G, Semenza C, Stoppa E, Lis A: Unilateral spatial neglect and recovery from hemiplegia: A follow-up study. *Brain* 105:543, 1982.

21. Paolucci S, Antonucci G, Gialloreti LE, Traballesi M, Lubich S, Pratesi L, Palombi L: Predicting stroke inpatient rehabilitation outcome: The prominent role of neuropsychological disorders. *Eur Neurol* 36:385, 1996.

22. Tatemichi TK, Desmond DW, Paik M, et al: Clinical determinants of dementia related to stroke. *Ann Neurol* 33:568, 1993.

23. Hanger HC, Walker G, Paterson LA, McBride S, Sainsbury R: What do patients and their carers want to know about stroke? A two-year follow-up study. *Clin Rehabil* 12:45, 1998.

24. Bamford J, Sandercock P, Dennis M, et al: Classification and natural history of clinical identifiable subtypes of cerebral infarction. *Lancet* 337:1521, 1991.

25. Beloosesky Y, Streifler JY, Burstin A, Grinblat J: The importance of brain infarct size and location in predicting outcome after stroke. *Age and Ageing* 24:515, 1995.

26. Ween JE, Alexander MP, D'Esposito M, Roberts M: Factors predictive of stroke outcome in a rehabilitation setting. *Neurology* 47:388, 1996.

27. Wade DT, Wood VA, Hewer RL: Recovery of cognitive function soon after stroke: A study of visual neglect, attention span, and verbal recall. *J Neurol Neurosurg Psychiatry* 51:10, 1988.

28. Desmond DW, Moroney JT, Sano M, Stern Y: Recovery of cognitive function after stroke. *Stroke* 27:1798, 1996.

29. Moroney JT, Bagiella E, Desmond DW, Paik MC, Stern Y, Tatemichi TK: Risk factors for incident dementia after stroke: Role of hypoxic and ischemic disorders. *Stroke* 27:1283, 1996.

30. Hajek VE, Gagnon S, Ruderman JE: Cognitive and functional assessments of stroke patients: An analysis of their relation. *Arch Phys Med Rehabil* 78:1331, 1997.

31. Lezak MD: *Neuropsychological Assessment.* New York, Oxford University Press, 1995.

32. Teng EL, Dick M, Kempler D, Taussig M: The Cross-Cultural Neuropsychological Test Battery (CCNB): Effects of education, age, and language on performance. *The Gerontologist* 35:219, 1995.

33. Folstein M, Folstein SE, McHugh PR: "Mini-mental state": A practical method for grading the cognitive state of patients for the clinicna. *J Psychiatric Res* 12:189, 1975.

34. Teng EL, Chui HC: The Modified Mini-Mental State (The 3MS) examination. *J Clin Psychiatry* 48:314, 1987.

35. Kaufman DM, Weinberger M, Stain JJ, et al: Detection of cognitive deficits by a brief mental status examination: The Cognitive Capacity Screening Examination: a reappraisal and a review. *Gen Hosp Psychiatry* 1:247, 1979.

36. Kiernan RJ, Mueller J, Langston JW, Van Dyke C: The Neurobehavioral Cognitive Status Examination: A brief but differentiated approach to cognitive assessment. *Ann Intern Med* 107:481, 1987.

37. Williams JM: *Memory Assessment Scales.* Odessa, FL, Psychological Assessment Resources, Inc., 1991.

38. Wechsler D: *Wechsler Memory Scale-Revised Manual.* San Antonio, TX, The Psychological Corporation, 1987.

39. Benton AL: *Revised Visual Retention Test,* 4th ed. New York, Psychological Corporation, 1974.

40. Goodglass H, Kaplan E: *Boston Diagnostic Aphasia Examination (BDAE).* Philadelphia, Lea and Febiger, 1983.

41. Kertesz A: *The Western Aphasia Battery.* San Antonio, TX, The Psychological Corporation, 1983.

42. Benton AL, Hamsher KDES: *Multilingual Aphasia Examination.* Iowa City, Iowa, AJA Associates, 1989.

43. Porch BE: *Porch Index of Communicative Ability. Manual.* Palo Alto, CA, Consulting Psychologists Press, 1983.

44. Wechsler D: *WAIS-R Manual.* New York, The Psychological Corporation, 1981.

45. Whiting SE, Lincoln NB, Bhavnani G, Cockburn J: *The Rivermead Perceptual Assessment Battery.* Windsor, UK, NEFR-Nelson, 1985.

46. Raven JC, Court JH, Raven J: *Manual for Raven's Progressive Matrices.* London, HK Lewis, 1976.

47. Berg EA: A simple objective treatment for measuring flexibility in thinking. *J Gen Psychology* 39:15, 1948.

48. Golden CJ: *Stroop Color and Word Test.* Chicago, IL, Stoelting, 1978.

49. Heaton RK, Grant I, Matthews CG: *Comprehensive norms for an expanded Halstead-Reitan battery.* Odessa, FL, Psychological Assessment Resources, 1991.

50. Kwan LY, Reed BR, Eberling JL, et al: Effects of subcortical cerebral infarction on cortical glucose metabolism and cognitive function: A PET study. *Arch Neurol,* in press.

51. Kitigawa Y, Meyer JS, Tachibana H, et al: CT-CBF correlations of cognitive deficits in multi-infarct dementia. *Stroke* 15:1000, 1984.

52. Mori S, Sadoshima S, Ibayashi S, Ilino K, Fujishima M: Relation of cerebral blood flow to motor and cognitive functions in chronic stroke patients. *Stroke* 25:309, 1994.

53. La Rue A: *Aging and Neuropsychological Assessment,* New York, Plenum Press, 1992.

54. Rubens AB: Caloric stimulation and unilateral neglect. *Neurology* 35:1019, 1985.

55. Pizzamiglio L, Frasca R, Guariglia C, Incoccia C, Antonucci G: Effect of opticokinetic stimulation in patients with visual neglect. *Cortex* 26:535, 1990.

56. Biguer B, Donaldson IM, Hein L, Jeannerod M: La vibration des muscles de la nuque modifie la position apparent d'une cible visuelle. *Compte Rendus de l'Academie des Sciences,* 1986.

57. Butter CM, Kirsch NL, Reeves G. The effect of lateralized stimuli on unilateral spatial neglect following right hemi-

sphere lesions. *Restorative Neurology and Neuroscience* 2:39–46, 1990.

58. Rossi PW, Kheyfets S, Reding MJ: Fresnel prisms improve visual perception in stroke patients with homonymous hemianopsia or unilateral visual neglect. *Neurology* 40:1597, 1990.

59. Butter CE, Kirsh N: Combined and separate effects of eye patching and visual stimulation on unilateral neglect following stroke. *Arch Phys Med Rehabil* 73:1133, 1992.

60. Lincoln NB, McGuirk E, Mulley GP, Lendrem W, Jones AC, Mitchell JR: Effectiveness of speech therapy for aphasic stroke patients: A randomised controlled trial. *Lancet* 1:1197, 1984.

61. Wertz RT, Weiss DG, Aten JL, et al: Comparison of clinic, home, and deferred language treatment for aphasia. A Veterans Administration Cooperative Study. *Arch Neurol* 43:653, 1986.

62. Shewan CM, Kertesz A: Effects of speech and language treatment on recovery from aphasia. *Brain Lang* 23: 272, 1984.

63. Wertz RT, Collins MJ, Weiss D, et al: Veterans Administration cooperative study on aphasia: A comparison of individual and group treatment. *J Speech Hear Res* 24: 580, 1981.

64. Hartmann J, Landau WM: Comparison of formal language therapy with supportive counseling for aphasia due to acute vascular accident. *Arch Neurol* 44:646, 1987.

65. Soderback I: The effectiveness of training intellectual functions in adults with acquired brain damage: An evaluation of occupational therapy methods. *Scan J Rehabil Med* 20:47, 1988.

66. Gordon WA, Hibbard MR, Egelko S, Diller L, Shaver MS, Lieberman A, Ragnarsson K: Perceptual remediation in patients with right brain damage: A comprehensive program. *Arch Phys Med Rehabil* 66:353, 1985.

67. AHCPR, 1995.

68. Hachinski VC, Iliff LD, Zilhka, et al: Cerebral blood flow in dementia. *Arch Neurol* 32:632, 1975.

69. Rosen WG, Terry RD, Fuld PA, Katzman R, Peck A: Pathological verification of ischemic score in differentiation of dementias. *Ann Neurol* 7:486, 1980.

70. Erkinjuntti R, Haltia M, Palo J, Sulkava R, Paetau A: Accuracy of the clinical diagnosis of vascular dementia: A prospective clinical and post-mortem neuropathological study. *J Neurol Neurosurg Psychiatry* 51:1037, 1988.

71. World Health Organization: *International Classification of Diseases, Tenth Revision.* Geneva, World Health Organization, 1993.

72. Chui HC, Victoroff JI, Margolin D, Jagust W, Shankle R, Katzman R: Criteria for the diagnosis of ischemic vascular dementia proposed by the State of California Alzheimer Disease Diagnostic and Treatment Centers (ADDTC). *Neurology* 42:473, 1992.

73. Román GC, Tatemichi TK, Erkinjuntti T, et al: Vascular dementia: Diagnostic criteria for research studies. Report of the NINDS-AIREN International Workshop. *Neurology* 43:250, 1993.

74. Wetterling T, Kanitz RD, Borgis KJ: Comparison of different diagnostic criteria for vascular dementia (ADDTC, DSM-IV, ICD-10, NINDS-AIREN). *Stroke* 27:30, 1996.

75. Verhey FRJ, Lodder J, Rozendaal N, Jolles J: Comparison of seven sets of criteria used for the diagnosis of vascular dementia. *Neuroepidemiology* 15:166, 1996.

76. Rockwood K, Parhad I, Hachinski V, et al: Diagnosis of vascular dementia: Consortium of Canadian Centres for clinical cognitive research consensus statement. *Can J Neurol Sci* 21:358, 1994.

77. Chui HC, Mack W, Jackson JE, et al: Clinical criteria for the diagnosis of vascular dementia: A multi-center study of comparability and inter-rates reliability. *Arch Neurol* (in press).

78. Knezevic S, Labs K-H, Kittner B, Rößner, Rother M: The treatment of vascular dementia: Problems and prospects, in Wade J, Knezevic S, Tatemichi T, Erkinjuntti T (eds): *Vascular Dementia: Current Concepts.* New York, John Wiley & Sons Ltd, 1996, pp 301–312.

79. Marler JR, Kozloff RC, Kunitz SC: The NINDS approach to vascular dementia and the ongoing nimodipine clinical trial, in Wade J, Knezevic S, Tatemichi T, Erkinjuntti T (eds): *Vascular Dementia: Current Concepts.* New York, John Wiley & Sons Ltd, 1996, pp 313–329.

80. Schneider LS, Olin JT: Overview of clinical trials of hydergine in dementia. *Arch Neurol* 51:787, 1994.

81. Battaglia A, Bruni G, Ardia A, Sacchetti G: Nicergoline in mild to moderate dementia: A multicenter, double-blind, placebo-controlled study. *J Am Ger Soc* 37:295, 1989.

82. Schneider LS, Olin JT: Meta-analysis of hydergine clinical trials in primary dementia. Neurobiology of Aging (suppl), 1992.

83. Black RS, Barclay LL, Nolan KA, Thaler HT, Hardiman ST, Blass JP. Pentoxifylline in cerebrovascular dementia. *Am Geriatr Soc* 40:237, 1992.

84. Blume J, Ruhlmann KU, De la Haye R, Rettig K: Treatment of chronic cerebrovascular disease in elderly patients with pentoxifylline. *J Med* 23:417, 1992.

85. Folnegovic-Smalc V, et al: European Pentoxifylline Multi-Infarct Dementia Trial (The EPMID) study. Fourth Meeting of the European Neurologial Society, Barcelona, Spain, 25-29 June 1994.

86. Saletu B, MIIller HJ, Grunberger J, et al: Propentofylline in adult-onset cognitive disorders: Double-blind, placebo-controlled, clinical, psychometric, and brain mapping studies. *Neuropsychobiology* 24:173, 1990.

87. Kittner B, for the European Propentofylline Study Group: Propentofylline (HWA 285): A subgroup analysis of phase III clinical studies in Alzheimer's disease and vascular dementia, in Becker R, Giacobini E (eds): *Alzheimer Disease: From Molecular Biology to Therapy.* Boston, Birkh user, 1996, p. 361–365.

88. Vernon MW, Sorkin EM: Piracetam: An overview of its

pharmacological properties and its therapeutic use in senile cognitive disorders. *Drugs Aging* 1:7, 1991.

89. Baumel B, Eisner L, Karukin M, et al: Oxiracetam in the treatment of multi-infarct dementia. *Prog Neuropsychopharmacol Biol Psychiatry* 13:673, 1989.

90. Bottini G, Vallar G, Cappa S, et al: Oxiracetam in dementia: A double-blind, placebo-controlled study. *Acta Neurol Scand* 86:237, 1992.

91. Dominguez K, de Cayaffia CL, Gomensoro J, Aparicio NJ: Modification of psychometric, practical and intellectual parameters in patients with diffuse cerebrovascular insufficiency during prolonged treatment with pentoxifylline: a double-blind, placebo-controlled trial. *Pharmatherapeutica* 1:498, 1977.

92. Harwart D: The treatment of chronic cerebrovascular insufficiency. A double-blind study with pentoxifylline ("Trental" 400). *Curr Med Res Opin* 6:73, 1979.

93. Ghose K: Oxipentfylline in dementia: A controlled study. *Arch Gerontol Geriatr* 6:19, 1987.

94. Maina G, Fiori L, Torta R, Fagiani MB, Ravizza L, Bonavita E, Ghiazza B, Teruzzi F, Zagnoni PG, Ferrario E, et al: Oxiracetam in the treatment of primary degenerative and multi-infarct dementia: A double-blind, placebo-controlled study. *Neuropsychobiology* 21:141, 1989.

95. Villardita C, Grioli S, Lomeo C, Cattaneo C, Parini J: Clinical studies of oxiracetam in patients with dementia of Alzheimer type and multi-infarct dementia of mild to moderate degree. *Neuropsychobiology* 25:24, 1992.

96. Dyksen MW, Katz R, Stallone F, Kuskowski M: Oxiracetam in the treatment of multi-infarct dementia and primary degenerative dementia. *J Neuropsych Clin Neurosci* 1:249, 1989.

97. Ban TA, Morey L, Aguglia E, Azzarelli O, Balsano F, Marigliano V, Caglieris N, Sterlicchio M, Capurso A, Tomasi NA, et al: Nimodipine in the treatment of old age dementias. *Prog Neuropsychopharmacol Biol Psychiatry* 14:525, 1990.

98. Ban TA, Morey LC, Aguglia E, Batista R, Campanella G, Conti L, Dreyfus JF, Fjetland OK, Grossi D, Modaferri A, et al: Glycosaminoglycan polysulfate in the treatment of old age dementias. *Prog Neuro Psychopharm Biol Psychiatr* 15:323, 1991.

99. Kanowski S, Fischhof PK, Grobe-Einsler R, Wagner G, Litschauer G: Efficacy of xantinolnicotinate in patients with dementia. *Pharmacopsychiatry* 23:118, 1990.

100. Passeri M, Cucinotta D: Ateroid in the clinical treatment of multi-infarct dementia. *Mod Prob Pharmacopsychiatry* 23:85, 1989.

101. Nicholson CS: Pharmacology of nootropics and metabolically active compounds in relation to their use in dementia. *Psychopharmacology* 101:147, 1990.

102. Hindmarch I, Fuchs HH, Erzigkeit J: Efficacy and tolerance of vinpocetine in ambulant patients suffering from mild to moderate organic psychosyndromes. *Int Clin Psychopharmacol* 1991; 6:31, 1991.

103. Larson EB, et al: Adverse drug reactions associated with global cognitive impairment in elderly persons. *Ann Intern Med* 107:169, 1987.

104. *Med Lett Drug Ther* 23:9, 1981.

105. Warlow CP, Dennis MS, van Gijn J, Hankey GJ, Sandercock PAG, Bamford JM, Wardlaw J: *Stroke: A Practical Guide to Management.* Oxford, Blackwell Science, 1996, pp 485.

106. Inouye SK, Charpentier PA: Precipitating factors for delirium in hospitalized elderly persons: Predictive model and interrelationship with baseline vulnerability. *JAMA* 275:852, 1996.

107. Wilkinson PR, Wolfe CD, Warbutron FG, et al: A long-term follow-up of stroke patients. *Stroke* 28:507, 1997.

108. Gueyffier F, Boissel J-P, Boutitie F, et al: Effect of antihypertensive treatment in patients having already suffered from stroke: Gathering the evidence. The INDANA (INdividual Data ANalysis of Antihypertensive intervention trials) Project Collaborators. *Stroke* 1997; 28:2557, 1997.

109. Meyer JS, Judd BW, Tawakina T, Rogers RL, Mortel KF: Improved cognition after control of risk factors for multi-infarct dementia. *JAMA* 256:2203, 1986.

110. Meyer JS, Rogers RL, McClintic K, Mortel KF: Controlled clinical trial of daily aspirin therapy in multi-infarct dementia. *Stroke* 19:148, 1988.

111. Wilkinson et al., 1997.

112. Dennis M, O'Rourke S, Lewis S, Sharpe M, Warlow C: A quantitative study of the emotional outcome of people caring for stroke survivors. *Stroke* 29:1867, 1998.

113. Nieboer AP, Schulz R, Matthews KA, Scheier MF, Ormel J, Lindenberg SM: Spousal caregivers' activity restriction and depression: A model for changes over time. *Soc Sci Med* 47:1361, 1998.

114. Scholte OP, Reimer WJ, de Haan RJ, Pijnenborg JM, Limburg M, van den Bos GA: Assessment of burden in partners of stroke patients with sense of competence questionnaires. *Stroke* 29:373, 1998.

115. Forster A, Young J: Specialist nurse support for patients with stroke in the community: A randomized controlled trial. *Brit Med J* 312:1642, 1996.

116. Kotila M, Numminen H, Waltimo O, Kaste M: Depression after stroke: Results of the FINNSTROKE study. *Stroke* 29:368, 1998.

117. Penrod JD, Kane RL, Finch MD, Kane RA: Effects of post-hospital Medicare home health and informal care on patient functional status. *Health Serv Res* 33:513, 1998.

Part 2
EVOLVING AND CONTROVERSIAL THERAPIES IN STROKE

Chapter 11

INTERVENTIONAL NEURORADIOLOGY IN ISCHEMIC STROKE

Y. Pierre Gobin
Fernando Viñuela

INTRODUCTION

The interventional neuroradiologist is responsible for the endovascular treatment of cerebrovascular diseases. The potential therapeutic alternatives offered by interventional neuroradiology in the management of ischemic stroke are enticing. Explosive progress in the development of catheters, microcatheters, angioplasty balloons, and stents has improved these devices for enhanced navigation and therapy of the brachiocephalic vessels.

Although endovascular techniques have never been studied in prospective randomized scientific trials, strong clinical evidence supports endovascular therapy as the first choice for symptomatic stenosis of proximal aortic arch lesions (subclavian, innominate, vertebral, and common carotid arteries). In the intracranial circulation, endovascular therapeutic techniques may be indicated for symptomatic stenoses resistant to medical therapy and emergency intra-arterial thrombolysis in the posterior circulation. On the other hand, percutaneous angioplasty of the carotid artery bifurcation and intra-arterial thrombolysis of embolic phenomena in the anterior circulation should be performed only in high-risk patients and/or in the context of a clinical trial. We will describe the role of interventional neuroradiology for the treatment of ischemic stroke in three sections: intra-arterial thrombolysis, angioplasty of brachiocephalic vessels, and intracranial angioplasty.

INTRA-ARTERIAL THROMBOLYSIS

Background

Cerebral angiography performed during the acute phase of an ischemic stroke will demonstrate an intracranial arterial occlusion in 75 to 80 percent of cases.[1,2] Arterial occlusions may be located in the cervical internal carotid artery (ICA) in one-third of cases, in the proximal M1 segment of middle cerebral artery (MCA) in another third, and in distal MCA branches in the remaining one third. The 20 to 25 percent of patients with a negative cerebral angiogram may be explained by early recanalization or occlusion of a small artery not visible on cerebral angiography.

Intracranial arterial occlusion is most often the result of an embolus originating from an atheromatous plaque in the common carotid artery bifurcation, the aortic arch, or the heart. These emboli rarely contain atheromatous material. More often, they are simply thrombi that potentially can be dissolved by thrombolytic agents. Less frequently, intracranial arterial occlusion is related to atherothrombosis in cerebral arteries.

The success of thrombolysis depends on the quality and age of the thrombus. Old thrombi are more difficult to treat than fresh thrombi. For example, intra-arterial thrombolysis of thrombi formed on the surface of catheters during vascular procedures is highly successful because the fresh clot is easily dissolved by thrombolytic agents.

The idea of treating ischemic stroke with thrombolysis has been known for a long time. Intravenous thrombolysis was first performed in the 1960's. Initial clinical trials had negative results, showing no clinical improvement and even deterioration because of hemorrhagic complications. In retrospect, those results are not unexpected given current knowledge that late thrombolysis, sometimes several days after the initial stroke, is associated with increased hemorrhagic complications. Furthermore, patients with hematomas were not excluded because computed tomography (CT) scan was not available. Interest in thrombolysis then dissipated, until several factors led to the recent rebirth of this therapy. First, experimental work proved the concept of the ischemic penumbra, the potentially salvable ischemic brain around an infarction, and showed that arterial revascularization was beneficial when performed early after onset of stroke in animal models. Second, CT scanners became widely available. In addition, thrombolysis was successfully used in myocardial infarction, pulmonary emboli, and ischemia in the peripheral arterial circulation.

There are both advantages and inconveniences when comparing intravenous vs. intra-arterial intracranial thrombolysis. The first advantage of intra-arterial thrombolysis is that a cerebral angiogram is automatically obtained as the first step of the procedure. The angiogram may demonstrate an intracranial arterial occlusion. If the angiogram is negative because the stroke is due to small vessel disease or the thrombus has already dissolved, the administration of potentially dangerous thrombolytic agent may be avoided. The cerebral angiogram may also identify the site and cause of the arterial occlusion (tandem lesion, dissection, partially thrombosed aneurysm) and therefore modify the indication and the technique of revascularization. A second advantage of the intra-arterial approach is that it allows selective delivery of highly concentrated thrombolytic agent into thrombus. Furthermore, the manipulation of the clot by the microcatheter-microguidewire combination allows mechanical disruption of the thrombus. Thus, it is not surprising that intra-arterial thrombolysis results in a 60 to 90 percent recanalization rate, whereas recanalization with intravenous thrombolysis succeeds in 30 to 50 percent of the cases.[3,4] An additional advantage of this technique is that during intra-arterial thrombolysis, the progression of recanalization can be followed by successive angiograms, and the infusion may be dis-

continued as soon as arterial recanalization occurs. Such a tailored dose of thrombolytic agent in the intra-arterial technique contrasts with the "one-dose-fits-all" method of intravenous thrombolysis.

Although intra-arterial thrombolysis provides many benefits over intravenous thrombolysis, there are drawbacks to this mode of administration. First, the intra-arterial approach is more invasive. However, very few complications, such as groin hematoma, arterial perforation, or dissection, have been attributed to the angiography and intracranial selective catheterization. Second, it takes more time to initiate thrombolytic administration (longer time to treatment). Intravenous thrombolysis can be initiated immediately after CT scan interpretation, whereas intra-arterial thrombolysis requires preparation of the patient and angiography suite. The patient needs to be brought to the angio room, and an emergency cerebral angiogram is performed. Then the site of the thrombus must be superselectively catheterized before actual administration of the thrombolytic agent. However, it is important to understand that the important time interval is the time to recanalization more than the time to initiation of treatment. A common misunderstanding is that clot dissolves during or soon after the 1-h intravenous infusion of recombinant tissue-type plasminogen activator (rt-Pa). Recanalization after thrombolysis may actually take several hours. The time to recanalization is 1 to 2 h for intra-arterial thrombolysis, and is most likely longer for intravenous thrombolysis. Therefore, the more effective and possibly faster recanalization obtained with the intra-arterial approach may outweigh the delay in time to treatment. Despite better recanalization rate, intra-arterial thrombolysis has not been proven to be more effective than intravenous thrombolysis in terms of clinical outcome, and both have the same rate of symptomatic intracranial hematoma (5 to 15 percent). The main advantage of intravenous thrombolysis is its simple technique, whereas intra-arterial thrombolysis requires a special infrastructure and personnel: an angiography suite with a radiology technician, an interventional neuroradiologist (or a physician well trained in cerebral catheterization), and an anesthetist must be available within 30 min of the patient's admission.

Intra-arterial thrombolysis may be the choice for recanalization of large vessels such as the ICA, the M1 segment of the middle cerebral artery, and the posterior circulation, whereas intravenous thrombolysis may be optimal for distal arterial occlusions.[5] A prospective trial randomizing intravenous vs. intra-arterial approach is necessary to evaluate better the benefits and disadvantages of both techniques.

Evidence

Several recent prospective randomized trials on the use of intravenous thrombolysis for stroke have been performed. Those trials performed with streptokinase were discontinued prematurely because of an increased incidence of hemorrhage in the treatment group. Two studies were performed with rt-PA.[6,7] The European ECASS study showed that in acute cerebral ischemia, intravenous thrombolysis performed within 6 h of onset with 1.1 mg/kg rt-PA did not improve clinical outcome in the overall (intention-to-treat) population because of an increased rate of hemorrhages in patients who received rt-PA. The clinical outcome was improved in the target population when patients with abnormal CT scans and other predetermined exclusions were omitted from the analysis. The National Institute of Neurological Disorders and Stroke (NINDS) study showed that intravenous thrombolysis with 0.9 mg/kg rt-PA administered within 3 h of onset resulted in a 12 percent increase in the number of patients with good recovery at 3 months. The hemorrhage rate in the treatment group was 20 percent in the ECASS study and 6.4 percent in the NINDS study. The positive results of the NINDS study led to the acceptance of clinical application of intravenous thrombolysis.[8]

The first intra-arterial thrombolysis for ischemic stroke was reported by Zeumer et al in patients with acute posterior circulation ischemia.[9] The natural history of posterior circulation strokes is so dismal that a placebo control study was not needed to prove that intra-arterial thrombolysis could improve patient outcome by recanalizing arteries in the vertebrobasilar circulation.[10] This preliminary clinical experience was followed by several small series of intra-arterial thrombolysis in posterior and also anterior circulations.[10–12] Many case series have been more recently reported, and finally, a randomized prospective trial tested intra-arterial infusion of recombinant pro-urokinase (rpro-UK) vs. placebo in middle cerebral artery occlusion.[13] In 46 patients, 58 percent recanalized with rpro-UK compared with 14 percent with placebo. There was a 42 percent rate of hemorrhage with a 15 percent rate of clinical deterioration. Recanalization was more likely when high doses of heparin were simultaneously given, an expected association, given the pharmacology of rpro-UK. However, higher heparin dose was also associated with higher rate of hemorrhage. All five patients with CT evidence of hypodensity involving more than one-third of the hemisphere developed hemorrhage at the ischemic site.

We have treated 26 patients with intra-arterial thrombolysis for acute ischemic stroke in the anterior circulation at UCLA Medical Center between 1993 and 1997. All patients had CT before the procedure to exclude hemorrhage. Fifteen patients had normal CT scan, whereas 11 patients had evidence of early stroke. Cerebral angiography showed nine patients with ICA occlusion, and of these, five also had clot migration into the MCA. Eight patients had clot in the proximal MCA, whereas nine had clot in the distal MCA branches. Urokinase, in doses ranging from 150,000 IU to 1.2 million IU, was used as thrombolytic agent. Time from onset to initiation of thrombolysis averaged 4 h, 30 min. Overall, recanalization was judged complete or near complete in 42 percent of patients, partial in 23 percent, and unsuccessful in 34 percent. There were 34 percent hemorrhages, of which one-third were symptomatic and one fatal. Post-thrombolysis hemorrhage was highly associated with early signs of stroke in the pre-procedure CT. Eight patients (30 percent) died. Of those, seven had minimal or no recanalization after thrombolysis, and the one patient with recanalization had a large cerebral hematoma. Ten patients (38 percent) had a good outcome. Of those, 7 had complete or near complete recanalization and 3 had no recanalization.

Our institution has also been involved in the EMS bridging trial (unpublished results) randomizing the administration of intravenous rt-PA vs. placebo followed by intra-arterial rt-PA. Two-thirds of the dose of rt-PA was given intravenously immediately after a negative CT scan, and one-third was given intra-arterially. This dual mode of administration aimed to combine the expediency offered by intravenous delivery with the better recanalization rate offered by intra-arterial delivery.

Therapeutic Recommendation

Indications The exclusion criteria for intra-arterial thrombolysis are the same as for intravenous thrombolysis. They include recent major surgery or trauma, active or recent hemorrhage in the previous 2 weeks, history of intracranial hemorrhage, recent major stroke, uncontrolled hypertension and bleeding disorders, and any kind of intracranial hemorrhage on the CT scan.

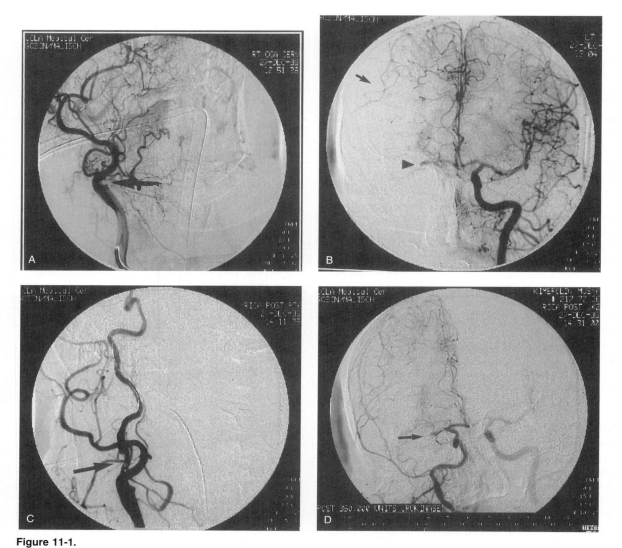

Figure 11-1.

Case 1. A 68-year-old female presented with sudden onset of left brachiofacial paralysis. The CT scan performed 4 h after onset was normal. Being outside the 3-h window for intravenous thrombolysis with rt-PA, the patient was immediately brought to the angiography suite for endovascular therapy. A   Right common carotid angiogram, cervical view, anteroposterior projection. The internal carotid artery is occluded at its origin (arrow), and only the external carotid artery and its branches are seen. Calcifications of the internal carotid artery origin were seen on the plain films (not shown). B   Left carotid injection, intracranial view, anteroposterior projection. There is partial filling of the right hemispheric arteries through the anterior communicating artery. The right middle cerebral artery is occluded (arrowhead) after the origins of the internal lenticulostriate arteries. The right anterior cerebral artery fills the distal middle cerebral artery branches via pial anastomoses (arrow). This angiogram allowed precise assessment of the situation; this patient had a longstanding silent atheromatous plaque of the internal carotid artery origin. When the atheromatous plaque thrombosed, an embolus migrated into the middle cerebral artery. The decision was to revascularize both the internal carotid and middle cerebral arteries. C   Common carotid injection, cervical view, anteroposterior projection, after revascularization of the internal carotid artery with injection of 350,000 IU urokinase and balloon angioplasty with a 3-mm-diameter balloon. There is a residual stenosis of the internal carotid artery origin (arrow). D   Common carotid injection, intracranial view, anteroposterior projection, after revascularization of the internal carotid artery. The middle cerebral artery occlusion is better seen (arrow). A microcatheter was navigated to contact the thrombus.

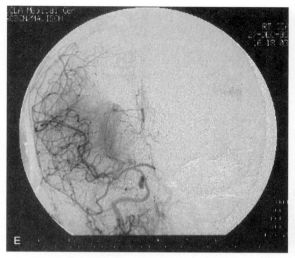
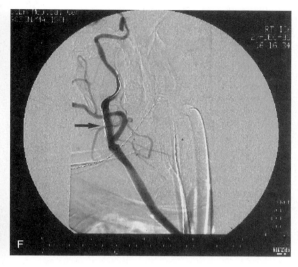

Figure 11-1. (*Continued*)
E   *Common carotid injection intracranial view, anteroposterior projection, after injection of 750,000 IU urokinase over 90 mins. There is complete reopening of the middle cerebral artery and its branches. F   Common carotid injection, cervical view, anteroposterior projection, after treatment of the residual stenosis with additional angioplasty and stenting* (arrow). *The patient recovered completely from her deficit.*

Early head CT signs of ischemic stroke such as hyperdense MCA sign, sulcal effacement, insular ribbon sign, loss of gray-white matter distinction, or hypodensity less than one-third of the hemisphere do not contraindicate intra-arterial thrombolysis. A large area of hypodensity involving more than one-third of the hemisphere[13,14] is a contraindication because it predicts a high incidence of post-treatment hemorrhage.

In our institution, intravenous thrombolysis is performed if treatment can be administered within 3 h of onset and the patient has a moderate stroke in the anterior circulation. Intra-arterial thrombolysis is used if the patient presents beyond 3 h of stroke onset, if he has a severe stroke, or if the stroke is in the posterior circulation. In addition, angiography may be required if the mechanism of stroke is uncertain. For example, if an intracranial dissection or aneurysm is suspected based on CT scan or clinical presentation, the angiogram may establish the cause of the stroke and may modify the indication or the technique of thrombolysis. Intra-arterial thrombolysis is also indicated for embolic complications of angiographic and neurointerventional procedures if the primary disease allows its safe administration.

In the posterior circulation, intra-arterial thrombolysis is performed for stroke in progression with moderate to severe neurologic deficit related to bilateral vertebral or basilar artery occlusion. The natural history of this type of ischemic stroke is so severe that intra-arterial thrombolysis is performed because it provides the best chance of rapid recanalization.[15] In addition, the intra-arterial approach allows for associated balloon angioplasty in atherothrombotic lesions. In contrast to the anterior circulation, there is no real time window, but intra-arterial thrombolysis is not indicated in cases of large cerebellar hypodensity, deep coma for more than 6 h, or loss of brainstem reflexes.

In the anterior circulation, intra-arterial thrombolysis is performed in cases of severe stroke associated with a hyperdense middle cerebral artery on the CT scan. In those circumstances, the embolus tends to be large, and the intra-arterial approach offers a better chance of faster recanalization. The suspicion of a tandem arterial lesion with occlusion of the cervical carotid artery by a plaque or dissection is also an indication for the intra-arterial approach because it allows simultaneous treatment of the carotid lesion with angioplasty and stenting (Fig. 11-1).

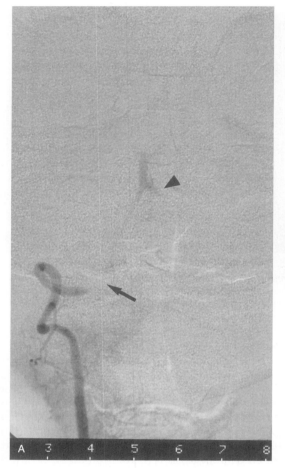

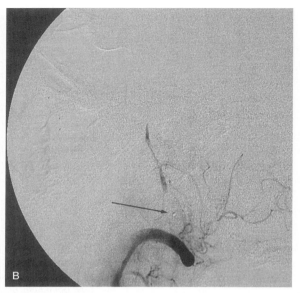

Figure 11-2.
Case 2. This 62-year-old male presented with recurrent episodes of tetraparesis and multiple cranial nerve palsy. A Right vertebral artery injection, anteroposterior view, showed a subtotal occlusion of the intracranial vertebral artery (arrow). There is a faint injection of the basilar artery (arrow) and reflux into the right vertebral artery (arrowhead). The complete cerebral angiogram (not shown) showed proximal occlusion of the left vertebral artery and partial filling of the distal basilar artery through the posterior communicating artery. The decision was to reopen the right vertebral artery. B Right vertebral artery angiogram, lateral view, showing the subtotal occlusion of the artery and the tip of the microcatheter within the thrombus (arrow).

Intra-arterial thrombolysis is also indicated if the patient presents after the 3-h therapeutic window for intravenous rt-PA therapy and the CT scan does not contraindicate thrombolysis. A small clinical series recently reported intra-arterial thrombolysis performed even later than six h after onset and showed benefits from intra-arterial thrombolysis if the initial CT scan was normal.[16]

Technique   A stroke code should be planned to minimize the time from patient arrival to the emergency room to initiation of treatment. At UCLA Medical Center, as soon as the patient presents to the ER with stroke symptoms, the stroke team is alerted, and a head CT scan is performed. The stroke neurologist examines the patient and reviews the CT scan. Intravenous thrombol-

ysis is administered if indicated. If intra-arterial thrombolysis is indicated (as described above), the interventional neuroradiologist is called, and the angiographic room is prepared. The patient or a close family member is consented for cerebral angiography and possible intra-arterial thrombolysis by the interventional neuroradiologist, and the patient is rapidly transported to the neuroangiography suite.

The presence of anesthesia coverage facilitates monitoring of vital signs, patient sedation, or the administration of general anesthesia if needed. The patient may be agitated, aphasic, or have trouble ventilating or swallowing. The management of arterial blood pressure during intra-arterial thrombolysis is very important. Approximately two-thirds of the patients are hypertensive. Moderate hypertension may be necessary to improve

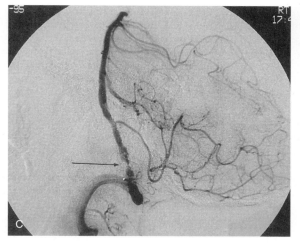

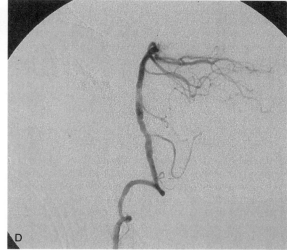

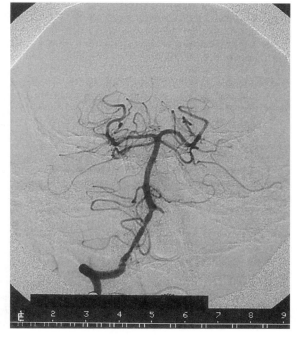

Figure 11-2. (*Continued*)
C *Right vertebral artery angiogram, lateral view, after infusion of 750,000 IU urokinase over 90 min, showing reopening of the vertebral artery with antegrade filling of the basilar artery and its branches, and a residual severe stenosis of the vertebral artery (arrow). Because of the risk of rethrombosis, balloon angioplasty was performed.* D *and* E *Right vertebral artery angiography, anteroposterior* (D) *and lateral* (E) *views after balloon angioplasty, showing a good angiographic result* (*compare with panels* A *and* B). *The patient made a complete recovery.*

cerebral perfusion, but uncontrollable hypertension is associated with a higher risk of hemorrhage when arterial recanalization and cerebral reperfusion occur. Our policy is not to treat moderate hypertension and to reduce severe hypertension to 150 to 170 mmHg systolic and 95 to 105 mmHg diastolic. If the patient is not hypertensive, we administer moderate fluid expansion with saline and macromolecules. Low-dose heparin is given, 3000 IU by intravenous bolus after the diagnostic angiogram, followed by 1000 IU/h.

The cerebral angiogram is performed by transfemoral approach. First, the suspected vessel (common carotid or vertebral artery) is catheterized, and cervical and intracranial views are obtained. Additional catheterizations to evaluate brain collateral circulation are also performed. Figures 11-1 and 11-2 are examples of intra-arterial thrombolysis in the anterior and posterior circulation.

After this angiogram, the stroke team selects the appropriate therapeutic management. If intra-arterial thrombolysis is selected, we frequently use urokinase, which is as effective as rt-PA for intra-arterial thrombolysis.[17] The urokinase solution is prepared by dissolving 500,000 IU in 60 cc of saline. A microcatheter and microguidewire combination is used to place the tip of the microcatheter immediately proximal to the clot. This placement generally takes no more than a few minutes. The urokinase is infused in small boluses of 0.1 cc at a rate of 1 cc/min over 5 min. Then, using the microguidewire, the microcatheter is passed distal to the clot, and urokinase is infused distal to and into the clot. Gentle manipulation of the microguidewire is performed within the thrombus to provide some mechanical disruption. Cerebral angiograms are performed through the guiding catheter every 10 to 15 min to check the progress of thrombolysis. If the clot partially dissolves, it may fragment and migrate distally. Then, the microcatheter is advanced to follow the clot, and the microcatheter tip is again placed in contact with the clot to repeat the process. When the clot fragments and migrates into several branches, the one serving the most eloquent territories is treated first. Thrombolysis is stopped when complete or subtotal revascularization is obtained or when the maximal dose of 1 million IU urokinase over 2 h has been given. In cases of cervical or intracranial artery stenosis, balloon angioplasty can be performed during the same procedure, especially if the stenosis is severe with risk of reocclusion.

After intra-arterial thrombolysis, the femoral sheath is left in place for 24 h. Heparin is discontinued but not reversed. A CT scan is always performed after the procedure before the patient is admitted to the neurology intensive care unit.

ANGIOPLASTY OF BRACHIOCEPHALIC ARTERIES

Background

Angioplasty has been the most important technique in the field of Interventional Radiology. Invented by Gruntzig in the early 1970's, inflation of a balloon at the site of an arterial stenosis is actually a "controlled and limited traumatic injury" to the artery. Angioplasty results in rupture of the intima and media, compression and rupture of the atheromatous plaque, and stretching of the artery. Healing occurs by formation of a neointima, smoother and less thrombogenic than the original atheromatous plaque. The first percutaneous transluminal angioplasty (PTA) of a brachiocephalic artery was performed in the early 1980's.[18,19] Since then, multiple case series have demonstrated that angioplasty of brachiocephalic arteries can be performed with a high technical success rate and few complications. Specifically, the most concerning complication was emboli from atheromatous debris fragmented from the plaque during angioplasty. This embolic complication was rarely clinically detected, probably because the emboli are small.

In the arterial circulation, atherosclerosis involves primarily bifurcations or origins, and plaques in the brachiocephalic arteries are no exception. Atheromatous lesions are commonly located at the carotid bifurcation and the origin of the common carotid, subclavian, innominate, and vertebral arteries. At the carotid bifurcation, plaques are frequently ulcerated and harbor thrombotic plugs, whereas in other sites, plaques are most often fibrous and uncomplicated. This explains the concern regarding cerebral emboli that might be associated with carotid bifurcation angioplasty but not with angioplasty in other locations of the brachiocephalic arteries. There are several reasons to perform angioplasty at a stenosis: (1) to enlarge the artery at the site of stenosis, thus increasing flow and distal perfusion pressure, and (2) to prevent distal embolization, first by enlarging the artery to provide smoother arterial flow with less turbulence and blood stagnation, and second by altering the characteristics of the atheromatous plaque with remodeling of the arterial wall and proliferation of a smooth, less thrombogenic neointima.

The most recent advance in angioplasty of brachiocephalic arteries has been the use of intravascular stents.[20] Stents improve short-term angioplasty results because they resist the arterial wall recoil, which tends to occur immediately after angioplasty and prevent the progression of dissection, which frequently complicates angioplasty. Eventually, the neointima that forms covers the stent, and the stent is incorporated into the arterial wall. Stents are also beneficial in the long term, as they decrease rate of restenosis.

Evidence

Because of the different pathophysiologic mechanisms, causes, treatment options, trials, and prognosis, it is logical to consider atherosclerosis of the carotid artery bifurcation separately from stenosis in other locations or nonatherosclerotic stenoses.

Atherosclerosis of the Carotid Artery Bifurcation A frequent condition and a major cause of strokes, carotid artery bifurcation atherosclerosis is a disease for which several prospective randomized trials have established level I evidence and guidelines for therapy. The two largest, the North American Symptomatic Carotid Endarterectomy trials (NASCET) and the Asymptomatic Carotid Atherosclerosis Study (ACAS), focused on comparing surgical and medical treatment. The NASCET trial demonstrated a dramatic benefit of surgery for patients with a greater than 70 percent stenosis and a significant but smaller benefit to patients with 50 to 69 percent stenosis. In the NASCET trial, there was a 7.5 percent risk of ipsilateral stroke or death in the perioperative period. The ACAS trial demonstrated the advantage of surgery over medical therapy in selected patients with greater than 60 percent stenosis when surgery could be performed with less than 3 percent perioperative morbidity and mortality. Both trials demonstrated the long-term efficacy of carotid endarterectomy in preventing stroke and death in selected (low-risk) patients when the surgery was performed by an expert surgeon. In contrast to carotid endarterectomy, carotid angioplasty has been reported only in case series, which may potentially be biased in patient selection, follow-up, and reporting.[21] Another consideration is that carotid bifurcation plaques have a more thrombogenic nature, which raises concern of cerebral embolic complications. Balloon protection of the internal carotid artery with a triple coaxial system to decrease untoward cerebral embolization[22] is a promising technique, but its procedural complexity prevents widespread application. Another example of the still evolving technical aspects of carotid angioplasty is the use of stents.[23] Although the idea is promising, a stent adapted to the carotid bifurcation, avoiding the risk of occlusion of the external carotid artery, still has to be developed. Furthermore, the long-term patency of stents in this location is unknown. In conclusion, current clinical evidence showing the benefit of carotid endarterectomy precludes performing carotid angioplasty for atherosclerosis in patients with low surgical risk, except perhaps in the context of a trial.

Stenosis in Other Locations or Nonatherosclerotic Lesions This category includes atheromatous and nonatheromatous stenoses of the subclavian, innominate, common carotid, and vertebral arteries, as well as nonatheromatous stenoses of the internal carotid artery. Causes of nonatheromatous stenosis include fibromuscular dysplasia, Takayasu's and other inflammatory ar-

teritis, and radiation therapy. In these locations, surgery is a more complicated procedure, using bypass or vessel transposition and sometimes an intrathoracic approach. Multiple case series have reported good results.[24–26] However, PTA has an equivalent excellent long-term patency rate and low morbidity and mortality with an added advantage, ability to treat several lesions at once. Furthermore, the time of arterial occlusion during PTA is limited to the period during which the balloon is inflated and lasts only 1 or 2 min, whereas during surgery, the duration of arterial occlusion is much longer. Patients with multiple occlusive disease may not tolerate lengthy occlusion during surgery, thus the use of a temporary shunt, a more complex procedure, may be required in conjunction with the operation. Because plaques in these regions are less thrombogenic than those at the carotid bifurcation, embolic complications are less of a concern during angioplasty. In cases of restenosis, repeating angioplasty is no more difficult than the first time, whereas the second surgery is more intricate. Finally, as angioplasty is performed under local anesthesia, the patient can return to his previous activities the following day. A recent review of the major reported cases series[27] found close to 1000 patients reported with a 95 percent technical success rate, 4 percent incidence of stroke, no deaths, and 5.7 percent restenosis rate at a mean follow-up of 54 months. Although these results are impressive, the results of these series must be interpreted with caution. One prospective study, the North American Cerebral Percutaneous Transluminal Angioplasty Registry (NACPTAR), which organized a multicenter database of angioplasty in patients with symptomatic, nonsurgical extracranial and intracranial atheromatous stenoses, reported a stroke rate of 7 percent and mortality of 1.8 percent, both of which are higher than any case series previously reported.[28] Another prospective trial, Carotid and Vertebral Artery Transluminal Angioplasty Study (CAVATAS), compares surgery with angioplasty for carotid and vertebral artery stenosis. This trial finished enrolling patients in 1997, and results should be available soon.

Therapeutic Recommendation

Indications The following indications for angioplasty of brachiocephalic arteries are based on the studies and other information presented in the "Evidence" section.

Atheromatous stenosis at the carotid bifurcation should be treated by carotid endarterectomy if the patient is a good surgical candidate and if the stenosis is

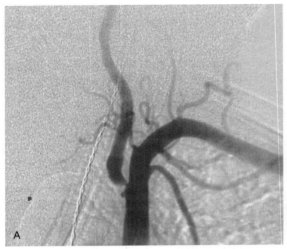
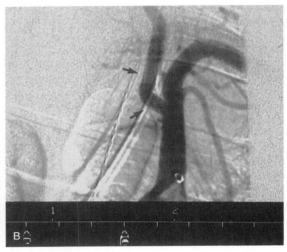

Figure 11-3.
Case 3. This 50-year-old male presented with transient ischemic attacks in the posterior circulation.
A Left subclavian artery angiogram, anteroposterior view, showed a severe and irregular stenosis
at the origin of the left vertebral artery. B Left subclavian artery angiogram, anteroposterior view,
after balloon angioplasty and stenting showing a good angiographic result (arrow *points to the two*
Palmaz stents). There was no recurrence of the TIA.

(1) more than 70 percent (symptomatic or asymptomatic), (2) symptomatic and greater than 50 percent, and (3) asymptomatic and 60 to 70 percent in males. Patients with a lesser degree of stenosis should be treated medically with 325 mg of aspirin per day. Unlike surgery, the indications for percutaneous carotid angioplasty are not well defined by a high degree of evidence based on prospective randomized trials. At our institution, angioplasty is performed in patients whose symptoms and degree of stenosis indicate surgical treatment but who are high surgical risk candidates (patients with severe medical conditions or patients with multiple vessel disease who cannot tolerate lengthy occlusion). Also, angioplasty may be preferred in cases of postsurgical restenosis or high internal carotid artery lesions because it is less invasive. The presence of tandem arterial stenoses, where the carotid bifurcation lesion is associated with a stenosis of the common carotid artery or the intracranial internal carotid artery, is also a good indication for angioplasty, as both lesions can be simultaneously treated endovascularly. Finally, we have on two occasions performed angioplasty with stent at the carotid artery bifurcation after intra-arterial thrombolysis of a middle cerebral artery embolus.

We recommend that angioplasty should be preferred to surgery for all stenoses of the brachiocephalic arteries except atheromatous stenosis of the carotid artery bifurcation. In our opinion, angioplasty is indicated in symptomatic patients with severe (greater than 70 percent) stenosis or in symptomatic patients resistant to medical therapy. In cases of multiple stenoses, we would treat first the symptomatic one and treat the asymptomatic (during the same session) only if it were severe.

Technique Figures 11-3 and 11-4 are examples of angioplasty of brachiocephalic arteries. Most patients are already on aspirin. If not, aspirin, 325 mg per day, is started the day before the procedure. The procedure is performed under mild sedation with local anesthesia at the puncture site, usually the groin. General anesthesia is necessary only in patients with multiple arterial occlusion, in whom temporary flow arrest during the 1 min of balloon inflation may not be tolerated. As soon as the arterial sheath is in place, anticoagulation is begun with 5000 IU, of heparin given IV followed by 1000 IU/h. A complete cerebral angiogram is performed to study all brachiocephalic arteries and the intracranial circulation to assess cerebral arterial collaterals. An 80-cm-long, 7F or 8F sheath is placed proximal to the stenosis. This large size sheath is necessary for stenting. The stenosis is traversed with a 0.035 guidewire and 5F cathe-

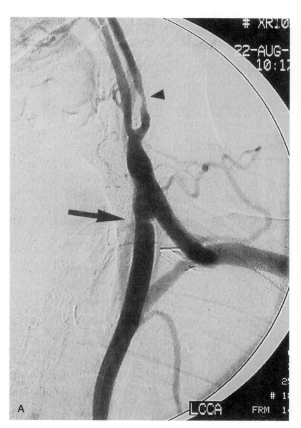
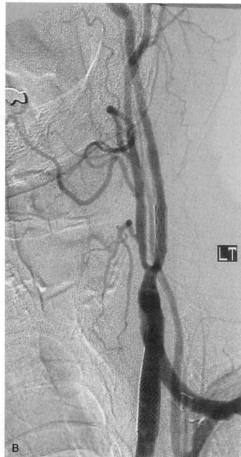

Figure 11-4.
Case 4. This 54-year-old female developed coldness in her left arm and vertigo due to subclavian steal syndrome secondary to left subclavian artery thrombosis. She was treated by a left common carotid to subclavian artery bypass. After temporary relief, her symptoms recurred. A   The left carotid angiogram, oblique view, demonstrated a dissection with severe stenosis of the common carotid artery below the bypass (arrow) *and severe stenosis of the left internal carotid artery* (arrowhead). B   *Control angiogram after angioplasty and stenting of the common carotid artery dissection and internal carotid artery stenosis demonstrated a good angiographic result with no residual stenosis. The patient became asymptomatic.*

ter, or, if very tight, it is crossed with a microcatheter and microguidewire before advancing the 5F catheter. A 0.025 I exchange guidewire is placed and will stay across the stenosis during the entire procedure. The catheter is exchanged for the balloon catheter. The balloon should be the diameter of the normal artery or up to 10 percent larger. The sizes used are 6 to 8 mm for the common carotid, 4 to 6 mm for the internal carotid, 3 to 6 mm for the vertebral, 7 to 10 mm for the subclavian, and 8 to 12 mm for the innominate artery. The length of the balloon should match the length of the stenosis and cover it entirely. If the balloon is too long, it will injure the normal artery, but if it is too short it will be unstable and slip during inflation. Both situations should be avoided as they increase intimal damage and risk of thrombosis. The length of the balloon is usually 20 mm, sometimes 40 mm. Under fluoroscopic control, the balloon is slowly inflated at a pressure of 8 to 12 atm and kept inflated for 1 min. When the stenosis is very severe, angioplasty is first performed with an undersized balloon (this is called pre-angioplasty) before angioplasty with the appropriately sized balloon. The balloon is deflated and removed with the guidewire still across the stenosis, and an angiogram is done. Then, an intravascular stent (Palmaz or Wallstents) is placed across the stenosis. Intravascular stents are indicated for most atherosclerotic lesions, especially when the result of angioplasty is imperfect because of residual stenosis or dissection. At the end of the procedure, heparin is not reversed but wears off over the next few hours, and the sheath is pulled out once the partial thromboplastin time (PTT) is back to normal. The patient is discharged the following day on aspirin.

Patients are followed at 3, 6, 12, and 24 months. The anatomic result of angioplasty is followed by Doppler ultrasound, MRA, or in cases of subclavian stenosis, comparative blood pressure on both arms. In case of restenosis (5 to 7 percent), a second angioplasty may be performed when the restenosis becomes symptomatic or anatomically severe (70 percent or more).

INTRACRANIAL ANGIOPLASTY

Background

Intracranial atheromatous stenosis develops in association with global atherosclerosis with a predilection for the Asian and African populations. The clinical presentation may be related to distal embolization, hemodynamic compromise owing to reduced distal blood flow, or compromise of the ostium of a perforating artery originating at the level of the stenosis. These mechanisms are difficult to distinguish and may coexist. In contrast to an embolus, which causes maximal symptoms at onset, an in situ thrombus manifests either by crescendo TIA or by progressive symptoms.[29] Intracranial stenoses evolve; a study with angiographic follow-up over 26.7 months demonstrated 20 percent regression, 40 percent stable lesions, and 40 percent progression of the stenosis.[30] Progression of the stenosis to complete occlusion can lead to a stroke if there are no collaterals. Yet the patient's symptoms may improve or disappear

if collateralization is adequate or if distal embolizations stopped with complete arterial occlusion.

The prognosis for an individual patient with intracranial stenosis is difficult to analyze because the stenosis may be asymptomatic for a long time, and transient ischemic events may occur in flurries. In the medical treatment arm of the extracranial to intracranial (EC/IC) bypass study group, patients treated with aspirin had a 7 to 8 percent ipsilateral stroke rate for stenoses and occlusions of the middle cerebral artery[31] and stenoses of the intracranial internal carotid artery.[32] Less data are available on the prognosis of posterior circulation stenosis. One study of patients with basilar and distal vertebral artery stenosis[33] showed 4.3 percent strokes per year in the vertebrobasilar territory. However, stenosis in the posterior circulation is, in our experience, more dangerous than in the anterior circulation. Reports on intracranial stenosis in the posterior circulation may be biased because of increased mortality at symptom onset, and only less aggressive stenoses can be followed in the retrospective studies reported.

Evidence

In the anterior circulation, intracranial stenoses have historically been treated surgically by EC/IC arterial bypass, until a prospective study randomizing patients to surgery vs. medical therapy failed to show a benefit from surgery.[32] Interestingly, even the group of patients expected to benefit most from surgery, those with middle cerebral artery or distal internal carotid artery occlusion, did not show improvement. Patients with stenosis in the posterior circulation and vertebrobasilar insufficiency treated with intracranial bypass demonstrated a high rate of morbidity and mortality, especially patients with stroke-in-evolution.[34] Currently, EC/IC bypass is rarely performed to treat intracranial stenosis, whereas case series of balloon angioplasty are increasingly being reported.

Balloon angioplasty in the intracranial circulation has problems specific to this vital location. The thin media of intracranial arteries are more vulnerable to rupture during balloon inflation than extracranial or coronary arteries. The stenoses are often located close to perforating arteries feeding critical territories, and these branches may be easily occluded due to displacement of the plaque or intimal dissection during angioplasty. Finally, although stents are an important part of angioplasty to avoid recoiling and treat dissections, they are extremely difficult to use in the intracranial

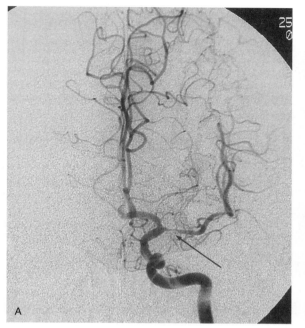

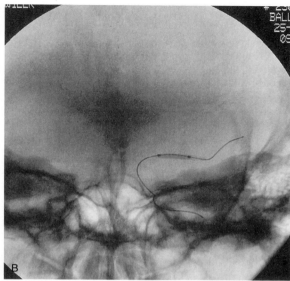

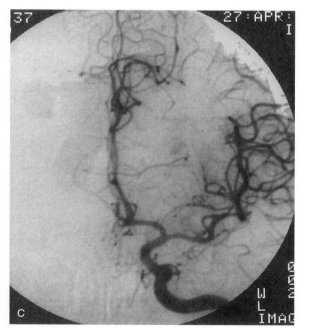

Figure 11-5.

Case 5. This 42-year-old male presented with recurrent episodes of right hemiparesis and aphasia. An outside angiogram showed a severe stenosis of the left middle cerebral artery. Symptoms persisted despite medical therapy, including anticoagulation with heparin, aspirin, and fluid expansion. It was decided to treat with balloon angioplasty. A The left internal carotid angiogram, anteroposterior view, showed a severe stenosis of the proximal M1 segment of the middle cerebral artery (arrow). B Unsubstracted anteroposterior view during balloon angioplasty of the stenosis. C Left internal carotid angiogram, anteroposterior view, after angioplasty showing good angiographic result with minimal residual stenosis. There was no recurrence of symptoms, and the patient was discharged 3 days after the procedure on 325 mg of aspirin daily.

arteries, and no specific stent for intracranial use has been developed yet.

The first angioplasty for intracranial artery stenosis was reported in 1980.[35] Since then, case reports and several small series have been published. Seven case series have reported 125 cases.[36–42] Angioplasty was anatomically successful in 82 percent, with a 10 percent permanent complication rate and 1 percent mortality. Successful angioplasty reversed symptoms in 80 percent of patients. Restenosis rates varied considerably, from 0 to 40 percent. Restenoses were observed early, usually within 6 months after angioplasty. Angioplasty can also be performed for revascularization of completely blocked arteries, a more challenging procedure. One recent series reported four successful recanalizations of six occluded middle cerebral arteries.[43]

Therapeutic Recommendation

Indications   As intracranial angioplasty carries a 10 percent risk and its long-term efficacy is not proven, it should be performed only in highly selected patients. In our institution, angioplasty is performed only in patients with severe (greater than 70 percent narrowing) intracranial stenosis, with recurrent symptoms despite medical therapy including antiplatelet agents, anticoagulants, and in certain cases volume expansion.

Technique   The procedure is performed under general anesthesia to avoid any movement, that could impair the necessary perfect substracted fluoroscopy critical for visualization of the small intracranial arteries and microballoon. Furthermore, flow arrest in the artery for 1 min during balloon inflation often leads to transient ischemic symptoms and movement if the patient is not asleep. Another essential factor is maintaining elevated blood pressure during induction of anesthesia and until the stenosis is treated, as these patients often suffer chronic cerebral hypoperfusion, and hypotension can lead to a permanent stroke. Most patients are already on aspirin and heparin, but additional heparinization is given with an intravenous bolus to reach a PTT of three times normal. From a transfemoral approach, a 6F guiding catheter is placed in the cervical internal carotid or vertebral artery. Figure 11-5 is an example of intracranial angioplasty. The balloon is chosen either to match the arterial diameter or to be slightly undersized for eccentric stenoses. Depending on the artery treated, the balloons have diameters of 1.5 to 3.5 mm and lengths of 1 to 2 cm. The catheterization is performed with

the balloon catheter over a microguidewire, and when across the stenosis the balloon is inflated very slowly to reach a pressure of 6 to 8 atm, which is maintained for 1 min. Then, the balloon is deflated and pulled proximal to the stenosis while the guidewire stays across the stenosis, and an angiogram is performed. A suboptimal result, with a mild to moderate residual stenosis, is satisfying, as it is enough to reverse the symptoms. Moreover, immediate re-angioplasty carries a high risk of dissection. If severe residual stenosis or dissection occurs, a stent can be used if the arterial segment is not too tortuous, such as the intrapetrous or intracavernous segment of the ICA or the vertebral artery termination. After the procedure, the patient is transferred to the ICU for 24 h, then to the regular ward for 48 h. Coumadin plus aspirin is given for 3 months. Coumadin is stopped at 3 months if there is a persistent good result of the angioplasty judged by clinical symptoms and a transcranial Doppler or an MRA. Follow-up is done at 3 and 6 months and then yearly because of possible restenosis. In case of restenosis, re-angioplasty is considered only if the patient is symptomatic or if there is progression to severe restenosis.

REFERENCES

1. Fieschi C, Argentino C, Lenzi G, et al: Clinical and instrumental evaluation in patients with ischemic stroke within the first six hours. *J Neurol Sci* 92:311, 1989.
2. Wolpert SM, Bruckmann H, Greenlee R: Neuroradiologic evaluation of patients with acute stroke treated with recombinant tissue plasminogen activator. *Am J Neuroradiol* 14:3, 1993.
3. Boysen G, Overgaard K: Thrombolysis in ischaemic stroke: How far from a clinical breakthrough? *J Intern Med* 237:95, 1995.
4. Brott T, Kothari R, Broderick J: Thrombolytic therapy for cerebral infarction, in Batjer HH (ed): *Cerebrovascular Disease.* Philadelphia, Lippincott-Raven, 1997, pp. 535–546.
5. Caplan L, Mohr JP, Kistler JP: Should thrombolytic therapy be the first-line treatment for acute ischemic stroke? *N Engl J Med* 337:1309, 1997.
6. Hacke W, Kaste M, Fieschi C, et al: Safety and efficacy of intravenous thrombolysis with a recombinant tissue plasminogen activator in the treatment of acute hemispheric stroke. *JAMA* 274:1017, 1995.
7. The National Institute of Neurological Disorders and Stroke rt-PA stroke study group: Tissue plasminogen activator for acute ischemic stroke. *N Engl J Med* 333:1581, 1995.

8. Chiu D, Krieger D, Villar-Cordova C, et al: Intravenous tissue plasminogen activator for acute ischemic stroke: Feasability, safety, and efficacy in the first year of clinical practice. *Stroke* 29:18, 1998.

9. Zeumer H, Hacke W, Ringelstein EB: Local intraarterial thrombolysis in vertebrobasilar thromboembolic disease. *Am J Neuroradiol* 4:401, 1983.

10. Hacke W, Zeumer H, Ferbert A, Bruckmann H, del Zoppo G: Intra-arterial thrombolytic therapy improves outcome in patients with acute vertebrobasilar occlusive disease. *Stroke* 19:1216, 1988.

11. Courtheoux P, Theron JG, Derlon JM, et al: In situ fibrinolysis in supra-aortic main vessels: A preliminary study. *J Neuroradiol* 13:111, 1986.

12. Mori T, Tabuchi M, Yoshida T: Intracarotid urokinase with thromboembolic occlusion of the middle cerebral artery. *Stroke* 19:802, 1988.

13. Del Zoppo G, Higashida RT, Furlan AJ, et al: Proact: A phase II randomized trial of recombinant pro-urokinase by direct arterial delivery in acute middle cerebral artery stroke. *Stroke* 29:4, 1998.

14. von Kummer R, Allen KL, Holle R, et al: Acute stroke: Usefulness of early CT findings before thrombolytic therapy. *Radiology* 205:327, 1997.

15. Becker KJ, Purcell LL, Hacke W, Hanley DF: Vertebrobasilar thrombosis: Diagnosis, management, and the use of intra-arterial thrombolytics. *Crit Care Med* 24:1729, 1996.

16. Barnwell SL, Clark WM, Nguyen TT, O'Neill OR, Wynn ML, Coull BM: Safety and efficacy of delayed intraarterial urokinase therapy with mechanical clot disruption for thromboembolic stroke. *Am J Neuroradiol* 15:1817, 1994.

17. Zeumer H, Freitag HJ, Zanella F, et al: Local intraarterial fibrinolytic therapy in patients with stroke: Urokinase versus recombinant tissue plasminogen activator (r-TPA). *Neuroradiology* 35:159, 1993.

18. Kerber CW, Cromwell LD: Catheter dilatation of proximal stenosis during distal bifurcation endarterectomy. *Am J Neuroradiol* 1:348, 1980.

19. Mullan S, Duda EE, Patro NA, et al: Some examples of balloon technology in neurosurgery. *J Neurosurg* 52:321, 1980.

20. Becker GJ: Should metallic vascular stents be used to treat cerebrovascular occlusive diseases? (Editorial; Comment). *Radiology* 191:309, 1994.

21. Ferguson RDG, Ferguson JG, Lee LI: Extracranial carotid and vertebral artery stenosis: The future of angioplasty, in Batjer HH (ed): *Cerebrovascular Diseases*. Philadelphia, Lippincott-Raven, 1997, pp. 445–450.

22. Theron JG, Payelle GG, Coskun O, Huet HF, Guimaraens L: Carotid artery stenosis: Treatment with protected balloon angioplasty and stent placement [Comments]. *Radiology* 201:627, 1996.

23. Roubin GS, Yadav S, Iyer SS, Vitek J: Carotid stent-supported angioplasty: A neurovascular intervention to prevent stroke. *Am J Cardiol* 78:8, 1996.

24. Edwards WJ, Tapper SS, Edwards WS, Mulherin JJ, Martin RR, Jenkins JM: Subclavian revascularization: A quarter century experience. *Ann Surg* 219:673, 1994.

25. Koskas F, Kieffer E, Rancurel G, Bahnini A, Ruotolo C, Illuminati G: Direct transposition of the distal cervical vertebral artery into the internal carotid artery. *Ann Vasc Surg* 9:515, 1995.

26. Law MM, Colburn MD, Moore WS, Quinones BW, Machleder HI, Gelabert HA: Carotid-subclavian bypass for brachiocephalic occlusive disease: Choice of conduit and long-term follow-up. *Stroke* 26:1565, 1995.

27. McNamara TO, Greaser LE, Fisher JR, et al: Initial and long-term results of treatment of brachiocephalic arterial stenoses and occlusions with balloon angioplasty, thrombolysis, stents. *J Invasive Cardiol* 9:372, 1997.

28. Ferguson R, Ferguson J, Schwarten D, et al: Immediate angiographic results and in-hospital central nervous system complications of cerebral percutaneous angioplasty. *Circulation* 88 (Suppl I):393, 1993.

29. Caplan L, Babikian V, Helgason C, et al: Occlusive disease of the middle cerebral artery. *Neurology* 35:975, 1985.

30. Akins PT, Pilgram TK, Cross DR, Moran CJ: Natural history of stenosis from intracranial atherosclerosis by serial angiography. *Stroke* 29:433, 1998.

31. Bogousslavsky J, Barnett HJM, Fox AJ, Hachinski VC, Taylor W: Atherosclerotic disease of the middle cerebral artery. *Stroke* 17:1112, 1986.

32. The EC/IC Bypass Study Group: Failure of extra-intracranial arterial bypass to reduce the risk of ischemic stroke. *N Engl J Med* 313:1191, 1985.

33. Moufarrij NA, Little JR, Furlan AJ, et al: Basilar and distal vertebral artery stenosis: Long term follow-up. *Stroke* 17:938, 1986.

34. Hopkins LN, Budny JL: Complications of intracranial bypass for vertebrobasilar insufficiency. *J Neurosurg* 70:207, 1989.

35. Sundt TMJ, Smith HC, Campbell JK, Vliestra RE, Cucchiara RF, Stanson A: Transluminal angioplasty for basilar artery stenosis. *Mayo Clin Proc* 55:673, 1980.

36. Callahan AR, Berger BL: Balloon angioplasty of intracranial arteries for stroke prevention. *Arterioscler Thromb Vasc Biol* 17:1872, 1997.

37. Clark WM, Barnwell SL, Nesbit G, O'Neill OR, Wynn ML, Coull BM: Safety and efficacy of percutaneous transluminal angioplasty for intracranial atherosclerotic stenosis. *Stroke* 26:1200, 1995.

38. McKenzie JD, Wallace RC, Dean BL, Flom RA, Khayata MH: Preliminary results of intracranial angioplasty for vascular stenosis caused by atherosclerosis and vasculitis. *Am J Neuroradiol* 17:263, 1996.

39. Mori T, Mori K, Fukuoka M, Arisawa M, Honda S: Percutaneous transluminal cerebral angioplasty: Serial angiographic follow-up after successful dilatation. *Neuroradiology* 39:111, 1997.

40. Takis C, Kwan ES, Pessin MS, Jacobs DH, Caplan LR: Intracranial angioplasty: Experience and complications. *J Vasc Interv Radiol* 8:997, 1997.

41. Terada T, Higashida RT, Halbach VV, et al: Transluminal angioplasty for arteriosclerotic disease of the distal vertebral and basilar arteries. *J Neurol Neurosurg Psychiatry* 60:377, 1996.

42. Touho H: Percutaneous transluminal angioplasty in the treatment of atherosclerotic disease of the anterior cerebral circulation and hemodynamic evaluation. *J Neurosurg* 82:953, 1995.

43. Mori T, Mori K, Fukuoka M, Honda S: Percutaneous transluminal angioplasty for total occlusion of middle cerebral arteries. *Neuroradiology* 39:71, 1997.

Chapter 12

RETROPERFUSION/ NEUROSURGICAL APPROACHES IN ISCHEMIC STROKE

John G. Frazee

INTRODUCTION

Early, effective treatment for stroke has been a quest of investigators and clinicians for decades. Traditional surgical therapies have been used to prevent strokes. These would include carotid endarterectomy and extracranial to intracranial arterial bypass. With the exception of acute embolectomy, surgical treatment has not been effective for acute stroke and could, in some instances, produce a more severe injury from reperfusion of the ischemic bed. Surgical therapies are generally slow to perform and therefore unsuitable for emergency stroke treatment. This has given rise to new therapies such as tissue-type plasminogen activator (t-PA) delivered intravenously or intra-arterially. These therapies are more quickly started and could potentially benefit the majority of ischemic stroke patients because cerebral vessel occlusion is most commonly the result of a blood clot. However, they do have important drawbacks. Although the time necessary to start intravenous thrombolysis with t-PA is very short, the number of patients who arrive in the emergency room within the 3-h therapeutic window is small, and treatment after this window results in a higher risk of intracerebral bleeding. Intra-arterial thrombolysis requires time to catheterize the appropriate arterial branch and commonly takes 1 to 2 h to lyse the clot. Both intravenous and intra-arterial therapies carry a risk of intraparenchymal bleeding. Therefore, there is room for another approach to acute stroke treatment.

RETROPERFUSION

Background

In the mid 1980's, reports appeared describing a new technique for the reversal of myocardial ischemia using autologous arterial blood pumped in a retrograde direction through the coronary sinus. The intent of this therapy was to provide arterial blood directly to the ischemic myocardium until the arterial obstruction could be cleared or bypassed. Reports from human trials suggested that it was both safe and effective.[1]

Early literature contains reports of surgical procedures designed to direct arterial blood retrograde to brain tissue. The earliest of these attempts was laboratory experiments in which the carotid artery and jugular vein were anastomosed.[2] Unfortunately, the arterial blood was not directed retrograde toward the brain, but instead passed directly back to the heart. Refining the technique by occluding the ipsilateral jugular vein, Beck et al[3] reported improvement in children with mental and convulsive disorders. However, the following year GurdJian et al[4] reported that there was no significant improvement in oxygenation of the superior sagittal sinus when this technique was used in monkeys. No further work for cerebral retrograde perfusion seems to have been done until reports began to appear in the cardiothoracic literature. Surgeons reported small experiences with completely reversing the flow of arterial blood during open heart surgery to wash out air and particulate emboli.[5] These historic reports of retrograde perfusion of the brain and the coronary sinus experiences led us to adapt and refine the coronary retroperfusion technique into what is now called retrograde transvenous neuroperfusion (RTN).

This technique was developed over the past 11 years at UCLA and involved more than 100 primate experiments. In its simplest form, RTN was meant to rapidly provide arterial blood to ischemic brain tissue temporarily until the original arterial obstruction spontaneously lysed, could be cleared with lytic therapy, or could be bypassed. The technique was to harvest autologous blood from a femoral artery using an external pump and to pass that blood through catheters located in the transverse sinuses. From there, the blood would pass into the veins of the brain and capillary bed (Fig. 12-1). It became obvious during experiments that catheter tip placement was crucial to the success of the procedure. Catheters located too far lateral obstructed crucial alternate venous outflow from the veins of Labbé and the superior petrosal sinuses. When the balloons on the tips of the RTN catheters were inflated to partially obstruct the outflow of blood from the transverse sinuses, they also obstructed these collateral pathways, resulting in high-resting venous pressures and even higher pressures when RTN flow was started. It was discovered that simply moving the catheters medially near to the torcular resulted in a dramatic drop in resting venous sinus pressures to near normal. When RTN was then started, pressures of only 10 to 20 mmHg were necessary to move blood retrograde into the venous system.

It was recognized that directing blood flow retrograde through veins and venules to the capillary bed was not an intuitively appealing concept. The first concern voiced by critics of RTN was for valves in the venous system that would obstruct the retrograde flow of blood. Thankfully, there are no valves in the cerebral venous system. The only valves that might cause obstruction are present in the proximal jugular system. Therefore, retrograde perfusion from the superior vena cava, as has been done in some cardiac surgery cases, may not reach the brain. This argues for the catheters to be placed intracranially.

A second and much greater concern of critics was that the superior sagittal sinus is the major outflow of blood from the brain. Obstructing this path would lead to serious consequences. This in part stemmed from the historic observation that superior sagittal sinus occlusion was accompanied by cerebral hemorrhage.[6] This

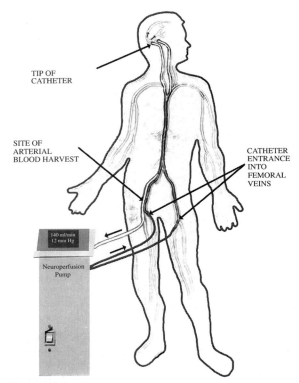

Figure 12-1.
This drawing shows the neuroperfusion pump and transfemorally placed intracranial catheters. Arterial blood is harvested from the femoral artery by the pump and then passed through two catheters located in the transverse sinuses near the torcular. The small inflated balloons at the tips of the catheters direct blood into the venous system. Flow rate is controlled by the speed of the neuroperfusion pump.

was underscored by neurosurgeons who found that occlusion of the superior sagittal sinus during surgery was accompanied by venous congestion and hemorrhagic infarction. Therefore, it was reasoned that directing blood flow through the superior sagittal sinus in a retrograde manner would likely cause similar consequences. The consequence was attributed to two factors. One, that pressure greater than normal sinus pressure would be required to bring about the retrograde flow. In turn, there would be pressure elevation in the venous and capillary beds, leading to hemorrhage from such fragile vessels. Two, an obstruction of the major venous outflow from the brain would lead to severe congestion, elevated capillary bed pressures, and ultimately cerebral hemorrhage. It must be remembered that our sampling of patients with superior sinus occlusion is biased. We only see those patients who are symptomatic from their sinus occlusion. There may be a larger proportion of patients with sinus occlusion who remain asymptomatic. The superior sagittal sinus may be occluded without serious consequences. It could be argued that the sinus occlusion may form slowly, allowing time for collateral venous outflow to develop and therefore patients remain asymptomatic. However, we believe that the collateral venous network is large and quite redundant and can readily handle the change in the outflow pattern that occurs when RTN forces blood through the superior sagittal sinus in a retrograde fashion. This concept is supported by the venous phase of angiography. Angiography shows such collateral paths that include the cavernous sinus, the basilar plexus, and the veins of Labbé.

It may also be that RTN and acute sinus occlusion are actually quite different and, therefore, not comparable. Acute sinus occlusion promotes stasis and clotting of blood within the sinus and connected veins and could indeed lead to hemorrhagic infarction in those areas with poor collateral venous outflow. On the other hand, RTN can be seen as promoting continued flow only in a retrograde direction. RTN does not promote stasis in areas with poor venous collateral flow. Instead, it helps to redirect flow from those areas to the collateral sites of outflow mentioned above. There is additional experimental data to suggest that RTN does not require unusual pressures to direct blood retrograde into the ischemic capillary bed. Symon[7] measured middle cerebral artery (MCA) pressures in primates before and after MCA occlusion. Prior to occlusion, the pressure measured in the proximal MCA averaged 94 mmHg, and middle cerebral venous (MCV) pressures averaged 14 mmHg. If one assumes that there is an approximately 80 percent drop in pressure across the arteriolar bed, then the normal capillary bed pressure should average 18 to 28 mmHg. This correlates well with actual measurements (18 to 22 mmHg) of an accessible capillary bed of the finger.[8] It would therefore be predicted that when RTN reached pressures near 20 mmHg, blood would flow into a normal capillary bed.

When Symon[7] measured pressures during occlusion of the MCA, he found that the mean arterial pressure distal to the occlusion was 20.6 mmHg and MCV pressures were 9.4 mmHg. The pressure in the capillary bed would be between these two and closest to the venous pressure owing to the drop in pressure across

the arteriolar bed. Thus, RTN pressures would likely need to be only slightly higher than the venous pressures for flow to move into the ischemic capillary bed. These pressures are in keeping with our own experimental results in baboons.[9]

There are additional primate experimental results that help to demonstrate that RTN can move arterial blood to the ischemic brain without hemorrhage or venous congestion. Early RTN research concentrated on venous angiography. It became apparent that dramatic filling of venous sinuses, along with deep and superficial veins, was possible when the pressure of retrograde perfusion was 30 mmHg or greater. However, these pressures were thought to be higher than was actually necessary to transport blood retrograde to the capillary bed as indicated above. Studies were performed that allowed for the direct observation of the cortical surface in both the ischemic and nonischemic hemispheres. It was possible to see that retrograde flow occurred in the surface veins at much lower pressures and that cortical capillary blood flow, as measured by laser Doppler, was increased to greater than normal levels in the ischemic area. Therefore, it was presumed that venous angiography did not fully demonstrate the penetration of RTN.

Additional early primate experiments demonstrated the penetration into brain tissue of RTN-transported dye. During occlusion of the right MCA, and with RTN being performed, red dye was injected into the arterial system and blue dye was mixed with the retroperfused blood. After approximately 30 s, the animal was sacrificed. These studies demonstrated excellent penetration of blue, RTN-perfused dye into the ischemic middle cerebral territory. Microscopic studies confirmed penetration to the capillary bed. There was no evidence of dye leaking from the capillaries, hemorrhage, or brain edema.

Evidence

The final evidence for both the safety and efficacy of RTN came from a series of 10 baboon survival experiments. The primates were divided into two equal groups and subjected to MCA occlusion for 3.5 h, after which time the animals were recovered, followed for 6 days, and then sacrificed. All animals were treated identically with the exception that five received RTN during the last 2.5 h of occlusion. The results of somatosensory-evoked potentials (SSEPs) during the ischemic period, clinical outcome during the 6 days of observation, and size of brain infarction were compared for the two groups.[9] The treated group clearly faired better than the untreated group. SSEPs, which demonstrated ischemia during the first hour of MCA occlusion, recovered to better than normal with RTN (103 percent) compared with 75 percent in the untreated group ($p < .01$). Clinical outcome scores were graded on a scale of 0 to 100, with the latter considered normal. Treated animals had an average score of 99, whereas the score for the untreated group was 66 ($p < .015$). The average infarction volume was 0.02 percent of the ipsilateral hemisphere in the RTN-treated group and 3.9 percent in the untreated group ($p < .05$). These data led us to propose opening a clinical trial at UCLA.

Clinical Trial This clinical trial was approved by the FDA and the UCLA Human Subjects Protection Committee and commenced in late 1994. The first patient was enrolled in September 1995. Since then, a total of eight patients have been enrolled at UCLA. Nine additional centers and a total of 30 patients have now been approved for inclusion in this ongoing phase I trial.

Inclusion Criteria Patients who may be included in this trial must be age 18 to 89 with an NIH stroke score of 2 or greater in one or more categories including arm, face, and leg motion, and language. These criteria mean that patients will present with partial or complete paralysis of face, arm, or leg and/or have difficulty talking or understanding speech or worse. The symptoms must be present longer than 1 h and less than 7 h, substantially reducing the chance of treating a transient ischemic attack (TIA) while not delaying treatment so long that recovery is unlikely. Each patient must have a CT scan to rule out hemorrhage. Hypodensity is not an exclusion criterion. However, patients are excluded if they are in coma, have a posterior fossa or brain stem injury, recent trauma, surgery, or nonhemorrhagic stroke, are candidates for intravenous t-PA, or have a contraindication to heparin use.

Procedure Once patients have been consented for RTN, they are taken to the angiography suite where a cerebral angiogram is completed. Patients are excluded at this point if no arterial obstruction is seen. Angiography also provides a view of the jugular veins and venous sinuses in preparation for sinus catheterization. The site of arterial catheterization is also used for harvesting arterial blood used in RTN. To proceed with RTN requires only the catheterization of both transverse si-

nuses using transfemoral approaches. The external bladder pump is then connected to the arterial source catheter and both sinus catheters, and the patient is fully heparinized. Activated clotting times (ACTs) are assessed every 30 min, and heparin boluses are given to maintain ACTs greater than 250 s. Once heparin is given, small balloons at the catheter tips are inflated to partially obstruct the transverse sinuses. This raises the sinus pressures 1 mmHg from a resting state of 5 to 12 mmHg. The RTN pump is started. The flow from the pump is gradually increased to a rate of between 100 and 200 mL/min. Flow rates are determined by intrasinus pressures. Pressures during RTN are between 10 and 20 mmHg and average 15 mmHg. RTN therapy is continued for 3 h under the current protocol. The first eight patients were treated for 6 h. The time was shortened because every patient that improved did so within the first 3 h. However, RTN therapy is not limited to 3 h or even 6 h. If there is evidence that the patient is continuing to improve, the therapy can be extended up to 24 h. During prolonged therapy, it is possible to move patients to other locations including the CT scanner and the intensive care unit. Throughout RTN, the patient currently remains in the angiography suite. If prolonged treatment is planned, this would be impractical, and patients would be transferred to the intensive care unit.

During the treatment, patients are examined at regular intervals by a neurologist. An anesthesiologist is constantly present to monitor vital signs and to administer small amounts of intravenous sedatives as patients become restless lying on the firm angiography table. The patients are not intubated. EEG monitoring has been used in each case of RTN but has not proven helpful. One person, who has undergone previous training, is assigned full time to manage the RTN pump. This person ensures that appropriate parameters are maintained during treatment and is available to troubleshoot any problems.

Once RTN therapy is completed, the pump is stopped after returning blood in the pumping circuit to the patient. The patient is observed for 30 min, and if there is no deterioration in the neurologic exam, anticoagulation is reversed if necessary and all catheters are removed. The patient undergoes a follow-up CT scan to rule-out an adverse reaction from RTN and is then taken to the intensive care unit or a monitored ward bed for observation.

Results The results from eight treated patients have been favorable. Six of our patients have shown some evidence of neurologic improvement with RTN. Three patients were normal at 3 months, two of these within 24 h. Only two patients did not improve. One patient was enrolled in the study but was not treated as the resting venous pressures were too high to allow for RTN therapy. There have been no significant adverse events that could be attributed to RTN. Two patients did develop hematomas at either the arterial or venous puncture site, but these resolved without sequelae. Follow-up CT scans showed no evidence of intracranial hemorrhage or brain edema.

Case Presentations   Two cases have been selected to provide a better understanding of the benefits of RTN.

Case I   This patient was a 61-year-old, right-handed, white male who had been in good health until the day of his treatment. While at home, he had one episode of complete left-side paralysis. Paramedics took him to the nearest emergency room, by which time his complaints had fully resolved. While in the emergency room, his left leg suddenly lost all strength. A CT scan was negative. The patient was transferred to UCLA and agreed to RTN treatment. Angiography was negative, but at that time the protocol did not require a visible angiographic defect. The patient remained unchanged to that point, and RTN was started 6 h, 40 min after the onset of his leg paralysis. Appropriate RTN flows were reached and continued for approximately 17 min, when the patient suddenly was less responsive. EEG was unchanged, but RTN was stopped. Within 13 min of stopping the pump, the patient again had a normal mental status exam, and the paralyzed left leg had recovered to normal strength. The patient remained normal during an observation period, and a follow-up CT scan was negative. The patient was anticoagulated for a new onset of atrial fibrillation, the presumed source of his emboli, and he was discharged with a normal neurologic exam. He returned to full-time work and remains normal more than 2 years later.

In retrospect, it is presumed that soon after starting RTN, a small embolus broke up and flow resumed in that vessel. It is unknown whether the embolus cleared spontaneously or whether the mild elevated backward pressure dislodged the clot. The close proximity of the improvement in neurologic state and the start of RTN hint at a role for RTN.

Case II   This patient was a 78-year-old, white, right-handed, retired male who was in good health and who played golf regularly. On the morning of this treatment, the patient suddenly became incoherent. He was immediately taken to the UCLA emergency room, where an examination found him very weak on the right side including the face, and he was unable to talk or understand speech. A CT scan was negative, and angiography demonstrated a large clot in the MCA immediately after its take-off from the left internal carotid artery. After obtaining consent from the patient's family, RTN was started 5 h, 47 min, after the onset of symptoms. Over the next 6 h, the patient regained strength in the extremities of his right side and he began to speak. An angiogram was repeated at the termination of the 6-h treatment, and the left MCA clot was no longer present. A follow-up CT scan was negative. The patient was observed overnight and the next morning was without a neurologic deficit. That evening, the patient began to develop myocardial ischemia and was emergently treated with a quadruple bypass. The patient had a complete recovery and was discharged, 6 days after the bypass surgery, neurologically normal. He remains normal 1.5 years after RTN treatment.

This patient's case demonstrates several important features about RTN. First, RTN can be associated with neurologic improvement even when an angiographically visible clot is present. Second, RTN can sustain that neurologic improvement until a clot either spontaneously clears or, as suggested in the first patient, is broken up by the retrograde flow of blood. Third, it is possible for RTN-treated patients to undergo major surgery following treatment without harm.

Future Studies   The nine additional centers for the phase I study are currently being chosen from major institutions across the United States. The stated objective is to continue to demonstrate the safety of RTN in the hands of others. Clearly, however, there has been a keen interest in the potential benefits of this treatment. Unlike intravenous t-PA, RTN offers rapid evidence of benefit. Whether there will be additional benefit at 3 months will require a larger controlled study. The rapid improvement seen in some patients is an exciting enticement for further studies.

Based upon current research, it is expected that in the future RTN will be a much simpler process. We recognize that RTN currently requires a substantial investment of manpower. Routinely, we have two interventional radiologists, one anesthesiologist, one neurologist, and both an EEG and RTN pump technician present. These people are present to do all that is possible to ensure the safety of the patient, to speed the setup of RTN, and to train other physicians. Our experience with the first eight patients has made it clear that fewer personnel can carry out the procedure. The catheters can be placed by one person. We also expect that in the future only one catheter, more centrally placed, may be necessary. This will certainly shorten the procedure. EEG, with a minor exception, has not been of value. However, anesthesia support certainly has been important. Some patients come to this procedure soon after a meal and are therefore at risk for aspiration. They must remain flat on the firm radiology table for several hours without much movement. They become uncomfortable and usually require some sedation, raising the risk of aspiration. Having an anesthesiologist present to prevent or manage these potential difficulties has been very helpful. In the future, it may be possible to shorten the stay in the radiology suite to the time necessary to place catheters and to then move the patient to the intensive care unit. This in turn might reduce or eliminate the need for an anesthesiologist.

Recent work in the research lab has suggested that we might be able to enhance the benefit of RTN by mildly cooling the patient's blood before returning it to the venous sinuses. There is a very large body of published data that suggests hypothermia is a very good cerebral protectant.[10] Hypothermia is used for just this reason during open heart surgery, as an adjunct in neurosurgery, and even in stroke patients. Ordinarily, producing hypothermia of the brain requires cooling of the body as well. This is usually time-consuming and may, as in the case of open heart surgery, require specialized equipment and personnel. Studies suggest that only a few degrees of cooling may provide significant benefit. Hypothermia slows the brain's metabolism, therefore presumably slowing the rate of injury in ischemic brain tissue. Reports suggest that temperatures lowered to only 32 or 33 degrees Centigrade may have marked benefit. Temperatures below that level may be more beneficial but can be accompanied by cardiac arrhythmias.

Our laboratory experience has led us to conclude that we can cool the retrograde perfused blood and lower the superficial and deep brain temperatures to 35 degrees Centigrade. The only difference from a normal RTN procedure is the inclusion of a refrigeration coil that cools the subject's blood as it passes in the external circuit to the RTN pump. Thermisters placed in the blood circuit just before reaching the patient monitor the degree of blood cooling. Tiny thermisters inserted into the brain in primates measure temperature changes

as the cooled blood reaches the brain. This system allows the brain and body of primates to be cooled to 35 degrees Centigrade in less than 1 h. Temperatures can then be held constant for whatever time is required.

Treatment Recommendation

At the present time, RTN is an experimental therapy. Despite the promise held out by the results of the animal experiments and the promising results of the pilot study, the results cannot be generalized, and it should not be used outside the setting of a research protocol with an experienced surgical team.

DECOMPRESSIVE CRANIOTOMY FOR SEVERE STROKE

Background

Severe brain swelling following cerebral infarction can lead to both tentorial and uncal herniation with subsequent death in the majority of patients. Those patients who do survive commonly have a severe disability or are in a persistent vegetative state. The current therapy for these patients has been aggressive, early medical management with intubation, paralysis, intracranial pressure monitoring, osmotic diuretics, and short-acting barbiturates. Mortality has been reported as high as 80 percent despite these measures.[11]

Evidence

Previous reports of surgical decompression have suggested that there may be improvement in outcome when this approach is taken.[12] Rieke et al[11] reported 53 patients, <70 years of age, who were suffering from malignant hemispheric infarction and who were treated with a wide surgical decompression or conservatively. Admission to this study was triggered by deterioration in the patient's clinical status as suggested by a progressing, severe hemiparesis or hemiplegia, impaired levels of consciousness, and rapid deterioration owing to rising intracranial pressure. The study was prospective but was not randomized. Thirty-two patients were treated with a large craniotomy and dural patch graft, without brain resection. Twenty-one patients received conservative treatment. The conservative group included patients who had extensive left hemisphere infarcts with global aphasia, severe medical problems, or for whom an informed consent could not be obtained. The two groups were similar for occlusion site, size of infarct, extent of perimesencephalic cistern effacement, midline shift, and time course. The surgically treated group was younger (mean age 48.8 years) than the conservatively treated group (mean age 58.4 years). Outcome was determined by a Glasgow Outcome Scale at discharge and a Barthel Index and Oxford Handicap Scale during follow-up. Twenty-one of 32 patients treated surgically survived compared with only 5 of 21 in the conservatively treated group. More important, follow-up showed 1 patient with an excellent outcome and 15 patients with dependency requiring minimal assistance following surgical treatment. Five patients were left with a severe disability. None of the surgical patients was left in a persistent vegetative state. Of the five surviving, conservatively treated patients, one had a moderate handicap and four had a moderately severe handicap.

This study suggests that it may be possible to dramatically improve the outcome for patients with malignant hemispheric infarction and dramatically decrease the mortality rate without increasing the number of patients who remain severely disabled or in a vegetative state.

Treatment Recommendation

The rationale for surgical decompression is to decrease intracranial pressure, reducing the risk of herniation and increasing the cerebral blood flow to ischemic regions. When decompressive surgery is chosen as a therapeutic option, early surgery is desirable. Surgery is indicated when intracranial pressures are higher than 30 mmHg or patients have fixed dilated pupils that are not responsive to aggressive antiedema therapy. Currently, removal of infarcted tissue is not recommended when surgical decompression is performed. This is because the infarction is poorly defined and resection might then include tissue that has the potential for recovery.

REFERENCES

1. Gore JM, Weiner BH, Benoti JR, et al: Preliminary experience with synchronized coronary sinus retroperfusion in humans. *Circulation* 74:381, 1986.
2. Carrel M: Anastomose bout a bout de la jugulaire et de la carotide primitive. *Lyon Med* 99:114, 1902.
3. Beck DS, Mekhann DF, Belnap WID: Revascularization of the brain through establishment of cervical arteriovenous fistula: Effects in children with mental retardation and convulsive disorders. *J Pediatr* 35:317, 1949.
4. GurdJian ES, Webster JE, Martin FA: Carotid-internal jugular anastomosis in the rhesus monkey. *J Neurosurg.* 7:467, 1950.
5. Mills NL, Ochsner JL: Massive air embolism during cardiopulmonary bypass. *J Thorac Cardiovasc Surg* 80:708, 1980.
6. Garcia JH, Joh K-L, Caccamo DV: Pathology of stroke, in Barnett HJM, Mohr JP, Stein EM, Yatsu FM (eds): *Stroke: Pathophysiology, Diagnosis, and Management,* 2nd ed. New York, Churchill-Livingstone, 1992, pp 125–145.
7. Symon L: Regional vascular reactivity in the middle cerebral arterial distribution: An experimental study in baboons. *J Neurosurg* 33:532, 1970.
8. Fagrell B, Intaglietta M: Microcirculation: Its significance in clinical and molecular medicine. *J Intern Med* 241:349, 1997.
9. Frazee JG, Luo X, Luan G, et al: Retrograde transvenous neuroperfusion: A back door treatment for stroke. *Stroke* 29, September 1998.
10. Ginsberg MD, Busto BS: Combating hyperthermia in acute stroke: A significant clinical concern. *Stroke* 29:529, 1998.
11. Rieke K, Schwab S, Krieger D, et al: Decompressive surgery in space-occupying hemispheric infarction: Results of an open prospective trial. *Crit Care Med* 23:1576, 1995.
12. Delashaw JB, Broaddus WC, Kassell NF, et al: Treatment of right hemispheric cerebral infarction by hemicraniectomy. *Stroke* 21:874, 1990.

Chapter 13

CYTOPROTECTIVE THERAPIES IN ISCHEMIC STROKE

Patrick D. Lyden
Justin A. Zivin

THEORY: PROTECTING IDLING NEURONS

After vascular occlusion, there is a heterogeneous depression of cerebral blood flow (CBF) in the territory of the occluded artery. The *penumbra* is identified as the brain region receiving regional CBF (rCBF) between two critical values.[1,2] The first, higher, critical value is associated with neuronal paralysis: brain areas receiving rCBF less than 18 to 20 mL/100 g/min do not function. The second, lower, critical value is associated with cell death: brain areas receiving less than 8 to 10 mL/100 mg/min do not survive, and this area becomes the *core* of the infarction. Neurons in the penumbra are sometimes identified as "idling" to suggest that they are salvageable, although the mechanism of such a phenomenon is unknown. The time course of cell death in the core is rapid, whereas cells in the penumbra may survive up to several hours. Therefore, cytoprotective therapy is often targeted at idling neurons rather than at the irretrievable core.

The sudden deprivation of oxygen and glucose sets into motion a set of events called the ischemic cascade. The use of the term cascade implies that ischemia proceeds in an orderly manner from the beginning of the cascade to the end. Alternatively, it is becoming clear that the several steps in the cascade occur simultaneously, rather than sequentially, and in addition there seem to be multiple feed-forward, feed-back, and amplification steps.[3–5] Space limitations dictate only a limited discussion of a few key observations, which are summarized in Fig. 13-1.

Glutamate exposure is associated with cell death and degeneration in cell culture (reviewed in Ref. 6), and glutamate receptor antagonists protect cultured cells from exposure to glutamate, hypoglycemia, and hypoxia.[7] At least three glutamate receptor subtypes are identified based on ligand-binding studies: N-methyl-D-aspartate (NMDA), α-amino-3-hydroxy-5-methyl-4-isoxazoleproionate (AMPA)-kainate, and metabotropic (See Table 13-1). Of these subtypes, the NMDA receptor seems to be critical in mediating the effects of ischemia, although interest in AMPA/kainate receptors continues, especially in studies of global ischemia,[7] and the role of the metabotropic receptor subtype remains unclear.[8]

Depolarization of the postsynaptic cell occurs in response to application of glutamate and seems to be a necessary step in the sequence of events leading to cell death.[9] During excitation of the postsynaptic membrane, there is an influx of sodium, chloride, calcium (via L-type, voltage-gated channels), and water into the cell.[7,10,11] Inflow of ions and water leads to edema, and if severe or prolonged such edema may lead to cell lysis and death.[11] Glutamate does not cause edema or lysis of mature neurons in culture unless sodium and/or chloride are present in the culture medium.[11] Inflow of calcium may lead to delayed neuronal death through unknown mechanisms after comparatively brief exposure to ischemia or excitotoxins.[10] There is some evidence, albeit preliminary and often contradictory, that this delayed cell death may be mediated through apoptotic mechanisms.[12] This effect persists in culture if sodium is not present in the medium but is blocked by MG^{+2} or by removing calcium from the medium.[11]

During ischemia, intracellular calcium concentrations increase through mechanisms other than the

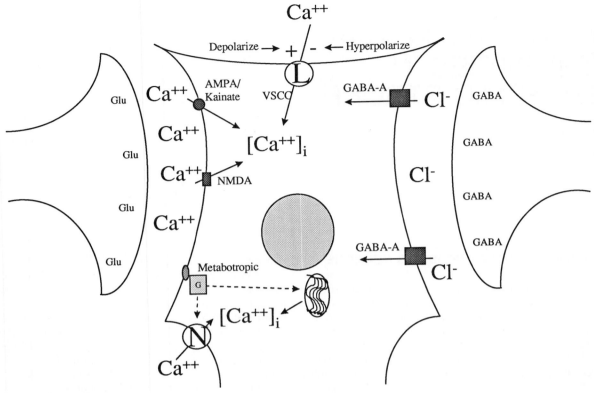

Figure 13-1.

Diagram of the complementary excitatory and inhibitory inputs on a schematized brain neuron. The excitatory neurotransmitter glutamate causes increased intracellular calcium via multiple sources. The NMDA and AMPA/kainate channels are ligand-gated calcium channels. The L-type calcium channel is a membrane voltage-gated channel. The metabotropic receptor is coupled to a second messenger transduction pathway that causes release of calcium from intracytoplasmic stores, as well as by activating the N-type calcium channel. All of these effects may be partially blocked by hyperpolarization arising from chloride influx via the GABA-A receptor, a ligand-gated channel.

Table 13-1.

Sites of action of drugs that are glutamate antagonists and have been evaluated for neuroprotective properties

Site	Receptors	Action	Drug
Ion channel	NMDA/AMPA	Block cation entry; inhibit membrane depolarization	MK-801, selfotel, eliprodil, cerestat, dextromethorphan
Glycine binding site	NMDA	Prevent binding of glutamate	ACEA 1021, GV15026, felbamate
??	Sodium channels	Inhibit glutamate release; may block depolarization	Lubeluzole, lamotrigine, fosphenytoin

ligand-gated channels described above. Some calcium channels are voltage gated, and depolarization to a membrane voltage that opens some of these channels may be a critical determinant of calcium influx.[10] However, as calcium seems to enter the cell through the NMDA receptor itself, ligand-gated influx seems to continue even in voltage-clamped cells. Nevertheless, it seems reasonable to suspect that prevention of glutamate-stimulated depolarization ought to prevent some of the early cellular edema due to sodium, chloride and water movement, and some of the calcium flow that leads to delayed toxicity. In support of this expectation, it was observed that hyperpolarization reduced or blocked calcium inflow into neurons[13] and reduced the probability of discharge.[14] Other routes of influx include the release of calcium from intracytoplasmic stores (mediated in part via metabotropic receptors linked to protein kinase C) and loss of ATP-dependent calcium extrusion mechanisms. Activation of the metabotropic receptor also may cause calcium influx via the N-type calcium channel. Also, with membrane damage there is influx of calcium down an electrochemical gradient.

There is now a growing consensus that the increase in intracellular calcium sets into motion a variety of events that lead to cell death, most especially the activation of cytosolic phospholipases and proteases.[3,15] Proteases may play a central role in activating programmed cell death; phospholipases may be critically involved in further excitotoxin release, and the generation of reactive oxygen species; as a direct result of early glutamate-mediated increases in intracellular calcium, a vicious cycle is created that causes spread of the core zone of infarction.[3]

Despite the obvious difference in blood flow between the core and the penumbra, the mechanisms of cell death in the two regions are not fully known. *Necrosis* is obviously one mechanism for cell death in both the penumbra and the core. During necrosis, the cell initially swells, then shrinks, and can be observed as a small, pyknotic form on sections.[16] Finally, microglia and macrophages remove the debris of the dead cell. If necrosis includes the adjacent glia and structural matrix, a cyst is formed and the process is termed *pannecrosis.* Recently, *apoptosis,* or programmed cell death, has been observed in ischemic brain.[17] In this type of cell death, ischemia is thought to activate "suicide" proteins that are latent in all cells. These proteins are normally expressed during embryogenesis and enable the organism to remove cells that will not be needed during further development. The morphometry of apoptosis is quite different than necrosis, and special techniques are available to study the two forms of cell death.[18] The role of

apoptotic cell death in the core and in the penumbra is not known. Figure 13-2 illustrates the factors involved in these two forms of cell death. How cells end up "choosing" one form of death over the other is not known.

THEORY: PREVENTING REPERFUSION INJURY

Restoration of arterial blood flow after several hours of occlusion may not result in complete tissue reperfusion, the so-called "no-reflow phenomenon."[19,20] The mechanism is not certain but may involve endothelial swelling, occlusion of microvessels with platelet-fibrin aggregates, red cell microthrombi, or perivascular swelling. The no-reflow effect does not occur if white blood cells are removed from the circulation.[20] Granulocytes may adhere to ischemic endothelium, blocking capillaries and stimulating platelet aggregation and formation of microthrombi, as illustrated in Fig. 13-3. The receptor complex on the granulocyte that mediates adherence is composed of the integrins CD18/CD11 (for review see Ref. 21). This complex binds to the intercellular adhesion molecule (ICAM) on the endothelial cell.

In addition to mediating the no-reflow phenomenon, granulocytes may have direct toxic effects in the brain. After adhesion, granulocytes migrate into the brain (diapedesis) and can be observed in the peri-ischemic zone within hours of permanent or transient arterial occlusion.[22] Once in the brain, granulocytes release phagocytic chemotactic factors as well as cytokines that may promote cellular destruction. Granulocytes also release enzymes that lead to the formation of free radicals, which leads to an increase in hypochlorous acid and chloramines.[23] These compounds then activate granulocytic serine proteases and metalloproteinases, which together begin to destroy surrounding tissue. These events proceed independent of the energy status of the brain cells and may be augmented by early reperfusion, the *reperfusion injury syndrome.* Granulocytes have been detected in the peri-infarction zone (penumbra) in multiple animal models.[24,25] There is very little evidence of reperfusion injury in humans after cerebral thrombolysis, however.

PRACTICE

Glutamate Antagonists

Background The best-studied cytoprotective agents modify glutamate, the most common excitatory neuro-

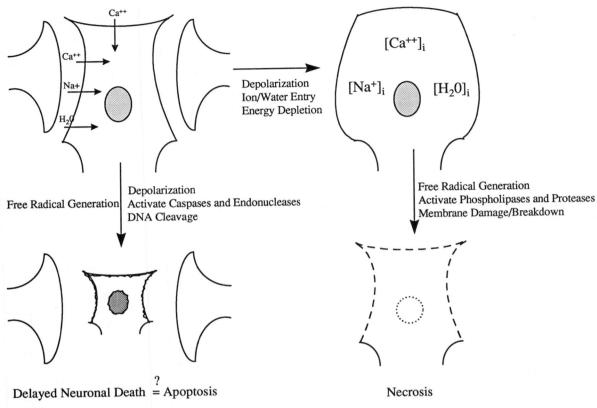

Figure 13-2.
Neuronal death proceeds by alternative pathways. Significant depolarization causes cellular swelling, energy depletion, and death. Histologically, this process has the characteristics of necrosis. Alternatively, intracellular calcium may initiate a process known as delayed neuronal death, or DND. This process may proceed by activation of programmed cell death, also known as apoptosis. The signals that tell the cell to die via necrosis or DND are not known. Further, the proportion of cells that die via the two pathways, and whether there may be other death pathways, are not known.

transmitter in the central nervous system, which is released in excess during ischemia.[26] Glutamate stimulates postsynaptic neurons by activating several types of receptors, and activation of these receptors permits influx of calcium through associated membrane channels, as shown in Fig. 13-1. Blockade of the NMDA type of glutamate receptor can decrease calcium influx into the cells and may reduce neuronal damage. Several direct glutamate antagonists (MK-801, CGS-19755, and dextrorphan) and indirect agents that bind at the NMDA glycine site (ACEA 1021, felbamate, GV150526a) seem to protect brain during focal ischemia.[27–32] The direct agents resemble dissociative anesthetics such as keta-

mine and phencyclidine, and humans experience significant side effects during treatment with NMDA antagonists. These side effects may have contributed to the demise of development efforts for some of these agents. Therefore, alternative strategies for brain protection during cerebral ischemia are being developed to block the effects of excitotoxins without causing severe side effects.

Evidence There was extensive preclinical development of several kinds of small molecules that block the NMDA receptors, and a few of these antagonists were evaluated in clinical trials. These drugs include Cerestat

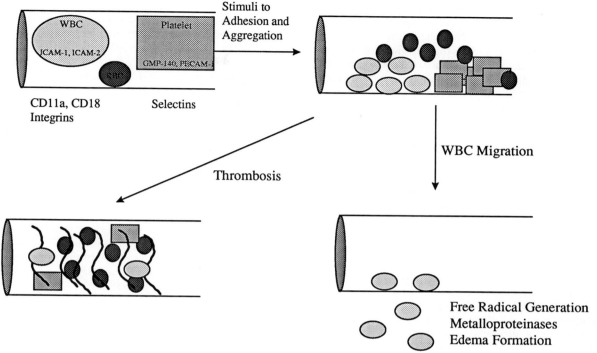

Figure 13-3.

Role of blood elements after ischemia. In microvessels distal to an arterial occlusion, white blood cells (WBC), red blood cells (RBC), and platelets all begin to collect and aggregate. WBCs adhere to the lumen wall using the integrins CD11a and CD18. Platelets adhere to the lumen wall via selectins. WBCs begin to migrate from the lumen, through the vessel wall and basement membrane, into the brain matrix. A variety of stimuli cause WBCs to generate active reactive oxygen species (free radicals). Also, WBCs release cytokines that activate matrix metalloproteinases, which facilitate WBC migration but also promote vasogenic edema. Platelets and WBCs release clotting factors that stimulate thrombus formation, which extends the thrombus distally.

(formerly called CNS 1102), selfotel (originally CGS 19755), and eliprodil. A series of phase I and II trials of selfotel were completed,[33] but soon after the phase III trials began, they were terminated because of unfavorable risk-benefit ratios. Similarly, a large, multinational, phase III trial of selfotel in head-injured patients was terminated early due to safety concerns. The phase III trial of eliprodil was prematurely stopped for similar reasons. The phase II trial of Cerestat suggested that it might have some efficacy without excessive side effects, and a phase III trial has been initiated.

All the NMDA antagonists identified to date, to varying degrees, cause phencyclidine-like side effects. Although these psychotic reactions are dose dependent and apparently reversible, they do create patient man-

agement difficulties.[34,35] In addition, a toxic side effect of moderate doses of some glutamate antagonists is the transient appearance of neuronal vacuoles in specific parts of the nonischemic brain.[36] The damage becomes permanent at higher doses.[37] The NMDA antagonists tested in clinical trials do not exhibit this property at the doses used. Of note, these vacuoles can be blocked with the simultaneous administration of a GABA agonist or other types of drugs.[38] Although the clinical development of these drugs has been difficult and expensive, the class as a whole has been highly effective in reducing neurologic damage in many stroke models. Therefore, the pharmaceutical companies and clinical investigators have been reluctant to abandon this line of investigation.

The glutamate receptor is quite complex. It can be modified by several related receptor sites that also gate cation influx into CNS cells. Classes of drugs in addition to NMDA blockers that can alter calcium entry into neurons include antagonists of glycine, which is required for glutamate binding to its receptor. Preclinical testing suggests drugs that block these sites may also have cytoprotective properties, and two of the glycine antagonists, ACEA 1021 and GV15026, have been tested in phase I clinical trials in stroke patients. Unfortunately, the development of ACEA 1021 is currently on hold due to safety concerns. A large phase III trial of GV15026 is currently under way. The hope is that the side-effect profile of these drugs differs from the NMDA antagonists, and in particular, the phencyclidine and neurotoxic actions may be minimized or eliminated.

Therapeutic Recommendations At this time, there are insufficient data to recommend any glutamate antagonists for use in patients. Because of recent lay press attention to this area of research, including reports that "cough syrup (dextromethorphan) cures strokes," many patients come to clinics with questions about these drugs. For the time being, patients should be counseled that these drugs cause more harm than benefit. Given the amount of development effort already expended, it is not clear whether any agent from this class will emerge as clinically useful. Hope remains for the glycine site antagonists, however.

GABA Agonists

Background In mammalian brain, GABA is considered the principal inhibitory neurotransmitter. Inhibitory neurotransmitters increase chloride conductance, lower the resting membrane potential of the neuron, and reduce the probability that glutamate stimulation leads to action potential.[14] GABA mediates its effects through two receptor subtypes, A and B. When GABA or a suitable analog occupies the postsynaptic GABA-A receptor, the resting membrane potential may not increase, and voltage-gated calcium channels are prevented from opening.[13,14] These events are illustrated in Fig. 13-1. Also, GABA-A agonists reduce the cerebral metabolic rate for glucose at doses that do not cause sedation or impair respiration or cardiac function.[39,40] GABA-A receptors are found on cerebral blood vessels and cause dilation of cerebral, but not extracranial, vessels. This effect is blocked by competitive antagonists of the GABA receptor.[41] GABA-B agonists reduce the presynaptic release of glutamate and ought to be cytoprotective via a presynaptic mechanism. Despite this rationale, and the preliminary work presented below, there may be conditions under which GABA is neurotoxic.

From the above considerations, we predicted that GABA-A agonists would prove to be neuroprotective for at least three reasons. First, increased chloride conductance could block voltage-mediated postsynaptic effects of glutamate by preventing induced action potentials and holding voltage-gated ligand channels closed. Second, in the face of ischemia, the reduced metabolic respiratory rate would preserve substrate and reduce the build-up of toxic by-products of anaerobic glycolysis. Third, vasodilation would improve blood flow into the ischemic penumbra via unobstructed collateral channels. We could not predict whether any or all of these mechanisms might serve our purpose, but the availability of several agonists led us to attempt simple pharmacologic observations of the effect of GABA-A agonists on outcome after focal ischemia.

Pharmacologic strategies to simulate GABA depend on a knowledge of the synthesis, storage, release, and reuptake of GABA. GABA is synthesized by the transamination of α-ketoglutarate to glutamic acid, which is then decarboxylated to GABA, by glutamic acid decarboxylase (GAD). As with most neurotransmitters, release from presynaptic storage vesicles requires energy, is calcium dependent, and is modulated by autoreceptors (GABA-B). There is an active reuptake mechanism that results in storage of GABA in the presynaptic neuron or in glia. The enzyme GABA amino transferase (GABA-T) catabolizes GABA into succinic semialdehyde. The differences and similarities between the neuronal and glial GABA reuptake transporter are not yet clear.

It is clear that there are several potential avenues to mimic the effects of GABA in the central nervous system (Table 13-2). A number of receptor agonists are available from natural or synthetic sources.[42,43] The most potent agonist of the GABA-A receptor is muscimol, derived from the mushroom *Amanita muscaria*. It is of interest to note that this plant is also the source of ibotenic acid (a potent neurotoxin) and muscaric acid (an anticholinergic). Muscimol causes sedation and other barbiturate-like psychic effects but has no effect on vital signs such as body temperature, pulse, or blood pressure. Muscimol is significantly more potent than GABA itself in terms of receptor-binding kinetics.[43,44] Related synthetic compounds include thiomuscimol, dihydromuscimol, and THIP (4,5,6,7-tetrahydroisoxa-

Table 13-2.

Sites of action of drugs that are GABA-mimetic and may prove to be neuroprotective in cerebral ischemia

Site	GABA-A or -B receptors	Action	Drug
Chloride channel	A	Increase chloride flux	Muscimol
Allosteric modulatory sites[a]	A	Modulate chloride flux when GABA occupies binding site	Benzodiazepines Barbiturates Neurosteroids Loreclezole Ethanol
? Site	A	Modulate chloride flux	Clomethiazole
Transporter	A/B	Block GABA reuptake	Nipecotic acid Tiagabine
GABA-transaminase	A/B	Block GABA catabolism	Vigabatrin
Presynaptic membrane	B	Inhibit excitatory neurotransmitter release	Baclofen

[a]Each compound has a distinct, but perhaps overlapping binding site.

zolo[5,4-c]pyridin-3-ol). These agents, and many like them, have been tested in seizure models; some have been selected for development as anticonvulsants. However, there is little work examining GABA agonists other than muscimol for anti-ischemia efficacy.

The metabolism of GABA can be directly inhibited with an agent such as vigabatrin, which irreversibly inactivates GABA-T. This results in a rapid increase in brain GABA concentration, as GABA-T controls the main degradative pathway for GABA. Vigabatrin may be a potent anticonvulsant, but it has not been studied for neuroprotection during ischemia.

GABA uptake can be inhibited by nipecotic acid, resulting in significant increases in synaptic concentrations. Recently, a lipophilic nipecotic acid derivative has been shown to possess significant anticonvulsant properties.[45] The compound [(-)-(R)-1-[4,4,-Bis(3-methyl-2-thienyl)-3-butenyl] nipecotic acid (tiagabine) is currently in clinical trials for epilepsy. Of note, tiagabine inhibits the glial as well as the neuronal GABA transporter. The consequence of this is a prolongation of the inhibitory effects of endogenous GABA release.

A new strategy for using GABAergic mechanisms emerged with the development of GABA modulators. Some steroid molecules have nongenomic actions on cells that seem to be mediated via binding sites on membrane-bound ionophores (for review see Refs. 46,47). Of particular relevance are the 5-reduced, 3α-hydroxylated pregnane steroids, which seem to be potent modulators of chloride flux through the GABA-A ion channel.[48]

On the other hand, other neurosteroids, such as pregnenolone sulfate, may have GABA-antagonist actions, and some have agonist or antagonist properties at the NMDA receptor. Pregnanolone and allopregnanolone are potent sedatives and anticonvulsants.[49]

Evidence Transient occlusion of both carotid and both vertebral arteries (4-vessel occlusion, 4VO) results in a reproducible hippocampus lesion in rats.[50] The lesion consists of neuron loss in the hippocampal CA1 and CA3 layers, a process that is mediated by glutamate. In this model, GABAergic neurons seem to resist ischemia, in that there is selective loss of glutamatergic neurons and relative sparing of GABAergic neurons. These neurons function during and after ischemia and seem to protect target neurons from excitotoxic cell death.[51] GABAergic neurons in the hippocampus show resistance to ischemia in other models as well.

Support for GABAergic-mediated neuroprotection comes from other sources as well. Elevated GABA after ischemia may explain the observation that adrenalectomy prior to ischemia reduces the extent of hippocampal cell loss.[52] In this experiment, GABA levels rose to high levels, compared with nonadrenalectomized controls, whereas glutamate levels were no different. The mechanism mediating the effect is unknown, but obviously the operated animals did not secrete any hydrocortisol. Steroids could alter the vulnerability of hippocampal cells by modulating GABA release, as was observed in this experiment, or by other speculative mechanisms.

The greater preservation of GABAergic neurons during ischemia in some brain regions suggests that GABA uptake inhibitors could be neuroprotective. Uptake inhibitors increase the synaptic concentration of a neurotransmitter by blocking reuptake without affecting release. Uptake inhibitors would be neuroprotective because release of the neurotransmitter is assured, i.e., some GABA-releasing neurons still function during and after ischemia. Unfortunately, as the active agent is GABA itself, receptor binding would occur at GABA-A as well as at presynaptic GABA-B sites. Presynaptic GABA-B receptors may be linked to release of other neurotransmitters, including glutamate. In the 4VO model, GABA uptake inhibitors are clearly protective when given before and after ischemia.[53]

Sternau et al published a provocative series of experiments involving GABA agonists.[54] A variety of agents were tested for neuroprotection against CA1 neuron loss. Many GABAergic agents were effective if given before the onset of ischemia, including diazepam, pentobarbital, valproic acid, baclofen, and muscimol. Pentobarbital, baclofen, and diazepam were given after the onset of ischemia and were not neuroprotective.

Also using the 2VO model, Shuaib and colleagues have studied GABA agonists extensively. Muscimol infused into the ventricle for 7 days protected cortex, hippocampus, substantia nigra, striatum, and thalamus from three episodes of 2-min ischemia.[55] In muscimol-treated animals, no degenerating neurons were seen in the cortex or hippocampus, areas where neurons receive both GABAergic and glutamatergic inputs. Madden used a model of spinal cord ischemia to show that muscimol, given 5 min after ischemia, significantly protected the animals, whereas, bicuculline (a GABA-A antagonist) significantly reduced the tolerance to ischemia.[56]

The most potent GABA-A agonist known is muscimol, which has been shown to be neuroprotective in a variety of experimental models.[55,57–59] Muscimol is effective, even if treatment is delayed several hours after ischemia onset (some data unpublished).[38,57,60] Similar results have now been published from two other laboratories.[55,56] Also, we have found that the combination of muscimol with glutamate antagonists may be synergistic. Thus, the combination affords protection that MK-801 (a glutamate antagonist) cannot when used alone, and muscimol can afford only if used at very high doses. Muscimol and neurosteroid GABA agonists are also effective in a model of intracerebral hematoma.[60] The GABA-B agonist baclofen 20 mg/kg i.p. was highly cytoprotective but caused an increase in blood pressure and brain hemorrhage, and intra-ischemic hypertension is associated with acute brain hemorrhage.[61,62]

A sedative/anticonvulsant that has been used in Europe for over 30 years was recently shown to possess neuroprotective properties. In 1991, clomethiazole was shown to protect against the delayed neuronal degeneration that occurs after transient ischemia.[63] Statistically significant protection was seen when the drug was given up to 3 h after the ischemic episode, and there was a trend toward a neuroprotective effect when it was given at 6 h. Intravenous administration of clomethiazole for 24 h was neuroprotective at plasma concentrations that produced little sedative effect.[64] Clomethiazole has also been shown to reduce the size of infarction in focal ischemia when given after permanent and after transient (1 h) ischemia.[65,66] Clomethiazole has recently been shown to be neuroprotective in an embolism model.[57] The precise mechanism of the neuroprotective effect of clomethiazole has not been elucidated, but one possibility involves an interaction with the GABA, receptor complex.[57,67,68]

Clomethiazole has been used clinically for a variety of indications including treatment of agitation and sleep disturbances in the elderly, during regional anesthesia, treatment of alcohol withdrawal symptoms, pre-eclamptic toxemia, eclampsia, delirium tremens, and status epilepticus. The drug is available in oral and intravenous preparations and has a very favorable side-effect profile. The most frequent side effect is sedation, as would be expected. In addition, there is a puzzling effect on nasal and tracheal epithelium resulting in sneezing and increased secretions, mainly during the loading phase. This effect is not blocked by antihistamines or anticholinergics.[69] Cardiovascular and respiratory effects are minimal or absent provided the drug is given in accordance with recommendations.

Pilot trials of clomethiazole for acute stroke have been completed. An open pilot study of three doses (50, 75, and 100 mg/kg) of intravenous clomethiazole (24-h infusion) has been completed in 17 acute ischemic stroke patients.[69] The most common adverse events were mild sedation, sneezing, and injection site thrombophlebitis. There was little or no effect on blood pressure. A dose of 75 mg/kg could be given without the need for dose reduction due to excessive sedation in most cases.[69]

The efficacy and safety of the 75 mg/kg dose given within 12 h of the onset of the stroke were evaluated in a large placebo-controlled study in Europe and Canada, the Clomethiazole Acute Stroke Study (CLASS).[69]

A total of 1356 patients with a mean age of 72 years and a mean score of 28 on the 58-point Scandinavian Neurological Stroke Scale (SSS) were treated within 12 h of their stroke. In the All Patients Treated analysis (APT), which included 94 patients (7 percent) with intracranial hemorrhage, the difference between clomethiazole and placebo-treated patients on the primary endpoint was not statistically significant. Safety analysis showed no difference in mortality between the two groups (19.4 percent vs. 19.6 percent). There were more serious adverse events reported in the clomethiazole-treated group during treatment, but these were related to the known sedative effects of the drug. A small, statistically significant decrease in blood pressure was observed in clomethiazole-treated patients, but this was not associated with a worse outcome. Safety data in patients with a diagnosis of hemorrhagic stroke were similar to that seen in patients with ischemic stroke.

A subgroup analysis of the efficacy data showed that the most important factors for outcome independent of treatment were age and severity of neurologic symptoms. The worst outcome was seen in the oldest and most severely ill patients. A positive effect of clomethiazole was seen in patients who had a total anterior cerebral syndrome (TACS) ($N = 545$ or 40 percent of the total in the study) according to the classification by Bamford et al.[70] These patients were characterized by having higher cortical dysfunction (e.g., aphasia), limb weakness, and visual field disturbances. In TACS patients, there were 11 percent more clomethiazole-treated patients scoring $\geq$60 on the Barthel Index (40.8 percent vs. 29.8 percent; $p = .008$ unadjusted), a 37 percent relative improvement over placebo. Mortality was slightly lower in this subgroup of clomethiazole-treated patients (28.6 percent vs. 32.2 percent). A second trial (CLASS-I) has been designed to focus specifically on TACS-like patients with ischemic stroke. This trial is powered to observe a beneficial effect of the same magnitude seen in CLASS.

Therapeutic Recommendations At this time, GABA agonists cannot be recommended for use in stroke patients. It is particularly important to continue research in this area, for there is some evidence that GABA agonists actually impede neurologic recovery if used chronically. Therefore, carefully controlled clinical trials with well-designed endpoints must continue to completion. The combination of GABA agonists with glutamate antagonists may be particularly useful, as this therapy may minimize side effects and optimize benefit.

Calcium Channel Blockers

Background Calcium plays a pivotal role in mediating cell death after ischemia as detailed above. A decade ago, there was great hope for calcium antagonists.[71] There were at least two mechanisms by which clinicians hoped calcium blockers would work. First, as calcium blockers were known to cause vasodilation, it was hoped that these agents would improve cerebral blood flow. Obviously, there was a preference for cerebroselective agents, as peripheral vasodilators might cause hypotension and actually reduce CBF. Second, it was hypothesized that antagonists of the voltage-gated calcium channel might block the glutamate-induced increase in intracellular calcium. Several candidate agents were studied and found to have both CBF effects and cytoprotective effects. As detailed under "Evidence," there was no protective effect of these agents found in human clinical stroke trials.

Recently, there has been a renewal of interest in calcium, for it plays a key role in activating cytoplasmic proteases. These enzymes may mediate alternative death pathways, such as an apoptotic-like phenomena. The key step seems to be an increase in intracytoplasmic calcium following excitotoxin stimulation of the postsynaptic cell.[72] Further, it is now clear that the delayed neuronal degeneration phenomenon is mediated by calcium, but not sodium influx. Finally, intracellular calcium concentration seems to regulate a number of enzymes involved in the final stages of ischemic cell death, including lipases, phospholipases, and free radical-generating pathways.

Evidence Calcium channel blockers reduce infarct volume in some, but not all animal models.[71,73–77] In general, the drugs seem more effective when the outcome measure is a morphometric estimate of lesion volume. When a behavioral outcome measure is used, there does not seem to be an impressive beneficial effect.[73,74] This is true for more recently developed calcium blockers as well.[78,79]

Calcium blockers did not work in clinical stroke trials. A controlled trial of flunarizine in acute stroke patients was conducted in Scandinavia and the Netherlands.[80] Three-hundred thirty-one patients who presented within 24 h after stroke onset were included. Patients received 50 mg of flunarizine or placebo by intravenous route daily for the first week after stroke. They then took oral flunarizine (tapering doses) for 3 more weeks. At the end of the 24-week follow-up period, there were no statistically significant differences in outcomes between the two groups. When the subgroup of patients who presented within 6 h of stroke onset was examined separately, there was again no benefit seen.

A trial of oral nimodipine was conducted in North America in patients who presented within 48 h of stroke onset.[81] Patients took nimodipine (various doses) or placebo for 21 days and were studied with several outcome measures. At the end of the 21 days, there were no statistically significant differences between the groups. After the study was completed the authors looked at many subgroups for an indication of efficacy but found none except in the group of patients who arrived at the hospital within 18 h of symptom onset and took 120 mg of nimodipine per day. This finding suggested to the authors that the study might have been positive if patients had begun therapy sooner after stroke onset. At the time of this writing, there are plans under way to examine nimodipine in another trial that focuses on such patients.

Oral nimodipine was also tested in a European study[82] including 1215 patients who presented within 48 h of stroke onset. In this study, the dose of 120 mg/day was used, and patients were followed for 6 months. At this time point, there were no statistically significant differences in the groups. Of concern, there were nonsignificant trends toward adverse outcome (higher mortality) in the group treated with nimodipine.

Nimodipine has been studied in other, smaller trials as well, but no benefit was found in the primary study groups.[83,84] Other agents have been studied, or are currently under study, but no pivotal, phase III trials have yet emerged.[85]

Therapeutic Recommendations Despite the elegant rationale for using calcium blockers, the evidence does not permit a recommendation for their use in stroke patients. One must acknowledge that the nimodipine clinical trials were conducted prior to our current understanding of the therapeutic time window. Thus, if these types of drugs were studied using a modern protocol, benefit might be found. Until such trials are completed and published, use of calcium blockers in stroke patients should be considered experimental.

White Blood Cell Inhibitors

Background It has been known for many years that when blood flow is transiently interrupted by vessel

occlusion, tissue damage may continue even if flow is restored. This "no-reflow" phenomenon has been observed in many organs, but is especially notable in brain.[86] The no-reflow phenomenon was essentially a laboratory curiosity in the stroke literature until the development of thrombolytic therapy. Recent evidence suggests that the process is an important contributor to ischemic injury. During ischemia, CD18 receptors on the surface of leukocytes can be stimulated and bind to the intracellular adhesion molecule (ICAM) on microvessel walls. This activation process produces adhesion of the white cells to the endothelial cells, which can cause occlusion of the microvessels.[20,24] Even if thrombolytic therapy reopens the large vessels, the occlusion of the small vessels may persist.[24] Subsequently, the activated leukocytes migrate across the endothelial walls into the brain substance. The white cells then release catabolic enzymes with resulting tissue destruction. Recently, several laboratories have shown that various antibodies to prevent leukocyte adhesion can reduce neurologic injury during CNS ischemia,[87–89] and a phase III clinical trial of enlimomab, an antibody to ICAM, was recently completed.

Evidence A monoclonal antibody directed against the ICAM receptor effectively blocks granulocyte adherence to endothelial cells and prevents the no-reflow phenomenon and trans-migration into brain.[24,25] In animal models, anti-ICAM reduces neurologic injury after focal ischemia.[25,90,91] The anti-ICAM-1 antibody (dose of 1 mg/kg given intravenously 2 h after ischemia onset, plus 0.5 mg/kg 24 h after ischemia onset) has been tested previously where it was effective in reducing infarction volume by 41 percent.[25] This was associated with a significant reduction in the numbers of granulocytes found in the cortex ipsilateral to the occlusion.

Focal ischemia can be temporary or permanent. Reversible ischemia in animals mimics the early reperfusion that might be seen in humans after thrombolysis. The importance of this distinction is illustrated by a recent study using the suture occlusion model.[92] The authors found that anti-ICAM-1 was effective after 2 h of reversible ischemia, but not if the occlusion was permanent. Because reperfusion did not occur in the permanently occluded group, fewer granulocytes entered the brain and its microcirculation, and there was no opportunity for the anti-ICAM-1 to exert benefit.

The combination of an antiadhesion antibody and t-PA has been tested.[93] The anti-ICAM-1 antibody was not neuroprotective when used alone 15 or 30 min following embolization. However, when given 15 min after embolization in combination with t-PA 2 h later, significant benefit was seen. The authors suggested that early blockade of white blood cell infiltration might prolong the therapeutic window for thrombolysis. Granulocyte infiltration can be blocked using other compounds as well. Small molecules that interfere with granulocyte adherence include synthetic peptides that interact with adhesion molecules.[94,95] These agents seem promising in single or small experimental studies, but large human trials have not begun.

A large clinical trial of anti-ICAM for acute stroke was recently stopped. The final data are not published as of this writing, but preliminary results have been presented (personal communication, W. Clark, MD). In this study of about 600 patients, a mouse monoclonal antibody against ICAM, or placebo, was randomly given in a double-blind fashion. Treatment continued over 4 days. According to the limited outcome data presented to date, the treated subjects suffered worse outcomes than those treated with placebo. For this reason, the safety committee halted the study prior to the planned completion. The explanation for the adverse outcomes is not clear.

Therapeutic Recommendations At this time, there are no data to support the use of white blood cell antagonists for acute stroke. The rationale for use of these types of agents is quite compelling, however, and further work will be needed to determine the final role for these agents in acute stroke therapy. The adverse outcomes seen with enlimomab may be due to a problem with the specific antibody, rather than a flaw in the basic conceptual approach. Further work, preferably guided by well-conducted experimental studies, is needed.

Free Radical Scavengers

Background During ischemia, reducing conditions develop in poorly perfused tissue. Highly reactive oxygen free radicals may be generated from several sources under these circumstances. For example, granulocytes enter the brain during and after ischemia (see above), where a variety of free radical-generating reactions are stimulated.[96,97] The endothelial cells contain the free radical-generating enzyme xanthine oxidase, which converts hypoxanthine to hydrogen peroxide and a superoxide radical during ischemia.[96] Inside the ischemic neuron, free radicals may arise if normal, energy-requiring free radical-scavenging mechanisms fail, again involving xanthine oxidase. If these free radicals are released, they

are potentially capable of starting chain reactions of further free radical generation that can destroy cell membranes, deoxyribonucleic acids, and proteins. Also, free radical generation seems to play a key role in mediating excitotoxic damage, including the initiation of apoptosis.[4,12,96,98] Free radicals are ordinarily "scavenged," i.e., bound into nonreactive compounds, by endogenous molecules such as ascorbate (vitamin C), α-tocopherol (vitamin E), glutathione, and catecholamines. There are also two enzymes found in large quantities in brain that are used to degrade superoxide and hydrogen peroxide: superoxide dismutase (SOD), and glutathione peroxidase. During ischemia, these energy-requiring enzymes fail. Free radicals react especially well with unsaturated lipid, which are found in high concentration in neuronal and glial cell membranes. The result is widespread lipid peroxidation, a reaction that amplifies itself when the conjugated dienes react with oxygen to form more peroxy radicals. Whether this chain of escalating events occurs to any appreciable extent during stroke has not been proven conclusively. However, preclinical studies of agents that have free radical-scavenging properties have been effective in reducing neurologic damage.[99] In particular, Tirilazad (originally designated U70046F) has been studied in a series of clinical trials for ischemic stroke, subarachnoid hemorrhage, and head injury.

Evidence That free radicals play a neurotoxic role is supported by the observation that SOD is neuroprotective. Mice that are deficient in SOD are markedly susceptible to ischemic damage.[100] Mice that overexpress SOD are markedly protected against ischemic damage.[101] The enzyme itself can be delivered to experimental subjects as an infusion. This requires either that the enzyme be dissolved in polyethylene glycol or that it be conjugated to a moiety that facilitates passage across the blood-brain barrier. Both of these treatments are neuroprotective.[102,103] Unfortunately, if the treatment with SOD is delayed too long after ischemia, there is no benefit. The reasons for this limitation are not clear, but this may markedly reduce the utility of these compounds in clinical practice.

Free radical spin-trapping agents combine with highly reactive oxygen species to form stable, and nontoxic, compounds. These agents ameliorate infarct size in a variety of animal models. A widely studied spin trap agent, N-tert-butyl-α-(2-sulfophenyl)-nitrone (S-PBN), and a related compound, α-phenyl-N-tert-butylnitrone (PBN), was shown to reduce damage after a variety of excitotoxic insults.[104] The combination of a glutamate blocker and PBN was found to provide synergistic neuroprotection.[105]

Recently, two unusual free radical scavengers have attracted notice as possible neuroprotectants. Melatonin, a neurohormone critically involved in regulating sleep/wake cycles, seems to act as an antioxidant and free radical scavenger. In a model of forebrain ischemia, intraperitoneally injected melatonin seemed to be neuroprotective.[106] An extract of Ginkgo biloba has also been suggested as possibly effective for acute and chronic ischemia.[107] Considerable further development is essential before either of these compounds can be used in stroke patients.

Extraordinary development effort has been put into a class of antioxidants known as 21-aminosteroids, or lazaroids.[108] The 21-aminosteroids were designed to provide the protective effects of steroids without the glucocorticoid side effects. The name "lazaroid" was coined after the drugs were found to possess remarkable resuscitative effects in experimental subjects, a Lazarus-like effect. Lazaroids act by multiple mechanisms. There is clearly an effect on cell membranes such that lipid peroxidation is inhibited. Also, it seems that lazaroids scavenge free radicals via a mechanism similar to α-tocopherol.

Lazaroids have been extensively studied in experimental models of stroke.[108–111] Many of these studies were done in subprimates using lesion size, rather than neurologic function, as the primary endpoint. As noted above, most compounds tend to show efficacy in models that emphasize morphometry. When neurologic recovery is measured with a behavioral or functional outcome, there is much less efficacy noted.[110] As with the other free radical and antioxidant strategies, these drugs are effective if given prior to, or soon after, the ischemia. However, lazaroids in general have not been shown to be effective when given after a clinically relevant delay time after ischemia.

Human trials of Tirilazad for stroke and subarachnoid hemorrhage have revealed conflicting results. A large, multicenter, international trial of Tirilazad in head injury has been completed, but results are not yet available (personal communication, L. Marshall, MD). In patients suffering subarachnoid hemorrhage two large, multicenter trials have been published. A study conducted at 41 centers in Europe, Australia, and New Zealand randomly treated 1023 patients with Tirilazad three doses; maximum = 6 mg/kg) or placebo. All patients also received intravenous nimodipine.[112] There was a statistically significant reduction in mortality (p=.01) and a greater chance of good recovery (p=.01)

in those patients who received 6 mg/kg Tirilazad, compared with placebo, but the effect was not significant in women. In 54 North American centers, a total of 902 patients randomly received Tirilazad (2 or 6 mg/kg) or placebo for 10 days beginning within 48 h of symptom onset.[113] All patients received oral nimodipine. By 3 months after the hemorrhage, there was no difference in mortality or recovery in the treated patients. When patients with only severe deficits were included in the analysis, there was a statistically significant benefit seen in men. The two trials conflict when compared on the primary hypotheses, and a variety of explanations have been offered for this discrepancy. One of the most intriguing problems was the observation that serum drug levels were markedly lower in women than in men. It was later found that the metabolism of the drug is increased in women. Therefore, two follow-up studies were launched to study a higher dose, 15 mg/kg, of Tirilazad. These studies are ongoing at this time, and the final answer on Tirilazad for subarachnoid hemorrhage-induced vasospasm and ischemia is unclear.

A large trial of Tirilazad for ischemic stroke was organized in North America, known as a Randomized Trial of Tirilazad in Patients with Acute Stroke, or RANTTAS.[114] The trial was conducted in 27 North American centers, and 660 patients were randomized. The study was properly blinded, and control patients received an infusion of vehicle. A preplanned interim analysis was done to examine the data for safety, early efficacy, or futility. RANTTAS is notable for being the first large stroke trial to contain preplanned stopping rules for futility. That is, the trial designers decided to abort the trial if at the interim analysis there was a low probability of having a positive result by the end of the trial. At the interim analysis, there were 556 fully eligible patients available with complete data. The odds of finding a significant benefit attributable to the drug was 0.87 with a 95 percent confidence interval that included 1.0, suggesting that there was no benefit. Therefore, as there was very little chance of finding a positive benefit due to the drug, even if the trial were completed, the trial was abandoned. A trial of a higher dose was organized, but later abandoned as well. For the moment, it seems that there is no evidence to suggest that Tirilazad should be used in patients with acute ischemic stroke.

Therapeutic Recommendations   At this time, Tirilazad is not available for any indications. However, the encouraging results in the subarachnoid hemorrhage trials, and the expected positive results from the follow-up trials, have led to considerable speculation that by the time this manuscript is in print, Tirilazad may be approved by FDA for preventing ischemic injury during vasospasm after subarachnoid hemorrhage. Because Tirilazad has few side effects, it will be tempting to try the drug in stroke patients. This cannot be endorsed. The preclinical data on Tirilazad, and antioxidants in general, suggested that if they are of value at all, therapy must begin within minutes following stroke onset. By the time most physicians encounter stroke patients, such therapy would be wasted effort. One hopes, however, that once the drug is available for some types of stroke, a trial can be organized to test the efficacy of Tirilazad if given by paramedics in the field to victims of acute stroke. Tirilazad would seem to be the ideal agent for use by paramedics as, alone among neuroprotectants, there are no sedative side effects.

CONCLUSIONS

Several drugs that have been evaluated in clinical trials are known to have multiple effects, and they are classified in a given category mainly for convenience. One such drug that has many types of actions is lubeluzole. It has been tested in several experimental stroke models and reduced neurologic damage. A series of phase I to III tests have been conducted, and there is suggestion of treatment efficacy, although the results are not yet conclusive.[115] Another drug, cytidine diphosphate choline (citicoline), has membrane-stabilization properties, but its actions are probably multiple. It was promising in a phase II trial and a more extensive phase III trial is in progress. Fosphenytoin, which is metabolized into phenytoin and has superior solubility properties, is also undergoing phase III testing for acute stroke. Phenytoin, of course, has been used as a first-line anticonvulsant for decades, but its tissue-sparing effects during ischemia seem to be unrelated to its anticonvulsant actions. Nalmefene, an opioid antagonist, has been evaluated recently, and the promising phase II results are likely to be investigated further. The reason for its ability to protect the nervous system is unclear.

At the present time, no cytoprotective agent is approved for use in acute stroke. After considerable effort, glutamate antagonists have not proven effective, although agents active at the glycine site may ultimately prove useful. GABA agonists are in an early stage of development, and considerable work remains to be done. In experimental preclinical work, GABA agonists are more potent at later time points than glutamate antagonists, making them possibly more likely to succeed in clinical trials. Calcium channel blockers do not work, although a proper trial using a short therapeutic window may elucidate a benefit missed in prior work. Antibodies of granulocytes may be ineffective, or perhaps even harmful, although this area of investigation remains open. Free radical strategies are not likely to be successful. To work in experimental studies, these drugs must be given before or soon after the onset of ischemia. Because some free radical scavengers have no sedative properties, however, such a drug may be ideal for use in the field by paramedics.

Ultimately, the most successful treatment for stroke is likely to be combinatorial. Such studies are just beginning, and considerable preclinical work should be done before human clinical trials are begun. It seems that cytoprotective agents may lengthen the therapeutic window for thrombolysis. If a combination of protective drugs could be used in the field, perhaps thrombolysis could be useful as late as 6 or 8 h after stroke. This would allow use of thrombolysis in far greater numbers of patients. Further, for patients unable to receive thrombolysis, cytoprotection may be the only available option.

This is an exciting time to be involved in neurology. Tremendous advances in stroke care have only just begun. The next breakthrough drug may be from one of the classes described above or may result from a novel strategy that is only now under investigation. It is quite clear, though, that further improvements in stroke treatment cannot proceed without properly designed clinical trials that are based on extensive, rigorous preclinical studies.

REFERENCES

1. Heiss W-D: Progress in cerebrovascular disease: Flow thresholds of functional and morphological damage of brain tissue. *Stroke* 14:329, 1983.
2. Astrup J, Symon L, Branston NM, Lassen NA: Cortical evoked potential and extracellular K+ and H+ at critical levels of brain ischemia. *Stroke* 8:51, 1977.
3. Strijbos PJLM, Leach MJ, Garthwaite J: Vicious cycle involving Na+ channels, glutamate release, and NMDA receptors mediates delayed neurodegeneration through nitric oxide formation. *J Neurosci* 16:5004, 1996.
4. Pellegrini-Giampietro DE, Cherici G, Alesiani M, Carla V, Moroni F: Excitatory amino acid release and free radical formation may cooperate in the genesis of ischemia-induced neuronal damage. *J Neurosci* 10:1035, 1990.
5. Lu YM, Yin HZ, Chiang J, Weiss JH: Ca^{2+}-permeable AMPA/kainate and NMDA channels: High rate of Ca^{2+}

influx underlies potent induction of injury. *J Neurosci* 16:5457, 1996.

6. Rothman SM, Olney JW: Glutamate and the pathophysiology of hypoxic-ischemic brain damage. *Ann Neurol* 19:105, 1986.

7. Hartley DM, Kurth MC, Bjerkness L, Weiss JH, Choi DW: Glutamate receptor-induced $^{45}Ca^{2+}$ accumulation in cortical cell culture correlates with subsequent neuronal degeneration. *J Neurosci* 13:1993, 1993.

8. Choi S, Lovinger DM: Metabotropic glutamate receptor modulation of voltage-gated Ca^{2+} channels involves multiple receptor subtypes in cortical neurons. *J Neurosci* 16:36, 1996.

9. Rothman SM: Synaptic activity mediates death of hypoxic neurons. *Science* 220:536, 1983.

10. Choi DW: Glutamate neurotoxicity in cortical cell culture is calcium-dependent. *Neurosci Lett* 58:293, 1985.

11. Choi DW: Ionic dependence of glutamate neurotoxicity. *J Neurosci* 7:369, 1987.

12. Schulz JB, Weller M, Klockgether T: Potassium deprivation-induced apoptosis of cerebellar granule neurons: A sequential requirement for new mRNA and protein synthesis, ICE-like protease activity, and reactive oxygen species. *J Neurosci* 16:4696, 1996.

13. Riveros N, Orrego F: N-Methylaspartate-activated calcium channels in rat brain cortex slices. Effect of calcium channel blockers and of inhibitory and depressant substances. *Neuroscience* 17:541, 1986.

14. Hirayama T, Ono H, Fukuda H: Effects of excitatory and inhibitory amino acid agonists and antagonists on ventral horn cells in slices of spinal cord isolated from adult rats. *Neuropharmacology* 29:1117, 1990.

15. O'Regan MH, Smith-Barbour M, Perkins LM, Phillis JW: A possible role for phospholipases in the release of neurotransmitter amino acids from ischemic rat cerebral cortex. *Neurosci Lett* 185:191, 1995.

16. Brown AW, Brierley JB: The nature, distribution, and earliest stages of anoxic-ischemic nerve cell damage in the rat brain as defined by the optical microscope. *Br J Exp Pathol* 49:87, 1968.

17. Linnik MD, Zobrist RH, Hatfield MD: Evidence supporting a role for programmed cell death in focal cerebral ischemia in rats. *Stroke* 24:2002, 1993.

18. Wyllie AH, Kerr JFR, Currie AR: Cell death: The significance of apoptosis. *Int Rev Cytol* 68:251, 1980.

19. Ames AI, Wright LW, Kowada M, Thurston JM, Majno G: Cerebral ischemia. II. The no-reflow phenomenon. *Am J Pathol* 52:437, 1968.

20. Schmid-Schönbein GW: Capillary plugging by granulocytes and the no-reflow phenomenon in the microcirculation. *Proc Fed Amer Soc Exp Biol* 46:2397, 1987.

21. Harlan JM, Vedder NB, Winn RK, Rice CL: Mechanisms and consequences of leukocyte-endothelial interaction. *West J Med* 155:365, 1991.

22. Hallenbeck JM, Dutka AJ, Tanishima T, et al: Polymorphonuclear leukocyte accumulation in brain regions with low blood flow during the early postischemic period. *Stroke* 17:246, 1986.

23. Menger MD, Lehr H-A, Messmer K: Role of oxygen radicals in the microcirculatory manifestations of postischemic injury. *Klin Wochenschr* 69:1050, 1991.

24. del Zoppo G, Schmid-Schönbein GW, Mori E, Copeland BR, Chang C-M: Polymorphonuclear leukocytes occlude capillaries following middle cerebral artery occlusion and reperfusion in baboons. *Stroke* 22:1276, 1991.

25. Zhang RL, Chopp M, Li Y, et al: Anti-ICAM-1 antibody reduces ischemic cell damage after transient middle cerebral artery occlusion in the rat. *Neurology* 44:1747, 1994.

26. Olney JW, Ho OL, Rhee V: Cytotoxic effects of acidic and sulphur containing amino acids on infant mouse central nervous system. *Exp Brain Res* 14:61, 1971.

27. Ozyurt E, Graham D, Woodruff G, McCullogh J: Protective effect of the glutamate antagonist MK-801 in focal cerebral ischemia in the cat. *J Cereb Blood Flow Metab* 8:138, 1988.

28. Park CK, Nehls DG, Graham DI, Teasdale GM, McCulloch J: The glutamate antagonist MK-801 reduces focal ischemic brain damage in the rat. *Ann Neurol* 24:543, 1988.

29. Boast CS, Gerhardt B, Pastor G, Lehmann J, Etienne PE, Liebman JM: The N-methyl-D-aspartate antagonist CGS19755 and CPP reduce ischemic brain damage in gerbils. *Brain Res* 442:345, 1988.

30. George CP, Goldberg MP, Choi DW, Steinberg GK: Dextromethorphan reduces neocortical ischemic neuronal damage in vivo. *Brain Res* 440:375, 1988.

31. Newell DW, Barth A, Malouf AT: Glycine site NMDA receptor antagonists provide protection against ischemia-induced neuronal damage in hippocampal slice cultures. *Brain Res* 675:38, 1995.

32. Tsuchida E, Bullock R: The effect of the glycine site-specific N-methyl-D-Aspartate antagonist ACEA1021 on ischemic brain damage caused by acute subdural hematoma in the rat. *J Neurotrauma* 12:279, 1995.

33. Grotta J: Safety and tolerability of the glutamate antagonist GCS19755 in acute stroke patients. *Stroke* 25:255, 1994.

34. Albers GW, Atkinson RP, Kelley RE, Rosenbaum DM: Safety, tolerability, and pharmacokinetics of the N-methyl-D-aspartate antagonist dextrorphan in patients with acute stroke. *Stroke* 26:254, 1995.

35. Grotta J, Clark W, Coull B, Pettigrew LC: Safety and tolerability of the glutamate antagonists CGS 19755 (Selfotel) in patients with acute ischemic stroke. *Stroke* 26:602, 1995.

36. Olney JW, Labruyere J, Price M: Pathological changes induced in cerebrocortical neurons by phencyclidine and related drugs. *Science* 244:1360, 1989.

37. Allen HL, Iversen LL: Phencyclidine, dizocilpine, and cerebrocortical neurons. *Science* 247:221, 1990.

38. Lyden PD, Lonzo L, Nunez S: Combination chemotherapy extends the therapeutic window to 60 minutes after stroke. *J Neurotrauma* 12:223, 1995.

39. Kelly PAT, McCulloch J: Effects of the putative GABAergic agonists, muscimol and THIP, upon local cerebral glucose utilisation. *J Neurochem* 39:613, 1982.

40. Kelly PT, McCulloch J: The effects of the GABAergic agonist muscimol upon the relationship between local cerebral blood flow and glucose utilization. *Brain Res* 258:338, 1983.

41. Edvinsson L, Krause DN: Pharmacological characterization of GABA receptors mediating vasodilation of cerebral arteries in vitro. *Brain Res* 173:89, 1979.

42. de Carolis SA, Lipparinai F, Longo VG: Neuropharmacological investigations on muscimol a psychotropic drug extracted from *Amanita muscaria. Psychopharmacology* 15:186, 1969.

43. Krogsgaard-Larsen P, Hjeds H, Curtis DR, Lodge D: Dihydromuscimol, thiomuscimol and related heterocyclic compounds as GABA analogues. *J Neurochem* 32:1717, 1979.

44. DeFeudis FV: Binding studies with muscimol; relation to synaptic γ-aminobutyrate receptors. *Neuroscience* 5:675, 1980.

45. Suzdak PD, Jansen JA: A review of the preclinical pharmacology of tiagabine: A potent and selective anticonvulsant GABA uptake inhibitor. *Epilepsia* 36:612, 1995.

46. Gee KW, McCauley LD, Lan NC: A putative receptor for neurosteroids on the GABA$_A$ receptor complex: The pharmacological properties and therapeutic potential of epalons. *Crit Rev Neurobiol* 9:207, 1995.

47. Lambert JJ, Belelli D, Hill-Venning C, Peters JA: Neurosteroids and GABA$_A$ receptor function. *Trends Pharmacol Sci* 16:295, 1995.

48. Devaud LL, Purdy RH, Morrow AL: The Neurosteroid, 3α-hydroxy-5α-pregnan-20-one, protects against bicuculline-induced seizures during ethanol withdrawal in rats. *Alcohol Clin Exp Resp* 19:350, 1995.

49. Hauser CAE, Wetzel CHR, Rupprecht R, Holsboer F: Allopregnanoline acts as an inhibitory modulator on α$_1$- and α$_6$-containing GABA$_A$ receptors. *Biochem Biophys Res Commun* 219:531, 1996.

50. Pulsinelli WA, Buchan AM: The four-vessel occlusion rat model: Method for complete occlusion of vertebral arteries and control of collateral circulation. *Stroke* 19:913, 1988.

51. Johansen FF, Christensen T, Jensen MS, et al: Inhibition in postischemic rat hippocampus: GABA receptors, GABA release, and inhibitory postsynaptic potentials. *Exp Brain Res* 84:529, 1991.

52. Ravindran J, Shuaib A, Ijaz S, et al: High extracellular GABA levels in hippocampus as a mechanism of neuronal protection in cerebral ischemia in adrenalectomized gerbils. *Neurosci Lett* 176:209, 1994.

53. Johansen FF, Diemer NH: Enhancement of GABA neurotransmission after cerebral ischemia in the rat reduces loss of hippocampal CA1 pyramidal cells. *Acta Neurol Scand* 84:1, 1991.

54. Stemau LL, Lust WD, Ricci AJ, Ratcheson R: Role for gamma-aminobutyric acid in selective vulnerability in gerbils. *Stroke* 20:281, 1989.

55. Shuaib A, Mazagri R, Ijaz S: GABA agonist "muscimol" is neuroprotective in repetitive transient forebrain ischemia in gerbils. *Exp Neurol* 123:284, 1993.

56. Madden K: Effect of gamma-aminobutyric acid modulation on neuronal ischemia in rabbits. *Stroke* 25:2271, 1994.

57. Lyden PD: GABA and neuroprotection, in Green AR, Cross AJ (eds): *Neuroprotective Agents and Cerebral Ischemia.* London, Academic Press Limited, 1997, pp 233–258.

58. Lyden PD, Hedges B: Protective effect of synaptic inhibition during cerebral ischemia. *Stroke* 23:1463, 1992.

59. Lyden PD, Lonzo L: Combination therapy protects ischemic brain in rats. *Stroke* 25:189, 1994.

60. Lyden PD, Jackson-Friedman C, Lonzo-Doktor L: Medical therapy for intracerebral hematoma with the gamma-aminobutyric acid-A agonist muscimol. *Stroke* 28:387, 1997.

61. Levy DE, Brott TG, Haley EC Jr, et al: Factors related to intracranial hematoma formation in patients receiving tissue-type plasminogen activator for acute ischemic stroke. *Stroke* 25:291, 1994.

62. Bowes MP, Zivin JA, Thomas GR, Thibodeaux H, Fagan SC: Acute hypertension, but not thrombolysis, increases the incidence and severity of hemorrhagic transformation following experimental stroke in rabbits. *Exp Neurol* 141:40, 1996.

63. Cross AJ, Jones JA, Baldwin HA, Green AR: Neuroprotective activity of chlormethiazole following transient forebrain ischaemia in the gerbil. *Br J Pharmacol* 104:406, 1991.

64. Cross AJ, Jones TA, Snares M, Jostell K, Bredberg U, Green AR: The protective action of chlormethiazole against ischemia-induced neurodegeneration in gerbils when infused at doses having little sedative or anticonvulsant activity. *Br J Pharmacol* 114:1625, 1995.

65. Sydserff SG, Cross AJ, Green AR: The neuroprotective effect of chlormethiazole on ischemic neuronal damage following permanent middle cerebral artery ischemia in the rat. *Neurodegeneration* 4:323, 1995.

66. Sydserff SG, Cross AJ, West KJ, Green AR: The effect of chlormethiazole on ischemic neuronal damage in a model of transient focal ischemia. *Br J Pharmacol* 114:1631, 1995.

67. Green AR, Cross AJ: The neuroprotective actions of chlormethiazole. *Prog Neurobiol* 44:463, 1994.

68. Cross AJ, Stirling JM, Robinson TN, Bowen DM, Francis PT, Green AR: The modulation by clomethiazole of the GABA-A receptor complex in rat brain. *Br J Pharmacol* 98:284, 1989.

69. Footitt D: Medical management of acute stroke. *Br J Cardiol* 4:104, 1997.

70. Bamford J, Sandercock P, Dennis M, Burn J, Warlow C: Classification and natural history of clinically identifiable subtypes of cerebral infarction. *Lancet* 337:1521, 1991.

71. Wong MCW, Haley CH: Calcium antagonists: Stroke therapy coming of age. *Stroke* 21:494, 1990.

72. Usachev YM, Thayer SA: All-or-none Ca^{2+} release from intracellular stores triggered by Ca^{2+} influx through voltage-gated Ca^{2+} channels in rat sensory neurons. *J Neurosci* 17:7404, 1997.

73. Grotta JC, Pettigrew LC, Rosenbaum D, Reid C, Rhoades H, McCandless D: Efficacy and mechanism of action of a calcium channel blocker after global cerebral ischemia in rats. *Stroke* 19:447, 1988.

74. Lyden PD, Zivin JA, Kochhar A, Mazzarella V: The effects of calcium channel blockers on neurological outcome following reversible and irreversible focal ischemia. *Stroke* 19:1020, 1988.

75. Kleiser B, Van Reempts J, Van Deuren B, et al: Favourable effect of flunarizine on the recovery from hemiparesis in rats with intracerebral hematomas. *Neurosci Lett* 103:225, 1989.

76. Madden KP, Clark WM, Marcoux RW, et al: Treatment with conotoxin an "N-type" calcium channel blocker in neuronal hypoxic-ischemic injury. *Brain Res* 537:256, 1990.

77. Snape MF, Baldwin HA, Cross AJ, Green AR: The effects of chlormethiazole and nimodipine on cortical infarct area after focal cerebral ischaemia in the rat. *Neuroscience* 53:837, 1993.

78. Campbell C, Mackay K, Patel S, et al: Effects of isradipine, an L-type calcium blocker on permanent and transient focal cerebral ischemia in spontaneously hypertensive rats. *Exp Neurol* 148:45, 1997.

79. Bowersox S, Singh T, Luther R: Selective blockade of N-type voltage-sensitive calcium channels protects against brain injury after transient focal cerebral ischemia in rats. *Brain Res* 747:343, 1997.

80. Franke C, Palm R, Dalby M, et al: Flunarizine in stroke treatment (FIST): A double-blind, placebo-controlled trial in Scandinavia and the Netherlands. *Acta Neurol Scand* 93:56, 1996.

81. The American Nimodipine Study Group: Clinical trial of nimodipine in acute ischemic stroke. *Stroke* 23:3, 1992.

82. The Trust Study Group: Randomised, double-blind, placebo-controlled trial of nimodipine in acute stroke. *Lancet* 336:1205, 1990.

83. Bogousslavsky J, Regli F, Zumstein V, Kobberling W: Double-blind study of nimodipine in non-severe stroke. *Eur Neurol* 30:23, 1990.

84. Martinez-Vila E, Guillen F, Villanueva J, et al: Placebo-controlled trial of nimodipine in the treatment of acute ischemic cerebral infarction. *Stroke* 21:1023, 1990.

85. Rosenbaum D, Zabramski JM, Frey J, et al: Early treatment of ischemic stroke with a calcium antagonist. *Stroke* 22:437, 1991.

86. Ames A III, Wright RL, Kowada M, Thurston JM, Majno G: Cerebral ischemia. II. The no-reflow phenomenon. *Am J Pathol* 52:437, 1968.

87. Clark WM, Madden KP, Rothlein R, Zivin JA: Reduction of central nervous system ischemic injury by monoclonal antibody to intercellular adhesion molecule. *J Neurosurg* 75:623, 1991.

88. Zhang RL, Chopp M, Li Y, et al: Anti-ICAM-1 antibody reduces ischemic cell damage after transient middle cerebral artery occlusion in the rat. *Neurology* 44:1747, 1994.

89. Lindsberg PJ, Sirén A-L, Feuerstein GZ, Hallenbeck JM: Antagonism of neutrophil adherence in the deteriorating stroke model in rabbits. *J Neurosurg* 82:269, 1995.

90. Bowes MP, Zivin JA, Rothlein R: Monoclonal antibody to the ICAM-1 adhesion site reduces neurological damage in a rabbit cerebral embolism stroke model. *Exp Neurol* 119:215, 1993.

91. Clark WM, Madden KP, Rothlein R, Zivin JA: Reduction of central nervous system ischemic injury by monoclonal antibody to intercellular adhesion molecule. *J Neurosurg* 75:623, 1991.

92. Zhang RL, Chopp M, Jiang N, et al: Anti-intercelluar adhesion molecule-1 antibody reduces ischemic cell damage after transient but not permanent middle cerebral artery occlusion in the Wistar rat. *Stroke* 26:1438, 1995.

93. Bowes MP, Rothlein R, Fagan SC, Zivin JA: Monoclonal antibodies preventing leukocyte activation reduce experimental neurologic injury and enhance efficacy of thrombolytic therapy. *Neurology* 45:815, 1995.

94. Yanaka K, Camarat P, Spellman S, et al: Neuronal protection from cerebral ischemia by synthetic fibronectin peptides to leukocyte adhesion molecules. *J Cereb Blood Flow Metab* 16:1120, 1996.

95. Morikawa E, Zhang S, Seko Y, Toyoda T, Kirino T: Treatment of focal cerebral ischemia with synthetic oligopeptide corresponding to the lectin domain of selection. *Stroke* 27:951, 1996.

96. Hallenbeck JM, Dutka AJ: Background review and current concepts of reperfusion injury. *Arch Neurol* 47:1245, 1990.

97. Fantone JC, Ward PA: Role of oxygen-derived free radicals and metabolites in leukocyte-dependent inflammatory reactions. *Am J Pathol* 107:397, 1982.

98. Oh SM, Betz AL: Interaction between free radicals and excitatory amino acids in the formation of ischemic brain edema in rats. *Stroke* 22:915, 1991.

99. Hall ED, Yonkers PA: Attenuation of postischemic cerebral hypoperfusion by the 21-aminosteroid U74006F. *Stroke* 19:340, 1988.

100. Kondo T, Reaume AG, Huang TT, et al: Reduction of CuZn-superoxide dismutase activity exacerbates neuronal cell injury and edema formation after transient focal cerebral ischemia. *Soc Neurosci* 17:4180, 1997.

101. Chan PH, Kinouchi H, Epstein CJ, et al: Role of superoxide dismutase in ischemic brain injury: Reduction of edema and infarction in transgenic mice following focal cerebral ischemia. *Prog Brain Res* 96:97, 1993.

102. Cerchiari EL, Hoel TM, Safar P, Sclabassi RJ: Protective effects of combined superoxide dismutase and deferoxa-

mine on recovery of cerebral blood flow and function after cardiac arrest in dogs. *Stroke* 18:869, 1987.

103. Matsumiya N, Koehler RC, Kirsch JR, Traystman RJ: Conjugated superoxide dismutase reduces extent of caudate injury after transient focal ischemia in cats. *Stroke* 22:1193, 1991.

104. Schulz JB, Henshaw DR, Siwek D, et al: Involvement of free radicals in excitotoxicity in vivo. *J Neurochem* 64:2239, 1995.

105. Barth A, Barth L, Newell DW: Combination therapy with MK-801 and α-phenyl-*tert*-butyl-nitrone enhances protection against ischemic neuronal damage in organotypic hippocampal slice cultures. *Exp Neurol* 141:330, 1998.

106. Cho S, Joh TH, Baik HH, Dibinis C, Volpe BT: Melatonin administration protects CA1 hippocampal neurons after transient forebrain ischemia in rats. *Brain Res* 755:335, 1997.

107. Garg RK, Nag G, Agrawal A: A double blind placebo controlled trial of ginkgo biloba extract in acute cerebral ischemia. *J Assoc Physicians India* 43:760, 1995.

108. Hall ED, Braughler JM, McCall JM: Role of oxygen radicals in stroke: Effects of the 21-aminosteroids (lazaroids). A novel class of antioxidants. *Curr Future Trends Antianxiety Stroke Ther* 351, 1990.

109. Xue D, Slivka A, Buchan AM: Tirilazad reduces cortical infarction after transient but not permanent focal cerebral ischemia in rats. *Stroke* 23:894, 1992.

110. Clark WM, Hotan T, Lauten J, Coull BM: Therapeutic efficacy of tirilazad in experimental multiple cerebral emboli. *Stroke* 24:175, 1993.

111. Auer RN: Combination therapy with U74006F (tirilazad mesylate), MK-801, insulin and diazepam in transient forebrain ischaemia. *Neurol Res* 17:132, 1995.

112. Kassell NF, Haley EC, Apperson-Hansen C, Alves WM: Randomized, double-blind, vehicle-controlled trial of Tirilazad mesylate in patients with aneurysmal subarachnoid hemorrhage: A cooperative study in Europe, Australia, and New Zealand. *J Neurosurg* 84:221, 1996.

113. Haley EC, Kassell NF, Apperson-Hansen C, Maile MH, Alves WM: A randomized, double-blind, vehicle-controlled trial of tirilazad mesylate in patients with aneurysmal subarachnoid hemorrhage: A cooperative study in North America. *J Neurosurg* 86:467, 1997.

114. The RANTTAS Investigators: A randomized trial of Tirilazad mesylate in patients with acute stroke (RANTTAS). *Stroke* 27:1453, 1996.

115. Diener HC, Hacke W, Hennerici M, Radberg J: Lubeluzole in acute ischemic stroke. A double-blind, placebo-controlled Phase II trial. *Stroke* 27:76, 1996.

Chapter 14

EMERGENCY CAROTID REVASCULARIZATION FOR ACUTE ISCHEMIC STROKE

Vikram S. Kashyap
Wesley S. Moore

BACKGROUND

Emergency carotid revascularization for acute stroke has been the interest of several investigators over the last three decades. The theoretical benefit of this procedure in the setting of acute neurologic dysfunction has only been inconsistently achieved. Because of early reports revealing poor outcomes, emergency carotid revascularization has never caught on as a widely used option in stroke treatment. However, with advances in diagnostic and therapeutic capability, recent reports have shown some benefit in carefully selected patients leading to a resurgence in interest in this modality. Specifically, properly selected patients treated for stroke-in-evolution or crescendo transient ischemic attacks (TIA) with emergency endarterectomy have had more favorable outcomes when compared with early reports evaluating heterogeneous patient groups presenting with varying levels of neurologic deficit.

Theoretically, immediate restoration of blood flow through a carotid artery responsible for an acute stroke has tremendous appeal. If the acute neurologic deterioration is the result of acute carotid occlusion, recurrent embolization, or extension of thrombus, revascularization of the ipsilateral carotid artery could provide (1) definitive treatment of the offending lesion with restoration of carotid patency before repair becomes impossible due to chronic occlusion, (2) immediate reversal of the acute deficit, and (3) late prevention of continued neurologic deterioration. With respect to the last, it is important to keep in mind that the chronically occluded internal carotid artery is not innocuous and the continuing ipsilateral stroke risk is on the order of 5 percent per year.[1,2] Multiple randomized prospective trials have documented the safety, benefit and durability of elective carotid revascularization in preventing stroke in both symptomatic and asymptomatic patients at risk for stroke.[3,4] However, no similar study has been attempted with patients with acute stroke. Substantial logistic hurdles, as well as a historic bias against emergency surgery on the carotid artery, must be overcome for a prospective study of this sort to come to fruition. The current and future expansion of emergency endarterectomy for acute stroke will rest on a few key variables: (1) the early identification of an ischemic stroke referable to an acutely occluded ipsilateral carotid artery, (2) the development of streamlined protocols that facilitate the expeditious movement of selected acute stroke patients from the emergency room to the operating room for surgical treatment, and most importantly, (3) the rigorous testing of these protocols for evidence of benefit in comparison with contemporary medical stroke management.

EVIDENCE

Early Experience

In the 1960's, the indications for carotid revascularization were being evaluated in patients with carotid artery atherosclerosis. Performing carotid revascularization for acute stroke was attempted, but postoperative cerebral hemorrhage was an unfortunately frequent occurrence. Rob had popularized carotid revascularization in the 1950's but reported a dismal experience with urgent carotid endarterectomy for internal carotid artery thrombosis.[5] He found that of 74 patients operated on, only 28 percent derived any benefit and 29 percent died. Wylie's early report in 1964 of nine patients undergoing urgent operation after acute stroke revealed that more than half of the patients died from delayed cerebral hemorrhage.[6] In 1969, the Joint Study of Extracranial Arterial Occlusion reported a 42 percent mortality rate for operations on totally occluded arteries following acute stroke.[7] Patients in this study had suffered acute, severe strokes within 2 weeks of endarterectomy. In retrospect, all of these studies were flawed by including results of delayed operations on patients with profound neurologic deficits, altered levels of consciousness, and uncontrolled hypertension. Other studies documented the hazards of operating on the carotid artery following acute stroke, leading the renowned neurologist W. S. Fields to conclude that a surgical mortality of up to 50 percent was to be expected if carotid surgery was performed during the acute neurologic deterioration of stroke.[8] Furthermore, he stated that a much higher percentage of these patients would recover from medical treatment alone. Taken together, these reports had a negative impact on the utility of carotid revascularization in the setting of acute stroke that has persisted today.

Postoperative cerebral hemorrhage was the condition that led to the majority of deaths in these studies. The etiology of postoperative cerebral hemorrhage is now thought to be a combination of the susceptibility of the ischemic cerebrum to hemorrhage coupled with hypertension. Meyer originally demonstrated ischemic damage to small vessels adjacent to ischemic brain lesions produced by middle cerebral artery occlusion in monkeys.[9] Capillary permeability is increased in areas surrounding ischemic cerebral tissue, which allows for massive intracerebral hemorrhage during reperfusion in areas of prior nonhemorrhagic infarction.

Another experimental observation with important clinical relevance is the concept of ischemic penumbra. This term implies a zone of neuronal electrical dysfunction without cellular death in the setting of oligemia surrounding a central infarction. Studies in primates suggest that up to 6 h of relative cerebral ischemia can be reversed without infarction.[10] Thus, tolerance of brain tissue to relative ischemia may allow the opportunity for therapeutic intervention to reverse the ischemic process. Similarly, some early reports did document that timing of emergency endarterectomy, if contemplated, should be done as soon as possible. In a report by Thompson

and colleagues of 100 occluded carotid arteries that underwent revascularization, cerebral blood flow was restored in only one-third of patients.[11] However, results were better in patients who were operated on within 6 to 12 h of symptom onset. In 1971, Najafi and colleagues reported on 53 patients undergoing emergency carotid surgery after stroke associated with cerebral angiography.[12] Half of the patients improved. The authors concluded that patients with acute stroke should be operated on within a few hours of symptom onset or not at all. Perhaps of greatest importance, these reports documented the dramatic and gratifying reversal of severe neurologic deficits in some patients undergoing carotid thromboembolectomy for acute stroke.

Recent Experience

The early retrospective reports did not have the benefit of formal neurologic severity scoring systems, and thus heterogeneous populations of patients were being analyzed for evidence of therapeutic benefit. However, recent advances in medical care make the early pessimistic reports on emergency carotid revascularization less relevant today. Perhaps most important in overall stroke management has been the advances in prehospital care with rapid transport of patients to organized emergency centers that allow for early diagnosis and intervention. Also, advanced in cerebral and arterial imaging, refinements in intraoperative management, and improved postoperative intensive care of these patients make the feasibility of emergency endarterectomy more valid today. One must keep in mind that the early studies were done in an era prior to the advent of CT scanning and the universal use of cardiovascular monitoring. Thus, in retrospect, the early reports on emergency endarterectomy were done in situations where an intracranial hemorrhage had not been definitively excluded preoperatively and the perioperative cardiovascular management (i.e., blood pressure control) may not have been ideal.

Recent experience with emergency carotid endarterectomy confirms that timing of operation has an important bearing on outcome. Kusunoki and colleagues found a marked difference in patency depending on the time of intervention.[13] In seven cases where the occluded internal carotid artery was operated on within 72 h, six had restoration of blood flow (86 percent). However, if the operation was delayed beyond 3 days, patency fell below 50 percent. Furthermore, of the patients with severe neurologic or medical risk factors undergoing this procedure, 65 percent suffered myocardial infarction, stroke, or death. A study using serial ultrasound or digital subtraction angiography postoperatively confirmed this relationship of early timing of operation with durable patency of the carotid artery.[14] Other recent studies include a series of 64 emergency endarterectomies performed at the Massachusetts General Hospital.[15] The selection of patients for surgery was based on level of consciousness and severity of neurologic deficit. The authors' conclusion was that a significantly altered level of consciousness was a contraindication for surgical treatment. A recent study evaluated operative vs. nonoperative management of angiographically verified acute internal carotid artery occlusion in 64 patients with ischemic stroke.[16] In this study, half underwent surgery emergently and half were treated medically. The groups were compared for functional recovery over 4 weeks and were found to have no significant differences, but mortality was lower in the medically treated group. However, this study was short-term and nonrandomized. McCormick's 1992 report on 42 patients with a history of stroke and internal artery occlusion included 12 cases that underwent emergent surgery for acute stroke.[17] In this series, profound preoperative neurologic deficit was considered a contraindication for operation. No postoperative deaths were reported, and all patients were stroke-free during a mean follow-up of 40 months.

Two distinct subgroups of patients with acute neurologic symptoms include those with stroke-in-evolution and crescendo TIA. Their response to surgical intervention may be quite different. Early reports often lumped patients with varying levels of neurologic compromise, representing a spectrum ranging from mild to dense, fixed neurologic deficits. In comparison, stroke-in-evolution, also called deteriorating stroke, progressing stroke, incomplete stroke, or stroke in progression, is an acute neurologic deficit, often mild to moderate, which progresses in a sequence of stepwise deteriorations to a major fixed neurologic deficit. Occasionally, this takes the form of a deficit that resolves partially only to come back again in a waxing and waning fashion. Crescendo TIA are characterized as episodes of transient ischemia that completely resolve, only to reappear in wider territory or increase in frequency. Patients with stroke-in-evolution and crescendo TIA have a poor prognosis, and previous studies have shown the natural history of these conditions is an eventual permanent moderate to severe deficit.[18] A recent study revealed that 36 percent of patients with progressive ischemic stroke continued to deteriorate despite being on heparin anticoagulation.[19]

Goldstone and Moore reviewed their experience with emergency CEA in 11 patients over an 18-month period.[20] Seven patients had gradually progressive deficits or waxing and waning deficits over 3 to 7 days. The other 4 patients had frequent TIA over 5 to 7 days. None of these patients had severe neurologic deficit or depressed level of consciousness, and none had carotid occlusions. Following CEA, all had complete recovery. A later report enlarged to 28 patients showed that 27 out of 28 patients improved, but the remaining one patient died of a brainstem stroke on the third postoperative day.[21] Mentzer and colleagues reviewed their experience with emergency endarterectomy in 24 patients with stroke-in-evolution or crescendo TIA and found that 79 percent improved, 17 percent remained unchanged, and one patient (4 percent) died.[22] In reviewing the reports dealing with surgery for fluctuating neurologic deficits up to 1980, they found 55 percent were improved, 25 percent remained unchanged, 10 percent were worse, and 10 percent died. The American Association of Neurological Surgeons performed a voluntary audit of CEA done in 1981. Of the 3328 operations reported from 46 centers, 38 were performed for stroke-in-evolution. In these patients, there was a 21 percent death or stroke rate.[23]

As stated for acute stroke, timing of surgery again is an important factor, with better results occurring early—rather than later—in the course of events. This allows the best opportunity for the definitive treatment of the lesion coupled with prevention of a permanent neurologic deficit. Recently, Gertler and associates reported 70 urgent operations in 68 patients with unstable neurologic conditions or anatomically compelling angiographic findings. Seventeen patients had stroke-in-evolution, and the rest had crescendo TIA or anatomically compelling angiograms. Grading results using a neurologic event severity scale, 86.5 percent of patients improved or stabilized, 3.8 percent worsened, and no deaths occurred.[24] Morgenstern and colleagues used the NASCET database to evaluate the necessity of emergency surgery in patients with symptoms and anatomically compelling angiograms.[25] Of 106 patients with near occlusion (95 to 99 percent) of the internal carotid artery, 29 had a string-like lumen. Of the 58 near occlusions treated medically, 14 had a "string sign." In the surgical group, 15 of 48 had a string sign. Three patients (6 percent) in the surgical group had a stroke in the first 30 days compared with one patient in the medical group (2 percent). These authors concluded that these results suggest emergency CEA is not needed for near occlusion of a symptomatic internal carotid artery.

THERAPEUTIC RECOMMENDATIONS

The Rand Corporation using an expert panel's opinions and rating the indications for operation[26] has published analysis of the appropriateness of carotid endarterectomy. There were internal inconsistencies with the methodology of this analysis, but a single episode of TIA and "acutely occluded" ipsilateral carotid artery was deemed a moderately strong indication for operation. Also, an atherothrombotic stroke associated with an acutely occluded ipsilateral artery of less than a 6-h duration was judged to be a weakly positive indication, but over 6 h was deemed extremely inappropriate. The Ad Hoc Committee of the Joint Council of the Society for Vascular Surgery and the North American Chapter of the International Society for Cardiovascular Surgery, a multidisciplinary group, published guidelines for carotid endarterectomy in 1992, some of which are relevant to emergency carotid endarterectomy.[27] A patient who is evaluated within 1 h of a neurologic event "may be considered a candidate for emergency intervention." However, an acute stroke was considered to be a contraindication for carotid endarterectomy because of the risk of increased mortality or reperfusion hemorrhage within the infarct. The conclusion was that a prospective, randomized trial was the only method of determining whether carotid endarterectomy, in addition to best medical management, was of benefit. Similarly, the American Heart Association concluded that acute carotid occlusions manifested by transient cerebral ischemia or mild stroke were classified as "uncertain indications" for carotid endarterectomy.[28]

An algorithm to identify individuals amenable to surgical intervention with stroke-in-evolution and crescendo TIA has been published.[29] It involves identifying individuals with acute unstable neurologic deficits, documenting the absence of a causal intracranial lesion (i.e., infarct, hemorrhage, tumor, arteriovenous malformation, etc.) with a CT or MR scan and proceeding with arteriography to try to identify an unstable arterial lesion that may be responsible for the condition. If an unstable lesion is discovered, emergency operation is considered. Many of the patients with stroke-in-evolution or crescendo TIA have critical lesions in the carotid bifurcation (>95 percent) that may be preocclusive. De-

spite many logistic hurdles inherent to this algorithm, it has been successfully applied in selected patients with mild to moderate neurologic deficit.

The recent effective use of thrombolytic therapy for an acute ischemic stroke adds validity to the belief that prompt restoration of cerebral blood flow is feasible and beneficial.[30] Furthermore, it underscores the theoretical benefit of surgical intervention in the acute setting as well. The increased utility of this regimen may lead to the finding of an underlying hemodynamically significant lesion in the ipsilateral carotid artery following lytic therapy in some patients. Carotid endarterectomy in this setting may be advocated during the same hospitalization as definitive therapy in stroke prevention. The role of combined thrombolysis and carotid endarterectomy is unknown, but its study should be entertained in the near future.[31]

In sum, the bias against emergency carotid revascularization in the setting of acute stroke is because of historical reports documenting poor results and the unavailability of a well-performed prospective trial documenting efficacy and benefit over medical management. A prospective trial has been advocated,[27,32] but it would be difficult to administer and keep well controlled.[33] The surgical arm of such a trial would disregard traditional categories such as TIA vs. stroke when the emergent operation is done within hours, thus underscoring the fact that surgery may be performed on patients that would improve regardless. Furthermore, distinguishing between an acute and chronic occlusion of the carotid artery could not be made preoperatively, leading to some patients having arterial exploration only.

Based on the available evidence, emergent carotid revascularization cannot be widely recommended for acute stroke. In rare cases, its performance should be done at institutions with documented expertise in cerebrovascular disease and the readily available resources to facilitate urgent operation. In general, patients with dense, fixed neurologic deficits, as well as patients being considered for thrombolytic therapy, should be excluded from consideration for emergency surgical revascularization. If emergency surgical revascularization is entertained, early timing of the operation is crucial. Recent evidence reveals that the subset of patients with stroke-in-evolution or crescendo transient ischemic attacks may have more favorable outcomes with emergency endarterectomy. Despite the lack of prospective data, experienced surgeons have documented the dramatic reversal in neurologic deficits following emergent revascularization in carefully selected patients.

REFERENCES

1. Cote R, Barnett H, Taylor D: Internal carotid occlusion: A prospective study. *Stroke* 14:898, 1983.
2. Makhoul R, Moore W, Colburn M, et al: Benefit of carotid endarterectomy after prior stroke. *J Vasc Surg* 18:666, 1993.
3. NASCET Collaborators: Beneficial effect of carotid endarterectomy in symptomatic patients with high-grade stenosis. *N Engl J Med* 325:445, 1991.
4. ACAS Executive Committee: Endarterectomy for asymptomatic carotid artery stenosis. *JAMA* 273:1421, 1995.
5. Rob C: Operation for acute completed stroke due to thrombosis of the internal carotid artery. *Surgery* 65:862, 1969.
6. Wylie E, Hein M, Adams J: Intracranial hemorrhage following surgical revascularization for treatment of acute strokes. *J Neurosurg* 21:212, 1964.
7. Blaisdell W, Clauss R, Galbraith J, et al: Joint study of extracranial arterial occlusion. *JAMA* 209:1889, 1969.
8. Fields W: Selection of stroke patients for arterial reconstructive surgery. *Am J Surg* 125:527, 1973.
9. Meyer J: Importance of ischemic damage to small vessels in experimental cerebral infarction. *J Neuropathol Exp Neurol* 17:571, 1958.
10. Watanabe O, Bremer A, West L: Experimental regional cerebral ischemia in the middle cerebral artery territory in primates: Part 1. Angioanatomy and description of an experimental model with selective embolization of the ICA bifurcation. *Stroke* 8:61, 1977.
11. Thompson J, Austin D, Patman R: Endarterectomy of the totally occluded carotid artery for stroke. *Arch Surg* 95:791, 1967.
12. Najafi H, Javid H, Dye W, et al: Emergency carotid thromboendarterectomy. *Arch Surg* 103:610, 1971.
13. Kusunoki T, Rowed D, Tator C, et al: Thromboendarterectomy for total occlusion of the internal carotid artery: A reappraisal of risks, success rate, and potential benefits. *Stroke* 9:34, 1978.
14. Welling R, Cranley J, Krause R, et al: Surgical therapy for recent total occlusion of the internal carotid artery. *J Vasc Surg* 1:57, 1984.
15. Walters B, Ojemann R, Heros R: Emergency carotid endarterectomy. *J Neurosurg* 66:817, 1987.
16. Bone G, Ladurner G, Waldstein N, Rendl K, Prenner K: Acute carotid artery occlusion: Operative or conservative management. *Eur Neurol* 30:214, 1990.
17. McCormick P, Spetzler R, Bailes J, et al: Thromboendarterectomy of the symptomatic occluded internal carotid artery. *J Neurosurg* 76:752, 1992.
18. Millikan C, McDowell F: Treatment of progressing stroke. *Stroke* 12:397, 1981.
19. Slivka A, Levy D: Natural history of progressive ischemic stroke in a population treated with heparin. *Stroke* 21:1657, 1990.
20. Goldstone J, Moore W: Emergency carotid surgery in neurologically unstable patients. *Arch Surg* 111:1284, 1976.
21. Goldstone J, Effeney D: The role of carotid endarterectomy in the treatment of acute neurologic deficits. *Prog Cardiovasc Dis* 22:415, 1980.
22. Mentzer R, Finkelmeir B, Crosby I, Wellons HJ: Emergency carotid endarterectomy for fluctuating neurologic deficits. *Surgery* 89:60, 1981.
23. Fode N, Sundt T, Robertson J, et al: Multicenter retrospective review of results and complications of carotid endarterectomy in 1981. *Stroke* 17:370, 1986.
24. Gertler J, Blankensteijn J, Brewster D, et al: Carotid endarterectomy for unstable and compelling neurologic conditions: Do results justify an aggressive approach. *J Vasc Surg* 19:32, 1994.
25. Morgenstern L, Fox A, Sharpe B, et al: The risks and benefits of carotid endarterectomy in patients with near occlusion of the carotid artery. *Neurology* 48:911, 1997.
26. Merrick N, Park R, Kosecoff J, et al: *A Review of the Literature and Ratings for the Appropriateness of Indications for Selected Medical and Surgical Procedures: Carotid Endarterectomy.* Santa Monica, CA, Rand Corporation, 1986.
27. Moore W, Mohr J, Najafi H, et al: Carotid endarterectomy: Practice guidelines. *J Vasc Surg* 15:469, 1992.
28. Moore W, Barnett H, Beebe H, et al: Guidelines for carotid endarterectomy: A multidisciplinary consensus statement from the Ad Hoc Committee, American Heart Association. *Circulation* 91:566, 1995.
29. Goldstone J: Emergency surgery for stroke in evolution and crescendo transient ischemic attacks, in Moore W (ed): *Surgery for Cerebrovascular Disease,* 2nd ed. Philadelphia, Saunders, 1996, p 302.
30. Grotta J: t-PA: The best current option for most patients. *N Engl J Med* 337:1310, 1997.
31. Beebe H: Surgery for acute stroke. *Semin Vasc Surg* 8:55, 1995.
32. Pritz M: Timing of carotid endarterectomy after stroke. *Stroke* 28:2563, 1997.
33. Beebe H: The natural history and current status of carotid endarterectomy for stroke secondary to acute carotid occlusion, in Moore W (ed): *Surgery for Cerebrovascular Disease,* 2nd ed. Philadelphia, Saunders, 1996, p 293.

Part 3
NONATHEROSCLEROTIC CAUSES OF STROKE

Chapter 15

DIAGNOSIS AND MANAGEMENT OF HYPERCOAGULABLE STATES

David Lee Gordon
William A. Rock, Jr.
Hartmut Uschmann

BACKGROUND

Introduction

Thrombosis and Thrombophilia Under normal conditions, blood is fluid within the vascular spaces, providing a means of transportation of nutrients to the body's organs, yet is able to gel quickly to plug leaks in the vascular system and thereby prevent blood loss. The blood and vessels achieve this delicate balance of fluidity and coagulation through the complex interplay of naturally occurring prothrombotic and antithrombotic properties (Table 15-1). The normal endothelium prevents thrombosis by producing inhibitors of platelet aggregation and coagulation factors. The intact endothelium inhibits platelet aggregation through its negative charge and production of prostacyclin, nitric oxide, and adenosine diphosphatase (ADPase). The endothelium also releases tissue plasminogen activator (t-PA) into the vessel lumen, which in turn converts plasminogen to plasmin, a fibrinolysing enzyme. The subendothelium, on the other hand, is generally prothrombotic. Subendothelial substances such as collagen and von Willebrand factor (vWF) adhere to platelets and promote platelet aggregation. Plasminogen activator inhibitor (PAI-1), produced by the endothelium but released into the subendothelium, inhibits t-PA and, by extension, does not allow the conversion of plasminogen to clot-dissolving plasmin. The liver produces circulating anticoagulants (e.g., protein C, protein S, and antithrombin III) that interact with endothelial substances (e.g., thrombomodulin and heparan sulfate) to prevent the activation of coagulation factors (e.g., factor V, factor VIII, thrombin, or factor X).

When the balance of hemostatic mechanisms is disrupted in favor of thrombosis, the patient is said to have "thrombophilia" or a "hypercoagulable state." In his classic treatise, Rudolf Virchow identified three possible mechanisms of thrombosis: (1) changes in the vascular wall, (2) changes in the blood itself, and (3) changes in blood flow.[1] If the endothelium is disrupted by traumatic injury, inflammation, or atherosclerosis, the prothrombotic subendothelium is exposed, resulting in platelet aggregation and formation of a platelet plug or "white clot." Platelets then bind to fibrinogen, and the platelet plug serves as a bench for the formation of the stronger fibrin thrombus or "red clot." Deficiencies of plasma-borne anticoagulants such as protein C, protein S, or antithrombin III may lead to a hypercoagulable state. When low flow or stasis occurs (such as in veins, abnormal cardiac chambers, or the vortex of blood distal to an arterial stenosis), the accumulation of platelets and activated clotting factors may overwhelm the endothelial anticoagulant and fibrinolytic mechanisms and result in a localized hypercoagulable state. Likewise, systemic elevations of clotting factors such as fibrinogen may result in a hypercoagulable state.

Table 15-1.

Summary of major participants in thrombosis and their primary roles

	Antithrombotic properties	Prothrombotic properties
Plasma	Protein C ⟶ Inhibits Va, VIIIa Protein S ⟶ Inhibits Va, VIIIa AT III ⟶ Inhibits thrombin, Xa, other factors Plasminogen ⟶ Breaks fibrin clot (as plasmin) Thrombin ⟶ Activates protein C	Fibrinogen ⟶ Binds platelets, forms fibrin clot Thrombin ⟶ Activates fibrinogen, platelet aggregant Factor Va ⟶ Activates prothrombin Factor VIIa ⟶ Activates X (extrinsic pathway) Factor VIIIa ⟶ Activates X (intrinsic pathway)
Platelet		TXA$_2$, ADP ⟶ Platelet aggregants GP receptors ⟶ Bind fibrinogen, platelets, subendothelium
Endothelium	PGI$_2$, NO, ADPase ⟶ Platelet antiaggregants Thrombomodulin ⟶ Activates protein C Heparin sulfate ⟶ Enhances AT III activity t-PA ⟶ Activates plasminogen	Tissue factor ⟶ Binds and activates VII
Subendothelium		Collagen, vWF ⟶ Platelet aggregants PAI-1 ⟶ Inhibits t-PA

AT III, antithrombin III; TXA$_2$, thromboxane; ADP, adenosine diphosphate; GP, glycoprotein; PGI$_2$, prostacyclin; NO, nitric oxide, ADPase, adenosine diphosphatase; t-PA, tissue plasminogen activator; vWF, von Willebrand factor, PAI-1, plasminogen activator inhibitor.

Determining Stroke Etiology It is likely that hypercoagulable states are an underrecognized cause of ischemic stroke, especially in young adults, primarily because hypercoagulable assessments are not performed routinely in stroke patients. The cost of the laboratory assessment of hypercoagulable states is of particular concern to clinicians and health-care systems. Yet, nearly half of the $40 billion a year spent on stroke patients in the United States is due to poststroke costs such as rehabilitation, nursing homes, lost wages, and lost productivity of patients or caregivers. Recent analyses have suggested that thrombolytic therapy for acute ischemic stroke patients will, in the long run, save money for the health-care system.[2] This is likely to be true, however, only if the patient does not suffer a recurrent, potentially more debilitating stroke. Secondary stroke prevention therapy is dependent on the cause of stroke, and one must perform diagnostic testing to determine the cause. Clinical criteria alone are not sufficient, as was demonstrated by a recent study in which stroke experts often changed their mind regarding the likely cause of stroke when asked on admission and then again after the diagnostic evaluation was completed.[3] Studies of carotid duplex testing, transesophageal echocardiography, and carotid endarterectomy have suggested that the expense of diagnostic testing and stroke prevention therapy is offset by the resultant decrease in the cost

of first or recurrent stroke.[4-7] Because the specific details of hypercoagulable testing are not yet standardized and the indications for such testing are not universally agreed upon, there is no equivalent cost-analysis study of the laboratory assessment for a hypercoagulable state in stroke patients. Still, it seems likely that the judicious use of laboratory testing for hypercoagulable states in stroke patients will save money in the long run by leading to fewer recurrent strokes.

Based on largely pathologic literature, the terms "thrombosis" and "embolism" have been used to delineate the two main causes of ischemic stroke. When one performs cerebral angiography within hours of ischemic stroke onset, however, it becomes clear that the vast majority of ischemic strokes are in fact due to "thromboembolism," i.e., the plugging of a cerebral artery by a clot that formed elsewhere. The pathophysiologic mechanism of clot initiation (i.e., via platelets or coagulation factors) depends on the site of origin of the clot. Clinical trials of antithrombotic medications have generally confirmed what one would expect—strokes caused by platelet-initiated thrombi on atherosclerotic arterial walls are best prevented by antiplatelet agents and strokes caused by coagulation factor-initiated thrombi in the cardiac chambers are best prevented by anticoagulant medications. Thus, it is less important to identify the cause of stroke as "thrombosis" or "embolism" and more important to determine the site of origin of the thromboembolus. For patients with stroke due to a thrombus that formed in the blood itself, i.e., those with a hypercoagulable state, there are currently no available clinical trials to guide therapy, yet, because the pathophysiology of clot initiation in these patients is similar to that in cardioembolic stroke patients and patients with deep vein thrombosis, it follows that anticoagulation is the most appropriate therapy.

The term "lacune" is also misleading. Although stroke physicians frequently use this term clinically and radiologists use it to describe findings on computed tomography (CT) or magnetic resonance imaging (MRI), in fact, lacune was originally a pathologic term meaning "little lake." Pathologists found small subcortical cerebral infarctions in autopsy specimens that seemed to be due to disease inherent to the small penetrating arteries in the brain. Specific clinical syndromes were then described that were consistent with small artery-territory ischemia. Yet, it is now clear that many small-artery "occlusions" are not due to small-artery "disease."[8] Hypercoagulable states (as well as atheroembolism, cardioembolism, and nonatherosclerotic vasculopathies) may cause strokes in small-artery territories, so that the finding of a small subcortical stroke should not preclude further investigation into the cause of stroke, especially in young patients and those without chronic hypertension or diabetes mellitus.

A "transient ischemic attack" (TIA) is part of the ischemic stroke continuum. The causes of TIA are the same as the causes of ischemic stroke. It is unfortunate that, unlike angina pectoris and myocardial infarction, TIA and cerebral infarction are often considered by clinicians to be two separate entities. In fact, the clinician should evaluate TIA and cerebral infarction patients in the same manner, and one should not treat a TIA patient with chronic aspirin without investigating the cause of the TIA. For patients whose TIA is due to cardioembolism or a hypercoagulable state, the proper stroke prevention therapy is likely to be warfarin, not aspirin.

Hypercoagulable States as the Cause of Stroke

The relationship between a hypercoagulable state and stroke is one of increased probability or risk. The presence of a hypercoagulable state increases the risk of a thrombotic event, thereby increasing the risk of cerebral infarction. Both venous and arterial thromboses are potential causes of stroke as venous thrombi may cross to the arterial circulation via a patent foramen ovale. Over the last 20 years, investigators have identified multiple abnormalities in the molecular biology of how clots form

and dissolve that are associated with an increased risk for thrombosis and stroke. Identification of thrombotic risk factors in a patient with stroke both explains the clinical event and determines the probability of recurrent stroke.

In asymptomatic persons, it is perhaps more correct to refer to these conditions as hypercoagulable "tendencies" rather than hypercoagulable "states." It is important to realize that often more than one thrombotic risk factor must be present to tip the scales in favor of thrombosis. Pathologic thrombosis may occur as a result of having two distinct and concurrent genetic hypercoagulable conditions, having an acquired condition superimposed on a pre-existing congenital condition, or having two acquired conditions.[9] This explains why a person with a congenital hypercoagulable state may not suffer a thromboembolic disease until adulthood or why a person with an isolated acquired thrombotic risk factor may be asymptomatic. The management of persons found to have an asymptomatic hypercoagulable "state" entails avoiding exposure to a second hypercoagulable state and taking special precaution when such exposure is inevitable. Thus, one should advise asymptomatic persons with an identified thrombotic risk factor to avoid oral contraceptives and dehydration, and it is reasonable to advise these patients to take some form of antithrombotic therapy during pregnancy (e.g., aspirin or subcutaneous heparin) or perioperatively (e.g., postoperative intravenous (IV) heparin).

As with any other thrombotic condition, ischemic stroke may occur as a result of two different mechanisms acting synergistically. Thus, a congenital condition such as protein C deficiency may go undetected for many years before an acquired condition such as anticardiolipin antibodies or pregnancy "triggers" the underlying predisposition. Similarly, a congenital cardiac condition such as patent foramen ovale or interatrial septal aneurysm may be asymptomatic until the patient obtains an acquired hypercoagulable state such as lupus anticoagulant. Especially among younger patients, finding one possible cause of stroke may not fully explain why the stroke occurred. Some authors recommend a stepwise evaluation for hypercoagulable states in patients with ischemic stroke. They argue that performing the entire battery of tests is too expensive in every individual, so it makes more sense to test for the more common conditions such as anticardiolipin antibodies first and to perform further testing only if the anticardiolipin antibodies are negative. This strategy, however, will not detect a possible multifactorial cause of thrombosis.

Determining a multifactorial cause of stroke is likely to affect decisions regarding the duration of anticoagulation; one is more likely to recommend anticoagulation for a limited period of time in patients with an isolated acquired hypercoagulable state, but indefinite anticoagulation may be more appropriate in patients with an inherited condition. Patients with an atrial septal abnormality such as patent foramen ovale or interatrial septal aneurysm should undergo a hypercoagulable evaluation before deciding on possible repair of the cardiac anomaly if the only reason for the repair is to prevent thromboembolism; if the patient has a hypercoagulable state, chronic anticoagulation is indicated in any event.

The incidence of hypercoagulable states as a cause of ischemic stroke is not known, and the many past stroke "data banks" or "registries" are of little help. Ischemic stroke registries from the late 1980's that included patients of all ages estimated that, at most, only 1 percent of patients have a hematologic cause of stroke.[8,10] Ischemic stroke registries of younger patients have found higher estimates of hematologic causes. As late as 1991, stroke registries estimated that hematologic conditions account for 5.8 percent to 8.1 percent of ischemic strokes in young patients.[11,12] More recently, investigators of stroke in young adults found that 7, 17, and 32 percent of their patients had hematologic causes of ischemic stroke.[13–15] Diagnostic testing for hypercoagulable abnormalities, however, has become more widely available only in the last decade, and even patients enrolled in current stroke registries do not routinely undergo hypercoagulable testing. Thus, many patients with "stroke of unknown cause" may in fact have hypercoagulable states. Furthermore, because new information about hypercoagulable states is discovered on a regular basis, it is quite likely that many patients with ischemic stroke of unknown cause despite undergoing a "complete" evaluation actually have a hypercoagulable state that we cannot yet detect. Although the current concern about the cost of performing hypercoagulable profiles in every stroke patient is valid, unless this testing is performed more frequently in academic stroke registries, we shall never have a true answer regarding the incidence of hypercoagulable states; thus, the indications for performing these laboratory assessments on a broader scale will not be known.

An example of the difficulty with past stroke data banks is the Lausanne stroke registry.[8] Published in 1988, it included 691 patients with first-ever CT-proven ischemic stroke. The average age of their patients was 61. The authors do not comment on the performance of specific hypercoagulable testing on any patient, yet they concluded that only 7 of their patients had stroke due to hematologic cause (polycythemia, thrombocythemia, and myeloma with viscosity). Even if one concludes that three of their patients had antiphospholipid antibodies rather than "systemic lupus erythematosus vasculitis without histologic proof," there were a total of only 10 patients (1 percent) with a hypercoagulable state. In the Iowa registry of stroke in young adults (ages 15 to 45), only 19 of 329 patients (5.8 percent) had ischemic stroke due to a hematologic disorder.[11] This study, however, included patients from 1977 to 1993, and the patients did not undergo routine hypercoagulable evaluations. A 1997 Swedish study of stroke in young adults concluded that 7 percent of patients (8 of 107) had a hematologic cause of ischemic stroke (10 percent, if one also includes oral contraceptive use as a hematologic cause).[13] The investigators performed hypercoagulable profiles in 102 patients, including IgG anticardiolipin antibodies, activated partial thromboplastin time (aPTT), Venereal Disease Research Laboratory test (VDRL), protein C, protein S, and antithrombin III. In a 1993 Mexican study, 60 patients under age 45 had blood drawn within 48 h of ischemic stroke onset.[14] The hypercoagulable profile included aPTT, syphilis serology, "autoantibody screen," lupus anticoagulant, fibrinogen, protein C, free protein S, and antithrombin III. They attributed a hematologic disorder as the cause of stroke in 10 of their patients (17 percent). In a 1994 Mexican study of 36 patients under age 40 with "idiopathic" ischemic stroke, 25 percent had a hypercoagulable state.[16] Their hypercoagulable profile included anticardiolipin antibodies, VDRL, protein C, protein S (free and total), antithrombin III, plasminogen, t-PA, and inhibitor of t-PA. We at the University of Mississippi Medical Center reported in 1995 that 18 of 55 (32.7 percent) ischemic stroke patients aged 18 to 50 had stroke due to a hypercoagulable state; our figures do not include patients with possible hyperhomocysteinemia or activated protein C deficiency, which we added to our testing at a later date.[15] A listing of the Mississippi hypercoagulable profile is shown in Table 15-2.

There are likely to be age-related differences in the incidence of hypercoagulable states as many of them are inherited, and there may be racial or regional variations as well, either due to genetic or environmental (e.g., autoimmune) factors. Although stroke is more common in elderly persons, it is such a common condition overall (third leading cause of death in the United States) that it is not rare among young adults. In the population of children and young adults with ischemic stroke, traditional causes such as atherosclerosis and

Table 15-2.

The hypercoagulable evaluation for acute ischemic stroke patients performed at the University of Mississippi Medical Center

	Initial testing	Specific testing
Indication(s)	1. AIS ≤ 55 years 2. AIS > 55 with normal arterial and cardiac evaluations	Positive corresponding initial testing
Blood elements	WBC count Hemoglobin Hematocrit Platelet count	
Coagulation factors	Fibrinogen Factor VII Factor VIII	
Natural anticoagulants	Protein C Protein S, total Protein S, free Antithrombin III	
Lupus anticoagulant	aPTT KCT DRVVT	DRVVT confirm HPN and PNP mixing studies
Anticardiolipin antibodies	VDRL IgG, IgM anticardiolipin antibodies	
Other antiphospholipid-protein antibodies	IgG, IgM anti-β_2-glycoprotein I antibodies IgG, IgM antiphosphatidylserine antibodies IgG, IgM antiphosphatidylinositol antibodies	
Fibrinolysis	Euglobulin clot lysis time (24 hours)	t-PA and PAI-1 plasminogen
Other	APCR ————————————→ Sickle cell screen ——————→ Homocysteine	Leiden factor V mutation hemoglobin electrophoresis

AIS, acute ischemic stroke; WBC, white blood cell; aPTT, activated partial thromboplastin time; VDRL, venereal disease research laboratory; Ig, immunoglobulin; KCT, kaolin clotting time; DRVVT, dilute Russell viper venom time; HPN, hexagonal phospholipid neutralization; PNP, platelet-neutralizing procedure; t-PA, tissue plasminogen activator; PAI-1, plasminogen activator inhibitor; APCR, activated protein C resistance.

small-artery disease are less likely, and "other" causes such as a hypercoagulable state or nonatherosclerotic vasculopathy occur more frequently.

Some ethnic groups, such as African Americans, have an increased incidence of stroke-related mortality. The reasons for this are not fully understood and are not explained solely by the traditional atherosclerotic risk factors. In some geographic regions, such as the southeastern United States, there is a higher incidence of death due to stroke. Epidemiologic studies exploring the incidence of traditional (i.e., atherosclerotic) risk factors in this so-called "Stroke Belt" have not explained this regional variation.[17] One plausible explanation requiring further investigation is an increased incidence of hypercoagulable states among African Americans or other persons living in the southeastern

United States. These ethnic or regional differences in the incidence and significance of various hypercoagulable states may very well extend beyond the issue of African Americans and the southeastern United States, so it is important to keep in mind the location and ethnicity of study populations when investigating the link between hematologic factors and risk of thrombosis.

The Hypercoagulable States

Hypercoagulable states may occur as inherited defects or acquired disease processes (Table 15-3). Inherited hypercoagulable states may be due to a new mutation or may be transferred from a similarly affected parent. Foremost among the acquired hematologic disorders that have been demonstrated to have a significant associ-

Table 15-3.
A classification of the causes of hypercoagulable states

Acquired conditions
  Acute-phase reactants
    Fibrinogen
    Thrombin
    Factor VII
    Factor VIII
    von Willebrand factor
  Altered inhibitors and procoagulants
    Factor VII (affected by diet)
    Activated protein C resistance
    Homocyst(e)ine (affected by diet)
  Autoimmune disorders (antibody-mediated
    thrombosis)
    Antiphospholipid-protein antibodies
      Lupus anticoagulant
      Anticardiolipin antibodies (IgG, IgM)
      Other antiphospholipid-protein antibodies
        Anti-β_2-glycoprotein I antibodies (IgG, IgM)
        Anti-phosphatidylserine antibodies (IgG, IgM)
        Anti-phosphatidylinositol antibodies (IgG, IgM)
      Heparin-induced thrombocytopenia
  Disorders of blood elements
    Myeloproliferative disorders
      Polycythemia vera
      Essential thrombocythemia
    Paroxysmal nocturnal hemoglobinuria
  Systemic disease
    Malignancy
    Nephrotic syndrome
    Inflammatory bowel disease
    Liver disease
    Infection/inflammation
  Estrogen-related conditions
    Pregnancy/puerperium
    Oral contraceptives (controversial with 3rd
      generation, low-estrogen pills)
    Hormone replacement therapy (controversial)
Inherited conditions
  Abnormal zymogen levels
    Protein C (decreased or dysfunctional)
    Protein S (decreased or dysfunctional)
    Antithrombin III (decreased or dysfunctional)
    Plasminogen (decreased)
    Tissue plasminogen activator (decreased)
    Plasminogen activator inhibitor I (elevated)
    Heparin cofactor II (decreased)
  Accumulation of hemostasis-interfering substances
    Hyperhomocyst(e)inemia
    Factor V Leiden mutation
    Factor II mutation
    Dysfibrinogenemia
  Sickle cell disease

ation with stroke are the acute-phase responders and the immune mechanisms. Some acquired conditions, such as malignancy, cause thrombosis by mechanisms that cannot currently be detected by hematologic testing. Knowing whether a hypercoagulable state is inherited or acquired has important clinical implications in terms of prognosis and treatment. Many conditions, however, can be inherited or acquired. Detection of a hypercoagulable state starts with suspicion by the clinician and performance of appropriate laboratory testing. Thus, for the clinician, rather than categorizing hypercoagulable states as inherited and acquired, it is perhaps more convenient to divide them on the basis of mechanism and laboratory findings into the following categories: (1) deficiencies of natural anticoagulants, (2) excessive or abnormal clotting factors, (3) antibody-mediated thrombosis, (4) abnormal fibrinolysis, (5) abnormal blood elements, and (6) other hematologic abnormalities.

Deficiencies of Natural Anticoagulants

Protein C Deficiency   Protein C is a vitamin K-dependent plasma glycoprotein produced in the liver as a zymogen (serine protease precursor). It is activated by thrombin in the presence of the endothelial protein, thrombomodulin. Activated protein C inhibits thrombosis by neutralizing the active forms of factors V and VIII (Va and VIIIa) with the assistance of protein S as a cofactor.[18] Inherited deficiencies of protein C occur in an autosomal dominant fashion; the heterozygote forms lead to a hypercoagulable state in adults, whereas the homozygous forms do not survive infancy.[19,20] The heterozygote deficiency is clearly associated with increased risk for deep vein thrombosis and in fact may account for up to 10 percent of venous thrombosis cases.[21,22] An association with stroke, however, has been limited to case reports and data from stroke registries.[11,14,16,23] Acquired protein C deficiency may occur as a result of inflammation, liver disease, disseminated intravascular coagulation (DIC), L-asparaginase therapy, and vitamin K antagonist therapy.[22,24,25]

Protein S Deficiency   Protein S is a vitamin K-dependent glycoprotein primarily produced in the liver and also produced in endothelial cells and platelets. Approximately 60 percent of protein S is bound to C4b-binding protein, and 40 percent is free in the plasma. It is the free form of protein S that acts as an anticoagulant by serving as a cofactor for protein C-induced inhibition of factors Va and VIIIa. C4b-binding protein increases as an acute-phase response; this may result in an increase in bound protein S and a decrease in functional free protein S. One can measure free protein S and total protein S separately, using both quantitative and qualitative assays. Total protein S levels may be normal despite the presence of a hypercoagulable state due to free protein S deficiency. When there is a deficiency in cofactor protein S, protein C is not activated, and there is an increased risk for thrombosis. The congenital deficiencies are transmitted in an autosomal dominant fashion, and the heterozygote form has a significant risk for venous thrombosis.[26,27] Protein S deficiency may be responsible for up to 5 percent of cases of venous thrombosis.[22,28] The relationship to stroke has been identified primarily through single case reports and stroke registries.[11,13,14,16,28–31] An acquired decrease in protein S may occur as a result of pregnancy, inflammation, liver disease, DIC, estrogen therapy, L-asparaginase therapy, and vitamin K antagonist therapy.[25] Not all decreases in protein S, however, are associated with thromboembolism as there are often parallel decreases in procoagulants such as occurs in liver disease and DIC.

Antithrombin III Deficiency Antithrombin III is a plasma glycoprotein produced primarily in the liver as well as the endothelium. It binds to and inhibits thrombin (factor IIa) and factors IXa, Xa, XIa, and XIIa; it exerts its greatest antithrombotic effect through the inhibition of thrombin and factor Xa. Antithrombin III is far more effective in its role as a serine-protease inhibitor when in the presence of the endothelial glycosaminoglycan, heparan sulfate, or the medication, heparin. Congenital antithrombin III deficiency is an autosomal dominant trait. Acquired forms occur as a result of pregnancy, liver disease, DIC, major surgery, nephrotic syndrome, estrogen therapy, and L-asparaginase therapy.[25] In nephrotic syndrome, antithrombin III is lost in the urine. Inherited antithrombin III deficiency carries a high risk of venous thrombosis, and several case reports and series link it to ischemic stroke.[11,14,16,22]

Excessive Clotting Factors

Fibrinogen Fibrinogen (factor I) is a large glycoprotein produced in the liver that circulates in the plasma. When activated by thrombin (factor IIa), fibrinogen becomes the insoluble protein fibrin. Fibrin strands then cross-link to form the fibrin clot, or thrombus. Fibrinogen also binds to activated platelets, enabling the transformation of the unstable white platelet clot into the stable red fibrin clot. Dissolution of the thrombus, or fibrinolysis, occurs when plasmin degrades fibrin. Fibrinolysis results in the release of solubilized fibrin degradation products and D-dimer. Elevation of D-dimer implies that thrombi are being formed and broken down in the circulation.

Several investigators have found that fibrinogen levels tend to be elevated during acute ischemic stroke as compared with control patients.[32–34] Fisher and Meiselman found that fibrinogen levels tended to normalize at 2 months postcerebral ischemia except when the patient suffered a severe stroke; they concluded that in most cases elevated fibrinogen at the time of acute stroke is a nonspecific finding.[32] Tohgi et al also found that fibrinogen levels were higher in patients with large ischemic strokes, and they found that fibrinogen levels remained elevated in ischemic stroke patients 28 days after the event as compared with control patients.[33] Tsuda and colleagues found that fibrinogen levels were significantly elevated in patients with lacunar infarction within 3 days of stroke, at 1 month poststroke, and at 12 months poststroke as compared with patients who had silent cerebral infarction seen on imaging studies or others who were at low risk for stroke.[34] Epidemiologic studies such as the Gothenburg study from Sweden and the American Framingham study have suggested that fibrinogen is in fact an independent risk factor for stroke.[35,36] The Swedes studied 792 54-year-old men and followed them for over 13 years; those who suffered a myocardial infarction or stroke had significantly higher levels of fibrinogen.[35] The Framingham investigators followed 1274 men and women aged 47 to 79 for 18 years; they found that fibrinogen was a significant risk factor for coronary artery disease and peripheral arterial disease in both sexes, but was a significant stroke risk factor in men only.[36] In both the Gothenburg and Framingham studies, fibrinogen was particularly elevated in those who smoked cigarettes, but remained a significant risk factor independent of smoking. Fibrinogen has also been found to be elevated in patients with TIA.[37–39] Coull et al found that fibrinogen levels were higher in stroke patients than in TIA patients, were higher in TIA patients than in those with stroke risk factors, and were higher in the at-risk patients than in healthy controls.[37] Resch et al followed 625 stroke survivors and found that those who suffered a second stroke, myocardial infarction, or cardiovascular death had significantly higher fibrinogen levels.[40] The authors concluded that hyperfibrinogenemia is an independent risk factor for cardiovascular events in stroke survivors. The exact mechanism by which hyperfibrinogenemia may cause thromboembolism is not clear; possibilities include promotion of atherosclerosis, enhanced platelet aggregation, increased likelihood of fibrin clot formation, and increased plasma viscosity.[41] In practical terms, fibrinogen levels are often increased at the time of acute thrombosis as an acute phase response, and hyperfibrinogenemia may often be an epiphenomenon rather than a cause of ischemic stroke, but persistently elevated fibrinogen levels (e.g., 6 weeks poststroke) may suggest that the fibrinogen itself is contributing to the occurrence of thromboembolism. Inherited dysfibrinogenemia is a rare disorder characterized by dysfunctional fibrinogen with usually decreased fibrinogen levels; it may cause thrombosis and, rarely, arterial ischemic stroke, and is best detected by an abnormal thrombin time.[91,101] Acquired dysfibrinogenemia, on the other hand, is usually due to liver disease and is associated with a bleeding tendency.

Factor VIII and von Willebrand Factor Factor VIII is a glycoprotein that is believed to be primarily synthesized in macrophages and endothelial cells in the liver (but not by hepatocytes). Factor VIII circulates in the plasma as a complex with vWF and facilitates clotting by accelerating the conversion of factor X to factor Xa in association with factor IXa. This is the last step of the "intrinsic pathway" of coagulation. The intrinsic and extrinsic pathways converge at the common pathway, which then leads to fibrin clot formation. A deficiency of factor VIII or factor IX results in hemophilia and excessive bleeding. VWF is a multimeric glycoprotein produced in the endothelium; it is either secreted into the plasma where it binds to factor VIII or deposited on the subendothelial surface where it binds to platelets. O'Donnell et al studied 260 patients who had had a thromboembolic event 3 to 24 months previously and who had no other hypercoagulable abnormality.[42] They found factor VIII activity was increased in 25.4 percent of the patients.[42] Over 90 percent of the time, the increased factor VIII activity was increased without corresponding elevations in recognized acute phase reactants such as C-reactive protein and fibrinogen. Catto and colleagues studied 171 ischemic stroke patients, categorized them into presumed large-vessel and small-vessel disease based on CT scan criteria, and compared them with 184 healthy controls.[43] They found that vWF and factor VIII were elevated in stroke patients acutely and decreased somewhat 3 months poststroke, but the acute and 3-month levels in stroke patients were both higher than those in the control subjects. Initial vWF and factor VIII activity levels were higher in the large-vessel group

than in the small-vessel group. In addition, Catto et al found that elevated vWF levels were associated with increased mortality 6 months poststroke.[43] Thus, as is likely the case with fibrinogen, factor VIII elevations may reflect an acute phase response in some stroke patients but may suggest an underlying hypercoagulable state in others.

Factor VII Factor VII is a vitamin K-dependent protein produced in the liver that circulates in the plasma. When the vessel wall is injured, factor VII binds to a tissue factor, a glycoprotein produced in the injured endothelium and adventitia. The factor VIIa:tissue factor complex in turn activates factor X. This is the last step of the "extrinsic pathway" of coagulation. Factor VII may play a particularly important role in arterial thrombosis because atherosclerotic plaques have a high content of membrane-bound tissue factor, which becomes exposed to flowing blood when plaques rupture.[44] Elevated factor VII was associated with increased risk for cardiovascular thrombosis in one study.[45] In other studies, however, elevated factor VII levels did not seem to be associated with increased risk for cardiovascular disease.[46,47,49] In an American cross-sectional study of 5201 subjects, there was a weak association of factor VII with cerebrovascular disease.[47] In the same study, elevated factor VII levels were associated with elevated cholesterol and triglyceride levels, and the lipid levels accounted for much of the fluctuation in factor VII levels, especially in women.[47] In a study of 18 healthy young men (mean age 27, range 22 to 33), consumption of high-fat meals led to elevations in levels of plasma factor VII, suggesting that high-fat meals may be prothrombotic.[48] More prospective data are necessary before one can make final conclusions regarding the association of factor VII levels and stroke.

Antibody-Mediated Thrombosis

Antiphospholipid-Protein Antibodies Antiphospholipid antibodies (aPLs) is the term for serum immunoglobulins that bind to charged phospholipids, have been associated with an increased risk of thrombosis, and are perhaps the most common acquired hematologic cause of stroke.[50,51] Although some authors use the terms "antiphospholipid antibody" and "anticardiolipin antibody" interchangeably, most consider aPL to be a broader term that includes both lupus anticoagulant (LA) and anticardiolipin antibodies (aCLs).[52] Investigators have also described antibodies against phospholipids other than cardiolipin, have found that there is extensive cross-reactivity of aCL with other negatively charged phospholipids, and have determined that these antibodies may actually bind to phospholipid-bound proteins rather than to phospholipids per se, so that the term "antiphospholipid-protein antibody" may be more accurate than antiphospholipid antibody.[155] Three antiphospholipid-protein antibodies other than aCL and LA that may cause thrombophilia include anti-beta-2-glycoprotein I, antiphosphatidylserine, and antiphosphatidylinositol antibodies (see Tables 15-2 and 15-3).[155]

The subsets of aPLs are defined by the laboratory methods used to detect their presence.[52] LA and aCLs may coexist in the same patient or they may occur independently. Approximately 80 percent of patients with LA have aCLs, and nearly 50 percent of patients with aCLs have LA.[51]

Although about 40 percent of patients with systemic lupus erythematosus (SLE) have aPLs, aPLs more commonly occur in the absence of any other autoimmune disease. By definition, the diagnosis of "primary aPL syndrome" requires positive IgG aCL or LA and at least one of three clinical features: thrombosis (venous or arterial), thrombocytopenia, or recurrent fetal wastage.[51] The aPLs have been associated with both venous and arterial thromboses in multiple case reports, patient series, and observational studies. The most common venous thromboses are deep vein thrombosis with or without pulmonary emboli, but thromboses may also occur in cerebral venous sinuses, hepatic veins, inferior vena cava, mesenteric veins, renal veins, and axillary veins.[53] Arterial thromboses due to aPL syndrome have been reported to occur in the coronary arteries, peripheral arteries, aorta, retinal arteries, mesenteric arteries, and cerebral arteries.[53,54] Fetal loss associated with aPL syndrome occurs as a result of placental vessel thrombosis and placental infarction; this results in recurrent spontaneous abortions in the first trimester, recurrent intrauterine death or growth retardation in the second and third trimesters, and maternal thrombocytopenia.[53]

The aPLs may also be found in patients with nonthrombotic conditions such as cancers, human immunodeficiency virus infection, childhood viral infections, syphilis, and migraine; in those taking certain drugs such as phenothiazines or procainamide; and even in asymptomatic, healthy people.[51,53,54] The finding of LA or aCL in such patients does not necessarily carry an increased risk for thrombosis.[51,53]

The exact mechanism by which LA or aCL leads to thrombosis is not clear. Theories have included interference with endothelial release of prostacyclin, inhibi-

tion of protein C or S activation, impaired degradation of factor Va by activated protein C, inhibition of antithrombin III activity, interaction with platelet membrane phospholipids, inhibition of prekallikrein activation, interference with endothelial release of t-PA, expression of monocyte tissue factor, and binding to prothrombin and beta-2-glycoprotein I.[51–53,55,56] Increasing evidence suggests that aPLs consist of a heterogeneous group of antibodies with different thrombotic propensities—and those that do promote thrombosis likely do so via multiple different mechanisms.[52,57,155] The finding of different classes of aPLs that carry different risks for thrombosis at least in part explains the variable clinical correlations of aPLs with thrombotic risk found by different authors.

Lupus Anticoagulant The identification of a hypercoagulable state with a circulating anticoagulant in lupus patients was first described in 1963 by Bowie et al.[58] LA is an antibody (IgG or IgM) that prolongs phospholipid-dependent coagulation tests such as the aPTT. The term "lupus anticoagulant" is misleading. Although it was first identified in patients with SLE, it can be found in patients with other conditions or in otherwise normal patients. Because LA prolongs the aPTT, it is termed an "anticoagulant," but in vivo it actually promotes thrombus formation. There are now methods for determining if a patient has LA that are more specific than the aPTT. Determination of the LA requires a positive screening test such as the kaolin clotting time or dilute Russell's viper venom time, demonstration of inhibition of anticoagulant activity using mixing studies with and without incubation, and demonstration of phospholipid dependence via the platelet neutralization procedure or hexagonal phospholipid neutralization.[59] The kaolin clotting time and the dilute Russell's viper venom time are good screening tests but may give false-positive results and so should be confirmed with the more specific testing (see Table 15-2). Approximately 10 percent of SLE patients have thromboembolic complications, but about 50 percent of patients with both SLE and LA have thromboembolism. The combination of abnormal vWF with LA may be responsible for many LA-related strokes.[60]

Anticardiolipin Antibodies The aCLs were first detected as a false-positive test for syphilis with beef heart cardiolipin and were later identified as a marker for thrombosis.[61] The aCLs bind to cardiolipins, thereby leading to false-positive results on cardiolipin-dependent tests such as the VDRL. There are three types of aCL: IgG, IgM, and IgA. These antibodies may be identified using an enzyme-linked immunosorbent assay (ELISA) method, which is not affected by heparin or warfarin. Most laboratories measure the IgG and IgM titers in terms of GPL or MPL units, respectively. Each unit equals 1 μg/mL in the ELISA. The assay results are usually designated as negative, indeterminate, positive, or high positive.[51] Positive results vary with each laboratory, but are usually greater than about 20 units. In general, IgG aCLs carry the greatest risk for thrombosis, IgM carry intermediate risk, and IgA carry minimal-to-no risk.[51] Hamsten et al found that 21 percent of 62 young patients with acute myocardial infarction had aCLs, and 62 percent of those with aCLs suffered a recurrent cardiovascular event (including two with cerebral infarction).[62] Morton et al found that patients with elevated aCLs preoperatively had an increased risk of coronary artery bypass graft occlusion postoperatively.[63] A subset of patients with Sneddon's syndrome (livedo reticularis and stroke) have elevated aCLs, and evidence is mounting that this syndrome is a clinical manifestation of small-vessel occlusions of multiple causes, one of which is aCLs.[54]

Antiphospholipid-Protein Antibodies and Stroke

Despite the abundant observational evidence that aPLs are associated with an increased risk of systemic thrombosis, there has been a reluctance among some stroke investigators to designate aPLs, especially aCLs, as a possible cause of stroke. The fact that aPLs are found in many otherwise normal persons and in many nonthrombotic conditions has led many investigators to believe that the finding of elevated serum aPLs at the time of stroke is an epiphenomenon, perhaps caused by damage to cerebral arterial endothelium during the stroke.[64] Adding to the difficulty in determining cause and effect, aCL titers can fluctuate significantly and may transiently decrease to normal levels at the time of thrombosis.[65] Many skeptics base their opinion that aPLs are not related to stroke on the basis of studies that include all age groups. Ischemic stroke, however, is a heterogenous entity with multiple possible causes. In the elderly population, atherosclerosis, small-artery disease, and cardioembolism due to atrial fibrillation are by far the most common identified causes of ischemic stroke, and one should not be surprised that hypercoagulable states in general are not commonly identified among elderly stroke patients. Increasing evidence suggests, however, that aPLs are an important cause of ischemic stroke in younger patients. Thus, one should interpret

with caution studies of an "unselected" population of stroke patients (i.e., including all age groups) that conclude aPLs are not an important cause or risk factor for stroke.

Studies from Canada and Scotland are examples of negative studies that included elderly stroke patients. In the Canadian study, Metz et al compared 151 ischemic stroke patients to 111 controls for the presence of aPLs.[66] Their patients were evaluated within 5 days of stroke and had an average age of 68. They found 12 percent of patients had aPLs and 10 percent of controls had aPLs, and concluded that aPLs are not an independent risk factor for stroke. The primary reason for their conclusion was that an unusually high number of their controls had positive aPLs. This is directly attributable to their definition of positive aPL—they included patients with prolonged aPTT, reactive VDRL, or any elevation of aCL by ELISA testing. The aPTT is a sensitive but not specific test for LA, whereas VDRL is neither sensitive nor specific for aCLs. No LA-specific testing was performed. In addition, they considered low titers (<20 GPL) of aCL to be positive. This definition of aPL is too broad. In fact they found six ischemic stroke patients (4 percent) and only two controls (1.8 percent) with >20 GPL titers of aCL.

In the Scottish study, Muir et al compared 262 consecutive stroke patients with a control group of 226 outpatient ophthalmologic patients for the presence of aCLs.[64] The patients were tested within 72 h of stroke onset. They concluded that aCLs are not a risk factor for stroke, but their study had many limitations. First, their study population was quite elderly (the youngest of three age groups included patients up to age 62). Second, their assessments included IgA aCLs, which likely carry no risk for thrombosis. If one eliminates the IgA results, 61 patients (23 percent) and only 34 controls (15 percent) had raised titers of either IgG or IgM aCLs; if one includes only the IgG aCLs (the subtype that carries the greatest risk for thrombosis), the titers were significantly greater in the patient population. Third, the inclusion criteria were too broad: among their "stroke" group, 13 percent had "transient ischemic attacks" (TIAs) and 7 percent had "reversible ischemic neurological deficits" (even experienced stroke clinicians have difficulty determining whether transient neurologic deficits are due to cerebral ischemia), 10 percent had primary intracerebral hemorrhage (there is no reason to expect a relationship between intracerebral hemorrhage and aCLs), and 2 percent did not have a CT scan (without a CT scan, one cannot determine with certainty whether a stroke is ischemic or hemorrhagic). Thus, nearly one-third of their target population may not actually have had cerebral ischemia. Fourth, they collected their samples within 72 h of stroke symptoms and did not obtain follow-up samples. Other investigators have reported that aCLs commonly fluctuate and may even decrease to normal levels at the time of thrombosis. Fifth, rather than comparing the number of aCL-positive (e.g., >20 GPL) patients to the number of aCL-positive controls as nearly every other investigator has done, they decided to base their primary analysis on the comparison of mean aCL titers in patients vs. controls. The result is a complicated statistical analysis with very little meaning. Muir and his colleagues are correct when they conclude that they found no evidence to suggest that aCLs are a cause of stroke, but, in light of the many design flaws in their study, neither did they disprove the existence of such a relationship.

In contrast to the above studies, a multicenter American study found that the frequency of aCLs was significantly increased in 248 patients with first-ever ischemic stroke (9.7 percent) vs. 255 control patients (4.3 percent).[67] The average age of their patients was 67 with a range of 25 to 93, and the aCL titers were drawn within 7 days of ischemic stroke. The authors concluded that aCL is an independent risk factor for first ischemic stroke in patients of both sexes and all ages.

There is increasing evidence that aPLs are associated with ischemic stroke in younger patients. In a Canadian study, Trimble et al found that 3 of 51 patients with stroke or TIA had LA.[68] The average age of their patients was 54 with a range of 17 to 84. The three patients with LA were aged 49, 50, and 51. Brey et al from San Antonio, Texas, compared 46 patients aged less than 50 who had stroke or TIA with 26 age- and sex-matched controls with some other neurologic disease.[69] Of the stroke/TIA patients, 21 (46 percent) had aPLs (8 IgG aCL, 2 IgM aCL, 3 IgG and IgM aCL, and 8 LA), whereas only 2 (8 percent) of the controls had an aPL (both IgM aCL). Hess et al from Medical College of Georgia evaluated 110 consecutive patients with recent (<14 days) ischemic stroke or TIA with average age 58.[70] They found that 9 (8.2 percent) had elevated IgG aCLs, a significantly greater prevalence than in the control group (2 of 122, 1.6 percent), whereas there was no difference in the prevalence of IgM aCLs (10 patients, 8 controls). The average age of their patients with elevated IgG aCL was 54 (range 17 to 72), but they

concluded that aCL screening be concentrated on the young. In a Polish study, Czlonkowska et al measured IgG and IgM aCL titers in 49 patients who were less than 50 years old with first-ever ischemic stroke or TIA.[71] Based on very liberal definitions of positive titers, they determined that 32 percent had positive IgG or IgM titers. However, only 3 of 49 (6 percent) had IgG aCL titers >20 GPL, and none of their patients had IgM titers >20 MPL. In an Italian study, Nencini et al sought to determine the frequency of aPLs in an unselected population of young adults with cerebral ischemia.[72] They tested 55 of 59 consecutive patients aged 15 to 44 years for LA and aCLs. Of 55 patients, 44 had ischemic stroke and 11 had TIA. They found either LA or aCLs in 10 (18 percent) of their patients. Of interest, all ten patients with aPLs had ischemic stroke rather than TIA, so that, among the cerebral infarction patients only, 23 percent (10 of 44) had aPLs. Only 2 of 55 controls who were tested for both LA and aCLs had positive findings. Among the ten aPL patients, 7 received antiplatelet therapy, 1 received anticoagulation, and 2 received antiplatelet therapy with corticosteroids. Among the 45 patients without aPLs, 34 received antiplatelet therapy, 5 received anticoagulation, 2 underwent carotid endarterectomy and then took antiplatelet therapy, and 4 received unspecified therapy. Nencini and her colleagues then followed their patients for an average of 35 months (range 14 to 47 months). They found that 40 percent of the aPL group had a recurrent thrombotic event and only 4 percent of the non-aPL group had a recurrent thrombotic event ($p<.005$). This implies that patients with stroke and aPLs are at increased risk for recurrent thrombosis and suggests that antiplatelet agents may not provide sufficient protection against recurrence in this population. Nagaraja et al compared 60 ischemic stroke patients aged 40 or less with 60 controls.[73] The stroke patients had IgG and IgM aCL titers drawn within 22 days of stroke onset. They found low- or medium-positive aCL titers in 14 patients (23 percent) and 2 controls (3 percent). Both positive controls were low positive. Further evidence that aPLs are related to cerebral ischemia comes from an autopsy study of four patients. Hughson et al compared cerebrovascular changes in two SLE patients without aPLs to one SLE patient with aPLs and one patient with primary aPL syndrome but not SLE.[74] They found that the two patients who had aPLs, with or without lupus, had evidence of a chronic thrombotic microangiopathy of the brain, whereas the two SLE patients without aPLs did not have evidence of cerebral vascular thrombosis.

Heparin-Induced Thrombocytopenia There are two types of heparin-induced thrombocytopenia (HIT). In the most common type, the platelet count decreases slightly 1 to 5 days after the onset of heparin therapy with no serious sequelae. This is likely caused by a direct effect of heparin on platelet activation.[56,75] In 1 to 3 percent of patients who receive heparin, however, there is a more serious, immune-mediated thrombocytopenia that occurs 6 to 12 days after the onset of therapy; immune-mediated HIT is associated with the formation of intravascular platelet thrombi and is therefore often called the "white-clot syndrome."[56,75,76] In these patients, heparin forms a complex with platelet factor 4 (a glycoprotein stored in platelet alpha granules that binds to a receptor on the platelet surface), thereby stimulating the formation of IgG antibodies; these antibodies then activate platelets via platelet Fc receptors with resultant platelet aggregation.[56,76] Past studies suggested that immune-mediated HIT primarily results in arterial thromboses, and there have been case reports of white-clot syndrome resulting in myocardial infarction, ischemic stroke, and limb amputation.[75] In a retrospective study of 127 patients with serologically proven HIT, however, 78 (61 percent) had venous thrombosis and 18 (14 percent) had arterial thrombosis.[76] In that study, approximately half of the patients were found to have HIT only after having suffered a thrombotic event. Among the 62 patients who did not suffer thrombosis initially, there was a subsequent 30-day cumulative risk of thrombosis of 52.8 percent; this risk was not affected by discontinuation of heparin alone or discontinuation of heparin with simultaneous warfarin therapy.

Abnormal Fibrinolysis

Plasminogen Deficiency Plasminogen is a circulating proenzyme that is cleaved by t-PA to form plasmin. Plasmin dissolves fibrin clots. Because t-PA activity is enhanced by binding to fibrin, the fibrinolytic activity of plasmin is isolated to the area of the clot. Theoretically, a deficiency of plasminogen might result in decreased fibrinolysis and a resultant hypercoagulable state. Hypoplasminogenemia, however, has rarely been reported to be the cause of thromboembolism. In 1985, Lottenberg et al concluded that a patient of theirs had recurrent venous thrombosis with pulmonary hypertension due to plasminogen deficiency.[77] Dolan et al reported four cases of symptomatic hypoplasminogenemia, three with venous thrombosis and one with ischemic stroke.[78] Furlan et al reported a case of a 29-year-old man with a cerebellar infarct and low plasminogen activity whose asymptomatic mother and son were also found to have low plasminogen activity.[79] In a Mexican study of young adults with ischemic stroke of unknown cause, one patient was reported to have stroke due to plasminogen deficiency.[16] Other investigators, however, studied 9611 blood donors and found that heterozygous plasminogen deficiency was not a significant thrombotic risk factor, at least in isolation.[80] Thus, current evidence suggests that hypoplasminogenemia is not an important cause of a hypercoagulable state. At the University of Mississippi, we no longer measure plasminogen as part of the initial testing for a hypercoagulable state. Instead, we perform a 24-h euglobulin clot lysis time, an inexpensive test of overall fibrinolytic activity. If this test is abnormal, we perform plasminogen levels to assist in clarifying the reason for the abnormal fibrinolysis.

Tissue Plasminogen Activator and Plasminogen Activator Inhibitor Endothelium-produced t-PA converts tissue-bound plasminogen to plasmin, the active enzyme that lyses fibrin clots. PAI-1, made in the endothelium and secreted into the subendothelial matrix, inhibits or modulates t-PA. A deficiency of t-PA activity or an excess in PAI-1 activity results in diminished fibrinolysis and a resultant persistence of fibrin thrombi. In 1981, Tengborn and colleagues found a deficiency in fibrinolysis in 38 percent of 101 patients with cerebral ischemia who were younger than age 45.[81] The same group then studied 100 patients with recurrent deep vein thrombosis or pulmonary embolism and identified 22 patients with increased PAI-1 activity and 11 patients with decreased t-PA activity.[82] In a British study, decreased fibrinolytic activity was found to be associated with an increased risk for ischemic heart disease in men aged 40 to 54.[83] Similarly, Hamsten et al found reduced fibrinolytic activity among 71 patients who had suffered a myocardial infarction before age 45 in comparison with 50 controls, primarily as a result of increased PAI-1 activity.[84] Complicating matters is the possibility that endothelial cell synthesis and release of both t-PA and PAI-1 occur as a result of a nonspecific acute-phase response to chronic vascular disease, as suggested by a French study of 67 patients with angina pectoris.[85] In a Swedish study, t-PA levels were significantly greater in ischemic stroke patients both within 7 days of stroke onset and 2 to 4 years later; the study compared 122 acute ischemic stroke patients with 77 controls and collected follow-up data on a subset of the subjects.[86] PAI-1 levels tended to be higher in the cerebral infarction patients both acutely and chronically, but the difference did not meet statistical significance. The elevation in t-PA at the time of ischemic stroke suggests that the fibrinolytic system is activated and that the patient is at increased risk for thrombosis from some other cause. Jorgensen and Bonnevie-Nielson described a family whose members had recurrent venous thrombosis and were found to have high PAI-1 levels and consequently low t-PA levels.[87] Macko et al demonstrated decreased t-PA levels in stroke patients who had had an infection or inflammatory process within 1 week before the stroke as compared with nonstroke controls; the stroke patients with infection/inflammation also had a lower t-PA to PAI-1 ratio when compared with either stroke patients without infection/inflammation or nonstroke controls.[88] Thus, congenitally abnormal fibrinolysis manifested by low t-PA or high PAI-1 activity may result in an increased tendency to clot in some patients, and, in others, infection or inflammation may cause transiently abnormal fibrinolysis and resultant thromboembolism. Measuring t-PA levels, however, is quite uncomfortable for the patient. One must compare pre-ischemic and ischemic samples from the patient, and this requires having a tourniquet on the arm for at least 15 min. As is the case with plasminogen, we use the 24-h euglobulin clot lysis time as a screen for fibrinolytic activity and perform t-PA and PAI-1 levels only in those with an abnormal screening test or in those with suspected thrombophilia but no other identifiable hypercoagulable abnormality.

Blood Element Abnormalities

Red Blood Cells

Polycythemia Vera   This myeloproliferative disorder is a neoplastic disease of the bone marrow manifested by excessive production of erythrocytes and resultant elevated hemoglobin and hematocrit. Polycythemia vera (PV) patients have increased serum viscosity and abnormal platelet function and are consequently at risk for thromboembolic complications. The presence of spontaneous erythroid colony growth and histopathologic findings on bone marrow biopsy help to distinguish PV (primary polycythemia) from secondary polycythemia (reactive erythrocytosis).[89] In general, PV patients with hematocrit greater than 60 percent are at particular risk for thrombosis due to hyperviscosity.[90]

Secondary polycythemia is an elevation of hematocrit that occurs as a response to some other condition such as cigarette smoking, chronic obstructive pulmonary disease, or cyanotic heart disease. In one study comparing 43 patients with PV to 27 patients with secondary polycythemia due to smoking, the patients with PV had a significantly greater risk of thromboembolic events.[97] Thus, in patients with secondary polycythemia, the risk of thromboembolism is relatively low, and one should investigate thoroughly for other causes of stroke and be hesitant to ascribe the cause of stroke to the erythrocytosis per se.

Paroxysmal Nocturnal Hemoglobinuria   In this rare, acquired disorder, red blood cells are prone to lysis by the complement system. The resultant chronic hemolytic anemia explains the clinical syndrome of iron-deficiency anemia, hemolysis, hemoglobinuria, and hemosiderinuria. For reasons that are yet unclear, these patients also have a propensity for thromboembolic events. Cerebral vein thrombosis is more common than arterial cerebral ischemia, but both have been reported.[98,99]

Sickle Cell Disease   In this inherited condition that primarily affects persons of African ancestry, abnormal hemoglobin results in a tendency for deoxygenated erythrocytes to form a sickle shape and occlude capillaries. This results in microinfarction of multiple organs, especially the spleen, bone, and kidneys. The occurrence of stroke in these patients, however, is due to intracranial large-artery disease. Sickled erythrocytes likely occlude the vaso vasorum of intracranial vessels (e.g., the internal carotid arteries) with resultant fibrotic, thickened arterial walls and arterial stenoses. Thus, cerebral infarction may occur as a consequence of acute platelet thrombus formation in large arteries previously affected by chronic sickling episodes. These patients typically have a moyamoya-like arteriopathy on angiography, but may also have cerebral aneurysms and thus are at risk for both ischemic and hemorrhagic stroke. The Cooperative Study of Sickle Cell Disease reported data on 4082 patients followed for an average of 5.2 years.[100] They found that all subtypes of sickle cell disease (SS, sickle cell anemia; SA, sickle trait; SC, sickle C disease) had an increased risk of stroke, with the highest prevalence (4.01 percent) and incidence (0.61 per 100 patient-years) among the SS patients. Previous estimates of stroke incidence in patients with SS disease were higher at 8 to 17 percent.[101] The cooperative study group found that the incidence of ischemic stroke among SS patients was greatest in children (<20 years old) and older adults (>29 years old), whereas the incidence of hemorrhagic stroke was greatest among SS patients aged 20 to 29.[100]

Platelets

Essential Thrombocythemia Primary or essential thrombocythemia (ET) is a myeloproliferative disorder in which platelet counts are consistently over 1 million/μL, and platelet function is abnormal as well. This disorder shares many features with polycythemia vera, and treatment is similar. Stroke occurs as a result of the abnormal platelet function rather than the elevated platelet count per se. Reactive or secondary thrombocytosis carries no increased risk of thromboembolism. Thromboxane A2 levels are increased in ET patients.[92] Migrainous symptoms such as headache and scintillating scotomata may occur in patients with ET.[104]

Thrombotic Thrombocytopenic Purpura Thrombotic thrombocytopenic purpura (TTP) is an acute, relapsing disease in which platelet thrombi form in the microcirculation. It is manifested by thrombocytopenia, hemolytic anemia, neurologic symptoms, renal dysfunction, and fever. It occurs more often in women. Although TTP most commonly results in microinfarcts of the cerebral cortex and subcortical white matter, it may on occasion be associated with large artery-territory ischemic strokes.[107]

Other Hematologic Conditions

Activated Protein C Resistance and Factor V Leiden Mutation
Inherited activated protein C resistance (APCR) was first described in 1993 by the Swedish team of Dahlback et al.[109] They identified a family with thrombophilia who had a poor anticoagulant response to activated protein C. Griffin et al from California tested 47 patients with venous thrombophilia for the presence of APCR and found that APCR was present in over half of the 25 patients who had been previously diagnosed as thrombophilia of unknown cause but was present in only 2 of 22 (9 percent) of those with some other identifiable cause of thrombosis.[110] In 1994, Bertina et al from Leiden in the Netherlands demonstrated that APCR can occur as a result of a mutation in the factor V gene (substitution of glutamine for arginine-506) that is inherited in an autosomal dominant fashion; they named this inherited defect the Leiden factor V mutation (FV Leiden).[111] Activated protein C inhibits thrombosis by inactivating factors Va and VIIIa. In pa-

tients with FV Leiden, one of the factor Va sites normally cleaved by activated protein C is eliminated, and unmodulated factor V results in the occurrence of inappropriate thrombosis.[111] APCR due to FV Leiden is now considered the most prevalent inherited cause of venous thrombosis, but the rates vary among different regions and ethnic groups. Reported prevalence rates of FV Leiden include 2 percent in the Netherlands, 7.8 percent in southern Germany, 3.56 percent in northeastern Germany, and 5.3 percent in Canada.[111-114] In an American study, prevalence rates were 5.27 percent for Caucasians, 2.21 percent for Hispanic Americans, 1.25 percent for Native Americans, 1.23 percent for African Americans, and 0.45 percent for Asian Americans.[115] For reasons that are as yet unclear, FV Leiden has a variable clinical presentation; unlike the inherited deficiencies of protein C and S, homozygotes for FV Leiden usually survive and may even be asymptomatic for many years. The Swedish investigators tested 308 members of 50 families with APCR for the presence of FV Leiden and found that, by age 33, venous thromboembolism had occurred in 8 percent of those not carrying the mutation, 20 percent of heterozygotes, and 40 percent of homozygotes.[116]

The APCR laboratory test per se has a functional clotting endpoint. It is a modified aPTT in which one measures the anticoagulant response to activated protein C; APCR is expressed as a ratio, and a positive diagnosis usually requires a value of less than or equal to 2.0.[116] In general, APCR is an effective screening test for the much more expensive FV Leiden, which is performed by polymerase chain reaction (PCR). APCR, however, can occur without the presence of FV Leiden.[116] The Dutch group found that 80 percent of patients with APCR had FV Leiden, and the Swedish group found that 47 of 50 families with APCR had FV Leiden.[111,116] APCR not due to FV Leiden has been associated with elevated factor VIIIa, IgG aCLs, LA, dysfunctional protein S, and oral contraceptives, though the cause-and-effect relationship between APCR and these conditions has not been established.[117-119] Hypercoagulability is often a multifactorial condition that occurs as a result of an acquired condition superimposed on a pre-existing condition. Zöller et al found that 25 (58 percent) of 43 heterozygotes and 7 (88 percent) of 8 homozygotes for FV Leiden had another thrombotic risk factor at the time of their initial thrombotic episode; the risk factors included pregnancy, puerperium, oral contraceptives, trauma, surgery, immobilization, and protein S deficiency.[116] APCR due to FV Leiden may be a particularly important cause of pregnancy-related thrombosis; Hallak et al found that 7 (47 percent) of 15 pregnant patients with thromboembolism had FV Leiden.[120]

An Italian study suggested that FV Leiden is the most frequent hypercoagulable cause of cerebral vein thrombosis.[121] Three studies from England and the United States suggested that FV Leiden is not associated with arterial ischemic stroke.[122–124] Two of these negative studies, however, included only elderly patients with median age of 74 (range 65 to 80) in one and mean age of 66 in the other.[122,124] The third study found that FV Leiden was not associated with ischemic stroke among men aged 60 or less, but further details regarding the age range of the patients are lacking.[123] Another American group, however, found that, among 114 patients with FV Leiden and a history of a thrombotic event, 11 (10 percent) had cerebral ischemia, 8 (7 percent) had retinal vascular occlusion, and 8 (7 percent) had myocardial infarction.[125] The mean age of patients with cerebral arterial ischemia was 45.2 years (range 30 to 58). Although this was a select population, the results suggest that, as is the case with other hypercoagulable states, FV Leiden may be an important cause of ischemic stroke among young adults. This is further supported by Simioni et al who reported the occurrence of ischemic stroke at young ages (42 years, 50 years, and 8 months) in three Italian families with FV Leiden.[126]

Although the association of FV Leiden and ischemic stroke is not yet clear, there is growing evidence that APCR not due to FV Leiden is associated with increased risk of cerebral ischemia, even among elderly patients. In a Dutch study of patients aged 55 and older, the odds ratio of cerebral ischemia (stroke and TIA) increased gradually with decreasing response to activated protein C; on the other hand, FV Leiden was not associated with cerebral ischemia in this population.[127] In a study of Hispanic Americans from California, Fisher et al found that 6 of 63 (9.5 percent) ischemic stroke patients had APCR, whereas none of 31 controls had APCR.[119] The average age of their patients was 57.

Hyperhomocyst(e)inemia The term "homocyst(e)ine" refers to several sulfur-containing amino acid by-products of methionine metabolism found in the plasma, including homocysteine, homocystine, mixed disulfides involving homocysteine, and homocysteine thiolactone.[128] Formerly, it was necessary to perform methionine loading before obtaining plasma homocyst(e)ine levels, but fasting levels are now accurate due to improved laboratory methods.[129] Homocyst(e)ine seems to promote atherosclerosis. Evidence to date suggests that hyperhomocyst(e)inemia induces endothelial dysfunction by generating hydrogen peroxide, resulting in oxidative injury to endothelial cells, exposure of the subendothelial matrix, and resultant platelet aggregation.[128] Homocyst(e)ine also induces a hypercoagulable environment by enhancing factor V, factor XII, and tissue factor and inhibiting protein C, thrombomodulin, and heparin sulfate.[128] As is typical of thrombophilia in general, there is likely a synergistic effect of hyperhomocyst(e)inemia with other hypercoagulable conditions such as APCR and FV Leiden.[130,131]

Congenital deficiencies in one of three enzymes may result in hyperhomocyst(e)inemia: (1) cystathionine synthase (vitamin B_6 dependent), (2) N^5-methyltetrahydrofolate methyltransferase (vitamin B_{12} dependent), and (3) N^5, N^{10}-methylenetetrahydrofolate reductase. Cystathionine synthase deficiency is the most common genetic cause of hyperhomocyst(e)inemia; the rare homozygous form results in congenital homocystinuria manifested by marked elevations in plasma homocyst(e)ine, premature severe atherosclerosis, thromboembolism, mental retardation, skeletal deformities, and dislocated lenses.[128] These patients tend to have ischemic strokes and myocardial infarctions in young adulthood with a resultant decreased life expectancy.

Mild elevations in plasma homocyst(e)ine are more common than marked elevations. Mild hyperhomocyst(e)inemia has multiple possible causes and has been found to be a marker for increased risk of vascular disease, including stroke.[129] Acquired causes of mild hyperhomocyst(e)inemia include nutritional deficiencies (vitamin B_6, vitamin B_{12}, and folate), chronic renal failure, hypothyroidism, pernicious anemia, cancer (e.g., breast, ovarian, and pancreatic), acute lymphoblastic leukemia, drugs (e.g., methotrexate, phenytoin, and theophylline), and cigarette smoking.[128]

Coull et al found that homocyst(e)ine was elevated in 99 patients with acute stroke, TIA, or vascular risk factors as compared with 31 normal controls.[132] In an Irish study, Clarke et al found hyperhomocyst(e)inemia in 42 percent of 38 cerebrovascular patients, 28 percent of 25 peripheral vascular disease patients, and 30 percent of 60 coronary artery disease patients, but in none of 27 normal controls.[133] In a British, nested, case-control study, Perry et al compared serum homocyst(e)ine in 107 men with a history of stroke to 118 men with no stroke history and concluded that homocyst(e)ine is a strong and independent risk factor for stroke.[134] Boushey et al performed a meta-analysis of 27 studies and concluded that an elevation of plasma homocyst(e)ine is an independent risk factor for vascular disease; they found an odds ratio of 1.7 for coronary artery disease (95 percent confidence interval (CI), 1.5 to 1.9), 2.5 for cerebrovascular disease (95 percent CI, 2.0 to 3.0), and 6.8 for peripheral arterial disease (95 percent CI, 2.9 to 15.8).[135] Graham et al performed a European, multicenter, case-control study of 750 patients with atherosclerosis (cardiac, cerebral, or peripheral) and 800 controls; they found that an increased plasma homocyst(e)ine level conferred an independent risk for vascular disease similar to that of smoking and hyperlipidemia that was particularly significant among patients who smoke or have hypertension.[136] The same European group later reported that low vitamin B_6 levels confer an increased risk of atherosclerosis independent of homocyst(e)ine levels, but that low folate levels confer an increased risk of atherosclerosis that is explained in part by increased homocyst(e)ine levels.[137] A 1998 multicenter American study using a prospective case-cohort design also found that serum levels of vitamin B_6 were independently associated with a risk of coronary artery disease, but they concluded that plasma homocyst(e)ine was not independently associated with a risk of coronary artery disease once one accounted for vitamin B_6 levels.[138] Confounding the interpretation of the stroke data is the finding by a Swedish team that homocyst(e)ine levels are lower in acute stroke patients (mean 2 days poststroke) than in controls and are higher than in controls 1 to 2 years after stroke.[139] Most investigators feel that homocyst(e)ine is an independent risk factor for vascular disease, including stroke.

Factor II (Prothrombin) Mutation   In 1996, the same group from the Netherlands that identified the FV Leiden mutation identified a mutation in the prothrombin gene; Poort et al found that this mutation (G20210A) resulted in elevated prothrombin levels and carried a nearly threefold increased risk of venous thrombosis.[140] In a 1997 study from New York, Kapur et al analyzed the DNA of 50 patients with a history of thrombosis and 50 normal controls.[141] They found that 19 percent of the 21 venous thrombosis patients, 0 percent of the 29 arterial thrombosis patients, and 2 percent of the 50 controls had the prothrombin gene mutation. In a 1998 study of women aged 18 to 45 years from Washington state, Longstreth et al found that neither FV Leiden nor the prothrombin variant were more common among 106 women with first stroke as compared with 391 normal women.[142] There has not yet been a reported case of stroke due to prothrombin gene mutation.

EVIDENCE

Deficiencies of Natural Anticoagulants

Based on an understanding of the underlying pathophysiology and numerous case reports, there is consensus that chronic anticoagulation with warfarin is the treatment of choice for patients with protein C deficiency, protein S deficiency, and antithrombin III deficiency.[18,21,23,25–81,150] Patients with protein C or S deficiency, however, may develop a clinical syndrome called coumarin skin necrosis when initiating warfarin therapy, manifested usually by eruptions and necrosis of areas with prominent subcutaneous adipose tissue such as the thighs, buttocks, or breasts.[144] Administering therapeutic IV heparin at the time of warfarin initiation and starting with lower doses of warfarin (e.g., 5 mg per day) lowers the risk of developing this rare but sometimes fatal condition. There has been a case report of successful treatment of a patient with homozygous protein C deficiency using low molecular weight heparin as chronic therapy.[151] There is not yet evidence for or against chronic anticoagulation in patients with transient free protein S deficiency due to infection or inflammation. Patients with antithrombin III deficiency will not respond to heparin therapy alone as heparin requires antithrombin III to function as an anticoagulant. These patients have been treated successfully with IV infusions of antithrombin III concentrate acutely and oral warfarin chronically.[25,150]

Excessive Clotting Factors

There is no specific clinical evidence to guide the acute or chronic treatment of hypercoagulability due to elevation in fibrinogen, factor VIII, or factor VII.

Antibody-Mediated Thrombosis

Because, over time, aCL levels may decrease to normal and the LA may become undetectable, some clinicians have concluded that patients with aPLs may not require anticoagulation indefinitely. Two retrospective studies, however, suggest that patients with aPLs and thromboembolism have a high recurrence rate and may require indefinite high-intensity warfarin. Rosove and Brewer reviewed the records of 70 patients with aCLs or LA who had a history of thrombosis.[147] They found that 53 percent of the patients had a recurrent thrombotic event and that warfarin with an international normalized ratio (INR) greater than or equal to 3.0 afforded the best protection against recurrence; patients who took no antithrombotic therapy, aspirin, or warfarin with INR <2.0 had significantly higher recurrence rates of thrombosis. Similarly, Khamashta et al, performed a retrospective study of 147 patients with aPL syndrome referred to a British lupus clinic and found that 69 percent of the patients suffered recurrent thrombosis and that high-intensity warfarin (INR ≥3.0) was more effective than either low-intensity warfarin (INR <3.0) or low-dose aspirin in preventing recurrent thrombosis.[148] The addition of aspirin 75 mg per day to warfarin therapy did not afford increased benefit for their patients. There has even been a case report in which the authors ascribe correction of aPL-associated thrombocytopenia to warfarin therapy.[149]

For the acute treatment of patients with HIT, both IV hirudin (a direct thrombin inhibitor) and IV danaparoid (a low molecular weight heparinoid) have been used successfully prior to initiation of a brief course of warfarin therapy.[146]

Abnormal Fibrinolysis

There is no specific clinical evidence to guide the acute or chronic treatment of hypercoagulability due to plasminogen deficiency, t-PA deficiency, or excessive PAI-1.

Blood Element Abnormalities

Treatment of PV generally consists of repeated phlebotomy, attempting to maintain a hematocrit of less than 45 percent.[90] The incidence of cerebral ischemia (stroke or TIA) in phlebotomy-treated PV patients is 4 to 5 percent per year.[91] The addition of myelosuppressive therapy to phlebotomy decreases the risk of thrombotic events, and hydroxyurea seems to be the least toxic choice for myelosuppressive therapy.[90] These patients also have persistently elevated thromboxane A2 levels independent of the platelet mass or serum viscosity, and it is possible that the resultant increased platelet activity may be at least partially responsible for the thromboembolic complications of PV.[92] Thus, one would expect aspirin, which inhibits the production of thromboxane A2 by inactivating platelet cyclo-oxygenase, to be effective in these patients. In a 1986 randomized trial of 166 PV patients, however, those who received repeated phlebotomy, aspirin 900 mg/day, and dipyridamole 225 mg/day had a greater incidence of both thrombotic events and major hemorrhage than those who received only radioactive phosphorus.[93] Bleeding complications

are particularly more frequent in PV patients who take high-dose aspirin and also have markedly elevated platelet counts.[94] An Italian group compared aspirin 40 mg/day with placebo in 112 PV patients with an average follow-up of 16 months.[95] They found that low-dose aspirin completely inhibited thromboxane A2 synthesis and did not result in increased bleeding complications. As a result of that study, a large, randomized, placebo-controlled trial is under way in Europe that aims to evaluate the efficacy and safety of aspirin 100 mg/day in 3500 PV patients for 3 to 4 years.[96]

In contrast to PV, patients with secondary polycythemia have a relatively low risk of thromboembolism, and there are no data to support phlebotomy as a treatment for these patients. Still many clinicians prescribe phlebotomy to maintain hematocrit values of less than 55 percent in patients with reactive erythrocytosis due to theoretical concerns of increased viscosity.

Based on case reports, anticoagulation, short-term with heparin and long-term with warfarin, is the treatment of choice for thromboembolism due to paroxysmal nocturnal hemoglobinuria.[98,99]

The primary treatment of sickle cell patients with SS disease and ischemic stroke is transfusion therapy aimed at maintaining the hemoglobin S concentration at 30 percent or less; this therapy decreases the risk of recurrent stroke.[101,152,153] Transfusion therapy has also been shown to decrease the risk of first-ever stroke in SS patients.[154] For primary prevention, serial transcranial Doppler studies were used successfully to determine the timing of transfusion therapy.[154] In addition, Charache and colleagues reported that hydroxyurea therapy decreases the crisis rate, number of hospitalizations, and number of transfusions in sickle cell anemia patients.[102] There has been no clinical trial of antiplatelet therapy in these patients, despite the fact that they have a large-vessel arteriopathy. Foulon and colleagues found that 49 patients with sickle cell disease had higher urinary metabolites of platelet and endothelial arachidonic acid than did 33 controls and that an analog of thromboxane A2 decreased ex vivo platelet aggregation more in the patients than in the controls.[103] The authors concluded that antiplatelet agents may be of benefit in the prophylaxis of thrombotic complications in sickle cell patients. A clinical trial of antiplatelet therapy (e.g., aspirin) would seem to be warranted in sickle cell patients who have suffered cerebral infarction or TIA.

Both transient migrainous symptoms and cerebral infarction due to ET may be prevented with low-dose aspirin therapy.[104] Dutch investigators studied 68 ET patients and found that patients taking aspirin 500 mg/day had a decreased incidence of thrombosis with an increase in minor bleeding complications; they also found that, as with PV patients, ET patients bled more if their platelet counts were markedly elevated.[105] The authors suggested that low-dose aspirin (100 mg/day) be used for thrombosis prophylaxis in ET patients whose platelet count is controlled. A single case report from France suggested that ADP-mediated platelet aggregation may be important in ET-induced thrombosis and that ticlopidine may be preferable to aspirin in these patients.[106] As in PV patients, the myelosuppressive agent hydroxyurea decreases the risk of thrombosis in ET patients, though in ET cytoreduction is generally reserved for patients who have suffered a thromboembolic event.[94]

Plasma exchange therapy has been shown to reduce mortality and complications due to TTP; the role of antiplatelet therapy is unknown in these patients.[108]

Other Hematologic Conditions

Based on an understanding of the underlying pathophysiology and few case reports, chronic anticoagulation with warfarin is the treatment of choice for patients with APCR, whether or not the APCR is due to FV Leiden.[110,111,120–122]

Studies have clearly shown that vitamin supplementation can result in decreased homocyst(e)ine levels, and folic acid, in particular, in doses as small as 650 micrograms, seems to be the most important agent in reducing fasting homocyst(e)ine levels.[135] What is not clear, however, is the therapeutic effect of such vitamin supplementation, i.e., does lowering plasma homocyst(e)ine result in a decreased risk of stroke or other vascular disease?[128,129] Clinical trials currently under way are attempting to answer this question.

There is no specific clinical evidence to guide the acute or chronic treatment of patients with factor II (prothrombin) mutation.

DIAGNOSTIC AND THERAPEUTIC RECOMMENDATIONS

Diagnostic Recommendations: The Laboratory Investigation

Routine laboratory testing will not uncover a hypercoagulable state. Detecting a hypercoagulable state requires both clinical suspicion and laboratory expertise.

It is imperative to keep in mind that the patient had cerebral ischemia for a reason and that the key to preventing a second event is identifying that reason. At the very least, one should perform a hypercoagulable profile on any patient (of any age) who has cerebral ischemia and no definitive arterial or cardiac thromboembolic source on etiologic evaluation. Suspicion should be greatest in patients under age 55 and those with recurrent venous thromboembolism. Table 15-2 summarizes an appropriate hypercoagulable evaluation for patients with acute ischemic stroke. Table 15-4 summarizes the laboratory caveats and considerations for the various hypercoagulable states.

When investigating a patient with suspected thrombophilia, one must realize that a single laboratory abnormality confers increased risk for thrombosis but may not be manifested clinically unless a second or third hypercoagulable state is introduced. The determination that a patient has concurrent hypercoagulable states will undoubtedly affect decisions regarding long-term therapy. For this reason, we recommend a comprehensive rather than a step-wise approach when performing a hypercoagulable evaluation.

Laboratory expertise is necessary both in the performance and interpretation of the hypercoagulable profile. Heparin or warfarin therapy should not preclude performing a hypercoagulable evaluation, though there are certain caveats (see Table 15-4). Anticoagulation does not affect ELISA or PCR methods, so it has no effect on aCLs or FV Leiden but does affect other testing (see Table 15-4). Protein C, protein S, and factor VII levels decrease with warfarin therapy, so that testing for these markers is best done when the patient is not taking warfarin. A clue that protein C deficiency exists beyond the effect of warfarin is a drop in protein C level out of proportion to the decreases in protein S and factor VII. Free protein S deficiency may occur in the setting of normal total protein S values, and infection or inflammation may cause a transient decrease in free protein S. Some methods of determining APCR are affected by heparin and warfarin, but there are other methods that compensate for the anticoagulant effect. Patients with elevations in fibrinogen or factor VIII at the time of acute ischemic stroke should have these tests repeated about 6 weeks later to determine whether the elevations are due to an acute-phase response or due to a persistent hypercoagulable state. Dysfibrinogenemia is rare but may result in a hypercoagulable state despite normal fibrinogen levels; an abnormal thrombin time is a clue that further investigation is necessary. Francis

Table 15-4.

Laboratory caveats and recommended therapy for hypercoagulable states associated with ischemic stroke

Hypercoagulable state	Laboratory caveats and considerations	Recommended secondary prevention therapy
Protein C deficiency	First antigen by ELISA, then functional assay; may be decreased with therapeutic warfarin	IV heparin, then chronic warfarin (coumarin skin necrosis may occur if warfarin started alone)
Protein S deficiency	Obtain total and free levels by ELISA; may be decreased with therapeutic warfarin	IV heparin, then chronic warfarin (coumarin skin necrosis may occur if warfarin started alone)
AT III deficiency	May be decreased with heparin, but not below 40–50% (chromogenic method)	IV AT III infusion and chronic warfarin (IV heparin not effective without IV AT III)
Fibrinogen	Not affected by anticoagulants (Claus method on fibrometer); repeat in 6 weeks to determine true elevation; dysfibrinogenemia suggested by abnormal thrombin time	Chronic warfarin if levels persistently elevated; ticlopidine is second choice
Factor VIII	Not affected by any therapeutic anticoagulant; repeat in 6 weeks to determine true elevation	Aspirin and avoid other thrombophilic states
Factor VII	Affected by warfarin and vitamin K deficiency	Aspirin and avoid other thrombophilic states
aCLs	Not affected by any anticoagulant (ELISA method); may be decreased acutely	Chronic warfarin
LA	KCT screen for LA (fibrometer); DRVVT with confirm for false (+) aPTT or KCT; HPN for false (+) aPTT, KCT, or DRVVT; mixing studies confirm LA, affected by anticoagulants	Chronic warfarin
HIT	Suggested by decreasing platelet counts while on heparin; may identify HIT antibody	IV danaparoid or IV hirudin followed by chronic warfarin for 3–6 month course
Plasminogen deficiency	Screen with euglobulin clot lysis time; clinical significance unclear	Evaluate for other possible causes; if this is only possible cause, chronic warfarin
t-PA deficiency	Screen with euglobulin clot lysis time; compare values pre- and posttourniquet on arm for 15 min; use tube with acidified anticoagulant	Chronic warfarin
PAI-I elevation	Screen with euglobulin clot lysis time; cool immediately and spin down to remove platelets	Chronic warfarin
Polycythemia vera	Spontaneous erythroid growth and bone marrow biopsy; confirm diagnosis	Phlebotomy to hematocrit <45%; hydroxyurea; perhaps aspirin 81 mg daily
PNH		Chronic warfarin
Sickle cell disease		Transfusion therapy to maintain hemoglobin S ≤30%; hydroxyurea; perhaps aspirin 81–325 mg qd
Essential thrombocythemia		Hydroxyurea; perhaps aspirin 81–100 mg daily
TTP		Plasma exchange therapy
APCR	Use method to neutralize heparin, compensate for warfarin therapy; 10% not due to FV Leiden	Chronic warfarin
FV Leiden	PCR method, not affected by anticoagulants	Chronic warfarin
Hyperhomocysteinemia	May be decreased acutely; marked elevations may be due to rare genetic condition	Folate, vitamin B_6, vitamin B_{12}; antiplatelet therapy; perhaps warfarin

has published a more detailed review of the laboratory investigation of hypercoagulability.[143]

Therapeutic Recommendations: Antithrombotic Therapy for Hypercoagulable States

In most cases, chronic anticoagulation with warfarin is the therapy of choice for patients who have suffered cerebral ischemia (infarction or TIA) due to a hypercoagulable state, though there are exceptions and caveats to this general principle (see Table 15-4). Anticoagulant therapy itself produces an altered state of coagulation with its own risk for serious complications. Chronic anticoagulation is not indicated unless a mechanism for continued risk for thrombosis exists. The manageable risk of hemorrhage due to anticoagulation, however, is preferable to the risk of suffering a recurrent, fatal or disabling stroke in a person with a hypercoagulable state. With proper support, the patient can learn to manage the antithrombotic therapy with minimal risk.

For patients with protein C deficiency or protein S deficiency, administer therapeutic IV heparin, simultaneously initiate warfarin therapy at 5 mg per day, and maintain the INR at 2.0 to 3.0 using chronic warfarin. Patients with transiently decreased free protein S due to an inflammatory process may not require chronic anticoagulation.

For patients with antithrombin III deficiency, treat urgently with replacement therapy using IV antithrombin III concentrates, with or without simultaneous IV heparin, and begin warfarin for chronic therapy, maintaining an INR of 2 to 3.

Persistent hyperfibrinogenemia (i.e., elevated fibrinogen levels 6 to 8 weeks after the stroke) carries a relatively high risk of recurrent thromboembolism, so we elect to treat these patients chronically with warfarin, maintaining an INR of 2 to 3. For those who cannot tolerate warfarin, ticlopidine is the second choice; some investigators have found that ticlopidine (but not clopidogrel or aspirin) lowers fibrinogen levels.[145]

Because the evidence linking factor VIII and factor VII with thromboembolic stroke is not quite as convincing as that for fibrinogen, we currently do not treat patients with stroke related to these conditions with chronic anticoagulation unless a second event occurs while taking aspirin and avoiding dehydration and other thrombophilic states.

For the acute treatment of patients with HIT, one can use either IV hirudin or IV danaparoid prior to initiation of a course of warfarin therapy for 3 to 6 months.

Warfarin is not indicated in patients with cerebral ischemia due to sickle cell disease, polycythemia vera, essential thrombocythemia, or thrombotic thrombocytopenic purpura. Patients with sickle cell disease are treated with transfusions to maintain hemoglobin S concentrations ≤30 percent. We also use hydroxyurea and aspirin 325 mg qd.

We treat patients with aPLs and thromboembolism with indefinite warfarin therapy, initially aiming for an INR of 2 to 3, but increasing the target INR to 3 to 4 if the patient should have any recurrent thromboembolic episodes.

Because clinical thromboembolism often does not occur in a person with an isolated hypercoagulable state unless a second condition is superimposed, it is important to advise the patient to avoid situations that may predispose to thrombosis. Thus, patients should be advised to avoid dehydration and to take prophylactic measures perioperatively (e.g., treat with heparin during the postoperative period). Women should be advised to avoid pregnancy if at all possible and to avoid hormonal contraception as well. Women who do become pregnant should receive aspirin 81 to 325 mg qd and subcutaneous heparin or low molecular weight heparin throughout the pregnancy, and soon after delivery should receive IV heparin and oral warfarin, as the postpartum period carries the greatest risk of thrombosis.

It is highly likely that hypercoagulable states as a cause of cerebral ischemia are underdiagnosed. Data from stroke registries are flawed due to selection bias and incomplete hypercoagulable evaluations. One must be careful when interpreting epidemiologic studies; although it is true that arterial ischemic stroke is most often due to either disease affecting the vessel walls or stasis in a diseased cardiac chamber, for the individual patient, one cannot assume that arterial or cardiac disease is present without performing diagnostic tests. If those tests are negative, one should perform a comprehensive hypercoagulable evaluation. Judicious use of hypercoagulable testing is likely to be cost-effective when one considers its effect on secondary prevention. In addition, our knowledge of thrombosis and thrombophilia is changing at a dramatic rate. It behooves the clinician to maintain contact with those patients who have cerebral ischemia of undetermined cause despite a complete evaluation; the definition of "complete evaluation" evolves continuously.

REFERENCES

1. Virchow R: Phlogose und thrombose, in Virchow R (ed): *Gesammelte Abhandlungen zur Wissenschaftlichen Medicin.* Frankfurt a.M., Meidinger, 1856, p 458.
2. Fagan SC, Morgenstern LB, Petitta A, et al: Cost-effectiveness of tissue plasminogen activator for acute ischemic stroke. NINDS rt-PA Stroke Study Group. *Neurology* 50:883, 1998.
3. Madden K, Karanjia P, Adams H, et al: Accuracy of initial stroke subtype diagnosis in the TOAST study. *Neurology* 45:1975, 1995.
4. Lavenson GS, Sharma D: Medical cost savings through stroke prevention from 100 consecutive new carotid duplex scans. *Cardiovasc Surg* 4:753, 1996.
5. McNamara RL, Lima JA, Whelton PK, et al: Echocardiographic identification of cardiovascular sources of emboli to guide clinical management of stroke: a cost-effectiveness analysis. *Ann Intern Med* 127:775, 1997.
6. Kuntz KM, Kent KC: Is carotid endarterectomy cost-

effective? An analysis of symptomatic and asymptomatic patients. *Circulation* 94:194, 1996.

7. Cronerwett, JL, Birkmeyer JD, Nackman GB: Cost-effectiveness of carotid endarterectomy in asymptomatic patients. *J Vasc Surg* 25:310, 1997.

8. Bogousslavsky J, Van Melle, G, Regli F: The Lausanne Stroke Registry: Analysis of 1,000 consecutive patients with first stroke. *Stroke* 19:1083, 1988.

9. Seligsohn U, Zivelin A: Thrombophilia as a multigenic disorder. *Thromb Haemost* 78:297, 1997.

10. Sandercock PA, Warlow CP, Jones LN: Predisposing factors for cerebral infarction: The Oxfordshire community stroke project. *BMJ* 298:75, 1989.

11. Adams HP, Kappell L, Biller J, et al: Ischemic stroke in young adults: *Arch Neurol* 52:491, 1995.

12. Lisovoski F, Rousseaux P: Cerebral infarction in young people: A study of 148 patients with early cerebral angiography. *J Neurol Neurosurg Psychiatry* 54:576, 1991.

13. Kristensen B, Malm J, Carlberg B: Epidemiology and etiology of ischemic stroke in young adults aged 18 to 44 years in northern Sweden. *Stroke* 28:1702, 1997.

14. Martinez HR, Rangel-Guerra RA, Marfil LJ: Ischemic stroke due to deficiency of coagulation inhibitors. *Stroke* 24:19, 1993.

15. Gordon DL, Ryder D, Rock WA Jr: Hypercoagulable states and stroke in young adults. *J Stroke Cerebrovasc Dis* 5:108, 1995.

16. Barinagarrementeria F, Cantu-Brito C, De La Pena A, et al: Prothrombotic states in young people with idiopathic stroke. *Stroke,* 25:287, 1994.

17. Howard G, Evans GW, Pearcek, et al: Is the stroke belt disappearing? An analysis of racial, temporal, and age effects. *Stroke* 26:1153, 1995.

18. Reitsma PH: Protein C deficiency: From gene defects to disease. *Thromb Haemost* 78:344, 1997.

19. Marciniak E, Wilson HD, Marlar RA: Neonatal purpura fulminans: A genetic disorder related to the absence of protein C in blood. *Blood* 65:15, 1985.

20. Witt I, Beck S, Seydewitz HH, et al: A novel homozygous missense mutation (val 325→ala) in the protein C gene causing neonatal purpura fulminans. *Blood Coagul Fibrinolysis* 5:651, 1994.

21. Koster T, Rosendaal FR, Briet E, et al: Protein C deficiency in a controlled series of unselected outpatients: An infrequent but clear risk factor for venous thrombosis. Leiden Thrombophilia Study. *Blood* 85:2756, 1995.

22. Tatlisumak T, Fisher M: Hematologic disorders associated with ischemic stroke. *J Neurol Sci* 140:1, 1996.

23. Kato H, Shirahama M, Ohmori K, et al: Cerebral infarction in a young adult associated with protein C deficiency. *Angiology* 46:169, 1995.

24. Esmon CT, Fukudome K: Cellular regulation of the protein C pathway. *Semin Cell Biol* 6:259, 1995.

25. Hirsh J, Prins MH, Samama M: Approach to the thrombophilic patient for hemostasis and thrombosis: Basic principles and clinical practice, in Colman RW, Hirsh J,

Marder VJ, Salzman EW (eds): *Hemostasis and Thrombosis: Basic Principles and Clinical Practice,* 3rd ed. Philadelphia, JB Lippincott, 1994, p 1543.

26. Comp PC, Esmon CT: Recurrent venous thromboembolism in patients with a partial deficiency of protein S. *N Engl J Med* 311:1525, 1984.

27. Schwarz HP, Fischer M, Hopmeier P, et al: Plasma protein S deficiency in familial thrombotic disease. *Blood* 64:1297, 1984.

28. Borgel D, Gandrille S, Aiach M: Protein S deficiency. *Thromb Haemost* 78:351, 1997.

29. Lagosky S, Witten CM: A case of cerebral infarction in association with free protein S deficiency and oral contraceptive use. *Arch Phys Med Rehabil* 74:98, 1993.

30. Simioni P, Battistella PA, Drigo P, et al: Childhood stroke associated with familial protein S deficiency. *Brain Dev* 16:241, 1994.

31. Nighoghossian N, Berruyer M, Getenet JC, et al: Free protein S spectrum in young patients with stroke. *Cerebrovasc Dis* 4:304, 1994.

32. Fisher M, Meiselman HJ: Hemorheological factors in cerebral ischemia. *Stroke* 22:1164, 1991.

33. Tohgi H, Kawashima M, Tamura K, et al: Coagulation-fibrinolysis abnormalities in acute and chronic phases of cerebral thrombosis and embolism. *Stroke* 21:1663, 1990.

34. Tsuda Y, Satoh K, Kitadai M, et al: Hemorheologic profiles of plasma fibrinogen and blood viscosity from silent to acute and chronic cerebral infarctions. *J Neurol Sci* 147:49, 1997.

35. Wilhelmsen L, Svardsudd K, Korsan-Bengtsen K, et al: Fibrinogen as a risk factor for stroke and myocardial infarction. *N Engl J Med* 311:501, 1984.

36. Kannel WB, D'Agostino RB, Belanger AJ: Update on fibrinogen as a cardiovascular risk factor. *Ann Epidemiol* 2:457, 1992.

37. Coull BM, Beamer N, de Garmo P, et al: Chronic hyperviscosity in subjects with acute stroke, transient ischemic attack, and risk factors for stroke. *Stroke* 22:162, 1991.

38. Ernst E, Matrai A, Marshall M: Blood rheology in patients with transient ischemic attacks. *Stroke* 19:634, 1988.

39. Qizilbash N, Jones L, Warlow C, et al: Fibrinogen and lipid concentrations as risk factors for transient ischaemic attacks and minor ischaemic strokes. *BMJ* 303:605, 1991.

40. Resch KL, Ernst E, Matrai A, et al: Fibrinogen and viscosity as risk factors for subsequent cardiovascular events in stroke survivors. *Ann Intern Med* 117:371, 1992.

41. Heinrich J, Assmann G: Fibrinogen and cardiovascular risk. *J Cardiovasc Risk* 2:197, 1995.

42. O'Donnell J, Tuddenham EGD, Manning R, et al: High prevalence of elevated factor VIII levels in patients referred for thrombophilia acreening: Role of increased synthesis and relationship to the acute phase reaction. *Thromb Haemost* 77:825, 1997.

43. Catto AJ, Carter AM, Barrett JH, et al: von Willebrand factor and factor VIII:C in acute cerebrovascular disease:

Relationship to stroke subtype and mortality. *Thromb Haemost* 77:1104, 1997.

44. Marckmann P, Bladbjerg EM, Jesperen J: Diet and blood coagulation factor VII: A key protein in arterial thrombosis. *Eur J Clin Nutr* 52:75, 1998.

45. Kelleher CC: Plasma fibrinogen and factor VII as risk factors for cardiovascular disease. *Eur J Epidemiol* 8:79, 1992.

46. Heinrich J, Balleisen L, Schulte H, et al: Fibrinogen and factor VII in the prediction of coronary risk: Results from the PROCAM study in healthy men. *Arterioscler Thromb* 14:54, 1994.

47. Cushman M, Yanez D, Psaty BM, et al: Association of fibrinogen and coagulation factors VII and VIII with cardiovascular risk factors in the elderly. The Cardiovascular Health Study. *Am J Epidemiol* 143:665, 1996.

48. Larsen LF, Bladbjerg EM, Jesperen J, et al: Effects of dietary fat quality and quantity on postprandial activation of blood coagulation factor VII. *Arterioscler Thromb Vasc Biol* 17:2904, 1997.

49. Folsom AR, Wu KK, Shahar E, et al: Association of hemostatic variables with prevalent cardiovascular disease and asymptomatic carotid artery atherosclerosis. *Arterioscler Thromb* 13:1829, 1993.

50. Long AA, Ginsberg JS, Brill-Edwards P, et al: The relationship of antiphospholipid antibodies to thromboembolic disease in systemic lupus erythematosus: A cross-sectional study. *Thromb Haemost* 66:520, 1991.

51. Feldmann E, Levine SR: Cerebrovascular disease with antiphospholipid antibodies: Immune mechanisms, significance, and therapeutic options. *Ann Neurol* 37:S114, 1995.

52. Esmon NL, Smirnov MD, Esmon CT: Thrombogenic mechanisms of antiphospholipid antibodies. *Thromb Haemost* 78:79, 1997.

53. Feinstein DI: Immune coagulation disorders, in Colman RW, Hirsh J, Marder VJ, Salzman EW (eds): *Hemostasis and Thrombosis: Basic Principles and Clinical Practice,* 3rd ed. Philadelphia, JB Lippincott, 1994, p 881.

54. Hess DC: Stroke associated with antiphospholipid antibodies. *Stroke* 23:I-23, 1992.

55. Triplett DA: Protean clinical presentation of antiphospholipid-protein antibodies (APA). *Thromb Haemost* 74:329, 1995.

56. Vermylen J, Hoylaerts MF, Arnout J: Antibody-mediated thrombosis. *Thromb Haemost* 78:420, 1997.

57. Brey RL, Coull BM: Antiphospholipid antibodies: Origin, specificity, and mechanism of action. *Stroke* 23:I-15, 1992.

58. Bowie EJW, Thompson JH, Pascuzzi CA, et al: Thrombosis in systemic lupus erythematosus despite circulating anticoagulants. *J Lab Clin Med* 62:416, 1963.

59. Brandt: JT, Barna LK, Triplett DA: Laboratory identification of lupus anticoagulants: Results of the Second International Workshop for Identification of Lupus Anticoagulants. *Thromb Haemost* 74:1597, 1995.

60. Schinco P, Borchiellini A, Tamponi G, et al. Lupus antico-

agulant and thrombosis: Role of von Willebrand factor multimeric forms. *Clin Exp Rheumatol* 15:5, 1997.

61. Harris EN, Gharavi AE, Boey ML, et al: Anticardiolipin antibodies: Detection by radioimmunoassay and association with thrombosis in lupus erythematosus. *Lancet* 2:1211, 1983.

62. Hamsten A, Norberg R, Bjorkholm M, et al: Antibodies to cardiolipin in young survivors of myocardial infarction: An association with recurrent cardiovascular events. *Lancet* 1:113, 1986.

63. Morton KE, Gavaghan TP, Krilis SA, et al: Coronary artery bypass graft failure: An autoimmune phenomenon. *Lancet* 2:977, 1987.

64. Muir KW, Squire IB, Alwan W, et al: Anticardiolipin antibodies in an unselected stroke population. *Lancet* 344:452, 1994.

65. Drenkard C, Sánchez-Guerrero J, Alarcón-Segovia D: Fall in antiphospholipid antibody at time of thromboocclusive episodes in systemic lupus erythematosus. *J Rheumatol* 16:614, 1989.

66. Metz LM, Edworthy S, Mydlarski R, et al: The frequency of phospholipid antibodies in an unselected stroke population. *Can J Neurol Sci* 25:64, 1998.

67. Antiphospholipid Antibodies in Stroke Study (APASS) Group: Anticardiolipin antibodies are an independent risk factor for first ischemic stroke. *Neurology* 43:2069, 1993.

68. Trimble M, Bell DA, Brien W, et al: The antiphospholipid syndrome: Prevalence among patients with stroke and transient ischemic attacks. *Am J Med* 88:593, 1990.

69. Brey RL, Hart RG, Sherman DG, et al: Antiphospholipid antibodies and cerebral ischemia in young people. *Neurology* 40:1190, 1990.

70. Hess DC, Krauss J, Adams RJ, et al: Anticardiolipin antibodies: A study of frequency in TIA and stroke. *Neurology* 41:525, 1991.

71. Czlonkowska A, Meurer M, Palasik W, et al: Anticardiolipin antibodies, a disease marker for ischemic cerebrovascular events in a younger population? *Acta Neurol Scand* 86:304, 1992.

72. Nencini P, Baruffi MC, Abbate R, et al: Lupus anticoagulant and anticardiolipin antibodies in young adults with cerebral ischemia. *Stroke* 23:189, 1992.

73. Nagaraja D, Christopher R, Manjari T: Anticardiolipin antibodies in ischemic stroke in the young: Indian experience. *J Neurol Sci* 150:137, 1997.

74. Hughson MD, McCarty GA, Sholer CM, et al: Thrombotic cerebral arteriopathy in patients with the antiphospholipid syndrome. *Mod Pathol* 6:644, 1993.

75. Gordon DL, Linhardt R, Adams HA Jr: Low-molecular-weight heparins and heparinoids and their use in acute or progressing ischemic stroke. *Clin Neuropharmacol* 13:522, 1990.

76. Warkentin TE, Kelton JG: A 14-year study of heparin-induced thrombocytopenia. *Am J Med* 101:502, 1996.

77. Lottenberg R, Dolly FR, Kitchens CS: Recurring throm-

boembolic disease and pulmonary hypertension associated with severe hypoplasminogenemia *Am J Hematol* 19:181, 1985.

78. Dolan G, Greaves M, Cooper P, et al: Thrombovascular disease and familial plasminogen deficiency: A report of three kindreds. *Br J Haematol* 70:417, 1988.

79. Furlan AJ, Lucas FV, Cracium R, et al: Stroke in a young adult with familial plasminogen disorder. *Stroke* 22:1598, 1991.

80. Tait RC, Walker ID, Conkie JA, et al: Isolated familial plasminogen deficiency may not be a risk factor for thrombosis. *Thromb Haemost* 76:1004, 1996.

81. Tengborn L, Larsson SA, Hedner U, et al: Coagulation studies in children and young adults with cerebral ischemic episodes. *Acta Neurol Scand* 63:351, 1981.

82. Nilsson IM, Ljungner H, Tengborn L: Two different mechanisms in patients with venous thrombosis and defective fibrinolysis: Low concentration of plasminogen activator or increased concentration of plasminogen activator inhibitor. *BMJ* 18:1453, 1985.

83. Meade TW, Ruddock V, Stirling Y, et al: Fibrinolytic activity, clotting factors, and long-term incidence of ischaemic heart disease in the Northwick Park Heart Study. *Lancet* 342:1076, 1993.

84. Hamsten A, Wiman B, de Faire U, et al: Increased plasma levels of a rapid inhibitor of tissue plasminogen activator in young survivors of myocardial infarction. *N Engl J Med* 313:1557, 1985.

85. Juhan-Vague I, Alessi MC, Joly P, et al: Plasma plasminogen activator inhibitor-1 in angina pectoris: Influence of plasma insulin and acute-phase response. *Arteriosclerosis* 9:362, 1989.

86. Lindgren A, Lindoff C, Norrving B, et al: Tissue plasminogen activator and plasminogen activator inhibitor-1 in stroke patients *Stroke* 27:1066, 1996.

87. Jorgensen M, Bonnevie-Nielson V: Increased concentration of the fast-acting plasminogen activator inhibitor in plasma associated with familial venous thrombosis. *Br J Haematol* 65:175, 1987.

88. Macko RF, Ameriso SF, Gruber A, et al: Impairments of the protein C system and fibrinolysis in infection-associated stroke. *Stroke* 27:2005, 1996.

89. Michiels JJ, Juvonen E: Proposal for revised diagnostic criteria of essential thrombocythemia and polycythemia vera by the Thrombocythemia Vera Study Group. *Semin Thromb Hemost* 23:339, 1997.

90. Rao AK, Carvalho ACA: Acquired qualitative platelet defects, in Colman RW, Hirsh J, Marder VJ, Salzman EW (eds): *Hemostasis and Thrombosis: Basic Principles and Clinical Practice,* 3rd ed. Philadelphia, JB Lippincott, 1994, p 685.

91. Hart RG, Kanter MC: Hematologic disorders and ischemic stroke: A selective review. *Stroke* 21:1111, 1990.

92. Landolfi R, Patrono C: Aspirin in polycythemia vera and essential thrombocythemia: Current facts and perspectives. *Leuk Lymphoma* 22 (Suppl 1):83, 1996.

93. Tartaglia AP, Goldberg JD, Berk PD, et al: Adverse effects of antiaggregating platelet therapy in the treatment of polycythemia vera. *Semin Hematol* 23:172, 1986.

94. Willoughby S, Pearson TC: The use of aspirin in polycythemia vera and primary thrombocythemia. *Blood Rev* 12:12, 1998.

95. Gruppo Italiano Studio Policitemia (GISP): Low-dose aspirin in polycythemia vera: A pilot study. *Br J Haemotol* 97:453, 1997.

96. Landolfi R, Marchioli R: European collaboration on low-dose aspirin in polycythemia vera (ECLAP): A randomized trial. *Semin Thromb Hemost* 23:473, 1997.

97. Schwarcz TH, Hogan LA, Endean ED, et al: Thromboembolic complications of polycythemia vera versus smokers' polycythemia. *J Vasc Surg* 17:518, 1993.

98. Al-Hakim M, Katirji B, Osorio I, et al: Cerebral venous thrombosis in paroxysmal nocturnal hemoglobinuria: Report of two cases. *Neurology* 43:742, 1993.

99. Al-Samman MB, Cuetter AC, Guerra LG, et al: Cerebral arterial thrombosis as a complication of paroxysmal nocturnal hemoglobinuria. *South Med J* 87:765, 1994.

100. Ohene-Frempong K, Weiner SJ, Sleeper LA, et al: Cerebrovascular accidents in sickle cell disease: Rates and risk factors. *Blood* 91:288, 1998.

101. Coull BM, Clark WM: Abnormalities of hemostasis in ischemic stroke. *Med Clin North Am* 77:77, 1993.

102. Charache S, Barton FB, Moore RD, et al: Hydroxyurea and sickle cell anemia: Clinical utility of a myelosuppressive "switching" agent. The Multicenter Study of Hydroxyurea in Sickle Cell Anemia. *Medicine* 75:300, 1996.

103. Foulon I, Bachir D, Galacteros F, et al: Increased in vivo production of thromboxane in patients with sickle cell disease is accompanied by an impairment of platelet functions to the thromboxane A2 agonist U46619. *Arterioscler Thromb* 13:421, 1993.

104. Koudstaal PJ, Koudstaal A: Neurologic and visual symptoms in essential thrombocythemia: Efficacy of low-dose aspirin. *Semin Thromb Hemost* 23:365, 1997.

105. Van Genderen PJ, Mulder PG, Waleboer M, et al: Prevention and treatment of thrombotic complications in essential thrombocythemia. *Br J Haemotol* 97:179, 1997.

106. Nurden P, Bihour C, Smith M, et al: Platelet activation and thrombosis: Studies in a patient with essential thrombocythemia. *Am J Hematol* 51:79, 1996.

107. Kelly PJ, McDonald CT, Neill GO, et al: Middle cerebral artery main stem thrombosis in two siblings with familial thrombotic thrombocytopenic purpura. *Neurology* 50:1157, 1998.

108. Marder VJ, Feinstein DI, Francis CW, et al: Consumptive thrombohemorrhagic disorders, in Colman RW, Hirsh J. Marder VJ, Salzman EW (eds): *Hemostasis and Thrombosis: Basic Principles and Clinical Practice,* 3rd ed. Philadelphia, JB Lippincott, 1994, p 1023.

109. Dahlback B, Carlsson M, Svensson PJ: Familial thrombophilia due to a previously unrecognized mechanism characterized by poor anticoagulant response to activated

protein C: Prediction of a cofactor to activated protein C. *Proc Natl Acad Sci USA* 90:1004, 1993.

110. Griffin JH, Evatt B, Wideman C, et al: Anticoagulant protein C pathway defective in majority of thrombophilic patients. *Blood* 82:1989, 1993.

111. Bertina RM, Koeleman BP, Koster T, et al: Mutation in blood coagulation factor V associated with resistance to activated protein C in venous thrombophilia. *Nature* 369:64, 1994.

112. Braun A, Müller B, Rosche AA: Population study of the G1691A mutation (R506Q, FV Leiden) in the human factor V gene that is associated with resistance to activated protein C. *Hum Genet* 97:263, 1996.

113. Schröder W, Koesling M, Wulff K, et al: Large-scale screening for factor V Leiden mutation in a north-eastern German population. *Haemostasis* 26:233, 1996.

114. Lee DH, Henderson PA, Blajchman MA: Prevalence of factor V Leiden in a Canadian blood donor population. *Can Med Assoc J* 155:285, 1996.

115. Ridker PM, Miletich JP, Hennekens CH, et al: Ethnic distribution of factor V Leiden in 4047 men and women: Implications for venous thromboembolism screening. *JAMA* 277:1305, 1997.

116. Zöller B, Svensson PJ, He X, et al: Identification of the same factor V gene mutation in 47 out of 50 thrombosis-prone families with inherited resistance to activated protein C. *J Clin Invest* 94:2521, 1994.

117. Laffan MA, Manning R: The influence of factor VIII on measurement of activated protein C resistance. *Blood Coagul Fibrinolysis* 7:761, 1996.

118. Ruiz-Argüelles GJ, Garcés-Eisele J, Alarcón-Segovia D, et al: Activated protein C resistance phenotype and genotype in patients with primary antiphospholipid syndrome. *Blood Coagul Fibrinolysis* 7:344, 1996.

119. Fisher M, Fernandez JA, Ameriso SF, et al: Activated protein C resistance in ischemic stroke not due to factor V arginine 506 → glutamine mutation. *Stroke* 27:1163, 1996.

120. Hallak M, Senderowicz J, Cassel A, et al: Activated protein C resistance (factor V Leiden) associated with thrombosis in pregnancy. *Am J Obstet Gynecol* 176:889, 1997.

121. Martinelli I, Landi G, Merati G, et al: Factor V gene mutation is a risk factor for cerebral venous thrombosis. *Thromb Haemost* 75:393, 1996.

122. Catto A, Carter A, Ireland H, et al: Factor V Leiden gene mutation and thrombin generation in relation to the development of acute stroke. *Arterioscler Thromb Vasc Biol* 15:783, 1995.

123. Ridker PM, Hennekens CH, Lindpaintner K, et al: Mutation in the gene coding for coagulation factor V and the risk of myocardial infarction, stroke, and venous thrombosis in apparently healthy men. *N Engl J Med* 332:912, 1995.

124. Press RD, Liu XY, Beamer N, et al: Ischemic stroke in the elderly: Role of the common factor V mutation causing resistance to activated protein C. *Stroke* 27:44, 1996.

125. Bontempo FA, Hassett AC, Faruki H, et al: The factor

V Leiden mutation: Spectrum of thrombotic events and laboratory evaluation. *J Vasc Surg* 25:271, 1997.

126. Simioni P, de Ronde H, Prandoni P, et al: Ischemic stroke in young patients with activated protein C resistance: A report of three cases belonging to three different kindreds. *Stroke* 26:885, 1995.

127. van der Bom JG, Bots ML, Haverkate F, et al: Reduced response to activated protein C is associated with increased risk for cerebrovascular disease. *Ann Intern Med* 125:265, 1996.

128. Welch GN, Loscalzo J: Homocysteine and athero-thrombosis. *N Engl J Med* 338:1042, 1998.

129. Boers GHJ: Hyperhomocysteinemia as a risk factor for arterial and venous disease: A review of evidence and relevance. *Thromb Haemost* 78:520, 1997.

130. Selhub J, D'Angelo A: Hyperhomocysteinemia and thrombosis: Acquired conditions. *Thromb Haemost* 78:527, 1997.

131. Mandel H, Brenner B, Berant M, et al: Coexistence of hereditary homocystinuria and factor V Leiden: Effect on thrombosis. *N Engl J Med* 334:763, 1996.

132. Coull BM, Malinow MR, Beamer N, et al: Elevated plasma homocyst(e)ine concentration as a possible independent risk factor for stroke. *Stroke* 21:572, 1990.

133. Clarke R, Daly L, Robinson K, et al: Hyperhomocysteinemia: An independent risk factor for vascular disease. *N Engl J Med* 324:1149, 1991.

134. Perry IJ, Refsum H, Morris RW, et al: Prospective study of serum total homocysteine concentration and risk of stroke in middle-aged British men. *Lancet* 346:1395, 1995.

135. Boushey CJ, Beresford SA, Omenn GS, et al: A quantitative assessment of plasma homocysteine as a risk factor for vascular disease: Probable benefits of increasing folic acid intakes. *JAMA* 274:1049, 1995.

136. Graham IM, Daly LE, Refsum HM, et al: Plasma homocysteine as a risk factor for vascular disease. The European Concerted Action Project. *JAMA* 277:1775, 1997.

137. Robinson K, Arheart K, Refsum H, et al: Low circulating folate and vitamin B6 concentrations: Risk factors for stroke, peripheral vascular disease, and coronary artery disease. European COMAC Group. *Circulation* 97:437, 1998.

138. Folsom AR, Nieto FJ, McGovern PG, et al: Prospective study of coronary artery disease incidence in relation to fasting total homocysteine, related genetic polymorphisms, and B vitamin. The Atherosclerosis Risk in Communities Study. *Circulation* 98:204, 1998.

139. Lindgren A, Brattstrom L, Norrving B, et al: Plasma homocysteine in the acute and convalescent phases after stroke. *Stroke* 26:795, 1995.

140. Poort SR, Rosendaal FR, Reitsma PH, et al: A common genetic variation in the 3'-untranslated region of the prothrombin gene is associated with elevated plasma prothrombin levels and an increase in venous thrombosis. *Blood* 88:3698, 1996.

141. Kapur RK, Mills LA, Spitzer SG, et al: A prothrombin

gene mutation is significantly associated with venous thrombosis. *Arterioscler Thromb Vasc Biol* 17:2875, 1997.

142. Longstreth WT Jr, Rosendaal FR, Siscovick DS, et al: Risk of stroke in young women and two prothrombotic mutations: Factor V Leiden and prothrombin gene variant. (G20210A). *Stroke* 29:577, 1998.

143. Francis JL: Laboratory investigation of hypercoagulability. *Semin Thromb Hemost* 24:111, 1998.

144. Levine MN, Hirsh J, Salzman EW: Side effects of antithrombotic therapy, in Colman RW, Hirsh J, Marder VJ, Salzman EW (eds): *Hemostasis and Thrombosis: Basic Principles and Clinical Practice,* 3rd ed. Philadelphia, JB Lippincott, 1994; p 936.

145. Lowe GDO: Agents lowering blood viscosity, including defibrinating agents, in Verstraete M, Fuster V, Topol EJ (eds): *Cardiovascular Thrombosis: Thrombocardiology and Thromboneurology,* 2nd ed. Philadelphia, Lippincott-Raven, 1998, p 321.

146. Sodian R, Loebe M, Gorman KF, et al: Heparin induced thrombocytopenia: Experiences in 12 heart surgery patients. *ASAIO J* 43:M430, 1997.

147. Rosove MH, Brewer PM: Antiphospholipid thrombosis: Clinical course after the first thrombotic event in 70 patients. *Ann Intern Med* 117:303, 1992.

148. Khamashta MA, Cuadrado MJ, Mujic F, et al: The management of thrombosis in the antiphospholipid-antibody syndrome. *N Engl J Med* 332:993, 1995.

149. Wisbey HL, Klestov AC: Thrombocytopenia corrected by warfarin in antiphospholipid syndrome. *J Rheumatol* 23:769, 1996.

150. Markus HS, Hambley H: Neurology and the blood: Haemotological abnormalities in ischemic stroke. *J Neurol Neurosurg Psychiatry* 64:150, 1998.

151. Monagle P, Andrew M, Halton J, et al: Homozygous protein C deficiency: Description of a new mutation and successful treatment with low molecular weight heparin. *Thromb Haemost* 79:756, 1998.

152. Russell MO, Goldberg HI, Hodson A, et al: Effect of transfusion therapy on arteriographic abnormalities and on recurrence of stroke in sickle cell disease. *Blood* 63:162, 1984.

153. Pegelow CH, Adams RJ, McKie V, et al: Risk of recurrent stroke in patients with sickle cell disease treated with erythrocyte transfusions. *J Pediatr* 126:896, 1995.

154. Adams RJ, McKie VC, Hsu L, et al: Prevention of a first stroke by transfusions in children with sickle cell anemia and abnormal results on transcranial Doppler ultrasonography. *N Engl J Med* 339:5, 1998.

155. Tanne D, Triplett DA, Levine SR: Antiphospholipid-protein antibodies and ischemic stroke: Not just cardiolipin any more. *Stroke* 29:1755, 1998.

Chapter 16

DIAGNOSIS AND MANAGEMENT OF DISSECTION

Hamid R. Salari-Namin
Stanley N. Cohen

BACKGROUND

Introduction

About 3 to 4 percent of cerebral ischemic infarcts occur in patients under the age of 45, and arterial dissection constitutes 6 to 22 percent of cerebral ischemic infarcts in this age group.[1-6] It represents the most important nonatherosclerotic arteriopathy of cervicocephalic arteries and is recognized with increasing frequency to be the cause of stroke in young adults. This is due, in part, to increasing familiarity with this clinical entity and the increasing application of noninvasive methods, particularly magnetic resonance imaging/magnetic resonance angiography (MRI/MRA), in diagnostic workup. Despite an increasing awareness, in the series reported by Sturzenegger, delay in diagnosis and treatment occurred in 38 of 44 patients with spontaneous internal carotid artery (ICA) dissection.[7]

Pathology

Dissection of cervicocephalic arteries is produced by penetration of blood into the arterial wall and formation of intramural hematoma. The intramural hematoma may extend for various lengths along the artery, often more distally than proximally. The hematoma may rupture back into the original arterial lumen and create a "double lumen."[8,14] The hematoma may be the consequence of the penetration of blood through an intimal tear or of a hemorrhage from the vasa vasorum.[9] Intramural hematoma may lie closer to either intima (subinti-

mal dissections) or adventitia (subadventitial dissections). Subintimal dissections are more likely to cause luminal stenosis or occlusion, whereas subadventitial dissections tend to cause arterial dilatation (dissecting aneurysms) (Fig. 16-1).[8] Either distal hypoperfusion or embolism may cause the ischemic symptoms, transient ischemic attack (TIA), or ischemic stroke. Reports on the pattern of infarction in patients with carotid dissection indicate that the majority of strokes are the result of distal embolization.[10-12] Subadventitial dissections extend outwardly and may induce compression of the surrounding structures. Horner's syndrome, less commonly single or multiple cranial nerve palsies, and only rarely cervical root or nerve palsies have been reported. Cranial neuropathies may be caused by compression or by ischemia owing to interruption of the supplying arteries.[13,34,35,52] Subadventitial dissections of vertebral arteries and less commonly the intracranial carotid system may rupture externally, giving rise to subarachnoid hemorrhage (SAH). The presence of only internal elastic lamina and a thin adventitia makes intracranial arteries vulnerable to subadventitial dissection and ultimately SAH. Bleeding is not a usual consequence of cervical artery dissections. The cervical segment of ICA, usually more than 2 cm distal to the carotid bifurcation, is the most common site of ICA dissection. The supraclinoid segment of the ICA is the most common intracranial site. About two-thirds of vertebral artery dissections are located in the V3 or V1 segments of the vertebral artery, and the intradural segment seems to be the next most common primary site (Table 16-1). Mechanical torsion and stretch on the vertebral artery is greatest at the C1

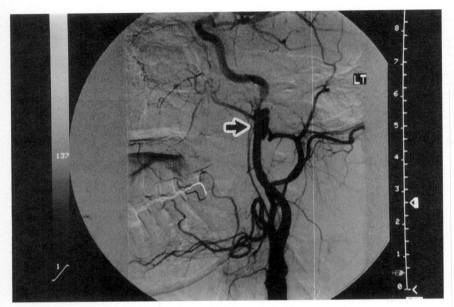

Figure 16-1.
Left common carotid angiogram showing an intracranial pseudoaneurysm associated with a dissection (arrow).

to C2 level, which is thought to be the reason most reported cases of dissection associated with chiropractic manipulation occur at this level.[53] Multiple simultaneous dissections might occur in up to 60 percent of patients. This seems to be more frequent when the dissection involves the vertebral artery.[14,37,39,40,50]

Epidemiology

The majority of cervicocephalic dissections occur in patients between 30 and 50 years of age, with a mean age of 40 years.[15,16] The incidence rate of nontraumatic cervical arterial dissection is 2.6 to 2.9 per 100,000 for all age groups.[17,18] Most reports indicate ICA dissection is slightly more common in males, whereas vertebral artery dissection is more common in females.

Major and minor traumas and various diseases of arterial wall have been implicated as main predisposing factors for dissection (Table 16-2). The role of minor or trivial trauma in pathogenesis of dissection is not clear. Chiropractic manipulation, neck extension and rotation (sports injuries, whiplash injuries), strenuous exercises (rock and roll performers), and straining maneuvers are activities that have been implicated. Underlying primary arteriopathies may also predispose to cervicocephalic dissection. Fibromuscular dysplasia (FMD) is present in up to 20 percent of patients with dissection.[8,14,21] Associations with cystic medial necrosis,[15,22] Ehlers-Danlos syndrome type IV,[23,24] osteogenesis imperfecta,[29] pseudoxanthoma elasticum,[29] Manfan's syndrome,[26–28] homocysteinemia,[29] and α_1-antitrypsin deficiency[30] have also been reported. Among other potential risk factors for dissection are oral contraceptives,[8] pregnancy,[54,55] hypertension,[8,40] migraine,[56,57] and smoking.[8,40] The occurrence of multivessel dissections, familial occurrence of spontaneous dissections, and familial aggregation of cervical artery dissections and cerebral aneurysms have also been reported.[15,19,20] Association

Table 16-1.
Location of dissections

Extracranial (90%)

ICA (75%): more than 2 cm distal to bifurcation

VA (25%): V3 segment/V1 segment

Intracranial (10%)

ICA: supraclinoid segment/MCA trunk

VA: V4 segment

Table 16-2.
Predisposing factors

Trauma
  Major (penetrating/nonpenetrating)
  Minor or trivial
    Chiropractic manipulation
    Neck extension and rotation
    Strenuous physical activity
    Straining maneuvers
    Others

Primary arteriopathies
  Fibromuscular dysplasia (FMD)
  Marfan's syndrome
  Ehlers-Danlos syndrome type IV
  Osteogenesis imperfecta
  Pseudoxanthoma elasticum
  Cystic medial necrosis (CMN)
  α_1-antitrypsin deficiency
  Homocystinuria
  ? Coiling/tortuosity/kinking

Others
  Hypertension
  Oral contraceptives
  Smoking
  Migraine
  Positive family history
  Congenital heart disorders
    Bicuspid aortic valve
    Pulmonic valve stenosis
    Aortic coarctation
  ? Recent infections

between a variety of congenital heart disorders and cervical arterial dissections has been reported by Schievink et al, and a neural crest abnormality has been suggested as a common pathogenic factor in the seemingly dissimilar cardiovascular disorders.[31]

Clinical Findings

ICA Dissection Pain is the most common symptom, occurring in more than 75 percent of patients. Pain is usually homolateral to the dissection and is localized to the anterior head, face, jaw, neck, or pharynx. ICA dissection is among the causes of carotidynia.[58] The pain is usually steady and nonthrobbing. The headache is severe in the majority of patients; however, it may fluctuate in intensity and last up to 3 months.[32,33]

Cerebral ischemia, including TIA, stroke, or both are the second most common symptoms. It occurs in approximately 70 percent of patients. Only a minority of strokes are preceded by TIAs. Transient monocular blindness (TMB), unilateral weakness, unilateral sensory loss, aphasia, and visual field defects have been reported. In a majority of these cases, the ischemic symptoms are delayed and follow unilateral headache by a period that ranges from minutes to days.[8,14]

Oculosympathetic paresis (Horner's syndrome), the third most common finding, is present in approximately half of the patients. It is homolateral to a carotid dissection and is not associated with anhidrosis because the external carotid plexus is spared. Although unilateral hemicranial headache and oculosympathetic paresis may be the only clinical manifestations of ICA dissection, in a majority of cases other symptoms are also present.[8,14]

Bruits, subjective, objective, or both, are noted in 30 percent of patients.[8,14] Single or multiple cranial nerve palsies have been reported in 5 to 12 percent of patients with spontaneous ICA dissection.[36] In order of frequency, the affected cranial nerves are 12th, 9th, 10th, 11th, 5th, 7th (corda tympani), 6th, and 3rd nerves. Cranial nerve palsies have been attributed to mechanical compression or stretching of these nerves by the expanded or aneurysmal ICA. However, another plausible mechanism for cranial nerve palsies is compromise of the blood supply to the cranial nerves.[8,34–36] Angiographic evaluation of cranial nerve palsies should include the extracranial ICA in addition to the intracranial circulation.

Nonarteritic ischemic optic neuropathy is reported to occur in about 4 percent of ICAD.[38] Light headedness, tinnitus, syncope, scalp tenderness, and neck swelling are other rare manifestations of ICA dissection (Table 16-3). In cases of intracranial dissection, SAH or seizure might occur.[8,13]

Vertebral Artery (VA) Dissection Headache with or without posterior neck pain is the most common manifestation of VA dissection, occurring in more than 75 percent of patients. The headache is usually occipital, ipsilateral to the dissection, but it can be in other head regions. Pain usually precedes ischemic symptoms from a few minutes to days. Vertebrobasilar territory TIA or stroke is the second most common manifestation occurring in approximately 70 percent of patients. TIAs are less frequent with vertebrobasilar than ICA dissections. Lateral medullary syndrome is the most frequent deficit, but various other brainstem syndromes involving cerebellum, pons, midbrain, and posterior cerebral artery territories have also been reported. Reporting on

Table 16-3.

Symptoms and signs of cervical ICA dissection

Headache	59–95%
Focal cerebral ischemia (TIA or stroke)	67–76%
Oculosympathetic paresis	30–55%
Cervical bruit	25–40%
Neck pain	3–65%
Amaurosis fugax	10%
Syncope	5%
Scalp tenderness	<5%
Neck swelling	<5%
Cranial nerve palsies	<5%
Dysgeusia	<5%
Tinnitus	<5%
Ischemic optic neuropathy	<5%

Adapted from Ref. 64.

a series of 37 patients under the age of 40 with cerebellar infarction, the most common cause was intracranial vertebral artery dissection.[25] Vertebral artery dissection can also lead to different patterns of spinal cord infarcts (Table 16-4). Multivessel dissections occur in a significant number of patients, and four-vessel angiography should always be attempted if a VA dissection is visualized. Intradural dissection may cause SAH because the muscularis and adventitial layers of intracranial arteries are less thick and lack external elastic membranes.[26,37,39,40,59,60]

Table 16-4.

Symptoms and signs of extracranial VA dissection

Neck pain	51%
Headache	56%
Neck or head pain	75%
Stroke	72%
TIA	32%
LMS[a]	34%

From Ref. 43.

[a]LMS, lateral medullary syndrome.

EVIDENCE

Diagnostic Testing

CT Scan Dynamic CT scan (single level slices), dynamic incremental CT scan (multilevel slices), and helical CT have been used to detect dissections. Zuber and colleagues[41] demonstrated that dynamic CT scan is a sensitive neuroimaging procedure for confirming the presence of the mural hematoma when angiography is not conclusive and MRI/MRA cannot be performed. The typical dynamic CT scan picture of dissection including an eccentric contrast enhancement (residual lumen) surrounded by a relative hypodensity (mural hematoma), itself surrounded by a thin annular enhancement, was noticed in 80 percent of dissected vessels. A major drawback of dynamic CT scan is that prior angiography is required to determine the appropriate level. Helical CT scan has the potential for providing sensitive imaging of the whole cervical portion of the ICA and does not need to be directed by prior angiography. However, more clinical experience with this technique is needed before its exact role is determined.[42]

Ultrasonography Multimodal ultrasonography (US), including carotid duplex (CD), extracranial Doppler (ECD), and transcranial Doppler (TCD), has a high sensitivity to detect dissections and is a useful screening and monitoring method.[44–47] It lacks specificity and cannot detect dissecting aneurysms.[43] Sturzenegger et al[44] performed combined US examination in 43 patients with ICA dissection. The overall sensitivity of the combined US examination was 95 percent. All three methods detected occlusions or high-graded stenoses in 100 percent of patients. However, the diagnostic sensitivity of US decreased to 80 percent for low or moderate degree stenoses. Steinke et al[46] reported initial abnormal Doppler sonographic findings in all 48 patients with angiographically confirmed ICA dissections. Because CD might miss high cervical stenosis, additional high cervical (retromandibular) TCD can be employed. Further, important information regarding adequacy of the collaterals and intracranial blood flow can be provided by the TCD. TCD offers the possibility of detecting those cases with persistent low flow that are at risk for infarction that might benefit from revascularization. TCD can also be used for emboli detection. Srinivasan and colleagues used TCD for microemboli detection in 17 cases of dissection.[48] They reported 70 percent of those with emboli presented with stroke compared with 14 percent of those without emboli ($p < .05$). Other US findings include an echogenic flap (the most specific sign), an echogenic thrombus, abrupt and smooth tapering luminal stenosis, double lumen, decreased or absent flow, and more characteristic high resistance biphasic systolic flow without diastolic flow (stump flow).[7,44]

MRI/MRA MRI/MRA play an increasingly important role in the detection of cervicocephalic arterial dissection. It is noninvasive, visualizes intramural hematoma, arterial wall expansion, and the relationship with the surrounding tissues.[16] The typical MRI finding is an eccentric or circumferential rim of hyperintense signal on T1-weighted and later T2-weighted images, surrounding narrowed hypointensity signal corresponding to the remaining flow in the lumen (crescent sign) (Fig. 16-2). The hyperintense signal corresponds to intramural hematoma with methemoglobin signal intensity. In some reports, all or part of the intramural hematoma appeared hypointense on T2-weighted images. In such cases, the hypointensities most likely represent acute clot deoxyhemoglobin or hemosiderin in the chronic stage.[61] Other MRI findings suggestive of dissection include (1) increased signal from the entire vessel, (2) poor or absent visualization of the vessel, and (3) significant compromise of the vessel lumen by adjacent abnormal signal tissue (also see Chap. 35 and Fig. 35-19).[62]

MRA can noninvasively display the same features of dissection as conventional angiography and increases the yield of MRI (Fig. 16-3C). MRA source images taken through the level of the dissection may show decreased true lumen diameter, blood in the false lumen, and a flap separating the two (Fig. 16-3A and B). Levy et al studied a total of 24 cervical dissections with three-dimensional time of flight (TOF) MRA, MRI, and cerebral angiography. In ICA dissection, they found that MRI had a sensitivity of 84 percent and a specificity of 99 percent. MRA was more accurate with 95 percent and 99 percent sensitivity and specificity, respectively. In the same study, MRI detected VA dissection with a sensitivity of 60 percent and a specificity of 98 percent, and MRA with a sensitivity of 20 percent, and specificity of 100 percent. Compared with standard cerebral angiography, MRI/MRA combined has a sensitivity of 95 percent and specificity of 99 percent for the diagnosis of carotid dissection. MRI/MRA is less sensitive for detecting vertebral artery dissection, leaving contrast angiography as the clear test of choice for this disorder.[43,47,49]

Catheter Angiography Catheter angiography (CA) is the gold standard technique for the diagnosis of cervicocephalic dissections, although MRI/MRAs play an increasingly important role. Angiography of all four vessels should be performed to detect multivessel dissections. The most common angiographic finding is smooth or irregularly tapered luminal stenosis (Fig. 16-4). The degree of stenosis can range from slight to severe narrowing (string sign) to complete occlusion. Other findings include abrupt or fairly abrupt reconstitution of lumen, which is usually seen at the carotid canal level, dissecting aneurysm, tapered stenosis with concomitant dissecting aneurysm, intimal flap, and double lumen.[47,49,50] In Mokri's series,[50] aneurysms occurred in more than one-third of the ICA dissections, and these were often located in the upper cervical and subcranial regions. At times, angiographic evidence of underlying FMD or complications of arterial dissection such as distal branch occlusions owing to embolization are detected. The characteristic location of extracranial carotid dissection is a few centimeters above the carotid bifurcation (Fig. 16-5). This differs from that of athero-

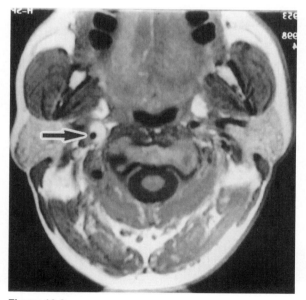

Figure 16-2.
T1-weighted MRI axial image through the neck showing a right carotid dissection with a flow void in a narrowed lumen surrounded by hyperintense crescent (arrow) consistent with intramural hematoma. Compare with the contralateral carotid, which has a larger flow void and is not surrounded by a hyperintensity.

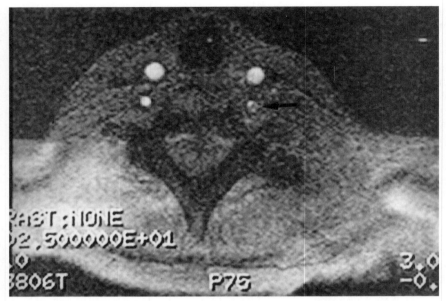

A

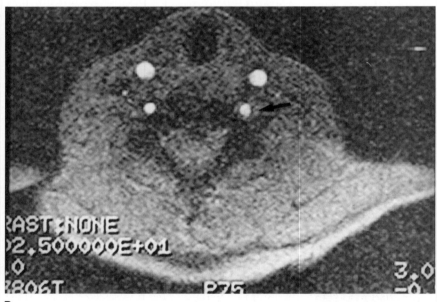

B

Figure 16-3.

MRI, MRA, and contrast angiogram of young woman with a left vertebral dissection. A   MRI source images showing an abnormal left vertebral artery (arrow). The lumen shows decreased flow with a dark line in the center suggestive of a flap. Compare with the normal contralateral vertebral artery in terms of size and signal intensity. B   MRI source images taken several centimeters above the image in 16-3A. The left vertebral artery lumen now appears normal in size with normal flow (arrow).

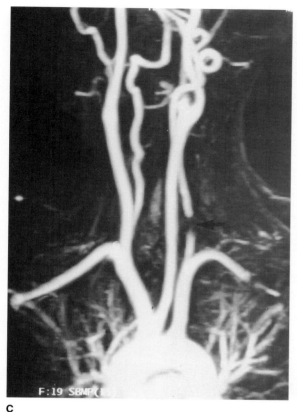

C

Figure 16-3 (Continued).
C Contrast-enhanced MRA of the aortic arch showing the inominate, subclavian, carotid, and vertebral arteries. There is a flow gap in the left vertebral artery (arrow) *corresponding to the level of the dissection. Both carotids and right vertebral are normal.*

sclerotic disease, which typically occurs at the carotid bifurcation. A stenosis that is long and tapered, rather than focal, also favors dissection. In the vertebral, dissection is often in the V3 section or distal to the origin of the vertebral, whereas atherosclerosis is most commonly at the origin (see Fig. 16-3D and E). See also Chapter 36, Figs. 36-10 and 36-11.

Course and Prognosis

Follow-up studies have shown a fairly good overall prognosis in extracranial dissections. Complete or excellent recovery occurs in 70 to 85 percent of patients. Major deficits remain in 10 to 20 percent and death occurs in 5 percent.[8,14,43] It should be kept in mind that the acute

prognosis of ischemic stroke reflects the extent of the brain lesion and is not specific to the arterial process. In 30 patients with ICA dissection, Bogousslavsky et al[5] reported seven deaths within 2 to 6 days after admission. These seven patients had the largest infarcts. Although both spontaneous and traumatic dissections of extracranial ICA tend to have a good prognosis, the outcome is somewhat less favorable for the traumatic group.[14] The overall prognosis in intracranial dissections, particularly when complicated by SAH, is less favorable.[26,37,39,40]

After the first month, the risk of recurrent dissection is 1 percent per year. Younger patients are more likely to have a recurrent dissection. Family history of arterial dissection is another important risk factor for the development of a recurrent arterial dissection.[15] At follow-up angiography, resolution or significant improvement of stenosis occurs in about 80 percent. Resolution of aneurysms occurs in only 40 percent. The remainder may diminish in size or remain the same size. Recanalization of total occlusions occurs in only 40 percent. Among the common clinical manifestations, oculosympathetic paresis resolution occurs less frequently. The residual partial Horner's syndrome is usually quite mild and not of concern. Headache and bruits resolve in the majority of patients. Persistent headache may indicate the presence of a residual dissecting aneurysm. Similarly, persistence of bruits may suggest the presence of a dissecting aneurysm, residual stenosis, or occlusion.[8,14,43]

Treatment

Treatment of cervicocephalic dissections remains controversial. A large randomized drug trial comparing treatment options in dissection would be very difficult because of the low rate of recurrent ischemic events.[63] Current recommendations are based on small, uncontrolled series, case studies, and personal experiences.[64] Following a review of the literature and an analysis of the Mayo Clinic experience, Mokri has suggested that there is no "infallible method for managing patients with spontaneous dissection of cervical arteries."[14] Anticoagulation with heparin followed by warfarin, antiplatelet agents, and various surgical and invasive endovascular procedures have been prescribed. The favorable natural history of dissections has shifted support to medical rather than surgical management.

Anticoagulation A number of important caveats regarding anticoagulation need to be taken into consideration: (1) there are no controlled clinical trials available that prove the benefit of anticoagulation in this setting,

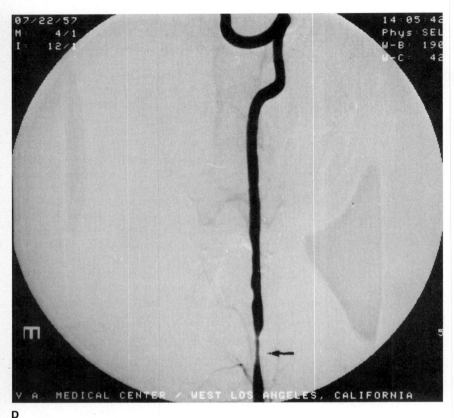

D

Figure 16-3 (Continued).
D *Contrast angiography of the left vertebral artery showing segmental narrowing in an area corresponding to the lesion on MRA.*

(2) reports of extension of dissection because of anticoagulation are rare,[1,7,14,21] and (3) early angiograms suggest that distal embolization of thrombotic fragments from the dissection site and in situ thrombus are the most common causes of neurologic worsening.[65,66] Clinical reports regarding the efficacy of anticoagulants are sparse. Sturzenegger[7] reported that none of 32 patients who received early heparin treatment showed any subsequent deterioration; yet, six young patients not immediately heparinized suffered severe stroke. Eljamel et al[67] anticoagulated seven patients with ICA dissection who did well. Others[69,70] found similar results. In their series of 80 carotid dissections, Biousse and colleagues reported five late strokes occurring after the diagnosis of dissection was established.[80] Four occurred in patients on anticoagulation. If there is no contraindication to anticoagulation, many experts recommend initial anti-coagulation with heparin followed by warfarin in patients with recurrent or progressive focal ischemic symptoms and signs and in patients who have angiographic evidence of distal embolization. In cases of intracranial dissection, prognosis is much less favorable; considering the higher chance of SAH, anticoagulation is probably not warranted, and heparin is best avoided[37,72] (Table 16-5). Some authors suggest anticoagulation of these patients if CT scan and examination of the spinal fluid show no evidence of SAH.[73] No solid data are available to determine optimal timing and duration of anticoagulation therapy. In one study of 80 extracranial ICA dissections, completed stroke occurred in 42 patients, most often (88 percent) during the first 7 days after onset of symptoms.[82] This suggests that any potential preventive treatment (anticoagulation) should be initiated as early as possible after the onset of symptoms.

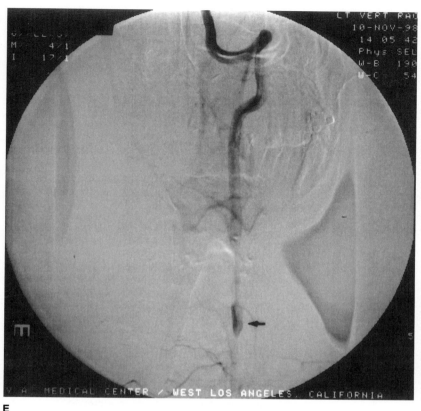

E

Figure 16-3 (Continued).
E *Contrast angiography of the left verterbral artery. This is a delayed image from the same injection
in Fig. 16-3D. At the* arrow, *there is delayed filling and emptying of the false lumen of the dissection.*

Duration of anticoagulation is also controversial. Some limited ultrasound (US) studies demonstrate that most of the dissections recover by 3 months, and beyond 6 months reconstitution of a normal lumen is highly unlikely. Therefore, anticoagulation should be continued for 3 months.[5,7] Beyond 3 months, persistence of the arterial lesion might influence selection of treatment, although there are no confirming data regarding follow-up treatment. If a follow-up MRI/MRA, CTA, or angiogram at 3 months shows hemodynamically significant stenosis or dissecting aneurysm, anticoagulation is continued for 3 more months.

Antiplatelet Antiplatelet agents, especially aspirin, have been prescribed in patients who present with only hemicranial headache and oculosympathetic paresis with angiographic evidence of mild stenosis and no dissecting aneurysm.[7,14,68,74] Antiplatelet therapy has also been suggested when warfarin is contraindicated.[76] The usefulness of aspirin in these patients is at best uncertain, as this group may do well with observation and no specific intervention. Biller et al found no difference in the rates of recurrent stroke between patients treated with aspirin and those treated with oral anticoagulants.[70] Josein reported two patients had recurrent symptoms when aspirin was discontinued.[71] In one study, antiplatelet agents did not stop the symptoms in three of four patients with ICA dissection, but anticoagulants did.[67] No reports are available with regard to usefulness of ticlopidine, clopidogrel, dipyridamole, or combinations of antiplatelet agents in patients with dissection.

Surgery Surgical intervention is recommended in patients with continuing ischemic symptoms despite anti-

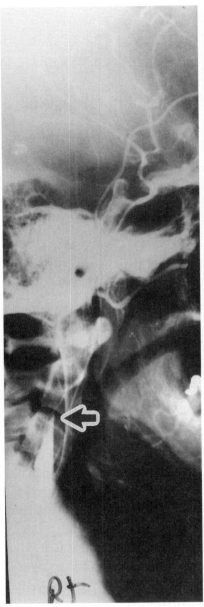

Figure 16-4.
*Right common carotid angiogram showing rapid tapering of
the internal carotid artery to a complete occlusion* (arrow).

coagulation, expanding dissecting aneurysm, or presenting with SAH caused by an intracranial dissection.
No trials have tested the efficacy of surgical procedures
in these settings. Surgical options include aneurysmal
resection and arterial reconstruction with interposition
grafting, proximal vessel ligation, trapping of the dissection or aneurysm, wrapping of the dissection, and augmentation of flow via extracranial-intracranial bypass
procedures.[51,72,77,78]

Interventional Radiology   Experience with interventional neuroradiologic techniques is limited. Hallbach
et al treated 16 patients with vertebral artery dissections
by endovascular techniques using detachable balloons,
electrolytically detachable coils, and platinum coils.[79] In
15 patients, angiography disclosed complete cure of the
dissection. They found balloon test occlusion and transluminal angioplasty as useful adjuncts in the management of their patients. Lefkowitz et al reported an interesting case of a fusiform aneurysm at the origin of the
posterior inferior cerebellar artery that was treated successfully with platinum microembolization coils.[80] The
use of stent placement to treat iatrogenic dissection has
been reported. The role of angioplasty and stent placement in spontaneous and traumatic dissection is still in
its infancy.

TREATMENT RECOMMENDATIONS

Diagnostic Testing

The evaluation of dissections includes imaging of the
brain and cervicocephalic arteries. An early CT scan
can show an ischemic stroke, a hyperdense artery sign
or SAH associated with intracranial dissections. If available, combined MRI/MRA allows early definite diagnosis in many cases, and therefore is the first diagnostic
test of choice. Ultrasonography is a quick and noninvasive test that may supplement the MRI/MRA findings.
If MRI/MRA is not available, the combined transcranial
Doppler and duplex examination is a quick way of sub-
stantiating clinical suspicion. However, issues concerning specificity and sensitivity, especially in the setting
of mild arterial occlusion, may limit its therapeutic usefulness. In the case of high-grade stenosis or occlusion,
TCD can provide more information regarding adequacy
of collaterals and also offers the possibility of detecting
those cases with persistent low flow that are at risk for
infarction. In addition, US is a very reliable method for
monitoring the necessity of continued anticoagulation.

Figure 16-5.
Arch angiogram showing an internal carotid occlusion several centimeters above the carotid bifurcation on one side (arrowhead) *and an intact internal carotid on the other side.*

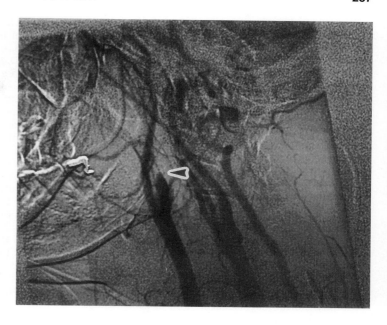

Although MRI/MRA can establish the diagnosis in the majority of cases, catheter angiography is the study of first choice when SAH is the initial manifestation arterial dissection. Catheter angiography is more sensitive when searching for aneurysms, an underlying arteriopathy (with or without multiple dissections), vertebral artery dissection, and intracranial extension of the dissection. In general, catheter angiography should also be done when clinical features strongly suggest dissection but the MRI/MRA findings are not conclusive. Applications of other examinations, such as cervical spine x-rays,

Table 16-5.
Anticoagulation in cervicocephalic arterial dissection

I. Proven indications: none

II. Widely accepted indications: extracranial arterial dissection with recurrent or progressive focal ischemic symptoms and signs; extracranial arterial dissection with transient ischemic attack; extracranial arterial dissection with small nonprogressing stroke

III. Uncertain indications: intracranial arterial dissection with negative CT and negative LP; extracranial dissection with pain and oculosympathetic paresis but without evidence of distal embolization; dissection with large nonprogressing stroke

IV. Contraindications: intracranial dissection with SAH

transesophageal echocardiography, and screening for underlying vascular disease need to be individualized.

Therapeutic Interventions

It must be remembered that the overwhelming majority of carotid and vertebral dissections have a favorable outcome (~80 to ~85 percent). Most of the patients with unfavorable outcome do poorly because of the presenting stroke rather than an event that occurs after diagnosis. There are no prospective randomized trials proving the benefit of anticoagulants. Anticoagulation is not without risk in the setting of acute stroke. Keeping this in mind, treatment for dissection is controversial and must be individualized.

Patients with dissection presenting with acute stroke in the first 6 h after symptom onset should be evaluated and treated as medical emergencies. The use of thrombolytic agents in acute stroke secondary to dissection has not been addressed in the clinical trials. No evidence-based recommendation can be made. There is theoretically increased risk of extending the intramural hemorrhage with a thrombolytic agent. In our experience, intravenous and intra-arterial thrombolytic therapy can be used in carefully selected extracranial dissections. Thrombolytic therapy should be used only as a treatment of last resort in intracranial dissection because of the risk of SAH.

In extracranial carotid dissection presenting with hemicranial headache and oculosympathetic paresis without evidence of hemodynamically significant stenosis or distal embolization or stroke, aspirin is recommended for 6 months. Most cases of intracranial dissection should not be treated with anticoagulation because of the risk of SAH.

Extracranial carotid or vertebral dissection presenting with recurrent, progressive, or transient cerebral ischemic symptoms or having evidence of hemodynamically significant stenosis should be considered for anticoagulation with heparin followed by warfarin unless there is a specific contraindication. The duration of therapy is determined by the time needed for recovery of the vessel wall. Because recanalization may occur within a few hours or take several months, the duration of anticoagulant treatment needs to be individualized. One common practice is to continue anticoagulation with warfarin for 3 months. A follow-up imaging study at 3 months will determine the subsequent treatment plan. If hemodynamically significant stenosis or pseudoaneurysm persist, anticoagulation is continued for 3 more months. If only mild luminal abnormalities persist, aspirin is administered for 3 additional months. Surgical and endovascular intervention is recommended when recurrent or progressive ischemic symptoms continue despite anticoagulation, when expanding dissecting aneurysm is causing compression of adjacent structures and when there is intracranial dissecting aneurysm with SAH.

REFERENCES

1. Hart RG, Sherman DG, Miller VT, et al: Diagnosis and management of ischemic stroke: II. Selected controversies. *Curr Probl Cardiol* 7:43, 1983.
2. Hart RG, Miller VT: Cerebral infarction in young adults: A practical approach. *Stroke* 14:110, 1983.
3. Chancellor AM, Glasgow GL, Ockelford PA, et al: Etiology, prognosis, and hemostatic function after cerebral infarction in young adults. *Stroke* 20:477, 1988.
4. Bevan H, Sharma K, Bradly W: Stroke in young adults. *Stroke* 21:382, 1990.
5. Bogousslavsky J, Despland PA, Regli F: Spontaneous carotid dissection with acute stroke. *Arch Neurol* 44:479, 1987.
6. Lisovoski F, Rousseux P: Cerebral infarction in young people: A study of 148 patients with cerebral angiography. *J Neurol Neurosurg Psychiatry* 54:576, 1991.
7. Sturzenegger M: Spontaneous internal carotid artery dissection: Early diagnosis and management in 44 patients. *J Neurol* 242:231, 1995.
8. Mokri B, Sundt TM, Houser OW, et al: Spontaneous dissection of the cervical internal carotid artery. *Ann Neurol* 19:126, 1986.
9. Leys D, Lucas C, Gobert M, et al: Cervical artery dissections. *Eur Neurol* 37:3, 1997.
10. Weiller C, Mullges W, Ringelstein EB, Buell V, Reich W: Patterns of brain infarction in internal carotid artery dissections. *Neurosurg Rev* 14:111, 1991.
11. Steinke W, Schwartz A, Hennerici M: Topography of cerebral infarction associated with carotid artery dissection. *J Neurol* 243:323, 1996.
12. Lucas C, Moulin T, Deplanque D, Tatu L, Chavot D, DONALD Investigators: Stroke patterns of internal carotid artery dissection in 40 patients. *Stroke* 29:2646, 1998.
13. Mokri B, Silbert PL, Schievink WI: Cranial nerve palsy in spontaneous dissection of the extracranial internal carotid artery. *Neurology* 46:356, 1996.
14. Mokri B: Dissections of cervical and cephalic arteries, in Sundt TM Jr (ed): *Occlusive Cerebrovascular Disease: Diagnostic and Surgical Management.* Philadelphia, Saunders, 1993, p 45.
15. Schievink WI, Mokri B, O'Fallon M: Recurrent spontaneous cervical-artery dissection. *N Engl J Med* B30:393, 1994.
16. Leys D, Moulinth M, Stojkovic T, et al: Long term course of cervical-artery dissection. *Cerebrovasc Dis* 5:43, 1995.
17. Shievink WI, Mokri B, Whisnant JP: Internal carotid artery dissection in a community: Rochester, Minnesota. *Stroke* 24:1673, 1993.
18. Giroud M, Fayolle H, André N: Incidence of internal carotid artery dissection in the community of Dijon. *J Neurol Neurosurg Psychiatry* 57:1443, 1994.
19. Mokri B, Stanson AW, Houser OW: Spontaneous dissection of the renal arteries in patients with previous spontaneous dissection of the internal carotid arteries. *Stroke* 16:959, 1985.
20. Mokri B, Houser OW, Stanson AW: Multivessel cervicocephalic and visceral arterial dissections: Pathogenic role of primary arterial disease in cervicocephalic arterial dissections. *J Stroke Cerebrovasc Dis* 1:117, 1991.
21. Hart RG, Easton JD: Dissections of cervical and cerebral arteries. *Neurol Clin* 1:155, 1983.
22. Brice JG, Crompton MR: Spontaneous dissecting aneurysms of the cervical internal carotid artery. *Br Med J* 2:790, 1964.
23. Schievink WI, Piepgras DG, Earnest F IV, et al: Spontaneous carotid cavernous fistulae in Ehlers-Danlos syndrome type IV: Case report. *J Neurosurg* 74:991, 1991.
24. Schievink WI, Limburg M, Oorthuys JWE, et al: Cerebrovascular disease in Ehlers-Danlos syndrome type IV. *Stroke* 21:626, 1996.
25. Barinagarrementeria F, Amaya LE, Cantu C: Causes and mechanisms of cerebellar infarction in young patients. *Stroke* 28:2400, 1997.
26. Youl BD, Coutellier A, Dubyis B, et al: Three cases of spontaneous extracranial vertebral artery dissection. *Stroke* 21:618, 1990.

27. Anstim MG, Schaefer RF: Marfan's syndrome with unusual blood vessel manifestations: Primary medionecrosis dissection of right inominate, right carotid, and left carotid arteries. *Arch Pathol* 64:205, 1957.
28. Mokri B, Okazaki H: Cystic medial necrosis and internal carotid artery dissection in a Marfan's sibling: Partial expression of Marfan's syndrome. *J Stroke Cerebrovasc Dis* 2:100, 1992.
29. Schievink WI, Michels W, Piepgras DG: Neurovascular manifestations of heritable connective tissue disorders: A review. *Stroke* 25:889, 1994.
30. Schievink WI, Pankash UBS, Piepgras DG, Mokri B: α_1-antitrypsin deficiency in intracranial aneurysms and cervical artery dissection. *Lancet* 343:452, 1994.
31. Schievink WI, Mokri B, Peipgras DG: Intracranial aneurysms and cervicocephalic arterial dissections associated with congenital heart disease. *Neurosurgery* 39:685, 1996.
32. Silbert PL, Mokri B, Shievink WI: Headache and neck pain in spontaneous internal carotid and vertebral dissections. *Neurology* 45:1517, 1995.
33. Bionsse V, D'Anglejan-Chatillan J, Massiou H: Head pain in non-traumatic carotid dissection: A series of 65 patients. *Cephalgia* 14:33, 1994.
34. Mokri B, Schievink WI, Olsen KD, et al: Spontaneous dissection of cervical internal carotid artery presentation with lower cranial nerve palsies. *Arch Otolaryngol Head Neck Surg* 118:431, 1992.
35. Schievink WI, Mokri B, Carrit JA: Ocular motor palsies in spontaneous dissections of the cervical internal carotid artery. *Neurology* 43:1938, 1993.
36. Mokri B, Silbert PL, Schievink WI: Cranial nerve palsy in spontaneous dissection of the extracranial internal carotid artery. *Neurology* 46:356, 1996.
37. Mokri B, Houser OW, Burton A: Spontaneous dissections of the vertebral arteries. *Neurology* 38:880, 1988.
38. Bioousse V, Schaison M, Touboul P-J, D'Anglejan-Chatillon J, Bousser M-G: Ischemic optic neuropathy associated with internal carotid artery dissection. *Arch Neurol* 55:715, 1998.
39. Caplan LR, Zarins CK, Hemmati M: Spontaneous dissection of the extracranial vertebral arteries. *Stroke* 16:6, 1985.
40. Mas JL, Bousser MG, Hasbaun D: Extracranial vertebral artery dissection: A review of 13 cases. *Stroke* 18:1037, 1987.
41. Zuber L, Meury E, Meder JF, et al: Magnetic resonance imaging and dynamic CT scan in cervical artery dissections. *Stroke* 25:576, 1994.
42. Leclerc X, Godefroy O, Salhi A, et al: Helical CT for the diagnosis of extracranial internal carotid artery dissection. *Stroke* 27:461, 1996.
43. Takis C, Saver JL: Cervicocephalic carotid and vertebral artery dissection: Management, in Batjer Hi (ed): *Cerebrovascular Disease*. Philadelphia, Lippincott-Raven, 1997, p 385.
44. Sturzenegger M, Mattle HP, Rivoir A, et al: Ultrasound findings in carotid artery dissection: Analysis of 43 patients. *Neurology* 45:691, 1995.
45. Müllges W, Rigelstein EB, Liebold M: Non-invasive diagnosis of internal carotid artery dissections. *J Neurol Neurosurg Psychiatry* 55:98, 1992.
46. Steinke W, Rautenbery W, Schwartz A: Non-invasive monitoring of internal carotid artery dissection. *Stroke* 25:998, 1994.
47. Provenzale JM: Dissection of the internal carotid and vertebral arteries: Imaging features *Am J Radiol* 165:1099, 1995.
48. Srinivasan J, Newell DW, Sturzenegger M, Mayberg MR, Winn HR: Transcranial Doppler in the evaluation of internal carotid artery dissection. *Stroke* 27:1226, 1996.
49. Levy C, Laissy JP, Raveun V, et al: Carotid and vertebral dissection: Three dimensional time-of-flight MR angiography and MR imaging versus conventional angiography. *Radiology* 190:97, 1994.
50. Houser OW, Mokri B, Sundt TM Jr, et al: Spontaneous cervical cephalic arterial dissection and its residuum: Angiographic spectrum. *Am J Neuroradiol* 5:27, 1984.
51. Schievink WI, Piepgras DG, McCaffrey TV, et al: Surgical treatment of extracranial internal carotid artery dissection aneurysms. *Neurosurgery* 35:804, 1994.
52. Dubard T, Ponchot J, Lamy C, et al: Upper limb peripheral motor deficits due to extracranial vertebral artery dissections. *Cerebrovasc Dis* 4:88, 1994.
53. Hart RG: Vertebral artery dissection. *Neurology* 38:987, 1988.
54. Wievers DO, Mokri B: Internal carotid artery dissection after child birth. *Stroke* 16:956, 1985.
55. Mas JL, Bousser MG, Corone P, et al: Dissecting aneurysm of the extracranial vertebral artery and pregnancy. *Rev Neurol (Paris)* 143:761, 1987.
56. D'Anglejan-Chatillon J, Ribeiro V, Mas JL, et al: Migraine: A risk factor for dissection of cervical arteries. *Headache* 29:560, 1989.
57. Fisher CM: The headache and pain of spontaneous carotid artery dissection. *Headache* 22:60, 1982.
58. Meligan JT, Cornelius O: Carotodynia associated with carotid artery disease and stroke. *Am J Surg* 142:210, 1981.
59. Gutowski NJ, Murphy RP, Beale DJ: Unilateral upper cervical posterior spinal artery syndrome following sneezing. *J Neurol Neurosurg Psychiatry* 55:841, 1992.
60. Pulliano P: Bilateral distal upper limb amyotrophy and watershed infarcts from vertebral dissection. *Stroke* 25:1870, 1994.
61. Kitanaka C, Tamka J, Kuwahana M, et al: Magnetic resonance imaging study of intracranial vetebrobasilar artery dissections. *Stroke* 25:571, 1994.
62. Sue DE, Brant-Zawadski MN, Chanle J: Dissections of cranial arteries in the neck: Correlation of MRI and angiography. *Neuroradiology* 34:1273, 1992.
63. Leys D, Moulin T, Stojkovic T, Gegey S, Chavot D, DONALD Investigators: Follow-up of patients with history of cervical artery dissection. *Cerebrovasc Dis* 5:43, 1995.
64. Adams HP, Love BB, Jacoby MR: Arterial dissections, in Ginsberg MD (ed): *Cerebrovascular Disease* (Vol. II). Boston, Blackwell Science, 1998, p 1430.

65. Torvik A: The pathogenesis of watershed infarcts in the brain. *Stroke* 21:1378, 1990.

66. Weiller C, Mullges W, Rinselstein EB, et al: Patterns of brain infarctions in internal carotid artery dissections. *Neurosurg Rev* 14:111, 1991.

67. Eljamel MSM, Humphry PRD, Shaw MDM: Dissection of the cervical internal carotid artery, the role of Doppler/Duplex and conservative management. *J Neurol Neurosurg Psychiatry* 53:379, 1990.

68. Sellier N, Chris J, Benhamons M, et al: Spontaneous dissection of the internal carotid artery. Clinical, radiological and evolutive features: A study of 46 cases. *J Neuroradiol* 10:243, 1983.

69. Charot D, Monlin T, Cattin F, et al: Cervical artery dissection. *Cerebrovasc Dis* 4:243, 1994.

70. Biller J, Barinaganementeria F, Gordon DL, et al: Cervicocephalic arterial dissections in young adults in Iowa City and Mexico City. *Ann Neurol* 30:284, 1991.

71. Josein E: Extracranial vertebral artery dissection: Nine cases. *J Neurol* 239:327, 1992.

72. Berger MS, Wilson CB: Intracranial dissecting aneurysms of the posterior circulation: Report of six cases and review of the literature. *J Neurosurg* 61:882, 1984.

73. Hart RG, Easton JD: Dissections (Editorial). *Stroke* 16:925, 1985.

74. Kline LB, Vitek JJ, Raymon BC: Painful Horner's syndrome due to spontaneous carotid dissection. *Ophthalmology* 94:226, 1987.

75. McCromik GF, Hallbach VV: Recurrent ischemic events in two patients with painless vertebral artery dissection. *Stroke* 24:598, 1989.

76. Hart RG, Easton JD: Dissections of cervical and cerebral arteries. *Neurol Clin North Am* 1:255, 1983.

77. Morgan MK, Sekron LHS: Extracranial-intracranial saphenous vein bypass for carotid or vertebral artery dissections: A report of six cases. *J Neurosurg* 80:237, 1994.

78. Anson J, Crowell RM: Cervicocranial arterial dissection. *Neurosurgery* 29:89, 1991.

79. Hallbach VV, Higashida RT, Dowd CF, et al: Endovascular treatment of vertebral artery dissections and pseudoaneurysms. *J Neurosurg* 79:183, 1993.

80. Lefkowitz MA, Teitelbaum GP, Giannotti BL: Endovascular treatment of a dissecting posteroinferior cerebellar artery aneurysm: Case report. *Neurosurgery* 39:1036, 1996.

81. Adams HP Jr, Brott TG, Crowell RM, et al: Guidelines for the management of patients with acute ischemic stroke: A statement for health care professionals from a special writing group of the stroke council, American Heart Association. *Stroke* 25:1901, 1994.

82. Biousse V, D'Angelian-Chatillon J, Toubone PM, et al: Time course of symptoms in extracranial artery dissection: A series of 80 patients. *Stroke* 26:235, 1995.

Chapter 17

DIAGNOSIS AND MANAGEMENT OF MOYAMOYA DISEASE

Glenn M. Fischberg
Amir Mohammadi
Shuichi Suzuki
Mark Fisher

BACKGROUND

Moyamoya disease (MMD) is characterized by spontaneous stenosis, and often eventual occlusion, of the distal internal carotid arteries and the basal cerebral vessels
of the circle of Willis. Dilated collateral vessels, including leptomeningeal and deep parenchymal arteries, particularly in the region of the basal ganglia, form as the
large-vessel lesions progress. "Moyamoya" is a Japanese term that signifies "cloudiness," which is the appearance produced by networks of these small vessels on
cerebral angiography. Manifestations include transient
ischemic attacks, infarctions, seizures, and intracerebral
hemorrhages. Symptoms may present in children or
adults, but the clinical profile tends to change with age.
Although this process occurs unilaterally, bilateral
involvement without a known underlying etiology of
vascular disease is generally required for a definitive diagnosis.

EPIDEMIOLOGY

MMD occurs worldwide but is concentrated in Japan.
A review by Fukui[1] estimated a total of 3800 patients
in Japan in 1994, with 100 new cases per year, and an
annual incidence of one per million. The predominant
presenting age was clearly under 10, fairly equally distributed above and below 5 years of age (Fig. 17-1). A
more modest peak was centered between the ages of
35 and 40, with an overall female-to-male ratio of 1.7:1.
The known familial incidence was 9 percent out of 474
families; however, more recent screening with magnetic
resonance imaging (MRI) has identified moyamoya vessels in family members who may be asymptomatic, and
this incidence may be greater.

This disease is seen with less prevalence in other
parts of the world. Goto and Yonekawa[2] reviewed cases
between 1972 and 1989, with a total of 1063 reported
outside of Japan. In that period, 625 cases were reported
in other parts of Asia, mostly in Korea and the People's
Republic of China. A total of 201 were reported in
Europe; the United States included 105 of the 176 cases
in the Americas. In Africa, 52 cases were reported,
mostly in the North, and Australia reported 9 cases. Of
note is that many patients on other continents are of
Asian origin. Reviews of patients from Yugoslavia[3] and
of Finno-Ugric origin[4] report a slight male predominance. These reviews in Europe, as well as in Singapore[5]
and Taiwan,[6] demonstrate an adult preponderance. A
review in Korea revealed a mean age of presentation
of 6.3 years in children and 36.8 years in adults, similar
to Japan.[7]

In the United States, a review of 98 cases revealed
a very large female predominance (71 percent), with
similar age peaks to those seen in the Japanese literature.[8] Three cases were unilateral, and some included

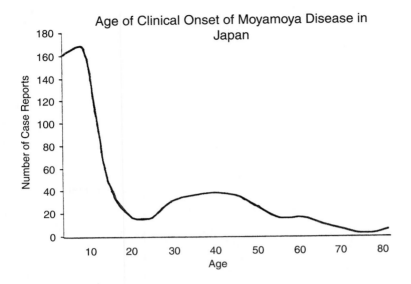

Figure 17-1.
Age of symptomatic presentation according to records of the Ministry of Health and Welfare of Japan through 1994. Adapted from Fukui, 1997.[1]

patients taking oral contraceptives or with atherosclerotic disease. Thirty-five of the 54 cases with known ethnic origin were Caucasians. Other ethnic backgrounds included 5 Japanese, 3 non-Japanese Asians, 5 African Americans, 3 Haitians, and 3 Hispanics. Two percent related a family history of the disease. A review of patients in Hawaii, where 22 percent of the population is Japanese, revealed 42 cases reported in a 10-year period from the mid 1980's to mid-1990's.[9] Of these, 21 were confirmed as definite cases; 9 were Japanese, with 4 Chinese, 3 Hawaiian, 2 Caucasian, 1 Filipino, and 2 unknown. The increase in the Japanese over the Caucasian, but not other Asian populations, was significant. There also seems to be no significant difference between the incidence in Japanese in Hawaii compared with Japan. A review of cases in the Midwest revealed most patients of East European background, with 6 of 30 being of Asian descent, and 3 cases in native Americans.[10]

ASSOCIATED DISORDERS AND ETIOLOGIC CONSIDERATIONS

The etiology of MMD is an unsettled issue. It is unclear whether MMD is a discrete entity or whether it is only a *syndrome* representing patterns of vascular change that may be common to numerous types of insults. For this reason, medical disorders found concomitantly with moyamoya findings are reported and scrutinized with respect to a possible linkage.

Genetic predisposition is suggested strongly by dominance in Japanese throughout the world and incidence among families, twins, and common haplotypes.[1,11,12] MMD has been reported in several patients with Fanconi's anemia (FA). In a genetic study of patients with FA, two were found to have MMD, and both were heterozygous for mutations in the FA complementation group C (FACC) not found in any other of the 174 FA families studied.[13]

Association with Down syndrome (DS) raises several issues, including genetics. Moyamoya patterns with histologic findings both similar and dissimilar to classic MMD have been reported.[14–16] Genetic linkage between the two entities may lie on chromosome 21, which encodes superoxide dismutase 1, interferon gamma receptors, cystathionine beta-synthase, and the alpha chain of collagen type VI. Excess collagen deposition in MMD could be related to collagen type VI overexpression.[15] Neurofibromatosis type 1 is another genetic disorder linked to clinical and histologic patterns of MMD.[17–19]

With regard to environmental influence in development of MMD as a possible secondary phenomenon, great attention has been paid to inflammatory factors. An association with leptospirosis in China and development after tuberculous meningitis have been noted, as well as reports of elevated antibody titers to *Propionibacterium acnes*.[2] Abnormal sympathetic activity with chronic respiratory infections has been proposed, but more extensive surveying has not identified consistent precipitants.[20] Mononuclear cell infiltration, macrophages and T cells in lesions, and presence of anti-Ro/SS-A and anti-La/SS-B antibodies have been described, but are not considered typical findings.[21–23] An experimental model of induction of MMD suggested that intrathecal antibodies or antigens could produce an initial arteritis.[24] MMD has occurred in several patients after receiving intracranial irradiation, particularly with sellar and parasellar tumors, and most notably with optic gliomas, but areas of multiple stenoses may occur outside the main focus of radiation.[25–28] These changes develop clearly more often in children, in whom abnormal net-like vessels and transdural anastomoses also usually appear. Even those adults who do develop carotid stenoses rarely demonstrate the latter features. Childhood predilection may reflect a greater susceptibility of the developing vessels to injury or the greater ability for prominent moyamoya-like collaterals to form in the immature system. Oral contraceptives have also gained considerable attention as an environmental factor, particularly in combination with smoking, in which mid-cervical and distal carotid lesions have demonstrated intimal and medial pathological findings reminiscent of MMD.[29]

MMD may be a manifestation of more widespread vascular disease. It has been reported with Raynaud's phenomenon, renovascular hypertension, sclerotic lesions of the coronary arteries, supravalvular aortic stenosis, renal artery fibromuscular dysplasia, primary pulmonary hypertension, beta-thalassemia, and antiphospholipid antibody syndrome. However, these reports are rare. Moyamoya patterns are even more notably absent in most children with sickle cell disease and most adults with atherosclerotic carotid disease. This scarcity still indicates that MMD development would require at least an innate predisposition, which would be lacking in most of these patients.

MMD has been considered as a developmental malady. Reports of MMD with other malformations, including midline craniofacial lesions with angiomata and skin aplasia, aplasia cutis congenita in siblings, and Noonan syndrome with cardiac and cerebrovascular disease, point to a central developmental role. Persistent primitive trigeminal arteries have been reported in at least eight MMD cases.[30] This artery is usually obliterated in embryonic development at a time when the anterior circulation resembles a moyamoya pattern; the middle cerebral artery circulation still exists as a plexiform network, and the anterior cerebral artery is incompletely formed. Although this supports the notion of MMD representing "suspended development," angiographic progression in patients, including extension from unilateral to bilateral disease, counters this concept. A persistent primitive hypoglossal artery has also been reported.[31]

Suzuki and colleagues suggested that pathologic carotid artery changes could be the result of increased sympathetic stimulation.[32] In children with intracranial carotid disease, they reported improved clinical results with superior cervical ganglionectomy and perivascular sympathectomy. Diseases related to sympathetic activity, including Harlequinism and several cases of Graves' thyrotoxicosis, have been reported with MMD.[33–35]

Increases in smooth muscle cell elastin, transforming growth factor-beta 1 and platelet-derived growth factor in arteries, as well as decreased responsiveness of smooth muscle cells to mitogens (including platelet-derived growth factor), are factors that may help provide etiologic clues.[36–38] Miscellaneous conditions and anomalies in which MMD has been reported include glycogen storage disorder-type 1, hypomelanosis of Ito, thrombotic thrombocytopenic purpura, Turner's syndrome, polycystic kidney disease and eosinophilic granuloma, Alagille syndrome, Sneddon's syndrome, Wilm's tumor, and precocious puberty with pustular psoriasis.

PATHOLOGY

More than 100 autopsy cases of MMD have been reported since Maki et al disclosed the first pathologic findings in 1965.[39] Most died from intracranial hemorrhage. Because of new imaging and improved prognosis, autopsy cases are now rather rare even in Japan.[40] The essential lesions are stenoses or occlusions of bilateral distal ends of the internal carotid arteries and the proximal portions of the middle and anterior cerebral arteries. Moyamoya vessels are recognized as collateral vessels.

Main Arteries

The stenotic or obstructive vascular lesions are predominantly in the anterior half of the circle of Willis.[40,41] A remarkable shrinkage of the outer diameter of internal carotid arteries is noted, which mostly occurs distal to the origin of the ophthalmic arteries and extends to the proximal portions of the anterior and middle cerebral and posterior communicating arteries. These arteries have a white, thread-like appearance (Fig. 17-2).[40] The basilar and vertebral arteries are usually normal in size. Reduction in the outer diameter of the affected arteries differs from characteristic findings of atherosclerotic stenoses, in which the size of the outer diameter is preserved. The principal pathologic findings of arterial narrowing or occlusion are from concentric fibrous intimal thickening. In the thickened intima, the elastic lamina is wavy and multilayered, but usually preserved all around the arterial wall.[40–42] The media are usually attenuated corresponding to the intimal changes. There is no significant adventitial thickening or inflammatory cell

reaction in the media or adventitia (Fig. 17-3). In the distal portion of the middle and anterior cerebral arteries, collapse of the lumen and folding of the elastic lamina gradually become more remarkable.[40–42]

Moyamoya Vessels

Numerous small or medium-sized, thin-walled, tortuous arteries form a dense network (moyamoya vessels), particularly at the base of the brain.[40–43] Moyamoya vessels frequently arise from the posterior half of the circle of Willis, anterior choroidal arteries, and internal carotid arteries. Some of them are perforating into the base of the brain, and some are connected to the proximal and distal patent portions of the major basal arteries, skipping the occluded portion. These collateral networks of vessels resemble fibrous roots of plants (Fig. 17-4) and correspond to the characteristic moyamoya pattern seen angiographically. Similar vessels are also often observed in the meninges of the Sylvian fissure.[40,41,43] In the cerebral parenchyma, they are commonly observed, especially in the basal ganglia and paraventricular regions, where cerebral hemorrhages and ischemic lesions frequently occur.[43] Histopathologic studies show that moyamoya vessels are composed of two types of arteries. In addition to the dilated thin-walled vessels, others are obstructed because of thrombi with laminar elastosis and fibrosis.[41] Some of these vessels have microaneurysmal formations.[44] The simultaneous presence of both extremely dilated and stenotic arteries in the brain parenchyma is characteristic. The rupture of these abnormal arteries is a major source of the intracranial hemorrhage of MMD.[44,45] Histopathologic study of intracerebral hemorrhage has revealed that the ruptured arteries are approximately 250 microns in diameter and not accompanied by fibrinoid necrosis. In contrast, with hypertensive intracerebral hemorrhage, the origin is usually from smaller perforating arteries (mean diameter, 150 microns) in the basal ganglia or thalamus, which are usually accompanied by fibrinoid necrosis.[43] Cerebral infarctions in MMD do not always correspond to the territories of the occluded main cerebral arteries and are multiple in nature, usually located in periventricular areas perfused by moyamoya vessels.[44]

Thrombotic lesions are frequently found.[39–41,45,46] Thrombi composed of platelets and fibrin are more frequent than those composed of erythrocytes and fibrin. They are predominantly located in the posterior portion of the circle of Willis but can be seen in the internal carotid arteries.[47] It is suggested that the recurrent thrombi and subsequent organization may contribute to the multilayered structures separated by multiple elastic

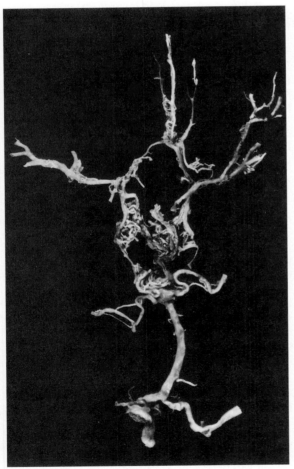

Figure 17-2.
Marked shrinkage of the outer diameter of the distal portion of the internal carotid arteries, and the proximal portions of the anterior and middle cerebral arteries, with a thread-like appearance. (Photo courtesy of Yasuhiro Hosoda.)

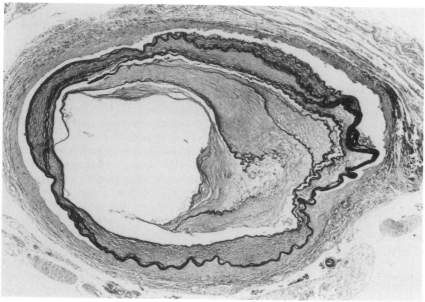

Figure 17-3.
The terminal portion of the internal carotid artery showing fibrous intimal thickening. (Photo courtesy of Yasuhiro Hosoda.)

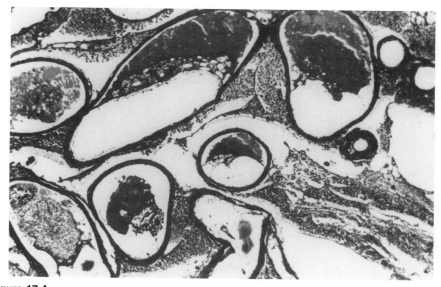

Figure 17-4.
Abnormal dilated vascular network around the circle of Willis showing coexistence of occluded small arteries. (Photo courtesy of Yasuhiro Hosoda.)

fibers in the thickened intima of MMD.[45,48] However, the possibility still remains that the thrombus formation is secondary to the preceding intimal thickening and arterial stenosis.[47]

Extracranial Vascular Lesions

The same morphologic changes observed in the main cerebral arteries of MMD (intimal thickening and folding of the internal elastic lamina) have also been reported in coronary arteries,[42] temporal arteries,[42,47] pulmonary arteries,[48] pancreatic arteries,[48] and renal arteries[49] in patients with MMD. These findings suggest the existence of systemic etiologic factors that lead to the formation of intimal lesions in this disease.

CLINICAL FEATURES

Ischemic Complications

Clinical onset is usually under the age of 10 (see Fig. 17-1).[1,50] A modest resurgence is seen from the mid-30's to mid-40's. The types of presenting or dominating symptoms differ depending on age (Fig. 17-5).[50] Ischemic symptoms predominate the pediatric population. For those under the age of 10, and particularly under the age of 5, transient ischemic symptoms are more commonly seen than are completed strokes.

Approximately 80 percent of ischemic events involve motor disturbances.[51] In older children, sensory or speech disturbances may be evident in approximately 15 to 40 percent of cases. A pattern of "alternating hemiplegia," with weakness occurring successively on opposite sides, has frequently been deemed a characteristic mode of ischemic presentation. In adults, although ischemic presentations are somewhat less frequent than hemorrhagic, the more common ischemic symptoms include transient paresis, dysphagia, hemianopsia, visual or tactile inattention, or dyspraxia.

Less common symptoms include visual disturbances, which are seen in approximately 20 percent of patients, and may be cortical or retinal in origin, including scintillating scotomata. Movement disorders, particularly chorea, may also be seen unilaterally or bilaterally, either from basal ganglia infarcts or more

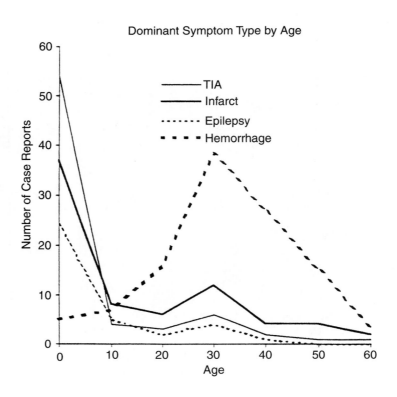

Figure 17-5.
Cases with clear predominant symptom types in Japan reported by Maki and Enomoto, 1984.[50] Unknown or mixed types accounted for approximately 10% of all registered Japanese cases through 1994.

commonly from chronic ischemia with a normal CT scan. Isolated torticollis has also been described. Continuous movements tend to cease during sleep. In children, these symptoms tend to last for several months.[51] Bilateral borderzone ischemia involving the paracentral frontal regions may also cause a paraparesis, which may prompt misguided investigations for spinal disease.

Bilateral involvement of the basal ganglia and anterior arterial borderzones may contribute to the neuropsychologic abnormalities in MMD, including an "athymhormic syndrome," with flattening of affect and loss of interest and drive. Personality disorders are not seen commonly in adult-onset disease. Mental disturbances, particularly low IQs, can be seen in subsets of children with MMD. IQs are seen to be lower with progressive degrees of ischemic symptom frequency or severity. This poverty of mental development or progressive deterioration (which may also be seen in adults) is one reason why children with this disease may benefit from early treatment rather than observing for angiographic progression or classic clinical deficits.

Seizures are seen in approximately 10 percent of patients. The mean age of onset is near 2 years. The term "epileptic type" moyamoya has been used, but seizures occur most often in those with cerebral infarcts by CT. Seizures usually improve spontaneously, but a substantial number, particularly with onset in infancy, develop lasting epilepsy.[52] Revascularization procedures, although improving other EEG patterns indicative of cerebral dysfunction, are not likely to improve or terminate epileptic discharges. Seizures may also occur in older patients following hemorrhages.

Headaches occur in less than 10 percent of children, and are seen in up to 40 percent of adults. They tend to present in those with less frequent or severe ischemia. This pattern suggests that headaches may be associated more with those who have established prominent vascular dilatation of collateral networks. In the series published by Matsushima et al,[51] children had cessation of headaches shortly after surgical revascularization.

Vascular Malformations and Hemorrhagic Complications

Arteriovenous malformations (AVMs) have been reported in at least 23 patients. Proximal arterial stenoses limiting blood flow could play a protective role with regard to the relatively low rate of hemorrhage compared with seizures. However, alternate feeding arteries may take over when a main feeder progresses from stenosis to complete occlusion. AVMs may actually contribute to intimal hyperplasia of the large vessels proximally by creating high, turbulent flow and provoking collateral formation by its low resistance demand,[53] or possible release of angiogenic factors.[54]

Aneurysms of the circle of Willis are seen in MMD in approximately 14 percent of cases.[55] Additionally, they may be found in the peripheral arteries that lead to moyamoya vessels, or in the moyamoya vessels themselves. The latter distribution occurs in approximately 9 percent of moyamoya patients and comprises 40 percent of aneurysms found in MMD. Many of these are actually pseudoaneurysms, caused after hemorrhage from small fragile vessels, with partially recanalized perivascular hematomas, giving the angiographic appearance of aneurysms. These are often seen to regress or disappear completely on follow-up studies, which is a virtual confirmation of a pseudoaneurysm diagnosis. Anterior and posterior choroidal arteries and their branches are the most commonly involved peripheral vessels. Ischemia in the region of these smaller distal vessels may play a role in precipitating hemorrhage. Bucciero et al[55] reported that out of 91 aneurysms in 75 patients, more than 29 percent were seen in the moyamoya vessels, and approximately 40 percent in total were seen in other collateral vessels. Regression of true saccular aneurysms may rarely occur, as intimal hyperplasia causes either occlusion of the neck or sufficient stenosis to allow thrombosis of the aneurysmal lumen. Saccular aneurysms are more likely to be seen at the basal cerebral arteries, particularly at the circle of Willis. With significant anterior circulation compromise, flow through the posterior circulation is increased; most aneurysms occur in the vertebrobasilar system, particularly at the basilar artery bifurcation.[56] In unilateral disease, the anterior communicating artery and posterior cerebral artery often carry the burden of collateral flow from the uninvolved regions and are frequent sites of aneurysms. This suggests that aneurysms may result from arterial wall damage from increased flow.

Hemorrhagic complications occur more frequently in adults than in children. They rarely occur before the age of 10, and predominate progressively with higher ages of onset in adults. For those who do present with symptoms as adults, hemorrhages dominate progressively with higher ages of onset. Bleeding may be intraventricular, intraparenchymal, subarachnoid, or in combination. In a series of 31 hemorrhagic cases reported by Kawaguchi et al,[57] 90 percent of patients had no neurologic symptoms prior to the hemorrhagic presentation. Earlier series reported an overwhelming predominance of subarachnoid bleeding, but later studies, which have used CT confirmation, have clearly shown that primary subarachnoid hemorrhage occurs in a minority of cases, mostly with saccular aneurysms. Intraparenchymal hemorrhages have been reported to occur in 40 to 65 percent of cases, with primary intraventricular hemorrhages occurring in 35 to 45 percent of cases. The majority of intracerebral bleeding occurs in the thalamus and basal ganglia.[58-60]

Hemorrhagic patterns depend on the source of bleeding. Subarachnoid hemorrhage may be relatively mild because aneurysms develop in the moyamoya vessels themselves, which are often small. Hemorrhage in the deep gray matter may be from degenerating, friable moyamoya vessels. Dilated vessels that serve the walls of the posterior portions of the ventricles, mainly from choroidal arteries and their medullary derivatives, may be responsible for intraventricular and periventricular hemorrhage by primary rupture or via microaneurysms. Dissection of blood may occur into the ventricles from these vessels. Inadequate blood supply in this region possibly could cause subependymal infarction, resulting in wall rupture and hemorrhage. Pseudoaneurysms found in the territory of peripheral vessls may be seen to dissipate in the course of approximately 6 weeks to 14 months. Although larger hemorrhages may occur with saccular aneurysms, surgical clipping or coiling generally ensures a lower rate of rebleeding as opposed to those who hemorrhage from fragile moyamoya vessels. Death may occur in 5 to 15 percent of patients with their first hemorrhagic event; this rate goes up disproportionately with rebleeding. A less common form of hemorrhage includes spontaneous, atraumatic subdural hematomas. This may occur from engorged transdural collateral vessels and may also make traumatic subdural hematomas easier to incite.

For aneurysmal hemorrhage, coil embolization or surgical clipping confers a favorable outcome with regard to rebleeding; however, surgery may be complicated by difficulty avoiding damage to delicate collateral networks. The same holds true for subdural hematomas, in which irrigation may initially be preferable to more invasive attempts at evacuation. Revascularization procedures may be attempted, not only to restore blood flow to ischemic areas but also to attempt to decrease engorgement of collateral vessels and stress on saccular aneurysms in those portions of the circle of Willis that carry compensatory augmented blood flow. Surgery performed for these aims, as well as for slowing the development of abnormal vessels, has been met with variable reported success in affecting recurrent hemorrahge.

Pregnancy

Complications of MMD during pregnancy have been reported in a few cases.[61] Intracranial hemorrhage has occurred as a presenting symptom within the second and third trimesters, which may reflect the hemodynamic changes of pregnancy. A number of those women reported with ischemic symptoms prior to pregnancy have had substantial alleviation during pregnancy. Fluctuation of blood pressure during and after delivery may contribute to hemorrhage. Control of hyperventilation or hypertension during delivery may be minimized by liberal pain control with a rapid vaginal delivery or use of a cesarean delivery.

Natural History and Prognosis

Mortality from MMD in children is approximately 5 percent. Cognitive deterioration or retardation, despite the lack of other overt neurologic events, is not unusual. Children presenting with ischemic symptoms typically will progress for 2 to 3 years before stabilizing, but approximately 40 percent of those with TIAs will advance to having completed infarctions. Olds et al reported that those presenting with strokes or hemorrhage tended to improve or remain unchanged, and those with initial TIAs had a greater tendency to develop cognitive decline or new strokes.[62] Kurokawa et al followed 27 pediatric patients from 4 to 15 years;[63] 19 percent (5 patients) were left with no symptoms, 33 percent (9 patients) had continued TIAs or headaches, 7 percent (2 patients) were dependent on constant care, and 3 percent (1 patient) died. Hypertension and young onset were prominent in those with poor outcomes. Angiographic disease progression often occurs in pediatric patients. Fukuyama et al reported 14 percent of 33 pediatric cases with unilateral to bilateral progression over nearly a 3-year period.[64] Despite 55 percent worsening by one or two stages angiographically, half of the patients after 7 years had no residual symptoms, with most of the others being clinically improved.

Adults have a higher rate of mortality, approximately 10 percent. Despite this being largely from hemorrhage, survivors have a relatively good prognosis. Rebleeding rates in most longitudinal studies range from 5 to 15 percent; however, Kawaguchi et al[57] in 1996 reported just over a 1 percent rebleed rate in 31 cases for up to 10 years. The authors attributed favorable rates to new surgical techniques. Adults who present with ischemic symptoms are more likely to experience continued difficulties. In a study of 18 adult patients (age greater than 16) by Nakada et al, 9 of the 10 patients with subarachnoid hemorrhage (SAH) survived. Seven of the nine surviving patients (78 percent) remained normal after a mean follow-up of 5 years, with a mortality of 10 percent.[65] Rebleeding occurred from 16 months to 7 years after initial presentation. Of the five patients with strokes, three (60 percent) remained disabled, and all three TIA patients had recurrent events, with two (67 percent) remaining severely disabled. There are few angiographic changes in adult follow-up. The Nakada study also emphasized a superior prognostic power of angiographic features. Ninety percent of those with only the anterior half of the circle of Willis involved remained clinically normal at the end of follow-up. Although most had SAH, even those with TIAs or strokes faired well despite a generally poor prognosis for ischemic presentations. In contrast, two-thirds of those with lesions extending to the posterior part of the circle of Willis were disabled; those with extension to the posterior cerebral arteries faired poorly clinically even with SAH, despite its generally good prognosis.

In the largest recent longitudinal study, Choi et al followed 88 patients for an average of 28.8 months (ranging from 6 to 86 months), 52 of whom had no surgical intervention.[66] Below age 6 ($n = 33$), 90 percent of those presenting with TIAs had repeated TIAs or infarctions. Of those below age 6 with initial infarctions, 25 percent had repeated infarcts, and 8 percent had subsequent hemorrhage. Twenty-seven percent of those at this age had no lesions on brain imaging initially but had infarcts by the end of follow-up. From the age of 6 to 15 ($n = 15$), 86 percent presenting with TIAs had repeated TIAs or infarctions, and 50 percent of those presenting with infarcts had more than one. None of the four in this age group presenting with hemorrhages had repeated episodes. One of them (7 percent) had no lesions on brain imaging initially but had an infarction on follow-up. In the group over age 15 ($n = 40$), those with TIAs had a 27 percent rate of repeated ischemic episodes, and 45 percent had subsequent hemorrhages. For those who presented with infarctions, 36 percent had repeated infarctions, and 27 percent followed with hemorrhages. Those with initial hemorrhages faired better, with only an 11 percent rebleed rate and no ischemic episodes. Of this older group, 15 percent had no brain lesions found initially but had evidence of infarctions (2.5 percent) or hemorrhage (12.5 percent) through the follow-up period. Overall, recurrent attacks, whether ischemic or hemorrhagic, occurred in 55 percent of patients. Activities of daily living scores improved for hemorrhagic patients and worsened for ischemic patients, based on initial symptomatic presentation.

DIAGNOSTIC TESTING

Angiography

Angiographic features are central to the diagnosis. The Ministry of Health and Welfare of Japan has suggested general angiographic diagnostic criteria, seen in Table 17-1.[67] Suzuki and Takaku[68] described six angiographic stages, which are still used for reference in grading severity and progression (Table 17-2). Most patients present clinically in either stage 3 or 4. In addition to the described cardinal features, transdural anastomotic vessels (*rete mirabile*) are also characteristic findings and may be seen in lieu of classic moyamoya vessels during later stages. Different terminology may be used depending on the predominant area of anastomotic networks. When in the region of the basal ganglia, the term *basal moyamoya* may be used (Fig. 17-6). *Ethmoidal moyamoya* shows a predominance of such vessels in the basal frontal region, which involve branches of the internal maxillary arteries feeding through the ethmoidal sinuses. *Vault moyamoya* demonstrates most prominent vessels in the basal parietal region and involves transdural anastomoses, with common supply via the superficial temporal arteries, the anterior facial arteries, the middle meningeal arteries, and the ethmoidal arteries (Fig. 17-7B). Any combination of these patterns may be seen. Repeated cerebral angiography may be used not only to follow disease progression but also to fill targeted receiving vessels, and to form new vessels, after revascularization and neovascularization procedures.

Table 17-1.
Angiographic diagnostic criteria[a]

1. Stenosis or occlusion of the terminal portion of the intracranial carotid arteries and/or the origins of the anterior or middle cerebral arteries.

2. Abnormal network of dilated basal intracerebral vessels in the arterial phase adjacent to the major stenoses.

3. Bilaterality of abnormal findings.

[a]From Ref. 67.

Table 17-2.
Angiographic staging[a]

Stage 1. Stenosis of the distal carotid arteries at their bifurcation.

Stage 2. Networks of moyamoya vessels, mostly dilated small intracerebral arteries, develop near the base of the brain.

Stage 3. Severe stenosis or occlusion of the trunks of the anterior and middle cerebral arteries; more prominent moyamoya vessels.

Stage 4. Progression of stenoses to the posterior cerebral arteries; intracerebral collateral vessels begin to diminish from reduced supply.

Stage 5. Disappearance of all major cerebral arteries; further diminution of moyamoya vessels.

Stage 6. Intracerebral moyamoya networks and major cerebral arteries have disappeared; blood supply is solely from external carotid artery branches.

[a]From Ref. 68.

Magnetic Resonance Imaging (MRI) and Magnetic Resonance Angiography (MRA)

These tests commonly provide diagnosis without angiography. MRI may show prominent flow voids, including dilated extracranial carotid vessels and leptomeningeal collaterals (Fig. 17-7A). Deep moyamoya vessels may be seen, particularly in the basal ganglia (Fig. 17-8). Gadolinium may improve sensitivity for these vessels and can produce an "ivy sign," which is diffuse meningeal enhancement representing a pervasive pial-arterial network.[71] MRA may show stenotic or occluded basal cerebral arteries, dilated extracranial vessels and their anastomoses to the intracranial circulation, and blushes that correspond to the networks of moyamoya vessels (Fig. 17-9).[69]

The diagnostic accuracy of MRI and MRA has been reported in several series. Yamada et al[72] reported accuracy of 100 percent using MRA to detect stenoocclusive lesions and 100 percent specificity for detecting

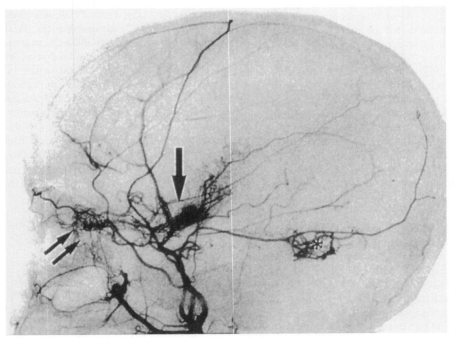

Figure 17-6.
Lateral view of a right internal carotid angiogram. Small basal (large arrow), *ethmoidal* (double arrow), *and vault* (asterisk) *moyamoya networks may be seen, supplied by external carotid artery branches. Reprinted with permission from Makiyama et al, 1994.*[69]

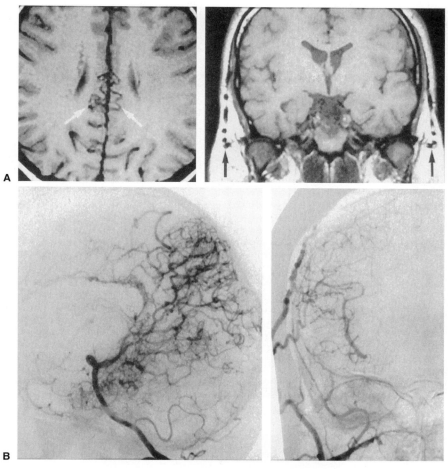

Figure 17-7.
A (Left) *T1-weighted MRI demonstrating leptomeningeal collaterals from the posterior cerebral to anterior cerebral artery territories, seen as flow voids in the medial aspects of the hemispheres.* (Right), *dilated superficial temporal arteries seen bilaterally* (arrows), *which serve transdural collateral vessels.* B (Left) *lateral projection of a left vertebral angiogram, corresponding to the MRI above, demonstrating moyamoya networks, with enlarged posterior cerebral artery branches sending collaterals to the anterior cerebral artery territory.* (Right), *frontal view of a right external carotid angiogram corresponding to the MRI above, demonstrating Sylvian branches of the middle cerebral artery receiving transdural flow via an enlarged superficial temporal artery. Reprinted with permission from Yamada et al, 1995.[70]*

moyamoya vessels. Sensitivity of detecting moyamoya vessels was 73 percent. Using MRI alone, evaluation of steno-occlusive lesions yielded 100 percent sensitivity and 71 percent specificity, with moyamoya vessel evaluation yielding 92 percent sensitivity and 100 percent specificity. Houkin et al[73] reported sensitivity for detecting moyamoya vessels of 93 percent in children and 69 per-

cent in adults with MRA, and 46 percent and 38 percent respectively, with MRI. Overestimation of large-vessel stenosis (due to signal loss produced by high velocity or turbulent blood flow) and insensitivity to small moyamoya vessels leads to a tendency to overestimate the disease stage by MR technology. The Houkin series reported 100 percent accuracy in patients with disease

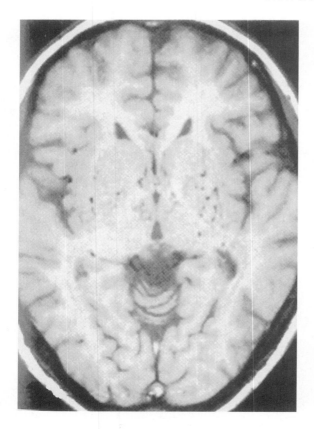

Figure 17-8.
T1-weighted MRI demonstrating numerous flow voids bilaterally from deep moyamoya vessels. Reprinted with permission from Yamada et al, 1995.[70]

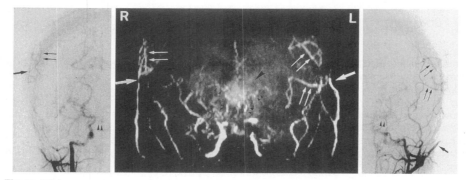

Figure 17-9.
Frontal views of left and right common carotid angiograms flanking a coronal MRA image. Large black arrows *bilaterally point to the cloud-like basal moyamoya network on MRA, with* small double arrows *on all images showing some of the more proximal dilated moyamoya vessels, which may be seen discretely.* Double arrows *on all images demonstrate cortical branches of the middle cerebral arteries receiving transdural collateral flow via dilated superficial temporal arteries* (single arrows). *MRA demonstrates truncated supraclinoid carotid signals and the absence of normal proximal middle cerebral artery signals. Reprinted with permission from Makiyama et al, 1994.*[69]

of stages 3 through 6 but reported overestimation in 25 percent of healthy subjects or patients with stage 1 angiograms, and 56 percent of those with stage 2 disease. MRA accuracy may be improved by using axial source images. Transdural collateral vessels were only well seen in 13 percent of cases with MRA and 4 percent with MRI in the Yamada series. This insensitivity may be improved somewhat with gadolinium. However, MRA is limiting with regard to evaluation of potential surgical candidates because the extracranial arterial supplies used as donors must be evaluated carefully. MRA may be used, however, to confirm the patency of extracranial-to-intracranial bypasses. Makayama et al detected anastomoses from encephaloduroarteriosynangiosis in 7 of 10 patients, but MRA more often fails to show postsurgical neovascularization visible by conventional angiography.

The frequency of infarcts (80 percent overall) increases significantly with progression of angiographic stages, particularly with compromise of the posterior cerebral arteries. Because the extent of infarcts may correlate with postsurgical prognosis of bypass procedures, MRI may still have an added benefit for surgical evaluation.[74,75] MRI may be a useful screen for family members of those who initially present with this disorder.

Computed Tomography (CT)

CT is a relatively insensitive modality for determination of MMD. Administration of intravenous contrast may show punctate hyperdensities corresponding to the basal moyamoya vessels in the middle stages of disease. Stenotic and occlusive lesions involving the distal carotid arteries and proximal middle cerebral arteries may be demarcated also with the use of contrast. In a series of cases by Hasuo et al[76] relative to MR, CT matched identification of steno-occlusive changes in the internal and middle cerebral arteries in only 38 percent of the cases. In 42 percent of the cases, CT was suggestive of disease where MR diagnosis was definitive. In 21 percent, the diagnosis was not at all suggested by CT. In the same 24 hemispheres, grading of moyamoya vessels matched between the two modalities in 79 percent of cases. In 21 percent, CT did not reveal the vessels identified by MR (which itself is not as sensitive as conventional angiography).

CT angiography may have greater success diagnostically. Detection of morphologic changes in vessels is aided by the ability to visualize them in any plane. Limitations do exist because of restricted resolution for detecting small vessels. In the series by Tsuchiya et al,[77] moyamoya vessels were only demonstrated in 2 of 7 patients with disease from stages 2 through 5. Also, enhancing veins in the choroid plexuses may be seen with contrast, in addition to the arteries of interest. The need for large amounts of contrast may limit the ability to cover the entire vasculature. CT angiography does have the ability to demonstrate leptomeningeal vessels and depicts stenoses or occlusions of the major arterial trunks well without the same degree of tendency to overestimate stenosis as MRA. It has been suggested that demonstration of superficial temporal artery to middle cerebral artery (STA-MCA) anastomoses can be depicted more clearly than with MRA.[78]

Other Diagnostic Testing

Single photon emission tomography (SPECT) and positron emission tomography (PET) allow for evaluation of regional cerebral tissue perfusion and use of oxygen. In general, abnormalities identified by SPECT or PET are larger than those seen by CT or MR imaging and may correlate better with symptoms, especially with transient ischemia. Iodoamphetamine (IMP) or ^{99m}TC-HMPAO (hexamethylpropyleneamine oxime) uptake, used in SPECT scanning, is proportional to regional blood flow. Baseline studies can reveal perfusion deficits, and vasodilation via acetazolamide helps to identify areas with inadequate functional reserve from limited further vasodilatory capacity or proximal obstruction. This technology may also be used to identify the success of revascularization.[79] Angiographic lesions of anterior and middle cerebral arteries correlate relatively well with decreased regional cerebral blood flow (rCBF) by SPECT or PET, but basal ganglia or posterior circulation territory rCBF does not correlate as well with specific angiographic lesions.[80] Posterior cerebral artery disease in later stages often parallels ischemia anteriorly when posterior-to-anterior collaterals have been prominent. In this way, functional imaging may be very useful in determining surgical targets not necessarily suggested by angiographic data.

Testing by PET has indicated that clinical recovery may occur without full recovery of baseline hemodynamic parameters and may occur largely from increased vasodilatory reserve.[81] Regional oxygen extraction fractions (rOEF) and regional metabolic rates of oxygen use (rCMRO$_2$) provided added value for determining the timing of surgery, as well as the most appropriate location of intervention. Induction of collateral vessels intended by revascularization procedures may not occur in areas where normal tissue perfusion already exists.

In areas in which rCMRO$_2$ has decreased significantly, new or collateral vessel formation may not occur because of decreased demand. Those with a reduction in rCBF, increased rOEF, and no significant rCMRO$_2$ decrease may be the best candidates for surgical benefit.

EEG may be used to diagnose or bring suspicion of diagnosis, particularly in children who present with seizures. A characteristic "re-buildup" phenomenon may be seen, which includes progressively decreasing frequency and activation of increased amplitude after cessation of hyperventilation. This fairly unique pattern is consistent with the delayed cerebral blood flow response to hyperventilation.[82]

Transcranial Doppler (TCD) is limited in its ability to provide diagnostic detail. It may be used to assess noninvasively the presence and direction of blood flow through potential collateral channels, particularly the anterior or posterior communicating arteries, reversed flow through the ophthalmic artery via the external carotid system, or the posterior cerebral artery flow to leptomeningeal collaterals running anteriorly. Patency of the terminal internal carotid and other major basal arteries may be monitored. Even barely opacified vessels by angiography may be identified by TCD.[83] As stages of disease progress angiographically, velocity patterns in the distal ICA and the MCA, respectively, tend to change from high-high to high-low and then finally low-low.[84] The high-low and low-low patterns are seen more commonly in patients with ischemic or hemorrhagic strokes, whereas the high-high pattern is more common in those who are asymptomatic. Functional monitoring with TCD has been used to help determine the need for bypass surgery.[85] For any particular artery, either its stenosis or function as a collateral channel may increase sampled velocities, whereas obstruction proximal to the sampled area may cause decreased velocities. The variable combination of these opposing factors may make standard velocity criteria for arterial stenoses difficult to follow. Carotid duplex may detect patterns of increased resistance in the internal carotid artery with stenosis distally.

MEDICAL TREATMENT

Medical management is usually directed toward patients with ischemic symptoms and is widely considered to be limited compared with surgical treatment. Antiplatelet agents are commonly used, particularly aspirin; however, there are no clinical trials or series regarding aspirin use in this particular population. Persantine and the newer antiplatelet agents, ticlopidine and clopidogrel, are also used for stroke prevention, either singly or as part of combination therapy. The combination of aspirin and 400 mg per day of persantine has been demonstrated to have an additive effect in secondary stroke prevention,[86] but comparative efficacy of any of these agents alone or as part of combination therapy relative to aspirin alone in MMD specifically is not known. Given an ever-present predisposition to hemorrhage, warfarin is generally contraindicated when significant moyamoya vessels are present.

Calcium channel blockers have gained considerable attention for their effects noted in small groups of patients. Flunarizine, a calcium ion blocker, has been shown to increase regional cerebral perfusion by SPECT analysis in combination with clinical efficacy.[87] Hosain et al reported that nicardipine, 10 mg three times a day, relieved two pediatric patients of ischemic symptoms for 3.5 to 4.5 years of follow-up.[88] Both patients had previously undergone revascularization procedures but continued with repeated and progressive courses before medical treatment. Intravenous verapamil injections of 10 mg were reported to reverse ischemic symptoms acutely in two children; both of them had also undergone bypass procedures within recent months.[89] Repeated injection during angiography was performed in one patient and demonstrated acutely improved filling of basal moyamoya vessels and the posterior branch of the middle cerebral artery. This patient was maintained successfully on 20 mg of oral verapamil three times daily for the next 1.5 years of follow-up. Success with nifedipine has also been reported,[90] and nimodipine use has been reported to be successful, including in adults.[91] Because of significantly less tendency to induce hypotension compared with other calcium channel blockers, nimodipine may, in the non-hypertensive patient, be considered the drug of choice. Calcium channel blockers are thought to be effective due to vasodilation. McLean et al speculated that the immediate effect of verapamil and angiographic findings implicated reversal of vasospasm, although spasm has not otherwise been clearly implicated in acute ischemic attacks.[89]

Dramatic success of steroids has been reported in treating a case of ischemia-induced chorea.[92,115] Symptoms recurred after discontinuing oral maintenance and again improved with reinstitution of prednisone. The mechanism in this case is unclear. Anectodal evidence has not generally supported efficacy of steroids in preventing disease progression, but no published data are available.

SURGICAL THERAPY

Surgical procedures have been used both in attempts to re-establish blood flow to ischemic areas and to reduce hemorrhages through relieving engorged collateral vessels. Surgical methods include direct and indirect revascularization procedures. The choice of surgical method depends on the age of the patient and availability of suitable donor and recipient arteries. The procedures that are most often used are superficial temporal artery–middle cerebral artery bypass (STA-MCA), encephaloduroarteriosynangiosis (EDAS), and encephalomyosynangiosis (EMS). Other variants are used less frequently.

STA-MCA bypass, a direct anastomotic method, is the most common procedure to revascularize the anterior cerebral circulation. The primary indication for this operation is for cerebral ischemic insults. This is a technically difficult procedure in young patients because the STA and MCA are very small and their walls are extremely vulnerable.

Nakashima et al reported on 18 STA-MCA anastomoses in which all patients had resolution of TIAs.[93] Houkin et al performed direct revascularization by STA-MCA bypass in 102 hemispheres in a series of 68 patients. Seventy-five percent had resolution of TIAs and no further cerebral infarctions.[94] Fujii et al, in a retrospective review of 455 patients, found a nonstatistically significant difference in rebleeding rates between patients medically treated (28 percent of 178 patients) and those treated by bypass (19 percent of 277).[95] A recent article by Okada et al[96] reported on results of STA-MCA anastomosis in a group of 15 adults with hemorrhagic presentations of MMD. Cerebral circulation was partially normalized as measured by SPECT, and moyamoya vessels decreased. Three patients presented with rebleeding within 2 to 4 years after surgery.

Encephaloduroarteriosynangiosis

In this indirect procedure, a patent superficial temporal artery is sutured along a longitudinal dural defect to approximate the artery to the brain surface.[97] In this method, one of the three main arteries of the scalp, the frontal or parietal branch of the superficial temporal artery or the occipital artery, is used as a donor. The donor vessel is exposed extensively. The galea is cut parallel to the artery so that a strip of galea is attached to the donor for its entire exposed length. The scalp artery with the strip of galea is freed from the pericra-

nium and is put aside. Then the fascia, the muscle, and the pericranium are cut just on the line where the donor artery was located. Two burr holes are made below the proximal and distal ends of the freed donor artery. A linear craniotomy, at least 20 mm wide, is made to connect the two burr holes. The dura mater is opened in a straight line trying to spare large dural vessels. The dural openings are closed by suturing the dural edge and galeal edge of the donor strip on each side. The artery and the strip of galea are merely laid on the arachnoid membrane.

Matsushima et al demonstrated gradual disappearance of TIAs and maintenance of intellectual function in all of 65 pediatric cases treated with EDAS, with mean follow-up of 6.4 years.[98] Ross et al reported no further neurologic events in 6 patients with previous strokes or recurrent TIAs during a mean follow-up of 67 months, ranging from 6 months to 9 years.[99] Hee et al, by combined clinical, angiographic, and SPECT criteria, reported excellent or good improvement in 10 patients, fair improvement in 2, no change in 2, and worsening in 1, with a follow-up of 4 to 29 months.[100] In 7 patients with continued frontal or occipital lobe ischemia after standard parietal STA branch use, multiple EDAS, using the addition of the frontal STA branch or occipital artery, showed good revascularization angiographically with no neurologic deterioration in 71 percent of 14 surgical sites.[101]

Encephalomyosynangiosis

With this indirect method, dura is removed along the meningeal artery, which is left intact. The temporalis muscle is detached from the bone flap and placed over the brain surface. The outer edge of the muscle's fascia is sewn to the dural margin. The bone flap is replaced over muscle. Neovascularization occurs from the muscle into the brain. The disadvantages of this method are disruption of spontaneous extra-to-intracranial collaterals and the risk of epilepsy (possibly related to electrical activity of muscle). Revascularization from indirect bypass begins to develop 2 weeks after surgery and becomes well developed by 3 months after surgery.[102] Takeuchi et al performed isolated EMS in a series of nine patients from age 7 to 16 with one to five ischemic events.[103] Postoperatively, 3 of 13 middle cerebral arteries studied angiographically showed faint signals; 10 of 13 had marked visualization. Six of 13 hemispheres studied demonstrated reduced moyamoya vessels. Cerebral blood flow did not increase in hemispheres with moderate or large preoperative lesions on CT. All patients had improvement or disappearance of TIAs and improvement of persisting neurologic deficits. Two patients had improved full IQ scores after 3 to 21 months. Three patients had complications of dysarthria or aphasia lasting from 3 days to 8 months. Karasawa et al[104] performed EMS on five patients with one to three ischemic events. Three had recovery of deficits and disappearance of TIAs after EMS alone. One had improvement of deficits and TIA severity. One underwent subsequent STA-MCA anastomosis with excellent results. This procedure is often used in combination with EDAS, termed encephaloduroarteriomyosynangiosis (EDAMS). It has also been reported that in children, STA-MCA bypass in combination with EMS in six patients shows better development of collateral circulation ($p<$ .05) and improvement in clinical condition ($p<$ .01) 1 year after surgery compared with EDAS alone in 10 patients.[105]

TREATMENT RECOMMENDATIONS

Medical Therapy

Medication should be considered for initial or immediate intervention, for those who are not candidates for surgery, or even as an augmentation of therapy for postsurgical patients. For nonhypertensive patients, nimodipine may be considered a first-line medication. Initial dosing to maintain a steady effect should be every 4 h while awake, starting with 30 mg for older children or adults. Administration three times per day has been used, in which case doubling the dose is preferable early if tolerated. Hypertensive patients may be treated with nicardipine, verapamil, or nifedipine orally at tolerated doses. A prudent regimen would include 325 mg of aspirin daily with persantine, 100 mg QID, or an alternative antiplatelet agent, in non-hemorrhagic cases. The authors' experience is that addition of these medications has improved continued postsurgical symptoms. Patients with a seizure history, particularly those with no cerebral lesions, should be re-evaluated periodically for need of continued antiepileptic medications.

Surgical Therapy

Surgical treatment is generally considered to be the mainstay of long-term treatment, particularly for ischemic disease. Hemodynamic improvement by surgery is best obtained in cases in which regional cerebral blood flow is low, oxygen extraction fraction is high, and there is decreased reactivity to acetazolamide.[106] Children who demonstrate cognitive impairment, even without discrete episodes of neurologic dysfunction, should be considered for early revascularization. The surgical effects for prevention of intracranial bleeding have been controversial; it is still not clear that bypass surgery can prevent or decrease rebleeding in patients with MMD.[107] According to a nationwide survey in Japan, it is estimated that approximately 18 percent of hemorrhagic patients will rebleed regardless of surgical or conservative therapy.[108] For predominantly ischemic disease in adults, STA-MCA bypass is most often effective.[104,109,110] In a young child it may be difficult to perform because of the small caliber of the STA, in which case indirect bypass methods (e.g., EDAS with EMS) are preferred.[1,111] For those in whom direct revascularization is possible, combined surgery (STA-MCA bypass with EDAMS) may be more effective in reducing postoperative ischemic attacks compared with indirect surgery alone and may be effective in preventing intellectual deterioration.[112] Recent data have suggested that advancing age negatively affects development of collateral vessels via indirect bypass.[113] Consequently, direct revascularization by STA-MCA is much more effective than indirect methods in adult MMD, particularly over the age of 40.

Surgical techniques with the STA and muscle flaps primarily revascularize the MCA territory and may not improve blood flow in the territories of the anterior and posterior cerebral arteries. In those cases, placement of bilateral burr holes, in addition to STA-MCA anastomosis, may be effective in the ischemic ACA territory by stimulating neovascularization from the meningeal arteries to recipient cerebral cortex.[109] Cortical branches in the posterior cerebral territory are very small in caliber, making the artificial formation of direct anastomosis between the superficial temporal artery or occipital artery and the cortical branch very difficult to achieve and ineffective in increasing the blood flow in the visual cortex. For this reason, indirect anastomosis using the omentum may be the first surgical choice to overcome ischemic symptoms in the posterior cerebral artery territory.[114]

REFERENCES

1. Fukui M: Current state of study on moyamoya disease in Japan. Surg *Neurol* 47:138, 1997.

2. Goto Y, Yonekawa Y: Worldwide distribution of moyamoya disease. *Neurol Med Chir (Tokyo)* 32:883, 1992.

3. Borota L, Bajic R, Marinkovic R, et al: Moyamoya disease in Yugoslavia: Angiographic study. *Neurol Med Chir* 37:512, 1997.

4. Fodstad H, Bodosi M, Forssell A, Perricane D: Moyamoya disease in patients of Finno-Ugric origin. *Br J Neurosurg* 10:179, 1996.

5. Peh WC, Kwok RK: Moyamoya disease in Singapore. *Ann Acad Med* 14:71, 1985.

6. Su CF, Shih CJ, Lin LS, Hung TP: Moyamoya disease in Taiwan. *J Formos Med Assoc* 93 (Suppl 2):90, 1994.

7. Yu GJ, Kim SY, Coe CJ: Moyamoya disease in Korea. *Yonsei Med J* 32:63, 1991.

8. Numaguchi Y, Gonzales CF, Davis PC, et al: Moyamoya disease in the United States. *Clin Neurol Neurosurg* 99 (Suppl 2):S26, 1997.

9. Graham JF, Matoba A: A survey of moyamoya disease in Hawaii. *Clin Neurol Neurosurg* 99 (Suppl 2):S31, 1997.

10. Edwards-Brown MK, Quets JP: Midwest experience with moyamoya disease. *Clin Neurol Neurosurg* 99 (Suppl 2):S36, 1997.

11. Aoyagi M, Ogami K, Matsushima Y, Shikata M, Yamamoto M, Yamamoto K: Human leukocyte antigen in patients with moyamoya disease. *Stroke* 26:415, 1995.

12. Sarenur T, Mehmet K, Vesile O, Nilgun Y, Yusuf D, Sabahattin K, Tugrul O: Twins with moyamoya disease. *Acta Paediatr Jpn* 36:705, 1994.

13. Pavlakis SG, Verlander PC, Gould RJ, Strimling BC, Auerbach AD: Fanconi anemia in moyamoya: Evidence for an association. *Neurology* 45:998, 1995.

14. Gaggero R, Tortori Donati P, Curia R, DeNegri M: Occlusion of unilateral carotid artery in Down syndrome. *Brain Dev* 18:81, 1996.

15. Cramer S, Robertson R, Dooling EC, Scott M: Moyamoya and Down syndrome: Clinical and radiological features. *Stroke* 27:2131, 1996.

16. Nito T, Becker LE: Vascular dysplasia in Down syndrome: A possible relationship to moyamoya disease. *Brain Dev* 14:248, 1992.

17. Sobata E, Ohkuma H, Suzuki S: Cerebrovascular disorders associated with von Recklinghausen's neurofibromatosis: A case report. *Neurosurgery* 22:544, 1988.

18. Reubi F: Neurofibromatose et lesions vasculaires. *Schweiz Med Wochenschr* 75:463, 1944.

19. Lamas E, Rabato RD, Carello A, Abad JM: Multiple intracranial arterial occlusions (moyamoya disease) in patients with neurofibromatosis: One case report with autopsy. *Acta Neurochi* 45:133, 1978.

20. Yamaguchi T, Matsushima Y, Takata Y, et al: Case-control study of moyamoya disease. *No To Shinkei* 41:485, 1989.

21. Panegyres PK, Morris JG, O'Neill PJ, Balleine R: Moyamoya-like disease with inflammation. *Eur Neurol* 33:260, 1993.

22. Minelli C, Takayangui OM, dos Santos AC, et al: Moyamoya disease in Brazil. *Acta Neurol Scand* 95:125, 1997.

23. Provost TT, Moses H, Morris EL, et al: Cerebral vasculopathy associated with collateralization resembling moyamoya phenomenon and with anti-Ro/SS-A and anti-La/SS-B antibodies. *Arthritis Rheum* 34:1052, 1991.

24. Ezura M, Fujiwara S, Nose M, Yoshimoto T, Kyogoku M: Attempts to induce immune-mediated cerebral arterial injury for an experimental model of moyamoya disease. *Childs Nervous System* 8:263, 1992.

25. Bitzer M, Topka H: Progressive cerebral occlusive disease after radiation therapy. *Stroke* 26:131, 1995.

26. Kestle JR, Hoffman HJ, Mock AR: Moyamoya phenomenon after radiation for optic glioma. *J Neurosurg* 79:32, 1993.

27. Tsuji N, Kuriyama T, Iwamoto M, Shizuki K: Moyamoya disease associated with craniopharyngioma. *Surg Neurol* 21:588, 1984.

28. Arita K, Uozumi T, Oki S, et al: Moyamoya disease associated with pituitary adenoma: Report of two cases. *Neurol Med Chir* 32:753, 1992.

29. Levine SR, Fagan SC, Pessin MS, et al: Accelerated intracranial occlusive disease, oral contraceptives, and cigarette use. *Neurology* 41:1893, 1991.

30. Tan E-C, Takagi T, Nagai H: Intracranial carotid artery occlusion with telangiectasia (moyamoya disease) associated with persistent primitive trigeminal artery. *Neurol Med Chir (Tokyo)* 31:800, 1991.

31. Kurose K, Kishi H, Sadatoh T: Moyamoya disease with persistent primitive hypoglossal artery: Case report. *Neurologia* 29:528, 1989.

32. Suzuki J, Takaku A, Kodama N, Sato S: An attempt to treat cerebrovascular moyamoya disease in children. *Child's Brain* 1:193, 1975.

33. Welch WC, McBride M, Kido DK, Nelson CN: Moyamoya disease in an infant with autonomic dysfunction: Angiographic and MRI findings. *J Child Neurol* 3:110, 1989.

34. Liu JS, Juo SH, Chen WH, Chang YY, Chen SS: A case of Grave's disease associated with intracranial moyamoya vessels and tubular stenosis of extracranial internal carotid arteries. *J Formos Med Assoc* 93:806, 1994.

35. Kushima K, Sato Y, Ban Y, Taniyama M, Ito K, Sugita K: Grave's thyrotoxicosis and moyamoya disease. *Can J Neurol Sci* 18:140, 1991.

36. Yamamoto M, Aoyagi M, Tajima S, et al: Increase in elastin gene expression and protein synthesis in arterial smooth muscle cells derived from patients with moyamoya disease. *Stroke* 28:1733, 1997.

37. Fukai N, Aoyagi M, Yamamoto M, et al: Human arterial smooth muscle cell strains derived from patients with moyamoya disease: Changes in biological characteristics and proliferative response during cellular aging in vitro. *Mech Aging Dev* 75:21, 1994.

38. Hoshimaru M, Takahashi JA, Kikuchi H, Nagata I, Hatanaka M: Possible roles of basic fibroblast growth factor

in the pathogenesis of moyamoya disease: An immunohistochemical study. *J Neurosurg* 75:267, 1991.

39. Maki Y, Nakata Y: Autopsy of a case with an anomalous hemangioma of the internal carotid artery at the skull base. *Brain Nerve (Tokyo)* 17:764, 1965.
40. Hosoda Y: Pathology of so-called "spontaneous occlusion of the circle of Willis." *Pathol Ann* 2:221, 1984.
41. Hosoda Y, Ikeda E, Hirose S: Histopathological studies on spontaneous occlusion of the circle of Wills (cerebrovascular Moyamoya disease). *Clin Neurol Surg* (Suppl 2): 203, 1997.
42. Haltia M, Iivanainen M, Majuri H, Puranen M: Spontaneous occlusion of the circle of Willis. *Clin Neuropathol* 1:11, 1982.
43. Yamashita M, Oka K, Tanaka K: Histopathology of the brain vascular network in moyamoya disease. *Stroke* 14:50, 1983.
44. Oka K, Yamashita M, Sadoshima S, Tanaka K: Cerebral haemorrhage in moyamoya disease at autopsy. *Pathol Anat* 392:247, 1981.
45. Yamashita M, Oka K, Tanaka K: Cervico-cephalic arterial thrombi and thromboemboli in moyamoya disease—possible correlation with progressive intimal thickening in the intracranial major arteries. *Stroke* 15:264, 1984.
46. Ikeda E, Hosoda Y: Distribution of thrombotic lesions in the cerebral arteries in spontaneous occlusion of the circle of Willis: Cerebrovascular moyamoya disease. *Clin Neuropathol* 12:44, 1993.
47. Aoyagi M, Fukai N, Yamamoto M, et al: Early development of intimal thickening in superficial temporal arteries in patients with moyamoya disease. *Stroke* 27:1750, 1996.
48. Ikeda E: Systemic vascular changes in "spontaneous occlusion of the circle of Willis." *Stroke* 22:1358, 1991.
49. Ellison PH, Largent JA, Popp AJ: Moya-moya disease associated with renal arterial stenosis. *Arch Neurol* 38:467, 1981.
50. Maki Y, Enomoto T: Moyamoya disease. *Childs Nervous System* 4:204, 1988.
51. Matsushima Y, Aoyagi M, Niimi Y, et al: Symptoms and their pattern of progression in childhood moyamoya disease. *Brain Dev* 12:784, 1990.
52. Nakase H, Ohnishi H, Touho H, et al: Clinical study of epileptic type moyamoya disease in children. *Jpn J Psychiatry Neurol* 46:419, 1992.
53. Mawad ME, Hilal SK, Michelsen WJ, et al: Occlusive vascular disease associated with cerebral arteriovenous malformations. *Radiology* 153:401, 1984.
54. Montanera W, Marotta TR, terBrugge KG, et al: Cerebral arteriovenous malformations associated with moyamoya phenomenon. *Am J Neuroradiol* 11:1153, 1990.
55. Bucciero A, Carangelo B, Vizioli L: Giant basilar artery aneurysm associated with moyamoya disease. Case report and review of the literature *Acta Neurol* 16:121, 1994.
56. Konishi Y, Kadowaki C, Hara M, Takeuchi K: Aneurysms associated with moyamoya disease. *Neurosurgery* 4:484, 1985.

57. Kawaguchi S, Sakaki T, Kakizaki T, et al: Clinical features of the hemorrhagic type moyamoya disease based on 31 cases. *Acta Neurochir* 138:1200, 1996.
58. Serdaru M, Gray F, Merland JJ, et al: Moyamoya disease and intracerebral hematoma. *Neuroradiology* 18:47, 1979.
59. Saeki N, Yamaura A, Hoshi S, et al: Hemorrhagic type of moyamoya disease. *No Shinkei Geka* 19:705, 1991.
60. Aoki N, Mizutani H: Does moyamoya disease cause subarachnoid hemorrhage? Review of 54 cases with intracranial hemorrhage confirmed by computerized tomography. *J Neurosurg* 60:348, 1984.
61. Hashimoto K, Fujii K, Nishimura K, et al: Occlusive cerebrovascular disease of moyamoya vessels and intracranial hemorrhage during pregnancy: Case report and review of the literature. *Neurol Med Chir (Tokyo)* 28:588, 1988.
62. Olds MV, Griebel RW, Hoffman HJ, et al: The surgical treatment of childhood moyamoya disease. *J Neurosurg* 66:675, 1987.
63. Kurokawa T, Tomita S, Ueda K, et al: Prognosis of occlusive disease of the circle of Willis (moyamoya disease) in children. 1:274, 1985.
64. Fukuyama Y, Umezu R: Clinical and cerebral angiographic evolutions of idiopathic progressive occlusive disease of the circle of Willis ("moyamoya" disease) in children. *Brain Dev* 7:21, 1985.
65. Nakada Y, Yoshii Y, Nose T, et al: Follow-up study of "moyamoya" in adult patients. *Neurol Med Chir* 18:75, 1978.
66. Choi JU, Kim DS, Kim EY, Lee KC: Natural history of moyamoya disease—comparison of activity of daily living in surgery and non-surgery groups. *Clin Neurol Neurosurg* 99 (Suppl 2):S11, 1997.
67. Nishimoto A: Moyamoya disease. *Neurol Med Chir* 19:221, 1979.
68. Suzuki J, Takaku A: Cerebrovascular moyamoya disease: Disease showing abnormal net-like vessels in base of brain. *Arch Neurol* 20:288, 1969.
69. Makiyama Y, Nishimoto H, Aihara T, Tsubokawa T: Magnetic resonance angiography in the management of childhood moyamoya disease: First choice for neurovascular scrutiny. *Surg Neurol* 42:32, 1994.
70. Yamada I, Suzuki S, Matsushima Y: Moyamoya disease: Diagnostic accuracy of MRI. *Neuroradiology* 37:356, 1995.
71. Ohta T, Tanaka H, Kuroiwa T: Diffuse leptomeningeal enhancement, "ivy sign" in magnetic resonance images of moyamoya disease in childhood: Case report. *Neurosurgery* 37:1009, 1995.
72. Yamada I, Suzuki S, Matsushima Y: Moyamoya disease: Comparison of assessment with MR angiography and MR imaging versus conventional angiography. *Radiology* 196:211, 1995.
73. Houkin K, Aoki T, Takahashi A, Abe H: Diagnosis of moyamoya disease with magnetic resonance angiography. *Stroke* 25:2159, 1994.
74. Yamada I, Matsushima Y, Suzuki S: Childhood moyamoya disease before and after encephaloduroarterio-

synangiosis: An angiographic study. *Neuroradiology* 34: 318, 1992.

75. Miyamoto S, Kikuchi H, Karasawa J, et al: Study of the posterior circulation in moyamoya disease: Clinical and neuroradiological evaluation. *J. Neurosurg* 61:1032, 1984.

76. Hasuo K, Yasumori K, Yoshida K, et al: Magnetic resonance imaging compared to computed tomography and angiography in moyamoya disease. *Acta Radiol* 31:191, 1990.

77. Tsuchiya K, Makita K, Furui S: Moyamoya disease: Diagnosis with three-dimensional CT angiography. *Neuroradiology* 36:432, 1994.

78. Kikuchi M, Asato M, Sugahara S, et al: Evaluation of surgically performed collateral circulation in moyamoya disease with 3D-CT angiography: Comparison with MR angiography and X-ray angiography. *Neuropediatrics* 27:45, 1996.

79. Touho H, Karasawa J, Ohnishi H: Preoperative and postoperative evaluation of cerebral perfusion and vasodilatory capacity with ^{99m}Tc-HMPAO SPECT and acetazolamide in childhood moyamoya disease. *Stroke* 27:282, 1996.

80. Hoshi H, Ohnishi T, Jinnouchi S, et al. Cerebral blood flow study in patients with moyamoya disease evaluated by IMP SPECT. *J Nucl Med* 35:44, 1994.

81. Ikezaki K, Matsushima T, Kuwabara Y, et al. Cerebral circulation and oxygen metabolism in childhood moyamoya disease: A perioperative positron emission tomography study. *J. Neurosurg* 81:843, 1994.

82. Touho H, Karasawa J, Shishido H, et al: Mechanism of the re-buildup phenomenon in moyamoya disease: Analysis of local cerebral hemodynamics with intra-arterial digital subtraction angiography. *Neurologia* 30:721, 1990.

83. Muttaqin Z, Ohba S, Arita K, et al: Cerebral circulation in moyamoya disease: A clinical study using transcranial Doppler sonography. *Surg Neurol* 40:306, 1993.

84. Takase K, Kashihara M, Hashimoto T: Transcranial Doppler ultrasonography in patients with moyamoya disease. *Clin Neurol Neurosurg* 99 (Suppl 2):S101, 1997.

85. Laborde G, Harders A, Klimek L, Hardenack M: Correlation between clinical, angiographic and transcranial Doppler sonographic findings in patients with moyamoya disease. *Neurol Res* 15:87, 1993.

86. Diener HC, Cunha L, Forbes C, et al: European Stroke Prevention Study 2: Dipyridamole and acetylsalicylic acid in the secondary prevention of stroke. *J Neurol Sci* 143:1, 1996.

87. Kuroki M, Nagamachi S, Hoshi H, et al: Cerebral perfusion imaging evaluates pharmacologic treatment of unilateral moyamoya disease. *J Nuclear Med* 37:84, 1996.

88. Hosain SA, Hughes JT, Forem SL, et al: Use of a calcium channel blocker (nicardipineHCl) in the treatment of childhood moyamoya disease. *J Child Neurol* 9:378, 1994.

89. McLean MJ, Gebarski SS, van der Spek AF, Goldstein GW: Reponse of moyamoya disease to verapamil (Letter). *Lancet* 1:163, 1985.

90. Sarenur T, Mehmet K, Vesile O, et al: Twins with moyamoya disease. *Acta Paediatr Jpn* 36:705, 1994.

91. Spittler JF, Smektala K: Pharmacotherapy in moyamoya disease. *Hokkaido Igaku Zasshi* 62:235, 1990.

92. Pavlakis SG, Schneider S, Black K, Gould RJ: Steroid-responsive chorea in moyamoya disease. *Mov Disord* 6(4) 347, 1991.

93. Nakashima H, Meguro T, Kawada S, et al: Long-term results of surgically treated moyamoya disease. *Clin Neurol Neurosurg* 99 (Suppl 2):S156, 1997.

94. Houkin K, Ishikawa T, Yoshimoto T, Abe H: Direct and indirect revascularization for moyamoya disease surgical techniques and peri-operative complications. *Clin Neurol Neurosurg* (Suppl 2):S142, 1997.

95. Fujii K, Ikezaki K, Irikura K, et al: The efficacy of bypass surgery for the patients with hemorrhagic moyamoya disease. *Clin Neurol Neurosurg* 99 (Suppl 2):S94, 1997.

96. Okada Y, Shima T, Nishida M, et al: Effectiveness of superficial temporal artery-middle cerebral artery anastomosis in adult moyamoya disease. *Stroke* 29:625, 1998.

97. Matsushima Y, Fukkai N, Tanaka K, et al: A new surgical treatment of moyamoya disease in children: A preliminary report. *Surg Neurol* 15:313, 1981.

98. Matsushima Y, Aoyagi M, Koumo Y, et al: Effects of encephalo-duro-arterio-synangiosis on childhood moyamoya patients: Swift disappearance of ischemic attacks and maintenance of mental capacity. *Neurologia* 31:708, 1991.

99. Ross IB, Shevell MI, Montes JL, et al: Encephaloduro-arteriosynangiosis (EDAS) for the treatment of childhood moyamoya disease. *Pediat Neurol* 10:199, 1994.

100. Han DH, Nam DH, Oh CW: Moyamoya disease in adults: Characteristics of clinical presentation and outcome after encephalo-duro-arterio-synangiosis. *Clin Neurol Neurosurg* 99 (Suppl 2):S151, 1997.

101. Tenjin H, Ueda S: Multiple EDAS (encephalo-duro-arterio-syangiosis): Additional EDAS using the frontal branch of the superficial temporal artery (STA) and the occipital artery for pediatric moyamoya patients in whom EDAS using the parietal branch of STA was insufficient. *Childs Nervous System* 13:220, 1997.

102. Kinugasa K, Mandai S, Kamata I, et al: Surgical treatment of moyamoya disease: Operative technique for encephalo-duro-arterio-myo-synangiosis, its follow-up, clinical results, and angiograms. *Neurosurgery* 32:527, 1993.

103. Takeuchi S, Tsuchida T, Kobayashi K, et al: Treatment of moyamoya disease by temporal muscle graft "encephalo-myo-synangiosis." *Child's Brain* 10:1, 1983.

104. Karasawa J, Kikuchi H, Furuse S, et al: A surgical treatment of moyamoya disease: "Encephalo-myo-synangiosis." *Neurol Med Chir* 17:29, 1977.

105. Matsushima T, Inoue T, Suzuki SO, et al: Surgical treatment of moyamoya disease in pediatric patients: Comparison between the results of indirect and direct revascularization procedures. *Neurosurgery* 31:401, 1992.

106. Iwama T, Hashimoto N, Takagi Y, et al: Predictability of extracranial/intracranial bypass function: A retrospective study of patients with occlusive cerebrovascular disease. *Neurosurgery* 40:53, 1997.

107. Houkin K, Kamiyama H, Abe H, et al: Surgical therapy for adult moyamoya disease: Can surgical revascularization prevent the recurrence of intracerebral hemorrhage? *Stroke* 27:1342, 1996.

108. Ikezaki K, Fukui M, Inamura T, et al: The current status of the treatment for hemorrhagic type moyamoya disease based on a 1995 nationwide survey in Japan. *Clin Neurol Neurosurg* (Suppl 2):S183, 1997.

109. Suzuki Y, Negoro M, Shibuya M, et al: Surgical treatment for pediatric moyamoya disease: Use of the superficial temporal artery for both areas supplied by the anterior and middle cerebral arteries. *Neurosurgery* 40:324, 1997.

110. Ishikawa T, Houkin K, Kamiyama H, Abe H: Effects of surgical revascularization on outcome of patients with pediatric moyamoya disease. *Stroke* 28:1170, 1997.

111. Matsushima T, Fujiwara S, Nagata S, et al: Surgical treatment for pediatric patients with moyamoya disease by indirect revascularization procedure (EDAS, EMS, EMAS). *Acta Neurochir* 98:135, 1989.

112. Ishikawa T, Houkin K, Kamiyama H, Abe H: Effects of surgical revascularization on outcome of patients with pediatric moyamoya disease. *Stroke* 28:1170, 1997.

113. Mizoi K, Kayama T, Yoshimoto T, Nagamine Y: Indirect revascularization for moyamoya disease: Is there a beneficial effect for adult patients? *Surg Neurol* 45:541, 1996.

114. Karasawa J, Touho H, Ohnishi H, et al: Cerebral revascularization using omental transplantation for childhood moyamoya disease. *J Neurosurg* 79:192, 1993.

115. Kuroki M, Nagamachi S, Hoshi H, et al: Cerebral perfusion imaging evaluates pharmacologic treatment of unilateral moyamoya disease. *J Nucl Med* 37:84, 1996.

Chapter 18

DIAGNOSIS AND MANAGEMENT OF SINOVENOUS THROMBOSIS

David Lefkowitz

BACKGROUND

The earliest description of cerebral vein and dural sinus thrombosis is attributed to Ribes in 1825. The true incidence of cerebral sinovenous occlusion is still unknown, but it is less common than arterial thrombosis. Towbin found cerebral venous thrombosis in 9.3 percent of 182 consecutive autopsies with a 2:1 female preponderance.[1] Sinovenous thrombosis was diagnosed in 3.75 percent of a pediatric population undergoing angiography.[2] The anatomy of the normal cerebral venous system has been reviewed elsewhere.[3,4]

CLINICAL CONSIDERATIONS

Sinovenous occlusion should be suspected whenever acute or subacute neurologic dysfunction presents with altered consciousness, focal deficits, seizures, or evidence of increased intracranial pressure. The differential diagnosis includes meningitis, intracranial abscess, arterial thrombosis, and tumor. Symptoms of sinovenous occlusion arise directly from the primary or underlying process, from venous obstruction, vascular inflammation, or secondary complications. Typical manifestations are headache, papilledema, seizures, focal deficits, and altered consciousness. Hyperacute headache may mimic subarachnoid hemorrhage and may occur without elevation of cerebral spinal fluid (CSF) pressure.[5]

In the majority of cases, thrombosis involves multiple dural sinuses or both sinuses and veins.[6] Isolated occlusion of one or more sinuses generally produces inceased intracranial pressure without localizing signs. Extension of thrombus into superficial cortical or deep veins more commonly leads to rapidly progressive, focal neurologic deficits. Venous infarction resulting from sinovenous thrombosis is likely to be hemorrhagic, and there may be bleeding in the brain parenchyma, subarachnoid, or subdural spaces.[7] Concomitant venous thrombosis may occur in other organ systems.

Superior Sagittal Sinus Thrombosis

The superior sagittal sinus is the most frequently involved and serves as the clinical prototype for sinovenous thrombosis. A well-defined syndrome of headache, papilledema, and intracranial hypertension, which is clinically indistinguishable from pseudotumor cerebri, occurs in approximately half of cases of superior sagittal sinus thrombosis.[6] Headache is usually persistent, unilateral, and may be limited to the forehead, temple, or occipital region.[8] Generalized or focal seizures frequently precede motor deficits. Findings characteristic of superior sagittal sinus thrombosis such as paraplegia and alternating or ascending paralysis are actually rare.[7] Cranial nerve involvement is also uncommon and usually results from elevated intracranial pressure or extension of thrombosis into the jugular vein or the cavernous or petrosal sinuses. Psychiatric dysfunction such as hallucinations and delusional thinking may be the primary or sole clinical manifestation.[8] Cortical blindness has also been reported.[9] The presentation is more severe when the superior sagittal sinus is occluded at or posterior to the Rolandic vein or the vein of Trolard.[10,11] Venous distention may cause scalp edema over the affected sinus, epistaxis from nasal collaterals, or dilatation of diploic veins, which may produce a caput medusae consisting of radially arranged, distended scalp veins.[8]

Lateral Sinus Thrombosis

Lateral sinus thrombosis was once a common complication of acute otitis media and mastoiditis in children but now is more often associated with chronic ear infections and petrous cholesteatomas in adults.[12] Symptoms are attributable either directly to the infection or to alterations in cerebrospinal fluid dynamics. High fever with acute otitis or intermittent fevers with a draining ear should suggest the diagnosis. Weight loss, fever, and anemia may be prominent, and sepsis may dominate the clinical picture.[12] Headache and ear pain are frequent complaints. Neck pain radiating along the margin of the sternocleidomastoid is often a sign of intracranial complications.[12] Edema over the site of the mastoid emissary vein is referred to as Greisinger's sign.[13] When the lateral sinus is occluded, compression of the contralateral jugular vein may lead to Crowe's sign, distention of the scalp and face veins. The presentation of lateral sinus thrombosis has changed since the introduction of antibiotics, with less fever and blood cultures more often sterile.[14] "Otogenic hydrocephalus," more appropriately referred to as otogenic intracranial hypertension, presents with headache, nausea, and papilledema associated with otitis or mastoiditis.[15] Involvement of the right transverse sinus, usually the dominant one, is more likely to be symptomatic.[16] Focal neurologic deficits are rare in lateral sinus thrombosis without intracranial abscess or spread into other sinuses or cortical veins. Brain abscesses usually occur in the temporal lobe or cerebellum from retrograde extension of infection through small veins draining the white matter. Extradural abscesses may also occur.[14] Infection may spread to the superior sagittal or cavernous sinuses. Dysphasia, hemianopia, or hemiparesis result from involvement of the posterior temporal or occipital lobes via the superior petrosal sinus or the inferior anastomotic vein.[17] Glossopharyngeal, vagus, and accessory nerve lesions arise from involvement of the jugular bulb, the hypoglossal from the vein of the hypoglossal canal, and the abducens nerve from the inferior petrosal sinus. Septic embolism involving lung, large joints, and subcutaneous tissue was common in the preantibiotic ear.[12]

Cavernous Sinus Thrombosis

Cavernous sinus thrombosis usually arises from infection of the middle third of the face, the sphenoid, ethmoid, or maxillary sinuses, and less commonly the oropharynx, teeth, neck, or ear.[13] The most important pathogens are *Staphylococcus aureus* in adults and *Hemophilus influenza* or *pneumococcus* in children.[18] Enteric Gram-negative organisms such as *Proteus* and *Pseudomonas, Mucor* and *Aspergillus,* or anaerobes may also be responsible, particularly in immunocompromised hosts. Headache is a common premonitory symptom. Mechanical obstruction to venous drainage results in proptosis and edema of the lids, conjunctiva, the bridge of the nose, pharynx, and tonsils with dilatation of facial veins.[18,19] Ophthalmoplegia and diplopia may arise from orbital congestion or inflammation of the intracavernous oculomotor, trochlear, and abducens nerves. The pupil is dilated and poorly reactive in about one-third of cases.[13] Facial numbness involves the first two divisions of the trigeminal nerve because of their intracavernous location, and sometimes the third division if thrombus or infection spreads to involve the inferior petrosal sinus.[20] Visual loss occurs in 10 to 20 percent of patients due to corneal ulceration, central retinal artery, or vein occlusion, arteritis, embolism, or ischemic optic neuropathy.[13,21] The opposite cavernous sinus is freqently affected due to communication across the midline through the circular or intracavernous sinuses.[22] Systemic signs include diaphoresis, tachycardia, and fever. Meningitis and septic embolism to the lung and other organs may occur.[18,21] Focal arteritis or infection of the intracavernous carotid artery may lead to cerebral infarction, internal carotid artery occlusion, mycotic aneurysms, or carotid cavernous fistulae.[19] Pituitary insufficiency may follow retrograde thrombosis, embolism, or direct intrasellar extension.[23] A Korsakoff-like amnesic syndrome with confabulation has been described with bilateral mesial temporal lobe infarction following bilateral cavernous sinus thrombosis.[24] The differential of cavernous sinus thrombosis includes dysthyroid ophthalmopathy, orbital cellulitis, superior orbital or orbital apex syndromes, and the Tolosa-Hunt syndrome. Bilateral involvement in cavernous sinus thrombosis is helpful in distinguishing it from these other conditions.

Thrombosis of Other Dural Sinuses

Thrombosis of the straight sinus may produce hemorrhagic infarction of the thalamus, subarachnoid hemorrhage, increased intracranial pressure, coma, seizures, or rigidity.[8,17] Although petrosal sinus thrombosis has been rare since the introduction of antibiotics, the sixth cranial nerve may be affected in Dorello's canal when the inferior sinus is thrombosed and the trigeminal nerve can be involved by contiguous spread from either the inferior or superior petrosal sinuses.[17] Seizures may follow extension of infection into the temporal lobe along veins draining into the superior petrosal sinus.

Cortical Vein Thrombosis

Solitary involvement of a single vein is unusual, making clinicoanatomic correlation difficult. Drainage of the central Rolandic vein is often bidirectional, into the superior sagittal sinus from the area above the representation of the hand on the homunculus and inferiorly into the middle cerebral vein and the cavernous sinus from below that level.[17] The clinical picture consists of spastic weakness of the proximal upper extremity and leg with relative sparing of the face and speech.[15,25] The arm may be adducted and internally rotated with the elbow flexed and pronated. The leg is more rigid than the arm and is extended, adducted, and internally rotated with spontaneous dorsiflexion of the toes. Involvement of the arm is usually transient. Sensory loss consists primarily of astereognosis. Both sides may be involved, and stepwise or alternating progression is not unusual. Monoplegia of the contralateral leg may follow occlusion of the superior cerebral vein,[25] and homonymous hemianopia has been reported following surgical ligation of the internal occipital vein.[26] Occlusion of the vein of Labbé produces hemiparesis with the face and arm affected more than the leg, with or without dysphasia or hemianopia.[15]

Deep Venous Thrombosis

Isolated spontaneous thrombosis of the deep venous system is relatively rare in adults.[26–28] In most cases, surgical sacrifice of one of the deep veins does not produce a specific clinical syndrome. Nevertheless, thrombosis of the internal cerebral vein may affect mesencephalic structures.[29] Infarction of the diencephalon and basal ganglia may lead to dystonia, tremor, or dyskinesia.[30] Vein of Galen thrombosis may produce intraventricular hemorrhage or hemorrhagic infarction of the medial basal ganglia and thalami with a residual movement disorder.[26] Both of these lesions carry a poor prognosis.

Venous Thrombosis of the Spinal Cord

Thrombosis of spinal cord veins typically produces a painful, rapidly progressive hemorrhagic infarction manifested by sensorimotor and sphincter disturbance.[31] When ischemic infarction occurs, the onset is more prolonged and pain is unusual.[32] Hemorrhagic infarctions tend to be more centrally located in the spinal cord than ischemic ones.

DIAGNOSIS

Early diagnosis of dural sinus or cerebral vein thrombosis is often elusive. Fever, peripheral leukocytosis, and elevated erythrocyte sedimentation rate occur more often when the etiology is infectious, inflammatory, or neoplastic. Cerebrospinal fluid abnormalities, including elevated pressure, moderate lymphocytic or mixed pleocytosis, and elevated protein, are nondiagnostic. There may be subarachnoid blood or xanthochromia. Cerebrospinal fluid cultures are usually sterile, even in septic cases.[12]

Electroencephalography is nonspecific. Generalized slowing is the most common electroencephalographic abnormality,[15] but slowing may be focal or asymmetric. A discrete epileptiform focus occurs in less than 20 percent of cases but often correlates with clinical seizures and cortical vein involvement.

Plain films may demonstrate an abnormality of the temporal bone in cases of septic lateral sinus thrombosis[12] or a fracture through a sinus groove when there is an injury or laceration of a dural sinus.[20] ^{99m}Technetium pertechnetate radionuclide brain scans have largely been replaced by other technologies. Increased radionuclide activity at the end of the thrombus and later involving the sinus diffusely has been reported with ^{111}Indium-labeled platelet scintigraphy.[33] Intracarotid ^{113}Xenon blood flow measurements in three patients were slightly reduced and were unresponsive to hypercarbia but decreased normally with hyperventilation.[34] Transcranial ultrasound may demonstrate increased flow in collateral venous channels[35–37] and can also be used to detect microembolic signals in the distal internal jugular vein in some patients with superior sagittal sinus thrombosis.[38]

Computed Tomography

The posterior 6 mm of the superior sagittal sinus, more anterior portions of this sinus, straight sinus, and the vein of Galen can be routinely imaged with computed tomography (CT). Basal venous structures such as the cavernous and petrosal sinuses are rarely visualized due to partial volume effect with adjacent bone.[39] The normal superior sagittal sinus may not be visualized on an unenhanced CT or may appear as a heterogenous hyperdensity.[40] After contrast administration, the superior sagittal sinus may enhance heterogeneously due to the presence of arachnoid granulations, fibrous bands, or septae. Discrete filling defects compatible with arachnoid granulations are imaged with CT in about one-quarter of contrast-enhanced studies and are most frequently seen in the transverse sinus.[41] If a central hypodensity occurs, it usually does not fill the entire cross-section of the sinus and is not present at consecutive levels.

CT findings in sinovenous occlusion are often nonspecific, and early scans may be normal. On the uninfused CT, the thrombosed sinus may appear as a dense triangle, sometimes referred to as the dense or filled delta sign[28,42,43] (Fig. 18-1). Spontaneous hyperden-sity has been described in all venous sinuses and is usually seen transiently as an early sign of venous thrombosis, occurring during the first 4 to 5 days after onset.[44–46] A similar appearance may also be seen with elevated hematocrit, interhemispheric subarchnoid hemorrhage, parasagittal subdural hematomas, and sometimes in normal children.[7,42] Analysis of attenuation units may help differentiate acute thrombus from flowing blood. The cord sign is a rounded hyperdensity representing intraluminal thrombus on sequential slices of an uninfused scan.[39,46,47] It is accentuated by an adjacent extra-axial collection displacing the vein from the inner table of the skull. Intraparenchymal linear hyperdensities representing thrombosed intracerebral veins have similar significance.[28] Precontrast CT may also demonstrate ischemic or hemorrhagic infarction, intraparenchymal hematoma, and evidence of increased intracranial pressure. As cerebral edema resolves over 1 to 2 weeks, the ventricles may enlarge.[11]

The use of intravenous contrast increases the utility of CT. One of the best documented signs of sagittal sinus thrombosis is the negative or empty delta sign on infused CT, consisting of a central hypodensity surrounded by a margin of contrast enhancement[40,47] (Fig. 18-2). The central lucency may arise from sluggish or absent blood flow within the sinus and the peripheral enhancement from peridural collaterals, granulation tissue, contrast containing blood flowing around the clot, inflammation of the sinus walls, or breakdown of the blood-brain barrier in surrounding tissue.[43] The negative delta sign is usually not seen for 3 to 4 days after the ictus[46] and persists for 2 to 3 months.[48] It should be seen on several contiguous slices. Varying the window settings may help visualize a filling defect within the sinus.[39,40,49] The negative delta sign may be confused with early splitting of the sinus (a normal variant),[28,39] the delayed delta sign in normal delayed postcontrast scans,[50] an extradural hypodensity such as abscess abutting the sinus,[39] and the pseudo-negative delta sign of subarachnoid blood outlining the superior sagittal sinus on precontrast studies. Similar filling defects have been reported in other venous sinuses. Other patterns of abnormal enhancement may result from collateral circulation, stasis, or hyperemia within dural venous structures, (Fig. 18-3). The presence of a dilated transcerebral medullary vein may be pathognomonic of sinovenous occlusion.[51] Tentorial enhancement is often considered a sign of straight sinus occlusion but may also be seen with occlusion of other sinuses.[6,52] Asymmetric meningeal enhancement over the cavernous sinus may be a sign of cavernous sinus thrombosis.[19] Gyral or linear enhance-

Figure 18-1.
Uninfused cranial computerized tomography demonstrating a dense delta sign in the superior sagittal sinus.

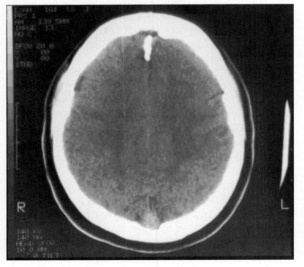

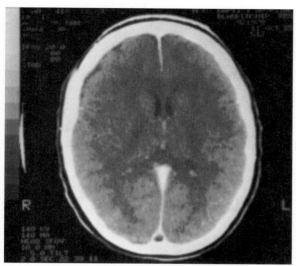

Figure 18-2.

Contrast enhanced cranial computerized tomography showing a central hypodensity in the superior sagittal sinus surrounded by contrast enhancement consistent with a negative delta sign.

ment may occur in areas of infarction. CT may occasionally be of value in identifying the etiology of sinovenous disease, such as sinus occlusion associated with meningioma.[47] Helical CT venography is an effective means of demonstrating the relationship of tumor to adjacent venous structures.[53]

Magnetic Resonance Imaging

Magnetic resonance (MR) imaging is an attractive option for diagnosis of sinovenous occlusion because of its ability to image flowing and stagnant blood without intravascular manipulation, exposure to iodinated contrast media, or ionizing radiation. MR is superior to CT in demonstrating the lateral sinuses and internal jugular veins due to the lack of bony artifact. The appearance of a thrombosed sinus varies with the stage of thrombosis and field strength. Macchi et al described initial loss of the normal flow void, T1 isointensity, and T2 hypointensity using a 1.5 Tessla magnet and spin-echo pulse sequences.[54] Flow void may be seen in collateral channels. Low-signal intensity of acute thrombus on T2-weighted images is more likely with high-field strength magnets, leading to the potential risk of mistaking decreased signal for the flow void of a patent vascular structure.[55] Flow-sensitive gradient-echo techniques

may help to avoid this pitfall.[56] A central area of nonenhancing, intermediate intensity (but not flow void) surrounded by an enhanced rim on contrast-enhanced T1-weighted scans represents the MR equivalent of the negative delta sign on CT[57] (Fig. 18-4). An intermediate stage of increased T1, and later T2, signal corresponds to conversion of deoxyhemoglobin within the thrombus to methemoglobin (Fig. 18-5). In later stages, the sinus appears isointense on T1 and hyperintense on T2-weighted images accompanied by restoration of the flow void, presumably due to recanalization of the thrombus. The first stage occurs during the first week, the intermediate stage during the first month, and the late stage thereafter, although dating of these stages is not precise due to the relative paucity of serial studies (Table 18-1). Parenchymal T2 hyperintensities may represent venous infarction or edema.[58] Abnormal enhancement patterns may also indicate collateral flow. Potential shortcomings of MR imaging include confusion of subdural hematoma

Figure 18-3.

Dilated collateral channels and tentorial enhancement on an infused computerized tomogram.

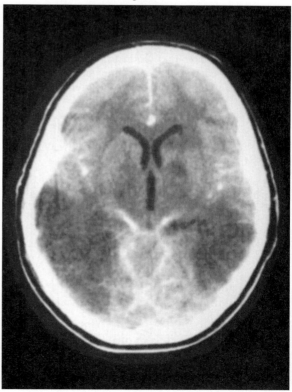

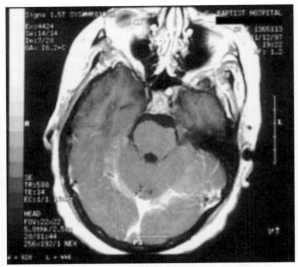

Figure 18-4.
Magnetic resonance imaging with gadolinium demonstrating a filling defect in the superior sagittal sinus and enhancement of the tentorium.

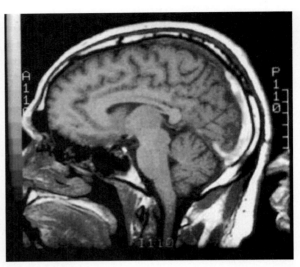

Figure 18-5.
Hyperintensity of thrombosed straight and superior sagittal sinuses on magnetic resonance imaging.

adjacent to the sinus or flow-related enhancement with intraluminal clot and misinterpretation of hypointensity from paramagnetic blood products as flow. Intense enhancement of chronic thrombus may mimic flow.[59] MR venography may demonstrate direct signs of venous thrombosis such as absent signal from a sinus or a frayed appearance of flow after recanalization, and indirect signs such as prominent venous collaterals, hemorrhage, or evidence of increased intracranial pressure[60] (Fig. 18-6).

Angiography and Other Contrast Studies

Angiography remains the definitive antemortem technique for diagnosis of sinovenous thrombosis. Radiographic findings include partial or complete nonvisual-

ization of the occluded sinus in 75 to 100 percent of cases, increased arteriovenous circulation time in 50 to 70 percent, dilatation or tortuosity of collateral veins in 50 to 60 percent, reversal of venous flow in 20 to 40 percent, and nonspecific mass effect in approximately 10 percent.[2,6,61,62] Abnormal-appearing cortical veins were seen in 25 percent of children in Scotti's series.[2] Krayenbühl stressed the importance of corkscrew-shaped capillaries and veins that fail to reach the cortical surface[27] (Fig. 18-7). Delayed venous films, subtraction techniques, bilateral simultaneous carotid injection, oblique projections, or cross-compression may be required to adequately visualize an occlusion. Submental views may facilitate visualization of the cavernous sinus. There are a number of pitfalls in the angiographic diagnosis of sinovenous thrombosis. Filling defects produced by mixed contrast and unopacified blood from the opposite hemisphere[25] may be avoided by aortic arch injections[44]

Table 18-1.
Evolution of signal characteristics of a thrombosed venous sinus

	Normal	Early	Intermediate	Late
T1 WI	Variable	Isointense	Hyperintense	Isointense
T2 WI	No signal	Hypointense	Hyperintense	Hypointense
Gradient echo	Hyperintense	Isointense	Hyperintense	Isointense

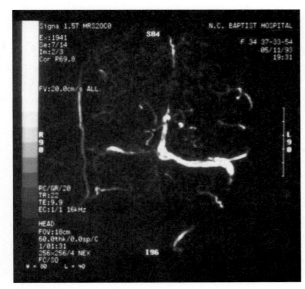

Figure 18-6.
Magnetic resonance venogram showing poor filling of the superior sagittal and right lateral sinuses.

or intravenous digital angiography,[63] as the contrast bolus reaches both hemispheres simultaneously. Opacification of intradural collaterals may mimic filling of the sinus itself if anteroposterior views are not assessed.[62] Cortical veins may fail to drain an area rendered ischemic by arterial occlusion.[25] Anatomic variants, such

Figure 18-7.
Angiogram demonstrating impaired drainage of a parietal cortical vein into the superior sagittal sinus.

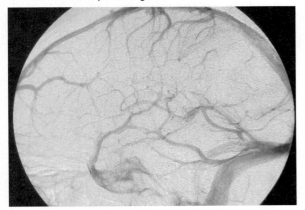

as atresia or hypoplasia of the anterior segment of the superior sagittal sinus, may also simulate occlusion.[27,62] Retrograde filling of the superior ophthalmic vein and delayed venous drainage may be nonspecific signs of increased intracranial pressure.[25,62] Delayed outflow of contrast through the venous system may not occur in venous or dural thrombosis if collateral channels are well developed.[25]

The superior sagittal, straight, and transverse sinuses and the vein of Galen are reliably imaged on lateral and anteroposterior views with intravenous digital angiography.[63] The cavernous and inferior petrosal sinuses are visualized better than with conventional angiography. Other veins are less consistently seen.

Retrograde jugular venography permits visualization of both lateral and cavernous sinuses as well as large portions of the straight and superior sagittal sinuses. Cortical veins and the vein of Galen are occasionally seen. Demonstration of intraluminal thrombus, abnormal collateral vessels, and failure to fill a dural sinus are signs of thrombosis.[62] Retrograde venography may give the false impression of sinus thrombosis if increased intracranial pressure leads to collapse of the sinuses and prevents reflux of dye past the jugular bulb. In cases of septic thrombophlebitis, there is an obvious risk of propagating infection intracranially. Orbital venography may also be useful in the diagnosis of cavernous sinus thrombosis.[18] Direct sinography is rarely performed now because of the need for a burr hole in adults and the risk of air embolism or extension of thrombus into adjacent cortical veins.[27,63] Sinography opacifies scalp veins and extracranial collaterals better than angiography,[8] but the deep venous system is not visualized.[61]

ETIOLOGIES

A number of conditions have been etiologically linked to dural sinus and cerebral venous thrombosis, although most are based on anecdote, and a causal relationship has not always been clear (Table 18-2). In most series, up to 25 percent of cases are idiopathic.[6,7,15,27]

Infection

There has been a dramatic decline since the introduction of antibiotics in the relative incidence of septic intracranial venous sinus disease. In recent publications, only about 10 percent of sinovenous occlusions are due to infection, although it is still the most common cause of cavernous sinus thrombosis and an important etiology

Table 18-2.
Potential etiologies of sinovenous thrombosis

Septic thrombosis	Bacterial (including syphilis), fungal (*Mucor, Aspergillus, Rhizopus*), viral (HIVÅCMV/primary CNS lymphoma), and parasitic (*Trichinella*) infections
Trauma	Penetrating and nonpenetrating head injuries, surgery, intravascular foreign bodies, iopamidol myelography
Hematologic disorders	Polycythemia vera, altitude-induced polycythemia, sickle cell anemia (and trait), cryofibrinogenemia, paroxysmal nocturnal hemoglobinuria, thrombocytosis, thrombocytopenia, severe anemia
Coagulopathy	Antithrombin III deficiency (hereditary or acquired from L-asparaginase or nephrotic syndrome), protein C deficiency, protein S deficiency, activated protein C resistance, 20210 G→A prothrombin mutation, antiphospholipid antibody syndrome, disseminated intravascular coagulation, twin transfusion reaction
Metabolic disorders	Diabetes, homocystinuria, carbon monoxide
Neoplasia	Metastatic (usually hematogenous malignancies), non-metastatic complications, meningioma
Inflammatory states	Behçet's syndrome, inflammatory bowel disease (ulcerative colitis, Crohn's), Wegener's granulomatosis, Cogan's syndrome, Köhlmeier-Degos, polyarteritis nodosa, systemic lupus erythematosus, sarcoidosis
Phakomatoses	Sturge-Weber syndrome
Hemodynamic states	Dehydration, fever, cardiac decompensation
Hormonal	Pregnancy and puerperium, thyrotoxicosis
Skull abnormalities	Osteopetrosis, achondroplasia, craniometaphyseal dysplasia
Vascular disorders	Arteriovenous malformations, arterial occlusions
Medications	Androgens, oral contraceptives, progestogens, L-asparaginase, ε-aminocaproic acid, inhalational agents, ecstasy (3,4-methylenedioxymethamphetamine)
Idiopathic	

of lateral sinus thrombosis.[6,15] Septic cavernous sinus thrombosis most commonly originates by hematogenous spread from the medial third of the face, nose, orbital contents, or paranasal sinuses, by contiguous spread from the ethmoid or sphenoid air cells, or through the lateral sinus from the ear. *Staphylococcus aureus* and *Streptococcal* species are the leading pathogens. Anaerobic and Gram-negative bacteria are more often responsible when the source of infection is the paranasal sinuses or abscessed tooth. The cavernous sinus is the one most frequently involved by fungal infection. *Aspergillus, Rhizopus,* and *Mucor* can involve venous sinuses by direct extension from paranasal sinusitis, meningitis, or hematogenous spread from the lungs or intestine. The bacteriology of lateral sinus thrombosis is similar to that of otitis media, primarily consisting of *Proteus* species, *Staphylococcus, Escherichia coli,* and anaerobes.[13] The superior sagittal sinus is the least often infected, but it can be involved by spread from the nose, paranasal sinuses, or via retrograde extension from the

transverse or cavernous sinuses through Batson's plexus and the vertebral veins, or through the bloodstream in septicemia or meningitis. Extension from osteomyelitis of the skull and extradural or subdural abscesses may also occur. Septic superior sagittal sinus thrombosis is usually due to Gram-positive organisms such as pneumococcus, *S. aureus,* and β-hemolytic *Streptococcus,* but *Klebsiella* and *Pseudomonas* species have also been isolated. Cerebral venous thrombosis may rarely complicate trichinosis,[64,65] syphilis,[10,40] and human immunodeficiency virus with cytomegalovirus coinfection[66] or multicentric primary CNS lymphoma[67] have also been implicated as causes of cerebral thrombophlebitis and dural sinus thrombosis.

Coagulopathy

There have been reports of nonspecific coagulation abnormalities such as increased fibrinogen levels or platelet hyperactivity in patients with sinovenous thrombosis, but several well-defined coagulopathies are clearly associated with sinovenous thrombosis.

Quantitative or qualitative familial antithrombin III deficiencies may produce heparin resistance and cortical vein or sinus thrombosis.[6,68,69] Acquired deficiencies may occur in the nephrotic syndrome as a result of excessive urinary excretion of antithrombin III[70] or after chemotherapy, particularly with L-asparaginase.[71,72] Cerebral venous thrombosis may occur with hereditary deficiencies of protein C or protein S.[73,74] Antigenic levels of protein S may be normal with a reduced free fraction.[75] Deficiencies of coagulation inhibitor protein deficiencies are best treated with warfarin. Activated protein C resistance has also been associated with cerebral venous thrombosis.[76] Most cases are due to a genetic defect referred to as the factor V Leiden mutation, which leads to absence of the protein C cleavage site on the activated factor V molecule.[77] A recently described G→A mutation at nucleotide 20210 of the prothrombin gene is a risk factor for venous but not arterial thrombosis.[78,79] In general, these abnormalities carry a relatively low spontaneous risk of thrombotic events.

Multiple or recurrent venous or arterial thromboses may also complicate the antiphospholipid antibody syndrome when there is either a high titer IgG anticardiolipin antibody or lupus anticoagulant. These antibodies inhibit phospholipid-dependent coagulation tests in vitro but promote thrombosis in vivo. The occurrence of arterial cerebral infarction in the antiphospholipid antibody syndrome and the high recurrence rate are well described.[80,81] Antiphospholipid antibodies may also be a significant predisposing factor for venous sinus thrombosis in patients with or without coexisting thrombotic risk factors.[82,83]

Other hypercoagulable states associated with sinovenous thrombosis include homocystinuria,[84] familial histidine-rich glycoprotein deficiency,[85] antifibrinolytic therapy with ε-aminocaproic acid,[86] and maternal twin transfusion reactions.[87]

Other Hematologic Disorders

Sinus thrombosis has been attributed in some cases to thrombocytosis[88] and thrombocytopenia.[87] Idiopathic cryofibrinogenemia and paraproteinemia may predispose to sinus thrombosis by altering plasma viscosity or coagulability.[89,90] Erythrocyte abnormalities, including polycythemia vera,[91] and erythrocytosis following high altitude exposure have been implicated in cerebral sinovenous occlusion.[92] Severe anemia, particularly iron deficiency and chlorosis, was historically a major reported

cause of sinus thrombosis.[93,94] Paroxysmal nocturnal hemoglobinuria (Marchiafava-Micheli syndrome) is a nonfamilial condition in which episodes of hemolysis are frequently associated with fever, pain, and venous thrombosis. The diagnosis rests on red cell lysis in the presence of acidified serum (Ham test), thrombin (Crosby test), or sucrose.[95] It is likely that sinus thrombosis in sickle cell disease or trait is related to increased viscosity in the face of relative hypoxemia and that the percent of hemoglobin-S is directly proportional to the risk.[96]

Inflammatory Disorders

Angiographically documented cerebral venous and dural sinus thrombosis have been reported in patients with ulcerative colitis and regional enteritis.[97] A history of systemic venous thrombosis has usually been present. Central nervous system venous complications do not necessarily correlate with the duration or severity of intestinal disease. These complications are postulated to arise from a hypercoagulable state, manifested by shortened partial thromboplastin times, increased factor VIII and fibrinogen levels, or thrombocytosis. In some of the published cases, other potential etiologies coexisted with inflammatory bowel disease.

Recent reports of Behçet's syndrome in 20 to 25 percent of Arab patients with sinovenous thrombosis may reflect a high prevalence of Behçet's in the Middle East.[98,99] Neurologic complications occur in 10 to 50 percent of patients with Behçet's syndrome.[100] Venous thrombosis is common but more often involves peripheral than intracranial veins. Benign intracranial hypertension may be the presenting manifestation. Increased fibrinogen levels suggest an abnormality of hemostasis, which may be related to the venous thrombosis.[101,102] Heparin, steroids, and immunosuppressant drugs have been recommended for cerebral venous thrombosis in patients with Behçet's syndrome. Angiographically proven occlusion of the left lateral and straight sinuses has been reported in a patient with meningeal sarcoidosis presenting with pseudotumor cerebri.[103]

Sinovenous occlusion has been reported with a variety of vasculitides. Gilbert and Talbott described a presumed cavernous sinus thrombosis in Cogan's syndrome, a systemic disorder manifested by nonsyphilitic interstitial keratitis, audiologic, and vestibular symptoms.[104] Superior sagittal sinus thrombosis may occur in Kohlmeier-Degos disease (malignant atrophic papulosis), a cutaneosystemic vasculopathy involving skin and intestine,[105] and may be the presenting manifestation.[106] Dural sinus and intracerebral venous thrombosis may also occur during the course of Wegener's granulomatosis,[107] polyarteritis nodosa,[108] or systemic lupus erythematosus.[109] Possible mechanisms of venous sinus thrombosis in systemic lupus include antiphospholipid antibodies, immune complex-mediated vascular damage, and nephrotic syndrome. Patients with nephrotic syndrome have a number of coagulation abnormalities including thrombocytosis, elevated factor V and VIII levels, and decreased factors XI and XII, plasminogen, and antithrombin III, which make them prone to thromboembolic complications, including cerebral sinovenous thrombosis.[70]

Phakomatoses

Sturge-Weber syndrome (trigeminofacial angiomatosis with cerebral calcifications) is a congenital disorder manifested by a port wine nevus in the distribution of the first division of the trigeminal nerve and ipsilateral cortical calcification. Seizures and hemiparesis are common clinical manifestations. Angiographic findings in Sturge-Weber syndrome may be indistinguishable from those of cortical vein or dural sinus thrombosis. Angiographic nonfilling of the superior sagittal sinus suggests agenesis or occlusion of the sinus.[110] There is frequently evidence of impaired superficial cortical venous drainage beneath the leptomeningeal angiomatosis and enlargement or tortuosity of deep venous collaterals.[111] The sagittal sinus may be filled from the contralateral side in patients with a unilateral venous abnormality. Whether the cortical veins are thrombosed or atretic is unclear. Segmental occlusion of the superior sagittal sinus and internal cerebral vein, suggestive of thrombosis, may also be noted. CT findings compatible with infarction in regions corresponding to nonfilling cortical veins on angiography in two patients led Garcia et al to postulate that clinical deterioration in Sturge-Weber results from recurrent venous thromboses in the area of the malformation.[112] Data suggesting that aspirin therapy may prevent neurologic deterioration supports this hypothesis.[113]

Trauma

Penetrating injuries, avulsion of tributary veins, or sinovenous occlusion may follow head trauma.[114] Depressed or compound skull fractures or tangential, nonpenetrating injuries to the vertex may directy damage the superior sagittal sinus or its bridging veins and produce an interhemispheric subdural hematoma. The vein linking the vein of Labbé with the lateral sinus and veins draining the temporal lobes into the petrosal sinuses are also susceptible to injury. Posterior fossa subdural hematomas may result from damage to the superior cerebellar veins. Epidural hematomas may follow trauma to the middle meningeal veins, superior sagittal, lateral, and superior petrosal sinuses.[25] Infratentorial epidural hematomas most frequently follow laceration of the transverse sinus, and carotid cavernous fistulae may arise from trauma to the cavernous sinuses. Laceration of a sinus may lead to air embolism. A syndrome of gait ataxia, headache and vomiting following blunt occipital head trauma may be associated with thrombosis of the sigmoid sinus.[115] Superior sagittal sinus thrombosis following closed head injury may be attributable to endothelial damage and intramural hemorrhage at the site of entry of draining veins.[116] A coagulopathy resulting from head trauma may also contribute to the pathogenesis.[114]

Intravascular Foreign Bodies

The presence of an intravenous foreign body may serve as a nidus for clot formation or extension. Multiple sinus thrombosis has been reported after the insertion of transvenous cardiac pacemakers,[117] central hyperalimentation,[118] and catheter-related subclavian vein thrombosis.[119]

Hormonal

Cerebral venous and dural sinus thrombosis is still a common complication of pregnancy in developing countries. In India, for instance, thrombosis of intracranial veins and dural sinuses is the most common cause of stroke in young women and accounts for 25 percent of maternal deaths.[120] Most cases occur in the first 3 weeks after delivery. Obstetric cases tend to be more acute in onset and self-limited than nonobstetric ones.[121]

Sinovenous thrombosis in a young woman on oral contraceptives was first described nearly 30 years ago. A diagnosis of intracranial sinovenous occlusive disease should be suspected whenever a young woman taking oral contraceptives presents with seizures, focal neurologic deficits, unexplained or persistent headache, or signs of increased intracranial pressure. Extracranial venous structures may be involved simultaneously. Sinus or vein thrombosis usually occurs within 1 year of the initiation of oral contraceptives but may occur after only a few days or weeks.[122,123] Potential mechanisms of this association include oral contraceptive-associated increases in platelet adhesiveness and aggregability, increased circulating coagulation factors, impaired antithrombin III activity, and cryofibrinogenemia. Endothelial proliferation observed in the lateral lacunae of intracranial veins may be of pathophysiologic significance.[124] Irey et al reported focal nodular intimal thickening and subendothelial fibrosis at the site of oral contraceptive-associated arterial thrombosis;[125] it is unknown whether similar pathologic findings exist in the venous system. It is likely that the risk of cerebral venous thrombosis from oral contraceptive use has been modified by the widespread use of low estrogen preparations. Recent studies suggest that low-dose oral contrceptives do not confer any appreciable increase in stroke risk.[126,127] Cerebral sinovenous thrombosis is rarely associated with postmenopausal estrogen replacement therapy.[128] Medroxyprogesterone acetate therapy for breast cancer[57] or the use of androgens[129,130] has also been linked to the development of intracranial venous thrombosis. An association between superior sagittal sinus thrombosis and thyrotoxicosis in Graves' disease has recently been reported.[131]

Neoplasia

A venous sinus can be compressed by adjacent tumor, such as meningioma or metastasis, with or without thrombosis. Solid neoplasms may invade the sinus, and hematogenous ones may infiltrate it. Glomus tumors may obstruct the jugular bulb and compromise venous drainage.[93] Sinus thrombosis can occur in cancer patients without any evidence of local tumor.[71,132] Sigsbee et al recognized two clinical syndromes.[132] The first, occurring early after initiation of chemotherapy, presents with seizures, focal deficits, headache, and altered consciousness and has a relatively good prognosis. The other, manifesting later with fluctuating mental status but no focal signs or seizures, has a poor outcome. Hypercoagulability secondary to the malignant process may be responsible for these nonmetastatic sinus occlusions. Four of the six patients studied by Sigsbee et al had abnormal coagulation parameters. In some cases, chemotherapy may contribute. Impairment of fibrinolysis by steroid therapy may play a significant role. There is frequently a history of recent intrathecal methotrexate therapy. Hemostatic abnormalities caused by L-asparaginase such as hypofibrinogenemia, acquired antithrombin III, and plasminogen deficiencies and depletion of factors IX and XI could conceivably be related to sinus thrombosis in children with acute leukemias receiving this agent.[72]

Miscellaneous Associations

Sinovenous thrombosis in infants and children has frequently been attributed to dehydration.[20] Congestive heart failure, debility, and dehydration have been cited as risks of intracranial venous thrombosis in older adults as well.[1] Dehydration may represent a common thread among cases complicating diabetic ketoacidosis,[133] fever therapy for syphilis, surgery, and use of inhalational drugs[134] or ecstasy.[135] Concomitant arterial and venous occlusion is well described, especially in the older literature. Venous thrombosis may result from ischemia of the sinus wall[91] or release of tissue thromboplastin from arterial cerebral infarction.[8] An underlying hypercoagulable state could provide a common mechanism for both arterial and venous occlusion. Amacher has reported occlusion of the posterior portion of the superior sagittal sinus in one of a set of twins with osteopetrosis, a rare bone dysplasia with failure of normal bone resorption, and persistent chondroid and primitive bony elements.[136] Jugular stenosis or obstruction in the jugular foramen is also common in osteopetrosis and in other disorders affecting the development of the skull base, such as achondroplasia and craniometaphyseal dysplasia.[137]

PROGNOSIS

Systematic data on the natural history of sinovenous thrombosis do not exist. Mortality rates in reported series range from 5 to 80 percent.[6,27,47,93,120,121,138] Early studies likely overestimate mortality due to the difficulty of antemortem diagnosis prior to introduction of modern imaging techniques.

The extent of angiographic involvement of the venous system may not predict outcome as accurately as the clinical assessment in predicting prognosis. The tempo of the clinical course may be a major prognostic factor. Early appearance of the "convulsoparalytic" phase and rapid generalization of seizures are thought to correlate with extension of thrombus into cortical veins and reflect poor outcome.[6,27] Rapid increases in intracranial pressure, increasing seizure frequency, fever, respiratory disturbance, tachycardia, hemorrhagic infarction, bilateral pyramidal signs, meningeal signs, and impairment of consciousness have also been suggested as poor prognostic signs.[7,20,139] Occlusion of deep veins seems to worsen prognosis but does not preclude good recovery.[28] The tendency to liquefaction of ischemic unmyelinated white matter and the delayed rise in intracranial pressure may contribute to the later diagnosis and worse prognosis in infants.

Clinical improvement probably reflects the adequacy of collateral channels rather than recanalization of the occluded lumen.[8] Complete recovery is the rule in survivors.[6,138,140] Residual disability was recorded in only 3 of 48 survivors in Krayenbühl's series[27] and 7 of 31 survivors in Bousser's.[6] In a series of 102 patients with angiographically proven venous sinus thrombosis reported by Villringer et al, 57 percent were neurologically normal on discharge compared with 7 percent of historic controls with arterial thrombosis from the Lausanne Stroke Registry.[141] Hemiparesis, optic atrophy, and subsequent seizures are the most commonly reported sequelae.[6,138] Residual deficit may correlate with chronic mode of onset.[6] Long-term prognosis and risk of recurrence are influenced by the nature of the underlying disease in patients with systemic disorders.

Prior to the introduction of antibiotics, septic venous sinus thrombosis was usually fatal. In reports since 1965, the mortality of cavernous sinus thrombosis has decreased to 13 to 29 percent and morbidity to 23 to 50 percent.[142] In contrast, the introduction of antibiotics has led to a decrease in the incidence of lateral sinus thrombosis with a less dramatic reduction in mortality.[12] A significant drop in mortality from lateral sinus thrombosis at the turn of the century prior to the introduction of antibiotics may be attributable to the development of surgical techniques for the treatment of this disorder.[16]

EVIDENCE

The treatment of sinovenous occlusions is controversial. General measures that are widely recommended include reduction of increased intracranial pressure, anticonvulsants, and antibiotics for infection. Steroids are usually employed for intracranial hypertension and cerebral edema. Fluid restriction, diuretics, and osmotherapy have also been recommended, although caution is advised as dehydration may predispose to venous stasis and further thrombosis. Barbiturates have also been used to lower intracranial pressure in patients with sinus thrombosis.[143,144] Serial lumbar punctures may benefit patients with the syndrome of pseudotumor cerebri. When possible, therapy should be directed at the underlying etiology. Management of hyperglycemia may be indicated.[145]

Antibiotics

Broad spectrum antibiotic coverage should be initiated prior to the return of culture reports when septic sino-

venous thrombosis is suspected. Lateral sinus thrombosis is treated initially with cefotaxime or ceftriaxone, a penicillinase-resistant penicillin such as nafcillin and metronidazole directed at the pathogens most likely to be associated with otitis media or mastoiditis, including *Proteus, E. coli, S. aureus,* and anaerobes. In cases of sagittal sinus thrombosis associated with meningitis, ceftriaxone or cefotaxime is recommended plus ampicillin if the patient is immunocompromised. Nafcillin and metronidazole should be added if the source of infection is dental or a brain abscess. If *Pseudomonas* is the primary organism, a third generation cephalosporin should be combined with an aminoglycoside. Appropriate management of cavernous sinus thrombosis begins with broad spectrum antibiotics having activity against anaerobes and Gram-positive cocci, including penicillinase-resistant *Staphylococci.* A penicillinase-resistant penicillin and either ceftriaxone or cefotaxime are usually recommended for 2 to 4 weeks after disappearance of local signs of infection. Metronidazole should be added if anaerobic infection from the paranasal sinuses or teeth is suspected.[13] In the immunocompromised host, empiric antifungal therapy should also be considered.

Anticoagulants

The primary rationale for heparin in sinovenous thrombosis is to prevent extension of thrombus into cortical veins. The main argument against anticoagulation has been the risks of hemorrhage and potential for heparin-induced thrombocytopenia. In an uncontrolled study, Krayenbühl found that 70 percent of untreated patients died compared with 37 percent of those treated with antibiotics alone and 7 percent of those receiving antibiotics plus oral anticoagulants.[27] Hemorrhagic complications were no more common in the anticoagulated patients. In another uncontrolled series of patients with sinovenous occlusion complicating pregnancy, 10 of 42 (24 percent) heparinized patients died compared with 21 of 47 (45 percent) untreated ones.[138] One fatal hemorrhage occurred in the anticoagulated group. There are anecdotal reports of prompt improvement with anticoagulants in patients who previously had failed to respond to conservative measures.[6,146,147] Hemorrhage during anticoagulation may not prevent satisfactory clinical recovery[6] but may also lead to significant deterioration[122] or death.[148] Anticoagulants are often employed in cavernous sinus thrombosis to prevent thrombosis of the intracavernous carotid artery, septic embolism, or extension of thrombus to contiguous dural sinuses. In a retrospective analysis, Levine et al reported that early institution of anticoagulants decreased morbidity but not mortality from cavernous sinus thrombosis.[149] Anticoagulants may be used for lateral sinus thrombosis to treat systemic embolic phenomena but are otherwise not recommended.[12,14,150]

Intravenous heparin has been subjected to a single randomized, placebo-controlled study in patients with sinovenous thrombosis.[151] The authors enrolled 20 patients with angiographically confirmed aseptic sinovenous occlusion who had no previous anticoagulant or antiplatelet therapy, no life-threatening medical disorders, and neither a contraindication nor a definite indication for heparin. After an initial bolus of 3000 units, heparin doses were adjusted to a target partial thromboplastin time of 80 to 100 s. Ratings were performed by blinded observers using a specially designed severity scale. The baseline characteristics of the two groups were comparable. Most patients had idiopathic superior sagittal sinus thrombosis. The median interval from onset of symptoms to randomization was 12 days. There was a statistically significant improvement in severity scores in the heparin-treated patients at days 7 and 21. After 90 days, there were no deaths and eight complete recoveries in the heparin group compared with three deaths and only one complete recovery in the placebo group. Intracranial hemorrhage was found in three patients randomized to heparin before the onset of anticoagulation and did not preclude clinical recovery. No hemorrhages occurred after starting heparin. Two patients receiving placebo had intracranial hemorrhage at the time of randomization, and an additional three patients in this group subsequently developed intracranial hemorrhage. The authors also did a retrospective study of 102 patients with angiographically verified sinovenous thrombosis during the previous 14 years to assess the effect of dose-adjusted heparin on intracerebral hemorrhage. The mortality rate in the 27 patients treated with heparin after hemorrhage was 15 percent compared with 69 percent among 13 patients not receiving heparin.

Fibrinolytic Therapy

The use of fibrinolytic therapy in sinovenous occlusion is based on anecdotal reports. Di Rocco et al treated five patients with sagittal, lateral, or cavernous sinus thrombosis treated with systemic urokinase followed by prolonged anticoagulation.[152] All improved within 5 days and the occluded venous structures recanalized on repeat angiography done 14 to 18 days after the ictus. Urokinase may be infused locally via direct percutaneous injection into the superior sagittal sinus[153,154] or through transjugular or transfemoral endovascular catheters.[155–158] The largest published experience with transvenous urokinase infusion is uncontrolled but demonstrated angiographic lysis and favorable clinical outcome in 92 percent of treated cases without significant hemorrhagic complications.[159] Good clinical results have also been reported with continuous intrathrombus infusion of recombinant tissue plasminogen activator.[160] Local fibrinolysis may be combined with surgical thrombectomy.[161,162]

Surgical Management

Surgery has a limited role in the treatment of sinovenous occlusion. Decompressive craniotomy or evacuation of hematoma may be beneficial in selected patients. Superior sagittal sinus thrombectomy in cases of nonseptic thrombosis is controversial. Thrombectomy has been recommended for rapid progressive visual loss from intracranial hypertension or life-threatening complications despite appropriate medical therapy.[140] This procedure is of limited benefit when tributary cortical veins are occluded or when there is hemorrhagic infarction. Complication rates are high when thrombus is removed from the posterior two-thirds of the superior sagittal sinus. Definitive surgical procedures in patients with septic lateral sinus thrombosis are aimed at the removal of infected tissue and thrombus. Sindou et al described an extra-anatomic, end-to-end saphenous vein bypass procedure from the lateral sinus to the superficial jugular vein for deteriorating patients in whom thrombectomy is not feasible or when reconstructive procedures are inadequate to repair a sinus invaded by tumor or damaged by trauma.[163] Jugular vein ligation is generally reserved for patients with lateral sinus thrombosis complicated by embolism or systemic sepsis despite adequate medical and surgical therapy. Jugular ligation does not prevent spread of infected thrombus via collaterals but may result in air embolism or injury to the tenth, eleventh, and twelfth cranial nerves.[17] The surgical indications in aseptic lateral sinus thrombosis are similar to those for superior sagittal sinus thrombosis.[16] Surgery is not usually recommended for cavernous sinus thrombosis unless it is intended to remove the source of infection.[18]

TREATMENT RECOMMENDATIONS

Standard therapy of sinovenous thrombosis consists of treatment of cerebral edema and anticonvulsant therapy. Antibiotics should be started immediately when infection is suspected. Broad spectrum coverage should include a third generation cephalosporin and a penicillinase-resistant penicillin with or without metronidazole for anaerobes.

Despite data suggesting the efficacy of anticoagulants in cerebral sinovenous thrombosis, it may still be prudent to withhold heparin from patients with large hematoma or hemorrhagic infarction and medical contraindications to anticoagulants such as active peptic ulcer disease or pulmonary manifestations of Behçet's syndrome.[164] Patients with seizures or focal deficits, suggesting cortical vein involvement, may also be at greater risk from anticoagulation, but heparinization prior to this stage may prevent extension of thrombus into cortical veins. Anticoagulants are advisable in patients who deteriorate during symptomatic or conservative management.[6,146] or who develop concomitant pelvic or deep vein thrombophlebitis.[7] Some authors recommend that all patients with sinovenous thrombosis be anticoagulated unless there is a definite medical contraindication.[15] There are no definitive guidelines regarding the duration of anticoagulation after sinovenous thrombosis. A 6-month course of oral anticoagulants might be appropriate in patients with idiopathic venous thrombosis, but indefinite therapy might be indicated for those with a continuing thrombophilic state.

Data are rare on the use of fibrinolytic therapy. Fibrinolysis may be considered when patients deteriorate despite anticoagulation or have resistant elevations of intracranial pressure. An experienced stroke team, including an interventional neuroradiologist, is necessary when fibrinolytic therapy is contemplated. The role of surgery is primarily limited to removal of a source of infection in cases of septic thrombosis.

ADDENDUM

Since submission of this manuscript, investigators in the Netherlands have completed a randomized, placebo controlled trial of subcutaneous low molecular weight heparin (nadroparin) followed by warfarin.[165] The primary outcome measure of death or a Barthel Index less than 15 after 3 weeks occurred in 20 percent of low molecular heparin patients and 24 percent in the placebo group; however, this difference was not statistically significant. In patients with baseline hemorrhages, poor outcome also occurred less often with nadroparin than placebo without reaching statistical significance.

REFERENCES

1. Towbin A: The syndrome of latent cerebral venous thrombosis: Its frequency and relation to age and congestive heart failure. *Stroke* 4:419, 1973.
2. Scotti LN, Goldman RL, Hardman DR, et al: Venous thrombosis in infants and children. *Radiology* 112:393, 1974.
3. Curé JK, Van Tassell P, Smith MT: Normal and variant anatomy of the dural venous sinuses. *Seminars in Ultrasound, CT and MRI* 15:499, 1994.
4. Meder JF, Chiras J, Roland J, et al: Venous territories of the brain. *J Neuroradiol* 21:118, 1994.
5. de Bruijn SF, Stam J, Kappelle LJ: Thunderclap headache as first symptom of cerebral venous sinus thrombosis: CVST Study Group. *Lancet* 348:1623, 1996.
6. Bousser MG, Chiras J, Bories J, et al: Cerebral venous thrombosis: A review of 38 cases. *Stroke* 16:199, 1985.
7. Gates PC, Barnett HJM: Venous disease: Cortical veins and sinuses, in Barnett HJM, Stein BM, Mohr JP, et al. (eds): *Stroke: Pathophysiology, Diagnosis, and Management.* New York, Churchill Livingstone, 1986, pp 731–746.
8. Kalbag RM: Cerebral venous thrombosis, in Kapp JP, Schmidek HH (eds): *The Cerebral Venous System and its Disorders.* Orlando, Grune and Stratten, 1984, pp 505–536.
9. Monteiro MLR, Hoyt WF, Imes RK: Puerperial cerebral blindness: Transient bilateral occipital blindness from presumed cerebral venous thrombosis. *Arch Neurol* 41:1300, 1984.
10. Lemmi H, Little SC: Occlusion of intracranial venous structures: A consideration of clinical and electro-encephalographic findings. *Arch Neurol* 3:252, 1960.
11. Munderloh S, Schnapf D, Coker S, et al: Changing ventricular size in dural sinus thrombosis. *Comput Tomogr* 5:11, 1981.
12. Teichgraeber JF, Per-Lee JH, Turner JS, Jr: Lateral sinus thrombosis: A modern perspective. *Laryngoscope* 92:744, 1982.
13. Southwick FS: Septic thrombophlebitis of major dural venous sinuses. *Curr Clin Topics Infect Dis* 15:179, 1995.
14. Sneed WF: Lateral sinus thrombosis. *Am J Otol* 4:258, 1983.
15. Bousser MG, Russell RR: *Cerebral Venous Thrombosis.* London, W. B. Saunders Company Ltd., 1997.
16. Goldenberg RA: Lateral sinus thrombosis: Medical or surgical treatment? *Arch Otolaryngol* 111:56, 1985.
17. Smith BH: Infections of the dura and its venous sinuses, in Baker AB, Baker LH, (eds): *Clinical Neurology,* 1984, pp 1–34.
18. Karlin RJ, Robinson WA: Septic cavernous sinus thrombosis. *Ann Emerg Med* 13:449, 1984.
19. Kaplan B, Mickle JP: Cavernous sinus thrombosis, in Kapp JP, Schmidek HH (eds): *The Cerebral Venous System and its Disorders,* Orlando, Grune and Stratten, 1984, pp 537–546.

20. Kalbag RML, Woolf AL: Thrombosis and thrombophlebitis of cerebral veins and dural sinuses, in Vinken PJ, Bruyn GW, (eds): *Handbook of Clinical Neurology,* Amsterdam, Elsevier, 1972, pp 422–446.

21. Geggel HS, Isenberg SJ: Cavernous sinus thrombosis as a cause of unilateral blindness. *Ann Ophthalmol* 14:569, 1982.

22. Zahller M, Spector RH, Skoglund RR, et al: Cavernous sinus thrombosis. *Western J Med* 133:44, 1980.

23. Oliven A, Harel D, Rosenfeld T, et al: Hypopituitarism after aseptic cavernous sinus thrombosis. *Neurology* 30:897, 1980.

24. Borgohain R, Radhakrishna H, Singh AK, et al: Bilateral cavernous sinus thrombosis causing Korsakoff's amnesic syndrome (Letter). *J Neurol Neurosurg Psychiatry* 58:514, 1995.

25. Schmidek HH, Auer LM, Kapp JP: The cerebral venous system. *Neurosurgery* 17:663, 1985.

26. Smith RR, Sanford RA: Disorders of the deep cerebral veins, in Kapp JP, Schmidek HH, (eds): *The Cerebral Venous System and its Disorders,* Orlando, Grune and Stratten, 1984, pp 547–555.

27. Krayenbuhl HA: Cerebral venous and sinus thrombosis. *Clin Neurosurg* 14:1, 1967.

28. Justich E, Lammer J, Fritsch G, et al: CT diagnosis of thrombosis of dural sinuses in childhood. *Eur J Radiol* 4:294, 1984.

29. Johnson S, Greenwood R, Fishman MA: Internal cerebral vein thrombosis. *Arch Neurol* 28:205, 1973.

30. Solomon GE, Engel M, Hecht HL, et al: Progressive dyskinesia due to internal cerebral vein thrombosis. *Neurology* 32:769, 1982.

31. Hughes JT: Venous infarction of the spinal cord. *Neurology* 21:794, 1971.

32. Kim RC, Smith HR, Henbest ML, et al: Nonhemorrhagic venous infarction of the spinal cord. *Ann Neurol* 15:379, 1984.

33. Bridgers SL, Strauss E, Smith EO, et al: Demonstration of superior sagittal sinus thrombosis by indium-111 platelet scintigraphy. *Arch Neurol* 43:1079, 1986.

34. Shinohara Y, Takagi S, Kobatake K, et al: Influence of cerebral venous obstruction on cerebral circulation in humans. *Arch Neurol* 39:479, 1982.

35. Wardlaw JM, Vaughan GT, Steers AJ, et al: Transcranial Doppler ultrasound findings in cerebral venous sinus thrombosis: Case report. *J Neurosurg* 80:332, 1994.

36. Valdueza JM, Schultz M, Harms L, et al: Venous transcranial Doppler ultrasound monitoring in acute dural sinus thrombosis: Report of two cases. *Stroke* 26:1196, 1995.

37. Becker G, Bogdahn U, Gehlberg C, et al: Transcranial color-coded real-time sonography of intracranial veins: Normal values of blood flow velocities and findings in superior sagittal sinus thrombosis. *J Neuroimag* 5:87, 1995.

38. Valdueza JM, Harms L, Doepp F, et al: Venous microembolic signals detected in patients with cerebral sinus thrombosis. *Stroke* 28:1607, 1997.

39. Ral KCVG, Knipp HC, Wagner EJ: Computed tomographic findings in cerebral sinus and venous thrombosis. *Radiology* 140:391, 1981.

40. Zilkha A, Daiz AS: Computed tomography in the diagnosis of superior sagittal sinus thrombosis. *J Comput Assist Tomogr* 4:124, 1980.

41. Leach JL, Jones BV, Tomsick TA, et al: Normal appearance of arachnoid granulations on contrast-enhanced CT and MR of the brain: Differentiation from dural sinus disease. *Am J Neuroradiol* 17:1523, 1996.

42. Patronas NJ, Duda EE, Mirfakhraee M, et al: Superior sagittal sinus thrombosis diagnosed by computed tomography. *Surg Neurol* 15:11, 1981.

43. Ford K, Sarwar M: Computed tomography of dural sinus thrombosis. *Am J Neuroradiol* 2:539, 1981.

44. Anxionnat R, Blanchet B, Dormont D, et al: Present status of computerized tomography and angiography in the diagnosis of cerebral thrombophlebitis cavernous sinus thrombosis excluded. *J Neuroradiol* 21:59, 1994.

45. Eick JJ, Miller KD, Bell KA, et al: Computed tomography of deep cerebral venous thrombosis in children. *Radiology* 140:399, 1981.

46. Chiras J, Bousser MG, Meder JF, et al: CT in cerebral thrombophlebitis. *Neuroradiology* 27:145, 1985.

47. Buonanno FS, Moody DM, Ball MR, et al: Computed cranial tomographic findings in cerebral sinovenous occlusion. *J Comput Assist Tomogr* 2:281, 1978.

48. Shinohara Y, Yoshitoshi M, Yoshii F: Appearance and disappearance of empty delta sign in superior sagittal sinus thrombosis. *Stroke* 17:1282, 1986.

49. Brant-Zawadzki M, Chang GY, McCarty GE: Computed tomography in dural sinus thrombosis. *Arch Neurol* 39:446, 1982.

50. Ulmer JL, Elster AD: Physiologic mechanisms underlying the delayed delta sign. *Am J Neuroradiol* 12:647, 1991.

51. Anderson SC, Shah CP, Murtagh FR: Congested deep subcortical veins as a sign of dural venous thrombosis: MR and CT correlations. *J Comput Assist Tomogr* 11:1059, 1987.

52. Ingstrup HM, Jorgensen PS: Case report: Tentorial changes in sigmoid sinus thrombosis. *J Comput Assist Tomogr* 5:760, 1981.

53. Casey SO, Alberico RA, Patel M, et al: Cerebral CT venography. *Radiology* 198:163, 1996.

54. Macchi PJ, Grossman RI, Gomori JM, et al: High field MR imaging of cerebral venous thrombosis. *J Comput Assist Tomogr* 10:10, 1986.

55. McMurdo SK, Brant-Zawadzki M, Bradley WG, et al: Dural sinus thrombosis: Study using intermediate field strength MR imaging. *Radiology* 161:83, 1986.

56. Dormont D, Anxionnat R, Evrard S, et al: MRI in cerebral venous thrombosis. *J Neuroradiol* 21:81, 1994.

57. Takahashi S, Higano S, Kurihara N, et al: Contrast-enhanced MR imaging of dural sinus thrombosis: Demonstration of the thrombosis and collateral venous channels. *Clin Radiol* 49:639, 1994.

58. Yuh WT, Simonson TM, Wang AM, et al: Venous sinus occlusive disease: MR findings. *Am J Neuroradiol* 15:309, 1994.

59. Dormont D, Sag K, Biondi A, et al: Gadolinium-enhanced MR of chronic dural sinus thrombosis. *Am J Neuroradiol* 16:1347, 1995.

60. Vogl TJ, Bergman C, Villringer A, et al: Dural sinus thrombosis: Value of venous MR angiography for diagnosis and follow-up. *Am J Roentgenol* 162:1191, 1994.

61. Askenasy HM, Kosary IZ, Braham J: Thrombosis of the longitudinal sinus: Diagnosis by carotid angiography. *Neurology* 12:288, 1962.

62. Vines F: Clinical radiologic correlates in cerebral venous occlusive disease. *Radiology* 98:9, 1971.

63. Modic MT, Weinstein MA, Starnes DL, et al: Intravenous digital angiography of the intracranial veins and dural sinuses. *Radiology* 146:383, 1983.

64. el Koussa S, Chemaly R, Fabre-Bou Abboud V, et al: Trichinosis and cerebral sinocavernous thrombosis. *Rev Neurol* 150:464, 1994.

65. Evans RW, Pattern BM: Trichinosis associated with superior sagittal sinus thrombosis (Letter). *Ann Neurol* 11:216, 1982.

66. Meyohas MC, Roullet E, Rouzioux C, et al: Cerebral venous thrombosis and dual primary infection with human immunodeficiency virus and cytomegalovirus. *J Neurol Neurosurg Psychiatry* 52:1010, 1989.

67. Doberson MJ, Kleinschmidt-DeMasters BK: Superior sagittal sinus thrombosis in a patient with acquired immunodeficiency syndrome. *Arch Pathol Lab Med* 118:844, 1994.

68. Ambruso DR, Jacobson LJ, Hathaway WE: Inherited antithrombin III deficiency and cerebral thrombosis in a child. *Pediatrics* 65:125, 1980.

69. Kobayashi S, Hino H, Tazaki Y: Superior sagittal sinus thrombosis due to familial antithrombin III deficiency: Case report of two families. *Rinsho Shinkeisaku* 20:904, 1980.

70. Lau SO, Bock GH, Edson JR, et al: Sagittal sinus thrombosis in the nephrotic syndrome. *J Pediatr* 97:948, 1980.

71. Lockman LA, Mastri A, Priest JR, et al: Dural venous sinus thrombosis in acute lymphoblastic leukemia. *Pediatrics* 66:943, 1980.

72. Steinherz PG, Miller LP, Ghavimi F, et al: Dural sinus thrombosis in children with acute lymphoblastic leukemia. *JAMA* 246:2837, 1981.

73. Confavreux C, Brunet P, Petiot P, et al: Congenital protein C deficiency and superior sagittal sinus thrombosis causing isolated intracranial hypertension. *J Neurol Neurosurg Psychiatry* 57:655, 1994.

74. Engesser L, Broekmans AW, Briet E, et al: Hereditary protein S deficiency: Clinical manifestations. *Ann Intern Med* 106:677, 1987.

75. Cros D, Comp PC, Beltran G, et al: Superior sagittal sinus thrombosis in a patient with protein S deficiency. *Stroke* 21:633, 1990.

76. Dulli DA, Luzzio CC, Williams EC, et al: Cerebral venous thrombosis and activated protein C resistance. *Stroke* 27:1731, 1996.

77. Svensson PJ, Dahlbäck B: Resistance to activated protein C as a basis for venous thrombosis. *N Engl J Med* 330:517, 1994.

78. Conard J, Brouzes C, Biousse V, et al: Frequency of the 20210 G→A mutation in the 3′-untranslated region of the prothrombin gene in 35 patients with cerebral venous thrombosis. *Stroke* 29:319, 1998.

79. Reuner KH, Ruf A, Grau A, et al: Prothrombin gene G20210 to A transition is a risk factor for cerebral venous thrombosis. *Stroke* 29:1765, 1998.

80. Levine SR, Brey RL, Sawaya KL, et al: Recurrent stroke and recurrent thrombo-occlusive events in the antiphospholipid antibody syndromee. *Neurology* 38:119, 1995.

81. The Antiphospholipid Antibodies in Stroke Study: Anticardiolipin antibodies are an independent risk factor for for first ischemic stroke. *Neurology* 1993:2069, 1993.

82. Carhuapoma JR, Panayiotis M, Levine SR: Cerebral venous thrombosis and anticardiolipin antibodies. *Stroke* 28:2363, 1997.

83. Levine SR, Kieran S, Puzio K, et al: Cerebral venous thrombosis with lupus anticoagulants: Report of two cases. *Stroke* 18:801, 1987.

84. Cochran FB, Packman S: Homocystinuria presenting as sagittal sinus thrombosis. *Eur Neurol* 32:1, 1992.

85. Shigekiyo T, Ohshima T, Oka H, et al: Congenital histidine-rich glycoprotein deficiency. *Thromb Haemost* 70:263, 1993.

86. Achiron A, Gornish M, Melamed E: Cerebral sinus thrombosis as a potential hazard of antifibrinolytic treatment in menorrhagia. *Stroke* 21:817, 1990.

87. Averback P: Primary cerebral venous thrombosis in young adults: The diverse manifestations of an under recognized disease. *Ann Neurol* 3:81, 1978.

88. Murphy MF, Clarke CR, Brearley RL: Superior sagittal sinus thrombosis and essential thrombocythaemia. *Br Med J Clin Res Ed* 287:1344, 1983.

89. Dunsker SB, Torres-Reyes E, Peden JC, Jr: Pseudotumor cerebri associated with idiopathic cryofibrinogenemia: Report of a case. *Arch Neurol* 23:120, 1970.

90. Gilman JK, Smith CH, Davis CE, et al: Benign intracranial hypertension, monoclonal gammopathy, and superior sagittal sinus thrombosis. *South Med J* 76:658, 1983.

91. Melamed E, Rachmilewitz EA, Reches A, et al: Aseptic cavernous sinus thrombosis after internal carotid arterial occlusion in polycythaemia vera. *J Neurol Neurosurg Psychiatry* 39:320, 1976.

92. Fujimaki T, Matsutani A, Asai A, et al: Dural venous sinus thrombosis due to high altitude polycythemia. *J Neurosurg* 64:148, 1986.

93. Kalbag RM: Dural sinus thrombosis. *J Neurol Neurosurg Psychiatry* 30:586, 1967.

94. Hartfield DS, Lowry NJ, Keene DL, et al: Iron deficiency: A cause of stroke in infants and children. *Pediatr Neurol* 16:50, 1997.

95. Johnson RV, Kaplan SR, Blailock ZR: Cerebral venous thrombosis in paroxysmal nocturnal hemoglobinuria: Marchiafava-Micheli syndrome. *Neurology* 20:681, 1970.

96. Oguz M, Aksungur EH, Soyupak SK, et al: Vein of Galen and sinus thrombosis with bilateral thalamic infarcts in sickle cell anaemia: CT follow-up and angiographic demonstration. *Neuroradiology* 36:155, 1994.

97. Schneiderman JH, Sharpe JA, Sutton DMC: Cerebral and retinal complications of inflammatory bowel disease. *Ann Neurol* 5:331, 1979.

98. Daif A, Awada A, al-Rajeh S, et al: Cerebral venous thrombosis in adults: A study of 40 cases from Saudi Arabia. *Stroke* 26:1193, 1995.

99. Najim al-Din AS, Mubaidin A, Wriekat AL, et al: Risk factors of aseptic intracranial venous occlusive disease. *Acta Neurol Scand* 90:412, 1994.

100. Bousser MG, Bletry O, Launay M, et al: Cerebral venous thrombosis in Behçet's disease *Rev Neurol* 136:753, 1980.

101. Imaizumi M, Nukada T, Yoneda S, et al: Behçet's disease with sinus thrombosis and arteriovenous malformation in brain. *J Neurol* 222:215, 1980.

102. Harper CM, Jr, O'Neil BP, O'Duffy JD, et al: Intracranial hypertension in Behçet's disease: Demonstration of sinus occlusion with use of digital subtraction angiography. *Mayo Clin Proc* 60:419, 1985.

103. Byrne JV, Lawton CA: Meningeal sarcoidosis causing intracranial hypertension secondary to dural sinus thrombosis. *Br J Radiol* 56:755, 1983.

104. Gilbert WS, Talbot FJ: Cogan's syndrome: Signs of periarteritis nodosa and cerebral venous sinus thrombosis. *Arch Ophthalmol* 82:633, 1969.

105. Dastur DK, Singhal BS, Schroff HJ: CNS involvement in malignant atrophic papulosis (Kohlmeier-Degos disease): Vasculopathy and coagulopathy. *J Neurol Neurosurg Psychiatry* 44:156, 1981.

106. Petiit WAHJ, Soso MJ, Higman H: Degos disease: Neurologic complications and cerebral angiography. *Neurology* 32:1305, 1982.

107. Mickle JP, McLennan JE, Chi JG, et al: Cortical vein thrombosis in Wegener's granulomatosis. *J Neurol Neurosurg Psychiatry* 46:248, 1977.

108. Kulawik H, Hoppe W: Thrombosis of intracranial veins and sinus in periarteritis nodos. *Schweizer Arch Neurol Neurochi Psychiatr* 109:237, 1971.

109. Vidailhet M, Piette JC, Wechsler B, et al: Cerebral venous thrombosis in systemic lupus erythematosus. *Stroke* 21:1226, 1990.

110. Poser CM, Taveras JM: Cerebral angiography in encephalo-trigeminal angiomatosis. *Radiology* 68:327, 1957.

111. Bentson JR, Wilson GH, Newton TH: Cerebral venous drainage patterns of the Sturge-Weber syndrome. *Radiology* 101:110, 1971.

112. Garcia JC, Roach ES, McLean WTJ: Recurrent thrombotic deterioration in the Sturge-Weber syndrome. *Child's Brain* 8:427, 1981.

113. Roach ES, Riela SR, McLean WTJ, et al: Aspirin therapy for Sturge-Weber syndrome (Abstract). *Ann Neurol* 18:387, 1985.

114. Hesselbrock R, Sawaya R, Tomsick T, et al: Superior sagittal sinus thrombosis after closed head injury. *Neurosurgery* 16:825, 1985.

115. Taha JM, Crone KR, Berger TS, et al: Sigmoid sinus thrombosis after closed head injury in children. *Neurosurgery* 32:541, 1993. Discussion, 545.

116. Carrie AW, Jaffé FA: Thrombosis of superior sagittal sinus caused by trauma without penetrating injury. *J Neurosurg* 11:173, 1954.

117. Girard DE, Reuler JB, Mayer BS, et al: Cerebral venous sinus thrombosis due to indwelling transvenous pacemaker catheter. *Arch Neurol* 37:113, 1980.

118. Souter RG, Mitchell A: Spreading cortical venous sinus thrombosis due to infusion of hyperosmolar solution into the internal jugular vein. *Br Med J* 285:935, 1982.

119. Birdwell BG, Yeager R, Whitsett TL: Pseudotumor cerebri: A complication of catheter-induced subclavian vein thrombosis. *Arch Intern Med* 154:808, 1994.

120. Bansal BC, Gupta RR, Prakash C: Stroke during pregnancy and puerperium in young females below the age of 40 years as a result of cerebral venous/venous sinus thrombosis. *Jpn Heart J* 21:171, 1980.

121. Cantu C, Barinagarrementeria F: Cerebral venous thrombosis associated with pregnancy and puerperium: Review of 67 cases. *Stroke* 24:1880, 1993.

122. Rousseaux P, Bernard MH, Scherpereel B, et al: Thrombose des sinus veineux intra-crâniens après prise d'estro-progestiffs-4 cas. *Nouv Presse Méd* 6:2049, 1977.

123. Dindar F, Platts ME: Intracranial venous thrombosis complicating oral contraception. *Can Med Assoc J* 111:545, 1974.

124. Poltera AA: The pathology of intracranial venous thrombosis in oral contraception. *J Pathol* 106:209, 1972.

125. Irey NS, Manion WC, Taylor HB: Vascular lesions in women taking oral contraceptives. *Arch Path* 89:1, 1970.

126. Schwartz SM, Petitti DB, Siscovick DS, et al: Stroke and risk of low-dose oral contraceptives in young women: A pooled analysis of two U.S. studies. *Stroke* 29:2277, 1998.

127. World Health Organization Collaborative Study of Cardiovascular Disease and Steroid Hormone Contraception: Ischemic stroke and combined oral contraceptives: Results of an international, multicenter, case-control study. *Lancet* 348:498, 1996.

128. Strachan R, Hughes D, Cowie R: Thrombosis of the straight sinus complicating hormone replacement therapy. *Br J Neurosurg* 9:805, 1995.

129. Shiozawa Z, Yamada H, Mabuchi C, et al: Superior sagittal sinus thrombosis associated with androgen therapy for hypoplastic anemia. *Ann Neurol* 12:578, 1982.

130. Jaillard AS, Hommel M, Mallaret M: Venous sinus thrombosis associated with androgens in a healthy young man. *Stroke* 25:212, 1994.

131. Siegert CE, Smelt AH, de Bruin TW: Superior sagittal

sinus thrombosis and thyrotoxicosis: Possible association in two cases. *Stroke* 26:496, 1995.

132. Sigsbee B, Deck MD, Posner JB: Nonmetastatic superior sagittal sinus thrombosis complicating systemic cancer. *Neurology* 29:139, 1979.

133. Ata M: Cerebral infarction due to intracranial sinus thrombosis. *Journal of Clinical Pathology* 18:636, 1965.

134. Murthy BV, Wenstone R: Cerebral venous thrombosis associated with inhalational drug abuse. *Rhinology* 34:188, 1996.

135. Rothwell PM, Grant R: Cerebral venous sinus thrombosis induced by 'ecstasy' (Letter). *J Neurol Neurosurg Psychiatry* 56:1035, 1993.

136. Amacher AL: Neurological complications of osteopetrosis. *Childs Brain* 3:257, 1977.

137. Curé JK, Van Tassel P: Congenital and acquired abnormalities of the dural venous sinuses. *Seminars in Ultrasound, CT and MR* 15:520, 1994.

138. Srinivasan K: Puerperal cerebral venous and arterial thrombosis. *Semin Neurol* 8:222, 1988.

139. Cantu C, Barinagarrementeria F: Cerebral venous thrombosis: Short-term prognosis. *Stroke* 29:316, 1998.

140. Estanol B, Rodriguez A, Conte G, et al: Intracranial venous thrombosis in young women. *Stroke* 10:680, 1979.

141. Villringer A, Mehraein S, Einhaupl KM: Pathophysiological aspects of cerebral sinus venous thrombosis (SVT). *J Neuroradiol* 21:72, 1994.

142. Yarington CT, Jr: Cavernous sinus thrombosis revisited. *Proc Royal Soc Med* 70:456, 1977.

143. Hanley DF, Feldman E, Borel CO, et al: Treatment of sagittal sinus thrombosis associated with cerebral hemorrhage and intracranial hypertension. *Stroke* 19:903, 1988.

144. Maruishi M, Kato H, Nawashiro H, et al: Successful treatment of increased intracranial pressure by barbiturate therapy in a patient with severe sinus thrombosis after failure of osmotic therapy: A case report. *Acta Neurochir* 120:88, 1993.

145. Jacewicz M, Plum F. Hyperglycemia: An important risk factor for cerebral infarction and early death in cerebral venous and dural thrombosis. *Stroke* 19:141, 1988.

146. Castaigne P, Laplane D, Bousser MG: Superior sagittal sinus thrombosis (Letter). *Arch Neurol* 34:788, 1977.

147. Fairburn B: Intracranial venous thrombosis complicating oral contraception: Treatment with anticoagulant drugs. *Br Med J* 2:647, 1973.

148. Gettelfinger DM, Kokmen E: Superior sagittal sinus thrombosis. *Arch Neurol* 34:2, 1977.

149. Levine SR, Twyman RE, Gilman S: The role of anticoagulation in cavernous sinus thrombosis. *Neurology* 38:517, 1988.

150. Hawkins DB: Lateral sinus thrombosis: A sometimes unexpected diagnosis. *Laryngoscope* 95:674, 1985.

151. Einhaupl KM, Villringer A, Meister W, et al: Heparin treatment in sinus venous thrombosis. *Lancet* 338:597, 1991. Erratum: *Lancet* 338:958, 1991.

152. Di Rocco C, Iannelli A, Leone G, et al: Heparin-urokinase treatment in aseptic dural sinus thrombosis. *Arch Neurol* 38:431, 1981.

153. Higashida RT, Helmer E, Halbach VV, et al: Direct thrombolytic therapy for superior sagittal sinus thrombosis. *Am J Neuroradiol* 10:S4, 1989.

154. Scott JA, Pascuzzi RM, Hall PV, et al: Treatment of dural sinus thrombosis with local urokinase infusion. *J Neurosurg* 68:284, 1988.

155. Smith TP, Higashida RT, Barnwell SL, et al: Treatment of dural sinus thrombosis by urokinase infusion. *Am J Neuroradiol* 15:801, 1994.

156. Khoo KB, Long FL, Tuck RR, et al: Cerebral venous sinus thrombosis associated with the primary antiphospholipid syndrome: Resolution with local thrombolytic therapy. *Med J Austr* 162:30, 1995.

157. Barnwell SL, Higashida RT, Halbach VV, et al: Direct endovascular thrombolytic therapy for dural sinus thrombosis. *Neurosurgery* 28:135, 1991.

158. Gurley MB, King TS, Tsai FY: Sigmoid sinus thrombosis associated with internal jugular venous occlusion: Direct thrombolytic treatment. *J Endovasc Surg* 3:306, 1996.

159. Horowitz M, Purdy P, Unwin H, et al: Treatment of dural sinus thrombosis using selective catheterization and urokinase. *Ann Neurol* 38:58, 1995.

160. Frey JL, Muro GJ, McDougall CG, et al: Intracranial venous thrombosis: Direct thrombolysis with rt-PA. *Stroke* 29:305, 1998.

161. Persson L, Lilja A: Extensive dural sinus thrombosis treated by surgical removal and local streptokinase infusion. *Neurosurgery* 26:117, 1990.

162. Kourtopoulos H, Christie M, Rath B: Open thrombectomy combined with thrombolysis in massive intracranial sinus thrombosis. *Acta Neurochir (Wien)* 128:171, 1994.

163. Sindou M, Mercier P, Bokor J, et al: Bilateral thrombosis of the transverse sinuses: Microsurgical revascularization with venous bypass. *Surg Neurol* 13:215, 1980.

164. Bank I, Weart C: Dural sinus thrombosis in Behçet's disease. *Arthritis Rheum* 27:816, 1984.

165. de Bruijn SF, Stam J: Randomized, placebo-controlled trial of anticoagulant treatment with low-molecular-weight heparin for cerebral sinus thrombosis. *Stroke* 30:484, 1999.

Chapter 19

DIAGNOSIS AND MANAGEMENT OF CENTRAL NERVOUS SYSTEM VASCULITIS

Chelsea S. Kidwell
David S. Liebeskind
Jeffrey L. Saver

INTRODUCTION

Vasculitis affecting the central nervous system remains an intriguing but poorly understood entity that poses diagnostic and treatment challenges for physicians and patients alike. Vasculitis (or angiitis) is defined as an inflammation of blood vessels that leads to ischemic tissue damage. Most experts prefer to distinguish primary (or isolated) angiitis of the central nervous system from secondary causes (systemic vasculitides, connective tissue disorders, drugs/toxins, malignancy, or infections).[1] Central nervous system (CNS) vasculitis can be classified by the size and the type of vessels affected or more commonly by the underlying pathogenic mechanism (Table 19-1). Many types display a characteristic histopathologic pattern. In the central nervous system, vasculitis has protean manifestations and multiple causes. Unfortunately, the nonspecific clinical presentations and lack of disease-specific markers often make diagnosis difficult. Although not a common cause of stroke, it is an important entity to identify. CNS vasculitis is treatable in most cases but is often devastating or fatal if not treated aggressively early in its course. This chapter will provide a general overview of vasculitis affecting the central nervous system including epidemiology, clinical manifestations, diagnosis and treatment, followed by more detailed discussion of specific entities.

CNS vasculitis, either primary or secondary to other disease states, is relatively rare. Overall incidence is not well documented in the general population. In series of patients with stroke under age 45, vasculitis is found in 0 to 19 percent of patients.[2] As major academic centers may only treat a few cases per year, much of the available data come from small case series. Both males and females of all ages may be affected, and it is an important entity to consider in the differential diagnosis of stroke in the young patient. Clinical manifestations of CNS vasculitis are varied and often nonspecific including ischemic or hemorrhagic stroke, encephalopathy, headache, cranial neuropathies, and occasionally myelopathy. The onset may be acute, subacute, or insidious and the course self-limiting, indolent, or fulminant. The presentation generally depends on the size, distribution, extent, and location of vessels involved. Other systemic signs or symptoms (fever, arthritis/arthralgias, rash, pulmonary or renal dysfunction) may provide clues to secondary causes (rheumatologic syndromes, infections).

On histologic analysis, involved vessels demonstrate infiltration of one or more layers by inflammatory cells including polymorphonuclear cells, mononuclear cells, giant cells, and occasionally eosinophils (Fig. 19-1, color inserts 2–3). The inflammatory response causes structural injury within the vessel wall, often with fibrinoid necrosis (Fig. 19-2, color insert 4). Luminal narrowing or obstruction (Fig. 19-3, color insert 5) results in ischemia or, alternatively, wall injury may lead to aneurysm formation with resultant hemorrhage.

Table 19-1.
Differential diagnosis/classification of CNS vasculitides

Primary CNS vasculitides		Primary angiitis of the central nervous system Cogan's syndrome Eales disease
Secondary CNS vasculitides	Systemic vasculitides	Polyarteritis nodosa Giant cell arteritis (temporal arteritis) Takayasu's arteritis Wegener's granulomatosis Henoch-Schonlein purpura Mixed essential cryoglobulinemia Churg-Strauss Other hypersensitivity vasculitides Behçet's disease Neurosarcoidosis
	Connective tissue diseases	Systemic lupus erythematosus Rheumatoid arthritis Scleroderma Mixed connective tissue disease Sjogren's syndrome Ankylosing spondylitis Reiter's syndrome
	Malignancy	Hodgkin's lymphoma Non-Hodgkin's lymphoma Leukemia Metastatic small cell lung cancer Lymphomatoid granulomatois
	Infections	Bacterial meningoencephalitis Basilar meningitis—fungal, AFB Syphilis Lyme disease Viral, retroviral Protozoal Mycoplasma Rickettsial
	Drug-induced/toxins	Cocaine Amphetamine Ephedrine Allopurinol Phenylpropanolamine Ergotamine Heroin
	Other	Inflammatory bowel disease Acute posterior multifocal placoid pigment epitheliopathy Cerebral amyloid angiopathy

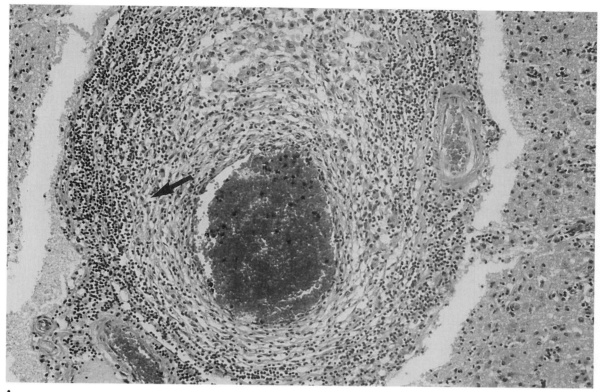

A

Figure 19-1.
A *perivascular inflammatory infiltrate in a patient with PACNS (10×) (See also color insert 2.)*

The size, location, and histologic features characteristic of some types of vasculitis may provide some clues to the underlying pathophysiologic mechanism. The final common pathway, however, in all CNS vasculitides is acute vascular inflammation leading to tissue ischemia. If severe or untreated, vessels may fibrose and scar, leading to irreversible injury. Proposed pathogenic mechanisms include antibody-mediated damage, cell-mediated immunity, direct vessel invasion, and injury by microbial pathogens or other cytotoxic mechanisms.

Immune complexes may circulate in the bloodstream or form in the vessel wall in situ and initiate an inflammatory response. Immune complexes play a role in hypersensitivity vasculitides, polyarteritis nodosa, and possibly some infectious and toxin-related vasculitic processes. Isolated antibodies expressed against vessel wall neoantigens may be the mechanism of vasculitis in Kawasaki's disease and Wegener's granulomatosis.[3] In

cell-mediated vasculitis, T cells interact with endothelial or other vessel wall cells leading to release of cytokines and induction of adhesion molecules, leading to further inflammatory responses. Nonspecific vascular inflammation may also occur in response to vessel injury. This mechanism may play a role in atherosclerosis, hypertension, infection, or toxin-induced processes.

Recently, increased understanding of mechanisms of immune-related injury has shed some light on the pathogenesis of some of these disorders. Three physiologic processes important in immune-mediated vascular injury are induction of adhesion molecules modulated by cytokines, modulation of vasomotor tone by nitric oxide and endothelins, and increased regional coagulation.[4]

Diagnosis of CNS vasculitis relies on a high index of suspicion based on the clinical presentation combined with thorough laboratory, radiographic, and tissue eval-

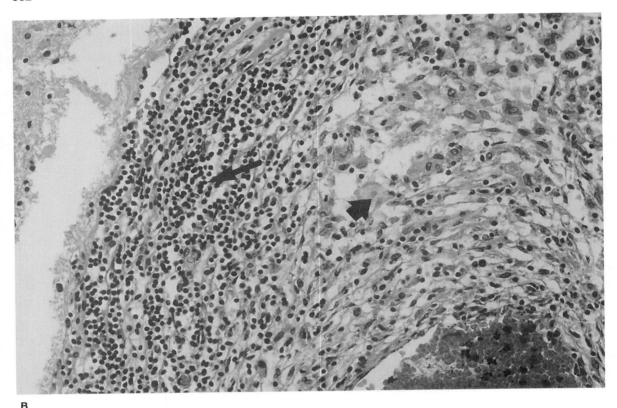

B

Figure 19-1 (*Continued*).
B   *detailed view of inflammatory infiltrate with polymorphonuclear cells* (long arrow) *and mononu-clear cells* (short arrow) *(20×). (See also color insert 3.)*

uation (Table 19-2). The diagnosis is often difficult to make, and no single test is both highly sensitive and specific. Nonspecific markers of a systemic inflammatory response are frequently elevated with secondary CNS vasculitides (erythrocyte sedimentation rate [ESR], complement levels, C-reactive protein). Positive auto-immune antibody titers (antineutrophilic cytoplasmic antibodies [ANCA], antinuclear antibodies [ANA], rheumatoid factor-RF) may suggest the presence of an underlying rheumatologic disorder. A test for human immunodeficiency virus (HIV) should be routinely performed as several cases of CNS angiitis have been found in HIV-positive patients. Patients should also be screened for lymphoma due to the association between Hodgkin's lymphoma and isolated CNS vasculitis.[5] In 50 to 90 percent of patients, cerebral spinal fluid (CSF) analysis reveals nonspecific inflammatory changes,[6] including increased protein (generally 100 to 150 mg/dL,

although much higher levels may occur)[7] and a mild-to-moderate leukocytosis (generally <50 to 80 cells per hpf, although higher counts may be observed). CSF analyses should include viral, fungal, and bacterial cultures, bacterial antigen assays, viral PCR (polymerized chain reaction) testing (varicella zoster virus—VZV, herpes simplex virus—HSV), and cytology to search for an underlying infectious or neoplastic process.

Information provided by neuroimaging studies is generally central to the diagnostic evaluation of patients with suspected CNS vasculitis. Brain computerized tomography (CT) demonstrates areas of ischemia (Fig. 19-4) or less commonly hemorrhage in up to 65 percent of patients.[6,8] Magnetic resonance imaging (MRI) is more sensitive (abnormalities seen in 75 to 90 percent of patients) than CT and frequently demonstrates both gray and white matter ischemic lesions (Figs. 19-5, 19-6, 19-7) as well as hemorrhages (Fig. 19-8). Subcortical

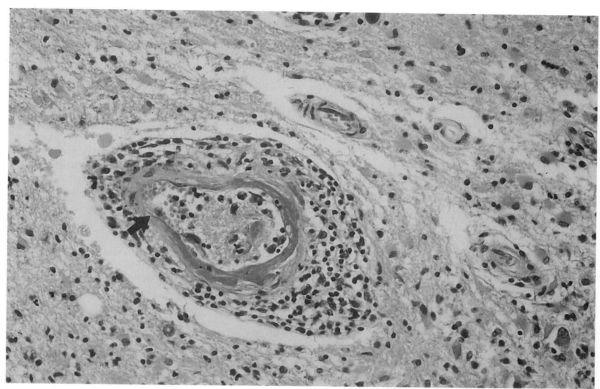

Figure 19-2.
Fibrinoid necrosis with focal destruction of the vessel wall in a patient with PACNS (20×). (See also color insert 4.)

white matter lesions are best visualized on T2-weighted or FLAIR sequences. Unlike multiple sclerosis plaques, vasculitic lesions usually do not have a predilection for the periventricular region and are unlikely to involve the corpus callosum. Vasculitic lesions may also be visualized in the brainstem and posterior fossa (see Fig. 19-7). Occasionally meningeal enhancement or mass lesions (likely due to inflammation and/or edema) are visualized. MRI is more sensitive than CT; however, both are nonspecific. In general, the probability of angiography or biopsy identifying an underlying CNS vasculitis is extremely low in the setting of a normal MRI scan, although a few such cases have been reported.[6,9]

Magnetic resonance angiography (MRA) may demonstrate abnormalities (vessel narrowings or occlusions) in patients with vasculitic involvement of the large basal vessels; however, these findings may again be nonspecific. In addition, MRA currently is not able to provide sufficient resolution to adequately visualize the medium or small intracranial vessels. Computerized tomographic angiography (CTA) is a newly emerging and evolving technique that offers promise as a means to evaluate both the large and medium-sized intracranial vessels. Although early experience suggests a high rate of sensitivity, further studies will be required to validate this technique (Fig. 19-9) (unpublished observations).[9a]

Cerebral angiography should be routinely performed in suspected cases of CNS vasculitis. Nondigital cut films are frequently preferred due to the superior spatial resolution for visualizing small vessel margins.[10] Abnormalities suggestive of a vasculitic or vasculopathic process occur in 70 to 75 percent of patients.[11,12] These abnormalities include segmental narrowings and dilatations that create a "beading" appearance (seen in 30 percent of cases) (Fig. 19-10). The vascular narrowings may be caused by vessel spasm, vessel wall infiltration and inflammation, or compression by meningeal or parenchymal infiltration of inflammatory cells.[13] Ultimately, some vessels may fibrose, leading to irreversible narrowing or occlusion. Vessel occlusions and aneurys-

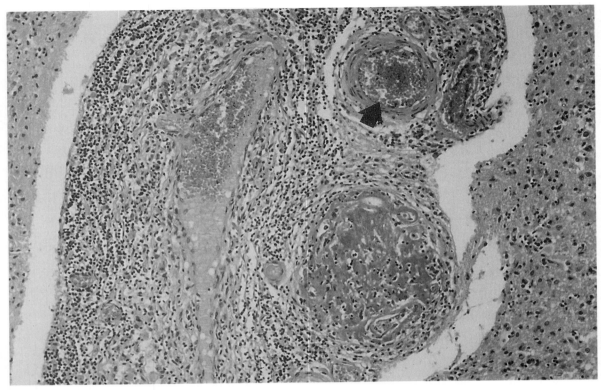

Figure 19-3.
Thrombosis of the microvasculature with surrounding inflammatory infiltrate in a patient with PACNS
(10×). (See also color insert 5.)

mal dilatations may also be visualized and likely result from weakening of the vessel wall or loss of autoregulation of vasomotor tone with subsequent vasoparalysis.[13] The study may be negative if the vasculitis primarily affects small vessels beyond the resolution of angiography. The complication risk of angiography is approximately 1 percent but depends on the experience and skill of the angiographer.[14,15] It is important to recognize that a specific diagnosis of CNS vasculitis cannot be made by angiography alone, as a variety of noninflammatory vasculopathies may mimic the radiographic appearance of vasculitis (Table 19-3).

Other diagnostic studies may be useful in individual cases. Diffuse or occasionally focal slowing is seen on electroencephalography (EEG) in the majority of patients with CNS vasculitis but is also a nonspecific finding.[16] One group has reported correlation between serial transcranial Doppler (TCD) abnormalities and proximal angiographic abnormalities and suggested that

TCD studies may be a useful imaging modality to follow patients over time.[17] Transthoracic or transesophageal echocardiography may rule out an underlying embolic source. Ophthalmologic examination may demonstrate evidence of ocular or retinal vasculitis, uveitis, or episcleritis. Single photon emission computed tomography (SPECT) or other cerebral blood flow studies may demonstrate areas of hypoperfusion. Chest x-rays may suggest the presence of an underlying pulmonary infection or autoimmune pulmonary disorder (e.g., Wegener's granulomatosis).

In general, histopathologic examination is required for a definitive diagnosis. However, even biopsy is positive in only 70 percent of cases due to the patchy nature of the disease.[18] The risk of serious morbidity or mortality with biopsy is small, approximately 1 to 2 percent.[19,20] The yield of a combined leptomeningeal and cortical biopsy is higher than sampling only one of these areas alone.[21,22] The nondominant temporal lobe is fre-

Table 19-2.

Diagnostic workup for CNS vasculitides

Serum
    CBC with platelets
    Chemistry panel
    Lipid panel[a]
    PT/PTT
    ESR
    ANA, dsDNA
    RNP (ribonucleoprotein)[a]
    Rheumatoid factor
    Cryocrit/cryoglobulins[a]
    ANCA
    C3/C4, CH-50
    C-reactive protein[a]
    Cold agglutinins[a]
    SCL70[a]
    Anti-Smith antibody[a]
    Anti-Ro and anti-La antibodies (SSA, SSB)[a]
    Circulating immunocomplexes (Raji test)[a]
    ACE[a] (angiotensin converting enzyme)
    VDRL
    HIV
    HTLV-1[a]
    Serum protein electrophoresis/immunoelectrophoresis[a]
    Hepatitis serology
    Coccidioides immitis titers[a]
    PEG (immune complex)[a]
    Hypercoagulable workup including antiphospholipid
        antibodies (DRVVT, ACL antibody)[a]
    Lyme titers
    Blood cultures
Urine
    Urinalysis
    Cultures
Chest x-ray
Lumbar puncture
    Cell count, glucose, protein
    VDRL
    Cytology
    ACE
    IgG synthesis, oligoclonal bands
    Cultures
    Viral titers and PCRs (VZV and HSV)
MRI with gadolinium
Angiogram
Brain biopsy
MRA or CTA
Ophthalmology exam including fluorescein
    angiography
Transthoracic and/or transesophageal echocardiography
Indium-labeled white cell scanning[a]
EEG (electroencephalography)[a]

[a]Select patients.

quently chosen, although it is often recommended to sample a region demonstrating radiographic abnormalities (but not frank infarction).[19] Some clinicians prefer the subtemporal tip to maximize the yield in patients with basal meningeal infections that might mimic primary angiitis of the central nervous system. Adequate tissue (at least 1 cc) including leptomeninges, cortex, and white matter should be obtained for light and electron microscopy, microbiology, and cytochemical studies.

In the majority of cases, vasculitis is related to autoimmune mechanisms or collagen vascular disease, and therefore corticosteroids and other immunosuppressive agents are the mainstays of therapy. Corticosteroids may, however, augment vessel constriction and platelet aggregation.[23] In addition, treatment with immunosuppressive agents and steroids can in turn lead to a new set of medical problems including infection or delayed malignancy.

In patients with an underlying secondary cause, treatment is aimed at eliminating any offending agent (drug) or treating the underlying disorder (infection or malignancy). Lack of clinical trials or even large-scale case series in most CNS vasculitic conditions precludes definitive evidence-based therapeutic recommendations. Future therapies may target specific events in the cascade of immune-mediated vascular injury, including use of monoclonal antibodies to adhesion molecules and cytokines.

Until the 1980's, most forms of CNS vasculitis, especially primary angiitis of the CNS, were thought to be routinely fatal. More recently, improved understanding of the underlying pathophysiologic processes combined with aggressive treatment have resulted in a more favorable prognosis for some patients.

PRIMARY ANGIITIS OF THE CENTRAL NERVOUS SYSTEM

BACKGROUND

Primary angiitis of the central nervous system (PACNS) is characterized by vascular inflammation within the CNS of unknown etiology that leads to diffuse ischemia, recurrent ischemic infarcts, or hemorrhages. In 1922, Harbitz described the first cases of probable PACNS reported in the medical literature.[24] However, it wasn't until 1959 that Cravioto and Feigin delineated this disorder as a new, distinct clinicopathologic syndrome.[25] Major advances in the diagnosis and treatment of PACNS occurred in the 1980's, prompted by a report of Cupps and colleagues of successful treatment of PACNS with

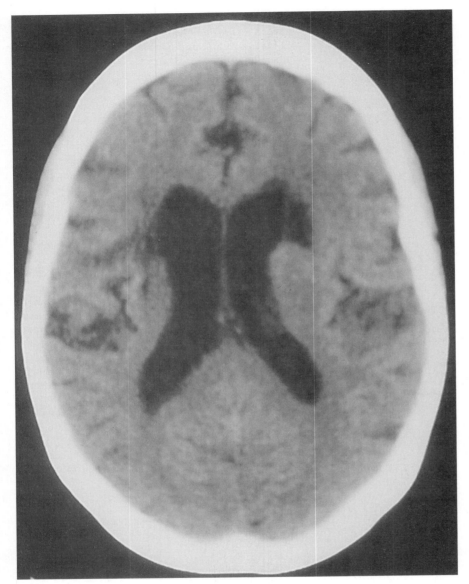

Figure 19-4.
*Noncontrast computed tomography of CNS vasculitis in a 66-year-old female with PACNS demon-
strating multiple subcortical infarcts.*

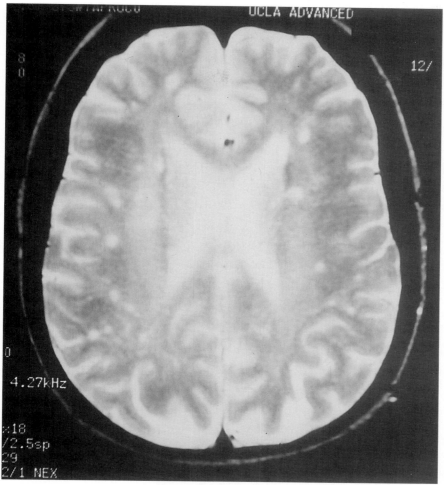

Figure 19-5.
Multiple gyriform hyperintensities evident on an axial T2-weighted MRI of a 13-year-old female with CNS vasculitis.

a combination of oral corticosteroids and cyclophosphamide.[26]

Nomenclature for primary angiitis of the central nervous system has been controversial and confusing. The term granulomatous angiitis of the central nervous system (GANS) was advocated early, but has come under attack, as only 20 to 50 percent[27] of cases exhibit granulomatous changes on pathologic examination. The term isolated angiitis of the central nervous system implies lack of vasculitic involvement outside the CNS, which is true in the majority but not all cases (some patients will have mild asymptomatic vasculitic changes found at autopsy in other organ systems as discussed below). Although some experts include cases associated with underlying diseases such as varicella zoster infection or Hodgkin's lymphoma, these cases do not meet the strict definition criteria for PACNS (requiring absence of underlying disorder). In Younger's series of 136 pathologically proven cases, 51 (37.5 percent) were associated with other diseases (11 systemic or temporal giant cell arteritis, 12 herpes zoster virus (HZV), 11 lymphoproliferative tumors (2 with HZV), 6 sarcoidosis, 10 cerebral amyloid angiopathy, 1 systemic lupus erythematosus and HZV, and 2 HIV without AIDS).[8]

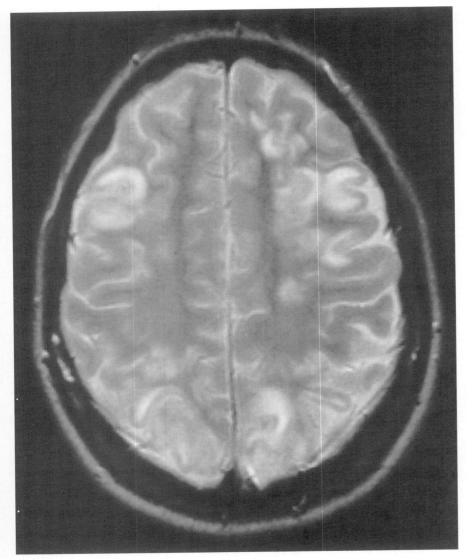

Figure 19-6.
Axial T2-weighted MRI of a 57-year-old female with CNS vasculitis demonstrating multifocal subcortical hyperintensities.

Clinical Presentation/Epidemiology Fewer than 200 cases of PACNS have been documented in the medical literature, and PACNS accounts for only 1 to 2 percent of all systemic vasculitides. PACNS most frequently affects the young to middle-aged with a mean age at onset of 45 (reported range in the literature 3 to 96). Men are affected slightly more frequently than women with a male to female ratio of 4:3.[27] There does not seem to be any particular ethnic propensity. Like all vasculitides affecting the central nervous system, the presentation of PACNS is variable and nonspecific. The onset may be insidious, subacute, or acute. There is often a long prodromal period (6 months or longer), and diagnosis may be delayed for months to years.[21,22]

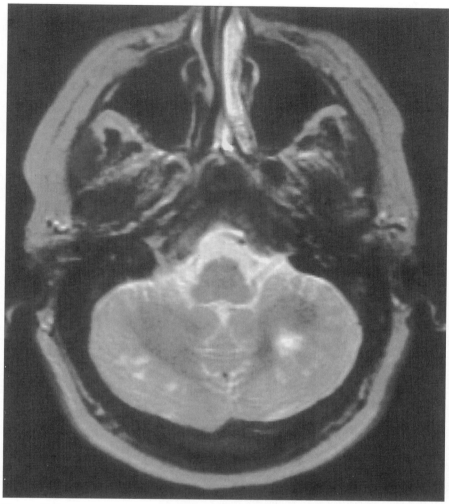

Figure 19-7.
T2-weighted magnetic resonance imaging demonstrating cerebellar hyperintensities due to CNS vasculitis displayed on an axial view.

Nonspecific constitutional symptoms including fevers and fatigue occur in 16 percent of patients.[8] However, symptoms of diffuse systemic autoimmune disease such as myalgias, arthralgias, or rash are generally absent. The most frequent presenting complaints of PACNS include focal neurologic symptoms such as monoparesis or hemiparesis, headache, confusion, and decreased or fluctuating level of consciousness (Table 19-4). Less common presenting symptoms include aphasia, nausea or vomiting, loss of memory, or seizure disorder. Other focal neurologic symptoms may occur later in the course of the illness and may not have a stroke-like onset.[16] Occasionally, patients may present with a dementing syndrome or a clinical and radiographic picture suggestive of a brain tumor. Spinal cord involvement characterized by paraparesis occurs in 11 to 23 percent of cases in various series[8,16,21] and occasionally may be the presenting or sole manifestation of the illness. In general, patients with PACNS have a chronic course punctuated by both focal and nonfocal CNS symptoms.

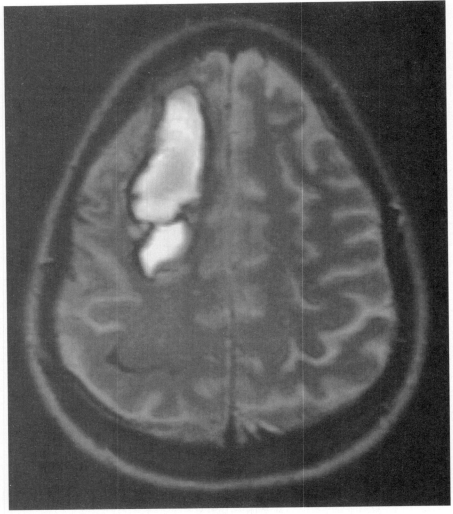

Figure 19-8.
Intraparenchymal hemorrhage of the right frontal lobe with surrounding edema secondary to CNS
vasculitis shown on an axial T2-weighted MRI.

Pathology PACNS preferentially affects the small and medium, but occasionally large, vessels within the central nervous system including both arteries and less commonly veins.[7] There is usually a predilection for leptomeningeal and cortical vessel involvement. Rarely, extracranial vessels in the aorta, heart, lungs, lymph nodes, kidney, or abdominal viscera may show subclinical vasculitic changes at autopsy.[26,28]

Gross pathologic examination reveals areas of small, and less commonly large, infarctions or hemorrhages. Histopathologic examination demonstrates a segmental or patchy vasculitis with frequent skip lesions. Lie described three histologic variants: (1) granulomatous, (2) necrotizing, or (3) lymphocytic; however, mixed forms are frequently found.[27] Only 20 to 50 percent of pathologically examined cases have demonstrated

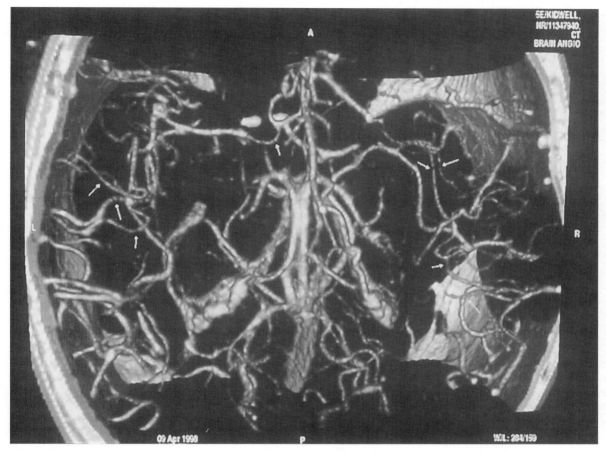

Figure 19-9.
Computed tomographic angiogram (CTA) of a 63-year-old female with giant cell arteritis. The arrows *indicate multifocal stenoses of the intracranial vasculature.*

granulomatous changes.[21,27] The inflammatory infiltrate is predominantly mononuclear (lymphocytes, plasma cells, histiocytes) (see Fig. 19-1). Eosinophils are rarely present. Multinucleated giant cells may be seen in the intima or media, usually in clusters. Lesions of different stages (acute, intermediate, healed) may occur simultaneously.[27] Vessels showing intimal fibrocellular proliferation most likely represent vessel healing. Vessel thrombosis has been reported in involved and uninvolved vessels (see Fig. 19-3).[27] In patients with spinal cord involvement, both granulomatous and nongranulomatous angiitis may be seen on histologic examination, either alone or in combination with vasculitis of the intracranial vessels.

Pathogenesis   The etiology of primary angiitis of the central nervous system is unknown. Theories regarding pathogenesis include autoimmune mechanisms and infectious causes. Moore speculated that cell-mediated immunity may be involved due to the absence of immune complexes and autoantibodies in pathologically examined cases.[22]

Diagnosis/Laboratory Workup   The first diagnostic criteria for PACNS were proposed by Calabrese and Mallek[12] in 1988 and Moore in 1989[22] and were later revised by Calabrese and Moore in 1995 to include: (1) history or clinical finding of an acquired neurologic deficit that remained unexplained after a thorough

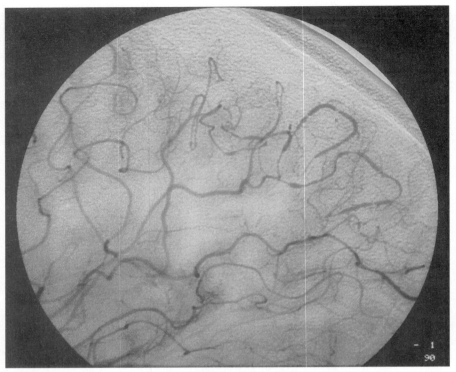

Figure 19-10.
Conventional angiography of a 13-year-old female with CNS vasculitis revealing alternating constrictions and dilatations of vessels with distal branch occlusions on a lateral view of a left carotid injection.

initial basic evaluation; (2) either classic angiographic or histopathologic features of angiitis within the CNS; and (3) no evidence of systemic vasculitis or any other condition to which angiographic or pathologic features could be secondary.[7] Biopsy has generally been recommended to make a definitive diagnosis in suspected cases.

The diagnosis of PACNS is frequently problematic due to lack of any routine laboratory or imaging study with a high degree of both sensitivity and specificity. In suspected cases, extensive laboratory workup should be performed to rule out other underlying processes (see Table 19-3). Mild elevation in the erythrocyte sedimentation rate (ESR) to the 30 to 40 mm/h range occurs in 60 percent of patients.[5] Serologic tests for collagen vascular disease are usually normal and if positive should raise suspicion for a separate process. A lumbar puncture should be performed to rule out infectious or malignant processes. Although nonspecific, CSF abnormalities are found in up to 90 percent of cases[21]

including a moderate elevation in CSF protein (70 percent of patients) to the 50 to 150 mg/dL range often with an associated lymphocytosis (60 percent of patients).[8,18,29] Opening pressure may be mildly elevated in 50 percent of patients,[18] whereas CSF glucose is usually within normal range.

EEG abnormalities occur in the majority of patients (93 percent in Vollmer's series)[16] and usually consist of diffuse slowing. In patients with moderate-to-large infarcts or hemorrhages, focal areas of slowing may be seen. Brain imaging studies are frequently abnormal but nonspecific. Head CT is abnormal in 63 to 68 percent of patients and may reveal frank ischemic infarcts, areas of diffuse white matter disease, hemorrhages, apparent mass, atrophy, or hydrocephalus.[16] Brain MRI is much more sensitive than CT, being abnormal in 76 to 100 percent of patients, but is also nonspecific. Abnormalities may include infarcts, hemorrhages, apparent masses, meningeal enhancement, and deep white matter disease.[9,16,30] Ehsan reported that changes

Table 19-3.

Differential diagnosis of multifocal vasculopathy on angiography (mimics of vasculitis)

Fibromuscular dysplasia
Moyamoya
Vasospasm (eclampsia, pheochromocytoma, postpartum angiopathy, subarachnoid hemorrhage, migraine headache, drug-induced)
Hypertensive encephalopathy
Antiphospholipid antibody syndrome
Thrombotic thrombocytopenic purpura
Radiation vasculopathy
Sickle cell disease
Angioendotheliomatosis
Acute meningoencephalitis or ADE
Myxomatous or SBE embolization
Neurofibromatosis
Diffuse cerebrovascular atherosclerosis
Neurosarcoidosis
Systemic lupus erythematosus vasculopathy

ADE, acute disseminated encephalomyelitis; SBE, subacute bacterial endocarditis.

in serial MRIs may correlate with clinical disease.[31] In small series, nuclear brain scans have been abnormal in two-thirds of cases, usually demonstrating areas of hypoperfusion.[16] In selected patients, other potentially useful tests include spinal cord imaging studies such as MRI or myelography. Reported abnormalities visualized on myelography include smooth extradural defects, incomplete obstruction to flow, irregularity of cauda equina and arachnoid, and enlargement of the conus medullaris.[16]

Catheter angiography may provide supportive evidence for a central nervous system vasculitis. However, angiography does not differentiate PACNS from other CNS vasculitides or from other nonvasculitic processes such as vasospasm, multiple emboli, or diffuse atherosclerosis. In addition, angiography may be normal in 10 to 47 percent of patients. In Vollmer's series, 56 percent of 41 angiograms in 31 cases of pure PACNS were abnormal, and 27 percent were diagnostic for vasculitis (abnormalities included: 1 aneurysm, 5 indeterminate, 6 mass effect, 11 diagnostic).[16]

Typical angiographic patterns of vasculitis may be seen in PACNS including irregularities of small and medium-sized leptomeningeal and cortical vessels char-

Table 19-4.

Clinical presentation PACNS

	Calabrese '92 n = 108	Vollmer '93 n = 40
	%	
Headache	62	68
Intracerebral hemorrhage	4	
Focal cerebral dysfunction		50
Paresis (hemiparesis, quadriparesis, paraparesis)	56	
Aphasia		
Hemianopia		
Brainstem dysfunction or cranial neuropathy		49
Decreased cognition	51	95
Decreased consciousness	29	
Seizure	21	25
Spinal cord dysfunction	18	23
Radiculopathy		20
Fever	19	
Weight loss	12	20
Increased intracranial pressure		43

acterized by beading (multifocal segmental stenoses), aneurysmal sausage-like dilatations, or vessel occlusions. Alternatively, angiography may be normal if vessels affected are beyond the size of angiographic resolution. Alhalabi and Moore reported that smooth narrowings in multiple vascular territories were the most frequent finding in their series of 19 patients.[9] Abnormalities of the large intracranial vessels including the distal internal carotid arteries, the middle cerebral arteries, and the vertebral arteries have frequently been reported at angiography. In a series of five patients with PACNS who underwent angiography reported by Moore, four of five had abnormalities of the large intracranial vessels as demonstrated on angiography.[22] Alterations in blood flow may also be seen including delayed vessel emptying and filling, evidence of new and anastomotic channels, or evidence of an associated mass effect. As opposed to systemic necrotizing vasculitis, there is not a predilection for vessel bifurcations in PACNS.[27]

Alhalabi and Moore also described the evolution of radiographic findings using serial angiography in 19 patients with PACNS.[9] They found segmental arterial narrowings and dilatations, vessel occlusions/thromboses, collateral formation, prolonged circulation time at baseline, and documented progression of changes prior to therapy and improvement or stabilization following therapy.

Pathologic examination is generally required for definitive diagnosis; however, even a biopsy may be falsely negative in 18 to 50 percent of cases of PACNS due to the patchy, multifocal nature of the disease.[16,18] In Younger's series of 44 patients (diagnosis verified at autopsy if biopsy was negative), biopsy was normal in 4 patients (9 percent), diagnostic in 34 (77 percent), and abnormal but nondiagnostic in 6 (14 percent).[30] The yield of biopsy is increased when both cortical and leptomeningeal tissues are sampled. In Calabrese's series, biopsy was diagnostic in 74 percent of cases (58 percent for cortical, 87 percent for leptomeningeal).[21] In general, a positive biopsy in the absence of secondary underlying causes is considered diagnostic. False-positive biopsy results are extremely rare and most commonly occur with stereotactic techniques in patients with lymphoproliferative processes. The recommended biopsy site is usually the nondominant temporal tip (or the rim of a radiographically identified involved region) including the leptomeninges as in other cases of CNS vasculitis.

Evidence

Steroids and cyclophosphamide are considered the mainstays of treatment of primary CNS vasculitis. Prior to the 1980's, the disease was considered to be routinely progressive and fatal. Following the report by Cupps and colleagues in 1983 of successful treatment with corticosteroids plus cyclophosphamide or azathioprine,[26] it has been increasingly recognized that long-term clinical remission and potential cure is possible in many patients. Successful treatment has been reported with steroids alone, or steroids in combination with other cytotoxic agents, most commonly cyclophosphamide and occasionally azathioprine.

No randomized, controlled trials have been performed comparing different therapeutic strategies for primary CNS vasculitis. Therapeutic recommendations generally arise from anecdotal reports and small case series. In Younger and colleagues' recent review, 11 of 17 patients treated with steroids alone improved or remained stable, whereas 13 of 17 patients treated with steroids and cyclophosphamide or azathioprine improved or remained stable, but only 1 of 20 patients not treated improved or remained stable.[30] Similarly, in Calabrese's series, an overall benefit occurred with treatment; however, there was no clear difference from steroids alone or in combination with cyclophosphamide.[32]

Prognosis for patients with PACNS seems less dismal than previously believed. Abu-Shakra and colleagues prospectively followed 16 patients with PACNS (median follow-up 28 months), 5 treated with steroids alone and 5 treated with steroids plus cyclophosphamide. Although half had a permanent neurologic deficit, all were still alive, suggesting that a majority of patients may have a nonprogressive, nonfatal course with treatment.[33]

Treatment Recommendations

Based on the limited data available, it seems that combination steroid and cyclophosphamide therapy is superior to steroids alone and should be initiated in most severe cases of PACNS. Moore recommended the following regimen for the first 6 weeks of therapy: prednisone 40 to 60 mg/day and cyclophosphamide 100 mg/day. Some experts recommend intravenous pulse cyclophosphamide, rather than oral, to decrease the incidence of sterility, hemorrhagic cystitis, and occurrence of late malignancies. Although the optimal duration of high-dose treatment is not known, it is generally recommended to treat for 6 to 12 months prior to drug taper.[22] Recurrence has been reported while tapering immunosuppressants and requires reinstitution of medications at higher doses.

It is unclear how the disease activity should best

be followed in patients with PACNS. Some authors advocate serial angiography in patients with an abnormal baseline angiogram. Serial MRI/MRA or serial CSF examinations may be sufficient in those patients with baseline abnormalities of these studies.

REVERSIBLE ANGIOPATHY OF THE CENTRAL NERVOUS SYSTEM

In the last decade, it has been suggested that a "benign" subset of PACNS may exist that primarily affects younger women. The term benign angiopathy of the CNS (BACNS) has been proposed by Calabrese[34] for this disorder as have the terms isolated benign cerebral vasculitis, isolated benign cerebral arteriopathy, and reversible cerebral segmental constriction. Clinical features of this putative entity include an acute, monophasic focal or multlifocal neurologic event (often intracerebral hemorrhage) usually associated with severe headache. We favor the term "reversible angiopathy of the central nervous system," as we do not consider a condition that can cause intracerebral hemorrhage benign, even if it is monophasic. Angiography demonstrates segmental narrowing, ectasia, and beading. CSF is routinely normal.

Evidence

In a review of 108 PACNS cases, Calabrese and colleagues found that those patients diagnosed by angiography alone, rather than histology, were younger, more often female, and tended to have a shorter course of disease activity.[34] From these data, they postulated that a subset of the patients diagnosed solely by angiography had the distinct condition of benign angiopathy of the central nervous system. Alternatively, this subset may better be considered to have been misreported under the rubric of PACNS and to actually have the well-known condition of reversible cerebral vasospasm, which can occur in migraine, the postpartum state, or pheochromocytoma. In a series of 10 patients meeting proposed initial diagnostic criteria for BACNS, Woolfenden and colleagues found none who actually had a benign course, arguing against the common occurrence of this entity.[35]

Treatment Recommendations

The monophasic course of this illness has been emphasized, and it is has been suggested that these patients do not need treatment with cytotoxic agents as prior cases have responded well to steroids alone. The use of calcium channel blockers has been advocated, but this recommendation is not supported by controlled clinical trials. All drugs that have sympathomimetic properties should be avoided, and patients may need to be educated regarding their presence in many over-the-counter drugs.

GIANT CELL (TEMPORAL) ARTERITIS

Background

Clinical Presentation/Epidemiology Temporal arteritis (TA) is a large and medium-vessel giant cell vasculitis that affects the elderly. The majority of patients develop symptoms in the 7th decade, with the diagnosis being extremely uncommon under the age of 50. Women are affected three times more frequently than men. Temporal arteritis can present with a variety of nonspecific symptoms. The onset is usually insidious but occasionally can be abrupt. Headache or neck pain is the most common symptom of TA and is usually severe, often throbbing, and may be unilateral or bilateral. New onset headache or a change in a chronic headache pattern in an older individual should raise suspicion for TA. The temporal arteries may be tender to palpation, swollen, red, or nodular on inspection. Scalp tenderness is common in this region but may spread to other areas. Pain or discomfort on chewing is caused by vascular claudication affecting the muscles of mastication. Polymyalgia rheumatica occurs in approximately 50 percent of patients with TA and consists of constitutional flu-like symptoms including malaise, fatigue, fevers, myalgias, backache, proximal arthralgias, and anorexia.[36]

Visual symptoms are a serious complication of temporal arteritis. Visual impairment occurs in approximately 8 to 23 percent of untreated patients and amaurosis fugax in 10 to 12 percent.[37] Total or partial monocular visual loss is caused by arteritic involvement of the posterior ciliary arteries supplying the optic nerve (leading to the arteritic form of anterior ischemic optic neuropathy), and less commonly by involvement of the central retinal artery or the ophthalmic artery. Visual field defects are most commonly altitudinal rather than central. Optic disc pallor with blurred disc margins may be seen on fundoscopy.

Temporal arteritis most commonly affects the medium and large extracranial vessels, especially the external carotid artery branches. Occasionally, TA may be accompanied by strokes caused by involvement of the extracranial carotids or vertebral arteries. A carotid bruit will be found on auscultation in 10 to 20 percent of patients. Slight encroachment of vasculitic changes from the extracranial to intracranial vasculature is not uncommon, whereas frank arteritic involvement of the large intracranial vessels is rare (less than 12 cases have been reported in the English literature).[37] Up to 15 percent of patients with TA have giant cell arteritis affecting the great vessels, most frequently the aorta. Epidemiologic studies, however, have demonstrated that there is not a statistically increased risk of stroke, myocardial infarction, or death in patients with TA,[38,39] although smaller case series suggest a greater stroke risk during the active phase of the disease.[40]

Pathology Histologic examination reveals multinucleated giant cells and an inflammatory response centered on the internal elastic lamina.[41] The general lack of involvement of the intracranial circulation likely due to the absence of elastica in these vessels. Recent reports implicate cell-mediated immunity in the pathogenesis of TA.[42,43]

Diagnosis Marked elevation of the erythrocyte sedimentation rate (ESR) occurs in the majority (90 to 97 percent) but not all patients.[37] Other nonspecific laboratory findings may include a mild normocytic anemia and a leukocytosis. Definitive diagnosis is based on temporal artery biopsy; however, even biopsy is not 100 percent sensitive due to the skip nature of the lesions. For this reason, a 4- to 5-cm specimen is recommended, preferably at the site of tenderness. Angiography of the branches of the external carotid artery, especially the superficial temporal artery, usually demonstrates areas of narrowing suggestive of arteritis and may help guide choice of biopsy site(s), although this test is not routinely recommended as part of the standard workup for patients with TA.

More recently, ultrasound techniques have demonstrated promise in the diagnosis of temporal arteritis. Schmidt and colleagues found that ultrasound can visualize a dark halo in the wall of an affected vessel in 73 percent of cases and that this finding was not present in control subjects.[44] If validated in confirmatory studies, this technique may allow diagnosis and institution of treatment in the appropriate patient without performing a temporal-artery biopsy.

Evidence

It is important to diagnose and treat temporal arteritis early because of its potentially devastating effects. The diagnosis should be considered in any patient over the age of 50 with new onset headaches, visual symptoms, or constitutional complaints suggestive of polymyalgia rheumatica. Steroids are the treatment of choice for temporal arteritis and have clearly been shown to arrest progression of the disease, including visual loss, when initiated promptly. Prior to the advent of steroids, case series demonstrated that 40 percent of patients developed visual loss in one or both eyes.[45] With steroid use, the probability of loss of vision developing after initiating oral glucocorticoid treatment was determined to be 1 percent, and the probability of additional loss was 13 percent in patients who had a visual deficit at the time therapy was begun.[46] With these compelling data, no randomized trials have been or are likely to be conducted comparing steroids with placebo.

Controversy has arisen regarding optimal steroid dose. Although some authors have suggested lower or even much higher intravenous doses initially (pulse steroids), there is no evidence that this regimen is more beneficial than the oral regimen. No trials or case series in the literature have tested high-dose intravenous or pulse steroids in temporal arteritis. Three retrospective analyses have in fact suggested that lower prednisone doses (20 to 40 mg/day) are as effective and less toxic than higher doses.[47-49] These findings have not yet been tested in a prospective randomized trial. Several small trials have been conducted with conflicting results to determine if other immunosuppressants could be substituted to avoid steroid side effects.[50,51]

Temporal arteritis is generally a self-limited process lasting months to years. Approximately 1 of 4 of patients will have a recurrence while tapering steroids often within the first few months of treatment. These patients should be treated with an increased steroid dose and a more gradual taper in the future.

Treatment Recommendations

The standard dose is prednisone 1 mg/kg/day orally or 40 to 60 mg/day. If there is a high index of suspicion, treatment should be initiated immediately and not be delayed for biopsy confirmation of the diagnosis (biopsy yield will not decrease with several days of steroid treatment).[52] Because 5 to 10 percent of patients will have a normal ESR and biopsy can occasionally miss the lesion, the patient should still be treated if there is a high index of suspicion despite a negative workup. Treatment with steroids usually prevents visual loss when started early and should be instituted even in patients who have already had visual symptoms in one eye to prevent involvement of the other eye. Duration of treatment varies and can be guided by following the ESR and presence of systemic symptoms while tapering steroid doses.

WEGENER'S GRANULOMATOSIS

Background

Wegener's granulomatosis is a systemic necrotizing vasculitis that primarily affects the respiratory tract in association with glomerulonephritis. Neurologic involvement occurs in approximately one-third of patients (range 13 to 54 percent).[53–55] Only 0 to 13 percent of patients in various series have developed central as opposed to peripheral nervous system dysfunction.[55–57] Two-thirds of cases with CNS dysfunction result from granulomatous inflammation within the brain (either contiguous extension from other sites or new granuloma formation) and one-third from vasculitis, which rarely can be the presenting symptom of the disease.[58]

Small and medium-sized arteries and veins are affected in the vasculitis associated with Wegener's granulomatosis. Fibrinoid necrosis and granulomas composed of giant cells are typically found. Ischemic infarcts, intracerebral hemorrhage, and commonly subarachnoid hemorrhage may occur in the CNS. Cerebral venous thrombosis has occasionally been reported.

Abnormal laboratory findings in patients with Wegener's granulomatosis include elevated ESR, hematuria and proteinuria, hypergammaglobulinemia, and occasionally circulating immune complexes. Antineutrophilic cytoplasmic antibodies (usually c-ANCA) are characteristically found. With CNS involvement, CSF may show increased WBCs, elevated protein, or evidence of SAH. CNS vasculitis or granulomatous inflammation within the brain should be considered if the patient develops focal CNS symptoms. A CT scan and/ or MRI should be performed to rule out granulomatous lesions and may demonstrate ischemic or hemorrhagic infarcts. A cerebral angiogram may show abnormalities characteristic of vasculitis of the small and medium-sized vessels.

Evidence

The combination of corticosteroids and cyclophosphamide has proven to be more effective than steroids alone in systemic Wegener's granulomatosis,[59,60] but no data are available regarding the optimal treatment for pa-

tients with CNS involvement. A recent randomized, placebo-controlled trial of trimethoprim and sulfamethoxazole vs. placebo given twice daily to patients with Wegener's granulomatosis in remission demonstrated a beneficial effect in preventing disease relapse.[61] Overall prognosis may be worse when CNS involvement occurs.[62]

Treatment Recommendations

Patients with CNS vasculitis in the setting of Wegener's granulomatosis should receive combination therapy with corticosteroids and cyclophosphamide to induce disease remission. Once remission is attained, maintenance therapy with trimethoprim and sulfamethoxazole should be considered.

POLYARTERITIS NODOSA

Polyarteritis nodosa (PAN) is a rare systemic necrotizing vasculitis that affects multiple organ systems throughout the body. In the series of Ford and Siekert, 46 percent of patients had evidence of CNS involvement, and 13 percent had ischemic infarct(s) or intracerebral hemorrhage(s).[63] CNS vasculitis occurs in approximately 20 to 40 percent of patients with PAN.[64] CNS vasculitis secondary to PAN can present with symptoms of a nonspecific encephalopathy, seizures, or focal symptoms secondary to stroke, either ischemic or hemorrhagic. Hypertension is often a feature of PAN due to renal compromise and may exacerbate neurologic symptoms if severe. Lesions in the cerebral hemispheres are the most common location, although the spinal cord may be affected. Visual complaints (blurring, visual loss) are common and may be due to vasculitis affecting the occipital cortices, optic nerves or tracts, or retinal and choroidal arteries. Cranial neuropathies affecting nerves III, IV, and VI have also been described. Some patients with PAN develop strokes caused by cardioembolism due to a cardiomyopathy. Intracranial saccular aneurysms may also develop in PAN, sometimes leading to SAH.

PAN is characterized by a necrotizing inflammatory vasculitis predominantly affecting the small and medium-sized blood vessels with a predilection for bifurcations. All layers of the vessel wall are infiltrated with PMNs followed by mononuclear cells. Intimal proliferation develops followed by fibrinoid and hyaline necrosis, thrombosis, and ischemia.

Laboratory abnormalities in PAN include elevated ESR, leukocytosis, anemia, thrombocytosis, circulating immune complexes, and low titers of rheumatoid factor or ANA. Some patients have a positive ANCA. Approximately one-third of patients have hepatitis B antigenemia, although this number is falling due to increasing use of hepatitis B vaccinations. Even with CNS involvement, CSF examination is usually normal. Brain imaging with CT or MRI often shows areas of ischemia, frank infarct, or hemorrhage. Cerebral angiography may show vasculitic abnormalities of the small and medium vessels or may be normal. Diagnosis of systemic disease is usually made by angiography and/or biopsy of muscle, nerve, skin, or kidney. CNS vasculitis secondary to PAN is suspected when there is evidence of CNS involvement in the setting of systemic PAN. Polyarteritis nodosa is treated with a combination of steroids and cytotoxic agents. No clinical trial data are available to guide therapeutic recommendations for CNS vasculitis associated with PAN. Five-year survival for treated patients is 80 percent.[64]

BEHÇET'S DISEASE

Behçet's disease is an inflammatory condition characterized by oral aphthous ulcers, uveitis, and genital ulcers. Males are affected more frequently than females (F:M = 1:4). There is an increased frequency of Behçet's disease in Japan, the Middle East, and Mediterranean countries. Neurologic involvement occurs in 4 to 49 percent of patients.[65,66] CNS involvement is variable and can include aseptic meningitis, meningoencephalitis, cerebral venous thrombosis, or vasculitis.[67] Clinical manifestations of CNS involvement include headaches, focal neurologic symptoms (often fluctuating), increased intracranial pressure, encephalopathy, or symptoms of spinal cord involvement.

Neuropathologic examinations of patients with neuro-Behçet's disease have demonstrated thickened meninges, intraparenchymal gliosis, and lymphocytic perivascular infiltration with areas of perivascular necrosis and scarring.[68] Occasionally, demyelinating lesions have been found. Less commonly, there is evidence of definite vasculitis and/or large infarctions. The brainstem is a frequent site of involvement. When vasculitis is seen, it most commonly affects the small vessels, especially venules.[69]

Patients with neuro-Behçet's usually have CSF abnormalities including elevated protein and pleocytosis. Anticardiolipin antibodies may be present. Brain imaging may demonstrate areas of increased T2 signal on MRI (most commonly in the white matter and brainstem) or hypodensities on CT. Occasionally, intraparenchymal hemorrhages may be seen. Cerebral angiography is typically normal due to involvement of small vessels beyond the resolution of angiography.[70] Treatment of Behçet's disease includes corticosteroids and cytotoxic agents. Evidence-based treatment strategies are limited due to the infrequency of reports in the literature of CNS vasculitis in the setting of Behçet's and the absence of controlled clinical trials. Although the prognosis for Behçet's disease is generally good, patients with CNS involvement seem to have a less benign course.[71,72]

CHURG-STRAUSS SYNDROME

Churg-Strauss syndrome (CSS) is an allergic granulomatous small and medium-vessel vasculitic disorder associated with eosinophilia that primarily affects the lungs and other systemic vessels and commonly occurs in patients with asthma and allergic rhinitis. Although neurologic involvement is common (62 to 75 percent),[73,74] CNS vasculitis is rare, occurring in only 6 percent of patients in one series of 47 patients.[75] The vasculitic lesions may be granulomatous or nongranulomatous, are usually necrotizing, and can affect both small arteries and veins. In addition to vasculitic lesions, patients with Churg-Strauss also demonstrate extravascular granulomas with eosinophilic infiltrates. Marked eosinophilia is a constant feature of CSS unless the patient has been treated with steroids. An elevated serum IgE level occurs in 75 percent of patients and a positive ANCA in 67 percent. Depending on disease severity, steroids and other immunosuppressive agents may be used alone or in combination. No data are available regarding optimal treatment of CNS vasculitis caused by CSS.

HYPERSENSITIVITY VASCULITIS

This group of disorders is characterized by cutaneous lesions and vasculitis caused by a hypersensitivity reaction and includes cutaneous vasculitis, drug-induced allergic vasculitis, postinfectious vasculitis, serum sickness, Henoch-Schonlein purpura, and some cases of essential mixed cryoglobulinemia.[4] Hypersensitivity vasculitides are characterized by inflammation of the small vessels, frequently the venules, in response to a precipitating antigen. Stroke and SAH have rarely been reported in patients with Henoch-Schonlein purpura, and there are several case reports of CNS vasculitis in the setting of other systemic hypersensitivity vasculitic disorders.[69] Drug-induced CNS vasculitis is discussed in a later section of this chapter. Evidence-based treatment strategies are limited due to the rarity of reports in the literature and the absence of controlled clinical trials.

CNS VASCULITIS ASSOCIATED WITH COLLAGEN VASCULAR DISEASES

System lupus erythematosus (SLE) is a multisystem connective tissue disorder that most commonly affects young women. Approximately 40 to 75 percent of patients with SLE develop some form of neurologic involvement.[76,77] Stroke and diffuse CNS dysfunction are frequent complications in patients with SLE often leading to suspicion of an underlying vasculitis. However, several pathologic and angiographic series have demonstrated that a true inflammatory vasculitis of the CNS is uncommon (0 to 12.5 percent) in the setting of SLE, with less than 10 histopathologically verified cases in the literature.[76,78–80] Instead, 65 to 83 percent of patients with SLE have a noninflammatory small vessel vasculopathy.[78] The most common mechanisms of stroke in the setting of SLE are hypercoagulable states secondary to antiphospholipid antibodies and cardioembolism secondary to noninfective valvular disease (Libman-Sacks endocarditis) rather than vasculitis.[76]

When a true CNS vasculitis does occur in the setting of SLE, symptoms include neuropsychiatric abnormalities, encephalopathy, seizures, aseptic meningitis, headache, stroke, cranial neuropathies, and, rarely, movement disorders, myelopathic symptoms, and hypothalamic-pituitary disorders. Brain imaging studies (CT or MRI) are not specific for vasculitis and may show evidence of small or large infarcts or hemorrhages. Angiographic abnormalities include beading, focal ectasia, occlusions, and aneurysms, both fusiform and saccular, which are often multiple.[78]

In patients with true CNS vasculitis and SLE, the optimal treatment regimen is unknown; however, a trial of high-dose immunosuppressants (cytotoxic agents and/or steroids) is the generally accepted treatment. Little data are available regarding prognosis for these patients. A review of a series of 11 patients with SLE and CNS vasculitis suggested a mortality rate of 67 percent; however, details on therapy were not provided for more than half of the patients.[81]

Rheumatoid arthritis is a deforming autoimmune disorder that has rarely been associated with a necrotizing CNS vasculitis.[82,83] When CNS vasculitis occurs, the small and medium-sized vessels are usually involved in isolation or in the setting of systemic vasculitis. Patients present with encephalopathic, or less commonly, focal neurologic symptoms. Small infarcts and occasional hematomas have been found at autopsy. In those patients reported in the literature, the course seems to be fulminant.

Scleroderma (progressive systemic sclerosis) is characterized by Raynaud's phenomenon, esophageal dysfunction, atrophic skin, pulmonary dysfunction, and renal failure. Although neurologic involvement is common (40 percent of patients),[84] CNS dysfunction is relatively rare (6 to 16 percent), and only a few cases of associated CNS vasculitis are reported in the literature.[84–87]

Sjogren's syndrome is characterized by keratoconjunctivitis sicca and xerostomia. It is frequently associated with Ro (SSA) and La (SSB) autoantibodies and commonly occurs in combination with other connective tissue disorders. CNS involvement may occur in up to 20 percent of patients, but only a few cases of associated vasculitis can be found in the literature. In Sjogren's patients with CNS disease and small vessel angiitis, antibodies against the Ro (SSA) antigen are present in an increased frequency.[88] These patients may have a more serious and extensive CNS disease than antibody-negative patients.

CNS vasculitis has rarely been reported in patients with a variety of other connective tissue diseases including ankylosing spondylitis, Reiter's syndrome, mixed connective tissue disease, and cryogobulinemia. Evidence-based treatment strategies are limited due to the infrequency of reports in the literature of CNS vasculitis in these settings and the absence of controlled clinical trials.

MALIGNANCY-ASSOCIATED VASCULITIS

Lymphomatoid granulomatosis (angioendotheliomatosis) is a rare disease previously considered under the category of vasculitis but now regarded as an angioinvasive lymphoreticular premalignant T or B cell lymphoma.[89] The lungs are the predominant site of involvement, although disease of the kidneys, skin, and central nervous system may be dramatic. CNS dysfunction occurs in approximately 20 to 30 percent of cases[90] and is caused by cellular infiltration of meninges, blood vessels, and brain parenchyma. Brain imaging may demonstrate apparent mass lesions or infarcts. Overall, the prognosis is poor; however, successful treatment in individuals has been reported with corticosteroids, cytotoxic agents, radiotherapy, and surgery.

The association of cerebral vasculitis and lymphoma, both Hodgkin's and non-Hodgkin's, has been firmly established. The nature of the association, however, is less clear. Some cases additionally have an underlying varicella zoster virus infection. The vasculitis may result from infection due to an immunocompromised state or may be a paraneoplastic or autoimmune phenomenon. Clinical presentation, histologic appearance and clinical course are similar to other patients with PACNS. Vasculitis cases have also been reported in association with hairy cell leukemia. Steroids and cytotoxic agents may treat both the underlying malignancy as well as the vasculitic process; however, there are no data available to guide specific treatment regimens.

DRUG-INDUCED CNS VASCULITIS

Drug-induced CNS vasculitis is a poorly delineated condition that has been attributed to multiple recreational drugs as well as over-the-counter preparations. Although a wide variety of agents have been implicated, the majority of cases have been described in association with sympathomimetic substances, such as amphetamines and cocaine. Clinical presentations include ischemic and hemorrhagic stroke or encephalopathic symptoms. Symptom onset may occur hours to months following drug use. Many cases of cerebral vasculitis attributable to drugs have shown angiographic patterns consistent with vasculopathy but lack histologic confirmation of vasculitis. Some of these cases may represent "reversible (referred to as 'benign' by Calabrese) angiopathy of the central nervous system" discussed earlier.[21,91]

In pathologically confirmed cases, an isolated non-necrotizing small vessel CNS angiitis devoid of fibrinoid degeneration, granulomas, giant cells, or foreign material is generally found, although a multi-organ systemic necrotizing angiitis can occur. Proposed pathophysiologic mechanisms of cerebrovascular complications associated with drugs include sympathomimetic pressor effects with multifocal vasospasm, direct toxicity to blood vessels, immune-mediated injury, hypersensitivity-related arterial hypotension, embolization of adulterants or foreign material, and enhanced platelet aggregation. Biopsy may be required for diagnosis as angiography may be negative. Diagnosis and identification of the offending agent is often hampered by simultaneous use of multiple drugs by individual patients or concomitant drug-related infections (hepatitis B, HIV, SBE). Initial treatment includes discontinuation of the inciting agent. Steroids and cytotoxic agents may be indicated in severe or refractory cases. Therapy aimed at ameliorating chronic vasoconstriction including antispasmodic therapy (e.g., papaverine, calcium channel blockers) and a limited course of corticosteroids has been recommended in sympathomimetic-induced cases.[7] McKenzie and colleagues treated five lesions caused by CNS vasculitis with angioplasty but found that all five lesions progressed to occlusion after initial improvement.[92]

Amphetamines and related compounds including ephedrine,[93] pseudoephedrine, phenylpropanolamine,[94] and phentermine[95] have been associated with CNS vasculitis. These substances may be obtained illegally or as over-the-counter preparations, as ingredients in diet pills and nasal decongestants, as well as by prescription, and may be taken orally, parenterally, inhaled, or smoked. Hypertension, vasoconstriction, and vasculitis are involved in stroke associated with abuse of these substances, but most cases lack clear evidence of one predominant pathophysiologic mechanism. Cerebral vasculopathy has frequently been demonstrated angiographically, but histologic evidence of true vasculitis has been reported in only six cases.[96]

Cocaine is increasingly recognized as a cause of cerebrovascular disease. The drug is abused by nasal inhalation, parenteral injection, or smoking the alkaloidal form, "crack." Postulated mechanisms of cerebrovascular injury include acute hypertension, vasospasm, a procoagulant platelet effect, and rarely vasculitis. A study by Peterson et al was the first to document a prospective series of complications related to cocaine, yet none of 33 patients studied was diagnosed with vasculitis.[97] Only seven cases of pathologically verified vasculitis have been reported in the setting of cocaine use.[98,99] Histologic examination usually reveals a small vessel infiltration with lymphocytes or polymorphonuclear cells. A pattern resembling PAN as well as hypersensitivity vasculitis has been noted in some patients.

Heroin-associated CNS vasculitis has rarely been reported. Parenteral injection of heroin raises the risk of embolization of foreign material, and CNS vasculitis resembling a hypersensitivity reaction with eosinophilia has been documented. These complications have also been described with the parenteral injection of crushed pentazocine and tripelennamine ("Ts and Blues").[98]

Opioid-associated vasculitis of the central nervous system has been inferred, although the evidence of a vasculitic component in these reported stroke cases is minimal.[98] CNS vasculitis has also been described in association with use or abuse of other drugs including allopurinol[100] and etodolac.[101] Stroke has been related to abuse of lysergic acid diethylamide (LSD) and phencyclidine (PCP), yet evidence of an underlying vasculitis attributable solely to these agents is lacking.[98]

INFECTIOUS CAUSES OF CNS VASCULITIS

Stroke associated with infection is frequently the consequence of CNS vasculitis. A diverse range of infectious agents, including bacteria, mycobacteria, spirochetes, viruses, fungi, parasites, rickettsiae, and mycoplasma, have been implicated in cases of CNS vasculitis. The clinical presentation is variable often including encephalopathy, fever, meningismus, seizures, behavioral problems, and elevated intracranial pressure resulting from a diffuse involvement of the cerebral vasculature, whereas focal neurologic deficits are caused by ischemia, infarction, or hemorrhage. Retinal vasculitis may cause blurred vision, decreased visual acuity, "floaters," or difficulty with color perception.

Both arteries and veins of varying sizes may be preferentially involved in CNS vasculitis associated with infection. Most agents have an affinity for particular types and sizes of vessels. Vessel injury and inflammation may be caused by direct invasion and subsequent damage to the vessel wall or indirectly through immune-mediated mechanisms. Cell-mediated immunity, autoantibodies, and immune complex deposition may be factors in particular infectious processes causing CNS vasculitis.

An accurate diagnosis is paramount in the immunocompromised patient, as a course of immunosuppressive therapy may carry even more than the usual substantial risks. Systemic symptoms such as fever and/or leukocytosis may be clues to an infectious process. A specific etiologic diagnosis is made by lumbar puncture including cultures, stains, antigen assays, PCRs plus serologic tests, and occasionally biopsy. Brain imaging may show infarctions, hemorrhage, or meningeal enhancement. Angiography may be normal or reveal intermittent narrowing of small and medium-sized arteries, prolonged circulation time of intracranial vessels, evidence of ectatic segments, and distal branch occlusions. Therapeutic interventions are principally focused on

specific antimicrobial regimens, although anti-inflammatory drugs, including steroids and immunosuppressive agents, may be beneficial in selected cases. Surgical debridement is necessary in a few conditions. Evidence-based strategies are limited due to the infrequent reports of these conditions in the literature.

Bacteria

Numerous bacteria, including *Streptococcus pneumonia, Escherichia coli*, Gram-negative species, *Listeria monocytogenes, Hemophilus influenzae, Nisseriae*, and *Staphylococci*, can cause acute septic meningitis, which may result in a pyogenic CNS arteritis. Stroke occurs in 10 percent of adults and up to 30 percent of neonates with bacterial meningitis.[102] The vasculitis generally affects the large vessels at the base of the brain as they pass through the subarachnoid space. Vascular injury may be due to direct spread of infection or to secondary inflammation and autoimmune processes. *Neisseria gonorrhea* and *Neisseria meningitidis* are particularly angioinvasive organisms. Venous sinus thrombosis and/or thrombophlebitis occur in 5 percent of cases of bacterial-induced CNS vasculitis. Although antibiotics are the mainstay of treatment, a short course of corticosteroids may decrease the inflammatory response.

Mycobacterium species can cause a prominent basilar meningitis affecting small and medium-sized arteries, especially the middle cerebral artery. Infarcts occur in up to 40 percent of patients with basilar meningitis secondary to *Mycobacterium tuberculosis*.[103] Histologic features of tuberculous angiitis include an inflammatory infiltration of blood vessel walls, fibrinoid and hyaline deterioration of the intima, subendothelial cellular proliferation, and perivascular cuffing of lymphocytes. Diagnosis is made by lumbar puncture, and treatment includes antituberculous agents. Steroids have been used empirically in severe cases.

Meningovascular syphilis develops in 10 to 12 percent of syphilitic infections.[104] Vessel injury is caused by direct vessel invasion by spirochetes. This entity can affect medium and large vessels (Heubner's arteritis) and arterioles (Nissl-Alzheimer's arteritis). The middle cerebral artery is most frequently affected. Syphilitic angiitis is a proliferative or obliterative endarteritis with transmural and perivascular infiltration of lymphocytes and plasma cells, subintimal fibroblastic proliferation, and irreversible damage of the elastica and media. Patients may present with an acute onset of a focal neurologic deficit or a slowly progressive encephalopathy. The peak incidence occurs approximately 7 years after initial infection. Diagnosis is confirmed by serum FTA-ABS (sensitive) and CSF VDRL (specific). Treatment is with penicillin. The use of corticosteroids in this setting is unsubstantiated.

Rickettsiae are small obligate intracellular Gram-negative coccobacilli that can rarely cause CNS vasculitis but are the most common presumed cause of "acute febrile cerebrovasculitis."[105] Invasion of endothelial cells and medial smooth muscle cells inciting cell injury and resultant inflammation cause a systemic microvascular angiitis.[106] Punctate cerebral hemorrhages may be seen. Clinical manifestations include fever, chills, myalgias, altered mentation, headache, and a macular rash. Definitive diagnosis relies on specific immunofluorescent antibody staining of biopsy specimens. Therapy includes tetracycline or chloramphenicol.

Mycoplasma pneumoniae can cause neurologic symptoms in up to 7 percent of patients.[107] Mycoplasmal particles have also been identified in vessels of patients with granulomatous angiitis of the CNS.[108] Both direct infection and autoimmune mechanisms may mediate the observed microangiopathy characterized by a mononuclear infiltrate and endothelial swelling. Definitive diagnosis requires CSF detection of the organisms or a fourfold rise in titers of serum cold hemagglutinins. Erythromycin and tetracycline are the antibiotics of choice, although these agents do not usually ameliorate the vasculitis when it is immune mediated.

A variety of other bacteria have been reported in the literature in association with CNS vasculitis. *Borrelia burgdorferi* is the causative agent of Lyme disease and has been associated with a segmental obliterative vasculopathy affecting all vessel sizes. *Borrelia recurrentis* usually causes relapsing fever but can lead to hemorrhagic lesions of the CNS and perivascular infiltrates. Leptospirosis may cause a severe angiitis with narrowing of major cerebral vessels and collateralization that angiographically appears similar to moyamoya. Brucellosis is caused by Gram-negative coccobacilli acquired through ingestion of unpasteurized dairy products. CNS involvement occurs after the acute phase of infection, causing a meningitis with extension to blood vessels. A panarteritis with formation of aneurysms and subsequent hemorrhage may be observed. Cat-scratch disease and Oroya fever, caused by *Bartonella* species, have rarely been associated with a cerebral arteritis.[109] Subacute bacterial endocarditis may result in CNS vasculitis via septic emboli and direct vessel invasion or by im-

mune complex deposition.[32] Successful treatment with steroids and antimicrobials has been reported.

Viruses and Retroviruses

Patients with herpes zoster ophthalmicus may develop a focal vasculitis of the ipsilateral intracranial arteries, most commonly the distal internal carotid or middle cerebral arteries, less commonly the vertebral or basilar arteries, weeks to months following the acute infection.[110] This syndrome typically presents with contralateral hemiparesis. A more diffuse form of CNS vasculitis has been described in association with systemic varicella zoster virus (VZV) infection. In either the focal or diffuse form, vessel inflammation may be caused by direct viral invasion of cerebral blood vessels from a hematogenous source[111,112] or by neural spread via the fifth cranial nerve branches.[113,114] In several cases, viral particles and antigens have been visualized in the medial layer of the vessel wall.[115] Up to 30 percent of patients have been found to have an underlying systemic disorder or malignancy.[113,116] The diagnosis is suggested by history and clinical presentation. CSF may show inflammatory changes, and diagnosis may be supported by a positive VZV PCR. The efficacy of acyclovir and corticosteroids is unproven in these cases, but these drugs are often used empirically. Eidelberg et al advocate the use of heparin in the setting of thrombotic cerebral vasculopathy associated with herpes zoster.[113]

Other viral infections including herpes simplex, cytomegalovirus, hepatitis, and lymphocytic choriomeningitis can cause vascular inflammatory changes in small intracranial arteries with perivascular cuffing of leukocytes. Cytomegalovirus has a specific tropism for vascular endothelium, and CMV-associated vasculitis has been documented in patients with AIDS.[117] Immunocompromised patients are at risk of CNS vasculitis related to an underlying secondary infection. In addition, an isolated AIDS-associated cerebral vasculitis (sometimes considered a form of PACNS) has been reported with features of eosinophilic vasculitis, granulomatous angiitis, necrotizing vasculitis, and intimal hyperplasia.[118,119] Therapy of this condition is difficult because of the degree of immunosuppression already present.

Fungi

A variety of fungal diseases can cause CNS vasculitis, often in association with an underlying immunocompromised state. Some fungal diseases (e.g., histoplasmosis, candidiasis, coccidiomycosis) may cause cerebrovascular complications due to occlusion of small subarachnoid blood vessels coincident with meningeal involvement.[120–123] Aspergillosis, cryptococcosis, and mucormycosis, however, cause specific stroke syndromes. Aspergillosis affects immunocompromised hosts, causing a necrotizing meningoencephalitis.[107] Hyphal angiitis of small and medium vessels can result in inflammation, aneurysm formation, and resultant hemorrhages. Immunocompromised and diabetic patients are particularly susceptible to mucormycosis. Hematogenous or direct spread may result in a necrotizing vasculitis resulting in cerebral infarction and/or hemorrhage. Diagnosis requires tissue biopsy. Cryptococcosis also affects immunocompromised individuals, occasionally with arachnoiditis causing leptomeningeal vascular inflammatory occlusions.[124] Diagnosis is made by CSF India ink visualization or by antigen detection in CSF. Treatment of CNS fungal infections is with amphotericin B, often in combination with flucytosine. Local debridement and possibly hyperbaric oxygen therapy have also been used in mucormycosis.

Parasites

Several parasitic diseases of the CNS have been associated with CNS vasculitis. In neurocysticercosis, the most common parasitic disease of the CNS, lacunar strokes may result from an inflammatory occlusion of small perforating arteries. The location, viability of the cysts and greater degree of immune reaction (arachnoiditis) were the most important features for development of cysticercotic vasculitis in a reported case series.[125] The role of antibiotic therapy in neurocysticercosis is controversial. Antibiotics may worsen the inflammatory response. There are no randomized trials or large case series specifically addressing the use of antibiotics in the setting of vasculitis secondary to neurocysticercosis. Some authors emphasize that the CSF findings and gadolinium-enhanced MRI can be used as markers of disease severity to guide therapy with corticosteroids.[125] Cerebral malaria due to *Plasmodium falciparum* causes endothelial damage and a diffuse encephalopathy with fever, generalized seizures, and altered level of consciousness. Treatment is with chloroquine. A double-blind study of steroids indicated a possible detrimental effect in this setting.[126] Paragonimiasis may produce small strokes due to an endarteritis or necrotizing vasculitis and requires treatment with praziquantel and steroids.[127] Other infectious agents including *Schistosoma*, *Trichinella*

spiralis, *Strongyloides stercoralis*, *Toxoplasma gondii*, *Acanthameba*, and *Naegleria fowleri* have been reported to induce CNS vasculitis.[101,107,128]

OTHER DISEASES ASSOCIATED WITH CNS VASCULITIS

Several miscellaneous conditions including neurosarcoidosis, cerebral amyloid angiopathy (CAA), retinal vasculitides, and inflammatory bowel disease (IBD) have been associated with CNS vasculitis. Angiitic neurosarcoidosis causes ischemic and hemorrhagic strokes, often in the setting of hypothalamic and pituitary dysfunction and meningitis. Granulomas form in perivascular areas and walls of small vessels. Brown and colleagues noted that although vascular involvement is a prominent feature of neurosarcoidosis, stroke is a rare complication.[129] CSF demonstrates mild lymphocytic pleocytosis and elevated protein. Treatment with steroids has met with success in some cases.[130]

Acute posterior multifocal placoid pigment epitheliopathy (APMPPE) is an idiopathic disease of young adults presenting with binocular visual blurring, metamorphopsia, and scotomas. Fundoscopy shows multiple yellow-white, flat lesions involving the choroid and pigment epithelium of the retina at the posterior fundus.[131] An autoimmune or infectious etiology is suspect as cases are sometimes preceded by a flu-like illness. The clinical course is usually self-limited, but occasional neurologic complications can be severe, including strokes that usually involve the posterior circulation and basal ganglia.[129,132] Fluorescein angiography may be helpful in confirming a diagnosis. Treatment with immunosupressive therapy for 6 to 12 months is advocated once a diagnosis of vasculitis is made,[131] but an evidence-based treatment strategy has yet to be established.[132]

Eales's disease is a retinal vasculitic syndrome that most commonly affects young males. Patients present with a variety of visual symptoms, often caused by retinal or vitreous hemorrhages.[133] Rare cases have been reported in which an associated CNS vasculitis occurs. Cogan's syndrome is characterized by interstitial keratitis (or scleritis/episcleritis) and vestibulocochlear symptoms and may involve an underlying vasculitic component.[134,135] Young adults are more frequently affected.

Cerebrovascular complications in the setting of inflammatory bowel disease may be the result of a hypercoagulable state, but a few cases of stroke secondary to biopsy-proven necrotizing CNS angiitis have been reported.

Several cases of CAA have been reported in association with a granulomatous angiitis.[136,137] Steroids and cyclophosphamide have been used with questionable benefit. An immune reaction to amyloid protein has been suggested as a causal mechanism.[138]

Radiation-induced angiopathy is not generally considered to be a true CNS vasculitic syndrome. Although perivascular lymphocytic infiltration occurs, it is probably not the primary mechanism of vessel injury. Symptoms usually occur years after radiation treatment.[139] If treatment has involved the neck or brainstem, a moyamoya type of angiographic pattern may occur.[140]

CONCLUSIONS

The CNS vasculitides are a heterogeneous and sometimes poorly understood group of disorders. The overall rarity of these disorders as well as the frequent challenges and difficulties in diagnosis have hampered large-scale studies and therapeutic clinical trials. Treatment recommendations are currently empiric, generally based on small case series and clinician experience. Multicenter trials will be necessary in the future to provide definitive data on the most appropriate therapeutic regimens.

REFERENCES

1. Lie JT: Classification and histopathologic spectrum of central nervous system vasculitis. *Neurol Clin* 15:805, 1997.
2. Biller J: Non-atherosclerotic vasculopathies, in Biller J, Mathews KD, Love BB (eds): *Stroke in Children and Young Adults*. Newton, MA, Butterworth-Heinemann, 1994, pp 66–72.
3. Sneller MC, Fauci AS: Pathogenesis of vasculitis syndromes. *Med Clin North Am* 81:221, 1997.
4. Moore PM: Neurological manifestation of vasculitis: Update on immunopathogenic mechanisms and clinical features. *Ann Neurol* 37 (Suppl1): S131, 1995.
5. Nadeau SE: Diagnostic approach to central and peripheral nervous system vasculitis. *Neurol Clin* 15:759, 1997.
6. Stone JH, Pomper MG, Roubenoff R, Miller TJ, Hellmann DB: Sensitivities of noninvasive tests for central nervous system vasculitis: A comparison of lumbar puncture, computed tomography, and magnetic resonance imaging. *J Rheumatol* 21:1277, 1994.
7. Calabrese LH: Vasculitis of the central nervous system. *Rheum Dis Clin North Am* 21:1059, 1995.
8. Younger DS, Kass RM: Vasculitis and the nervous system: Historical perspective and overview. *Neurol Clin* 15:737, 1997.

9. Alhalabi M, Moore PM: Serial angiography in isolated angiitis of the central nervous system. *Neurology* 44:1221, 1994.
9a. Liebeskind DS, Koral K, Hardart M, Villablanca JP: CT angiography of CNS vasculitis. *ASNR Proceedings,* 1999, p. 273.
10. Stein RL, Martino CR, Weinert DM, Hueftle M, Kammer GM: Cerebral angiography as a guide for therapy in isolated central nervous system vasculitis. *JAMA* 257:2193, 1987.
11. Harris KG, Tran DD, Sickels WJ, Comell SH, Yuh WT: Diagnosing intracranial vasculitis: The roles of MR and angiography. *AJNR Am J Neuroradiol* 15:317, 1994.
12. Calabrese LH, Mallek JA: Primary angiitis of the central nervous system: Report of 8 new cases, review of the literature, and proposal for diagnostic criteria. *Medicine* 67:20, 1988.
13. Greenan TJ, Grossman RI, Goldberg HI: Cerebral vasculitis: MR imaging and angiographic correlation. *Radiology* 182:65, 1992.
14. Hurst RW, Grossman RI: Neuroradiology of central nervous system vasculitis. *Semin Neurol* 14:320, 1994.
15. Hellmann DB, Roubenoff R, Healy RA, Wang H: Central nervous system angiography: Safety and predictors of a positive result in 125 consecutive patients evaluated for possible vasculitis. *J Rheumatol* 19:568, 1992.
16. Vollmer TL, Guamaccia, J, Harrington W, Pacia SV, Petroff OA: Idiopathic granulomatous angiitis of the central nervous system: Diagnostic challenges. *Arch Neurol* 50:925, 1993.
17. Morgenlander JC, McCallum RM, Devlin T, Moore MS, Gray L, Alberts MJ: Transcranial Doppler sonography to monitor cerebral vasculitis. *J Rheumatol* 23:561, 1996.
18. Hankey GJ: Isolated angiitis/angiopathy of the central nervous system. *Cerebrovasc Dis* 1:2, 1991.
19. Parisi JE, Moore PM: The role of biopsy in vasculitis of the central nervous system. *Semin Neurol* 14:341, 1994.
20. Whitley RJ, Cobbs CG, Alford CA Jr, et al: Diseases that mimic herpes simplex encephalitis: diagnosis, presentation, and outcome. NIAD Collaborative Antiviral Study Group. *JAMA* 262:234, 1989.
21. Calabrese LH, Furlan AJ, Gragg LA, Ropos TJ: Primary angiitis of the central nervous system: Diagnostic criteria and clinical approach. *Cleve Clin J Med* 59:293, 1992.
22. Moore PM: Diagnosis and management of isolated angiitis of the central nervous system. *Neurology* 39:167, 1989.
23. Villringer A, Moore P: Vasculitides and other nonatherosclerotic vasculopathies of the nervous system, in Brandt T, Caplan LR, Dichgens J, et al (eds): *Neurological Disorders*. New York, Academic Press, 1996.
24. Harbitz F: Unknown forms of arteritis with special reference to their relation to syphilitic arteritis and periarteritis nodosa. *Am J Med Sci* 163:250, 1922.
25. Cravioto H, Fegin I: Noninfectious granulomatous angiitis with a predilection for the nervous system. *Neurology* 9:599, 1959.

26. Cupps TR, Moore PM, Fauci AS: Isolated angiitis of the central nervous system: Prospective diagnostic and therapeutic experience. *Am J Med* 74:97, 1983.

27. Lie JT: Primary (granulomatous) angiitis of the central nervous system: A clinicopathologic analysis of 15 new cases and a review of the literature. *Hum Pathol* 23:164, 1992.

28. Reik L Jr, Grunnet ML, Spencer RP, Donaldson JO: Granulomatous angiitis presenting as chronic meningitis and ventriculitis. *Neurology* 33:1609, 1983.

29. Yuen RW, Johnson PC: Primary angiitis of the central nervous system associated with Hodgkin's disease. *Arch Pathol Lab Med* 120:573, 1996.

30. Younger DS, Calabrese LH, Hays AP: Granulomatous angiitis of the nervous system. *Neurol Clin* 15:821, 1997.

31. Ehsan T, Hasan S, Powers JM, Heiserman JE: Serial magnetic resonance imaging in isolated angiitis of the central nervous system. *Neurology* 45:1462, 1995.

32. Calabrese LH, Duna GF: Evaluation and treatment of central nervous system vasculitis. *Curr Opin Rheumatol* 7:37, 1995.

33. Abu-Shakra M, Khraishi M, Grosman H, Lewtas J, Cividino A, Keystone EC: Primary angiitis of the CNS diagnosed by angiography. *Q J Med* 87:351, 1994.

34. Calabrese LH, Gragg LA, Furlan AJ: Benign angiopathy: A distinct subset of angiographically defined primary angiitis of the central nervous system. *J Rheumatol* 20:2046, 1993.

35. Woolfenden AR, Tong DC, Marks MP, Ali AO, Albers GW: Angiographically defined primary angiitis of the CNS: Is it really benign? *Neurology* 51:183, 1998.

36. Berlit P: Clinical and laboratory findings with giant cell arteritis. *J Neurol Sci* 111:1, 1992.

37. Caselli RJ, Hunder GG: Giant cell (temporal) arteritis. *Neurol Clin* 15:893, 1997.

38. Jonasson F, Cullen JF, Elton RA: Temporal arteritis: A 14-year epidemiological, clinical and prognostic study. *Scott Med J* 24:111, 1979.

39. Bengtsson BA, Malmvall BE: Prognosis of giant cell arteritis including temporal arteritis and polymyalgia rheumatica: A follow-up study on ninety patients treated with corticosteroids. *Acta Med Scand* 209:337, 1981.

40. Paulley JW, Hughes JP: Giant cell arteritis or arteritis of the aged. *BMJ* 2:1562, 1960.

41. Hinchey JA, Sila CA: Cerebrovascular complications of rheumatic disease. *Rheum Dis Clin North Am* 23:293, 1997.

42. Brack A, Geisler A, Martinez-Taboada VM, Younge BR, Goronzy JJ, Weyand CM: Giant cell vasculitis is a T cell-dependent disease. *Mol Med* 3:530, 1997.

43. Elling P, Olsson AT, Elling H: A reduced CD8+ lymphocyte subset distinguishes patients with polymyalgia rheumatica and temporal arteritis from patients with other diseases. *Clin Exp Rheumatol* 16:155, 1998.

44. Schmidt WA, Kraft HE, Vorpahl K, Volker L, Gromnica-Ihle EJ: Color duplex ultrasonography in the diagnosis of temporal arteritis. *N Engl J Med* 337:1336, 1997.

45. Birkhead NC, Wagner JP, Shick RM: Treatment of temporal arteritis with adrenal corticosteroids: Results in fifty-five cases in which lesion was proved at biopsy. *JAMA* 163:821, 1957.

46. Aiello PD, Trautmann JC, McPhee TJ, Kunselman AR, Hunder GG: Visual prognosis in giant cell arteritis. *Ophthalmology* 100:550, 1993.

47. Myles AB, Perera T, Ridley MG: Prevention of blindness in giant cell arteritis by corticosteroid treatment. *Br J Rheumatol* 31:103, 1992.

48. Lundberg I, Hedfors E: Restricted dose and duration of corticosteroid treatment in patients with polymyalgia rheumatica and temporal arteritis. *J Rheumatol* 17:1340, 1990.

49. Nesher G, Rubinow A, Sonnenblick M: Efficacy and adverse effects of different corticosteroid dose regimens in temporal arteritis: A retrospective study. *Clin Exp Rheumatol* 15:303, 1997.

50. van der Veen MJ, Dinant HJ, van Booma-Frankfort C, van Albada-Kuipers GA, Bijlsma JW: Can methotrexate be used as a steroid sparing agent in the treatment of polymyalgia rheumatica and giant cell arteritis? *Ann Rheum Dis* 55:218, 1996.

51. Krall PL, Mazanec DJ, Wilke WS: Methotrexate for corticosteroid-resistant polymyalgia rheumatica and giant cell arteritis. *Cleve Clin J Med* 56:253, 1989.

52. Achkar AA, Lie JT, Hunder GG, O'Fallon WM, Gabriel SE: How does previous corticosteroid treatment affect the biopsy findings in giant cell (temporal) arteritis? *Ann Intern Med* 120:987, 1994.

53. Nishino H, Rubino FA, DeRemee RA, Swanson JW, Parisi JE: Neurological involvement in Wegener's granulomatosis: An analysis of 324 consecutive patients at the Mayo Clinic. *Ann Neurol* 33:4, 1993.

54. Hoffman GS, Kerr GS, Leavitt RY, et al: Wegener granulomatosis: An analysis of 158 patients. *Ann Intern Med* 116:488, 1992.

55. Fauci AS, Haynes BF, Katz P, Wolff SM: Wegener's granulomatosis: Prospective clinical and therapeutic experience with 85 patients for 21 years. *Ann Intern Med* 98:76, 1983.

56. Cruz DN, Segal AS: A patient with Wegener's granulomatosis presenting with a subarachnoid hemorrhage: Case report and review of CNS disease associated with Wegener's granulomatosis. *Am J Nephrol* 17:181, 1997.

57. Falk RJ, Jennette JC: Wegener's granulomatosis, systemic vasculitis, and antineutrophil cytoplasmic autoantibodies. *Annu Rev Med* 42:459, 1991.

58. Nishino H, Rubino FA, Parisi JE: The spectrum of neurologic involvement in Wegener's granulomatosis. *Neurology* 43:1334, 1993.

59. Calabrese LH, Hoffman GS, Guillevin L: Therapy of resistant systemic necrotizing vasculitis: Polyarteritis, Churg-Strauss syndrome, Wegener's granulomatosis, and

hypersensitivity vasculitis group disorders. *Rheum Dis Clin North Am* 21:41, 1995.

60. Hoffman GS, Leavitt RY, Kerr GS, Fauci AS: The treatment of Wegener's granulomatosis with glucocorticoids and methotrexate. *Arthritis Rheum* 35:1322, 1992.

61. Stegeman CA, Cohen Tervaert JW, DeJong PE: Trimethoprim-sulfamethoxazole (co-trimoxazole) for the prevention of relapses of Wegener's granulomatosis. *N Engl J Med* 335:16, 1996.

62. Bajema IM, Hagen EC, Weverling-Rijnsburger AW, et al: Cerebral involvement in two patients with Wegener's granulomatosis. *Clin Nephrol* 47:401, 1997.

63. Ford R, Siekert R: Central nervous system manifestation of periarteritis nodosa. *Neurology* 15:115, 1965.

64. Moore PM, Cupps TR: Neurological complications of vasculitis. *Ann Neurol* 14:155, 1983.

65. Allen NB: Miscellaneous vasculitic syndromes including Behcet's disease and central nervous system vasculitis. *Curr Opin Rheumatol* 5:51, 1993.

66. Banna M, el-Ramahl K: Neurologic involvement in Behcet disease: Imaging findings in 16 patients. *AJNR Am J Neuroradiol* 12:791, 1991.

67. Shakir RA, Sulaiman K, Kahn RA, Rudwan M: Neurological presentation of neuro-Behcet's syndrome: Clinical categories. *Eur Neurol* 30:249, 1990.

68. Nishimura M, Satoh K, Suga M, Oda M: Cerebral angio- and neuro-Behcet's syndrome: Neuroradiological and pathological study of one case. *J Neurol Sci* 106:19, 1991.

69. Moore PM, Calabrese LH: Neurologic manifestations of systemic vasculitides. *Semin Neurol* 14:300, 1994.

70. O'Duffy JD: Vasculitis in Behcet's disease. *Rheum Dis Clin North Am* 16:423, 1990.

71. Gerber S, Biondi A, Dormont D, Wechsler B, Marsault C: Long-term MR follow-up of cerebral lesions in neuro-Behcet's disease. *Neuroradiology* 38:761, 1996.

72. Akman-Demir G, Baykan-Kurt B, Serdaroglu P, et al: Seven-year follow-up of neurologic involvement in Behcet syndrome. *Arch Neurol* 53:691, 1996.

73. Chumbley LC, Harrison EG Jr, DeRemee RA: Allergic granulomatosis and angiitis (Churg-Strauss syndrome): Report and analysis of 30 cases. *Mayo Clin Proc* 52:477, 1977.

74. Lanham JG, Elkon KB, Pusey CD, Hughes GR: Systemic vasculitis with asthma and eosinophilia: A clinical approach to the Churg-Strauss syndrome. *Medicine* 63:65, 1984.

75. Sehgal M, Swanson JW, DeRemee RA, Colby TV: Neurologic manifestations of Churg-Strauss syndrome. *Mayo Clin Proc* 70:337, 1995.

76. Devinsky O, Petito CK, Alonso DR: Clinical and neuropathological findings in systemic lupus erythematosus: The role of vasculitis, heart emboli, and thrombotic thrombocytopenic purpura. *Ann Neurol* 23:380, 1988.

77. van Dam AP: Diagnosis and pathogenesis of CNS lupus. *Rheumatol Int* 11:1, 1991.

78. Liem MD, Gzesh DJ, Flanders AE: MRI and angio-graphic diagnosis of lupus cerebral vasculitis. *Neuroradiology* 38:134, 1996.

79. Ellis SG, Verity MA: Central nervous system involvement in systemic lupus erythematosus: A review of neuropathologic findings in 57 cases, 1955–1977. *Semin Arthritis Rheum* 8:212, 1979.

80. Johnson RT, Richardson EP: The neurological manifestations of systemic lupus erythematosus. *Medicine* 47:337, 1968.

81. Weiner DK, Allen NB: Large vessel vasculitis of the central nervous system in systemic lupus erythematosus: Report and review of the literature. *J Rheumatol* 18:748, 1991.

82. Watson P, Fekete J, Deck J: Central nervous system vasculitis in rheumatoid arthritis. *Can J Neurol Sci* 4:269, 1977.

83. Ramos M, Mandybur TI: Cerebral vasculitis in rheumatoid arthritis. *Arch Neurol* 32:271, 1975.

84. Averbuch-Heller L, Steiner I, Abramsky O: Neurologic manifestations of progressive systemic sclerosis. *Arch Neurol* 49:1292, 1992.

85. Pathak R, Gabor AJ: Scleroderma and central nervous system vasculitis. *Stroke* 22:410, 1991.

86. Hietaharju A, Jaaskelainen S, Hietarinta M, Frey H: Central nervous system involvement and psychiatric manifestations in systemic sclerosis (scleroderma): Clinical and neurophysiological evaluation. *Acta Neurol Scand* 87:382, 1993.

87. Estey E, Lieberman A, Pinto R, Meltzer M, Ransohoff J: Cerebral arteritis in scleroderma. *Stroke* 10:595, 1979.

88. Alexander EL, Ranzenbach MR, Kumar AJ, et al: Anti-Ro(SS-A) autoantibodies in central nervous system disease associated with Sjogren's syndrome (CNS-SS): Clinical, neuroimaging, and angiographic correlates. *Neurology* 44:899, 1994.

89. Donner LR, Dobin S, Harrington D, Bassion S, Rappaport ES, Peterson RF: Angiocentric immunoproliferative lesion (lymphomatoid granulomatosis): A cytogenetic, immunophenotypic, and genotypic study. *Cancer* 65:249, 1990.

90. Katzenstein AL, Carrington CB, Liebow AA: Lymphomatoid granulomatosis: A clinicopathologic study of 152 cases. *Cancer* 43:360, 1979.

91. Martin K, Rogers T, Kavanaugh A: Central nervous system angiopathy associated with cocaine abuse. *J Rheumatol* 22:780, 1995.

92. McKenzie JD, Wallace RC, Dean BL, Flom RA, Khayata MH: Preliminary results of intracranial angioplasty for vascular stenosis caused by atherosclerosis and vasculitis. *AJNR Am J Neuroradiol* 17:263-8, 1996.

93. Wooten MR, Khangure MS, Murphy MJ: Intracerebral hemorrhage and vasculitis related to ephedrine abuse. *Ann Neurol* 13:337, 1983.

94. Glick R, Hoying J, Cerullo L, Periman S: Phenylpropanolamine: An over-the-counter drug causing central

nervous system vasculitis and intracerebral hemorrhage. Case report and review. *Neurosurgery* 20:969, 1987.

95. Kokkinos J, Levine SR: Possible association of ischemic stroke with phentermine. *Stroke* 24:310, 1993.

96. Giang DW: Central nervous system vasculitis secondary to infections, toxins, and neoplasms. *Semin Neurol* 14:313, 1994.

97. Peterson PL, Roszler M, Jacobs I, Wilner HI: Neurovascular complications of cocaine abuse. *J Neuropsychiatry Clin Neurosci* 3:143, 1991.

98. Brust JC: Vasculitis owing to substance abuse. *Neurol Clin* 15:945, 1997.

99. Merkel PA, Koroshetz WJ, Irizarry MC, Cudkowicz ME: Cocaine-associated cerebral vasculitis. *Semin Arthritis Rheum* 25:172, 1995.

100. Rothwell PM, Grant R: Cerebral vasculitis following allopurinol treatment. *Postgrad Med J* 72:119, 1996.

101. Lie JT: Vasculitis associated with infectious agents. *Curr Opin Rheumatol* 8:26, 1996.

102. Chang CWJ: The acute management of neurologic complications associated with CNS infections, in *Central Nervous System Infectious Diseases and Therapy*. New York, Marcel Dekker, 1997, pp 691–709.

103. Leiguarda R, Berthier M, Starkstein S, Nogues M, Lylyk P: Ischemic infarction in 25 children with tuberculous meningitis. *Stroke* 19:200, 1988.

104. Holland BA, Perrett LV, Mills CM: Meningovascular syphilis: CT and MR findings. *Radiology* 158:439, 1986.

105. Wenzel RP, Hayden FG, Groschel DH, et al: Acute febrile cerebrovasculitis: A syndrome of unknown, perhaps rickettsial, cause. *Ann Intern Med* 104:606, 1986.

106. Jennette JC, Falk RJ, Milling DM: Pathogenesis of vasculitis. *Semin Neurol* 14:291, 1994.

107. Gerber O, Roque C, Coyle PK: Vasculitis owing to infection. *Neurol Clin* 15:903, 1997.

108. Arthur G, Margolis G: Mycoplasma-like structures in granulomatous angiitis of the central nervous system: Case reports with light and electron microscopic studies. *Arch Pathol Lab Med* 101:382, 1977.

109. Selby G, Walker GL: Cerebral arteritis in cat-scratch disease. *Neurology* 29:1413, 1979.

110. Patrick JT, Russell E, Meyer J, Biller J, Saver JL: Cervical (C2) herpes zoster infection followed by pontine infarction. *J Neuroimaging* 5:192, 1995.

111. Caekebeke JF, Peters AC, Vandvik B, Brouwer OF, de Bakker HM: Cerebral vasculopathy associated with primary varicella infection. *Arch Neurol* 47:1033, 1990.

112. Doyle PW, Gibson G, Dolman CL: Herpes zoster ophthalmicus with contralateral hemiplegia: Identification of cause. *Ann Neurol* 14:84, 1983.

113. Eidelberg D, Sotrel A, Horoupian DS, Neumann PE, Pumarola-Sune T, Price RW: Thrombotic cerebral vasculopathy associated with herpes zoster. *Ann Neurol* 19:7, 1986.

114. MacKenzie RA, Forbes GS, Kames WE: Angiographic findings in herpes zoster arteritis. *Ann Neurol* 10:458, 1981.

115. Gilden DH, Kleinschmidt-DeMasters BK, Wellish M, Hedley-Whyte ET, Rentier B, Mahalingam R: Varicella zoster virus, a cause of waxing and waning vasculitis: The *New England Journal of Medicine* case 5-1995 revisited. *Neurology* 47:1441, 1996.

116. Reshef E, Greenberg SB, Jankovic J: Herpes zoster ophthalmicus followed by contralateral hemiparesis: Report of two cases and review of literature. *J Neurol Neurosurg Psychiatry* 48:122, 1985.

117. Golden JA: Cytomegalovirus infection or disease (Letter). *Ann Intern Med* 101:882, 1984.

118. Vinters HV, Guerra WF, Eppolito L, Keith PED: Necrotizing vasculitis of the nervous system in a patient with AIDS-related complex. *Neuropathol Appl Neurobiol* 14:417, 1988.

119. Brannagan TH 3rd: Retroviral-associated vasculitis of the nervous system. *Neurol Clin* 15:927, 1997.

120. Kobayashi RM, Coel M, Niwayama G, Trauner D: Cerebral vasculitis in coccidioidal meningitis, *Ann Neurol* 1:281, 1977.

121. Einstein HE, Johnson RH: Coccidioidomycosis: New aspects of epidemiology and therapy. *Clin Infect Dis* 16:349, 1993.

122. Burgert SJ, Classen DC, Burke JP, Blatter DD: Candidal brain abscess associated with vascular invasion: A devastating complication of vascular catheter-related candidemia. *Clin Infect Dis* 21:202, 1995.

123. Kieburtz KD, Eskin TA, Ketonen L, Tuite MJ: Opportunistic cerebral vasculopathy and stroke in patients with the acquired immunodeficiency syndrome. *Arch Neurol* 50:430, 1993.

124. Scalzini A, Castelnuovo F, Puoti M, Cristini G: A case of cryptococcal meningoencephalitis and focal cerebral vasculitis with transient immunodeficiency. *Acta Neurol* 12:301, 1990.

125. Cantu C, Barinagarrementeria F: Cerebrovascular complications of neurocysticercosis: Clinical and neuroimaging spectrum. *Arch Neurol* 53:233, 1996.

126. Warrell DA, Looareesuwan S, Warrell MJ, et al: Dexamethasone proves deleterious in cerebral malaria: A double-blind trial in 100 comatose patients. *N Engl J Med* 306:313, 1982.

127. Kusner DJ, King CH: Cerebral paragonimiasis. *Semin Neurol* 13:201, 1993.

128. Wachter RM, Burke AM, MacGregor RR: *Strongyloides stercoralis* hyperinfection masquerading as cerebral vasculitis. *Arch Neurol* 41:1213, 1984.

129. Brown MM, Thompson AJ, Wedzicha JA, Swash M: Sarcoidosis presenting with stroke. *Stroke* 20:400, 1989.

130. Futrell N: Connective tissue disease and sarcoidosis of the central nervous system. *Curr Opin Neurol* 7:201, 1994.

131. Comu S, Verstraeten T, Rinkoff JS, Busis NA: Neurological manifestations of acute posterior multifocal placoid pigment epitheliopathy. *Stroke* 27:996, 1996.

132. Bewermeyer H, Nelles G, Huber M, Althaus C, Neuen-Jacob E, Assheuer J: Pontine infarction in acute posterior multifocal placoid pigment epitheliopathy. *J Neurol* 241:22, 1993.

133. Das T, Biswas J, Kumar A, et al: Eales' disease. *Indian J Ophthalmol* 42:3, 1994.

134. Haynes BF, Kaiser-Kupfer MI, Mason P, Fauci AS: Cogan syndrome: Studies in thirteen patients, long-term follow-up, and a review of the literature. *Medicine* 59:426, 1980.

135. Bicknell JM, Holland JV: Neurologic manifestations of Cogan syndrome. *Neurology* 28:278, 1978.

136. Fountain NB, Eberhard DA: Primary angiitis of the central nervous system associated with cerebral amyloid angiopathy: Report of two cases and review of the literature. *Neurology* 46:190, 1996.

137. Kidwell CS, Vinters H, Saver JL: Cerebral amyloid angiopathy, in *Neurobase* 1997.

138. Gray F, Vinters HV, Le Noan H, Salama J, Delaporte P, Poirier J: Cerebral amyloid angiopathy and granulomatous angiitis: Immunohistochemical study using antibodies to the Alzheimer A4 peptide. *Hum Pathol* 21:1290, 1990.

139. Omura M, Aida N, Sekido K, Kakehi M, Matsubara S: Large intracranial vessel occlusive vasculopathy after radiation therapy in children: Clinical features and usefulness of magnetic resonance imaging. *Int J Radiat Oncol Biol Phys* 38:241, 1997.

140. Bitzer M, Topka H: Progressive cerebral occlusive disease after radiation therapy. *Stroke* 26:131, 1995.

Chapter 20

DIAGNOSIS AND MANAGEMENT OF NONATHEROSCLEROTIC LARGE VESSEL DISEASE

Ravinder Singh

INTRODUCTION

There are a variety of nonatherosclerotic arterial diseases that cause cerebrovascular disease, including inflammatory and noninflammatory etiologies. The blood vessels supplying the brain can be pathologically affected by a heterogeneous group of inflammatory processes, collectively known as arteritis (angiitis, vasculitis). Arteritis is an inflammatory disease that results in structural damage (necrosis, fibrosis) to the vessel wall (intima and media). Blood vessels of any type and size can be affected. The cerebral arteries can be affected preferentially or as part of a systemic process. These vasculitides all share a common etiology of inflammation and necrosis as proven by histologic evidence.

In this chapter, we will focus our discussion on two specific etiologies: Takayasu's arteritis and fibromuscular dysplasia.

TAKAYASU'S ARTERITIS

Background

Background and Epidemiology Takayasu's arteritis (TA) is a nonspecific, chronic, idiopathic, inflammatory arteritis, affecting primarily the large vessels, primarily the aorta and its major branches. Known by various names ("pulseless disease," aortic branch disease, idiopathic aortitis, occlusive thromboaortopathy, obliterative brachiocephalic arteritis), it was originally described in young Japanese females by Takayasu, an ophthalmologist, in 1908.[1] Most cases have been reported from Asian countries, but it is now known to be more widespread, affecting patients of any age, race, or gender. Patients with TA are increasingly being recognized in Western countries. It tends to be more common in females during their reproductive years.[2-4] The estimated incidence rate of TA is 2.6 cases per million persons per year.[5]

Classification The Takayasu Conference, held in 1994, devised the current classification of TA (Table 20-1):[6]

Type I: Primarily involves branches from the aortic arch

Type IIa: Involves the ascending aorta, aortic arch, and its branches

Type IIb: Involves the ascending aorta, aortic arch and its branches, and the thoracic descending aorta

Type III: Involves the thoracic descending aorta, abdominal aorta, and/or the renal arteries

Type IV: Involves only the abdominal aorta and/or the renal arteries

Type V: Combination of type IIb and IV.

Involvement of coronary or pulmonary artery is designated as C(+) or P(+).

Table 20-1.

Classification of nonatherosclerotic causes according to the predominant vessel affected

Large arteries	Large and medium-sized arteries

Inflammatory
  Takayasu's arteritis
	Inflammatory
	  Giant cell arteritis

Noninflammatory
  Arterial dissection
	Noninflammatory
	  Fibromuscular dysplasia (FMD)

Medium-sized and small arteries	Small vessels

Inflammatory
  Primary systemic angiitides
    PAN group
      Polyarteritis nodosa
      Kawasaki's disease
    Churg-Strauss syndrome
    Wegener's granulomatosis
  Angiitis associated with other systemic diseases
    Behçet's disease
    Buerger's disease
    Sarcoidosis
  Angiitis associated with connective tissue disorder
    Rheumatoid arthritis
    Sjogren's syndrome
    Scleroderma
    Systemic lupus erythematosus
  Primary isolated angiitis of the central nervous system
	Inflammatory
	  Hypersensitivity angiitis

Pathology The most common sites of involvement are the aortic arch, innominate, common carotid, and the subclavian arteries.[7,8] It is a recurrent vasculitis, with active and quiescent phases. The pathologic process in the arterial wall begins initially with lymphocytic infiltration along the vasa vasorum, followed by involvement of the media. The acute period is characterized by a fulminant inflammatory reaction. The process culminates in segmental intimal thickening due to hyperplasia and fibrosis, leading to multiple areas of stenosis, poststenotic dilatation, irregularity, localized aneurysmal dilatation, and calcification in the arterial walls.[9] Vessel rupture and dissection are uncommon.[10] Thrombosis of the involved vessel is a common next step, followed by eventual recanalization. A specific etiology for TA has not been found, although the overall bulk of the evidence favors an immunopathogenic mechanism.[11] An association between TA and some autoimmune disorders (e.g., systemic lupus erythematosus and inflammatory bowel disease) has been noted.[12,13] Anecdotal re-

ports suggest association of TA with antiphospholipid antibodies (lupus anticoagulant and anticardiolipin antibodies) in the absence of other connective tissue diseases.[14]

Histologically, the arterial changes found in TA are similar to those of giant cell arteritis—scattered foreign bodies, occasional Langhan's giant cells, inflammatory mononuclear cell infiltrates, intimal proliferation and fibrosis, and disruption of the elastic lamina.[15] The ethnic predilection of TA has led investigators to postulate association with specific human leukocyte antigen (HLA) antigens. However, in the North American experience, there were no significant differences in the distribution of HLA antigens in TA patients and the general population.[5] Similarly, no consistent association with antibodies such as rheumatoid factor, antinuclear antibodies, circulating immune complexes, etc. has been found.[8,16] Antiaortic antibodies have been detected in TA patients, and one study found a preponderance of antiendothelial cell antibodies in patients with TA compared with controls.[11] The significance of these antibodies to the pathogenesis of TA is not clear; they may just be a marker of vasculitis.

Clinical Features   TA affects mainly young women during their reproductive years, although males can be affected in varying numbers in different populations (Table 20-2). In one study. Japanese patients were almost exclusively females (96 percent), whereas males comprised 37 percent of Indian patients with TA.[6] The median age of onset is 25 years.[5] Classically, patients with TA are felt to have a "triphasic" clinical course. The initial *systemic inflammatory phase* is characterized by the presence of systemic features. This is followed by the *vessel inflammatory phase,* characterized by painful ischemic vessels and symptoms of vascular insufficiency. The final phase is the *"burnt out" phase,* where patients experience symptoms of ischemia of major organs due to arterial involvement.[17,18] However, not all patients follow this classical course. There are many clinical presentations of TA, reflecting preferential involvement of

different vascular sites in different populations.[6] Almost all of the patients with TA have multiple sites of arterial involvement. Patients with TA have a diverse course. Japanese and North American patients tend to have involvement of the ascending aorta, the aortic arch, and its branches, resulting in symptoms of neurologic and upper extremity involvement.[5,6] Involvement of the abdominal aorta and its branches (renal and iliac arteries) can lead to symptoms such as hypertension and lower limb claudication. Clinical manifestations vary depending on the site and severity of the vascular lesions and the amount of collateral circulation. Characteristic systemic features such as fever, malaise, arthralgias, night sweats, and weight loss are present in only one-third of patients as their initial symptoms and may not be present in up to 57 percent of patients during their entire course of the disease.[5] Vascular ischemic symptoms are the hallmark of the disease, although in certain populations, hypertension and headache tend to be more common.[5,6] This diversity in the initial presentation, disease severity and the pace of disease progres-

Table 20-2.
Typical clinical features of Takayasu's arteritis

Clinical features		
Gender	Female (96%)	Male (4%)
Median age at onset	25 Years	Range 7–64 years
Median delay between onset of symptoms and diagnosis of disease	10 Months	Range 0–13 years
Neurologic symptoms	Generalized cerebral ischemia vertigo, dizziness	30–40%
	Focal cerebral ischemia	
	TIA or stroke	<10%
	Visual symptoms	20–30%
	Seizures	2–5%
	Encephalopathy	<5%
Other vascular symptoms		
	Claudication	60% (upper limbs)
		32% (lower limbs)
	Loss of pulse	53% (upper limbs)
		15% (lower limbs)
	Hypertension	33%
Other systemic symptoms		
	Myalgias, joint pain	40–50%
	Malaise	30–40%
	Fever	20–30%
	Weight loss	10–20%
	Cardiac disease	30–40%

sion, can result in a delay in the diagnosis of TA for several months and even years.[5]

Vascular and Neurologic Symptoms and Signs

Symptoms Although any of the aortic branches can be affected, the most common site is the common carotid arteries. CNS symptoms reflect progressive involvement of the extracranial cerebral arteries (carotid and/or vertebral arteries), causing stenosis and occlusion. Eighty percent of patients with cerebral vascular symptoms (stroke or TIA) have angiographic evidence of carotid or vertebral artery disease (or both).[5] However, symptoms of focal cerebral and ocular involvement are not as common as would be expected, given the extent of angiographically proven cervical arterial disease. Stroke and TIA tend to occur in less than 20 percent of patients. Using positron emission tomography (PET) to assess cerebral hemodynamics in TA patients, one study found no significant differences.[19] The development of focal brain ischemia might depend more on the degree of development of the collateral circulation. Gradual onset and progression of proximal arterial disease can lead to extensive extracranial and intracranial collateral circulation, thereby reducing the incidence and recurrence rate of stroke. Additionally, some of the focal neurologic symptoms may be due to global hypoperfusion, causing border-zone infarcts.[19] Lightheadedness, vertigo, and other posterior circulation symptoms may represent subclavian steal phenomenon or vertebral artery stenosis.

Other neurologic symptoms include headache, visual blurring, paresthesias in the upper extremities, confusion, and jaw claudication.[11,20] Retinal perfusion depends on a balance between central retinal artery pressure and intraocular pressure. Compromise in the cervical carotid artery circulation can affect the retinal circulation, leading to retinal ischemia. Chronic ocular ischemia may lead to visual loss. Anterior ischemic optic neuropathy (AION) and amaurosis fugax have been reported rarely.[15,21] Visual disturbances more often tend to be bilateral and are related to the presence of carotid and/or vertebral artery disease. Rarely, TA can present with bilateral blindness.[22]

Signs The most common clinical finding is a bruit, most commonly in the carotid arteries, followed by claudication and diminished or absent pulses.[5] Claudication and diminished or absent pulses, especially in the upper extremities, can result from progressive involvement of the aortic branches. Hypertension is a frequent clinical finding, affecting up to 50 percent of patients.[6] The majority of the patients with hypertension have unilateral or bilateral renal artery stenosis. Seventy-four percent of patients with renal artery stenosis have hypertension, whereas only 8 percent without renal artery stenosis have hypertension. Hypertension may be difficult to diagnose in the setting of upper limb claudication, causing delay in treatment. In these cases, only central, systemic pressures obtained during angiography are reliable. In advanced TA, hypertension can lead to chronically reduced cerebral hemodynamic reserve, predisposing patients to cerebral ischemia with any small reductions in blood pressure.[19] Hypertension in these cases should be treated with caution. In hypertensive TA patients who show evidence of significant cerebral ischemia, in the form of infarction, treating hypertension may lower the cerebral perfusion pressure below the autoregulatory lower limit.

Musculoskeletal and Constitutional Findings
Muscle and joint symptoms occur in less than 50 percent of patients. In many cases, symptoms are initially attributed to other connective tissue diseases, especially in the early stages of the disease, prior to the development of the classic angiographic lesions of the aorta. In some cases, other rheumatologic conditions may occur concurrently with TA.[5]

Cardiac Findings
The most common cardiac finding is aortic regurgitation, resulting from a dilated aortic root.[5,6] Cardiomegaly and congestive heart failure are common complications of aortic regurgitation or hypertension.[4] Involvement of the proximal segments of the coronary arteries is an important and potentially fatal complication.[10] Fortunately, the coronary arteries are seldom involved.[23] However, cardiac complications (ischemia regurgitation, and systemic and pulmonary hypertension) are the most common causes of death in patients with TA.[23,24]

Natural History of TA
TA is associated with a significant incidence of premature deaths and major morbidity. The 5-year survival rate after diagnosis is approximately 80 percent, with a worse prognosis if TA is accompanied by one or more complications (i.e., hypertension, retinopathy, aortic regurgitation, or aneurysm formation).[3–5] Hypertension has been found to be the most common contributing factor to the occurrence of strokes, renal failure, and cardiac failure. Other predictive factors in the long-term outcome are the degree

of functional disability and evidence of cardiac involvement.[3,5] Patients with none of these factors have a good long-term prognosis. Younger patients may show spontaneous clinical improvement.

Angiographic Features   Contrast angiography (CA) is highly sensitive and is considered the gold standard in detecting the anatomic abnormalities in the vasculature in patients with TA. Although the location of the involved arterial segment can be predicted on the basis of clinical presentation, the classic angiographic features help to differentiate TA from other vascular diseases and to assess the extent of collateral circulation. The majority of the patients have long, stenotic lesions ranging from mild narrowing to multifocal stenoses in the affected arterial segments. The most common arterial segments involved are the branches of the aortic arch, i.e., the innominate, common carotids, and the subclavian arteries, with relative preservation of the internal and external carotid, and the vertebral arteries. A small percentage of patients (12 to 17 percent) have poststenotic dilatation.[6] Aneurysms are noted in up to 27 percent of patients.[5] Other findings on CA include occlusion and the extent of intracranial and extracranial cerebral collateral circulation.[19] The relative sparing of the vertebral arteries, even in the most advanced cases of TA, provides an important intracranial collateral pathway.[18] Branches of the external carotid artery may also provide collaterals linking the branches of the subclavian and the vertebral circulation. In some cases of advanced TA, where all the brachiocephalic arteries may be totally occluded, collaterals can develop in the mediastinum, using the intercostal arteries to provide linkage to the vertebral circulation.[18] (Please see Chap. 36 and Fig. 36-8.)

Recent small studies with no control groups have attempted to evaluate the utility of various noninvasive modalities, such as carotid ultrasound (US), computerized tomographic angiography (CTA), and magnetic resonance imaging (MRI), comparing the results with angiographic findings, in the diagnosis and long-term follow-up of TA.[25-33] Among the purported advantages of US over CA are higher two-dimensional resolution and its ability to measure wall thickness.[26] Correlation between the two is not perfect, with cases of both false positives and false negatives.[26] However, sequential duplex scanning can provide information on progression of the disease and a simple, safe, and relatively accurate long-term means of follow-up.[25,27] Finding of long-segment stenoses in the common carotid arteries on US is suggestive of TA.[27,28] Transcranial Doppler has also

recently been used experimentally in TA, although the clinical utility has not been established.[29]

In other studies, cross-sectional scanning, such as with CT or MRI, has been used as a noninvasive tool to demonstrate the morphologic changes of the vessel walls, especially to facilitate in the early diagnosis of TA.[30,31] Most of the studies have evaluated the vertical sections of the aorta, with poor visualization of the aortic arch and the vessels of the proximal arch. Both modalities have claimed excellent visualization of the arteries, identifying stenoses, dilatations, aneurysms, and wall thickenings. In a comparative study of CTA and CA in 20 patients with documented TA, CTA was found to have a sensitivity of 95 percent and a specificity of 100 percent.[32] In fact, CTA has been purported to have advantages over CA by providing additional mural information.[33] A recent study compared MR angiography (MRA) findings with CA in 16 patients with TA.[34] MRA was also found to have good correlation with CA. However, false positives and false negatives were found as well. Although these various noninvasive tools are promising, angiography remains the gold standard for the initial diagnosis of TA.

Laboratory Investigations   Since an autoimmune etiology is suspected as the cause of TA, it is reasonable to examine for evidence of an autoimmune mechanism. Current laboratory parameters in TA have a low sensitivity. The laboratory evaluation can include complete blood count, erythrocyte sedimentation rate (ESR), serum electrolytes, serum creatinine and urea concentrations, serum tests for rheumatoid factor, antinuclear antibodies (ANA), anti-DNA antibodies, antibodies to extractable nuclear antigens (ENA), anti-Ro antibodies, anticardiolipin antibodies (ACLA), circulating immune complexes, antiendothelial cell antibodies (AECA), and antineutrophil cytoplasmic antibodies (ANCA). Characteristic laboratory findings include an elevated ESR in a vast majority of patients, mild anemia, and elevated immunoglobulin levels. The elevated ESR does not necessarily indicate histologically active disease.[1] In one study, the only consistent laboratory abnormality was the presence of AECA, although it did not correlate with the ESR or clinical activity of the disease.[11] The significance of AECA in the pathogenesis of TA is not known. One case report described two patients with an elevated titer of ACLA and lupus anticoagulant.[14] No other surrogate markers of active disease have been studied adequately. No antigen has been found on endothelial calls to which the antibody in sera from TA patients is directed.

Differential Diagnosis of TA   Ross and McKusick, in their classic paper,[35] described the differential diagnosis of the aortic arch syndrome. The clinical context and systemic considerations of the differential diagnosis will help to facilitate the diagnosis and subsequent treatment of TA (Table 20-3). Localization of the disease to the aortic arch is initially suspected on the basis of absent or diminished pulses in the arms and neck. The typical

clinical and angiographic features of these diseases help to differentiate them from TA.

Evidence

Medical Therapy   There have been no reported randomized controlled trials assessing the efficacy of any

Table 20-3.
Differential diagnosis of TA

Differential diagnosis	Typical differentiating factor(s) from TA
Inflammatory/infectious	
Sarcoidosis	Affects multiple organ systems, esp. lungs, high ACE levels; meningeal enhancement on MRI; biopsy of affected organ diagnostic
Syphilis	Positive serology
Systemic lupus erythematosus	Polyarthritis and dermatitis most common symptoms; common CNS symptoms include chronic fatigue, disturbances of cognition and affect (generalized encephalopathy); positive ANA and DNA antibodies
Rheumatoid arthritis	CNS involvement rare, positive serology; arteritis restricted to rheumatoid nodules
Rheumatic arteritis	Must be accompanied by endocarditis, and most often involves the coronary arteries
Thromboangiitis obliterans	Affects males exclusively, predilection for lower extremities
Polyarteritis nodosa	Affects males > females; diffuse encephalopathy and PNS involvement more common, CNS involvement late, seizures more frequent than stroke
Isolated angiitis of the CNS	Multifocal neurologic symptoms, headache, nausea, vomiting, dementia, amnesia, encephalopathy occur early on, systemic features uncommon
Temporal arteritis	Older patients (females > males), temporal headache, jaw claudication, and scalp tenderness common
Developmental anomalies	
Ehler-Danlos syndrome	Congenital disease causing joint hypermobility, hyperextensibility, and hyperelasticity of skin, associated with carotid dissection
Marfan syndrome	Inherited autosomal dominant disorder, affects skeletal, ocular, cardiovascular, and CNS, aortic involvement causes arterial dissection
Noninflammatory	
Extrinsic compression	Angiographic evidence
Thrombotic and embolic occlusion	Angiographic evidence
Coarctation of the aorta	Angiographic evidence
Congenital anomalies of the aorta	Angiographic evidence
Aortic trauma	History of neck trauma, no systemic features, angiographic evidence
Atherosclerosis	Angiographic evidence
Aortic dissection	May have a history of neck trauma, no systematic features, angiographic evidence

treatment modality in TA. Medical treatment with glucocorticoids and/or cytotoxic agents, and surgical treatment, ranging from angioplasty and endarterectomy, to bypass procedures have been tried with varying success. The North American study was the largest cohort of patients with TA studied in the United States.[5] In this study, 60 patients with active disease were treated with oral glucocorticoids at a dose of 1 mg/kg per day for 3 months. If patients could not be tapered to an alternate-day regimen without disease exacerbation, a cytotoxic agent was added (cyclophosphamide 1 to 2 mg/kg per day, azathioprine 1 to 2 mg/kg per day, or methotrexate 0.15 to 0.35 mg/kg once weekly, up to a maximum of 25 mg). Eighty percent (48 of 60) patients received glucocorticoids alone or in combination with a cytotoxic agent for active disease. Remission was achieved once in 60 percent of patients treated with glucocorticoids alone, with a median time to remission of 22 months. Addition of a cytotoxic agent caused remission in 40 percent of 25 patients receiving combination therapy, with a median time to remission of 20 months. Regardless of therapy, 45 percent of patients in remission had at least one relapse. Glucocorticoids and cytotoxic agents can lead to further complications. In the North American study, five patients treated with cyclophosphamide developed hemorrhagic cystitis. All patients treated with glucocorticoids became cushingoid.

In one case report of one patient presenting with AION as a manifestation of TA, intravenous methylprednisolone was given for 6 days, followed by oral prednisone.[15] There was only minimal improvement in the patient's vision with this treatment regimen. In another case record, one patient was treated initially with high-dose prednisone only.[23] Tapering of the dose of prednisone resulted in re-emergence of the patient's symptoms and elevation of the ESR, which responded to increasing the dose. Further deterioration of symptoms while on a stable dose of prednisone resulted in the addition of cyclosporine, which caused resolution of the symptoms.

The National Institutes of Health (NIH) conducted a prospective study of TA.[36] These investigators studied 60 patients with TA over a period of 20 years. The study required angiographic proof of diagnosis, with sequential angiographic follow-up in all patients, regardless of disease activity status. All patients received standardized treatment consisting of daily prednisone in doses of 1 mg/kg, up to 60 mg/day, for 1 to 3 months, followed by a slow taper to an alternate-day schedule during the next 4 to 8 weeks, if the disease remained quiescent. Subsequent tapering was continued to discontinuation over the next 6 to 12 months, barring exacerbation of symptoms. If discontinuation was not successful, or the disease relapsed, the patient became eligible for daily cyclophosphamide (2 mg/kg) or weekly methotrexate (0.15 to 0.3 mg/kg) therapy. Out of the 60 patients who entered the study 20 percent did not require any immunosuppressive therapy. Of the 48 patients who had active TA, 60 percent achieved remission with prednisone alone. Only 40 percent of patients requiring additional cytotoxic therapy achieved remission. Twenty-three percent of patients never achieved drug-free remission, and 45 percent with remissions experienced at least one relapse. Twenty-five percent of patients did not experience any significant disability in their activities of daily living.

Surgical Therapy As with medical therapy, there have been no reported controlled trials for surgical treatment in TA. Surgical treatments include bypass procedures, most commonly in the carotid circulation, but also for coronary artery disease, aneurysm repair, anastomotic repair, aortic valve replacement, thrombectomy, and balloon angioplasty. In the North American trial,[5] surgical treatment was reserved for patients who had (1) hypertension associated with critical stenosis of the renal vessels, (2) extremity ischemia limiting activities of daily living, (3) clinical features of cerebrovascular ischemia and/or critical (>70 percent) stenosis of at least three cerebral vessels, (4) moderate aortic regurgitation, or (5) cardiac ischemia with proven coronary artery stenosis. Patients underwent a variety of vascular procedures, including 50 bypass procedures with a 30 percent complication rate. The majority of these complications were due to restenosis, followed by thrombosis, hemorrhage, and infection. Nine patients underwent bypass procedures for critical stenoses in the carotid arteries for prophylaxis against stroke. During a median follow-up of 44 months, there was only 1 stroke in this group of patients. In another group of 19 patients who did not undergo carotid bypass, only 1 patient suffered a TIA during a mean follow-up of 35 months. Coronary artery bypass surgery was performed on three patients with coronary artery stenosis and angina, and aortic valve replacement in two patients with aortic regurgitation, all with good success. Twenty angioplasty procedures, most often on the subclavian and renal vessels, were performed with a 56 percent success on the first attempt. Restenosis occurred between 3 and 13 months, with three patients eventually requiring a bypass procedure. In one study of anastomotic surgery for TA, the surgical procedure led to the development of postanastomotic aneurysms.[37] The incidence of these aneurysms was 12 percent over 20 years and tended to occur more often after operations for aneurysmal lesions.

Percutaneous transluminal angioplasty (PTA) is an emerging treatment for arterial stenosis in TA.[38-40] However, the extensive fibrosis and thickening of the arterial wall produces a tough, noncompliant and rigid vessel wall, producing a higher resistance to balloon inflation. This can result in post-PTA complications. Patients with short stenotic lesions experience more relief with PTA than patients with long segment stenoses.[41] Angioplasty can lead to large intimal flaps and, occasionally, dissection. Use of a vascular stent has shown promise in case reports in treating dissection.[42] There are no reported studies comparing different modalities for the treatment of dissection, however. A recent study compared subclavian artery stenting in patients with TA to patients with stenosis due to atherosclerosis. The stenotic lesions in TA patients required higher balloon inflation pressures, with a more residual stenosis after PTA. During a mean follow-up of 43 months, restenosis was more often observed in patients with TA.[39]

Treatment Recommendations

Glucocorticoids remain the most commonly used and effective palliative agents for most patients with TA. The response to glucocorticoids ranges from 20 to 100 percent.[5] Addition of a cytotoxic agent is reserved for patients demonstrating clinical worsening or unresponsiveness to steroid therapy. In the absence of data from randomized trials, a stepwise approach, based upon the North American study, is recommended, as outlined in Table 20-4. Surgical treatment is reserved for patients failing medical therapy or for prevention of complications from the disease (see "Evidence"). For bypass surgery, the patency rate is less than ideal, with development of stenosis in the bypass graft the most common complication. Although angioplasty has a high rate of restenosis (approximately 45 percent), it may be beneficial in patients with short, proximal stenotic lesions requiring urgent relief.[5]

FIBROMUSCULAR DYSPLASIA

Background

Background and Epidemiology   Fibromuscular dysplasia (FMD, fibrous dysplasia) is an uncommon, segmental, noninflammatory, nonatherosclerotic arteriopathy. It occurs predominantly in middle-aged Caucasian women, especially in their fourth and fifth decades of life.[43] This group accounts for approximately 90 percent of cases.[44] Involvement in children is unusual, although it should be considered as an uncommon cause of stroke in children.[44] It is the most frequent arterial dysplasia

Table 20-4.
Medical treatment of TA

	Patients with active disease	
Medication	Dose & duration	
Oral glucocorticoids[a]	1 mg/kg/day for 3 months	
Cyclophosphamide[b]	1–2 mg/kg/day	
Azathioprine	1–2 mg/kg/day	
Methotrexate	0.15–0.35 mg/kg/week Starting dose: 15 mg/week 2.5-mg increments every 1 to 2 weeks; Maximum weekly dose of up to 25 mg	

[a]If active disease improves, taper daily glucocorticoid therapy to alternative-day regimen. If disease remains inactive, taper glucocorticoids further and stop. If patients cannot be tapered to an alternate-day regimen without disease exacerbating, add a cytotoxic agent (cyclophosphamide, azathioprine, or methotrexate).

[b]Continue the cytotoxic agent alone for 1 year after remission, then taper (cyclophosphamide and azathioprine at 25 mg/mo, methotrexate at 2.5 mg/mo) until discontinued. If disease recurs, increase or restart both glucocorticoids and cytotoxic agent.

and is estimated to have a frequency of less than 1 percent.[45] It is a common feature on renal arteries, but it is rarely responsible for occlusive disease of extracranial arteries supplying the brain.[46] The exact incidence of FMD involving the cervicocephalic arteries is not known. It has been reported to be between 2.5 and 6.5 percent of patients undergoing carotid artery angiography for evaluation of cerebrovascular disease.[47] In patients presenting with dissection of the ICA, angiographic evidence of FMD can be found in up to 23 percent of cases.[48] However, it was found in only 0.02 percent of 20,244 consecutive autopsies done at the Mayo Clinic over a 25-year period.[49] It affects primarily medium-sized arteries. FMD was initially described in the renal arteries and is the most common location, but it is now known to also involve the extracranial carotid and vertebral arteries and, less commonly, the splanchnic circulation.[45,50] FMD may be widespread or may involve one or two arterial territories. In the carotid and vertebral circulation, it is most commonly localized to the distal extracranial segments adjacent to the first and second cervical vertebra.[45] The internal carotid artery is involved in approximately 95 percent of patients with cephalic FMD. Bilateral carotid artery involvement is common, affecting as many as 60 to 80 percent of patients with carotid involvement.[43] The intracranial arteries are rarely affected.[51] The prevalence of familial FMD is not known; however, in one study of renal FMD, the prevalence of familial FMD was found to be 11 percent.[52] Familial cases tended to exhibit more multifocal pathology and were more commonly bilateral.

Pathology The pathologic process consists of fibrodysplasia of smooth muscles leading to formation of rings of fibrous tissue and smooth muscle. This occurs most commonly in the tunica media (90 to 95 percent of cases and much more commonly in women), although the other layers, the intima and the adventitia, can also be affected.[45] Four histologic types have been described: medial, intimal, perimedial or subadventitial dysplasia, and medial hyperplasia without associated fibrotic changes.[53] Medial fibroplasia (type 1) is the most common type. The rings of fibrous tissue alternate with areas of medial thickening and destruction of the elastic layer, leading to areas of arterial lumen widening and narrowing. When the process involves the intima, the proliferation of fibrous cells in this layer leads to tubular stenosis and focal stenosis. Intimal fibrodysplasia is more common in children and young adults.[45]

The etiology of FMD is unclear. Familial occurrence, association with intracranial aneurysmal disease and other congenital anomalies, suggests a congenital

disorder as the underlying etiology.[53] In addition, humoral factors, mechanical trauma, immunologic factors, and more recently, an association with α_1 antitrypsin deficiency have all been implicated.[49,54]

Clinical Features Patients with cervicocephalic FMD may be asymptomatic or may present with a variety of neurologic symptoms. Cerebrovascular symptoms and pulsatile tinnitus are the most common manifestations.[46,49] The neurologic abnormalities can be attributed to global cerebral hypoperfusion, focal ischemia, or direct compressive effects of the arterial wall lesion. The symptoms may be nonspecific, nonlocalizing ones such as headaches, syncope, episodic dizziness and vertigo, pulsatile tinnitus, and cervical bruit. The patient may also have focal symptoms of vascular insufficiency, such as transient ischemic attacks or cerebral infarction.[46] This may be due to a thromboembolic phenomenon or arterial dissection. The specific clinical manifestations of vascular insufficiency provide a clue to the specific vessels involved and the degree of impairment of blood flow. In most cases, however, the relationship between FMD and focal as well as global ischemic symptoms is unclear. Cervical bruits and pulsatile tinnitus may be caused by the direct effects of the arterial wall lesions and their complications, such as turbulent flow, and may be the only neurologic abnormality.

A well-known complication of FMD is arterial dissection in the extracranial carotid arteries. Most cases of "spontaneous" dissection are attributed to an underlying vasculopathy, of which FMD is the most common.[48,55] The dissection most often occurs between the intima and media, but may also occur between the media and adventitia. The dissection can cause ischemic lesions either by compromise of the vascular lumen by the intramural hematoma or a thrombus formed over the fibrosed intima (see Chap. 16).[56]

FMD may result in extracranial ICA aneurysm formation. Literature has shown a range from 20 to 50 percent.[57,58] FMD of the intracranial arteries is rare, although the exact incidence of asymptomatic FMD is unknown.[59] It is estimated that almost two-thirds of the patients have had definite cerebrovascular symptoms. Patients with FMD are also at a higher risk of harboring an intracranial aneurysm, although the exact magnitude is not known. The incidence of aneurysms associated with FMD ranges from 3 to 50 percent.[51,60] In a recent meta-analysis of 17 angiographic series of ICA/vertebral artery (VA) FMD, the incidence of incidental, asymptomatic intracranial cerebral aneurysms was found to be approximately 7 percent.[61] The presence of an intracranial aneurysm increases the likelihood of subarachnoid hemorrhage or intracerebral hematoma. The aneurysms have the same distribution and histology as in patients without FMD. Most of the aneurysms are located at the junction of the internal carotid artery and the posterior communicating artery, at the bifurcation of the middle cerebral artery, or at the junction between the anterior communicating artery and the anterior cerebral artery. Many cases of FMD, however, are an incidental finding at CA or autopsy.

The mechanisms underlying neurologic symptoms in patients with FMD are unclear. Several mechanisms have been proposed. These include artery-to-artery emboli, local thrombosis, emboli arising from a pseudo-aneurysmal sac, and relative hypoperfusion distal to the stenosis. A hemodynamic mechanism, however, is considered to be much less common.[49] Arterial dissection is a frequent cause.[62] Patients with FMD also have associated atherosclerosis, which may be a contributory factor.

Diagnosis   The diagnosis of FMD is based mainly on the classic angiographic findings of "string of beads" pattern, which is caused by alternating zones of dilatation (due to thinned vascular walls), which are always wider than the normal lumen, and narrowing (due to thickened fibromuscular ridges), which usually reduce the caliber of the lumen to less than 40 percent.[45,51] This feature, the most common angiographic appearance, is considered pathognomonic for FMD and is seen in 80 to 90 percent of patients (see Chap. 36 and Fig. 36-8). Two other angiographic patterns have been described. Some patients exhibit a relatively smooth unifocal or multifocal tubular stenosis. This pattern may be associated with any histologic type of FMD. A third pattern is termed "atypical FMD." One wall of the affected segment demonstrates a diverticulum-like outpouching that may progress into an aneurysm.[59,63]

The natural history of FMD is not known, although serial angiograms have revealed increasing severity of a particular pattern. However, one case report suggested that these angiographic patterns are not necessarily fixed and may change from a "string-of-beads" appearance to a tubular pattern.[53] Extracranial ICA aneurysms due to FMD are uncommon, constituting only 3 percent of all ICA aneurysms. Most of the aneurysms are true saccular aneurysms involving all three layers of the vessel wall. However, dissecting aneurysms with associated focal stenosis have been described.[63] The natural history of aneurysms in FMD is also not known. The diagnosis of intracranial FMD is also based on angiographic demonstration of the typical appearance.

MRA has been shown to exhibit the "string-of-beads" sign in case reports of FMD, although the sensitivity and specificity are not known.[44,64,65] MR imaging can be helpful in distinguishing arterial dissection from tubular FMD or arterial dysplasia.[51] Another noninvasive technique, CTA is being used more frequently to study arterial disease. In a comparison study of CTA and CA of the carotid bifurcation, the overall agreement between the two was 45 percent.[66] CTA tended to overestimate stenoses and erroneously interpreted marked stenoses as occluded. In the two patients with FMD in this study, long stenotic segments of FMD of the ICA were interpreted as occluded on CTA.[66] All the noninvasive techniques, including CTA, duplex imaging, and MRA, may suggest the diagnosis, although they carry the risk of misdiagnosis.[67]

Evidence

There have been no large prospective trials concerning the clinical and angiographic natural history of untreated FMD of arteries supplying the brain. No randomized controlled trials of medical or surgical treatments have been undertaken in the treatment of FMD. In a retrospective clinical outcome study, 79 patients with FMD were followed for 5 years.[68] In this group, 64 patients did not receive any treatment, 11 patients received either antiplatelet therapy or anticoagulation, and 3 patients had surgical treatment. In the untreated group, 1 patient suffered a stroke in the arterial distribution of the affected artery, and 2 patients suffered a stroke in the nonaffected circulation. Stroke or TIA did not occur in the treated group. According to this study, the incidence of focal symptoms in untreated patients seems to be low. In a retrospective study of 30 patients with symptomatic cerebrovascular FMD, patients receiving surgical (arterial dilation) or medical therapy (antiplatelet agents) showed significant benefit compared with patients not receiving any therapy at all.[69] In a recent trial of surgical treatment in FMD, 70 patients underwent surgery in a nonrandomized fashion with no control group.[46] Patients underwent unilateral or bilateral revascularization of the involved carotid and/or vertebral arteries, alone or in association with another procedure (endarterectomy, resection anastomosis, shortening- or patch-angioplasty, and embolectomy). Some patients underwent carotid bifurcation to distal internal carotid bypass. The incidence of postoperative death was 1.4 percent and nonlethal stroke was 2.8 percent. Long-term follow-up revealed actual survival rates at 5 and 10 years of 96.4 and 82.1, respectively. Despite the overall favorable outcome, the lack of knowledge about the natural history of FMD limits generalization

Color Plates

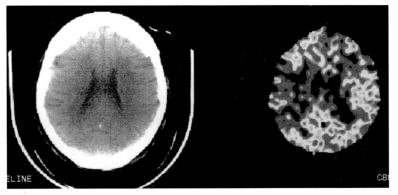

Plate 1 (see Figure 2-4).
Simultaneous CT and xenon CT Left. CT scan without evidence of ischemia. Right. Xenon CT with significantly decreased blood flow in right middle cerebral artery territory shown in blue (range 27–38 ml/ 100 g/min). Normal blood flow in homologous area in left middle cerebral artery territory shown as yellow-orange (range 45–72 ml/100 g/min).

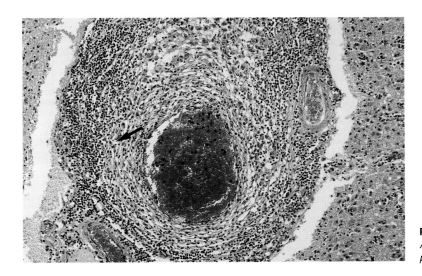

Plate 2 (see Figure 19-1A).
A perivascular inflammatory infiltrate in a patient with PACNS (10×).

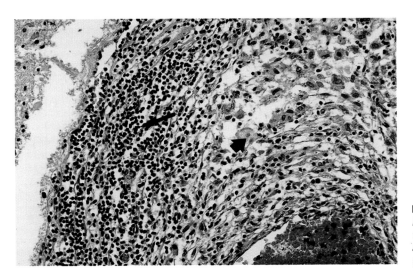

Plate 3 (see Figure 19-1B).
Detailed view of inflammatory infiltrate with polymorphonuclear cells (long arrow) and mononuclear cells (short arrow) (20×).

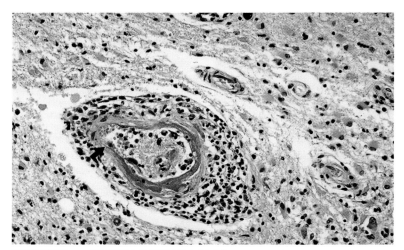

Plate 4 (see Figure 19-2).
Fibrinoid necrosis with focal destruction of the vessel wall in a patient with PACNS (20×).

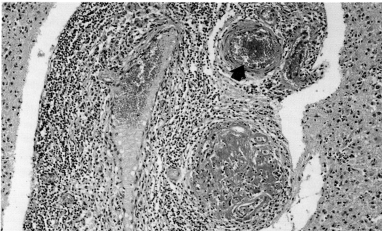

Plate 5 (see Figure 19-3).
Thrombosis of the microvasculature with surrounding inflammatory infiltrate in a patient with PACNS (10×).

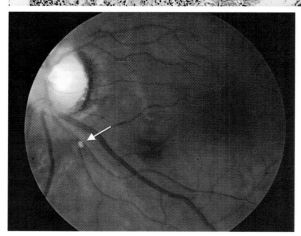

Plate 6 (see Figure 31-1).
Hollenhorst plaque. Note presence of intra-arterial plaque at a bifurcation point (arrow).

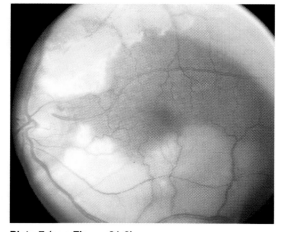

Plate 7 (see Figure 31-2).
CRAO. Central retinal artery occlusion demonstrating white retinal swelling with sparring of a portion of the macular area supplied by a cilioretinal artery.

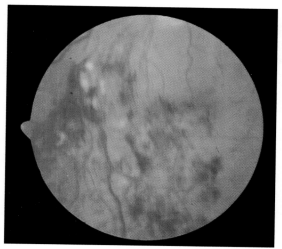

Plate 8 (see Figure 31-3).
BRVO. Branch retinal vein occlusion showing dilation of the vein and associated hemorrhage.

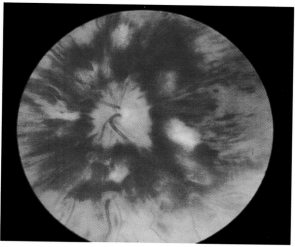

Plate 9 (see Figure 31-4).
CRVO. Typical appearance of a central retinal vein occlusion with diffuse hemorrhage.

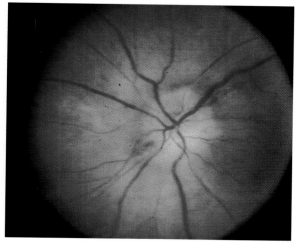

Plate 10 (see Figure 31-5).
AION. The optic disc in anterior ischemic optic neuropathy is swollen and often has associated nerve fiber layer hemorrhages.

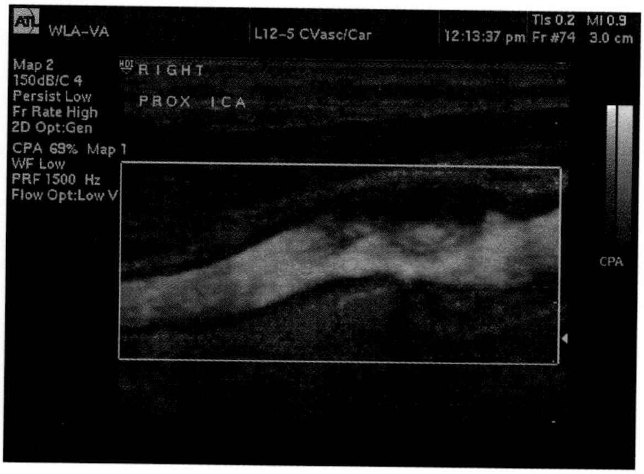

Plate 11 (see Figure 33-1).
Non-hemodynamically significant lesions. Color power Doppler image of the right proximal internal carotid artery reveals a well-defined, hypoechoic plaque that narrows the vessel lumen less than 50 percent. Non-hemodynamically significant lesions may be screened for using only power imaging in the future. Further investigation needs to confirm the efficacy of this technique prior to widespread use.

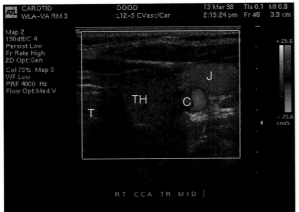

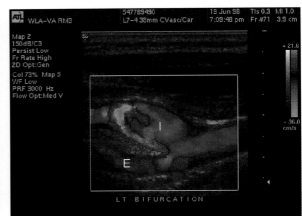

Plate 12 (see Figure 33-3).

Normal anatomy. Transverse image through mid-neck depicts normal sonographic anatomy. The trachea (T) lies in the midline adjacent to the low-level gray-scale echoes of the thyroid (TH). Lateral the thyroid lies the common carotid artery (C) and jugular vein (J). The sternocleidomastoid muscle (S) lies anteriorly.

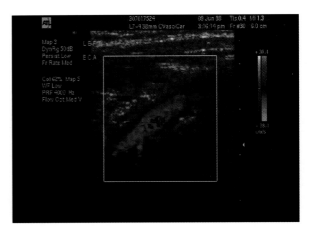

Plates 13–15 (see Figure 33-4 A–C).

*Normal carotid bifurcation: **Plate 13.** With proper angulation, images of both bifurcation vessels can often be obtained in a single plane. Note that color assignment is totally angle dependent. Flow in the external carotid artery (E) is displayed in blue beyond its immediate bifurcation as flow has turned toward the transducer. Areas of flow in the ICA (I), which are displayed in various shades of blue and shade into yellow, are likely due to the presence of boundary separation layers. Boundary separation layers are areas of flow reversal and slow flow and are normal at vascular bifurcations. The stress factors imposed by boundary separation layers on the vessel walls may be an associated factor in the development of atherosclerotic plaquing. **Plate 14.** The external and internal carotid arteries frequently are scanned individually, in separate scan planes. The ECA can be differentiated from the ICA by means of identifying branches (arrows). The ICA gives off no branches in the neck. The most commonly identified branch is the superior thyroidal artery, which is typically identified at or near the origin of the ECA. **Plate 15.** The internal external carotid arteries are also able to be differentiated by means of their spectral Doppler signatures. The internal carotid artery is a typical low resistance vessel with a large amount of diastolic flow. Flow continues in a forward direction throughout the cardiac cycle.*

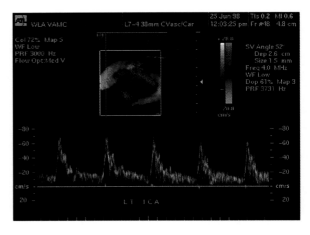

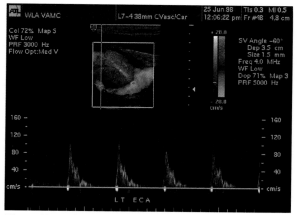
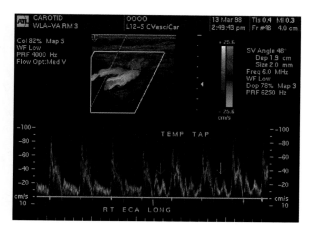

Plates 16–17 (see Figure 33-4 D–E).

Plate 16. The spectral pattern of the ECA can be readily differentiated from that of the ICA by virtue of a high resistance spectral signal. In this particular patient, the ECA demonstrates no diastolic flow. Note brief period of flow reversal, which is the hallmark of high resistance arteries supplying muscular beds. **Plate 17.** A third method of differentiating the ICA from the ECA is the temporal tap. In this maneuver, one taps lightly over the temporomandibular joint where a large branch of the external carotid artery (the temporal artery) lies in a superficial location. Tapping over the temporal artery will produce oscillations in the ECA, which are particularly prominent in diastole (arrows). This maneuver may be used as further supportive evidence that the spectral Doppler cursor is the external carotid artery as shown.

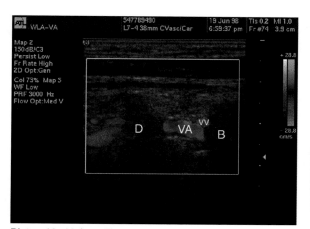
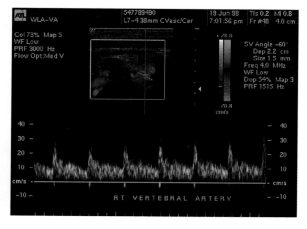

Plates 18–19 (see Figure 33-5 A–B).

Normal vertebral vessels. **Plate 18.** The normal vertebral artery courses through the transverse foramina of the cervical spine producing areas of periodic shadowing as the vessel passes through bone (B). Note the varying Doppler angle relationships as the vessel changes direction in relation to the linear array transducer. The more inferior portion of the vertebral artery is directed toward the transducer and displayed in red (VA). The more distal portion is displayed in blue as flow is directed away from the transducer. The vertebral vein is displayed in the opposite colors (VV). **Plate 19.** The spectral pattern of the normal vertebral artery is that of a low resistance artery; it supplies the posterior fossa with blood. The vertebral arteries join to form the basilar artery within the skull.

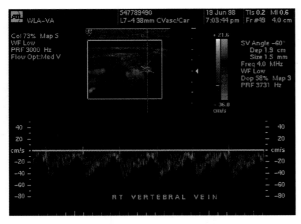

Plate 20 (see Figure 33-5C).
Spectral patterns from the vertebral vein may be confused with those of the accompanying artery. The two must be carefully differentiated to avoid a misdiagnosis of subclavian steal. In this particular subject, the venous patterns are fairly similar to those from an artery. If a question exists, breath-holding and other physiologic maneuvers may allow differentiation, as arterial flow is usually unaffected. In most cases, the venous wave forms display a more typical triphasic pattern, which is present but somewhat subtle in this case. The differentiation of vein from artery can also often be made by listening to the Doppler sounds.

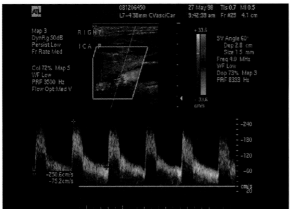

Plate 21 (see Figure 33-10A).
Moderate (≥60 percent) internal carotid artery stenosis. Color Doppler imaging reveals an area of intense aliasing (note mixture of color) suggesting a region of high-speed flow in association with a significant stenosis. Spectral Doppler demonstrates the peak systolic velocity was 250 cm/s; end diastolic velocity was 75 cm/s. The ratio in this case measured 2.9.

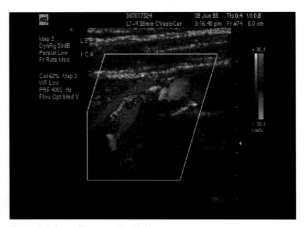

Plate 22 (see Figure 33-11A).
Severe (≥70 percent) internal carotid artery stenosis. Color Doppler imaging reveals an area of marked vessel narrowing at the origin of the left internal carotid artery (arrow). Note aliasing and flow reversal distal to the region of stenosis. The superficial vessel (arrowheads) represents the jugular vein.

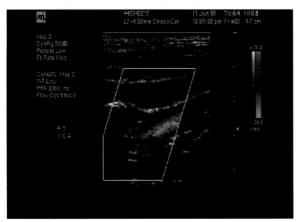

Plate 23 (see Figure 33-12A).
Total internal carotid occlusion. Color Doppler imaging reveals an abrupt cessation of flow just beyond the origin of the internal carotic artery. Note focal area of flow reversal (arrow) as forward-moving flow strikes occluding plaque and direction/color are reversed.

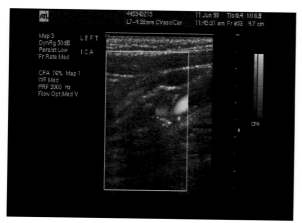

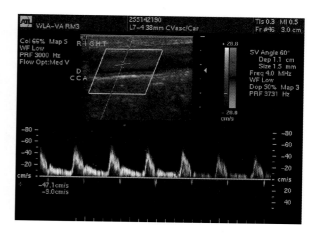

Plates 24–25 (see Figure 33-12 B–C).
Plate 24. *Color power Doppler confirms presence of complete occlusion. No evidence of a minute flow channel is depicted. The original occluded vessel (arrows) is well defined in this patient; solid plaque fills lumen.* **Plate 25.** *Spectral tracing from the common carotid artery of the same patient reveals an externalized wave form typical of patients with ICA occlusion in whom all flow in the common carotid artery is directed toward the ECA. Note, typical periods of flow reversal in early diastole.*

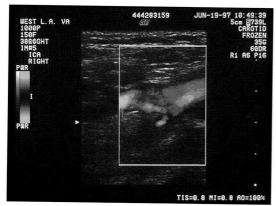

Plate 26 (see Figure 33-13A).
Subtotal internal carotid occlusion. Conventional color Doppler imaging failed to reveal evidence of flow in the internal carotid artery; complete occlusion was suspected. Color power imaging demonstrated a small vascular channel (arrow) suggesting subtotal occlusion.

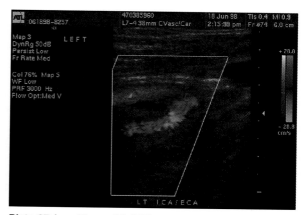

Plate 27 (see Figure 33-15B).
Scanning at the carotid bifurcation reveals two patent vessels with differing color/flow direction. Flow in the ECA (shown in blue) was reversed and toward the transducer. The artery was serving as a feeding collateral to the ICA (shown in red) which maintains normally directed flow. In patients with common carotid artery occlusion, it is essential to scan at the bifurcation to identify such collateral pathways.

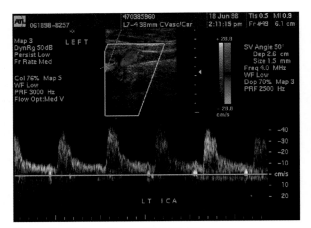 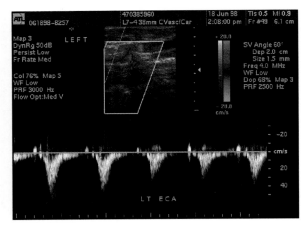

Plates 28–29 (see Figure 33-15 C–D).

Plate 28. *Spectral Doppler of the internal carotid artery reveals normally directed flow with a typical low resistance pattern.* **Plate 29.** *Scanning in the external carotid artery demonstrates reversed flow with a higher resistance pattern than was identified in the internal carotid.*

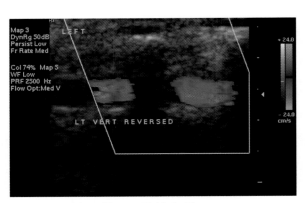 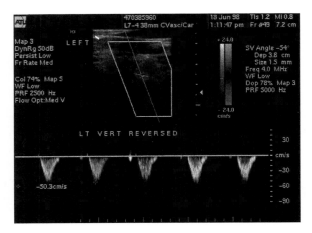

Plates 30–31 (see Figure 33-16 A–B).

Subclavian steal syndrome. **Plate 30.** *Color Doppler imaging demonstrates reversed flow in the left vertebral artery. Flow is toward the feet and displayed in blue. Note periodic areas of shadowing from the lateral masses of the cervical spine confirming that this vessel represents the vertebral artery.* **Plate 31.** *Spectral evaluation of the same vessel confirms reversal of flow and that vessel is an artery. Note absence of diastolic flow component. This finding is typical of spectral patterns from the vertebral arteries of patients with subclavian steal. It is most likely caused by the vertebral artery serving the high resistance vasculature of the arm.*

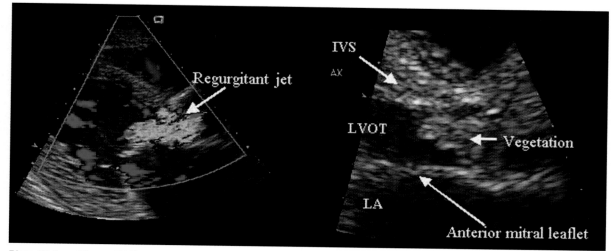

Plate 32 (see Figure 37-2).
Large aortic vegetation detected by two-dimensional transthoracic echocardiography in patient with endocarditis and cerebral embolism. LVOT = interventricular septum; IVS = interventricular septum; LA = left atrium.

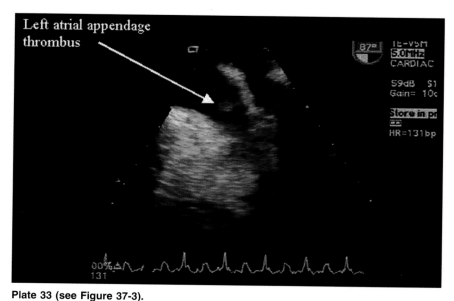

Plate 33 (see Figure 37-3).
Left atrial appendage thrombus in patient with atrial fibrillation. Left atrial and ventricular enlargement and ejection fraction of 15 percent.

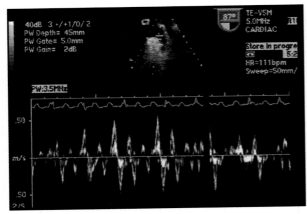 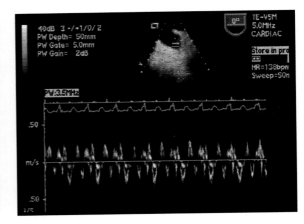

Plates 34–35 (see Figure 37-4 A–B).
Plate 34. *Pulsed doppler of the left atrial appendage in a patient with atrial fibrillation and no atrial appendage thrombus; velocities vary from 0.25 to 0.50 m/s.* **Plate 35.** *Atrial fibrillation with atrial appendage flow velocities less than 0.25 m/s in patient with left atrial appendage thrombus.*

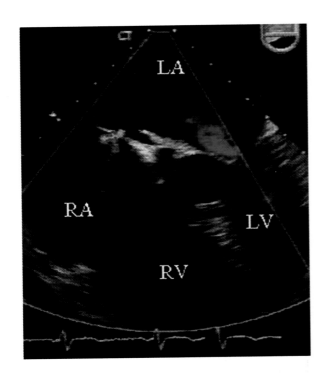

Plate 36 (see Figure 37-8).
Color flow jet across the interatrial septum demonstrating the presence of a patent foramen ovale.

of the results of this trial to individual patients with FMD.

PTA has been reported to be safe and efficacious in the treatment of FMD.[70-72] No controlled trials using this technique have been reported, however. Case reports of treatment with self-expanding endovascular stents, coil embolization, and surgical ligation have been described with good clinical outcome.[71,73] These techniques have been used more often for patients presenting with carotid dissection as a complication of FMD. One retrospective study of PTA of supra-aortic vessels demonstrated excellent immediate and long-term results for the common, external and internal carotid arteries (100 percent success rate), and vertebral arteries (93 percent success rate). Subclavian PTA resulted in approximately 50 percent restenosis rate.[74]

Treatment Recommendations

In the absence of specific clinical data in FMD, treatment is based upon extrapolation of available clinical data from stroke treatment trials. In uncomplicated patients, antiplatelet therapy is suggested. The high association of FMD with intracranial aneurysms limits the use of anticoagulants because of the increased risk of aneurysm rupture and bleeding. In patients who have tight stenotic disease in the extracranial carotid circulation, various surgical procedures have been used, such as PTA, extracranial/intracranial bypass, resection anastomosis, and patch grafting. Graduated intraluminal dilation is the most frequently performed surgical procedure for FMD lesions. Because atherosclerosis is frequently found in association with the FMD, endarterectomy has also been performed in conjunction with these procedures. In the absence of data from well-controlled clinical trials and the low incidence of focal, serious neurologic outcomes in untreated or medically treated patients, a conservative approach is recommended. Surgical treatment should be reserved for patients who continue to have symptoms despite medical treatment. Given the lack of randomized clinical trials of surgical procedures such as endarterectomy in FMD, the decision regarding surgical treatment should be based upon available data on surgical management of carotid stenosis, regardless of the etiology.

REFERENCES

1. Shimizu K, Sano K: Pulseless disease. *J Neuropath Clin Neurol* 1:37, 1951.

2. Nakao K, Ikeda M, Kimata S, Niitani H, et al: Takayasu's arteritis: Clinical report of eighty-four cases and immunological study of seven cases. *Circulation* 35:1141, 1967.

3. Ishikawa K: Diagnostic approach and proposed criteria for the clinical diagnosis of Takayasu's arteriopathy. *J Am Col Cardiol* 12:964, 1988.

4. Subramanyan R, Joy J, Balakrishnan KG: Natural history of aortoarteritis (Takayasu's disease). *Circulation* 80:429, 1989.

5. Kerr GS, Hallahan CW, Giordano J, et al: Takayasu arteritis. *Ann Intern Med* 120:919, 1994.

6. Moriwaki R, Noda M, Yajima M, Sharma BK, Numano F: Clinical manifestations of Takayasu arteritis in India and Japan: New classification of angiographic findings. *Angiology* 48:369, 1997.

7. Sano K, Alga T, Saito I: Angiography in pulseless disease. *Radiology* 94:69, 1970.

8. Hall S, Barr W, Lee JT, et al: Takayasu arteritis: A study of 32 North American patients. *Medicine* 54:89, 1985.

9. Wada T, Kodaira K, Fujishiro K, et al: Common carotid artery wall properties in Takayasu's arteritis. *Angiology* 47:669, 1996.

10. Parums DV: The arteritides. *Histopathology* 25:1, 1994.

11. Eichhorn J, Sima D, Thiele B, et al: Anti-endothelial cell antibodies in Takayasu arteritis. *Circulation* 94:2396, 1996.

12. Saxe PA, Altman RD: Aortitis syndrome (Takayasu's arteritis) associated with SLE. *J Rheumatol* 17:1251, 1990.

13. Ikenaga H, Ogihara T, Iyori S, et al: Does a common pathophysiological basis exist in the association of ulcerative colitis and Takayasu's aortitis? Report of a case. *Postgrad Med J* 65:761, 1989.

14. Yokoi K, Hosoi E, Akaike M, et al: Takayasu's arteritis associated with antiphospholipid antibodies: Report of two cases. *Angiology* 47:315, 1996.

15. Schmidt MH, Fox AJ, Nicolle DA: Bilateral anterior ischemic optic neuropathy as a presentation of Takayasu's disease. *J Neuroophthalmol* 17:156, 1997.

16. Gyotoku Y, Kakiuchi T, Nonaka Y, et al: Immune complexes in Takayasu's arteritis. *Clin Exp Immunol* 45:246, 1981.

17. Shelhamer JH, Volkman DJ, Parrillo JE, et al: Takayasu's arteritis and its therapy. *Ann Intern Med* 103:121, 1985.

18. Lupi-Herrera E, Sanchez-Torres G, Marcushamer J, et al: Takayasu's arteritis: Clinical study of 107 cases. *Am Heart J* 93:94, 1977.

19. Takano K, Sadoshima S, Ibayashi S, et al: Altered cerebral hemodynamics and metabolism in Takayasu's arteritis with neurological deficits. *Stroke* 24:1501, 1993.

20. Hankey GJ: Necrotizing and granulomatous angiitis of the CNS, in Ginsberg MD, Bogousslavsky J, (ed): *Cerebrovascular Disease: Pathophysiology, Diagnosis, and Management.* Massachusetts, Blackwell Science, 1998, pp 1659–1660.

21. Charlton JF, Dalla K: Amaurosis and pulselessness in a young white woman: A case of Takayasu disease. *J Am Board Fam Pra* 10:227, 1997.

22. Rodriguez-Pla A, de Miguel G, Lopez-Contreras J, et al: Bilateral blindness in Takayasu's disease. *Scand J Rheumatol* 25:394, 1996.

23. Case records of the Massachusetts General Hospital: Case 4-1995. *N Engl J Med* 332:380, 1995.

24. Hashimoto Y, Tanaka M, Hata A, et al: Four year follow-up study in patients with Takayasu arteritis and severe aortic regurgitation: Assessment by echocardiography. *Intern J Cardiol* 54(Suppl): S143, 1996.

25. Sun Y, Yip PK, Jeng JS, et al: Ultrasonographic study and long-term follow-up of Takayasu's arteritis. *Stroke* 27: 2178, 1996.

26. Taniguchi N, Itoh K, Honda M, et al: Comparative ultrasonographic and angiographic study of carotid arterial lesions in Takayasu's arteritis. *Angiology* 48:9, 1997.

27. Wang HT, Chou YH, Teng MM, et al: Duplex ultrasound of extracranial carotid artery in a male patient of Takayasu's arteritis: A case report. *Chung-Hua i Hsueh Tsa Chih Chin Med J* 53:243, 1994.

28. Matsumura Y, Morimoto K, Ishikawa M, et al: Images in Cardiovascular Medicine. Ultrasonographic images of Takayasu's arteritis. *Circulation* 98:1585, 1998.

29. Egido JA, Castrillo C, Sanchez M, et al: Takayasu's arteritis: Transcranial Doppler findings and follow-up. *J Neurosurg Sci* 40:121, 1996.

30. Hata A, Numano F: Magnetic resonance imaging of vascular changes in Takayasu's arteritis. *Intern J Cardiol* 52: 45, 1995.

31. Matsunaga N, Hayashi K, Sakamoto I, et al: Takayasu arteritis: MR manifestations and diagnosis of acute and chronic phase. *J Magn Reson Imag* 8:406, 1998.

32. Yamada I, Nakagawa T, Himeno Y, et al: Takayasu arteritis: Evaluation of the thoracic aorta with CT angiography. *Radiology* 209:103, 1998.

33. Park JH, Chung JW, Lee KW, et al: CT angiography of Takayasu arteritis: Comparison with conventional angiography. *J Vasc Interv Radiol* 8:393, 1997.

34. Kumar S, Radhakrishnan S, Phadke RV, et al: Takayasu's arteritis: Evaluation with three-dimensional time-of-flight MR angiography. *Eur Radiol* 7:44, 1997.

35. Ross RS, McKusick VA: Aortic arch syndromes: Diminished or absent pulses in arteries arising from arch of aorta. *Arch Intern Med* 92:701, 1953.

36. Hoffman GS: Takayasu arteritis: Lessons from the American National Institutes of Health experience. *Intern J Cardiol* 54(Suppl):S99, 1997.

37. Miyata T, Sato O, Deguchi J, et al: Anastomotic aneurysms after surgical treatment of Takayasu's arteritis: A 40-year experience. *J Vasc Surg* 27:438, 1998.

38. Tyagi S, Kaul VA, Nair M, et al: Balloon angioplasty of the aorta in Takayasu's arteritis: Initial and long-term results. *Am Heart J* 124:876, 1992.

39. Tyagi S, Verma PK, Gambhir DS, et al: Early and long-term results of subclavian angioplasty in aortoarteritis (Takayasu disease): Comparison with atherosclerosis. *Cardiovasc Interv Radio* 21:219, 1998.

40. Murakami R, Korogi Y, Matsuno Y, et al: Percutaneous transluminal angioplasty for carotid artery stenosis in Takayasu arteritis: Persistent benefit over 10 years. *Cardiovasc Interv Radiol* 20:219, 1997.

41. Lee HY, Rao PS: Percutaneous transluminal coronary angioplasty in Takayasu's arteritis. *Am Heart J* 132:1084, 1996.

42. Sharma S, Bahl VK, Rajani M: Stent treatment of obstructing dissection after percutaneous transluminal angioplasty of aortic stenosis caused by nonspecific aortitis. *Cardiovasc Interv Radiol* 20:377, 1997.

43. Chiu NC, DeLong GR, Heinz EL: Intracranial fibromuscular dysplasia in a five-year old child. *Pediatr Neurol* 14:262, 1996.

44. Zurin AA, Houkin K, Asano T, et al: Childhood ischemic stroke caused by fibromuscular dysplasia of the intracranial artery: Case report. *Neurologia Medico-Chirurgica* 37: 542, 1997.

45. Wolpert SM, Caplan LR: Current role of cerebral angiography in the diagnosis of cerebrovascular diseases. *Am J Roengenol* 159:191, 1992.

46. Chiche L, Bahnini A, Koskas F, et al: Occlusive fibromuscular disease of arteries supplying the brain: Results of surgical treatment. *Ann Vasc Surg* 11:496, 1997.

47. Natuzzi ES, Stoney RJ: Fibromuscular dysplasia of the carotid artery, in Ernst CB, Stanley JC, (ed): *Current Therapy in Vascular Surgery*. St Louis, Mosby-Year Book, Inc., 1995, pp 114–118.

48. Desfontaines P, Despland PA: Dissection of the internal carotid artery: Aetiology, symptomatology, clinical and neurosonological follow-up, and treatment in 60 consecutive cases. *Acta Neurol Belgi* 95:226, 1995.

49. Schievink WL, Bjornsson J: Fibromuscular dysplasia of the internal carotid artery: A clinicopathological study. *Clin Neuropath* 15:2, 1996.

50. Leadbetter WF, Berkland CE: Hypertension in unilateral renal disease. *J Urol* 39:611, 1938.

51. Furie DM, Tien RD: Fibromuscular dysplasia of the arteries of the head and neck: Imaging findings. *Am J Roentgenol* 162:1205, 1994.

52. Pannier-Moreau I, Grimbert P, Fiquet-Kempf B, et al: Possible familial origin of multifocal renal artery fibromuscular dysplasia. *J Hyperten* 15:1797, 1997.

53. Sell JJ, Seigel RS, Orrison WW, et al: Angiographic pattern change in fibromuscular dysplasia: A case report. *Angiology* 46:165, 1995.

54. Schievink WI, Meyer FB, Parisi JE, et al: Fibromuscular dysplasia of the internal carotid artery associated with alpha1-antitrypsin deficiency. *Neurosurgery* 43:229, 1998.

55. Goldstein LB, Gray L, Hullette CM: Stroke due to recurrent ipsilateral carotid artery dissection in a young adult. *Stroke* 26:480, 1995.

56. Arunodaya GR, Vani S, Shankar SK, et al: Fibromuscular dysplasia with dissection of basilar artery presenting as "locked-in-syndrome." *Neurology* 48:1605, 1997.

57. Moreau P, Albat B, Thevenet A: Surgical treatment of

extracranial internal carotid artery aneurysm. *Ann Vasc Surg* 8:409, 1994.

58. Faggioli GL, Freyrie A, Stella A, et al: Extracranial internal carotid artery aneurysms: Results of a surgical series with long-term follow-up. *J Vasc Surg* 23:587, 1996.

59. Belen D, Bolay H, Firat M, et al: Unusual appearance of intracranial fibromuscular dysplasia: A case report. *Angiology* 47:627, 1996.

60. George B, Mourier KL, Gelbert F, et al: Vascular abnormalities in the neck associated with intracranial aneurysms. *Neurosurgery* 24:499, 1989.

61. Cloft HJ, Kallmes DF, Kallmes MH, et al: Prevalence of cerebral aneurysms in patients with fibromuscular dysplasia: A reassessment. *J Neurosurg* 88:436, 1998.

62. Galitica Z, Gibas Z, Martinez-Hernandez A: Dissecting aneurysm as a complication of generalized fibromuscular dysplasia. *Hum Pathol* 23:568, 1998.

63. Rhee RY, Gloviczki P, Cherry KJ Jr, et al: Two unusual variants of internal carotid artery aneurysms due to fibromuscular dysplasia. *Ann Vasc Surg* 10:481, 1996.

64. Leventer RJ, Kornberg AJ, Coleman LT, et al: Stroke and fibromuscular dysplasia: Confirmation by renal magnetic resonance angiography. *Pediat Neurol* 18:172, 1998.

65. Russo CP, Smoker WRK: Nonatheromatous carotid artery disease. *Neuroimag Clin N Am* 6:811, 1996.

66. Castillo M, Wilson JD: CT angiography of the common carotid artery bifurcation: Comparison between two techniques and conventional angiography. *Neuroradiology* 36:602, 1994.

67. Heiserman JE, Drayer BP, Fram EK, Keller PJ: MR angiography of cervical fibromuscular dysplasia. *Am J Neuroradiol* 13:1454, 1992.

68. Wells RP, Smith RR: Fibromuscular dysplasia of the internal carotid artery: A long-term follow-up. *Neurosurgery* 10:39, 1982.

69. Wesen CA, Elliott BM: Fibromuscular dysplasia of the carotid arteries. *Am J Surg* 151:488, 1986.

70. Kellogg JX, Nesbit GM, Clark WM, et al: The role of angioplasty in the treatment of cerebrovascular disease. *Neurosurgery* 43:549, 1998.

71. DeOcampo J, Brillman J, Levy DI: Stenting: A new approach to carotid dissection. *J Neuroimag* 7:187, 1997.

72. Ballard JL, Guinn JE, Killeen JD, et al: Open operative balloon angioplasty of the internal carotid artery: A technique in evolution. *Ann Vasc Surg* 9:390, 1990.

73. Manninen HI, Koivisto T, Saari T, et al: Dissecting aneurysms of all four cervicocranial arteries in fibromuscular dysplasia: Treatment with self-expanding endovascular stents, coil embolization, and surgical ligation. *Am J Neuroradiol* 18:1216, 1997.

74. Motarjeme A: Percutaneous transluminal angioplasty of supra-aortic vessels. *J Endovasc Surg* 3:171, 1996.

Chapter 21

INFECTIOUS CAUSES OF STROKE

Elyse J. Singer

INTRODUCTION

Infections of the heart, great vessels, and central nervous system (CNS) are well-known causes of ischemic stroke. Recent studies indicate that infections that do not directly involve the heart, great vessels, or CNS also increase the risk of ischemic stroke through mechanisms such as the acceleration of atherosclerosis, up-regulating the levels of procoagulant cytokines, the development of autoimmune vasculitis, and the formation of antibodies to circulating anticoagulants. This chapter reviews the role of infectious diseases in stroke, with an emphasis on human immunodeficiency virus type 1 (HIV-1) and related illnesses.

Stroke Associated with Infective Endocarditis

Background   In infective endocarditis (IE), the heart and great vessels are directly infected. Most often, the pathogen is a bacteria, but fungi, rickettsia, and other atypical organisms can cause IE. In IE, infected thrombi (vegetations) form within the mural cavities or on the heart valves. These vegetations can break off and enter the arterial circulation. Although most such emboli are clinically silent, they can occlude any artery. The most common neurologic sequelae of an infected embolism that reaches the cerebral arteries is an ischemic stroke. Additionally, brain abscess, infected (mycotic) cerebral aneurysms, and meningitis are possible sequelae of IE. These latter complications can also cause localized cerebral ischemia or hemorrhage.

IE is a relatively common syndrome. Conditions that predispose to the development of IE include: rheumatic heart disease, congenital heart disease, prosthetic valves, implanted pacemakers, degenerative heart disease (e.g., calcified atheromatous deposits on the valves), intravenous drug use (IDU), and indwelling central intravenous (IV) catheters. The incidence of IE is increasing[1] as the population ages, and as the numbers of persons with prosthetic valves, implanted pacemakers, and indwelling IV catheters expands. Additionally, HIV disease increases the susceptibility of IV drug users to IE.[2]

It is theorized that noninfectious lesions of the cardiac endothelium initiate IE. Such injuries, which may be microscopic, can result from abnormal blood flow caused by structural abnormalities of the heart. This sterile injury results in the activation of circulating procoagulants and platelets, localized platelet and fibrin deposition, and the formation of a sterile thrombus on the endothelium. Fibrin and platelets continue to accumulate over time, resulting in a nonbacterial thrombotic endocarditis (NBTE). Circulating microbes attach to this NBTE and proliferate first within the thrombus, then the surrounding cardiac tissue. As the thrombus is propagated, an infected vegetation forms on the cardiac valves or within the cavities of the heart. Portions of infected vegetations can be flicked off into the arterial circulation, causing stroke and other ischemic symptoms. As IE progresses, patients may develop cardiac abscesses, intraventricular conduction defects, valvular destruction, and acute cardiac failure.

Some investigators have reported that vegetations over 10 mm in diameter and mobile vegetations present a greater risk for embolization and stroke, although these observations are not universally agreed upon.[3–6] The chronic release of micro-organisms into the circulation can stimulate the formation of immune complexes that also damage vascular endothelium.

The bacteria that cause IE can be introduced after minor mucosal trauma such as dental prophylaxis, invasive dental procedures, invasive medical procedures, IDU, the insertion of chronic indwelling IV catheters, and hospital-acquired infections. The most common pathogens are Gram-positive cocci such as streptococcus, staphylococcus, and enterococcus. *Staphylococcus aureus* is associated with a particularly virulent course of IE, characterized by a high incidence of cerebral embolism, large infarcts, and cerebral hemorrhage.[4,7,8] Gram-negative bacteria are often associated with IE of prosthetic valves, IDU, and nosocomial infection. The most common fungus that causes IE is *Candida* species. Severe immunosuppression, IDU, diabetes mellitus, and previous antibiotic treatment that has wiped out the normal flora tend to predispose to fungal IE. The rickettsia *Coxiella burnetii,* which causes Q fever, can present with IE and stroke.

The reader is referred elsewhere for a detailed discussion of the criteria for the diagnosis of IE.[9] Briefly, IE is confirmed by a constellation of clinical, microbiological, and echocardiographic findings. The clinical signs and symptoms of IE include fever, tachycardia, shortness of breath, a new or changed murmur, splinter hemorrhages, and petechiae.[10] Cerebral emboli occur in approximately 15 to 30 percent of cases of IE. When present, these emboli tend to lodge in the middle cerebral artery distribution and are associated with a high degree of mortality.[11,12] Stroke may be the first sign of IE. In a study of native valve endocarditis, 74 percent of ischemic strokes occurred by the time of presentation and an additional 13 percent occurred within 48 h after diagnosis.[7] Embolic stroke recurred at a rate of 0.5 percent per day and was often associated with relapse or uncontrolled infection.[7]

Positive blood cultures can be obtained in over 90 percent of cases of bacterial IE. The detection of the causative organism by blood cultures is key to the establishment of this diagnosis. In some cases, if an organism cannot be cultured, it may be identified by serology (e.g., *Coxiella burnetii, Brucella, Legionella,* and *Bartonella*) or by biopsy and direct examination of a cardiac abcess or peripheral embolic material. Determination of the organism's sensitivity to antibiotics is also essential to proper treatment of IE and control of embolization. If an organism cannot be identified, but the other criteria for IE can be established, the physician may select an empiric treatment regimen for IE.

Echocardiography is a crucial part of the investigation of suspected IE and is particularly useful to differentiate IE from sepsis.[13] The major echocardiographic findings of IE include mobile, echo-dense masses attached to valvular leaflets or mural endocardium, periannular cardiac abscesses, new dehiscence of a prosthetic valve, and new valvular regurgitation.[9,14] The technique of transthoracic echocardiography has a sensitivity of 50 to 60 percent and is suboptimal for prosthetic valves but is often performed as a first step because it is less costly and complicated. Transesophageal echocardiograms have a sensitivity of 76 to 100 percent in series of IE and are better to detect small vegetations and prosthetic valve disease.[15,16]

A lumbar puncture (LP) that demonstrates an abnormal cerebrospinal fluid (CSF) profile (such as pleocytosis, or a low CSF glucose) should be a "red flag" signaling an infectious etiology of stroke. The CSF profile tends to reflect the nature of the underlying infectious pathogen in IE with cerebral emboli. However, in some cases of CNS infection, the routine CSF profile (cell count, glucose, protein) may be unremarkable.[11] This is especially likely in severely immunosuppressed patients.[17]

Therapeutic Recommendations   Infective endocarditis is associated with a high degree of mortality (up to 35 percent) even with appropriate therapy.[10] Effective antibiotic treatment is usually the most important factor in stopping further embolization. Equally important, the detection of IE allows the physician to avoid potentially harmful therapeutic manuvers such as rapid anticoagulation with IV heparin or thrombolysis with tissue plasminogen activation factor (TPA), which could convert an ischemic stroke into a cerebral hemorrhage.

The main objective of medical treatment of infective endocarditis is to sterilize the vegetative lesions and allow the endothelium to heal. This requires high doses of intravenous antibiotics over a long period of time with bacteriocidal therapy, often with two or more synergistic drugs.[18] Treatment is typically continued for 4 to 6 weeks. Follow-up blood cultures off treatment must be monitored for possible relapse.

Anticoagulation is not indicated to treat IE of native valves. Numerous investigators have reported cases of IE and cerebral embolism in which anticoagulation (especially heparin) converted an ischemic infarct into a cerebral hemorrhage.[19] However, the issue of anticoagulation is more complex in patients with IE of a prosthetic valve, which requires chronic anticoagulation. Such patients may actually form more emboli if they are not anticoagulated and may need to continue anticoagulation unless there is a cerebral hemorrhage.[14]

Cardiac surgery is indicated in a subset of patients with IE. This subset of patients may also include cases in which IE is caused by yeast or fungi that form bulky vegetations that are difficult to sterilize with antibiotic drugs.[12,14] These fungal infections tend to embolize to large blood vessels and cause severe, life-threatening strokes. Surgery may also be performed in cases of cardiac abscess, acute valvular regurgitation with hemodynamic failure, to replace a prosthetic valve, for uncontrolled infection with recurrent emboli, or if direct biopsy or culture is necessary to identify the causative microbe.

The type of organism identified, the in vitro antibiotic sensitivity, and the patient's other medical conditions guide the choice of an antibiotic regimen. The recommended treatment regimens are updated frequently and are published by the American Heart Association in its journals and on its website.[14,20]

Stroke Associated with Direct Infection of the CNS

Background Stroke frequently complicates the course of cerebral infections. Approximately 15 to 37 percent of cases of bacterial meningitis are complicated by stroke.[21–23] These strokes can be caused by the direct infiltration of blood vessels by an organism, with subsequent thrombosis and ischemia, or by the indirect effects of infection on hemocoagulation.

Many bacteria, rickettsia, and viruses infect human endothelial cells and/or vascular smooth muscle in vitro and/or in vivo. Examples include (but are not limited to) the bacteria *Chlamydia pneumoniae,* the rickettsia *Coxiella burnetii,* and viruses such as herpes simplex virus (HSV), varicella zoster virus (VZV), cytomegalovirus (CMV), HIV, adenovirus type 7, measles, mumps, poliovirus type 1, echovirus type 9, parainfluenza virus type 3, and coxsackie B virus.[24–28] Direct infection of the blood vessel walls can lead to vasculitis, characterized by inflammation, necrosis of blood vessel walls, thrombosis, and ischemia. In addition, the indirect effects of a systemic infection can also cause vasculitis, as described in Chap. 19.

The host inflammatory response to infection is characterized by the increased synthesis of proinflammatory cytokines such as tumor necrosis factor-alpha (TNF-α), interleukin (IL)-1, and IL-6, prostaglandins,

arachidonic acid, and nitric oxide (NO).[23] These products of inflammation can cause tissue injury that directly contributes to the morbidity and mortality of CNS infections. Further, this inflammatory response may temporarily be exacerbated during the early stages of treatment by the use of antimicrobial drugs. This can occur when large amounts of a pathogenic microbe are lysed within the CNS, resulting in the release of large quantities of endotoxin and other antigens. Endotoxin and other foreign antigens further increase the synthesis of proinflammatory cytokines, creating a positive feedback cycle.[29]

Foreign antigens also activate resident CNS cells such as endothelial cells, microglia, macrophages, and astrocytes. These activated CNS cells synthesize chemotactic factors that attract activated leukocytes. They also synthesize TNF-α, which directly increases the permeability of the blood-brain barrier (BBB) and upregulates the synthesis of leukocyte-endothelial cell adhesion factors. Endothelial cell adhesion factors increase the migration of polymorphonuclear leukocytes (PMNS) across the BBB. These PMNs release cytotoxic substances and reactive oxygen species within the CNS, causing the death of resident CNS cells as well as of bacteria.

In addition to causing vasculitis, bacterial meningitis can cause arterial stenoses, venous thrombosis, cerebral edema, increased intracranial pressure, and reduced cerebral blood flow.[30,31] Arterial stenoses and reduced cerebral blood flow have been demonstrated in both animal and human subjects with bacterial meningitis.[32–34] The human subjects were studied with cerebral Doppler and single photon emission computed tomography (SPECT). One study found that 51 percent of patients with bacterial or fungal meningitis had one or more cerebral arterial stenoses during their infection. Patients with such stenoses had worse Glasgow Coma Scale scores and exhibited more focal cerebral signs.[33] This research supports the notion that stroke in patients with bacterial meningitis is associated with a poor prognosis.[21]

Whenever bacterial meningitis is suspected, patients are treated empirically pending laboratory confirmation of the causative pathogens(s). In 1995, the most common causes of bacterial meningitis in the United States were *S. pneumoniae*, *N. meningitis*, group B streptococcus, *Listeria* monocytogenes, and *H. influenzae*.[35] These pathogens can usually be identified by CSF culture unless the patient has been partially treated with antibiotics.[29] Immunologic assays that detect capsular polysaccharide antigens in the CSF are available and are helpful in such cases.[36–38] Serologic tests have limited use, but can identify organisms such as *Coxiella burnetii*, *Brucella*, *Bartonella*, and other organisms that are too difficult or too dangerous to culture.

In some instances, infection of the CNS presents with an isolated CNS vasculitis and stroke rather than a generalized infection or a systemic vasculitis. The clinical presentation of CNS vasculitis is described elsewhere in this volume. However, the differentiation of infectious from noninfectious vasculitis is crucial. Infectious vasculitis is managed by treating the underlying infection, giving supportive care, and if needed by the limited use of steroids. Noninfectious vasculitis is usually treated with steroids and immunosuppressive or cytotoxic therapies that could worsen the course of an infection and could be dangerous in patients with HIV or other immunosuppressive conditions.

Until the advent of modern molecular techniques, it has often been difficult to identify the cause of an infectious vasculitis. The culture of CSF is suboptimal to detect pathogens that are rare, fastidious, slow-growing, present in minute quantities, or dangerous to culture in a clinical laboratory. For example, such relatively common viral infections of the CNS such as HSV, VZV, and CMV can be difficult to culture from CSF even in cases of encephalitis.[39] The rickettsia that causes Q fever is too dangerous to grow in most laboratories. Tuberculosis may require up to 6 weeks for growth in culture. Techniques such as PCR[6,40,41] and serologic assays are preferable to identify these pathogens.

The polymerase chain reaction (PCR) technique amplifies minute amounts of DNA (or RNA, from which a DNA copy can be made) using genetic sequences that are unique to a particular organism. The PCR technique is useful to detect viruses, fatidious or slow-growing pathogens, in cases of early disease, when there are low volumes of a specimen sample, a nonviable organism, or in cases where an organism is dangerous to culture in the laboratory.[42,43] Examples of organisms that can be detected by PCR include: *Bartonella henselae* (the etiologic agent of bacillary angiomatosis, or cat scratch fever), *Chlamydia pneumoniae*, the Whipple's disease bacterium, mycobacterium tuberculosis, hepatitis viruses B, C, D, E, and G; human papilloma virus: HIV, HTLV I and II, the herpesviruses HSV-1, HSV-2, CMV, Epstein-Barr virus, human herpes virus (HHV) 6 and HHV 8 (the agent that causes Kaposi's sarcoma and some cases of primary CNS lymphoma), enterovirus, human parvovirus B19, and others.[42]

Treatment Recommendations The treatment of bacterial meningitis is based on correct identification of the causative organism, selecting the correct antimicrobial regimen, and curbing the deleterious effects of CNS inflammation. When bacterial, tuberculous, or fungal meningitis is suspected on the basis of the clinical picture and/or CSF profile, empirical treatment is started immediately.

Corticosteroids such as dexamethasone have been used to reduce the neurologic sequelae of bacterial meningitis, such as hearing loss.[44] However, their use for this purpose is controversial and is not universally supported.[45] Most of these studies were conducted on children with community-acquired bacterial meningitis. In some of these studies, the addition of dexamethasone to antibiotic therapy decreased the incidence and severity of sequelae such as hearing loss.[29,44] However, the cerebrovascular complications of bacterial meningitis were not evaluated in these studies.

Increased Stroke Risk Associated with Extracerebral Infection

Background Extracerebral infection seems to play a role in the pathogenesis of stroke, myocardial infarction (MI), and other vascular diseases.[46–49] It is postulated that infection may accelerate atherosclerosis, increase procoagulant activity and thrombosis, and trigger the formation of immune complexes that damage the vascular endothelium. Infectious illnesses such as influenza may explain the observed seasonal variation in stroke incidence and the increased mortality from cardiovascular diseases during the winter months.[50,51]

The association between stroke and infection was first observed in children.[47] In one series of pediatric strokes, 15 of 44 (34 percent) of children with ischemic stroke had an infection in the preceding 3 weeks, vs. 11 percent of control cases.[52] The most common antecedent was an unidentified upper respiratory infection, followed by infections such as *Varicella*, *Borrelia*, and gastroenteritis.

A recent infectious illness occurring in the period of 1 week to 1 month prior to the event was significantly more common in adults with ischemic stroke than in matched controls.[53–55] This association was more pronounced in patients under the age of fifty years.[46,50] Both acute bacterial and viral infections have been associated with subsequent stroke, despite frequent lack of associated fever.[46] Most patients who suffered a stroke after an infection had other risk factors, suggesting that infection further, or temporarily, increased their risk.[56]

Chronic and recurrent infections have also been associated with an increased risk of stroke.[57] The most commonly cited infections are *Chlamydia pneumoniae*,[58,59] *Helicobacter pylori*,[60] CMV[61,62] and chronic dental infections.[53,57] These observations are controversial and have been disputed on the basis that these relationships were confounded by other risk factors, or that these infections were an epiphenomena.[63–66]

Chlamydia pneumoniae is an obligate intracellular Gram-negative bacterium, which is a common cause of respiratory infections, sinusitis, and pneumonia in adults. Two cross-sectional studies found that persons with stroke or transient cerebral ischemia were significantly more likely to have serologic evidence of acute or chronic *Chlamydia pneumoniae* infections than were controls.[58,59] Antibodies to *Chlamydia* were also more common in persons with other atherosclerotic diseases, such as coronary artery disease (CAD) and abdominal aortic aneurysms.[66–68] *Chlamydia* is more likely to be detected in the walls of atherosclerotic vessels than normal arteries.

Helicobacter pylori is a Gram-negative rod-shaped bacteria that is associated with peptic ulcer disease and gastric lymphoma. *Helicobacter* has also been implicated in the pathogenesis of MI and stroke,[60,64] although less evidence is available for *Helicobacter* than for *Chlamydia*. Some investigators have found no association when factors such as social class, smoking, and blood pressure were taken into account.[63,65]

Cytomegalovirus (and to a lesser extent other herpes viruses) has been associated with accelerated atherosclerosis and subsequent ischemia.[61,69–73] Antibodies to CMV are more common in patients with atherosclerosis.[74] The presence of CMV antibodies is correlated with intimal thickening of the carotid arteries. CMV infection is also associated with the restenosis of arterial grafts, due to accelerated atherosclerosis in patients with CAD and in patients with transplants.[72,75]

Several reports have found an association between chronic periodontal disease and other dental infections and an increased risk for ischemic stroke.[57,76]

Pathologic studies indicate that the "fatty streak" (a precursor of mature atherosclerotic lesions) is inflammatory in nature.[77] The precise series of events that initiate the formation of the "fatty streak" remain unclear; however, *Chlamydia*, CMV, and other microbes have been detected within atherosclerotic plaques, which suggests that infection of the vascular endothelium instigates inflammation and possibly contributes to atherogenesis.[58a,78–80] However, these organisms may have simply colonized previously existing lesions.[80]

Chickens infected with Marek's virus (an avian DNA herpes virus) develop atherosclerotic lesions similar to those seen in humans.[81] This animal model has been used to study the relationship between infection and atherosclerotic disease. Marek's virus can be detected in the arterial walls of infected birds. Atherosclerotic lesions develop in normocholestremic chickens. However, the lesions progress more rapidly in birds fed a high-cholesterol diet. In another animal model, rabbits infected with *Chlamydia pneumoniae* and fed cholesterol-enriched chow developed atherosclerosis more rapidly than uninfected controls.[56]

Many pathogens can directly infect vascular cells in vitro, including monocytes, macrophages, vascular smooth muscle cells, and endothelial cells.[24,28,56,60,67,80,82,83] Although productive viral infection of vascular tissue can occur, latent viral infections can also initiate a chain of events that predispose to thrombosis. It is hypothesized that in vivo, infection causes increased adherence of granulocytes to the endothelial cells; these granulocytes can release toxic products, including oxygen radicals, which can damage the endothelium, especially after exposure to immune complexes, endotoxin, or activated complement.[48] Immune complexes can also induce production of tissue factor, which initiates the extrinsic coagulation pathway, in endothelial cells.[48] Further, herpes can make the vascular endothelium prone to thrombus formation by causing loss of surface heparans and thrombomodulin and reduced prostacyclin.

In bacterial infection, substances such as LPS induce the synthesis of cytokines such as TNF-α and IL-1 in monocytes and endothelial cells.[48] These cytokines induce procoagulant activity in endothelial cells, attract polymorphonuclear cells and monocytes, and stimulate production of platelet-activating factor and the release of tissue factor, and other substances that increase coagulation. LPS also stimulates secretion of growth factor for smooth muscle cells and fibroblasts. The proliferation of fibroblasts, thickening of the vessel walls, and increased adhesion of inflammatory cells and platelets may gradually result in a "remodeled" vessel with a narrowed lumen. Further cycles of inflammation may narrow the arterial lumen and restrict blood flow, causing ischemia.

In still other studies, bacteria themselves have been shown to induce aggregation of platelets and to activate the extrinsic pathway of blood coagulation.[48]

Treatment Recommendations In one animal study, azithromycin treatment blunted the atherogenic effect of *Chlamydia pneumoniae* infection.[56] In a large case-control study, persons with a first-time acute MI were significantly less likely to have used tetracycline antibiotics or quinolones in the previous 3 years than matched controls without MI.[84] Although these observations do not warrant the use of antibiotics to treat atherosclerosis or stroke at this time, controlled clinical trials would be welcomed.

Infection As a Cause of a Hypercoagulable State

Reduction of endogenous anticoagulants

Background The host immune response is increasingly appreciated as a factor in producing the symptoms and signs of an illness, such as fever, headache, sleep disturbances, anorexia, and wasting.[85–87] The degree of the host inflammatory response is influenced by gender, heredity, and concurrent medications.

Infection activates the immune system, resulting in an up-regulation of proinflammatory cytokines. For example, during sepsis, the levels of TNF-α, IL-1, IL-6, and IL-8 rise. This rise is paralleled by a rise in the levels of biologic markers for thrombin activation, such as fibrinopeptide A and prothrombin fragments. Exposure to endotoxin, or inflammatory cytokines, activates endothelial cells to synthesize leukocyte adhesion molecules, platelet-aggregating factor (PAF), and tissue factor. Tissue factor can activate coagulation in the extrinsic pathway and reduce thrombomodulin secretion, diminishing the anticoagulant power of protein C. It increases plasminogen activator inhibitor type 1 synthesis by endothelial cells, reducing their fibrinolytic capacity. Both coagulation activation and reduction in fibrinolysis result in fibrin deposition in the microvascular system. The increase in procoagulant activity represents a possible mechanism for infection-associated ischemic stroke.

Acute inflammation is also associated with elevated levels of acute-phase proteins such as fibrinogen, C-reactive protein, and with leukocytosis. These factors may have a causal role in stroke.[88] Persons who suffered an ischemic stroke within 1 week after an infection were found to have higher level of C-reactive protein (a marker for a hypercoagulable state) than stroke patients without such history.[88,90] Elevated plasma fibrinogen levels, which increase blood viscosity, are associated with new events in stroke patients.[88]

In summary, infection and subsequent inflamma-

tion initiate a chain of events that reduce the levels of naturally occuring anticoagulant substances and impair the function of the fibrinolytic system. This in turn predisposes to thrombosis and ischemic stroke. The biologic purpose of this chain of events may be the trapping of bacteria in fibrinous deposits.

Treatment Recommendations In a study of MI, it was observed that the protective effect of aspirin was associated with a reduction in the levels of C-reactive protein. No studies have been performed to determine if a similar association exists for patients with cerebral ischemia. However, in ischemic stroke precipitated by a hypercoagulable state, the current treatment includes anticoagulation.

Induction of Endogenous Procoagulants

Background Autoantibodies, such as anticardiolipin antibody and lupus anticoagulant, have been reported to occur more frequently in young persons with cerebral ischemia.[91] Such autoantibodies can appear after common illnesses such as viral infections.[92] In most instances, postinfectious autoantibodies are transient, low-titer, poly-specific, and are not associated with clinical symptoms. However, viruses such as hepatitis C and B, HIV, VZV, and parvovirus B19 frequently trigger the synthesis of high titers of autoantibodies that have subtype specificity and are associated with clinical symptoms.[92] In particular, HIV infection is associated with the development of antibodies to cardiolipin, phospholipids, and coagulation proteins.[93] Some patients with these HIV-induced autoantibodies have been reported to manifest lupus-like symptoms and coagulopathies.[92] Hepatitis viruses A, B, and C, as well as HIV, can trigger cryoglobulinemia, which is associated with vasculitis.[92] Elevated titers of other virus-induced antibodies have been reported in persons with venous thrombosis and stroke, e.g., autoantibodies in an HIV-seronegative individual with CMV infection were associated with venous thrombosis.[94] However, there is debate as to whether these antibodies actually cause disease or represent an epiphenomena.

Anticardiolipin antibodies have been found in up to 86 percent of HIV-infected men.[93,95,96] The effect of these antibodies on thrombosis is controversial. In some series of HIV-infected individuals, such autoantibodies were not associated with thrombosis,[95] whereas other authors reported a correlation between antiphospholipid antibodies and cerebral thrombosis.[97] In another series of HIV-infected persons, the presence of anticardiolipin antibodies was correlated with acquired deficiency of free protein S.[96] Many of these patients developed clinical thrombosis. Although the presence of anticardiolipin antibodies and protein S deficiency did not predict who would develop thrombosis in this particular group, a stronger association might have been seen in a larger sample.[96] Autoantibodies to phospholipids have also been reported in persons with hepatitis C and other viral illnesses; but, association between these infections and hypercoagulability is less well established.[92,98]

Recommendations Patients with hypercoagulable states due to autoantibodies, who suffer ischemic or thrombotic clinical events, are usually fully anticoagulated.

Selected Pathogens Associated with Ischemic Stroke

Mycobacterium Tuberculosis Tuberculosis is a common disease worldwide. A chronic tuberculous meningitis can occur in persons with disseminated tuberculosis. This meningitis is frequently associated with ischemic infarcts. In one series 66 percent of patients with intracranial tuberculosis had radiographic evidence of a stroke.[99] The cerebral infarctions associated with tuberculosis meningitis are described as bilateral and symmetric, with a predilection for the medial striate and thalamoperforating arteries.[100] Stroke in children with intracranial tuberculosis is particularly common and is associated with a poor prognosis.[101]

Neurosyphilis Syphilis, caused by the spirochete *Treponema pallidum,* is a well-known cause of stroke. The spirochetes enter the CNS early in syphilitic infection, usually without producing any neurologic symptoms. Left untreated, the spirochetes may disappear spontaneously from the CNS. However, a small number of patients develop a syphilitic meningitis about 2 years after infection. This "aseptic" meningitis can be associated with ischemic stroke. Meningovascular syphilis, which is associated with an arteritis of small and medium arteries, tends to occur within 5 to 7 years after infection. The most severe neurological diseases occur in a minority of patients, usually at least 10 to 20 years after an untreated infection.[102] The progression of syphilis in untreated, HIV-seronegative persons is usually quite slow, and less than 10 percent of such individuals with tertiary syphilis develop neurologic disease.[103] In contrast, in HIV-infected persons the natural history of syphilis may be accelerated.[104,105] Coinfection with HIV and syphilis is not uncommon, as these infections have similar risk factors and modes of transmission. Some HIV-infected persons have also been reported to have nonreactive syphilis serology despite positive clinical evidence of the disease and to be more likely to fail the standard antibiotic treatments for syphilis.[104–111] Neurosyphilis may be particularly difficult to diagnose in HIV-infected persons because *Treponema pallidum* is extremely difficult to culture,[108] false-negative CSF VDRL tests are common (up to 25 percent of cases in which spirochetes can be recovered from CSF),[108] and because the presence of HIV can confound other abnormal CSF findings, such as pleocytosis and elevated total protein.[108,109] These observations are not universally accepted and require further study.[112]

The most common neurologic abnormalities in persons with neurosyphilis are cerebral infarcts secondary to arteritis.[113] The arteritis that involves medium and large arteries in meningovascular syphilis is called "Heubner's arteritis" and is characterized by the infiltration of vessels by lymphocytes and plasma cells, damage to the arterial muscle fibers, proliferation of subendothelial fibrous material, and occlusion of the vessel.[102]

The precise mechanism for the arteritis caused by syphilis is unclear. *T. pallidum* can adhere to and penetrate between vascular endothelium in vitro[114]; however, intracellular *T. pallidum* was not observed in these studies. *T. pallidum c* has been reported to activate endothelial cells, to induce the expression of intercellular adhesion molecule-1 (ICAM-1), and to induce adherence of lymphocytes and monocytes to vascular endothelium.[115,116] *T. pallidum* also induces procoagulant activity on the surface of vascular endothelial cells, which may promote stroke.[115] Finally, *T. pallidum* may induce an autoimmune response[117] and the formation of circulating immune complexes,[118] which could potentially induce an arteritis.

A lumbar puncture is recommended for all HIV-infected persons with serologic evidence of syphilis. In contrast, lumbar puncture is recommended for HIV-1 seronegative persons with syphilis only if they have symptomatic syphilis, a high titer RPR or VDRL, a history of treatment failure, or if treatment with antibiotics other than penicillin is planned.[119]

The recommended treatment regimen for neurosyphilis is intravenous aqueous penicillin G, 2 to 4 million units every 4 h for 10 to 14 days, or procaine penicillin, 2.4 million units intramuscularly once daily, plus probenecid, 500 mg per mouth 4 times a day, both for

10 to 14 days. The CDC has recommended that HIV-infected persons receive monthly serum VDRL or RPR tests for 3 months, and then once every 3 to 6 months, until the tests are nonreactive or the titers have stabilized at <1:8. The CSF should be examined at 3 months post-treatment and then every 6 months thereafter until normal.[119] Retreatment is recommended if the patient worsens neurologically, the CSF pleocytosis increases after 6 months, the CSF VDRL increases, or the serum RPR or VDRL increases by fourfold or more.

Lyme Disease   Lyme disease is caused by the spirochete *Borrelia burgdorferi*, which is transmitted by *Ixodes dammini* ticks. The first sign of an infection may be a skin lesion called erythema chronicum migrans, which occurs at the site of the tick bite. Other early symptoms include musculoskeletal pain and arthritis. Neurologic symptoms are rare in early infection. When present, such symptoms might include aseptic meningitis, facial palsy, peripheral neuropathy, or radiculopathy. Frequently, the symptoms of Lyme disease will subside without treatment. In the minority of cases, it will progress to cause clinical disease of the heart and CNS. In the late stages of disease, neuroborreliosis may be characterized by chronic encephalitis, dementia, cerebral atrophy, vasculitis, stroke, and TIA.[120–122] The cerebrovascular manifestations of *Borrelia* seem to be due to an indirect effect of the infection, as spirochetes have not been demonstrated to directly infect cells.[123]

Borrelia infection can be detected by a reactive enzyme-linked immunosorbent assay (ELISA) test, which is confirmed by a Western blot. However, a reactive serology does not necessarily imply active CNS disease.[124] In some cases, the spirochetes can be cultured from the CSF. Because *Borrelia* can be difficult to culture, especially in late disease, CSF PCR is often used to detect CNS infection. Neuroborreliosis is treated with intravenous ceftiaxone, 2 grams per day for 30 days.

Cryptococcal Meningitis   *Cryptococcus neoformans* is an encapsulated yeast, which is transmitted by the inhalation of *Cryptococcus* spores. In healthy persons, this causes a self-limited pulmonary infection. In immunosuppressed persons (e.g., persons with AIDS, cancer, or who are post-organ transplant), *Cryptococcus* can cause a disseminated infection, which frequently involves the CNS. Such dissemination may occur after a primary infection but is usually a reactivation of an old infection during immune suppression.

The symptoms of cryptococcal meningitis develop over a few days to 3 weeks. Early symptoms are nonspecific, such as low-grade fever, lethargy, and headache.

They are followed by severe headache, delirium, seizures, and coma. If untreated, cryptococcal infection of the brain can lead to brain herniation.[125,126] Meningismus is relatively uncommon. Some patients develop focal deficits, which may be due to intraparenchymal brain abscesses (called cryptococcomas)[126] or due to cerebral infarcts.

Both stroke and TIA can be seen in cryptococcal meningitis. The author has reported a patient witnessed to have classic TIAs with complete resolution of his neurologic findings, caused by previously undiagnosed cryptococcal meningitis and AIDS.[127]

Cryptococcal antigen is the most rapid and sensitive test to diagnose cryptococcal disease. It has a 90 to 95 percent sensitivity and specificity in CSF.[128] Serum cryptococcal antigen is positive in 99 percent of patients with meningitis but does not indicate CNS disease.[129] The CSF India ink test, which demonstrates the encapsulated yeast, is positive in 50 percent of non-AIDS and 82 percent of AIDS patients.[125] Elevated CSF pressure, CSF pleocytosis, elevated CSF total protein, and low CSF glucose are common and nondiagnostic findings. Some AIDS patients with cryptococcal meningitis have "normal" CSF profiles.[125]

The most commonly used first-line treatment is intravenous amphotericin B, 0.5 to 0.7 mg/kg/day.[125,130,131] This dose may be reduced if the patient has kidney disease. Recently, less toxic liposomal formulations of intravenous amphotericin B have been released, but they are not generally recommended as initial therapy for cryptococcoal meningitis. Another intravenous antifungal drug, 5-flucytosine, may be given with amphotericin B at a dose of 100 to 150 mg/kg/day in divided doses.[132]

These drugs are continued until the CSF is sterilized, generally 2 to 4 weeks. Increased intracranial pressure should be monitored carefully and may require lumbar drainage for management. Fluconazole, an oral antifungal drug, 200 to 400 mg/day PO, is used for maintenance therapy and secondary prophylaxis.[133]

Coccidioides immitis   *Coccidioides immitis* is a fungal infection, which is prevalent in specific geographic areas such as the American Southwest. Healthy patients who inhale the organism typically develop a self-limited pulmonary infection. Disseminated disease is relatively uncommon in previously healthy individuals; however, immunocompromised persons are more likely to have disseminated infection.

Disseminated coccidioidomycosis can cause a chronic fungal meningitis. Patients with CNS coccidioidomycosis often develop cerebral vasculitis and stroke. In an autopsy series of eight patients who died of CNS coccidioidomycosis, four (50 percent) had endarteritis obliterans and two (25 percent) had infarcts.[134] In another clinical-pathologic study, 17 of 32 subjects (53 percent) had endarteritis, and 31 percent had cerebral infarcts.[135]

C. immitis can be especially difficult to culture from CSF, and currently there are no direct antigen detection methods or PCR tests. The most commonly used diagnostic test is the complement-fixing antibody (CFA) titer, which detects IgG. However, complement-fixing antibodies may fail to develop in immunodeficient patients.[136] Aggressive empiric treatment of suspected *Coccidioides meningitis* with amphotericin B and possibly with concomitant use of dexamethasone may be warranted in situations in which this diagnosis seems likely, even before laboratory confirmation is available.

Candida *Candida albicans* is the most common pathogenic *Candida* species in humans. This yeast is a normal inhabitant of the human body. In immunosuppressed persons (AIDS, cancer, chemotherapy, high doses of immunosuppressive drugs, diabetes mellitus, persons treated with hyperalimentation, IDUs, and persons treated with high doses of broad-spectrum antibiotics), *Candida* can disseminate, causing IE, meningitis, and visceral disease.

Candida albicans infection can cause ischemic stroke as a consequence of infected cardiac emboli in persons with IE, or by causing the thrombosis of both large and small cerebral vessels as a direct result of CNS infection.[137]

In *Candida meningitis,* low glucose and mild pleocytosis characterize the CSF. The recommended treatment is amphotericin B, with or without flucytosine.[136] Despite therapy with amphotericin B, the mortality rates are over 30 percent.

HIV-1

Background Human immunodeficiency virus is a pathogenic retrovirus that is well known as a cause of immunodeficiency, malignancy, and neurologic disease. As a consequence of the immune deficiency, patients develop opportunistic infections caused by bacteria, fungi, parasites, and other viruses. Less well known but equally important consequences of HIV infection include the development of autoantibodies, which cause a wide variety of clinical diseases, and the effects of HIV and HIV medications on metabolism, such as elevated

levels of triglycerides, and the development of diabetes mellitus.

Clinical series suggest that the prevalence of stroke in persons with HIV-1/AIDS is higher than that expected in HIV-seronegatives of similar age.[138] The prevalence of cerebrovascular disease of all types in clinical series of HIV-1-infected adults ranges from 0.75 to 4.0,[138,139] and in HIV-infected children the incidence of stroke in a longitudinal study has been reported to be 1.3 percent per year.[140]

Most strokes in HIV-infected persons are ischemic infarcts.[141] These infarcts are usually small, frequently multiple, and tend to be localized in the basal ganglia.[142] In some cases, stroke is associated with calcification of surrounding brain tissue and the vessel wall.[143] In addition to cerebral thrombosis, HIV/AIDS patients may develop strokes from IE, NBTE, thickening of the blood vessel walls, granulomatous angiitis, and development of aneurysmal dilatation of the arteries.[144-147] Many of the opportunistic CNS diseases that occur in AIDS patients will also cause ischemic stroke. HIV-infected patients often develop acquired protein S deficiency, protein C deficiency, and other acquired coagulopathies that predispose to ischemic stroke.[96,148,149]

Cerebral hemorrhages also occur at an increased rate in HIV/AIDS patients, especially if there are predisposing factors such as thrombocytopenia, other HIV-associated coagulopathies, and toxoplasmosis.[141,146,150]

Most HIV-infected patients with cerebrovascular disease are severely immunosuppressed, with CD4+ counts below 50 cells/mm^3, an opportunistic infection, or HIV-1-associated dementia complex.[145,151,152] One series reported more cerebrovascular lesions in HIV-infected transfusion and hemophiliac patients than in other risk groups.[153] However, HIV-1-associated cerebrovascular disease has been reported in all risk groups and at all stages of infection.[154]

Neuroimaging studies have found a higher incidence of stroke in HIV-1-infected persons than have clinical series, suggesting that the diagnosis of stroke may be overlooked during life. In a review of 71 consecutive abnormal MRIs performed on AIDS patients over a 2-year period at a single institution 22 infarcts were observed in 13 of the 71 patients (frequency of 18 percent).[155] The most common site was the basal ganglia, but stroke has been observed in all locations.

Autopsy series of HIV-1-infected patients have also found a higher number of strokes in HIV and AIDS patients than have clinical series, ranging from 1.5 to 34 percent of cases.[142,156-158] Some of the subjects studied may have been selected for a neuropathologic examination because they had been neurologically symptomatic during life. However, the higher prevalence of cerebrovascular lesions in autopsy studies adds evidence to the notion that many strokes in HIV/AIDS patients go undiagnosed during life.

Mechanisms   HIV invades the CNS early, during the time of primary infection.[159] In most instances, HIV remains neurologically silent until the late stages of disease, when it may cause encephalitis, myelopathy, neuropathy, and stroke, among many other neurologic problems. Within the CNS, HIV infects monocytes, macrophages, multinucleated giant cells, endothelial cells, astrocytes, choroid plexus cells, and ependyma. Neurons and oligodendrocytes rarely if ever seem to be infected.

There are multiple mechanisms by which HIV can cause cerebrovascular disease. The most obvious is the direct infection of endothelial cells in the brain.[27] In addition, HIV has been noted to cause a diffuse arteriopathy with aneurysmal dilatations, particularly in children.[140] HIV causes progressive immunodeficiency, which promotes the development of opportunistic CNS infections (such as herpes viruses) that may cause CNS vasculitis and stroke.[147,160] Chronic HIV infection causes an inflammatory response that is characterized by the production of proinflammatory cytokines, which are known to predispose to cerebral thrombosis. HIV is associated with the presence of antibodies to phospholipids, preprothrombin, and/or lupus anticoagulant.[93] HIV/AIDS patients with these antibodies may develop TIAs and/or an ischemic stroke.[97,161]

Recommendations   There are no studies on the treatment of HIV-associated ischemic infarctions. A stroke in an HIV-infected person may be caused by HIV alone, by a CNS opportunistic infection, by an indirect complication of HIV infection, or even by unrelated problems. In the absence of formal studies, the author recommends that the most important maneuver is to search for a treatable second infection, such as herpes simplex, varicella, or IE. Patients who have poorly controlled HIV infection, as evidenced by a rising HIV viral load in plasma or CSF, or a falling CD4+ count, should have their medications reviewed by a specialist in HIV, with the goal of reducing viral replication as quickly as possible. Quantitative HIV RNA PCR in the CSF may be helpful in determining if medications are adequately treating this compartment. HIV-infected patients with acquired coagulopathies should be anticoagulated if possible.

Herpes Viruses   The herpes viruses are ubiquitous human pathogens. They include herpes simplex 1 (HSV-1), herpes simplex 2 (HSV-2), varicella zoster virus (VZV), Epstein-Barr Virus (EBV), cytomegalovirus (CMV), and human herpes viruses (HHV)-6, HHV-7, and HHV-8 (also known as the Kaposi's sarcoma virus). Other herpes viruses infect animals and are used as experimental models for human diseases.

Herpes viruses can infect most tissues but have a predilection for neurons, particularly the cells of the dorsal root ganglia and their cranial nerve equivalents, such as the trigeminal ganglion. After a primary infection, herpes viruses persist in a latent state within the nervous system and can be reactivated by stress or immunosuppression. Some herpes viruses can directly infect capillary endothelium as well. Since the development of molecular techniques to detect viral genome, HSV, VZV, EBV, HHV-6, and CMV have all been demonstrated to cause CNS vasculitis, and CMV has been associated with hypercoagulable states.

Herpes Simplex 1 & 2   HSV-1 causes oral ulcers, ocular infections, meningitis, and facial palsy. It is also the most common cause of sporadic encephalitis in the HIV-1-seronegative, adult general population. HSV-2 is less common, and infection is correlated with sexual activity. HSV-2 causes genital ulcers and can also cause "aseptic" meningitis.

In immunocompetent patients, HSV-1 encephalitis has a well-characterized clinical course and neuropathologic features. Patients typically present with seizures and altered mental status. If untreated, HSV-1 encephalitis can lead to coma and death. HSV-1 encephalitis is relatively uncommon in AIDS patients, considering the high exposure rate to this pathogen. When it occurs, the clinical and pathologic features of HSV-1 encephalitis often differ from those seen in HIV-1-seronegative persons. In HIV-infected persons, HSV-1 encephalitis tends to present with a more diffuse CNS disease and is characterized by less CNS necrosis and hemorrhage.[162]

Herpes simplex 1 can infect vascular endothelium and initiate the sequence of events that promote thrombosis.[62] It has also been detected in atherosclerotic plaques and is implicated in altering local cholesterol trafficking.[69]

Prior to the advent of PCR, the diagnosis of HSV-1 in the CNS usually required a brain biopsy. However, CSF HSV-1 PCR is a less invasive and equally satisfactory method for establishing a diagnosis.[163]

The treatment for HSV-1 or HSV-2 infections of

the CNS is acyclovir [9-(2-hydroxyethoxymethyl)guanine]. The dose for AIDS patients with CNS disease is 10 mg/kg every 8 h for 10 to 14 days, given intravenously.[164]

Varicella Zoster Virus Varicella zoster virus (VZV) causes the childhood disease varicella (chickenpox). After the primary infection, VZV lies dormant within dorsal root or cranial nerve ganglia cells. The VZV can reactivate in persons with impaired cell-mediated immunity. The localized reactivation of VZV in a nerve root is called herpes zoster or "shingles." Neuropathic pain, sensory loss, and vesicular eruption in a dermatomal distribution characterize zoster. The VZV may also reactivate without a rash in both HIV-infected and in HIV-seronegative persons.[165] Of all the herpes viruses, VZV is the most frequently associated with angiitis and stroke. Apparently, VZV can spread from reactivation sites in the ganglia of cranial nerves, particularly the trigeminal nerve, to the arterial wall by neural pathways. There, VZV can directly infect the walls of CNS arteries, causing an inflammatory process that can lead to stroke. Visible zoster skin lesions in the trigeminal or upper cervical areas often precede such stroke.[26,166] In particular, VZV infections of the trigeminal distribution have been noted to cause a delayed stroke with contralateral hemiparesis, which may occur days to weeks after the appearance of vesicles. Recently, investigators have reported that herpes viruses such as VZV can be identified in the affected blood vessel walls and/or CSF of some persons with stroke and idiopathic CNS vasculitis syndromes, such as granulomatous angiitis.[25,26,160,166,167]

A positive CSF VZV PCR is the least invasive method of diagnosing VZV infection of the CNS.[168,169] However, if the CSF is not diagnostic, a brain biopsy and direct examination of the affected vessel may be necessary to establish the diagnosis.

Cytomegalovirus CMV is a ubiquitous herpes virus spread by oral and respiratory routes, blood, genital secretions, transplants, and from mother to child. The primary infection is typically a self-limited viral syndrome that may resemble mononucleosis. CMV persists in a latent state in many cell lines and can reactivate during immunosuppression, causing end-organ disease in the retina, CNS, lungs, and gastrointestinal tract. CMV can infect the arterial walls,[70] causing a vasculitis.[170] Strokes due to CMV infection in immunosuppressed patients typically occur in the setting of a meningitis or encephalitis. In addition, CMV infection can be associated with a hypercoagulable state, even in otherwise healthy persons, and CMV has been implicated in the genesis of atherosclerosis as described above.[28,71,75]

The CSF profile in CMV infection may show a polymorphonuclear pleocytosis, hypoglycorrhachia, and elevated total protein.[171-174] This profile is not uniformly present and is not diagnostic for CMV.[175] Detection of CMV by CSF viral culture is specific but the sensitivity is poor, even in documented infection.[175] Serologic tests for CMV are rarely helpful, because most adults have been previously infected and have positive CMV serology. Further, the levels of CMV IgG may rise as part of a nonspecific response to immune activation. Likewise, the mere presence CMV in blood does not guarantee an active CNS infection, particularly in AIDS patients.[176] The preferred method to diagnose and follow CNS CMV infection is a CSF CMV PCR.[177]

No controlled trials have yet been published for the treatment of CMV within the CNS. Case reports indicate that intravenous ganciclovir may be an effective therapy for the CNS complications of CMV and that treatment can be followed with quantitative CSF CMV PCR.[163,171] If the patient cannot tolerate ganciclovir or if his/her CMV becomes ganciclovir-resistant, intravenous foscavir or cidofovir can be used. These drugs are nephrotoxic, and little has been published about their use in neurologic disease.[171,172]

Parasitic Diseases and Stroke

Trichinosis Trichinosis is a zoonotic disease caused by a parasitic nematode. Humans are infected by eating undercooked meat containing infective, encysted *Trichinella* larvae. The adult parasites inhabit the mammalian small bowel, where the female releases tiny worm-like larvae that can enter the blood vessels, heart, and arterial circulation. These larvae can penetrate any organ; however, they can only reach maturity in skeletal muscle, where they become encysted.

The main clinical features of trichinosis include diarrhea, fever, myalgias, oculopalpebral signs, and eosinophilia. Involvement of the CNS and heart is limited to severe cases of infestation. In such instances, the larvae can cause thrombosis of cerebral vessels, ischemic stroke, encephalitis, or cerebral hemorrhage. The mechanisms include obstruction of the cerebral arteries, the release of toxic antigens, which cause a severe inflammatory response, and eosinophilic infiltration. DNA probes and PCR technology may help to identify *Trichinella* spp., and muscle biopsy may disclose encapsulated *Trichinella spiralis* larvae coiled within a muscle fiber host cell. This disease is treated with oral thiabendazole,

25 mg/kg bid for 7 days, but this will not kill encysted parasites. Corticosteroids may be necessary to manage severe CNS disease.

Neurocysticercosis The tapeworm *Taenia solium* is a common intestinal parasite that is widely distributed throughout the world. It is transmitted by eating infected pork that contains the tissue larvae (cysticerci) or by the ingestion of eggs that hatch in the small intestine. In the latter case, the embryos migrate through the mucosa into the circulation, where they migrate to various tissues. In most instances, the invasion of the CNS by *T. solium* is clinically silent. Most CNS symptoms generally develop within 1 to 30 years (median of 5 to 7 years) after the initial infection.[178] In general, few symptoms occur while the parasite remains alive. However, when the cystercerci begin to die, larval antigens are released, which incite a powerful CNS inflammatory response.[179] This process that may be accelerated by treatment.[180] This inflammatory response is associated with features such as headache, seizures, increased intracranial pressure, meningismus, nausea, vomiting, and a cerebral arteritis of both large and small vessels, and ischemic stroke.[181,182] The diagnosis of neurocysticercosis can be made by the characteristic appearance of the cysts on neuroimaging (MRI or CT). They appear as rounded lesions, with or without enhancement and edema. The dead (inactive) cysts are typically calcified. Serology (antibody tests) have a high rate of sensitivity and specificity for cysticercosis.

Therapy for neurocysticercosis is controversial. In cases of neurocysticercosis with few or inactive symptoms, treatment may be deferred. Treatment for symptomatic disease with albendazole can cause an exacerbation of the neurologic symptoms because of the release of antigen from the dying larva, with resultant inflammation and CNS complications. This may require the addition of steroids for management.

Strongyloidiasis *Strongyloides stercoralis* is a parasitic nematode that can live free in soil or can inhabit the human small intestine. The infective (filariform) larvae can enter the human host by penetrating the skin. They travel through the lymphatics to the venous system and lungs, are coughed up into the glottis, swallowed, and enter the gastrointestinal tract, where they attach to the duodenum and jejeunum. Mature forms can reproduce therein, and the eggs pass out of the body via the feces.

Rarely, *Strongyloides* disseminates to other body organs. This occurs when there is an unusually large number of infecting invasive filariform larvae or if the eggs produced within the host's intestines are able to mature into the infective (filariform) larvae before leaving the bowel. In such cases, they can invade other organs by penetrating the bowel wall, or by penetrating the skin around the anus after they are expelled in the feces. This process, "autoinfection," allows the parasite to cycle for many years without returning to the environment. It is relatively uncommon and involves relatively few larvae, unless the host has compromised cell-mediated immunity. In such cases, the number of larvae increases rapidly and produces a "hyperinfection" syndrome, involving multiple organs including the CNS. This process has been reported to occur in patients treated with immunosuppressive drugs and in AIDS patients.

Within the CNS, *Strongyloides* can obstruct cerebral vessels, causing thrombosis and ischemic stroke. These parasites also carry enteric bacteria with them and may cause bacteremia and meningitis. *Strongyloides* can be treated with albendazole.

Toxoplasmosis Toxoplasmosis is caused by a parasitic protozoa, *Toxoplasma gondii*. Humans acquire toxoplasmosis by vertical transmission, or by ingestion of *T. gondii* cysts from inadequately cooked, infected meat, contaminated soil, and human or cat feces. The primary infection in healthy persons is characterized by lymphadenopathy and a mononucleosis-type illness. In immunosuppressed individuals, toxoplasmosis can disseminate to the CNS, where it causes an encephalitis characterized by focal abscesses or masses surrounded by relatively intact tissue. Toxoplasmosis is the most common cause of a brain mass in adult AIDS patients, accounting for up to 70 percent of such lesions.[183]

Depending upon the stage of the illness and the location of the lesions, patients may present with nonfocal symptoms such as headache, fever, malaise, lethargy, and delirium. They may also present with focal signs and symptoms that can be localized to specific abscesses such as hemiparesis, hemisensory loss, hemianopsia, aphasia, and focal or generalized seizures. Untreated, patients develop cerebral edema, increased intracranial pressure, coma, and brain herniation. Toxoplasmosis is relevant to this discussion of stroke because it is occasionally associated with cerebral hemmorhage,[100] and because the focal signs can sometimes be mistaken for cerebral infarcts.

Using modern assays, serum toxoplasmosis titers (IgG and IgM antibodies) are positive in almost 100 percent of AIDs patients with CNS toxoplasmosis.[184,185]

A negative serum toxoplasmosis titer makes toxoplasmosis very unlikely. However, serum antibodies to toxoplasmosis are so common that they cannot be used as the sole measure to diagnose CNS disease. In addition, CSF toxoplasmosis titers are very unreliable.[186,187] Consequently, additional confirmation is usually required to confirm this diagnosis. Most often, the diagnosis is confirmed by clinical and or radiologic response to empiric treatment under close observation over a 2-week period. If the patient fails to improve or continues to deteriorate, a brain biopsy is warranted.

The recommended treatment for adults is oral pyrimethamine (50 to 100 mg PO per day), along with oral folinic acid 10 mg/day (to prevent megaloblastic anemia), and oral sulfadiazine (1 to 1.5 every 6 h). Patients who are allergic to sulfonamides can be treated with clindamycin, 600 mg intravenously or orally every 6 h, and pyrimethamine (200 mg PO at onset followed by 75 to 100 mg PO every day).[188]

REFERENCES

1. Sanabria T, Alpert J, Goldberg R, Pape L: Increasing frequency of staphylococcal infective endocarditis: Experience at a university hospital, 1981 through 1988. *Arch Intern Med* 150:1305, 1990.
2. Manoff S, Vlahov D, Herskowitz A, et al: Human immunodeficiency virus infection and infective endocarditis among injecting drug users. *Epidemiology* 7:566, 1996.
3. De Castro S, Magni G, Beni SCD, et al: Role of transthoracic and transesophageal echocardiography in predicting embolic events in patients with active infective endocarditis involving native cardiac valves. *Am J Cardiol* 80:1030, 1997.
4. Erbel R, Liu F, Ge J, Rohmann S, Kupferwasser, I: Identification of high-risk subgroups in infective endocarditis and the role of echocardiography. *Eur Heart J* 16:588, 1995.
5. Heinle S, Wilderman N, Harrison J, et al: Value of transthoracic echocardiography in predicting embolic events in active infective endocarditis. Duke Endocarditis Service. *Am J Cardiol* 74:799, 1994.
6. Mugge A, Daniel W: Echocardiographic assessment of vegetations in patients with infective endocarditis: Prognostic implications. *Echocardiography* 12:651, 1995.
7. Hart R, Foster J, Luther M, Kanter M: Stroke in infective endocarditis. *Stroke* 21:695, 1990.
8. Kanter, M, Hart, R: Neurologic complications of infective endocarditis. *Neurology* 41:1015, 1991.
9. Durack D, Lukes A, Bright D: New criteria for the diagnosis of infective endocarditis: Utilization of specific echocardiographic findings. Duke Endocarditis Service [see comments]. *Am J Med* 96:200, 1994.

10. Benn M, Hagelskjaer, L, Tvede M: Infective endocarditis, 1984 through 1993: A clinical and microbiological survey. *J Int Med* 242:15, 1997.
11. Pruitt A, Rubin R, Karchmer Al Duncan G: Neurologic complications of bacterial endocarditis. *Medicine* 57:329, 1978.
12. Weinstein L: Life-threatening complications of infective endocarditis and their management. *Arch Intern Med* 146:953, 1986.
13. Bayer A, Ward J, Ginzton L, Shapiro S: Evaluation of new clinical criteria for the diagnosis of infective endocarditis. *Am J Med* 96:211, 1994.
14. Bayer A, Bolger A, Taubert K, et al: Diagnosis and management of infective endocarditis and its complications. *Circulation* 98:2936, 1998.
15. Liu F, Ge J, Kupferwasser I, et al: Has transesophageal echocardiography changed the approach to patients with suspected or known infective endocarditis? *Echocardiography* 12:637, 1995.
16. Lowry R, Zoghbi W, Baker W, Wray R, Quinones M: Clinical impact of transesophageal echocardiography in the diagnosis and management of infective endocarditis. *Am J Cardiol* 73:1089, 1994.
17. Singer E, Synduklo K, Tourtellotte W: Neurodiagnostic testing in HIV infection: Cerebrospinal fluid, in Berger J, Levy R (eds): *AIDS and the Nervous System,* 2nd ed. New York, Raven Press, 1996.
18. Besnier J, Choutet P: Medical treatment of infective endocarditis: General principles. *Eur Heart J* 16 (Suppl B): 72, 1995.
19. Bitsch A, Nau R, Hilgers R, Verheggen R, Werner G, Prange H: Focal neurologic deficits in infective endocarditis and other septic diseases. *Acta Neurol Scand* 94:279, 1996.
20. Wilson W, Karchmer A, Dajani A, et al: Antibiotic treatment of adults with infective endocarditis due to streptococci, enterococci, staphylococci, and HACEK microorganisms. American Heart Association. *JAMA* 274:1706, 1995.
21. Pfister H, Borasio GD, Dirnagl U, Bauer M, Einhaupl K: Cerebrovascular complications of bacterial meningitis in adults. *Neurology* 42:1497, 1992.
22. Pfister H, Feiden W, Einhaupl K: Spectrum of complications during bacterial meningitis in adults: Results of a prospective clinical study. *Arch Neurol* 50:575, 1993.
23. Pfister H, Fontana A, Tauber M, Tomasz A, Scheld W: Mechanisms of brain injury in bacterial meningitis: Workshop summary. *Clin Infect Dis* 19:463, 1994.
24. Conaldi P, Serra C, Mossa A, et al: Persistent infection of human vascular endothelial cells by group B coxsackie viruses. *J Infect Dis* 175:693, 1997.
25. Martin J, Mitchell W, Henken D: Neurotropic herpesviruses, neural mechanisms and arteritis. *Brain Pathol* 1:6, 1990.
26. Melanson M, Chalk, C, Georgevich L, et al: Varicella-zoster virus DNA in CSF and arteries in delayed contralat-

eral hemiplegia: Evidence for viral invasion of cerebral arteries. *Neurology* 47:569, 1996.

27. Poland S, Rice G, Dekaban G: HIV-1 infection of human brain-derived microvascular endothelial cells in vitro. *J Acquir Immune Defic Syndr Hum Retrovirol* 8:437, 1995.

28. Yonemitsu Y, Komori K, Sueishi K, Sugimachi K: Possible role of cytomegalovirus infection in the pathogenesis of human vascular diseases. *Jpn J Clin Med* 56:102, 1998.

29. Lambert H: Meningitis. *J Neurol Neurosurg Psych* 57:405, 1994.

30. Dosquet C, Weill D, Wautier J: Cytokines and thrombosis. *J Cardiovasc Pharmacol* 25 (Suppl 2): S13, 1995.

31. Goh D, Minns R: Cerebral blood flow velocity monitoring in pyogenic meningitis. *Arch Dis Childhood* 68:111, 1993.

32. Forderreuther S, Tatsch K, Einhaupl K, Pfister H: Abnormalities of cerebral blood flow in the acute phase of meningitis in adults. *J Neurol* 239:431, 1992.

33. Muller M, Merkelbach S, Huss G, Schimrigk K: Clinical relevance and frequency of transient stenoses of the middle and anterior cerebral arteries in bacterial meningitis [see comments]. *Stroke* 26:1399, 1995.

34. Ries S, Schminke U, Fassbender K, Daffertshofer M, Steinke W, Hennerici M: Cerebrovascular involvement in the acute phase of bacterial meningitis. *J Neurol* 244:51, 1997.

35. Schuchat A, Robinson K, Wenger J, et al: Bacterial meningitis in the United States in 1995. *N Engl J Med* 337:970, 1997.

36. Bhisitkul D, Hogan A, Tanz R: The role of bacterial antigen detection tests in the diagnosis of bacterial meningitis. *Pediat Emerg Care* 10:67, 1994.

37. Gray L, Fedorko D: Laboratory diagnosis of bacterial meningitis. *Clin Microbiol Rev* 5:130, 1992.

38. Yang Y, Leng Z, Shen X, et al: Acute bacterial meningitis in children in Hefei, China 1990–1992. *Chin Med J* 109:385, 1996.

39. Shoji H, Honda Y, Murai I, Sato Y, Oizumi K, Hondo R: Detection of varicella-zoster virus DNA by polymerase chain reaction in cerebrospinal fluid of patients with herpes zoster meningitis. *J Neurol* 239:69, 1992.

40. Mullis K, Faloona F, Scharf S, Saiki R, Horn G, Erlich H: Specific enzymatic amplification of DNA in vitro. The polymerase chain reaction. *Symp Quant Biol* 51(1):263, 1986.

41. Mullis KB, Faloona FA: Specific synthesis of DNA in vitro via a polymerase-catalyzed chain reaction. New York, Academic Press, 1987.

42. Weidbrauk D, Hodinka R: Applications of the polymerase chain reaction, in Specter S, Bendinelli M, Friedman H, (eds): *Rapid Detection of Infectious Agents*. New York, Plenum Press, 1998, pp 97–116.

43. Zheng X, Persing D: Genetic amplification techniques for diagnosing infectious diseases, in Specter S, Bendinelli M, Friedman H (eds): *Rapid Detection of Infectious Agents*. New York, Plenum Press, 1998, pp 69–82.

44. Girgis N, Farid Z, Mikhail I, Farrag I, Sultan Y, Kilpatrick M: Dexamethasone treatment for bacterial meningitis in children and adults. *Pediat Infect Dis J* 8:848, 1989.

45. Wald E, Kaplan S, Mason EJ, et al: Dexamethasone therapy for children with bacterial meningitis. Meningitis Study Group *Pediatrics* 95:21, 1995.

46. Grau A, Buggle F, Becher H, et al: Recent bacterial and viral infection is a risk factor for cerebrovascular ischemia: Clinical and biochemical studies. *Neurology* 50:196, 1998.

47. Janak S, Baruah J, Jayaram S, Saxena V, Sharma S, Gulati M: Stroke in the young: A four-year study, 1968–1972. *Stroke* 55:318, 1975.

48. Mattila K, Valtonen V, Nieinen M, Asikainene S: Role of infection as a risk factor for atherosclerosis, myocardial infarction, and stroke. *Clin Infect Dis* 26:719, 1998.

49. Valtonen V: Infection as a risk factor for infarction and atherosclerosis. *Ann Med* 23:539, 1991.

50. Hindfelt B, Nilsson O: Brain infarction in young adults (with particular reference to pathogenesis). *Acta Neurol Scand* 55:145, 1977.

51. Woodhouse P, Khaw K, Plummer M, Foley A, Meade T: Seasonal variations of plasma fibrinogen and factor VII activity in the elderly: Winter infections and death from cardiovascular disease. *Lancet* 343:435, 1994.

52. Riikonen R, Santavuori P: Hereditary and acquired risk factors for childhood stroke. *Neuropediatrics* 25:227, 1994.

53. Bova I, Bornstein N, Korczyn A: Acute infection as a risk factor for ischemic stroke. *Stroke* 27:2204, 1996.

54. Macko R, Ameriso S, Gruber A, et al: Impairments of the protein C system and fibrinolysis in infection-associated stroke. *Stroke* 27:2005, 1996.

55. Syrjanen J, Valtonen V, Iivanainen M, Hovi T, Malkamaki M, Makela P: Association between cerebral infarction and increased serum bacterial antibody levels in young adults. *Acta Neurol Scand* 73:273, 1986.

56. Muhlestein J, Anderson J, Hammond, E et al: Infection with *Chlamydia pneumoniae* accelerates the development of atherosclerosis and treatment with azithromycin prevents it in a rabbit model. *Circulation* 97:633, 1998.

57. Grau A, Buggle F, Ziegler C, et al: Association between acute cerebrovascular ischemia and chronic and recurrent infection. *Stroke* 28:1724, 1997.

58. Cook P, Honeybourne D, Lip G, Beevers D, Wise R, Davies P: *Chlamydia pneumoniae* antibody titers are significantly associated with acute stroke and transient cerebral ischemia: The West Birmingham Stroke Project. *Stroke* 29:404, 1998.

58a. Cook P, Lip G: Infectious agents and atherosclerotic vascular disease. *Q J Med* 89:727, 1996.

59. Wimmer M, Sandmann-Strupp R, Saikku P, Haberl R: Association of chlamydial infection with cerebrovascular disease. *Stroke* 27:2207, 1996.

60. Markus H, Mendall M: *Helicobacter pylori* infection: A risk factor for ischaemic cerebrovascular disease and carotid atheroma. *J Neurol Neurosurg Psych* 64:104, 1998.

61. Mehta J, Saldeen T Rand K: Interactive role of infection, inflammation and traditional risk factors in atherosclero-

sis and coronary artery disease. *J Am Coll Cardiol* 31: 1217, 1998.

62. Vercellotti G: Effects of viral activation of the vessel wall on inflammation and thrombosis. *Blood Coagul Fibrinolysis* 9 (Suppl 2): S3, 1998.

63. Danesh J, Peto R: Risk factors for coronary heart disease and infection with *Helicobacter pylori*: Meta-analysis of 18 studies. *Br Med J* 316:1130, 1998.

64. Parente F, Porro G: The association between *Helicobacter pylori* infection and ischemic heart disease: Facts or fancy? *Helicobacter* 2 (Suppl 1): S67, 1997.

65. Whincup P, Mendall M, Perry I, Strachan D, Walker M: Prospective relations between *Helicobacter pylori* infection, coronary heart disease, and stroke in middle aged men. *Heart* 75:568, 1996.

66. Juvonen J, Juvonen T, Laurila A, et al: Demonstration of *Chlamydia pneumoniae* in the walls of abdominal aortic aneurysms. *J Vasc Surg* 25:499, 1997.

67. Laurila A, Bloigu A, Nayha S, Hassi J, Leinonen M, Saikku P: Chronic *Chlamydia pneumoniae* infection is associated with a serum lipid profile known to be a risk factor for atherosclerosis. *Arterioscler Thromb Vasc Biol* 17:2910, 1997.

68. Muhlestein J, Hammond E, Carlquist J, et al: Increased incidence of *Chlamydia* species within the coronary arteries of patients with symptomatic atherosclerotic versus other forms of cardiovascular disease. *J Am Coll Cardiol* 27:1555, 1996.

69. Hsu H, Nicholson A, Pomerantz K, Kaner R, Hajjar D: Altered cholesterol trafficking in herpesvirus-infected arterial cells. Evidence for viral protein kinase-mediated cholesterol accumulation. *J Biol Chem* 270:19630, 1995.

70. Melnick J, Hu C, Burek J, Adam E, DeBakey M: Cytomegalovirus DNA in arterial walls of patients with atherosclerosis. *J Med Virol* 42:170, 1994.

71. Nieto F, Sorlie P, Comstock G, Wu K, Adam E, Melnick J, Szklo M: Cytomegalovirus infection, liprotein (a), and hypercoagulability: An atherogenic link? *Arterioscler Thromb Vasc Biol* 17:1780, 1997.

72. Pouria S, State O, Wong W, Hendry B: CMV infection is associated with transplant renal artery stenosis. *Q J Med* 91:185, 1998.

73. Raza-Ahmad A, Kiassen G, Murphy D, et al: Evidence of type 2 herpes simplex infection in human coronary arteries at the time of coronary artery bypass surgery. *Can J Cardiol* 11:1025, 1995.

73a. Ridker P, Cushman M, Stamper M, Tracy R, Hennekens C: Inflammation, aspirin, and the risk of cardiovascular disease in apparently healthy men. *N Engl J Med* 336: 973, 1997.

74. Libby, P, Egan D, Skariatos S: Roles of infectious agents in atherosclerosis and restenosis. An assessment of the evidence and need for future research. *Circulation* 96: 4095, 1997.

75. Koskinen P, Lemstrom K, Mattila S, Hayry P, MS, N: Cytomegalovirus infection associated accelerated heart allograft arteriosclerosis may impair the late function of the graft. *Clin Transplant* 10:487, 1996.

76. Seymour R, Steele J: Is there a link between periodontal disease and coronary heart disease? *Br Dent J* 184:33, 1998.

77. Stary H, Chandler A, Glagov S, et al: A definition of initial, fatty streak, and intermediate lesions of atherosclerosis: A report from the Committee on Vascular Lesions of the Council on Arteriosclerosis, American Heart Association. *Circulation* 89:2462, 1994.

78. Hendrix M, Salimens M, van Bowen C, Bruggeman C: High prevalence of latently present cytomegalovirus in arterial walls of patients suffering from grade III atherosclerosis. *Am J Pathol* 136:23, 1990.

79. Jackson L, Campbell L, Schmidt R, et al: Specificity of detection of *Chlamydia pneumoniae* in cardiovascular atheroma: Evaluation of the innocent bystander hypothesis. *Am J Pathol* 150:1785, 1997.

80. Saikku P: *Chlamydia pneumoniae* and atherosclerosis: an update. *Scand J Infect Dis Suppl* 104:53, 1997.

81. Fabricant C, Fabricant J, Minick C, Litrena M: Herpesvirus-induced atherosclerosis in chickens. *Fed Proc* 42:2476, 1983.

82. Fryer R, Schwobe E, Woods M, Rodgers G: *Chlamydia* species infect human vascular endothelial cells and induce procoagulant activity. *J Invest Med* 45:168, 1997.

83. Gaydos C, Summersgill J, Sahney N, Ramirez J, Quinn T: Replication of *Chlamydia pneumoniae* in vitro in human macrophages, endothelial cells, and aortic artery smooth muscle cells. *Infect Immun* 64:1614, 1996.

84. Meier C, Derby L, Jick S, Vasilakis C, Jick H: Antibiotics and risk of subsequent first-time myocardial infarction. *JAMA* 281:427, 1999.

85. Besedovsky H, del Rey A: Immune-neuroendocrine circuits: Integrative role of cytokines, in Ganong W, Luciano M (eds): *Frontiers in Neuroendocrinology,* New York, Raven, 1992, pp 61–94.

86. Blatteis C: Neuromodulative actions of cytokines. *Yale J Biol Med* 63:133, 1990.

87. Hanisch U, Seto D, Quirion R: Modulation of hippocampal acetylcholine release release: A potent central action of IL-2. *J Neurosci* 14:3368, 1993.

88. Breamer N, Coull B, Clark W, Briley D, Wynn D, Sexton G: Persistent inflammatory response in stroke survivors. *Neurology* 50:1722, 1998.

89. Grau A, Buggle F, Steichen-Wiehn C, et al. Clinical and biochemical analysis in infection-associated stroke. *Stroke* 26:1520, 1995.

90. Macko R, Ameriso S, Barndt R, Clough W, Weiner, J, Fisher M: Precipitants of brain infarction. Roles of preceding infection/inflammation and recent psychological stress [see comments]. *Stroke* 27:1999, 1996.

91. Brey R, Hart R, Sherman D, Tegeler C: Antiphospholipid antibodies and cerebral ischemia in young people. *Neurology* 40:1190, 1990.

92. Hansen K, Arnason J, Bridges A: Autoantibodies and

common viral illnesses. *Semin Arthritis Rheum* 27:263, 1998.

93. Abuaf N, Laperche S, Rajoely B, et al: Autoantibodies to phospholipids and to the coagulation proteins in AIDS. *Thromb Haemost* 77:856, 1997.

94. Labarca, J, Rabaggliati, R, Radrigan, F, et al: Antiphospholipid syndrome associated with cytomegalovirus infection: Case report and review. *Clin Infect Dis* 24:197, 1997.

95. Canoso R, Zon L, Groopman J: Anticardiolipin antibodies associated with HTLV-III infection. *Br J Haematol* 65:495, 1987.

96. Hassell K, Kressin D, Neumann A, Ellison R, Marlar R: Correlation of antiphospholipid antibodies and protein S deficiency with thrombosis in HIV-infected men. *Blood Coagul Fibrinol* 5:455, 1994.

97. Keeling D, Birley H, Machin S: Multiple transient ischaemic attacks and a mild thrombotic stroke in a HIV-positive patient with anticardiolipin antibodies. *Blood Coagul Fibrinol* 1:333, 1990.

98. Loizou S, Cazabon J, Walport M, Tait D, So A: Similarities of specificity and cofactor dependence in serum antiphospholipid antibodies from patients with human parvovirus B19 infection and from those with systemic lupus erythematosus. *Arthritis Rheumatism* 40:103, 1997.

99. Jinkins J: Computed tomography of intracranial tuberculosis. *Neuroradiology* 33:126, 1991.

100. Hsieh F, Chia L, Shen W: Locations of cerebral infarctions in tuberculous meningitis. *Neuroradiology* 34:197, 1992.

101. Leiguarda R, Berthier M, Starkstein S, Nogues M, Lylyk P: Ischemic infarction in 25 children with tuberculous meningitis. *Stroke* 19:200, 1988.

102. Hook E: Central nervous system syphilis, in Scheld W, Whitley R, Durack D (eds): *Infections of the Central Nervous System*. New York, Raven, 1991 pp, 639–656.

103. Clark E, Danbolt N: The Oslo study of the natural history of untreated syphilis: An epidemiological investigation based on a restudy of the Boeck-Bruusgaard material. A review and appraisal. *J Chronic Dis* 2:311, 1955.

104. Johns DR, Tierney M, Felsenstein D: Alteration in the natural history of neurosyphilis by concurrent infection with the human immunodeficiency virus. *N Engl J Med* 316:1569, 1987.

105. Marra C, Handsfield H, Kuller L, Morton W, Lukehart S: Alterations in the course of experimental syphilis associated with concurrent simian immunodeficiency virus infection. *J Infect Dis* 165:1020, 1992.

106. Erbelding E, Vlahov D, Nelson K, et al: Syphilis serology in human immunodeficiency virus infection: Evidence for false-negative fluorescent treponemal testing. *J Infect Dis* 176:1397, 1997.

107. Gordon S, Eaton, M, George R, et al: The response of symptomatic neurosyphilis to high-dose intravenous penicillin G in patients with human immunodeficiency virus infection (see comments). *N Engl J Med* 331:1469, 1994.

108. Lukehart S, Hook ED, Baker-Zander S, Collier A, Critchlow C, Handsfield H: Invasion of the central ner-

vous system by *Treponema pallidum*: Implications for diagnosis and treatment. *Ann Intern Med* 109:855, 1988.

109. Malessa R, Agelink M, Hengge U, Mertins L, Gastpar M, Brockmeyer N: Oligosymptomatic neurosyphilis with false negative CSF-VDRL in HIV-infected individuals? *Eur J Med Res* 1:299, 1996.

110. Malone J, Wallace M, Hendrick B, et al: Syphilis and neurosyphilis in a human immunodeficiency virus type-1 seropositive population: Evidence for frequent serologic relapse after therapy. *Am J Med* 99:55, 1995.

111. Musher D, Hamill R, Baughn R: Effect of human immunodeficiency virus (HIV) infection on the course of syphilis and on the response to treatment. *Ann Intern Med* 113:872-871, 1990.

112. Marra C, Gary D, Kuypers J, Jacobson M: Diagnosis of neurosyphilis in patients infected with human immunodeficiency virus type 1. *J Infect Dis* 174:219, 1996.

113. Brightbill T, Ihmeidan I, Post M, Berger J, Katz D: Neurosyphilis in HIV-positive and HIV-negative patients: Neuroimaging findings. *Am J Neuroradiol* 16:703, 1995.

114. Thomas D, Fogelman A, Miller J, Lovett M: Interactions of *Treponema pallidum* with endothelial cell monolayers. *Eur J Epidemiol* 5:15, 1989.

115. Riley B, Oppenheimer-Marks N, Hansen E, Radolf J, Norgard M: Virulent *Treponema pallidum* activates human vascular endothelial cells. *J Infect Dis* 165:484, 1992.

116. Riley B, Oppenheimer-Marks N, Radolf J, Norgard M: Virulent *Treponema pallidum* promotes adhesion of leukocytes to human vascular endothelial cells. *Infect Immun* 62:4622, 1994.

117. Wicher K, Wicher V: Autoimmunity in syphilis, *Immunol Ser* 52:101, 1990.

118. Jorizzo J, McNeely M, Baughn R, Solomon A, Cavallo T, Smith E: Role of circulating immune complexes in human secondary syphilis. *J Infect Dis* 153:1014, 1986.

119. Centers for Disease Control and Prevention: 1993 Sexually transmitted diseases treatment guidelines. *Morb Mortal Weekly Rep* 42 (RR-14):1, 1993.

120. May E, Jabbari B: Stroke in neuroborreliosis. *Stroke* 21:1232, 1990.

121. Pachner A: Neurologic manifestations of Lyme disease, the new "great imitator." *Rev Infect Dis* 11 (Suppl 6): S1482, 1989.

122. Uldri P-A, Regli F, Bogousslavsky J: Cerebral angiopathy and recurrent strokes following *Borrelia burgdorferi* infection. *J Neurol Neurosurg Psychiatry* 50:1703, 1987.

123. Duray P, Johnson R: The histopathology of experimentally infected hamsters with the Lyme disease spirochete, *Borrelia burgdorferi* (422251). *Proc Soc Exp Biol Med* 181:263, 1986.

124. Steere A: Diagnosis and treatment of Lyme arthritis. *Med Clin North Am* 81:179, 1997.

125. Kovacs JA, Kovacs AA, Polis M, et al: Cryptococcosis in the acquired immunodeficiency syndrome. *Ann Intern Med* 103:533, 1985.

126. Matthews V, Alo P, Glass J, et al: AIDS-related CNS

cryptococcosis: Radiologic-pathologic correlation. *Am J Neuroradiol* 13:1477, 1992.

127. Davies D, Singer E, McGill L, Baumhefner R, Tourtellotte W: Cryptococcal meningitis/AIDS presenting as a transient neurologic deficit. *J Stroke Cerebrovasc Dis* 2:189, 1992.

128. Darras-Joly C, Chevret S, Wolff M, et al: *Cryptococcus neoformans* infection in France: Epidemiologic features of and early prognostic parameters for 76 patients who were infected with human immunodeficiency virus. *Clin Infect Dis* 23:369, 1996.

128a. Nelson M, Bower M, Smith D, Reed C, Shanson D, Gazzard B: The value of serum cryptococcal antigen in the diagnosis of cryptococcal infection in patients infected with the human immunodeficiency virus. *J Infect* 21:175, 1990.

129. Nelson M, Bower M, Smith D, Reed C, Shanson D, Gazzard B: The value of serum cryptococcal antigen in the diagnosis of cryptococcal infection in patients infected with the human immunodeficiency virus. *J Infect* 21:175, 1990.

130. van der Horst C, Saag M, Cloud G, Hamill R, Graybill J, Sobel J: Treatment of cryptococcal meningitis associated with the acquired immunodeficiency syndrome. National Institute of Allergy and Infectious Diseases Mycoses Study Group and AIDS Clinical Trials Group. *N Engl J Med* 337:15, 1997.

131. Zuger A, Louie E, Holzman RS, Simberkoff MS, Rahal JJ: Cryptococcal disease in patients with the acquired immunodeficiency syndrome: Diagnostic features and outcome of treatment. *Ann Intern Med* 104:234, 1986.

132. van der Horst C, Saag M, Cloud G, et al: Treatment of cryptococcal meningitis associated with the acquired immunodeficiency syndrome. National Institute of Allergy and Infectious Diseases Mycoses Study Group and AIDS Clinical Trials Group. *N Engl J Med* 337:15, 1997.

133. Sugar A, Saunders C: Oral fluconazole as suppressive therapy of disseminated cryptococcosis in patients with acquired immunodeficiency syndrome. *Am J Med* 85:481, 1988.

134. Mischel P, Vinters V: Coccidioidomycosis of the central nervous system: Neuropathological and vasculopathic manifestions and clinical correlates. *Clin Infect Dis* 20:400, 1995.

135. Sobel R, Ellis W, Nielson S, Davis R: Central nervous system coccidiomycosis: A clinicopathologic study of treatment with and without amphotericin B. *Hum Pathol* 15:980, 1984.

136. Slavoski L, Tunkel A: Therapy of fungal meningitis. *Clin Neuropharmacol* 18:95, 1995.

137. Grimes D, Lach B, Bourque P: Vasculitic basilar artery thrombosis in chronic *Candida albicans* meningitis. *Can J Neurol Sci* 25:76, 1998.

138. Engstrom J, Lowenstein D, Bredesen D: Cerebral infarctions and transient neurologic deficits associated with ac-

quired immunodeficiency syndrome. *Am J Med* 86:528, 1989.

139. Perriens J, Mussa M, Luabeya M, et al: Neurologic complications of HIV-1-seropositive internal medicine inpatients in Kinshasa, Zaire. *J Acquir Immune Defic Syndr* 5:333, 1992.

140. Park Y, Belman A, Kim T, et al: Stroke in pediatric acquired immunodeficiency syndrome. *Ann Neurol* 28:303, 1990.

141. Pinto A: AIDS and cerebrovascular disease. *Stroke* 27:538, 1996.

142. Mizusawa H, Hirano A, Llena J, Shintaku M: Cerebrovascular lesions in acquired immune deficiency syndrome (AIDS). *Acta Neuropathol* 76:451, 1988.

143. Bode H, Rudin C: Calcifying arteriopathy in the basal ganglia in human immunodeficiency virus infection. *Pediat Radiol* 25:72, 1995.

144. Husson R, Saini R, Lewis L, Butler K, Patronas N, Pizzo P: Cerebral artery aneurysms in children affected with human immunodeficiency virus. *J Pediatr* 121:927, 1992.

145. Philippet P, Blanche S, Sebag G, Rodesch G, Griscelli C, Tardieu M: Stroke and cerebral infarcts in children infected with human immunodeficiency virus. *Arch Pediatr Adolesc Med* 148:965, 1994.

146. Snider WD, Simpson DM, Nielson S, Gold JWM, Metroka C, Posner JB: Neurological complications of acquired immune deficiency syndrome: Analysis of 50 patients. *Ann Neurol* 14:403, 1983.

147. Yankner B, Skolnik P, Shoukimas G, Gabuzda D, Sobel R, Ho D: Cerebral granulomatous angiitis associated with isolation of human immunodeficiency virus type III from the central nervous system. *Ann Neurol* 20:362, 1986.

148. Sorice M, Griggi T, Arcieri P, et al: Protein S and HIV infection: The role of anticardiolipin and anti-protein S antibodies. *Thromb Res* 73:165, 1994.

149. Sugerman R, Church J, Goldsmith J, Ens G: Acquired protein S deficiency in children infected with human immunodeficiency virus. *Pediatr Infect Dis J* 15:106, 1996.

150. Roquer J, Palomeras E, Knobel H, Pou A: Intracerebral haemorrhage in AIDS. *Cerebrovasc Dis* 8:222, 1998.

151. Brew B, Miller J: Human immunodeficiency virus type 1-related transient neurological deficits. *Am J Med* 101:257, 1996.

152. Palomeras E, Roquer J: Cerebrovascular disease as a form of presentation of HIV infection. *Neurologic* 11:346, 1996.

153. Davies J, Everall I, Weich S, McLaughlin J, Scaravilli F, Lantos P: HIV-associated brain pathology in the United Kingdom: An epidemiological study. *AIDS* 11:1145, 1997.

154. Card T, Wathen C, Luzzi G: Primary HIV-1 infection presenting with transient neurological deficit [letter]. *J Neurol Neurosurg Psych* 64:281, 1998.

155. Gillams A, Allen E, Hrieb K, Venna N, Craven D, Carter A: Cerebral infarction in patients with AIDS. *Am J Neuroradiol* 18:1581, 1997.

156. Anders K, Guerra WF, Tomiyasu U, Verity AM, Vinters

HV: The neuropathology of AIDS: UCLA experience and review. *Am J Pathol* 124:537, 1986.

157. Kibayashi K, Mastri A, Hirsch C: Neuropathology of human immunodeficiency virus infection at different disease stages. *Human Pathol* 27:637, 1996.

158. Rosenberg S, Lopes MB, Tsanaclis AM: Neuropathology of acquired immunodeficiency syndrome (AIDS): Analysis of 22 Brazilian cases. *J Neurol Sci* 76:187, 1986.

158a. Ross R: Atherosclerosis. An inflammatory disease. *N Engl J Med* 340:115, 1990.

159. Davis LE, Hjelle BL, Miller VE, et al: Early viral brain invasion in iatrogenic human immunodeficiency virus infection. *Neurology* 42:1736, 1992.

160. Verghese A, Sugar A: Herpes zoster ophthalmicus and granulomatous angiitis: An ill-appreciated cause of stroke. *J Am Geriatr Soc* 34:309, 1986.

161. Rubbert A, Bock E, Schwab J, et al: Anticardiolipin antibodies in HIV infection: Association with cerebral perfusion defects as detected by 99m Tc-HMPAO SPECT. *Clin Exp Immunol* 98:361, 1994.

162. Chretien F, Belec L, Hilton D, et al: Herpes simplex virus type 1 encephalitis in acquired immunodeficiency syndrome. *Neuropathol Appl Neurobiol* 22:394, 1996.

163. Cinque P, Cleator G, Weber T, Monteyne P, Sindic C, van Loon A: The role of laboratory investigation in the diagnosis and management of patients with suspected herpes simplex encephalitis: A consensus report. The EU Concerted Action on Virus Meningitis and Encephalitis. 61:339, 1996.

164. Holland N, Power C, Mathews V, et al: CMV encephalitis in acquired immunodeficiency syndrome. *Neurology* 44:507, 1994.

165. Gilden, D, Wright R, Schneck S, Gwaltney J, Mahalingam R: Zoster sine herpete, a clinical variant. *Ann Neurol* 35:530, 1994.

166. Patrick J, Russell E, Meyer J, Biller J, Saver J: Cervical (C2) herpes zoster infection followed by pontine infarction. *J Neuroimaging* 5:192, 1995.

167. Amlie-Lefond C, Kleinschmidt-DeMasters B, Mahalingam R, Davis L, Gilden D: The vasculopathy of varicella-zoster virus encephalitis. *Ann Neurol* 37:784, 1995.

168. Bergstrom T: Polymerase chain reaction for diagnosis of varicella zoster virus central nervous system infections without skin manifestations. *Scand J Infect Dis Suppl* 100:41, 1996.

169. Burke D, Kalayjian R, Vann V, Madreperla S, Shick H, Leonard D: Polymerase chain reaction detection and clinical significance of varicella-zoster virus in cerebrospinal fluid from human immunodeficiency virus-infected patients. *J Infect Dis* 176:1080, 1997.

170. Golden M, Hammer S, Wanke C, Albrecht M: Cytomegalovirus vasculitis. Case reports and review of the literature. *Medicine* 73:246, 1994.

171. Cohen B: Prognosis and response to therapy of cytomega-

lovirus encephalitis and meningomyelitis in AIDS. *Neurology* 46:444, 1996.

172. Cohen B, McArthur J, Grohman S, et al: Neurological prognosis of cytomegalovirus polyradiculomyelopathy in AIDS. *Neurology* 43:493, 1993.

173. de Gans J, Tiessens G, Portegies P, Tutuarima J, Troost D: Predominance of polymorphonuclear leukocytes in cerebrospinal fluid of AIDS patients with cytomegalovirus polyradiculomyelitis. *J Aquir Immune Defic Syndr* 3:1155, 1990.

174. Kalayjian R, Cohen M, Bonomo R, Flanigan T: Cytomegalovirus ventriculoencephalitis in AIDS. A syndrome with distinct clinical and pathologic features. *Medicine* 72:67, 1993.

175. McCutchan J: Cytomegalovirus infections of the nervous system in patients with AIDS. *Clin Infect Dis* 20:747, 1994.

176. Zurlo J, O'Neill D, Polis M, et al: Lack of clinical utility of cytomegalovirus blood and urine cultures in patients with HIV infection. *Ann Intern Med* 118:12, 1993.

177. Clifford DB, Buller, RS, Mohammed S, Robison L, Storch GA: Use of polymerase chain reaction to demonstrate cytomegalovirus DNA in CSF of patients with human immunodeficiency virus infection. *Neurology* 43:75, 1993.

178. Dixon H, Lipscomb F: Cysticercosis: An analysis and follow-up of 450 cases. *Med Res Counc Spec Rep Ser* 299:1, 1961.

179. Pittella J: Neurocysticercosis. *Brain Pathol* 7:681, 1997.

180. Soltero I, Liu K, Cooper R, Stamler J, Garside D: Trends in mortality from cerebrovascular diseases in the United States, 1960 to 1975. *Stroke* 9:549, 1978.

181. Barinagarrementeria F, Cantu C: Frequency of cerebral arteritis in subarachnoid cysticercosis: An angiographic study. *Stroke* 29:123, 1998.

182. Cantu C, Barinagarrementeria F: Cerebrovascular complications of neurocysticercosis. Clinical and neuroimaging spectrum. *Arch Neurol* 53:233, 1996.

183. Luft BJ, Hafner R: Toxoplasmic encephalitis. *AIDS* 4:593, 1990.

184. Laing R, Flegg P, Brettle R, Leen C, Burns S: Clinical features, outcome and survival from cerebral toxoplasmosis in Edinburgh AIDS patients. *Int J STD AIDS* 7:258, 1996.

185. Orefice G, Carrieri PB, Chirianni A, et al: Cerebral toxoplasmosis in subjects with acquired immunodeficiency syndrome [Ita]. *Riv Neurol* 59:89, 1989.

186. Eggers C, Gross U, Klinker H, Schalke B, Stellbrink H, Kunze K: Limited value of cerebrospinal fluid for direct detection of Toxoplasma gondii in toxoplasmic encephalitis associated with AIDS. *J Neurol* 242:644, 1995.

187. Potasman L, Resnik L, Luft B, Remington J: Intrathecal production of antibodies against Toxoplasma gondii in patients with toxoplasma encephalitis and the acquired immunodeficiency syndrome (AIDS). *Ann Intern Med* 108:49, 1988.

188. Rolston K, Hoy J: Role of clindamycin in the treatment of central nervous system toxoplasmosis. *Am J Med* 83:551, 1987.

Chapter 22

MIGRAINE AND STROKE

Panayiotis N. Varelas
Pierre B. Fayad

INTRODUCTION

Migraine and stroke are two conditions with high prevalence in the general population. The first report of an association between them dates as remotely as 167 B.C., but the earliest comprehensive writings are credited to Charcot.[1] More than a century after his observations, the problem of causative relationship between these two conditions remains one of the most perplexing and intriguing problems encountered in neurology. They are separated by a prevalence of stroke in an older age group and of migraine in a younger age group. Nonetheless, migraine and stroke overlap at the distal ends of their peak age prevalence, creating difficulties in extricating or defining them. We review in this chapter the information necessary to a better understanding of the issues connecting migraine and stroke and the features that distinguish them. We discuss separately the characteristics and treatment of the familial syndromes where migraine and stroke coexist or are connected.

DEFINITIONS AND CLASSIFICATION

One of the most difficult aspects in dealing with stroke and migraine is classifying the spectrum of clinical syndromes in categories that are accurate, reliable, and predictive for outcome and treatment. Because there are no objective tests to help distinguish the syndromes, the clinical features provide the only and most important clues. According to the International Headache Society (IHS) classification,[2] for the term *migrainous infarction* to be used, the patient had to previously have fulfilled the criteria for *migraine with aura* (Table 22-1). These

definitions replaced previously used terms such as "classical migraine," "complicated migraine," "hemiplegic," "hemiparesthetic," "ophthalmic," or "aphasic migraine," which have added confusion to the definition of migraine-related stroke. The 1989 IHS classification, however, retained the terms "ophthalmoplegic and retinal migraine" as separate diagnostic categories.

In 1990, Welch and Levine[3] suggested the expansion of the IHS classification, introducing four categories of "migraine-related stroke" (Table 22-2). In the first category, "coexisting stroke and migraine," the stroke symptoms must occur remotely in time from a typical migraine attack. Therefore, two common diseases are occurring in one individual with no causal relationship. In the second category, stroke with clinical features of migraine, a structural lesion (i.e., arteriovenous malformation) causes episodic symptoms typical of migraine attacks with aura, which finally lead to a stroke ("symptomatic migraine"). The same category includes a stroke that is caused by an acute and progressive structural disease or that presents with headache and progressive neurologic signs and symptoms difficult to distinguish from those of migraine ("migraine mimic"). The third category, "migraine-induced stroke," defines the strictest etiologic connection between the two conditions and encompasses the IHS definition of migrainous infarction with the modifier that stroke risk factors might be present, although other causes of stroke should be excluded. The last category, "uncertain," includes all the migraine-related strokes that do not fit well in one of the previous categories. Examples may include (1) migraine without an aura, (2) stroke associated with treatment of a migraine attack, (3) cerebral angiography-induced migraine progressing to stroke, (4) late-onset migraine

Table 22-1.
Criteria for migraine with aura and migrainous infarction[a]

Migraine with aura

At least two attacks having three of the following four characteristics:

One or more fully reversible aura symptoms, which are neurologic deficits indicating cerebral cortical and/or brainstem dysfunction

Gradual development of one aura symptom over more than 4 min, or two or more aura symptoms developing in succession

Each aura symptom lasts for less than 60 min. If there is more than one symptom, the duration may be proportionally increased

The headache may begin before or simultaneously with the aura. If it follows the aura, the free interval in between should be less than 60 min

One of the following:

History, physical, and neurologic examination do not suggest several other disorders having headache as a prominent feature

If they do suggest such a disorder, it is ruled out by appropriate investigations

If such disorder is present, the migraine attacks do not occur for the first time in close temporal relation to the disorder

Migrainous infarction

Previously fulfilled criteria for migraine with aura, as per migraine with aura

The present attack is typical of previous attacks, but the deficit did not reverse within 7 days and was confirmed as an ischemic stroke in a relevant area by neuroimaging studies

Other causes of infarction have been ruled out by appropriate investigation

[a] According to IHS.[2]

Table 22-2.
Classification of migraine-related stroke[a]

Category	Feature
I	Coexisting stroke and migraine
II	Stroke with clinical features of migraine Symptomatic migraine Migraine mimic
III	Migraine-induced stroke Without risk factors With risk factors
IV	Uncertain

[a] According to Welch and Levine.[3]

studied) that migraine history may be positive in up to 10 to 30 percent of stroke patients just by mere coexistence of these two common disorders.[5,6] Because most migraineurs have less than one attack of migraine a month,[7] stroke during an attack of migraine should be rare.[8,9] The incidence of migrainous stroke has been estimated at 3.4/100,000 per year, or 1.44/100,000 per year when other stroke risk factors are excluded.[5] Some studies implicated migraine in up to 25 percent of patients with stroke that are younger than 50 years.[9–12]

Although women have a high proportion of "migrainous stroke,"[9,13] no significant differences distinguish them when compared with migraine sufferers in general (60 to 70 percent).[14] Similarly, no differences are identifiable in patients affected with "migraine stroke" compared with patients with migraine in many variables such as mean patient age, mean age of migraine onset, family history of migraine, or history of hypertension.[9,15] Patients with a history of migraine with aura, however, have more than a twofold increased risk for ischemic stroke.[16,17] Age and gender are also important variables. With advancing age, migraine prevalence decreases, whereas stroke incidence increases.[18] No association between migraine and stroke was found in one study, except in the subgroup of women younger than 45 years, where there is a fourfold risk increase.[19] In another case-controlled study, a history of migraine was an independent risk factor for cerebral ischemia in patients below the age of 45 and in women below the age of 35.[20] The attributable risk of cerebral ischemia to migraine was 6 and 20 percent, respectively. Merikangas et al reported that the risk for stroke associated with migraine (after controlling for stroke risk factors) decreases as the age of stroke events increases.[18] The migraine stroke risk

accompaniments, (5) migraine with intracerebral hemorrhage, and (6) monocular migraine or ophthalmoplegic migraine among others.[4]

EPIDEMIOLOGY

Migraine has such a high prevalence in the general population (4 to 29 percent depending on the population ratio at age 40 years was 2.8, compared with 1.7 at age 60 years.

PATHOGENESIS AND RISK FACTORS

The pathophysiologic mechanisms that underlie migraine-associated stroke are unclear. Structural lesions and/or physiologic changes, in the context of inherited individual differences, form the background on which environmental risk factors could precipitate an infarction in the course of a migrainous attack. Hemodynamic, neuronal, coagulation, and metabolic factors have been postulated to play the greatest roles.

Arterial vasospasm, presumed to be implicated in the pathogenesis of migraine, may also play a causative role in migraine stroke. Normal[9,21,22] and abnormal[21,23] cerebral arteriographic findings in migraineurs have been reported. In a controlled study by Bogousslavsky et al, three equal groups of 22 patients underwent cerebral angiography and echocardiography.[9] Ninety-one percent of patients with migraine with aura who had a stroke during a migrainous attack had no arterial or cardiac anomalies. This is compared with only 9 percent of patients who had a stroke remotely from the migrainous attack and with 18 percent of patients who had a stroke without a history of migraine. These findings suggested that an occlusive or vasospastic cause is unlikely in migraine stroke.

Reduction of regional cerebral blood flow (rCBF) crossing over the boundaries of the major cerebral arterial territories has been reported almost exclusively in patients suffering from migraine with aura or migraine aura without headache ("migraine equivalent"). This hypoperfusion, dubbed "spreading oligemia," progressed anteriorly from the occipital lobes with a rate of 2 to 5 mm/min.[24–28] Woods et al reported a patient who developed migraine with hazy vision during positron-emission tomography (PET).[29] A bilateral decrease in rCBF, presumed to be spreading depression, started at the occipital regions and progressed anteriorly, crossing specific arterial territories. Borderline perfusion at the penumbra zone may lower the threshold for developing spreading cortical depression and lead to a flurry of migraine attacks in middle-aged or elderly patients who had infrequent or no migraine attacks before the stroke.[30] A primary neurogenic mechanism from hypothalamic or brainstem dysfunction, mediated by neuropeptides, has been also implicated in the development of spreading oligemia. This spontaneous depolarization of intrinsic neurons may lead to vasoconstriction and flow reduction.[31,32]

In situ thrombosis of small vessels in the context of ischemia triggered by spreading oligemia may also contribute to migrainous stroke.[14] Disturbance in the clotting cascade or platelet dysfunction has been previously reported in migraineurs.[9,33,34] The relationship between migraine and antiphospholipid antibodies (i.e., anticardiolipin antibodies or lupus anticoagulant), which are associated with an increased risk of thrombosis, has been both supported[35–37] and challenged[38–40] in different studies. Silvestrini et al[41] reported that patients with migrainous infarction and antiphospholipid antibodies had migraine attacks that were particularly frequent, long-lasting, and severe, with a poor response to specific therapy. Olesen et al,[30] suggested that a marked reduction of rCBF superimposed on other factors frequently present during a migraine attack, such as hypovolemia from dehydration, platelet activation, or vasoactive medications, may eventually lead to ischemic damage.

Abnormalities in brain or muscle energy metabolism, in the context of a systemic mitochondrial dysfunction, have been also reported in patients suffering from migraine with aura[42,43] or migraine without aura.[44] Controversy exists whether the transient or permanent neurologic deficits in these migraine patients are due to vasospasm-induced cerebral ischemia, a failure of brain energy metabolism, or both, under stressful conditions.[45]

Several risk factors, either for migraine or for stroke, some of them common to both, have been implicated in the development of migrainous infarction. A prospective study conducted by Rothrock et al did not find any difference in the stroke risk factors between migraineurs who had a stroke and those without a stroke.[15] Nevertheless, an association between ischemic stroke and oral contraceptive use or smoking in young women with migraine has been suggested.[20,46,47] Mitral valve prolapse (MVP) that is associated with migraine[48,49] may be a source for microembolic stroke in young adults.[50–52] Bogousslavsky et al, however, did not find such an association.[9] Migraine may be a risk factor for arterial dissection,[53] thus predisposing patients to cerebral infarction, although no such association was found in well-controlled studies.[9,15] In multivariate analysis of 140 patients with stroke and patent foramen ovale, Bogousslavsky et al found that a history of recently active migraine was an independent risk factor for recurrent stroke.[54]

CLINICAL FEATURES

We discuss in this section the clinical characteristics associated with migrainous stroke that could help in the differential diagnosis. In a review of the literature between 1950 and 1983, 73 percent of patients with available data reported an increased frequency or intensity of migraine attacks that accompanied the stroke.[55] In a controlled study, the mean number of migraine attacks preceding the stroke was similar to that in patients with migraine who did not develop a stroke.[9] However, the mean duration of the attacks preceding the stroke was longer (6 h in the migraine stroke group vs. 4 h in the migraine without stroke group). A history of previous stroke is more likely in patients with acute migrainous stroke (even after exclusion of patients with no history of migraine prior to stroke) compared with patients with migraine only.[15]

The progression of the neurologic deficits in migrainous stroke is often slower than in patients with stroke that is unrelated to a migraine attack. Usually, this gradual build-up of symptoms develops over 1 to 2 h.[9,47] Visual disturbances are by far the most frequent neurologic manifestations of the aura. Stars, expanding geometric patterns, fortification spectra, scotomata, hemianopsia, or even more complex visual disturbances such as micropsia or dysmetropsia, are the most common visual aura symptoms. Next in frequency are dysesthesias, often in the lower face or hand (cheiro-oral distribution), and less frequent are motor symptoms, such as hemiparesis or clumsiness, and aphasia or slurred speech. The onset of the nonvisual symptoms often follows the visual symptoms.[9,31]

The headache associated with migraine stroke was throbbing[47] and contralateral to the side of the neurologic deficits in 65 percent of the cases reviewed by Featherstone.[55] The most commonly involved arterial territory in patients with migraine stroke seems to be that of the posterior cerebral artery.[9,47,56] The posterior cerebral artery territory is more frequently involved in these patients compared with nonmigraineurs with stroke (41 vs. 14 percent), and the global middle cerebral artery territory is less frequently involved (5 percent vs. 18 percent, respectively).[9]

HEREDITARY DISEASES WITH FEATURES OF MIGRAINE AND STROKE

The identification of a familial pattern in a patient with migraine and stroke narrows the diagnostic possibilities.

We review some of the unique familial entities that combine migraine and stroke as prominent features.

Familial Hemiplegic Migraine (FHM)

Background Familial hemiplegic migraine is an autosomal dominant disorder with incomplete penetrance. Linkage to the short arm of chromosome 19p has been reported in some families but not in others, indicating nonallelic genetic heterogeneity.[57] The onset is generally before the age of 30 and most commonly in childhood (mean age, 10 years). The attacks may be precipitated by minor head trauma or cerebral angiography, and the symptoms resolve without residual deficits. The hemiplegia may precede or follow the headache and may last for hours or days. Patients do not develop strokes, however, and based on neuroimaging studies the most likely explanations are cerebral ischemia due to vasospasm[58] or transient cerebral edema.[59] Within a family, some members may have hemiplegic attacks, whereas others have migraine with nonhemiplegic aura or even without aura.[60,61]

In some families with FHM, ataxia may be an additional feature. Ataxia that recurs in paroxysms lasting from 15 min to several days and may improve with acetazolamide has also been described (acetazolamide-responsive hereditary paroxysmal cerebellar ataxia, HPCA). Some of these patients develop nonhemiplegic migraine attacks after the onset of the ataxia.[62] Seven mutations in a calcium channel α1-subunit gene on chromosome 19p have been reported in chromosome 19-linked FHM families.[63] The possibility that FHM, HPCA, and other types of migraine with or without aura are ion channel disorders raises the potential for new therapeutic options.

Evidence The value of treatment during an attack of hemiplegic migraine, aiming at reversing the hemiplegia, is debatable.[64] Flunarizine, a calcium channel blocker, has been shown to reverse symptoms in a case of hemiplegic migraine.[65] Two other patients were successfully treated with acetazolamide.[66]

Recommendations for Treatment Neuroimaging studies (see below) and family history are essential to establish the diagnosis. No specific treatment is proven effective, but the general guidelines for migraine treatment are recommended.[67] Acetazolamide and flunarizine (outside the United States) should be tried prophylactically.

Cerebral Autosomal Dominant Arteriopathy with Subcortical Infarcts and Leukoencephalopathy (CADASIL)

Background CADASIL is characterized by transient ischemic attacks (TIA) and subcortical ischemic strokes. Migraine, with or without aura, that usually starts during adolescence is a prominent feature in 13 to 80 percent of CADASIL families (CADASILM).[68] Sixty percent of the patients have migraine with typical aura, 20 percent have basilar migraine, and 20 percent have hemiplegic migraine or migraine with prolonged aura. Stroke or TIA may present early but will have a peak incidence in adult life, affecting 50 to 84 percent of patients. Two-thirds of these events have features of subcortical small vessel strokes. Psychiatric disorders, particularly monopolar or bipolar psychosis, occur in 35 percent of patients. Subcortical dementia occurs in 12 to 35 percent, especially later in life. Cranial magnetic resonance imaging (MRI) shows initially well-delineated lesions in the white matter that later coalesce or involve the basal ganglia. After the age of 60 years, diffuse leukoencephalopathy is prominent.[69] By electron microscopy, the pathology responsible for this disease is a granular osmiophilic material (GOM) deposition in vascular smooth muscle cells of cerebral or extracerebral vessels in families with CADASIL. These findings can be demonstrated from skin biopsies of symptomatic patients, asymptomatic patients with abnormal MRI, or patients with migraine and normal MRI, making the pathologic diagnosis more accessible.[70] CADASIL was mapped to chromosome 19q13.1, and mutations in the human Notch 3 gene have been identified as its cause.[68,71]

Evidence No specific treatment is available. One patient with CADASIL showed marked reduction of the frequency of the migraine attacks after treatment with acetazolamide.[72]

Recommendations for Treatment MRI of the head is useful to screen asymptomatic members of CADASIL families. Even if MRI is negative, skin or muscle biopsy is recommended to establish the diagnosis in patients younger than 35 years.[73] Genetic analysis seems a very promising diagnostic tool.[74] Symptomatic treatment of the stroke-like episodes with rehabilitation, stroke risk factor modification, and stroke prophylaxis is recommended. Acetazolamide may be tried as a prophylactic treatment for migraine attacks.

Mitochondrial Myopathy, Encephalopathy, Lactic Acidosis, and Stroke-like Episodes (MELAS)

Background MELAS has a usual onset before age 40 and is characterized by exercise intolerance, seizures, lactic acidosis, stroke-like symptoms, and ragged-red muscle fibers.[75] Virtually all patients suffer from severe migraine attacks that are prolonged, occur in clusters, and are accompanied by severe nausea and vomiting.[76] Many members in MELAS families have a history of migraine with or without aura. These attacks usually precede the strokes. Signs, such as ophthalmoplegia, ptosis, or neuropathy, common in other mitochondrial encephalomyopathies, are not frequently encountered in these patients.[77,78] On MRI, the lesions are mainly cortical, with adjacent subcortical white matter involvement, enhance with contrast, do not conform to arterial territories, and have a migratory evolution (tend to disappear and reappear in another area) with predilection for the posterior parts of the hemispheres.[78] Cerebral angiography is usually normal, consistent with nonocclusive, nonvascular pathogenesis of the stroke-like episodes.[77]

Increased number of abnormal mitochondria in the cytoplasm of smooth muscle cells found in small pial arteries hypertrophy of endothelial cells with increased number of mitochondria and narrowing of the capillary lumen[79] support a "mitochondrial angiopathy."[80] A point mutation was first reported in the tRNA$^{Leu(UUR)}$ gene of mtDNA at nucleotide pair (np) 3243. This leads to an A-to-G substitution and is present in 80 percent of MELAS patients. A second point mutation was found in 8 percent of MELAS patients at np 3271 of the tRNA$^{Leu(UUR)}$ gene. No phenotypic or clinical difference was found between patients with either mutation. A third point mutation was discovered in a Japanese patient at np 3291 of the tRNA$^{Leu(UUR)}$ gene, indicating the genetic heterogeneity of the syndrome.[80]

Evidence Coenzyme Q10, which moves electrons in the respiratory chain from complexes I and II to complex III, improves muscle weakness in patients with MELAS. The addition of idebenone to coenzyme Q improved further the CNS symptoms in one MELAS patient.[81] Some authors also proposed high doses of multivitamins, particularly nicotinamide, riboflavin, and vitamin C, that may be helpful by donating electrons directly to complex IV, enhancing mitochondrial energy production and scavenging free radicals.[82,83]

Four patients with MELAS had less fatigability, motor disability, and frequency of stroke-like episodes and headaches after they were started on a combination of cytochrome *c,* flavin mononucleotide, and thiamine diphosphate.[84] Three other patients showed improvement of cognitive functions and decreased levels of lactate and pyruvate in the serum and CSF on dichloroacetate regimen.[85] Nicotinamide treatment after the first stroke-like episode in another patient lead to clinical improvement and a decrease in the lesion volume on MRI within the first month.[86] Steroids and carnitine-supplement therapy improved the symptoms in one patient with MELAS and chronic progressive external ophthalmoplegia, found to have carnitine deficiency.[87]

Recommendations for Treatment   MRI is useful in the delineation of the lesions and the follow-up of the migratory patterns, although the final diagnosis is made by genetic analysis. A combination of coenzyme Q, idebenone, and vitamins B_1, B_2, C, E, K_3, and nicotinamide in high doses may improve the clinical picture. Dichloroacetate may also be used, and the effect can be monitored by magnetic resonance spectroscopy.[88]

Hereditary Hemorrhagic Telangiectasia (HHT)

Background   Hereditary hemorrhagic telangiectasia is an autosomal dominant disorder with systemic angiomatosis affecting several organs. The diagnosis requires the presence of two elements of the triad; (1) telangiectasias (mainly in the orofacial area and fingertips), (2) family history of HHT, and (3) recurrent bleeding episodes (mainly epistaxis and enteric bleed). Telangiectasias are the hallmark and are present on the oral mucosa, skin, lungs, or gastrointestinal tract, leading to recurrent bleeding or blood shunting. Paradoxic embolism, through pulmonary arteriovenous malformations (AVMs) present in 15 to 40 percent of patients with HHT, leads to cerebral ischemic events or brain abscess. Hemorrhagic stroke may result from a rupture of the intracranial vascular malformations.[89] Migraine may be present in up to 50 percent of patients. The majority has migraine with aura, in contrast to the higher prevalence of migraine without aura in non-HHT migraineurs.[90] Unusual neurologic symptoms mimicking stroke and migraine are also quite common. Linkage analyses have indicated at least three different HHT loci. Several mutations have been identified in the endoglin gene on chromosome 9q33-q34 in families with higher incidence of pulmonary AVMs and in the gene for activin receptor-like kinase (ALK1) on chromosome 12.[91]

Evidence   There is no evidence that migraine attacks in patients with HHT should be treated differently than attacks in migraineurs. Long-term use of nonsteroidal anti-inflammatory agents, however, should be used cautiously in patients with HHT, as they can worsen their bleeding tendency.[89]

Recommendations for Treatment   A detailed examination of the tongue, lips, and fingertips in every patient with migraine who has a positive family history of migraine or epistaxis along with the history of epistaxis can yield the diagnosis. Chest radiography in combination with arterial gases on room air and 100% oxygen inhalation or spiral chest CT are sensitive tests for the detection of pulmonary AVMs. Balloon obliteration of pulmonary AVMs decreases the risk of stroke and brain abscess and may improve migraine by improving oxygenation and decreasing hypercarbia.[89] MRI of the head with and without contrast and MRA are a good screen in patients and family members, but cerebral angiography may be necessary in some to exclude intracranial vascular malformations that can be very small at times. Genetic analysis should always be considered. Migraine treatment in these patients is otherwise similar to the treatment of other migraineurs except for the avoidance of long-term nonsteroidal anti-inflammatory agents.

DIFFERENTIAL DIAGNOSIS

If no familial history is available for migraine and stroke, a search for other causes of stroke, through clinical features and diagnostic tests, should be undertaken to classify the type of migraine stroke for prognostic and treatment implications.

Clinical Features

The diagnosis of migrainous infarction may not be difficult when one adheres to the criteria proposed by the IHS[2] or the expanded criteria of Welch and Levine.[3] Controversy exists as to whether a distinction should be made between migraine-induced stroke and migraine-related stroke. Migraine-induced stroke usually implies causality, is rare, and is a diagnosis of exclusion when no other mechanism can be found. Migraine-related stroke, on the other hand, implies coexistence and the presence of comorbid factors.[12,92] A third possibility may represent nonmigrainous ischemic cerebrovascular disease, causing single or recurrent migraine attacks.[27,30,56]

When faced with a patient presenting with both migraine and stroke, one has to ask a number of important questions that potentially can lead to the correct diagnosis. A suggested algorithm in Fig. 22-1 covers the major steps in the diagnostic differential.

A detailed history is always the most important first step upon which all other clues are built. The temporal relation between the migrainous attack and the development of the neurologic deficit is very important. One hour or less is the free interval needed between the onset of the neurologic deficit (that usually antedates) and the headache (that usually follows) in a migrainous infarction.[2] The characteristics of both the aura and the headache are also helpful. The differentiation of migraine aura (which may occur without headache, termed acephalgic migraine, migraine sine hemicrania, or migraine equivalent) from ischemic cerebrovascular disease relies heavily on the slow march of aural symptoms vs. the sudden maximal deficit during an embolic or (most of the times) ischemic cerebrovascular event. The duration of the symptoms is less reliable. Although typical migraine aura symptoms last for less than 60 min, they may be occasionally prolonged. In that latter case, if the neuroimaging studies are normal, a diagnosis of migraine with prolonged aura is entertained.[2] The combination of a neurologic deficit with the onset of headache and vomiting is not distinctive, as these are well known symptoms of hemorrhagic stroke.[93] In ischemic stroke, the headache may also be associated with nausea, vomiting, or both.[94] Although the characteristics of the headache in ischemic stroke can be quite variable,[95] continuous or non-throbbing headache is reported in 92 to 96 percent of patients with ischemic stroke.[96] The headache in migraine stroke, however, is throbbing.[47]

The age of the patient may be helpful, as the prevalence of common types of headache declines with aging and that of stroke increases.[97] If the patient is older than 60, other causes of stroke beyond migraine have to be ruled out first (Table 22-3).

Familial aggregation of cases of migraine, stroke, and especially atypical clinical features and absence of other risk factors may lead the differential to the group of familial disorders that includes FHM, CADASIL, MELAS, and HHT discussed earlier. Even if these conditions are excluded, other disorders listed in Table 22-3 need to be addressed before a diagnosis of migrainous infarction is made.

The clinical and radiologic localization of the stroke seems to be helpful in deciding if migraine is the most likely cause. The mere existence of headache related to the neurologic deficits may or may not add to the localization. Headache is less common with small vessels than with large artery strokes. It is twice as frequent with vertebrobasilar than with carotid artery distribution ischemic events. Moreover, in acute stroke, headache may often be a reactivation of the usual type of headache that the patient was experiencing before.[98,99] The posterior cerebral artery territory is more frequently involved in patients with migraine stroke, who develop homonymous hemianopia at the beginning of their stroke. On the other hand, the anterior circulation territory is more frequently involved in younger patients with stroke.[9,11,47,100] Migraine stroke is uncommon in the territory of the anterior cerebral artery; therefore, other disorders (refer to Table 22-3) have to be excluded first.[101] The same is true if the stroke can be localized in the middle cerebral artery or the vertebrobasilar circulation territory but still does not conform to the IHS criteria. Additionally, lacunar strokes are rarely migraine-related. It is obvious that the diagnosis of migrainous infarction may be quite arduous and one of exclusion.

Diagnostic Evaluation

After a careful historical and physical evaluation, neuroimaging forms the next step toward diagnosis of migrainous infarction and is required by the IHS classification for confirmation of ischemic infarction and exclusion of other causes of stroke (Table 22-3). Stroke attributed to migraine does not have a different imaging appearance than ischemic stroke from other causes. Head CT is useful to exclude parenchymal or subarachnoid hemorrhage. MRI is the neuroimaging study of choice because it is more sensitive to ischemia, particularly with diffusion techniques. When migraine with aura is present, and particularly when atypical features (onset in mid-adulthood, basilar or prolonged aura, with hemiplegia, depression, or dementia) and a strong family history of stroke are present, MRI should be considered first. MR angiography is a noninvasive test helpful to evaluate for cerebral aneurysm, AVM, or arterial dissection. When these pathologies are strongly suspected, despite a negative MRI/MRA, cerebral angiography should be performed. Cerebral angiography may show an arterial occlusion in patients with migraine stroke, but it can itself precipitate vasospasm in patients with migraine.[100] Noninvasive cardiac and carotid artery

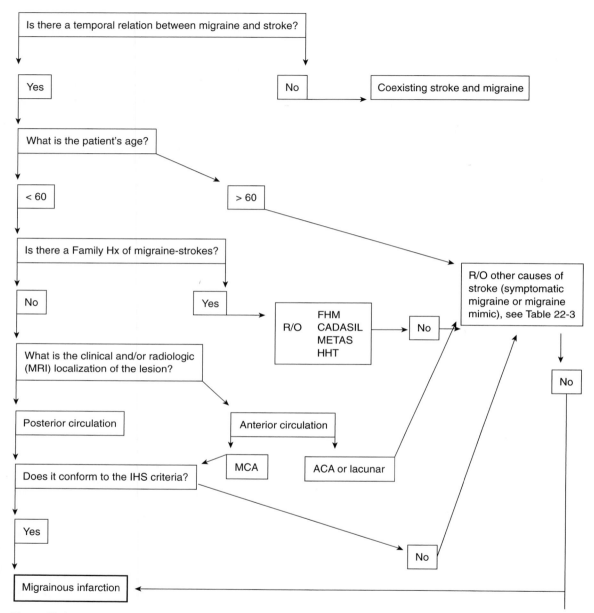

Figure 22-1.
Suggested algorithm for migraine-stroke evaluation and diagnosis.

Table 22-3.
Disorders presenting as stroke and headache

Angiopathies

   Infectious: syphilis, borreliosis, tuberculosis, malaria, *Chlamydia pneumoniae*, herpes zoster, mycoses

Inflammatory: collagen disorders, granulomatous angiitis of nervous system, sarcoidosis

   Noninflammatory: dissection, moyamoya, fibromuscular dysplasia, venous thrombosis, subarachnoid hemorrhage, vascular malformation

Hematologic diseases

   Protein C, S, antithrombin III deficiency, factor V Leiden, paraneoplastic coagulopathy, disseminated intravascular coagulation, thrombotic thrombocytopenic purpura, sickle cell disease, antiphospholipid antibodies

Cardiac or pulmonary disorders

   Infective or marantic endocarditis, atrial myxoma, fibroelastoma, mitral valve prolapse, prosthetic valve, patent foramen ovale, atrial septal aneurysm, atrial fibrillation, acute myocardial infarct, dilated cardiomyopathy, hereditary hemorrhagic telengiectasia

Metabolic or channel dysfunction

   Familial hemiplegic migraine, acetazolamide-responsive hereditary paroxysmal cerebellar ataxia, CADASIL MELAS, alternating hemiplegia of childhood

studies should also be performed to exclude sources of embolism.

Other serologic or diagnostic tests can be helpful. Routine blood tests, serum lactate (before and after exercise), and hypercoagulability screen (especially with a history of thrombotic events, collagen disorder, or spontaneous abortions) seem appropriate. Cerebrospinal fluid examination is usually normal but sometimes reveals pleocytosis or elevated protein[55] and helps exclude subarachnoid bleeding or infection when clinical suspicion exists. Skin biopsy may be positive in families with CADASIL.[70] DNA analysis for FHM, CADASIL, MELAS, or HHT mutations should be considered in cases with a family history of migraine and strokes for diagnostic purposes and genetic counseling.

PROGNOSIS

Although the number of patients with migraine stroke reported so far is small and the natural course of the disease unknown, the short-term outcome seems similar to that of stroke without migraine. The presence of a stroke attributable to migraine was a relatively poor prognostic factor for the recurrence of stroke in one study. Nine out of 30 patients with migrainous stroke (30 percent) had a history of previous stroke compared with 4 out of 310 patients with migraine (1.3 percent). Within a year of follow-up, five patients in the migrainous stroke group had six new strokes (18 percent) compared with none in the migraine group.[15] Not all studies have corroborated this bad prognosis, however. Mild or no neurologic deficit and minimal disability (Rankin grade 2) have been reported,[11,47] and the prognosis seemed not to differ after a stroke according to the presence or absence of migraine.[9,17]

EVIDENCE

The treatment of migraine stroke is mainly based on empiric or anecdotal reports as its low incidence, combined with a lack of good systematic use of a classification scheme, did not allow a thorough assessment of therapies with prospective treatment trials.

Medications that are commonly used in acute migraine attacks or acute stroke may not be suitable in the setting of migrainous infarction. Some reports associated ergotamine to transient monocular blindness or other focal neurologic deficits.[102,103] On the other hand, the use of calcium channel blockers, such as flunarizine,[65] or IV naloxone has been advocated[104] No data exist about r-tPA use in case of migrainous infarction.

The long-term plan may be also different, as preventive treatment is aimed at both migraine and stroke. Nonselective beta-1 blockers (which increase platelet aggregation), like propranolol, have been implicated in migrainous stroke in one case.[105] In another patient with migraine-associated ischemic stroke causing amnesia, treatment with propranolol was thought to be contributory.[106] Some authors suggest that calcium channel blockers are a better choice than propranolol.[64] Preventive treatment with aspirin may reduce both stroke risk and frequency of the migraine attacks.[91] Aspirin treatment assignment in the U.S. Physician's health study, however, did not modify the association found between migraine and stroke, although the numbers were too small to reach solid conclusions.[17]

Modification of possible stroke risk factors other than migraine may be another field of intervention. Migraine with aura does not increase the risk for ischemic stroke when hypertension, diabetes, or smoking is present.[16] Gender, smoking, hypertension, estrogen use, mitral valve prolapse, or family history of migraine frequency is not different in patients with migrainous infarction compared with migraineurs.[15] Other studies found heavy smoking or use of oral contraceptives to increase the risk of ischemic stroke in young women.[46,47] Discontinuing or restarting the use of ovarian hormones in patients with stroke is very controversial, and no data exist in migrainous infarction. Low-dose estrogen may carry a small risk for stroke but seems to carry many overall benefits for osteoporosis and cardiovascular prevention.[108] In postmenopausal women, hormone replacement either has no significant effect on the risk for stroke[109,110] or decreases the risk of stroke incidence and mortality in selected populations.[111] An ongoing randomized, double-blind study is trying to assess the benefit of estrogen supplementation in secondary stroke prevention in postmenopausal women after TIA or minor stroke.[112]

TREATMENT

The treatment of migraine stroke should address both migraine and stroke management perspectives.

The options for acute treatment of migraine stroke are limited. It may be wise to avoid abortive migraine medications with vasoconstrictive properties, like ergotamine or tryptan preparations, because there is no evidence for benefit in resolving a migraine stroke, whereas their role in worsening ischemia through their vasocontrictive properties is controversial. Tryptans are ineffective at aborting visual migraine aura and therefore unlikely to help resolve deficits from acute migraine stroke. Intravenous thrombolytic therapy with r-tPA is indicated for acute ischemic stroke within 3 h but should probably be avoided when a strong clinical suspicion of migraine stroke exists, as its benefit is unproven in this specific situation. Nonetheless, the accurate diagnosis of migraine stroke acutely would be almost impossible unless previous similar diagnostic episodes have been well documented. Calcium channel blockers, such as flunarizine or IV naloxone, seem to be a better choice. The intravascular volume should be replenished from the dehydration related to nausea and vomiting. The acute use of estrogen can be entertained in patients with known recurrent neurologic deficits associated with migraine and documented changes in serum estrogen levels when no other causes can be found.

For secondary prevention of migraine stroke, modification of all possible stroke risk factors in addition to medications would be helpful.[113] Cigarette smoking should be stopped in smokers.[46] Discontinuing birth control pills after a migraine stroke should not be automatic. Its risks for provoking a recurrence should be balanced with the risk of pregnancy or the availability and effectiveness of other birth control methods.

For long-term prophylaxis, patients with migraine only should not be treated for potential future stroke. Platelet inhibitors or anticoagulants can be used for stroke prevention in patients with transient or permanent neurologic deficits during the migraine attack, especially if intrinsic stroke risk factors, such as anticardiolipin antibodies or mitral valve prolapse are discovered.[31,50] If migrainous infarction has occurred or migraine attacks with aura are very frequent, particularly with hemiplegia, aphasia, or brainstem symptoms, preventive treatment with aspirin may reduce both the stroke risk and the frequency of the migraine attacks.[107] More selective beta-1 blockers (which do not increase platelet aggregation), calcium channel blockers (verapamil or flunarizine), or valproic acid may be preferable to beta-2 blockers.

REFERENCES

1. Ramadan NM. Migrainous infarction: The Charcot-Fere syndrome? *Cephalalgia* 13:249, 1993.
2. International Headache Society: Classification and diagnostic criteria for headache disorders, cranial neuralgias, and facial pain. *Cephalalgia* 8 (Suppl 7):10, 1988.
3. Welch KMA, Levine SR: Migraine-related stroke in the context of the International Headache Society classification of head pain. *Arch Neurol* 47:458, 1990.
4. Welch KMA: Relationship of stroke and migraine. *Neurology* 44 (Suppl 7):S33, 1994.
5. Henrich JB, Sandercock PAG, Warlow CP, et al: Stroke and migraine in the Oxfordshire Community Stroke Project. *J Neurol* 233:257, 1986.
6. Olesen J, Friberg L, Olsen TS, et al: Ischaemia-induced (symptomatic) migraine attacks may be more frequent than migraine-induced ischaemic insults. *Brain* 116:187, 1993.
7. Rasmussen BK, Jensen R, Olesen J: A population-based analysis of the diagnostic criteria of the International Headache Society. *Cephalalgia* 11:129, 1991.
8. Linet MS, Stewart WF: Migraine headache: Epidemiological perspectives. *Epidemiol Rev* 6:107, 1984.
9. Bogousslavsky J, Regli F, VanMelle G, et al: Migraine stroke. *Neurology* 38:223, 1998.
10. Alvarez J, Matias-Guiu J, Sumalla, et al: Ischemic stroke in young adults: I. Analysis of etiologic subgroups. *Acta Neurol Scand* 80:29, 1989.
11. Broderick JP, Swanson JW: Migraine-related strokes. *Arch Neurol* 44:868, 1987.

12. Fernandez-Beer E, Biller J: Cerebral infarction and migraine, in Biller J (ed): *Stroke in Children and Young Adults.* Newton, MA, Butterworth-Heinemann, 1994, pp 103–111.

13. Logan WR, Tegeler CH, Keniston WD, Hart RG: Migraine and stroke in young adults. *Neurology* 34 (Suppl 1):206, 1984.

14. Tatemichi TK, Mohr JP: Migraine and stroke, in Barnett HJM, Stein BM, Mohr JP, Yatsu FM (eds): *Stroke: Pathophysiology, Diagnosis and Management,* vol 2. New York, Churchill-Livingstone, 1992, pp 761–785.

15. Rothrock J, North J, Madden K, et al: Migraine and migrainous stroke: Risk factors and prognosis. *Neurology* 43:2473, 1993.

16. Henrich JB, Horowitz RI: A controlled study of ischemic stroke risk in migraine patients. *J Clin Epidemiol* 42:773, 1989.

17. Buring JE, Hebert P, Romero J, et al: Migraine and subsequent risk of stroke in the physicians' health study. *Arch Neurol* 52:129, 1995.

18. Merikangas KR, Fenton, BT, Cheng SH, et al: Association between migraine and stroke in a large-scale epidemiological study of United States. *Arch Neurol* 54:362, 1997.

19. Tzourio C, Iglesias S, Hubert J-B, et al: Migraine and risk of ischemic stroke: A case-controlled study. *Br Med J* 307:289, 1993.

20. Carolei A, Marini C, De Matteis G, the Italian National Research Council Study Group on Stroke in the Young: History of migraine and risk of cerebral ischemia in young adults. *Lancet* 347:1503, 1996.

21. Dorfman LJ, Marshall WH, Enzmann DR: Cerebral infarction and migraine: Clinical and radiologic correlations. *Neurology* 29:317, 1979.

22. Pereira Monteiro JM, Leite Carneiro A, Bastos Lima AT, et al: Migraine and cerebral infarction: Three case studies. *Headache* 25:429, 1985.

23. Rascol A, Cambier J, Guiraud B, et al: Accidents ischemiques cerebraux au cours de crises migraineuses: A propos des migraines compliquees. *Rev Neurol (Paris)* 135:867, 1979.

24. Olesen J, Larsen B, Lauritzen M: Focal hyperemia followed by spreading oligemia and impaired activation of rCBF in classic migraine. *Ann Neurol* 9:344, 1981.

25. Lauritzen M, Olesen J: Regional cerebral blood flow during migraine attacks by Xenon-133 inhalation and emission tomography. *Brain* 107:447, 1984.

26. Anderson AR, Friberg L, Olsen TS, et al: Delayed hyperemia following hypoperfusion in classic migraine: Single photon emission computed tomographic demonstration. *Arch Neurol* 45:154, 1988.

27. Olesen J: Cerebral and extracranial circulatory disturbances in migraine: Pathophysiologic implications. *Cerebrovasc Brain Metab Rev.* 3:1, 1991.

28. Frieberg L, Olesen J, Iversen HK, et al: Migraine pain associated with middle cerebral artery dilatation: Reversal by sumatriptan. *Lancet* 338:13, 1991.

29. Woods RP, Iacoboni M, Mazziota JC: Bilateral spreading cerebral hypoperfusion during spontaneous migraine headache. *N Engl J Med* 331:1689, 1994.

30. Olesen J, Friberg L, Olsen TS, et al: Ischaemia-induced (symptomatic) migraine attacks may be more frequent than migraine-induced ischaemic insults. *Brain* 116:187, 1993.

31. Welch KMA: Migraine and stroke, in Olesen J, Tfelt-Hansen P, Welch KMA (eds): *The Headaches,* New York, Raven Press, 1993, pp 427–436.

32. Nicholson C: Volume transmission and the propagation of spreading depression, in Lehmenkuhler A, Grotemeyer K, Tegtmeier F (eds): *Migraine: Basic Mechanisms and Treatment.* Munich, Urban and Schwarzenberg, 1993, pp 293–308.

33. Kalendovsky Z, Austin JH: Changes in blood clotting systems during migraine attacks. *Headache* 16:293, 1977.

34. Riddle JM, D'Andrea G, Welch KMA, et al: Platelet activation and analysis of organelles in migraineurs. *Headache* 29:28, 1989.

35. Briley DP, Coull BM, Goodnight SH: Neurological disease associated with antiphospholipid antibodies. *Ann Neurol* 25:221, 1989.

36. Shuaib A, Barklay L, Lee MA: Migraine and antiphospholipid antibodies. *Headache* 29:42, 1989.

37. Levine SR, Deegan MJ, Futrell N, et al: Cerebrovascular and neurologic disease associated with antiphospholipid antibodies: 48 cases. *Neurology* 40:1181, 1990.

38. Hering R, Couturier EGM, Steiner TJ, et al: Antiphospholipid antibodies in migraine patients. *Cephalalgia* 11:19, 1991.

39. Markus HS, Hopkinson N: Migraine and headache in systemic lupus erythematosus and their relationship with antibodies against phospholipids. *J Neurol* 239:39, 1992.

40. Tietjen GE, Day M, Norris RN, et al: Role of anticardiolipin antibodies in young persons with migraine and transient neurologic events: A prospective study. *Neurology* 50:1433, 1998.

41. Silvestrini M, Matteis M, Troisi E, et al: Migrainous stroke and the antiphospholipid antibodies. *Eur Neurol* 34:316, 1994.

42. Barbiroli B, Montagna P, Cortelli P, et al: Abnormal brain and muscle energy metabolism shown by 31P magnetic resonance spectroscopy in patients affected by migraine with aura. *Neurology* 42:1209, 1992.

43. Sacquegna T, Lodi R, De Carolis P, et al: Brain energy metabolism studied by 31P-MR spectroscopy in a case with migraine with prolonged aura. *Acta Neurol Scand* 86:376, 1992.

44. Montagna P, Cortelli P, Monari L, et al: 31P magnetic resonance spectroscopy in migraine without aura. *Neurology* 44:666, 1994.

45. Montagna P, Cortelli P, Barbiroli B: Magnetic resonance spectroscopy studies in migraine. *Cephalalgia* 14:184, 1994.

46. Tzourio C, Tehindrazanarivelo A, Iglesias S, et al: Case-

control study of migraine and risk of ischemic stroke in young women. *Br Med J* 310:830, 1995.

47. Hoekstra-van-Dalen RAH, Cillessen JPM, Kappelle LJ, et al: Cerebral infarcts associated with migraine: Clinical features, risk factors and follow-up. *J Neurol* 243:511, 1996.

48. Litman GI, Freidman HM: Migraine and the mitral valve prolapse syndrome. *Am Heart J* 96:610, 1978.

49. Spence JD, Wong DG, Melendez LJ, et al: Increased prevalence of MVP in patients with migraine. *Can Med Assoc J* 131:1457, 1984.

50. Centonze V, Amat G, Loisy C, et al: Considerations sur les accidents vasculaires cerebraux chez les migraineux. *Sem Hop Paris* 56:1908, 1980.

51. Conomy JP, Hanson MR, McFarling D: Does migraine increase the risk of cerebral ischemic events in persons with mitral valve prolapse? *Ann Neurol* 12:83, 1982.

52. Amat G, Jean Louis P, Lorsy C et al: Migraine and the mitral valve prolapse syndrome. *Ady Neurol* 33:27, 1983.

53. D'Anglejan-Chatillon J, Ribeiro V, Youl BD, et al: Migraine-a risk factor for dissection of cervical arteries. *Headache* 29:560, 1989.

54. Bogousslavsky J, Garazi S, Jeanrenaud X, et al: Stroke recurrence in patients with patent foramen ovale: The Lausanne Study. *Neurology* 46:1301, 1996.

55. Featherstone HJ: Clinical features of stroke in migraine: A review. *Headache* 26:128, 1986.

56. Broderick JP, Swanson JW: Migraine-related strokes. *Arch Neurol* 44:868, 1987.

57. Terwindt GM, Ophoff RA, Haan J, et al: Familial hemiplegic migraine: A clinical comparison of families linked and unlinked to chromosome 19. *Cephalalgia* 16:153, 1996.

58. Pierelli F, Pauri F, Cupini LM, et al: Transcranial Doppler sonography in familial hemiplegic migraine. *Cephalalgia* 11:29, 1991.

59. Goldstein JM, Shaywitz BA, Sze G, et al: Migraine associated with focal cerebral edema, cerebrospinal fluid pleocytosis and progressive cerebellar ataxia: MRI documentation. *Ann Neurol* 40:1284, 1990.

60. Whitty CWM: Familial hemiplegic migraine, in Vinken PJ, Bruyn GW, Klawans HL, Clifford Rose F (eds): *Headache, Handbook of Clinical Neurology,* vol 4. Amsterdam, Elsevier, 1986, pp 141–153.

61. Haan J, Terwindt GM, Ferrari MD: Genetics of migraine. *Neurol Clin* 15:43, 1997.

62. Ophoff RA, Van Eijk R, Sandkuijl LA, et al: Genetic heterogeneity of familial hemiplegic migraine. *Genomics* 22:21, 1994.

63. Ophoff RA, Terwindt GM, Vergouwe MM, et al: Familial hemiplegic migraine and episodic ataxia type 2 are caused by mutations in the P-Q-type calcium channel a1—subunit gene (CACNL1A4) on chromosome 19P13. *Cell* 87:543, 1996.

64. Campbell JK, Zagami A: Hemiplegic migraine, in Olesen J, Tfelt-Hansen P, Welch KMA (eds): *The Headaches.* New York, Raven Press, 1993, pp 409–411.

65. Tobita M, Masatoshi H, Ichikawa N, et al: A case of hemiplegic migraine treated with flunarizine. *Headache* 27:487, 1987.

66. Athwal BS, Lennox GG: Acetazolamide responsiveness in Familial Hemiplegic Migraine. *Ann Neurol* 40:820, 1996.

67. Rajput V, Kramer ED: Adult onset familial hemiplegic migraine. *Headache* 35:423, 1995.

68. Verin M, Rolland Y, Landgraf F, et al: New phenotype of the cerebral autosomal dominant arteriopathy mapped to chromosome 19: Migraine as a prominent clinical feature. *J Neurol Neurosurg Psychiatry* 59:579, 1995.

69. Chabriat H, Vahedi K, Iba-Zizen MT, et al: Clinical spectrum of CADASIL: A study of 7 families. *Lancet* 346:934, 1995.

70. Ebke M, Dichgans M, Bergmann M, et al: CADASIL: Skin biopsy allows diagnosis in early stages. *Acta Neurol Scand* 95:351, 1997.

71. Joutel A, Corpechot C, Ducros A, et al: Notch3 mutations in cerebral autosomal dominant arteriopathy with subcortical infarcts and leukoencephalopathy (CADASIL), a Mendelian condition causing stroke and vascular dementia. *Ann NY Acad Sci* 826:213, 1997.

72. Weller M, Dichgans J, Klockgether T: Acetazolamide-responsive migraine in CADASIL. *Neurology* 50:1505, 1998.

73. Goebel HH, Meyermann R, Rosin R, et al: Characteristic morphologic manifestation of CADASIL, cerebral autosomal dominant arteriopathy with subcortical infarcts and leukoencephalopathy, in skeletal muscle and skin. *Muscle Nerve* 20:625, 1997.

74. Goate AM, Morris JC: Notch 3 mutations and the potential for diagnostic testing for CADASIL. *Lancet* 350:1490, 1997.

75. Hirano M, Pavlakis SG: Mitochondrial myopathy, encephalopathy, lactic acidosis and stroke-like episodes (MELAS): Current concepts. *J Child Neurol* 9:4, 1994.

76. Montagna P, Gallassi R, Medori R, et al: MELAS syndrome: Characteristic migrainous and epileptic features and maternal transmission. *Neurology* 38:751, 1988.

77. Hasuo K, Tamura S, Yasumori K, et al: Computed tomography and angiography in MELAS (mitochondrial myopathy, encephalopathy, lactic acidosis and stroke-like episodes). *Neuroradiology* 29:393, 1987.

78. Satoh M, Ishikawa N, Yoshizawa T, et al: *N*-isopropyl-*p*-(123-l)iodoamphetamine SPECT in MELAS syndrome: Comparison with CT and MRI imaging. *J Comput Assist Tomogr* 15:77, 1991.

79. Kishi M, Yamamura Y, Kurihara T, et al: An autopsy case of mitochondrial encephalomyopathy: Biochemical and electron microscopic studies of the brain. *J Neurol Sci* 86:31, 1988.

80. Goto Y: Clinical features of MELAS and mitochondrial DNA mutations. *Muscle Nerve* Suppl 3:S107, 1995.

81. Ihara Y, Namba R, Kuroda S, et al: Mitochondrial encephalomyopathy (MELAS): Pathological study and success-

ful therapy with coenzyme Q10 and idebenone. *J Neurol Sci* 90:263, 1989.

82. Penn A, Lee J, Thuillier P, et al: MELAS syndrome with mitochondrial tRNA Leu (UUR) mutation: Correlation of clinical state, nerve conduction, and muscle 31P magnetic resonance spectroscopy during treatment with nicotinamide and rivoflavin. *Neurology* 42:2147, 1992.

83. Silbert L, Durocher A, Biller J: The "S" in MELAS. *J Stroke Cerbrovasc Dis* 6:67, 1996.

84. Tanaka J, Nagai T, Arai H, et al: Treatment of mitochondrial encephalomyopathy with a combination of cytochrome C and vitamins B1 and B2. *Brain Dev* 19:262, 1997.

85. Saitoh S, Momoi MY, Yamagata T, et al: Effects of dichloroacetate in three patients with MELAS. *Neurology* 50:531, 1998.

86. Majamaa K, Rusanen H, Remes AM, et al: Increase of blood NAD+ and attenuation of lactacidemia during nicotinamide treatment of a patient with the MELAS syndrome. *Life Sci* 58:691, 1996.

87. Hsu CC, Chuang YH, Tsai JL, et al: CPEO and carnitine deficiency overlapping in MELAS syndrome. *Acta Neurol Scand* 92:252, 1995.

88. Pavlakis SG, Kingsley PB, Kaplan GP, et al: Magnetic resonance spectroscopy: Use in monitoring MELAS treatment. *Arch Neurol* 55:849, 1998.

89. Fayad P: Neurologic manifestations of heredirary hemorrhagic telangiectasia, in Gillman S, Goldstein GW, Waxman SG (eds): *Neurobase,* 2nd ed. La Jolla, CA, Arbor, 1995.

90. Steele JG, Narh PU, Burn J, Porteous ME: An association between migrainous aura and heredirary hemorrhagic telangiectasia. *Headache* 33:145, 1993.

91. Shovlin CL: Molecular defects in rare bleeding disorders: Hereditary hemorrhagic telangiectasia. *Thrombosis Haemostasis* 78:145, 1997.

92. Dayno JM, Silberstein SD: Migraine-related stroke versus migraine-induced stroke. *Headache* 37:463, 1997.

93. Gorelick PB, Hier DB, Caplan LR, Langenberg P: Headache in acute cerebrovascular disease. *Neurology* 36:1445, 1986.

94. Ferro LM, Melo TP, Oliveira V, Salgado AV, Crespo M, Canhao P, Pinto AN: A multivariate study of headache associated with ischemic stroke. *Headache* 35:315, 1995.

95. Mitsias P, Ramadan NM: Headache in ischemic cerebrovascular disease: Part II. Mechanisms and predictive value. *Cephalalgia* 12:341, 1992.

96. Koudstaal PJ, Van Gijn J, Kappelle LJ: Headache in transient or permanent cerebral ischemia. *Stroke* 22:754, 1991.

97. Rasmussen BK, Jensen R, Schroll M, Olesen J: Epidemiology of headache in a general population: A prevalence study. *J Clin Epidemiol* 44:1147, 1991.

98. Saito K, Moskowitz MA: Contributions of the upper cervical dorsal roots and trigeminal ganglia to the feline circle of Willis. *Stroke* 20:524, 1989.

99. Vestergaard K, Andersen G, Nielsen MI, Jensen TS: Headache in stroke. *Stroke* 24:1621, 1993.

100. Chambers BR, Bladin PF, McGrath K, et al: Stroke syndromes in young people. *Clin Exp Neurol* 18:132, 1982.

101. Levine SR, Ramadan NM: The relationship of stroke and migraine, in Adams HP (ed): Handbook of cerebrovascular diseases. New York, Marcel Dekker, 1993, pp 221–231.

102. Brohult J, Forsberg O, Hellstrom R: Multiple arterial thrombosis after oral contraceptives and ergotamine. *Acta Med Scand* 181:483, 1967.

103. Merhoff GC, Porter JM: Ergot intoxication: Historical review and description. *Ann Surg* 180:773, 1974.

104. Centrozone V, Brucoli C, Macinagrossa G, et al: Nonfamilial hemiplegic migraine responsive to nalaxone. *Cephalalgia* 3:125, 1983.

105. Bardwell A, Trott JA: Stroke in migraine as a consequence of propranolol. *Headache* 27:381, 1987.

106. Mendizabal JE, Greiner F, Hamilton WJ, Rothrock JF: Migrainous stroke causing thalamic infarction and amnesia during treatment with propranolol. *Headache* 37:594, 1997.

107. Olesen J, Welch KMA, Carolei A: Treatment to prevent migraine-related stroke. *Cerebrovasc Dis* 3:244, 1993.

108. Lidegaard O: Oral contraception and the risk of a cerebral thromboembolic attack: Results of a case-control study. *Br Med J* 306:956, 1993.

109. Grodstein F, Stampfer MJ, Manson JE, et al: Postmenopausal estrogen and progestin use and the risk of cardiovascular disease. *N Engl J Med* 335:453, 1996.

110. Petitti DB, Sidney S, Quesenberry CP, et al: Ischemic stroke and use of estrogen and estrogen/progestogen as hormone replacement therapy. *Stroke* 29:23, 1998.

111. Finucane FF, Madans JH, Bush TL, Wolf PH, Kleinman JC: Decreased risk of stroke among postmenopausal hormone users. *Arch Intern Med* 153:73, 1993.

112. Kernan WN, Brass LM, Viscoli CM, Sarrel PM, Macuch R, Horwitz RI: Estrogen after ischemic stroke: Clinical basis and design of the Women's Estrogen for Stroke Trial. *J Stroke Cerebrovasc Dis* 7:85, 1998.

113. Matias Guiu J, Alvarez J, Insa R, et al: Ischemic stroke in young adults: II. Analysis of risk factors in the etiological subgroups. *Acta Neurol Scand* 81:314, 1990.

Chapter 23

ATRIAL FIBRILLATION AND STROKE

Helmi L. Lutsep
Gregory W. Albers

BACKGROUND

History

Wright and Foley advocated the use of dicumarol, a blood thinner synthesized by Karl Paul Link, for the prevention of cardiac emboli in patients with rheumatic atrial fibrillation (AF) in 1947.[1,2] Until 1978, when the Framingham Study was reported, the risk of stroke in patients with chronic AF unassociated with valvular or rheumatic disease was generally believed to be too low to require medication.[3] The Framingham Study documented that stroke incidence was increased in patients with chronic nonrheumatic AF.[4] Since the landmark Framingham Study, multiple clinical trials have sought to identify those AF patient subgroups who are at particularly low or high risk for thromboembolism in an effort to optimize stroke prevention therapies.

Biologic Basis

Cardiac thrombi form in the presence of AF, embolizing to cerebral vessels to cause stroke. The thrombi most frequently occur in the left atrial appendage or, less commonly, in the left atrium.[5] Although left atrial appendage thrombi develop primarily because weak atrial contractions result in sluggish blood flow, other factors may contribute to the formation of thromboemboli. Advanced age, a prior embolic event, hypertension, and diabetes increase the stroke rate in AF.[6] Associated cardiac disease, such as congestive heart failure, coronary artery disease, mitral stenosis, or prosthetic heart valves, also seems to augment stroke risk in AF patients. The echocardiographic finding of decreased left ventric-

ular function has been shown to be another risk factor for AF-associated stroke.[7,8]

Transesophageal echocardiographic studies have shed light on the mechanisms underlying the increased rate of thromboembolism seen in patients with a history of hypertension and atrial fibrillation. Patients with a history of hypertension and AF are more likely to have atrial appendage thrombi, reduced atrial appendage velocity, and dense spontaneous echo contrast than AF patients without associated vascular risk factors, suggesting that in these cases the emboli are more likely to originate in the left atrial appendage.[9] In AF patients at high risk for thromboembolic events, extra-cardiac pathology may also mediate thromboembolism. Transesophageal echocardiographic studies show aortic plaque, particularly complex plaque, more frequently in patients predicted to be at high risk of stroke based on clinical criteria than in those in low or moderate risk groups.[9]

Epidemiology

Epidemiologic studies have shown that the prevalence of atrial fibrillation increases with age. Four large population-based surveys have provided a prevalence estimate of AF. These prevalence figures have been applied to United States census data to calculate absolute numbers of people with the dysrhythmia.[10] The prevalence of AF in the United States is 0.89 percent, which suggests that there are approximately 2.23 million people with AF. In people over the age of 40, the prevalence of AF is 2.3 percent, and in those over the age of 65 it is 5.9 percent. Eighty-four percent of the AF population is over age 65. Despite a higher prevalence of AF in men than in women at all ages, there is little difference in the absolute number of men and women with AF. This apparent paradox occurs because there are almost twice as many women as men in the older age groups. At ages greater than 75, approximately 60 percent of persons with AF are women.

In 1978, epidemiologic data confirmed the association of AF with stroke. By assessing stroke occurrence in 5184 men and women with chronic AF over a period of 24 years, the Framingham Study delineated the risks of stroke in chronic AF.[4] When AF was associated with rheumatic heart disease, stroke incidence increased 17-fold. In the absence of rheumatic heart disease, stroke incidence still increased more than fivefold in the context of chronic AF. As the duration of AF increased, stroke occurrence increased. Although previous studies had suggested that strokes cluster at the time of AF onset, recent analyses from pooled data have shown a nearly constant rate of stroke over time in patients with AF.[6,11,12] Moreover, paroxysmal AF seems to confer a risk of stroke similar to that of constant AF.[6]

Clinical Manifestations

The clinical manifestations of stroke occurring in the context of atrial fibrillation are relatively nonspecific, although more patients may display depressed consciousness than in other forms of stroke. Of the cerebral infarctions that occur in AF patients, approximately 70 percent are believed to be the result of emboli from the heart.[13] Atrial fibrillation-associated emboli may be larger than those of other sources, such as emboli of valvular origin.[14] The large size of the emboli in AF may contribute to the occurrence of a decreased level of consciousness at the time of the stroke, which is seen in almost 20 percent of cardioembolic strokes.[15] The neurologic deficit occurs suddenly in three-fourths of patients with presumed cardioembolism and is maximal at onset.[16] However, symptoms with an abrupt, maximal onset occur almost as frequently in other mechanisms of stroke.[15] Cardiac emboli most often cause infarctions in the middle cerebral artery territory and only rarely cause lacunar infarcts by occluding deep penetrating arteries in isolation.[17]

Diagnosis

Most cerebral ischemic events in patients with atrial fibrillation are due to emboli from the heart. However, about 30 percent of the cerebral infarctions in these patients are caused by intracranial or extracranial ath-

erosclerosis.[13] About 12 percent of elderly patients with AF have moderate or severe carotid stenosis.[18] About half of the patients with AF have hypertension, which may contribute to small vessel ischemic disease.[6] The diagnostic evaluation in patients presenting with ischemic stroke and AF, therefore, should attempt to exclude coexistent causes of stroke and identify any cardiac abnormalities that may affect management.

In patients with cardioembolic stroke, imaging studies of the brain frequently reveal clinically unsuspected cortical infarctions in other arterial territories.[19] Most cardioembolic infarcts reveal some degree of hemorrhagic transformation on magnetic resonance imaging (MRI).[20] Not only does hemorrhagic transformation occur more frequently in cardioembolic strokes than with other stroke mechanisms, it is generally more dense.[21] Figure 23-1 shows the apperance of hemorrhagic transformation on computed tomography (CT) in a patient with two cardioembolic strokes.

In one-fourth of patients with AF who present with stroke, the AF is discovered on admission.[16] The dysrhythmia may be intermittent, or paroxysmal, in one-third of patients with AF.[22]

Evaluation

Because about 12 percent of elderly patients with AF have carotid stenosis of at least moderate degree, Hart et al have recommended assessing the carotid arteries for stenosis if the patient is an endarterectomy candidate and the stroke is in the anterior circulation.[14,18] Transthoracic echocardiography is recommended if previous studies have not been obtained to exclude occult mitral stenosis or atrial tumor, or to determine a cause for unexplained heart failure.

Echocardiography may also be considered in those patients in whom evidence supporting a cardioembolic etiology of stroke may influence treatment decisions, such as those in whom anticoagulation is relatively contraindicated.[14] In a pooled analysis of three randomized clinical trials, left ventricular systolic dysfunction emerged as an independent predictor of stroke risk in patients with AF even in those without a clinical history of heart failure.[8] On the other hand, neither mitral regurgitation nor left atrial diameter was found to be significantly associated with stroke risk in the analysis.

Because most patients with AF and stroke are anticoagulated with warfarin irrespective of findings on cardiac studies, the value of transesophageal echocardiography (TEE) in these patients has been disputed.[23,24] TEE has, however, shown promise in investigations of stroke pathophysiology and treatment effects in AF pa-

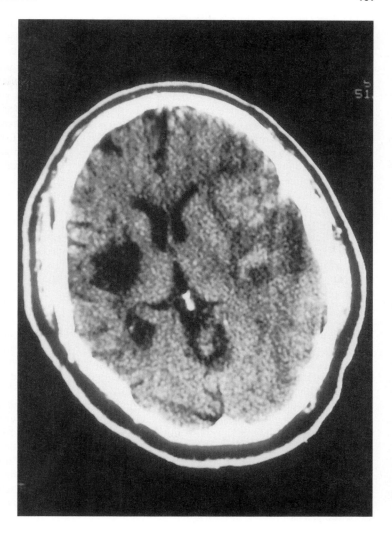

Figure 23-1.

Computed tomography scan from a patient with two cardioembolic strokes. The scan illustrates the hemorrhagic transformation that has complicated the patient's subacute left middle cerebral artery infarct (brighter regions within gray wedge on right side of figure) and reveals the presence of an older stroke in the middle cerebral artery territory in the opposite hemisphere (round dark area on left side of figure).

tients. TEE data were collected in 786 patients entering the Stroke Prevention in Atrial Fibrillation (SPAF) III trial who were stratified into stroke risk groups by clinical criteria.[9]

The SPAF III TEE study provided a preliminary assessment of the safety and efficacy of warfarin for treatment of patients with AF who have aortic plaque. Despite early reports that warfarin could precipitate cholesterol crystal embolization from aortic plaques, the SPAF III substudy found cholesterol embolization in only one patient during 127 person-years of warfarin treatment.[25] High-risk AF patients with thoracic aortic plaque randomized to adjusted dose warfarin (international normalized ratio (INR) 2.0 to 3.0) showed a trend toward

lower embolic event rates than patients randomized to fixed low-dose warfarin plus coated aspirin (325 mg). In patients with complex aortic plaque, treatment with adjusted dose warfarin significantly reduced event rates to 4.0 percent per year compared with an event rate of 15.8 percent per year on fixed dose warfarin and aspirin.[26]

EVIDENCE

Stroke Prevention Trials in Atrial Fibrillation

Five trials compared oral anticoagulant therapy with placebo in the late 1980's and early 1990's.[6] Warfarin decreased the overall frequency of ischemic strokes by 68 percent. All subgroups of patients who were treated with warfarin showed a lower stroke rate except those younger than 65 years of age with no other risk factors (history of hypertension, previous stroke or transient ischemic attack, or diabetes), in whom the annual risk of stroke was very low (1 percent).

In the three trials in which aspirin therapy was evaluated, aspirin showed a less consistent benefit than warfarin for stroke prevention when compared with placebo. Pooled data from these studies showed a mean stroke risk reduction of 21 percent.[12] No subgroup of patients with AF has been identified, which shows a particularly large reduction in stroke incidence with aspirin therapy.[27]

In the Stroke Prevention in Atrial Fibrillation (SPAF I and II) trials, 854 patients were randomly assigned to aspirin treatment at a dose of 325 mg per day. Multivariate analysis of these patients suggested that aspirin was inadequate for stroke prevention in four AF subgroups: women over 75 years of age, patients with systolic hypertension (greater than 160), recent congestive heart failure or impaired left ventricular function, or a history of prior thromboembolism.[28] Table 23-1 shows the thromboembolic rate per year for each of these four risk factors in aspirin-treated patients. Although aspirin-treated patients with one of these risk factors had an overall thromboembolic rate of 5.9 percent per year, patients taking aspirin without these risks had a thromboembolic rate of 1.9 percent per year.

Table 23-1.

Thromboembolic risk in aspirin-treated AF patients with a single risk factor[a]

Risk factor	Thromboembolic rate per year
	%
Woman >75 years old	6.9
History of thromboembolism	5.9
Systolic hypertension (>160 mmHg)	5.7
Recent congestive heart failure or impaired left ventricular function	2.6
None of the above	1.9

[a]Data from Prevention in Atrial Fibrillation Investigators: Risk factors for thromboembolism during aspirin therapy in patients with atrial fibrillation: The stroke prevention in atrial fibrillation study. *J Stroke Cerebrovasc Dis,* 5:150, 1995.

Although warfarin (INR 2.0 to 3.0) has consistently been shown to be effective in preventing stroke in patients with atrial fibrillation, the cumbersome monitoring requirements and associated risk of hemorrhage encouraged the investigation of alternative therapies. SPAF III sought alternative therapy to adjusted-dose warfarin for those AF patients determined to be at high risk for stroke on aspirin alone in the previous SPAF studies.[29] Low-intensity (INR 1.2 to 1.5), fixed-dose warfarin with aspirin, 325 mg per day, was compared with adjusted-dose warfarin in patients with at least one stroke risk factor. However, when the rate of embolism was discovered to be significantly higher in the patients on the combination therapy (7.9 percent per year) compared with those on adjusted-dose warfarin (1.9 percent per year), the trial was stopped. A case-control study has also suggested that lower intensities of anticoagulation (INR less than 2.0) are less effective for preventing stroke.[30] In this study, INR obtained at the time of ischemic stroke revealed that the risk of stroke rose sharply at INR below 2.0, nearly doubling at an INR of 1.7 and tripling at an INR of 1.5.

An additional phase of the SPAF III study evaluated the efficacy of aspirin therapy alone in those AF patients without any of the four risk factors for stroke in aspirin-treated patients identified in the previous SPAF studies.[31] In this low-risk group, the rate of ischemic stroke and systemic emboli (primary events) was 2.2 percent per year on 325 mg of aspirin per day. Although previous SPAF studies had not found that a history of hypertension, without current systolic hypertension, predicted high stroke risk in patients taking aspirin, this study found that previous hypertension was an independent predictor of primary events.[6,7,28] The rate of thromboembolic events among those with a history of hypertension was 3.6 percent per year, compared with a rate of 1.1 percent per year in the patients without this risk factor. The presence of diabetes or a history of coronary artery disease (without recent congestive heart failure or reduced left ventricular function) did not seem to substantially increase the risk of thromboembolic events in the group as a whole. However, these clinical factors were not individually assessed for their ability to predict stroke risk.

Risks of Preventative Therapies

Warfarin can significantly reduce the risk of stroke in patients with AF and is generally associated with an acceptably low risk of hemorrhage. An analysis of five randomized trials comparing warfarin with control in

AF patients with a mean age of 69 has found an annual stroke risk of 1.4 percent for patients treated with warfarin and a stroke rate of 4.5 percent for the control group.[6] The annual rate of major hemorrhage (one requiring hospitalization, two units of blood, or occurring intracranially) was 1.3 percent in the warfarin group and 1.0 percent in the control group. The risk of intracranial hemorrhage (ICH) in the warfarin group was only 0.3 percent per year. In an analysis of the pooled data from three randomized trials, aspirin, which is less efficacious than warfarin, was associated with an annual major hemorrhage rate of 1.0 percent.

Although no difference was seen in the mean age of the patients with intracranial bleeding when compared with those without ICH in the first five randomized trials, the number of patients with intracranial bleeds (six) was small. In the SPAF II trial, patients older than 75 years of age had a major hemorrhage rate of 4.2 percent per year, compared with a rate of 1.7 percent per year in younger patients.[32,33] The intracranial hemorrhage rate in those older than 75 years was 1.8 percent per year, compared with a rate of 0.6 percent per year in younger patients. These findings questioned the safety of anticoagulation use in the very elderly. However, the target levels of anticoagulation were higher in this study, INR 2.0 to 4.5, than in earlier trials. Both the SPAF II study and others have found the intensity of anticoagulation to be a powerful independent risk factor for bleeding.[34] Patients with marked hypertension (systolic pressures greater than 180 mmHg or diastolic pressures of more than 100 mmHg despite treatment), dementia, previous intracranial hemorrhage, and other bleeding abnormalities were excluded from the atrial fibrillation trials. Therefore, the risk of bleeding cannot be accurately determined in patients with these characteristics.

THERAPEUTIC RECOMMENDATIONS

Prevention of Stroke in Atrial Fibrillation

Oral anticoagulation (INR 2.0 to 3.0) is generally recommended for patients with AF and other clinical risk factors for stroke, including a history of hypertension, previous thromboembolism, diabetes, advanced age, heart failure, coronary artery disease, mitral stenosis, prosthetic heart valves, or thyrotoxicosis.[35] AF patients without any of these risk factors are at low risk of stroke and can be treated with aspirin. Aspirin is also appropriate for patients who are at high bleeding risk from warfarin or are opposed to warfarin therapy.

In a group of patients treated with aspirin alone for stroke prevention in the SPAF III study, the presence of diabetes or coronary artery disease did not increase the risk of stroke in the group as a whole.[31] However, a history of hypertension was associated with a significant increase in stroke risk. The risk of stroke among patients with diabetes or coronary artery disease was not individually assessed. Additional data will be necessary to clarify if either of these patient subgroups can be safely treated with aspirin.

AF patients over the age of 75 fall into a high-risk group for stroke. Older age has been associated with increased rates of stroke in AF patients, even if they do not have any other risk factors.[28] Although the SPAF studies suggest that elderly women with AF are at considerably higher stroke risk than elderly men, warfarin has also been recommended for men greater than 75 years of age if they are good candidates for anticoagulation. On the contrary, patients less than 65 years of age with no clinical risk factors have such a low stroke rate, 1 percent per year or less, that warfarin is not recommended. Either aspirin or no antithrombotic therapy is appropriate in these risk-free, younger patients. Patients between the ages of 65 and 75 years of age who have no risk factors seem to have stroke rates of only 1 to 2 percent per year. They can be treated with either aspirin or warfarin. These treatment recommendations are summarized in Table 23-2.

When selecting an agent for stroke prophylaxis, patient preferences as well as medical predictors of stroke risk should be incorporated into the decision.

Table 23-2.
American College of Chest Physicians Consensus Conference on Antithrombotic Therapy recommendations for stroke prevention in atrial fibrillation[a]

Age	Recommendation
<65 years	
No risk factors	Aspirin or nothing
Risk factors	Warfarin INR 2-3
65 to 75 years	
No risk factors	Warfarin or aspirin
Risk factors	Warfarin INR 2-3
>75 years	Warfarin INR 2-3

[a]Modified from Laupacis A, Albers G, Dalen J, et al: Antithrombotic therapy in atrial fibrillation. *Chest* 108(Suppl):358S, 1995.

Patient ratings of anticipated quality of life after a stroke as well as their perception of the inconveniences involved with warfarin or aspirin therapy vary considerably.[36] In the majority of patients, however, quality of life estimates for taking either warfarin or aspirin are quite high, whereas major stroke is rated as being equal to or worse than death.

Anticoagulation in the Context of Acute Stroke

Few data are available to assist with the timing of anticoagulation therapy in a patient with AF who has incurred an acute stroke. The risks of immediate anticoagulation of cardioembolic stroke may include a higher likelihood of hemorrhagic transformation and neurologic deterioration.[21,37] However, one small randomized trial comparing immediate anticoagulation with placebo in acute cardioembolic stroke did not show delayed clinical deterioration from hemorrhage in any patient.[38] Strokes that are moderate or large in size may increase the risk of hemorrhagic transformation, as may excessive anticoagulation.[34,37,39] In several reported patients, a heparin bolus of 5000 to 7000 units preceded the appearance of hemorrhage. The avoidance of anticoagulation in the first days after an ischemic event may not place all patients at increased risk for stroke recurrence, as two recent studies suggest that strokes recur in only 2 to 5 percent of patients in the first 2 weeks after cardioembolism.[40,41]

For patients at high risk of embolism, including those with mechanical heart valves, known intracardiac thrombus, mitral stenosis, or congestive heart failure, early anticoagulation of ischemic infarcts is generally recommended. Conversely, in those patients with large infarcts or uncontrolled hypertension or in whom the risk for early recurrence of thromboembolism is low, delaying anticoagulation for several days to a week may reduce the risk of hemorrhagic complications. The initial administration of a large heparin bolus should be avoided.

After significant hemorrhagic infarction, anticoagulation should generally be delayed.[42] In many reported cases, however, patients remained clinically stable, and hemorrhagic regions resolved despite continued anticoagulation. Therefore, hemorrhagic infarction is not an absolute contraindication to anticoagulation and may be considered in those patients with high-risk embolic sources.[43]

Particularly difficult are decisions regarding the resumption of anticoagulants in patients who have developed a primary intracerebral hemorrhage but are also at high risk of thromboembolism as a result of AF. Although prospective trials are lacking, anecdotal reports have suggested that in some cases anticoagulants may be resumed safely after intracranial hemorrhage has occurred. In patients at risk of thromboembolism from prosthetic heart valves, anticoagulants were resumed from 8 to 27 days after intraparenchymal hemorrhage and 5 to 42 days after subdural hematoma without neurologic deterioration.[44,45]

The timing of anticoagulation may be guided by the probable cause of the hemorrhage. If the hemorrhage has characteristics of a hypertensive bleed, it is reasonable to resume anticoagulants for high-risk patients after allowing the hemorrhage to resolve. Because ongoing hypertension may increase the risk of intracranial hemorrhage, anticoagulants should not be restarted until blood pressures are well controlled.[46] We usually recommend that anticoagulants be withheld for at least 4 to 6 weeks in patients with small hypertensive hemorrhages and longer in patients with larger bleeds.

If the brain hemorrhage seems to be associated with amyloid angiopathy, we recommend that anticoagulants be permanently discontinued. In amyloid angiopathy, noncontractile amyloid protein replaces the contractile elements of the arterial wall.[47] In addition, local endothelial dysfunction causes alterations in the chemical mediators of hemostasis. Both of these processes may contribute to hematoma enlargement, which could be exacerbated by anticoagulants. Brain hemorrhages may also recur in as many as 20 percent of patients with amyloid angiopathy within weeks of the initial hemorrhage.[48] For these reasons, the risk of significant recurrent hemorrhage in patients with amyloid angiopathy will likely cancel the benefits of using anticoagulants to prevent ischemic stroke.

REFERENCES

1. Stahmann MA, Heubner CF, Link KP: Studies on the hemorrhagic sweet clover disease: V. Identification and synthesis of the hemorrhagic agent. *J Biol Chem* 138: 513, 1941.
2. Wright IS, Foley WT: Use of anticoagulants in the treatment of heart disease. *Am J Med* 3:718, 1947.
3. Phillips E, Levine SA: Auricular fibrillation without other evidence of heart disease. *Am J Med* 7:478, 1949.
4. Wolf PA, Dawber TR, Thomas HE, Kannel WB: Epidemiologic assessment of chronic atrial fibrillation and risk of stroke: The Framingham study. *Neurology* 28:973, 1978.
5. Hart RG, Coull BM, Hart D: Early recurrent embolism

associated with nonvalvular atrial fibrillation: A retrospective study. *Stroke* 14:688, 1983.

6. Atrial Fibrillation Investigators: Risk factors for stroke and efficacy of antithrombotic therapy in atrial fibrillation: Analysis of pooled data from five randomized controlled trials. *Arch Intern Med* 154:1449, 1994.

7. Stroke Prevention in Atrial Fibrillation Investigators: Predictors of thromboembolism in atrial fibrillation: II. Echocardiographic features of patients at risk. *Ann Intern Med* 116:6, 1992.

8. Atrial Fibrillation Investigators: Echocardiographic predictors of stroke in patients with atrial fibrillation: A prospective study of 1,066 patients from three clinical trials. *Arch Intern Med* 158:1316, 1998.

9. Zabalgoitia M, Halperin JL, Pearce LA, et al for the Stroke Prevention in Atrial Fibrillation III Investigators: Transesophageal echocardiographic correlates of thromboembolic risk in nonvalvular atrial fibrillation. *J Am College Cardiol* 31:1622, 1998.

10. Feinberg WM, Blackshear JL, Laupacis A, et al: Prevalence, age distribution, and gender of patients with atrial fibrillation. *Arch Intern Med* 155:469, 1995.

11. Wolf PA, Kannel WB, McGee DL, et al: Duration of atrial fibrillation and imminence of stroke: The Framingham study. *Stroke* 14:664, 1983.

12. Albers GW: Atrial fibrillation and stroke: Three new studies, three remaining questions. *Arch Intern Med* 154: 1443, 1994.

13. Foulkes MA, Wolf PA, price TR, et al: The Stroke Data Bank: Design, methods and baseline characteristics. *Stroke* 19:547, 1988.

14. Hart RG, Albers GW, Koudstaal PJ: Cardioembolic stroke, in Bogousslavsky J, Ginsberg M (eds): *Cerebrovascular Disease.* Cambridge, MA, Blackwell Science, Inc., 1995, pp 2–49.

15. Ramirez-Lassepas M, Cipolle RJ, Bjork RJ: Can embolic stroke be diagnosed on the basis of neurologic clinical criteria? *Arch Neurol* 44:87, 1987.

16. Bogousslavsky J, Cachin C, Regli F, et al: Cardiac sources of embolism and cerebral infarction: Clinical consequences and vascular concomitants. *Neurology* 41:855, 1991.

17. Ringelstein EB, Koseborke S, Holling A, et al: Computed tomographic patterns of proven embolic brain infarctions. *Ann Neurol* 26:759, 1989.

18. Kanter MC, Tegeler CH, Pearce LA, et al on behalf of the SPAF Investigators: Carotid stenosis in patients with atrial fibrillation: Prevalence, risk factors and relationship to stroke. *Arch Intern Med* 154:1372, 1994.

19. Boon A, Lodder J, Heuts-van Raak L, Kessels F: Silent brain infarcts in 755 consecutive patients with acute cerebrovascular disease. *Stroke* 25:2384, 1994.

20. Hornig CR, Bauer T, Simon C, et al: Hemorrhagic transformation in cardioembolic cerebral infarction. *Stroke* 24:465, 1993.

21. Hart RG, Easton JD: Hemorrhagic infarcts. *Stroke* 17:586, 1986.

22. Lindgren A, Roijer A, Norrving B, et al: Carotid artery and heart disease in subtypes of cerebral infarction. *Stroke* 25:2356, 1994.

23. Warner MF, Momah KI. Routine transesophageal echocardiography for cerebral ischemia: Is it really necessary? *Arch Intern Med* 156:1719, 1996.

24. Manning WJ: Role of transesophageal echocardiography in the management of thromboembolic stroke. *Am J Cardiol* 80:19D, 1997.

25. Blackshear JL, Zabalgoitia M, Pennock G, et al: Warfarin safety and efficacy in patients with thoracic aortic plaque and atrial fibrillation. *Am J Cardiol* 83:453, 1999.

26. The Stroke Prevention in Atrial Fibrillation Investigators Committee on Echocardiography: Transesophageal echocardiographic correlates of thromboembolism in high-risk patients with nonvalvular atrial fibrillation. *Ann Intern Med* 28:639, 1998.

27. The Atrial Fibrillation Investigators: The efficacy of aspirin in patients with atrial fibrillation: Analysis of pooled data from 3 randomized trials. *Arch Intern Med* 157:1237, 1997.

28. Stroke Prevention in Atrial Fibrillation Investigators: Risk factors for thromboembolism during aspirin therapy in patients with atrial fibrillation: The stroke prevention in atrial fibrillation study. *J Stroke Cerebrovasc Dis* 5:147, 1995.

29. Stroke Prevention in Atrial Fibrillation Investigators: Superiority of adjusted-dose warfarin over low-intensity, fixed-dose warfarin plus aspirin for high-risk patients with atrial fibrillation: The stroke prevention in atrial fibrillation III randomized clinical trial. *Lancet* 348:633, 1996.

30. Hylek EM, Skates SJ, Sheehan MA, Singer DE: An analysis of the lowest effective intensity of prophylactic anticoagulation for patients with nonrheumatic atrial fibrillation. *N Engl J Med* 335:540, 1996.

31. Stroke Prevention in Atrial Fibrillation Investigators: Patients with nonvalvular atrial fibrillation at low risk of stroke during treatment with aspirin: Stroke prevention in atrial fibrillation III study. *JAMA* 279:1273, 1998.

32. Stroke Prevention in Atrial Fibrillation Investigators: Bleeding during antithrombotic therapy in patients with atrial fibrillation. *Arch Intern Med* 156:409, 1996.

33. Stroke Prevention in Atrial Fibrillation Investigators: Warfarin versus aspirin for prevention of thromboembolism in atrial fibrillation: Stroke Prevention in Atrial Fibrillation II Study. *Lancet* 343:687, 1994.

34. Hylek EM, Singer DE: Risk factors for intracranial hemorrhage in outpatients taking warfarin. *Ann Intern Med* 120:897, 1994.

35. Laupacis A, Albers G, Dalen J, et al: Antithrombotic therapy in atrial fibrillation. *Chest* Oct 108 (Suppl):352S, 1995.

36. Gage BF, Cardinalli AB, Owens DK: The effect of stroke and stroke prophylaxis with aspirin or warfarin on quality of life. *Arch Intern Med* 156:1829, 1996.

37. Babikian VL, Kase CS, Pessin MS, et al: Intracerebral hemorrhage in stroke patients anticoagulated with heparin. *Stroke* 20:1500, 1989.

38. Cerebral Embolism Study Group: Immediate anticoagula-

tion of embolic stroke: A randomized trial. *Stroke* 14:668, 1983.

39. Cerebral Embolism Study Group: Immediate anticoagulation of embolic stroke: Brain hemorrhage and management options. *Stroke* 15:779, 1984.

40. International Stroke Trial Collaborative Group: The International Stroke Trial (IST): A randomised trial of aspirin, subcutaneous heparin, both, or neither among 19,435 patients with acute ischaemic stroke. *Lancet* 349:1569, 1997.

41. The Publications Committee for the Trial of ORG10172 in Acute Stroke Treatment (TOAST) Investigators: Low molecular weight heparinoid, ORG 10172 (danaparoid), and outcome after acute ischemic stroke. *JAMA* 279: 1265, 1998.

42. Yatsu FM, Hart RG, Mohr JP, Grotta JC: Anticoagulation of embolic strokes of cardiac origin: An update. *Neurology* 38:314, 1988.

43. Pessin MS, Estol CJ, Lafranchise F, Caplan LR: Safety of anticoagulation after hemorrhagic infarction. *Neurology* 43:1298, 1993.

44. Gomez CR, Sandhu J, Mehta P: Resumption of anticoagulation during hypertensive cerebral hemorrhage with prosthetic heart valve. *Stroke* 19:407, 1988.

45. Babikian VL, Kase CS, Pessin MS, et al: Resumption of anticoagulation after intracranial bleeding in patients with prosthetic heart valves. *Stroke* 19:407, 1988.

46. Lyden PD, Zivin JA: Hemorrhagic transformation after cerebral ischemia: Mechanisms and incidence. *Cerebrovasc Brain Metab Rev* 5:1, 1993.

47. Leblanc R, Carpenter S, Stewart J, Pokrupa R: Subacute enlarging cerebral hematoma from amyloid angiopathy: Case report. *Neurosurgery* 36:403, 1995.

48. Kalyan-Raman UP, Kalyan-Raman K: Cerebral amyloid angiopathy causing intracranial hemorrhage. *Ann Neurol* 16:321, 1984.

Chapter 24

SUBSTANCE ABUSE AND STROKE

John C.M. Brust

INTRODUCTION

Recreational substance use can result in two types of drug dependence. "Psychic dependence" refers to psychic drive—craving—that requires periodic or continuous administration of the drug to achieve pleasure or to avoid discomfort. "Physical dependence" is an adaptive state in which cessation of drug intake or administration of an antagonist produces physical symptoms and signs. "Addiction" is psychic dependence and can be present in the absence of physical dependence. "Tolerance" is the need for increasing doses of a drug to achieve desired effects or to avoid psychic or physical symptoms of withdrawal. "Drug abuse" is a social judgment, whether the drug is taken continuously or intermittently and whether or not it is legally available.[1]

In developed countries, a large number of substances are used recreationally (Table 24-1). Of these, ethanol, tobacco, and caffeine are readily and legally available. Household products, such as aerosols and glues or-over-the-counter drugs such as phenylpropanolamine, are also readily available but used in a manner usually unintended by their manufacturers. Others, for example, morphine, amphetamine, and barbiturates, require a physician's prescription. Still others, for example, marijuana, LSD, and alkaloidal cocaine, are not legally available. With the exception of anticholinergics and caffeine, each of the categories of drugs listed in Table 24-1 has been implicated in ischemic or hemorrhagic stroke. With some, the evidence for a causal relationship is epidemiologic. With others it is anecdotal. In this chapter, we will briefly review different agents under the several categories given in Table 24-1, examine the evidence for risk of stroke, and address implications for stroke management.

OPIOIDS

Background

Opioids comprise many drugs with agonist, antagonist, or mixed agonist-antagonist actions on specific receptors in the central and peripheral nervous systems. The opioid most widely used recreationally is heroin, which is injected intravenously ("mainlining") or subcutaneously ("skinpopping") or snorted or smoked. Taken in intended dosage, heroin, morphine, and other opioid agonists produce euphoria, drowsiness, analgesia, nausea and vomiting, miosis, and respiratory depression; parenteral injection or smoking produces a brief ecstatic "rush." Overdose produces coma, respiratory depression, and pinpoint pupils and is treated with ventilatory support and the opioid antagonist naloxone. Withdrawal produces flu-like symptoms—nausea, vomiting, diarrhea, myalgia, muscle spasms, rhinorrhea, and sweating alternating with chills—plus intense craving. Treatment of withdrawal consists of administering an opioid agonist, usually methadone. In adults, opioid withdrawal does not produce hallucinations, seizures, or delirium, and the condition is not life threatening. In neonates, opioid withdrawal is much more severe and sometimes fatal.[1]

Evidence for Stroke Risk

Opioid users are at risk for stroke by at least two different mechanisms, namely, indirectly through infection and more directly from effects of the drug itself or its contaminants.

Parenteral abusers of any drug are subject to a host of infections, of which endocarditis, hepatitis, and

Table 24-1.
Categories of recreationally used drugs

Opioids

Psychostimulants

Sedatives

Cannabis

Hallucinogens

Inhalants

Acylcyclohexylamines

Anticholinergics

Ethanol

Tobacco

Caffeine

HIV can result in stroke. Infectious endocarditis, especially associated with *Staphylococcus aureus* and *Candida,* but sometimes with *Pseudomonas* or more unusual organisms, causes bland embolic infarction, meningitis with secondary infarction, intraparenchymal or extraparenchymal brain or spinal cord abscess (which can be mistaken for infarction), and intracerebral or subarachnoid hemorrhage from diffuse cerebral vasculitis or rupture of a septic ("mycotic") aneurysm. Unlike subarachnoid hemorrhage from rupture of a saccular aneurysm, septic aneurysm rupture can initially produce subtle or insidiously progressive neurologic or systemic symptoms, such as mild headache, fever, syncope, hemiparesis, or aphasia, and cerebrospinal fluid (CSF) pleocytosis can precede rupture. Although they may disappear with antimicrobial therapy, they can also persist, enlarge, or rupture. The high mortality associated with their rupture and the relative ease (compared with saccular aneurysms) of their surgical removal has led some clinicians to recommend that cerebral angiography be performed in endocarditis patients with unexplained neurologic symptoms or abnormal CSF. Once a mycotic aneurysm is identified, surgically accessible aneurysms should be promptly excised.[2,3]

Hepatitis and liver failure with deranged clotting theoretically predispose to hemorrhagic stroke, but the actual prevalence of such a complication among parenteral drug abusers is unknown.

HIV infection causes stroke by diverse mechanisms, including infectious and noninfectious endocarditis, myocarditis, infectious and noninfectious vasculitis, coagulopathy, cachexia, hypotension, thrombocytopenia, and hemorrhage into an intracranial neoplasm.[4]

Although a case-control study did not find an increased risk for stroke among patients with AIDS,[5] anecdotal reports and case series, including autopsies, are persuasive that a causal association exists. In young children, HIV causes large vessel intracranial vasculopathy.

A number of reports describe ischemic stroke in young heroin users without endocarditis, hepatitis, HIV infection, or other apparent risk factors such as hypertension. Some strokes were associated with loss of consciousness following intravenous heroin; others affected active users but were not related to overdose or recent injection. In some, cerebral angiography was normal; in others, there was irregular intracranial arterial narrowing ("beading"), consistent with—but not pathognomonic for—vasculitis. Suggesting hypersensitivity, patients have variably demonstrated eosinophilia, serum hypergammaglobulinemia, positive direct Coombs test, elevated erythrocyte sedimentation rate (ESR), and positive Latex fixation test.[6–9] One patient's stroke was preceded by dyspnea and symptoms suggestive of anaphylaxis.[8] Some heroin strokes have followed the first injection in weeks or months. Occlusive stroke has also followed heroin snorting and sniffing.[10,11] A young adult developed intracerebral hemorrhage within minutes of intravenous heroin,[12] and a middle-aged woman who habitually snorted heroin had rupture of a cerebellar vascular malformation.[13]

Mechanisms other than hypersensitivity could underlie some opioid-related strokes.[14] Overdose produces hypoventilation and hypotension, and hemiplegia has appeared on awakening from antagonist-responsive coma. Bilateral globus pallidus infarction, presumably secondary to shock, is a common finding at autopsies of heroin users, and hemichorea was a feature of one heroin-related stroke.[6] Awkward postures of the neck after overdose could kink the carotid artery.[9]

Also possible is direct toxic injury from drug or adulterant. In the United States, heroin is usually mixed with lactose or mannitol and often with quinine. Mixtures have contained talc, starch, curry powder, caffeine, Vim, Ajax, and strychnine,[14] and heroin is frequently combined with cocaine or amphetamine ("speedball"). Quinine is suspected as contributing to heroin-induced pulmonary edema and sudden death,[15] but evidence is lacking to implicate it in stroke.

Embolization of foreign material to the brain has been observed in abusers of opioids other than heroin.[16–18] During the 1970's, parenteral abuse of pentazocine (Talwin) combined with tripelennamine (Pyribenzamine) ("Ts and blues") was popular in the American Midwest. Crushed oral tablets, suspended in water and injected intravenously, produce talc and cellulose microemboli, which reach the brain, causing occlusive or hemorrhagic stroke.[19] Their passage through the pulmonary vasculature is abetted by prior pulmonary emboli, pulmonary hypertension, and functional pulmonary arteriovenous shunts. "Beaded" and occluded cerebral vessels seen angiographically could reflect either multiple emboli or reactive vasculitis.

Foreign body embolic stroke has also been reported in parenteral abusers of paregoric,[20] meperidine tablets,[21] and hydromorphone suppositories.[22]

Probably vascular are some cases of heroin myelopathy.[23] A number of case reports describe acute paraparesis, sensory loss, and urinary retention occurring shortly after injection. In some, preserved proprioception suggested anterior cerebral artery territory infarction, and an autopsy showed thoracic level necrosis affecting gray more than white matter. If these lesions are infarcts, their cause could be hypotension with "border-zone" damage, hypersensitivity, or direct toxicity. In one case, abrupt paraplegia followed injection of heroin into a vein overlying the mid-thoracic spine.[1] In another case, cord biopsy revealed vasculitis with double-refractile particles in vessel walls.[24]

AMPHETAMINE AND RELATED PSYCHOSTIMULANTS

Background

These indirect bioamine agonists, which release dopamine and norepinephrine at central and peripheral nervous system synapses, are sold both by prescription and over-the-counter for treatment of narcolepsy and attention-deficit hyperactivity disorder and as appetite suppressants and decongestants.[1] There are different patterns of abuse, orally for increased alertness and mood elevation and parenterally or by inhalation for a "rush" qualitatively different from that experienced by opioid abusers. Smokable methamphetamine is known as "ice." Chronic use of these drugs produces paranoia progressing to psychosis and stereotypic movements progressing to frank dyskinesias. Overdose causes excitement, hypertension, tachycardia, sweating, myoglobinuria, shock, coma, and death. Withdrawal causes depression (sometimes suicidal) and increased appetite.[1]

Evidence for Stroke Risk

Parenteral psychostimulant abusers are subject to the same infectious complications—and indirect stroke risks—discussed above. Numerous anecdotal reports additionally describe strokes related to the drugs themselves.

Over 30 patients have had intracranial hemorrhage after use of amphetamine, methamphetamine, or, in single instances, diethylpropion or pseudoephedrine. Several also used methylphenidate, cocaine, heroin, or other nonpsychostimulant drugs. Routes of administration were oral, nasal, or parenteral.[1,25-35] Most were chronic users, but in some, stroke followed a first exposure. Blood pressures were elevated in 15 of the 26 cases in which it was recorded. Computerized tomography (CT) in 14 patients showed, variably, intracerebral or subarachnoid hemorrhage, or was normal. In 12 patients, there was angiographic "beading" of intracranial vessels, and in 3 of these patients the drug had been taken orally. Three patients had vasculitis at autopsy, and in one of these angiography had shown only an avascular mass. Thus, some of these psychostimulant-related intracranial hemorrhages were plausibly secondary to acute hypertension, others to vasculitis, and some to a combination of the two, but in others neither feature was evident. A drug-induced hypertensive surge could of course be evanescent enough to be missed. Conversely, acute hypertension could be a transient result of hemorrhagic stroke rather than its cause. Brain hemorrhage is sometimes a complication of human heat stroke, but extreme hyperpyrexia does not seem to have been present in any of these cases.

Brain infarction in users of amphetamine-like drugs is also described anecdotally. Necrotizing angiitis affected 14 Los Angeles abusers of multiple drugs, of which methamphetamine was used in all but two.[36] Symptoms and signs, variably present, included skin rash, hypertension, arthralgia, pneumonitis, renal failure, peripheral neuropathy, and anemia. Two had "encephalopathic" symptoms; autopsy in one showed arteriolar vasculitis in the pons and in the other brainstem infarcts and cerebellar hemorrhage. The vascular changes were typical for polyarteritis nodosa; hepatitis antigen was not present.[37]

Similar brain lesions have been found pathologically in other polydrug abusers (including amphetamine), but their pathophysiology, and whether they are caused by either the drug itself or a contaminant, are unknown.[33,38] More often, cerebral vasculitis has been presumed on the basis of cerebral angiography, and the relation to amphetamine has in some cases been tenuous.[25,34,39] In one such report, 19 young drug abusers (mostly intravenous methamphetamine), admitted for stroke or coma, had angiographic "beading" of cerebral arteries, with multiple occlusions, consistent with either multiple emboli or vasculitis.[40] In other reports, ischemic stroke followed intranasal methamphetamine use, and angiography, performed in three, showed supraclinoid "beading" of the internal carotid artery, occlusion of the proximal internal carotid artery, and occlusion of the supraclinoid internal carotid artery.[41,42]

Animal studies confirm that amphetamine and related psychostimulants can cause vasculitis. Monkeys studied angiographically within 10 min of receiving single doses of intravenous methamphetamine had irregularly decreased caliber of small cerebral vessels; in some, there was a return to normal at 24 h, consistent with acute vasospasm. In others, narrowing occurred in both small and large vessels and persisted for 2 weeks, sometimes actually worsening, and postmortem examination revealed subarachnoid hemorrhage, brain petechial hemorrhages, infarcts, microaneurysms, and perivascular leukocyte cuffing.[43] Monkeys receiving methamphetamine repeatedly for up to a year showed, angiographically, brain vessel occlusions and, pathologically, microaneurysms, fragmented arterioles and capillaries, dilated venules, neuronal loss, and gliosis.[44] Rats receiving intravenous methamphetamine for 2 weeks developed vesicular abnormalities in the endothelium of vessels too small to be seen angiographically.[44] These lesions differ from polyarteritis, in which elastic arteries, capillaries, and veins are spared. Whether they signify hypersensitivity angiitis or a direct toxic effect, and the possible contribution of subarachnoid hemorrhage, is uncertain.[45]

An adolescent amphetamine abuser developed mononeuropathy multiplex, and sural nerve biopsy showed changes consistent with hypersensitivity angiitis, including fibrinoid necrosis and infiltration by polymorphonuclear leukocytes, lymphocytes, and plasma cells. The central nervous system, however, was clinically unaffected.[46]

Phenylpropanolamine (PPA) is sold over-the-counter as a decongestant (e.g., Contac) or diet pill (e.g., Dexatrim, Maxi-slim) and in "legal stimulants" sometimes deliberately made to resemble amphetamine ("look-alike pills"). A small margin of safety exists between recommended and toxic dose, and complications include hypertension, agitation, hallucinations, seizures, cardiac arrhythmia, hemorrhagic stroke, and death.[47–53] In one case, "cerebral arteritis" was based on angiographic "beading"[53]; in another, intracerebral hemorrhage with biopsy-confirmed cerebral vasculitis occurred 3 weeks postpartum after a single dose of Dexatrim.[52] PPA with caffeine in a commercial diet preparation caused subarachnoid hemorrhage in rats receiving it parenterally in several times the recommended dose.[54]

Ephedrine and pseudoephedrine, also available over-the-counter as decongestants and bronchodilators, have each been anecdotally associated with hypertensive emergencies, myocardial infarction, and hemorrhagic stroke.[51,55–59] In one case, subarachnoid hemorrhage occurred 1 h after ingesting ephedrine. Although the initial angiogram was normal, a week later it showed "beading" and branch occlusions; biopsy of normal-appearing skin showed deposits of IgM and the C3 component of complement, consistent with circulating immune complexes.[57] During the 1990's, popularity of "legal stimulants" made from the herb Ephedra (ma huang), which contains ephedrine, resulted in numerous complications, including stroke and death. In 1996, such products were banned in several states.

A young woman developed right hemiplegia after attempted injection of crushed methylphenidate tablets into her left jugular vein, and 2 weeks later left hemiplegia followed similar right injection.[60] Talc microemboli have been observed in retina and brain of intravenous methylphenidate abusers.[16,61] A young woman had infarction of the medulla following intravenous methylphenidate, and at autopsy talc deposits were seen in small vessels around the infarct.[17] A 12-year-old boy taking methylphenidate in prescribed oral dosage for attention-deficit hyperactivity disorder developed hemiparesis and aphasia; angiography revealed vessel irregularities and occlusions suggestive of arteritis.[62] Rats receiving intravenous methylphenidate developed cerebrovascular lesions similar to those receiving methamphetamine.[44]

Subclavian and carotid mycotic aneurysms developed in a parenteral abuser of the diet pill phentermine,[63] and occlusive stroke was reported in two daily users of oral phentermine, one of whom also used phendimetrazine.[64] In 1997, reports of valvular heart disease and pulmonary hypertension in people using fenfluramine, dexfenfluramine, and phentermine lead to removal of these drugs from the U.S. market.[65]

A popular recreational drug on college campuses, methylenedioxymethamphetamine (MDMA, "ecstasy") produces both stimulatory effects as seen with amphetamine and illusions and hallucinations more often encountered with agents such as LSD. At least one case of cerebral infarction has been reported in a young man without other risk factors.[66]

Chronic use of the most widely used psychostimulant—caffeine—is inversely related to nonfatal stroke.

Unlike amphetamine, caffeine's actions include inhibition of brain adenosine, and up-regulation of adenosine receptors might have neuronal protective effects during ischemia.[67,68]

COCAINE

Background

Like amphetamine, cocaine is an indirect bioamine agonist; by binding to dopamine, norepinephrine, and serotonin transporter proteins, it blocks re-uptake of these neurotransmitters into their synaptic nerve endings. Cocaine is also the only naturally occurring local anesthetic. It produces symptoms—intended, overdose, and withdrawal—similar to those of amphetamine. Two forms of cocaine are used recreationally. Cocaine hydrochloride is taken nasally or parenterally; alkaloidal cocaine ("crack") is smoked, allowing more sustained delivery of higher doses.[1]

Evidence for Stroke Risk

Parenteral cocaine users are subject to the same infectious complications described for opioids and other psychostimulants. In addition, because of promiscuity and the culture of "drugs for sex," female crack smokers are at increased risk for AIDS. The risk of stroke in such patients would theoretically be the same as in other HIV-infected subjects. Cocaine causes myocardial infarction, arrhythmia, and cardiomyopathy, which indirectly predispose to stroke.

Like amphetamine, cocaine also causes stroke by more direct mechanisms. Although one case control series failed to identify cocaine as a risk factor for stroke,[69] numerous case reports of stroke in young cocaine users with neither cardiac disease, infection, nor other risk factors make it difficult to dismiss a causal role for cocaine. By the mid-1990's, more than 400 cases had been described, about half ischemic and half hemorrhagic, especially in "crack" cocaine users, but also in association with intranasal, intramuscular, and intravenous use.[70–89]

Ischemic CNS disease includes transient ischemic attacks and infarction of the cerebrum, thalamus, brainstem, spinal cord, and retina.[84,90–94] Reports include neonates and pregnant women,[95,96] and an ultrasound study of 26 newborns exposed in utero to cocaine found "periventricular leukomalacia" in 5, cerebral infarction in 8, intraventricular hemorrhage in 7, and intracerebral hemorrhage in 6.[97] Angiographic abnormalities have been interpreted as either vasculitis or sympathomimetic vasospasm; some of these cases probably represented cerebral vasospasm secondary to undetected subarachnoid hemorrhage.[98–100] Autopsies have usually shown normal cerebral vessels, but in five cases biopsy revealed mild cerebral vasculitis (round cell infiltration without vessel wall necrosis).[45,101–104]

Intraparenchymal or subarachnoid hemorrhage has occurred during or within hours of cocaine use or has had less clear temporal relationship.[14,105–112] Of patients subjected to angiography, nearly half had saccular aneurysms or vascular malformations.[14,105,106,108,112–114] Cases include hemorrhagic embolic infarction and bleeding into an astrocytoma,[115] and cerebral hemorrhages have occurred in neonates and pregnant women.[95,96,116–119] In a woman with multiple cerebral hemorrhages after smoking crack, cerebral vessels at autopsy were histologically normal.[120] Spontaneous acute subdural hematoma and spontaneous spinal epidural hematoma are described.[74,121]

A considerable amount of literature addresses possible mechanisms of cocaine-related stroke. For reasons unclear, hemorrhagic stroke occurs more often than occlusive stroke in users of cocaine hydrochloride, whereas hemorrhagic and occlusive strokes occur with roughly equal frequency in "crack" cocaine users.[122] The rising prevalence of stroke since the introduction of "crack" cocaine probably reflects widespread use and high dosage rather than a particular pharmacologic feature of "crack" cocaine itself.

Cocaine is a vasoconstrictor, acting both at sympathetic nerve endings and at vascular calcium channels. Surges of systemic hypertension could cause hemorrhagic stroke, especially in subjects with underlying vascular malformations or aneurysms. Cervical or intracranial vasoconstriction could result in ischemic stroke, which in the presence of cocaine-induced hypertension would have a propensity to become hemorrhagic.[123–125] Relevant to strokes that occur after other acute effects of cocaine have worn off, cocaine metabolites also cause cerebral vasoconstriction.[126]

Human, animal, and in vitro studies describe cocaine effects on platelets, atherosclerosis, clotting factors, and anticardiolipin antibodies.[127–130] Some patients have had strokes while taking cocaine with ethanol; a metabolite, cocaethylene, binds to synaptic bioamine transporters more powerfully than cocaine itself and thus might increase the risk of stroke.

It is controversial whether cocaine use results in lasting cognitive impairment and, if so, whether the damage is ischemic in origin.[130–134] Similar controversy exists over the nature and degree of cocaine-induced fetal damage.[135–138]

PHENCYCLIDINE

Background

Acylcyclohexylamine compounds, which include phencyclidine (PCP, "angel dust") and ketamine, are called "dissociative anesthetics" because of a tendency of patients during anesthesia to keep their eyes open and seem "disconnected" from the environment. Phencyclidine antagonizes excitatory N-methyl-D-aspartate (NMDA) receptors and also binds to brain sigma receptors. Recreationally, the drug is eaten, snorted, and injected, but most often smoked, sometimes combined with marijuana or cocaine. Low doses cause euphoria or dysphoria and a sense of numbness; higher doses cause sensory distortions, hallucinations, paranoia, agitation, psychosis, hypertension, nystagmus, myoglobinuria, respiratory depression, and shock.[139] Mental symptoms can last for days, and hypertension can occur either acutely or after a delay of days. Addiction occurs, but there is little evidence of physical dependence.[1]

Evidence for Stroke Risk

Anecdotal reports of stroke in PCP users are few, but they are plausible as to causality, especially in view of PCP's cardiovascular effects. A 13-year-old boy became comatose with normal blood pressure after taking PCP; 3 days later, although he was more alert, blood pressure rose to 220/130 mmHg, and he suffered a fatal cerebral hemorrhage.[140] A 6-year-old boy developed seizures and parieto-occipital lucency on CT; his urine contained PCP.[141] Subarachnoid hemorrhage has followed PCP smoking.[13,142,143] In one case, a 17-year-old boy died following perforation of his basilar artery.[142] Single photon emission computed tomography (SPECT) studies on PCP users revealed asymmetric perfusion abnormalities in the cerebral cortex; each subject had used other drugs, however, including ethanol and cocaine.[144]

PCP-induced hypertension might be related to enhancement of catecholamine or serotonin action.[145] In vitro studies, however, suggest direct contractile responses of cerebral vessels to PCP.[146]

LSD

Background

Taken orally, the synthetic ergot lysergic acid diethylamide (LSD) causes sensory distortions and hallucinations (especially visual and formed), derealization, depersonalization, ataxia, tremor, tachycardia, and hypertension. Adverse reactions consist of paranoia or panic, which can result in fatal accidents or suicide, and very high doses cause severe hypertension, obtundation, and seizures. Withdrawal symptoms do not occur. LSD (and other hallucinogenic indolealkylamines) act through serotonergic pathways, but their precise mechanism of action is uncertain.[1]

Evidence for Stroke Risk

As with phencyclidine, evidence that LSD can cause stroke is limited to a few case reports, but the drug's cardiovascular effects make causality plausible. A 14-year-old boy had seizures after ingesting LSD, and 4 days later he developed hemiplegia; carotid angiography showed progressive narrowing of the internal carotid artery from its origin to the siphon, with occlusion at its bifurcation.[147] A young woman developed hemiplegia a day after ingesting LSD; angiography showed marked narrowing of the internal carotid artery at the siphon, which 9 days later was occluded.[148] A 19-year-old with acute aphasia and cerebral angiographic findings of segmental arterial narrowing had used both LSD and heroin.[149] Another patient with similar angiographic findings had used both LSD and "diet pills."[40]

Cerebral vessel strips immersed in solution containing LSD develop spasm; the effect is prevented or reversed by methysergide.[146]

CANNABIS

Background

The hemp plant, *Cannabis sativa*, contains numerous cannabinoid compounds, of which Δ-9-tetrahydrocannabinol (Δ-9-THC) is responsible for the desired psychic effects, acting at cannabinoid receptors in the brain. Marijuana, from leaves and flowers of the plant, is smoked or eaten. Hashish, made from the resin covering the leaves and flowers, has a higher concentration of Δ-9-THC. In addition to producing dreamy euphoria, marijuana impairs judgement, memory, and coordination and causes tachycardia, increased systolic blood pressure, and postural hypotension. Adverse effects include paranoia or panic, and high doses produce hallucinations, psychosis, bradycardia, and hypotension, but fatal overdose has not been documented. Withdrawal symptoms and signs are usually mild—jitteriness, headache, anorexia, and tremor.[1]

Evidence for Stroke Risk

Marijuana is the most widely used illicit drug in the United States, and it is therefore not surprising that occlusive stroke affects some users. In some case reports, causality is doubtful.[150–152] Other reports are more persuasive. While smoking marijuana, two young men developed hemiparesis, and CT confirmed cerebral infarction.[153] Another young marijuana smoker had TIAs followed by hemiparesis and aphasia, and CT showed a striatocapsular infarct.[154] Systemic hypotension and cerebral vasospasm might account for marijuana-induced stroke, but neither has been documented in clinical reports. In rats, delta-9-THC has vasoconstrictor actions on systemic vessels.[155] In humans, marijuana has unpredictable effects on cerebral blood flow, either increasing or decreasing it.[156]

SEDATIVES

Background

Usually abused orally, sedatives/tranquilizers in overdose cause coma and respiratory depression, and withdrawal symptoms, as with ethanol, include tremor, hallucinosis, and delirium tremens.[1]

Evidence for Stroke Risk

Brain or spinal cord infarction can follow shock accompanying sedative overdose, but occlusive or hemorrhagic stroke has not otherwise been documented. In rare reports of angiographic "vasculitis" affecting barbiturate users, other drugs were used as well.[40]

INHALANTS

Background

A large number of household and industrial products—including aerosols, cleansers, glues, lighter fluid, paints, paint thinners, gasoline, volatile anesthetics, and nitrites—produce euphoria-inducing vapors, and they are widely abused in the United States, especially by children, who inhale the vapors from a plastic bag, pan, or soaked rag. Effects are similar to those produced by ethanol, and inhalants are addicting, but physical dependence is not evident. Death can be the result of asphyxiation, aspiration, cardiac arrhythmia, or accidents.[1]

Evidence for Stroke Risk

A 12-year-old glue sniffer developed hemiplegia after a period of inhalation, and angiography showed occlusion of the middle cerebral artery. A proposed mechanism was vasospasm secondary to trichlorethylene-induced sensitization of catecholamine receptors on brain vessels.[157] Radioisotope brain scan in a boy with status epilepticus after toluene sniffing showed wedge-shaped areas of increased uptake in both cerebral hemispheres, consistent with infarction.[158]

ETHANOL

Background

In the United States, roughly two-thirds of adults drink alcoholic beverages, half infrequently and half with some regularity. How many regular drinkers should be considered "alcoholic" is difficult to say, for the term is not consistently defined. If "alcoholism" includes not only those who are psychically or physically dependent on ethanol but also those who periodically drink excessively with harmful consequences, then nearly 7 percent of American adults and 19 percent of American adolescents are alcoholic.[1]

Evidence for Stroke Risk

There is good evidence that mild-to-moderate intake of ethanol reduces the risk of coronary artery disease, whereas heavy intake increases it.[159] Myocardial infarction, by causing cardiac hypokinesia or arrhythmia, is a risk factor for cardioembolic stroke. In addition, ethanol intoxication and withdrawal are associated with cardiac arrhythmia ("holiday heart"), and alcoholic cardiomyopathy frequently results in cardioembolism.[160]

A large amount of literature addresses whether ethanol increases the risk of stroke independently of cardiac disease or other risk factors. In contrast to studies of stroke and illicit drugs, which consist largely of anecdotal case reports and case series, the literature on ethanol and stroke consists of numerous case-control and cohort studies (i.e., epidemiologic evidence).

Retrospective studies from Finland, using population prevalence data as controls, described an association between recent heavy ethanol use and both occlusive and hemorrhagic stroke.[161,162] Other similarly designed analyses found no such association,[163] an association that disappeared when corrected for tobacco,[164] or an association only for intracerebral hemorrhage.[165]

Not surprisingly, studies addressing the relationship of stroke to chronic ethanol use have differed in endpoint (e.g., total stroke, occlusive or hemorrhagic stroke, or stroke mortality), amount and duration of ethanol consumption, correction for other risk factors (especially hypertension and tobacco), ethnicity and socioeconomics, and selection of controls. Case-control studies have found low doses of ethanol protective against both ischemic stroke and intracerebral hemorrhage,[166] no protective effect when corrected for obesity and exercise,[167] no risk when corrected for hypertension, diabetes, obesity, and hyperlipidemia,[168] and increased risk from moderate drinking of "spirits," reduced risk from moderate drinking of wine, and no effect from moderate drinking of beer.[169]

Among cohort studies, the Yugoslavia Cardiovascular Disease Study found increased stroke mortality among drinkers overall but reduced risk for modest drinkers.[170] The Honolulu Heart Study found an increased risk for hemorrhagic stroke in heavy drinkers but no increased risk for occlusive stroke.[171,172] The Framingham Study found lower than expected stroke incidence among "moderate" drinkers and higher incidence among both heavy drinkers and nondrinkers.[173] In the Nurses' Health Study, there was an inverse association between modest ethanol intake and occlusive stroke, with a positive association at higher intake, and both low and high intake increased the risk for subarachnoid hemorrhage.[174] In the Lausanne Stroke Registry, severity of internal carotid artery stenosis inversely correlated with "light-to-moderate" ethanol intake; there were too few patients to assess heavy intake.[175] Different Japanese studies found either no independent association between ethanol and occlusive or hemorrhagic stroke[176]; reduced risk of cerebral infarction in light drinkers and increased risk of cerebral hemorrhage in heavy drinkers with hypertension[177]; positive association between drinking and hemorrhagic but not occlusive stroke[178]; and a "J-shaped relationship" between ethanol intake and occlusive stroke. Drinkers of less than 42

g/day ethanol had a lower risk than nondrinkers, but heavier drinkers had a higher risk.[179]

A review of 62 epidemiologic studies that examined the relation between stroke and "moderate" ethanol consumption (less than 2 drinks, or 1 oz. of absolute ethanol) found that ethnicity influenced results.[180] Among whites, moderate doses of ethanol were protective against ischemic stroke, whereas higher doses increased risk. Among Japanese, there was little association between ethanol and ischemic stroke. In both populations, any dose of ethanol increased the risk of both intracerebral and subarachnoid hemorrhage.

Ultrasound and angiographic studies have found positive association between heavy drinking and carotid atherosclerosis, with mild drinking lowering the risk.[181] A CT study found that leukoaraiosis correlated positively with heavy drinking and inversely with mild drinking,[182] and a Japanese study found ethanol an independent risk factor for "vascular dementia."[183]

Several mechanisms underlie the positive and negative associations between ethanol and stroke. Acutely and chronically, ethanol raises blood pressure,[184–186] perhaps related to increased adrenergic activity and increased blood levels of cortisol, aldosterone, renin, and vasopressin.[187] With abstinence, blood pressure may become normal.

Ethanol lowers blood levels of low-density lipoproteins and raises levels of high-density lipoproteins (although not necessarily of the more protective HDL-2 subfraction).[188,189] Ethanol preferentially protects large vessels from atherosclerosis, perhaps accounting for ethnic differences in patterns of risk.[190]

In different studies, ethanol decreased fibrinolytic activity, increased factor VII levels, increased platelet reactivity to ADP,[71,191] shortened bleeding time, increased endogenous tissue plasminogen activator,[192] decreased plasma fibrinogen levels,[193] increased blood prostacyclin levels,[194] decreased platelet function,[195] and stimulated release of endothelin from endothelial cells.[196] Ethanol-induced liver disease has its own effects on clotting.[187] During withdrawal, rebound "thrombostasis" and platelet hyperaggregability are observed,[197] and dehydration leads to hemoconcentration.[187] Acute ethanol intoxication produces cerebral vasodilatation,[198] and increased cerebral blood flow has been described during withdrawal.[199] By contrast, animal and in vitro studies show that ethanol constricts cerebral arterial strips and brain arterioles.[200] Ethanol depletes magnesium ion from cultured canine vascular smooth muscle cells, and pretreatment of animals with magnesium ion prevents ethanol-induced stroke.[201]

TOBACCO

Background

In the United States each year, tobacco is responsible for roughly 450,000 premature deaths, more than 20 percent of all mortality. The addictive substance is nicotine, which, along with carbon monoxide, is also a major contributor to heart disease in smokers. The "tar" in cigarette smoke contains numerous other chemicals, some of which are responsible for tobacco-induced cancer. Psychic dependence on tobacco is powerful; following withdrawal, some smokers describe nausea, fatigue, irritability, or insomnia, but in most there is little evidence of physical dependence.[1]

Evidence for Stroke Risk

Some tobacco-related diseases are themselves risk factors for stroke. Coronary artery disease predisposes to cardioembolism, and lung cancer can cause hypercoagulability and nonbacterial thrombotic endocarditis. As with ethanol, case-control and cohort studies demonstrate that tobacco is also a direct risk for both occlusive and hemorrhagic stroke.[70,71,164,202–206] In women, this risk is greater in those also taking oral contraceptives. In a cohort study, the risk increased in a dose-dependent fashion; for those smoking more than 25 cigarettes daily, the relative risk for stroke was 3.7 and for subarachnoid hemorrhage 9.8, independent of other risk factors including hypertension, ethanol, and oral contraceptives.[207] In another cohort study, smoking increased the risk of occlusive and hemorrhagic stroke independent of coronary artery disease.[208] Several studies found that stroke risk declines with cessation of smoking.[209] One study found that for subarachnoid hemorrhage, maximal stroke risk occurred within 3 h of smoking a cigarette.[210]

Multifocal symptoms developed in four young women who smoked and used oral contraceptives; cerebral angiography showed moyamoya, and abnormal ESR, antinuclear antibodies, and CSF IgG suggested an immunologic basis. No new symptoms occurred after reduction in smoking and discontinuation of oral contraceptives.[211]

Cigarette smoking correlates with MRI periventricular signal abnormalities (equivalent to CT leukoaraiosis) independently of hypertension and age.[212]

Stroke was reported following application of a nicotine patch.[213]

Smoking aggravates atherosclerosis.[214,215] Nicotine damages endothelium, and circulating endothelial cells increase after smoking.[216] Acutely, smoking raises blood pressure and causes tachycardia.[217] Chronically, it accelerates the progression of hypertension to malignant hypertension.[218] Smoking increases platelet reactivity,[219] inhibits prostacyclin formation,[220] raises blood fibrinogen levels,[221] causes secondary polycythemia,[222] and increases levels of F_2-isoprostones in the circulation, suggesting oxidative damage by free radicals.[223]

THERAPEUTIC RECOMMENDATIONS

1. Substance abuse in a stroke patient, licit or illicit, does not in itself alter management. Controversial treatment decisions such as thrombolytic therapy, anticoagulation for embolic stroke, or the timing of antihypertensive therapy are based on the same considerations whether the patient is or is not an alcoholic, a heroin addict, a middle-aged "crack" smoker, or an adolescent taking over-the-counter "diet" pills. Thrombolytics and anticoagulants are contraindicated in patients with infective endocarditis.

2. Withdrawal symptoms and signs must be anticipated. Abstinence syndromes of ethanol and sedative drugs can be fatal in their own right, and the presence of agitation, seizures, or autonomic instability should obviously be avoided in someone with an ischemic or hemorrhagic stroke, especially subarachnoid hemorrhage. Appropriate treatment includes titrated doses of benzodiazopines. Although opioid withdrawal is less dangerous, agitation can be considerable, and diarrhea and vomiting can lead to hypovolemia or aspiration. Prevention and treatment are quite simple with methadone. Cocaine, amphetamine, and other psychostimulants produce little in the way of objective withdrawal signs, but depression—already present in many stroke patients—calls for early identification and appropriate intervention. With other classes of abused drugs (tobacco, marijuana, hallucinogens, inhalants, or phencyclidine), withdrawal symptoms are unlikely to be a problem.

3. Less often a problem is continuing intoxication, but some drugs—for example, ethanol, some sedatives, some opioids, and phencyclidine—are pharmacologically active for many hours, producing symptoms that can mask another diagnosis. All-too-familiar in emergency rooms is the patient inebriated from ethanol who hours later turns out to have meningitis, a subdural hematoma, or a stroke.

4. Substance abuse in a stroke patient might dictate diagnostic measures. If the result were to influence treatment, cerebral angiography would be indicated in a patient with endocarditis and either occlusive or hemorrhagic stroke. MR angiography, conventional angiography, or both should be seriously considered in a cocaine user with intracranial hemorrhage.

5. Although some amphetamine-related strokes (and possibly some heroin- and cocaine-related strokes) are vasculitic in origin, angiographic "beading" is nonspecific. Many patients with cerebral vasculitis do not have "beading," and there are no data on immunosuppressant therapy, including corticosteroids, in such patients. Immunosuppressant treatment is therefore not indicated.

6. Substance abuse treatment is part of the long-term management of any substance-abusing stroke patient. This includes ethanol and tobacco.

REFERENCES

1. Brust JCM: *Neurological Aspects of Substance Abuse.* Boston, Butterworth-Heinemann, 1993.
2. Brust JCM, Dickinson PCT, Hughes JEO, Holtzman RNN: The diagnosis and treatment of cerebral mycotic aneurysms. *Ann Neurol* 27:238, 1990.
3. Gattell JM, Miro JM, Pare C, et al: Infective endocarditis in drug addicts. *Lancet* 1:228, 1984.
4. Brust JCM: AIDS and stroke, in Welch KMA, Caplan LR, Reis DJ, Siesjo BK, Weir B (eds): *Primer on Cerebrovascular Diseases.* San Diego, Academic Press, 1997, p 423.
5. Pinto AN: AIDS and cerebrovascular disease. *Stroke* 27:538, 1996.
6. Brust JCM, Richter RW: Stroke associated with addiction to heroin. *J Neurol Neurosurg Psychiatry* 39:194, 1976.
7. Lignelli GJ, Buchheit WA: Angiitis in drug abusers. *N Engl J Med* 284:112, 1971
8. Woods BT, Strewler GJ: Hemiparesis occurring six hours after intravenous heroin injection. *Neurology* 22:863, 1972.
9. Jensen R, Olsen TS, Winther BB: Severe non-occlusive ischemic stroke in young heroin addicts. *Acta Neurol Scand* 81:354, 1990.
10. Bartolomei F, Nicoli F, Swiader L, Gastaut JL: Accident vasculaire cérébral ischémic apres prise nasale d'héroine. *Presse Med* 21:983, 1992.
11. Herskowitz A, Gross E: Cerebral infarction associated with heroin sniffing. *South Med J* 66:778, 1973.
12. Knoblauch AL, Buchholz M, Koller MG, Kistler H:
13. Sloan MS, Kittner SJ, Rigamonti D, Price TR: Occurrence of stroke associated with use/abuse of drugs. *Neurology* 41:1358, 1991.
14. Caplan LR, Hier DB, Banks G: Stroke and drug abuse. *Stroke* 13:869, 1982.
15. Levine LH, Hirsch CS, White LW: Quinine cardiotoxicity: A mechanism for sudden death in narcotic addicts. *J Forensic Sci* 18:167, 1973.
16. Atlee W: Talc and cornstarch emboli in eyes of drug abusers. *JAMA* 219:49, 1972.
17. Mizutami T, Lewis R, Gonatas N: Medial medullary syndrome in a drug abuser. *Arch Neurol* 37:425, 1980.
18. Sapira JD: The narcotic addict as a medical patient. *Am J Med* 45:555, 1968.
19. Caplan LR, Thomas C, Banks G: Central nervous system complications of addiction to "T's and Blues." *Neurology* 32:623, 1982.
20. Butz WC: Disseminated magnesium and silicate associated with paregoric addiction. *J Forensic Sci* 15:58, 1970.
21. Lee J, Sapira JD: Retinal and cerebral microembolization of talc in a drug abuser. *Am J Med* 265:75, 1973.
22. Biter S, Gomez CR: Stroke following injection of a melted suppository. *Stroke* 24:74, 1993.
23. Pearson J, Richter RW, Baden MM, et al: Tranverse myelopathy as an illustration of the neurologic and neuropathologic features of heroin addiction. *Hum Pathol* 3:109, 1972.
24. Judice DJ, LeBlanc HJ, McGarry PA: Spinal cord vasculitis presenting as spinal cord tumor in a heroin addict. *J Neurosurg* 48:13, 1978.
25. Cahill DW, Knipp H, Mosser J: Intracranial hemorrhage with amphetamine abuse. *Neurology* 31:1058, 1981.
26. Delaney P, Estes M: Intracranial hemorrhage with amphetamine abuse. *Neurology* 30:1125, 1980.
27. D'Souza T, Shraberg D: Intracranial hemorrhage associated with amphetamine use. *Neurology* 31:922, 1981.
28. Gericke OL: Suicide by ingestion of amphetamine sulfate. *JAMA* 128:1125, 1980.
29. Harrington H, Heller HA, Dawson D, et al: Intracerebral hemorrhage and oral amphetamine. *Arch Neurol* 40:503, 1983.
30. Lukes SA: Intracerebral hemorrhage from an arteriovenous malformation after amphetamine injection. *Arch Neurol* 40:60, 1983.
31. Matick H, Anderson D, Brumlik J: Cerebral vasculitis associated with oral amphetamine overdose. *Arch Neurol* 40:253, 1983.
32. Salanova V, Taubner R: Intracerebral hemorrhage and vasculitis secondary to amphetamine use. *Postgrad Med J* 60:429, 1984.
33. Shukla D: Intracranial hemorrhage associated with amphetamine use. *Neurology* 32: 917, 1982.
34. Yu YJ, Cooper DR, Wallenstein DE, et al: Cerebral angi-

Hemiplegie nach Injektion von Heroin. *Schweiz Med Wochenschr* 113:402, 1983.

itis and intracerebral hemorrhage associated with meth-amphetamine abuse. *J Neurosurg* 58:1009, 1983.

35. Imanse J, Vanneste J: Intraventricular hemorrhage following amphetamine abuse. *Neurology* 40:1318, 1990.

36. Citron BP, Halpern M, McCarron M, et al: Necrotizing angiitis associated with drug abuse. *N Engl J Med* 283:1003, 1970.

37. Citron BP, Peters RL: Angiitis in drug abusers. *N Engl J Med* 284:112, 1971.

38. Kessler JT, Jortner BS, Adapon BD: Cerebral vasculitis in a drug abuser. *J Clin Psychiatry* 39:559, 1978.

39. Bostwick DG: Amphetamine induced cerebral vasculitis. *Hum Pathol* 12:1031, 1981.

40. Rumbaugh CL, Bergeron RT, Fang HHC, et al: Cerebral angiographic changes in the drug abuse patient. *Radiology* 101:335, 1971.

41. Rothrock JF, Rubenstein R, Lyden PD: Ischemic stroke associated with methamphetamine inhalation. *Neurology* 38:589, 1988.

42. Sachdeva K, Woodward KG: Caudal thalamic infarction following intranasal methamphetamine use. *Neurology* 39:305, 1989.

43. Rumbaugh CL, Bergeron T, Scanlon RL, et al: Cerebral vascular changes secondary to amphetamine abuse in the experimental animal. *Radiology* 101:345, 1971.

44. Rumbaugh CL, Fang HCH, Higgins RE, et al: Cerebral microvascular injury in experimental drug abuse. *Invest Radiol* 11:282, 1976.

45. Brust JCM: Vasculitis owing to substance abuse. *Neurol Clin* 15:945, 1997.

46. Stafford CR, Bogdanoff BM, Green L, et al: Mononeuropathy multiplex as a complication of amphetamine angiitis. *Neurology* 25:570, 1975.

47. Forman HP, Levin S, Stewart B, et al: Cerebral vasculitis and hemorrhage in an adolescent taking diet pills containing phenylpropanolamine: Case report and review of the literature. *Pediatrics* 83:737, 1989.

48. Kase CS, Foster TE, Reed JE, et al: Intracebral hemorrhage and phenylpropanolamine use. *Neurology* 37:399, 1987.

49. Kikta DG, Devereaux MW, Chandar K: Intracranial hemorrhages due to phenylpropanolamine. *Stroke* 16:510, 1985.

50. Maertens P, Lum G, Williams JP, et al: Intracerebral hemorrhage and cerebral angiopathic changes in a suicidal phenylpropanolamine poisoning. *South Med J* 80:1584, 1987.

51. Stoessl AJ, Young GB, Feasby TE: Intracerebral hemorrhage and angiographic beading following ingestion of catecholaminergics. *Stroke* 16:734, 1985.

52. Fallis RJ, Fisher M: Cerebral vasculitis and hemorrhage associated with phenylpropanolamine. *Neurology* 35:405, 1985.

53. Ryu SJ, Lin SK: Cerebral arteritis associated with oral use of phenylpropanolamine: Report of a case. *J Formos Med Assoc* 94:53, 1995.

54. Mueller SM, Ertel PJ: Subarachnoid hemorrhage associated with over-the-counter diet medications. *Stroke* 14:16, 1983.

55. Garcia-Albea E: Subarachnoid hemorrhage and nasal vasoconstrictor abuse. *J Neurol Neurosurg Psychiatry* 46:875, 1983.

56. Mariani PJ: Pseudoephedrine-induced hypertensive emergency: Treatment with labetalol. *Am J Emerg Med* 4:141, 1986.

57. Wooten MR, Khangure MS, Murphy MJ: Intracerebral hemorrhage and vasculitis related to ephedrine abuse. *Ann Neurol* 13:337, 1983.

58. Loizou LA, Hamilton JG, Tsementzis SA: Intracranial hemorrhage in association with pseudoephedrine overdose. *J Neurol Neurosurg Psychiatry* 45:471, 1982.

59. Cockings JG, Brown M: Ephedrine abuse causing acute myocardial infarction. *Med J Aust* 167:199, 1997.

60. Chillar RK, Jackson AL: Reversible hemiplegia after presumed intracarotid injection of Ritalin. *N Engl J Med* 304:1305, 1981.

61. Tse DT, Ober RR: Talc retinopathy. *Am J Ophthalmol* 90:624, 1980.

62. Trugman JM: Cerebral arteritis and oral methylphenidate. *Lancet* 1:584, 1988.

63. Hamer R, Phelp D: Inadvertent intra-arterial injection of phentermine: A complication of drug abuse. *Ann Emerg Med* 10:148, 1981.

64. Kokkinos J, Levine SR: Possible association of ischemic stroke with phentermine. *Stroke* 24:310, 1993.

65. Connolly HM, Crary JL, McGoon MD, et al: Valvular heart disease associated with fenfluramine-phentermine. *N Engl J Med* 337:581, 1997.

66. Manchanda S, Connolly MJ: Cerebral infarction in association with Ecstasy abuse. *Postgrad Med J* 69:874, 1993.

67. Grobbee DE, Rimm EB, Giovannucci E, et al: Coffee, caffeine, and cardiovascular disease. *N Engl J Med* 323:1026, 1990.

68. Sutherland GR, Peeling J, Lesiuk HJ, et al: The effects of caffeine on ischemic neuronal injury as determined by magnetic resonance imaging and histopathology. *Neuroscience* 42:171, 1991.

69. Qureshi AI, Akbar MS, Czander E, et al: Crack cocaine use and stroke in young patients. *Neurology* 48:341, 1997.

70. Brust JCM: Drug dependence, in Joynt RJ, Griggs RC (eds): *Baker's Clinical Neurology,* vol 2. Philadelphia, Lippincott-Raven, 1998, pp 1–121.

71. Brust JCM: Stroke and substance abuse, in Barnett HJM, Mohr JP, Yatsu FM, Stein BM (eds): *Stroke, Pathophysiology, Diagnosis, and Management* 3rd ed. Philadelphia, Saunders, 1998, pp 979–1000.

72. Sloan MA, Kittner SJ, Feeser BR, et al: Illicit drug-associated ischemic stroke in the Baltimore-Washington Stroke Study. *Neurology* 50:1688, 1998.

73. Tuchman AJ, Marks S, Daras M: Recurring strokes with repeated cocaine use. *Cerebrovasc Dis* 2:369, 1992.

74. Samkoff LM, Daras M, Kleiman AR, Koppell BS: Sponta-

neous spinal epidural hematoma: Another neurologic complication of cocaine? *Arch Neurol* 53:819, 1996.

75. Daras M, Tuchman AJ, Koppell BS, et al: Neurovascular complications of cocaine. *Acta Neurol Scand* 90:124, 1994.

76. Martinez N, Diaz-Tjedor E, Frank A: Vasospasm/thrombus in cerebral ischemia related to cocaine abuse. *Stroke* 27:148, 1996.

77. Konzen J, Levine S, Garcia J: Vasospasm and thrombus formation as possible mechanism of stroke related to alkaloidal cocaine. *Stroke* 26:114, 1995.

78. Aggarwal S, Williams V, Levine SR, et al: Cocaine associated intracranial hemorrhage: Absence of vasculitis in fourteen cases. *Neurology* (in press)

79. Kibayashi K, Mastri AR, Hirsch CS: Cocaine induced intracerebral hemorrhage: An analysis of predisposing factors and mechanisms causing hemorrhagic stroke. *Hum Pathol* 26:659, 1995.

80. Martin K, Rogers T, Kavanaugh A: Central nervous system angiopathy associated with cocaine abuse. *J Rheumatol* 22:780, 1995.

81. Berger JR, Romano J, Menkin M, et al: Benign focal cerebral vasculitis: Case report. *Neurology* 45:1731, 1995.

82. Reeves RR, McWilliams ME, Fitzgerald MJ: Cocaine-induced ischemic cerebral infarction mistaken for a psychiatric syndrome. *South Med J* 88:352, 1995.

83. Fessler RD, Esshaki CM, Stankewitz RC, et al: The neurovascular complications of cocaine. *Surg Neurol* 47:339, 1997.

84. DiLazzaro V, Restuccia D, Oliviero A, et al: Ischemic myelopathy associated with cocaine: Clinical, neurophysiological, and neuroradiological features. *J Neurol Neurosurg Psychiatry* 63:531, 1997.

85. Egido-Herrero JA, Gonzalez JL: Pontine hemorrhage after abuse of cocaine. *Rev Neurol* 25:137, 1997.

86. Nolte KB, Brass LM, Fletterick CF: Intracranial hemorrhage associated with cocaine abuse: A prospective autopsy study. *Neurology* 46:1291, 1996.

87. Baquero M, Alfaro A: Progressive bleeding in spontaneous thalamic hemorrhage. *Neurologia* 9:364, 1994.

88. Casas Perera I, Gatto E, Fernandez Pardal MM, et al: Complicaciones neurologicas por abuso de cocaina. *Medicina* 54:35, 1994.

89. Diaz-Calderone, A, Del Brutto O, Aguirre R, et al: Bilateral internuclear ophthalmoplegia after smoking "crack" cocaine. *J Neuroophthalmol* 11:297, 1991.

90. Peterson PL, Rozzler M, Jacobs I, Wilner HI: Neurovascular complications of cocaine abuse. *J Neuropsychiatr* 3:143, 1991.

91. Daras M, Tuchman AJ, Marks S: Central nervous system infarction related to cocaine abuse. *Stroke* 22:1320, 1991.

92. Brust JCM, Richter RW: Stroke associated with cocaine abuse? *NY State J Med* 77:1473, 1977.

93. Devenyi P, Schneiderman JF, Devenyi RG, et al: Cocaine-induced central retinal artery occlusion. *Can Med Assoc J* 138:129, 1988.

94. Rowley HA, Lowenstein DH, Rowbothan MC, et al:

95. Levine SR, Brust JCM, Futrell N, et al: Cerebrovascular complications of the use of the "crack" form of alkaloidal cocaine. *N Engl J Med* 323:69, 1990.

96. Hoyme HE, Jones KL, Dixon SD, et al: Prenatal cocaine exposure and fetal vascular disruption. *Pediatrics* 85:743, 1990.

97. Dixon SD, Bejar R: Echoencephalographic findings in neonates associated with maternal cocaine and methamphetamine use: Incidence and clinical correlates. *J Pediatr* 115:770, 1989.

98. Golbe LI, Merkin MD: Cerebral infarction in a user of free-base cocaine ("crack") *Neurology* 36:1602, 1986.

99. Kaye BR, Feinstat M: Cerebral vasculitis associated with cocaine abuse. *JAMA* 258:2104, 1987.

100. Levine SR, Welch KMA, Brust JCM: Cerebral vasculitis associated with cocaine abuse or subarachnoid hemorrhage? *JAMA* 259:1648, 1988.

101. Fredericks RK, Lefkowitz DS, Challa VER, et al: Cerebral vasculitis associated with cocaine abuse. *Stroke* 22:1437, 1991.

102. Krendel DA, Ditter SM, Frankel MR, et al: Biopsy-proven cerebral vasculitis associated with cocaine abuse. *Neurology* 40:1092, 1990.

103. Case Records of the Massachusetts General Hospital: Cocaine vasculitis. *N Engl J Med* 329:117, 1993.

104. Morrow PL, McQuillan JB: Cerebral vasculitis associated with cocaine abuse. *J Forensic Sci* 38:732, 1993.

105. Lowenstein DH, Massa SM, Rowbotham MC, et al: Acute neurologic and psychiatric complications associated with cocaine abuse. *Am J Med* 83:841, 1987.

106. Cregler LL, Mark H: Relation of stroke to cocaine abuse. *NY State J Med* 87:128, 1987.

107. Lehman LB: Intracerebral hemorrhage after intranasal cocaine use. *Hosp Physician* 7:69, 1987.

108. Lichtenfield PJ, Rubin DB, Feldman RS: Subarachnoid hemorrhage precipitated by cocaine snorting. *Arch Neurol* 41:223, 1984.

109. Lundberg GD, Garriott JC, Reynolds PC: Cocaine-related death. *J Forensic Sci* 22:402, 1977.

110. Nails G, Disher A, Daryabagi J, et al: Subcortical cerebral hemorrhages associated with cocaine abuse: CT and MR findings. *J Comput Assist Tomogr* 13:1, 1989.

111. Peterson PL, Moore PM: Hemorrhagic cerebrovascular complications of crack cocaine abuse. *Neurology* 39 (Suppl 1):302, 1989.

112. Schwartz KA, Cohen JA: Subarachnoid hemorrhage precipitated by cocaine snorting. *Arch Neurol* 41:705, 1984.

113. Mody CK, Miller BL, McIntyre HB, et al: Neurologic complications of cocaine abuse. *Neurology* 38:1189, 1988.

114. Mangiardi JR, Daras M, Gellet ME, et al: Cocaine-related intracranial hemorrhage: Report of nine cases and reviews. *Acta Neurol Scand* 77:177, 1988.

115. Wojak JC, Flamm ES: Intracranial hemorrhage and cocaine use. *Stroke* 18:712, 1987.

116. Spires MC, Gordon EF, Choudhuri M, et al: Intracranial hemorrhage in a neonate following prenatal cocaine exposure. *Pediatr Neurol* 5:324, 1989.

117. Henderson CE, Torbey M: Rupture of intracranial aneurysm associated with cocaine use during pregnancy. *Am J Perinatol* 5:142, 1988.

118. Mast J, Carpanzano CR, Hier L: Maternal cocaine use: Neurologic effects on the offspring. *Neurology* 39 (Suppl 1):187, 1989.

119. Mercado A, Johnson G, Calver D, et al: Cocaine, pregnancy, and postpartum intracerebral hemorrhage. *Obstet Gynecol* 73:467, 1989.

120. Green R, Kelly KM, Gabrielson T, et al: Multiple intracerebral hemorrhages after smoking "crack" cocaine. *Stroke* 21:957, 1990.

121. Keller TM, Chappell ET: Spontaneous acute subdural hematoma precipitated by cocaine abuse: Case report. *Surg Neurol* 47:12, 1997.

122. Levine SR, Brust JCM, Futrell N, et al: A comparative study of the cerebrovascular complications of cocaine: Alkaloidal vs. hydrochloride. A review. *Neurology* 41:1173, 1991.

123. Konzen JP, Levine SR, Charbel FT, Garcia JH: The mechanisms of alkaloidal cocaine-related stroke. *Neurology* 42 (Suppl 3):249, 1992.

124. Libman RB, Masters SR, dePaola A, et al: Transient monocular blindness associated with cocaine abuse. *Neurology* 43:228, 1993.

125. Fayad PB, Price LH, McDougle CJ, et al: Acute hemodynamic effects of intranasal cocaine on the cerebral and cardiovascular systems. *Stroke* 23:26, 1992.

126. Powers RH, Madden JA: Vasoconstrictive effects of cocaine metabolites and structural analogs on rat cerebral arteries. *FASEB J* 4:A1095, 1990.

127. Togna G, Tempesta E, Togna AR, et al: Platelet responsiveness and biosynthesis of thromboxane and prostacyclin in response to in vitro cocaine treatment. *Hemostasis* 15:100, 1985.

128. Zurbano MJ, Heras M, Rigol M, et al: Cocaine administration enhances platelet reactivity to subendothelial components: Studies in a pig model. *Eur J Clin Invest* 27:116, 1997.

129. Langner RO, Bement CL, Perry LE: Arteriosclerotic toxicity of cocaine. *NIDA Res Monogr* 88:325, 1987.

130. Toler KA, Anderson B: Stroke in an intravenous drug user secondary to lupus anticoagulant. *Stroke* 19:274, 1988.

131. Weinreib RM, O'Brien CP: Persistent cognitive deficits attributed to substance abuse. *Neurol Clin* 11:663, 1993.

132. Pascual-Leone A, Dhuna A, Anderson DC: Cerebral atrophy in habitual cocaine abusers: A planimetric CT study. *Neurology* 41:34, 1991.

133. Holman BL, Carvalho PA, Mendelson J, et al: Brain perfusion is abnormal in cocaine-dependent polydrug users: A study using technetium-99m-HMPAO and ASPECT. *J Nucl Med* 32:1206, 1991.

134. Strickland TL, Stein R: Cocaine-induced cerebrovascular impairment: Challenges to neuropsychological assessment. *Neuropsychol Rev* 5:69, 1995.

135. Chiriboga CA, Bateman D, Brust JCM, et al: Neurologic findings in cocaine-exposed infants. *Pediatr Neurol* 9:115, 1993.

136. Chiriboga CA, Vibbert M, Malouf R, et al: Neurological correlates in high risk infants with cocaine positive urine toxicology: Transient hypertonia of infancy and in early childhood. *Pediatrics* 96:1070, 1995.

137. Hier LA, Carpanzano CR, Mast J, et al: Maternal cocaine abuse: The spectrum of radiologic abnormalities in the neonatal CNS. *Am J Radiol* 157:1105, 1991.

138. Volpe BJ: Effect of cocaine use on the fetus. *N Engl J Med* 327:399, 1992.

139. McCarron MM, Schultze BW, Thompson CA, et al: Acute phencyclidine intoxication: Incidence of clinical findings in 1000 cases. *Ann Emerg Med* 10:237, 1981.

140. Eastman JW, Cohen SN: Hypertensive crises and death associated with phencyclidine poisoning. *JAMA* 231:1270, 1975.

141. Crosley CJ, Binet EP: Cerebrovascular complications in phencyclidine intoxication. *J Pediatr* 94:316, 1979.

142. Boyko OB, Burger PC, Heinz ER: Pathological and radiological correlation of subarachnoid hemorrhage in phencyclidine abuse: A case report. *J Neurosurg* 67:446, 1987.

143. Besson HA: Intracranial hemorrhage associated with phencyclidine abuse. *JAMA* 248:585, 1982.

144. Hertzman M, Reba RC, Kotyarov EV: Single photon emission computed tomography in phencyclidine and related drug abuse. *Am J Psychiatry* 147:255, 1990.

145. Illet KF, Jarrott B, O'Donnell SR, et al: Mechanism of cardiovascular actions of 1(phenylcyclohexyl)-piperidine hydrochloride (phencyclidine). *Br J Pharmacol* 28:73, 1966.

146. Altura B, Altura BM: Phencyclidine, lysergic acid diethylamide, and mescaline: Cerebral artery spasms and hallucinogenic activity. *Science* 212:1051, 1981.

147. Sobel J, Espinas OE, Friedman SA: Carotid artery obstruction following LSD capsule ingestion. *Arch Intern Med* 127:290, 1971.

148. Lieberman AN, Bloom W, Kishore PS, et al: Carotid artery occlusion following ingestion of LSD. *Stroke* 5:213, 1974.

149. Lignelli GJ, Buchheit WA: Angiitis in drug abusers. *N Engl J Med* 284:112, 1971.

150. Barrett CP, Braithwaite RA, Teale JD: Unusual case of tetrahydrocannabinol intoxication confirmed by radioimmunoassay. *Br Med J* 2:166, 1977.

151. Cooles P: Stroke after heavy cannabis smoking. *Postgrad Med J* 63:51, 1987.

152. Mohan H, Sood GC: Conjugate deviation of the eyes after cannabis intoxication. *Br J Ophthalmol* 48:160, 1964.

153. Zachariah SB: Stroke after heavy marijuana smoking. *Stroke* 22:406, 1991.

154. Barnes D, Palace J, O'Brien MD: Stroke following marijuana smoking. *Stroke* 9:138, 1992.

155. Adams MD, Earnhardt JT, Dewey WL, et al: Vasoconstrictor actions of delta-8 and delta-9-tetrahydrocannabinol in the rat. *J Pharmacol Exp Ther* 196:649, 1976.

156. Mathew RJ, Wilson WH: Substance abuse and cerebral blood flow. *Am J Psychiatry* 148:292, 1991.

157. Parker MJ, Tarlow MJ, Milne-Anderson J: Glue-sniffing and cerebral infarction. *Arch Dis Child* 59:675, 1984.

158. Lamont CM, Adams FG: Glue-sniffing as a cause of positive radio-isotope brain scan. *Eur J Nucl Med* 7:387, 1982.

159. Ahlawat SK, Siwach SB: Alcohol and coronary artery disease. *Int J Cardiol* 44:157, 1994.

160. Thornton JR: Atrial fibrillation in healthy non-alcoholic people after an alcoholic binge. *Lancet* 2:1013, 1984.

161. Hillbom M, Kaste M: Alcohol intoxication: A risk factor for primary subarachnoid hemorrhage. *Neurology* 32:706, 1982.

162. Hillbom M, Kaste M: Ethanol intoxication: A risk factor for ischemic brain infarction. *Stroke* 14:694, 1983.

163. Hilton-Jones O, Warlow CP: The cause of stroke in the young. *J Neurol* 232:137, 1985.

164. Gorelick PB, Rodin MB, Langenberg P, et al: Weekly alcohol consumption, cigarette smoking, and the risk of ischemic stroke: Results of a case-control study at three urban medical centers in Chicago, Illinois. *Neurology* 39:339, 1989.

165. Moorthy G, Price TR, Tuhrim S, et al: Relationship between recent alcohol intake and stroke type? The NINCDS Stroke Data Bank. *Stroke* 17:14, 1986.

166. Jamrozik K, Broadhurst RJ, Anderson CS, et al: The role of lifestyle factors in the etiology of stroke: A population-based case-control study in Perth, Western Australia. *Stroke* 25:5, 1994.

167. Shinton R, Sagar G, Beevers G: The relation of alcohol consumption to cardiovascular risk factors and stroke: The West Birmingham stroke project. *J Neurol Neurosurg Psychiatry* 56:458, 1993.

168. Beghi E, Bobliun G, Cosso P, et al: Stroke and alcohol intake in a hospital population: A case-control study. *Stroke* 26:169, 1995.

169. Gronback M, Deis A, Sorensen TL, et al: Mortality associated with moderate intakes of wine, beer, or spirits. *Br Med J* 10:1165, 1995.

170. Kozarevic DJ, Vodvodic N, Gordon T, et al: Drinking habits and death: The Yugoslavia Cardiovascular Disease Study. *Int J Epidemiol* 12:145, 1983.

171. Kagan A, Popper JS, Rhoads GG, et al: Dietary and other risk factors for stroke in Hawaiian-Japanese men. *Stroke* 16:390, 1985.

172. Donahue RP, Abbott RD, Reed DM, et al: Alcohol and hemorrhagic stroke: The Honolulu Heart Study. *JAMA* 255:231, 1986.

173. Wolf PA, D'Agostino RB, Odell P, et al: Alcohol consumption as a risk factor for stroke: The Framingham Study. *Ann Neurol* 24:177, 1988.

174. Stamfer MJ, Coditz GA, Willett WC, et al: A prospective study of moderate alcohol consumption and the risk of coronary disease and stroke in women. *N Engl J Med* 319:267, 1988.

175. Bogousslavsky J, Van Melle G, Despland PA, et al: Alcohol consumption and carotid atherosclerosis in the Lausanne Stroke Registry. *Stroke* 21:715, 1990.

176. Ueda K, Hasuo Y, Kiyohara Y, et al: Hisayama: Incidence, changing pattern during long-term follow up, and related factors. *Stroke* 19:48, 1988.

177. Kiyohara Y, Kato I, Iwamoto H, et al: The impact of alcohol and hypertension on stroke incidence in a general Japanese population: The Hisayama Study. *Stroke* 26:368, 1995.

178. Tanaka H, Ueda Y, Hayashi M, et al: Risk factors for cerebral hemorrhage and cerebral infarction in a Japanese rural community. *Stroke* 13:62, 1982.

179. Iso H, Kitamara A, Shimamoto T, et al: Alcohol intake and the risk of cardiovascular disease in middle-aged Japanese men. *Stroke* 26:767, 1995.

180. Camargo CA: Moderate alcohol consumption and stroke: The epidemiologic evidence. *Stroke* 20:161, 1989.

181. Palomaki H, Kaste M, Raininko R, et al: Risk factors for cervical atherosclerosis in patients with transient ischemic attack or minor ischemic stroke. *Stroke* 24:970, 1993.

182. Jorgensen HS, Nakagama H, Raaschou HO, et al: Leukoaraiosis in stroke patients: The Copenhagen Stroke Study. *Stroke* 26:588, 1995.

183. Yoshitake T, Kiyohara Y, Kato L, et al: Incidence and risk factors of vascular dementia and Alzheimer's disease in a defined elderly Japanese population: The Hisayama Study. *Neurology* 45:116, 1995.

184. Beilin LJ: Alcohol and hypertension. *Clin Exp Pharmacol Physiol* 22:185, 1995.

185. Brackett DJ, Gauvin DV, Lerner MR, et al: Dose- and time-dependent cardiovascular responses induced by ethanol. *J Pharmacol Exp Ther* 268:78, 1994.

186. Lip GY, Beevers DG: Alcohol, hypertension, coronary disease, and stroke. *Clin Exp Pharmacol Physiol* 22:189, 1995.

187. Gorelick PB: Alcohol and stroke. *Stroke* 18:268, 1987.

188. Gorelick PB: The status of alcohol as a risk factor for stroke. *Stroke* 20:1607, 1989.

189. Haskell WJ, Camargo C, Williams PT, et al: The effect of cessation and resumption of moderate alcohol intake on serum high-density lipoprotein subfractions: A controlled study. *N Engl J Med* 310:805, 1984.

190. Reed DM, Resch JA, Hayashi T, et al: A prospective study of cerebral artery atherosclerosis. *Stroke* 19:820, 1988.

191. Hillbom M, Kaste M, et al: Acute ethanol ingestion increases platelet reactivity: Is there a relationship to stroke? *Stroke* 16:19, 1985.

192. Ricker PM, Vaughn DE, Stampfer MJ, et al: Association of moderate alcohol consumption and plasma concentration of endogenous tissue-type plasminogen activator. *JAMA* 272:929, 1994.

193. DiMinno G, Mancini M: Drugs affecting plasma fibrinogen levels. *Cardiovasc Drugs Ther* 6:25, 1992.

194. Jakubowski JA, Vaillancourt R, Deykin D: Interaction of ethanol, prostacyclin, and aspirin in determining human platelet reactivity in vitro. *Arteriosclerosis* 8:436, 1988.

195. Fenn CG, Littleton JM: Inhibition of platelet aggregation by ethanol: The role of plasma and platelet membrane lipids. *Br J Pharmacol* 73:305P, 1981.

196. Tsaji S, Kawano S, Michida T, et al: Ethanol stimulates immunoreactive endothelin-1 and -2 release from cultured human umbilical vein endothelial cells. *Alcohol Clin Exp Res* 16:347, 1992.

197. Hutton RA, Fink FR, Wilson DT, et al: Platelet hyperaggregability during alcohol withdrawal. *Clin Lab Haematol* 3:223, 1981.

198. McQueen JD, Sklar FK, Posey JB: Autoregulation of cerebral blood flow during alcohol infusion. *J Stud Alcohol* 39:1477, 1978.

199. Hemmingsen R, Barry DL, Hertz MM, et al: Cerebral blood flow and oxygen consumption during ethanol withdrawal in the rat. *Brain Res* 173:259, 1979.

200. Gordon EL, Nguyen TS, Ngai AC, et al: Differential effects of alcohol on intracerebral arterioles: Ethanol alone causes vasoconstriction. *J Cerebral Blood Flow Metab* 15:532, 1995.

201. Altura BM, Gebrewold A, Altura BT, et al: Role of brain $[Mg^{2+}]$ in alcohol-induced hemorrhagic stroke in a rat model: A 31P-NMR in vivo study. *Alcohol* 12:13, 1995.

202. Fogelholm R: Cigarette smoking and subarachnoid hemorrhage: A population based case-control study. *J Neurol Neurosurg Psychiatry* 50:78, 1987.

203. Shinton R, Beebers G: Meta-analysis of relation between cigarette smoking and stroke. *Br Med J* 298:789, 1989.

204. Donnan GA, Adena MA, O'Malley HM, et al: Smoking as a risk for cerebral ischemia. *Lancet* 2:643, 1989.

205. Harmsen P, Rosengren A, Tsipogianni A, et al: Risk factors for stroke in middle-aged men in Goteborg, Sweden. *Stroke* 21:223, 1990.

206. Love BB, Biller J, Jones MP, et al: Cigarette smoking: A risk factor for cerebral infarction in young adults. *Arch Neurol* 47:693, 1990.

207. Colditz GA, Bonita R, Stamplet MJ, et al: Cigarette smoking and risk of stroke in middle-aged women. *N Engl J Med* 318:937, 1988.

208. Abbott RD, Reed DM, Yano K: Risk of stroke in male cigarette smokers. *N Engl J Med* 315:717, 1986.

209. Wolf PA, D'Agostino RB, Kannel WB, et al: Cigarette smoking as a risk factor for stroke: The Framingham Study. *JAMA* 259:1025, 1988.

210. Longstreth WT, Nelson LM, Koepsell TD, et al: Cigarette smoking, alcohol use, and subarachnoid hemorrhage. *Stroke* 23:1242, 1992.

211. Levine SR, Fagan SC, Floberg J, et al: Moyamoya, oral contraceptives, and cigarette use. *Ann Neurol* 24:155, 1988.

212. Fukada H, Kitani M: Cigarette smoking is correlated with the periventricular hyperintensity grade on brain magnetic resonance imaging. *Stroke* 27:645, 1996.

213. Pierce JR: Stroke following application of a nicotine patch. *Ann Pharmacol* 28:402, 1994.

214. Dempsey RJ, Moore RW: Amount of smoking independently predicts carotid artery atherosclerosis severity. *Stroke* 23:693, 1992.

215. Wilson PWF, Hoeg JM, D'Agostino RB, et al: Cumulative effects of high cholesterol levels, high blood pressure, and cigarette smoking on carotid stenosis. *N Engl J Med* 337:516, 1997

216. Zimmerman M, McGreachie J: The effect of nicotine on aortic endothelium: A quantitative ultrastructural study. *Atherosclerosis* 63:33, 1987.

217. Benowitz NL: Pharmacological aspects of cigarette smoking and nicotine addiction. *N Engl J Med* 319:1318, 1988.

218. Green MS, Jucha E, Luz Y: Blood pressure in smokers and non-smokers: Epidemiologic findings. *Am Heart J* 111:932, 1986.

219. Sharp DS, Benowitz NL, Bath PMW, et al: Cigarette smoking sensitizes and desensitizes impedance-measured ADP-induced platelet aggregation in whole blood. *Thromb Haemost* 74:730, 1995.

220. Nadler JL, Velasco JS, Hotton R: Cigarette smoking inhibits prostacyclin formation. *Lancet* 1:1248, 1983.

221. Kannel WB, D'Agostino RB, Belanger AL: Fibrinogen, cigarette smoking, and risk of cardiovascular disease: Insights from the Framingham Study. *Am Heart J* 113:1006, 1987.

222. Schwarcz TH, Hogan LA, Endean ED, et al: Thromboembolic complications of polycythemia: Polycythemia vera vs. smokers' polycythemia. *J Vasc Surg* 17:518, 1993.

223. Morrow JD, Frei B, Longmire AW, et al: Increase in circulating products of lipid peroxidation (F_2-isoprostanes) in smokers. *N Engl J Med* 332:1198, 1995.

Part 4
OTHER ISSUES IN STROKE MANAGEMENT

Chapter 25

DIAGNOSIS AND MANAGEMENT OF INTRACRANIAL STENOSIS AND STROKE

Owen B. Samuels
Marc I. Chimowitz

BACKGROUND

Introduction

Of the 700,000 patients suffering a stroke annually in the United States, approximately 595,000 (85 percent) patients suffer an ischemic stroke.[1,2] Atherosclerosis of a major intracranial artery is estimated to account for 6 to 29 percent of all ischemic strokes, with blacks, Hispanics, and Asians at highest risk.[3] Overall, intracranial large-artery occlusive disease is estimated to cause over 40,000 strokes per year in the United States alone. The importance of intracranial atherosclerosis as a cause of stroke is underscored when one considers that two other common causes of stroke, nonvalvular atrial fibrillation and extracranial carotid stenosis, account for approximately 70,000 and 85,000 strokes, respectively, in the United States each year.[4,5]

Over the last 10 years, much has been learned about the epidemiology, clinical presentation, and prognosis of intracranial large-artery disease. The recent development of transcranial Doppler ultrasound (TCD) and magnetic resonance angiography (MRA) has enabled noninvasive diagnosis of intracranial large-artery disease. Although treatment remains empiric, therapeutic studies comparing the efficacy of medical therapies such as antiplatelet agents and anticoagulants for stroke prevention in patients with intracranial large artery disease are in progress. The role of angioplasty for high-grade intracranial stenotic lesions is evolving. In this article, we review the epidemiology, clinical presentation, and prognosis of intracranial large-artery occlusive disease and discuss diagnostic and therapeutic options for managing patients with this disease.

Epidemiology

Studies performed in the 1960's established the importance of atherosclerotic intracranial large-artery occlusive disease as a cause of stroke.[6–10] In the Joint Study of Extracranial Arterial Occlusion, 3788 patients with signs and symptoms of ischemic cerebrovascular disease underwent four-vessel angiography. Stenotic lesions were identified in 7.7 percent of basilar arteries, 4.4 percent of intracranial vertebral arteries, 6.7 percent intracranial carotid arteries, 3.8 percent of middle cerebral arteries (MCA), 3.2 percent anterior cerebral arteries (ACA), and 2.6 percent of posterior cerebral (PCA) arteries. Overall, 6.1 percent of patients in the study (84 percent of whom were white) had isolated intracranial occlusive disease.[6] Subsequent studies have confirmed that at least 6 to 10 percent of ischemic strokes in whites are caused by intracranial stenosis.[11–15] In the largest of these studies,[15] isolated intracranial stenosis ≥ 50 was the cause of stroke in 199 (7 percent) of 3000 patients enrolled in an ongoing prospective study (J. Bogousslavsky, personal communication, 1996). These studies underestimate the true frequency of intracranial stenosis as a cause of stroke because angiography, the most reliable method for establishing this diagnosis, was only performed in 38 to 75 percent of patients.

Several studies have suggested that blacks are more likely to develop intracranial large-artery atherosclerosis than extracranial carotid artery atherosclerosis and have a higher frequency of intracranial atherosclerosis than whites.[7,8,10,11,16,17] In a study of patients with anterior circulation ischemia, the rates of MCA occlusion were significantly higher in black males than in white males.[18] In another study of patients with posterior circulation ischemia, distal basilar artery and intracranial branch lesions were significantly more frequent in blacks, whereas severe extracranial vertebral artery disease was five times more common in whites.[19] Recent studies have shown that 6 to 29 percent of TIAs or strokes in blacks are caused by stenosis of a major intracranial artery.[11,16,17] In one study in which angiography was performed in 45 consecutive blacks with carotid distribution TIA, 13 patients (29 percent) had isolated intracranial stenosis involving the ipsilateral carotid siphon (6 patients), MCA stem (4 patients), or an MCA branch (3 patients).[17] In comparison, 12 patients (24 percent) had extracranial internal carotid artery stenosis.[17] Japanese, Chinese, and Hispanics are also at high risk of developing intracranial stenosis.[11,20–22] Studies of these racial groups have shown that 11 percent of strokes in Hispanics and 22 to 26 percent of strokes in Asians are caused by intracranial large artery atherosclerosis.[11,20,23] One study of patients with symptomatic intracranial anterior circulation ischemia showed that 83 percent of severely stenotic lesions in Japanese-Asians involved the intracranial arteries, whereas 85 percent of severe lesions in American whites involved the extracranial internal carotid artery.[21] In another study comparing Chinese-Americans with American whites, the Chinese-American patients had significantly higher rates of intracranial carotid artery and MCA stenoses.[22] The explanation for the variance in the distribution of cerebral atherosclerosis in different races is uncertain. Some studies have suggested that genetic susceptibility to intracranial large-artery disease in blacks, Hispanics, and Asians play a major role,[22,24] whereas other studies suggest that the influence of lifestyle and risk profiles on the distribution of atherosclerosis may be important.[11,25]

Support for the latter is provided by the results of studies showing a lower frequency of intracranial large-artery disease in black Africans than in black Americans,[25] and a strong correlation between the high rate of intracranial large-artery disease in Hispanics and the presence of diabetes.[3] Most studies, however, that have controlled for the presence of traditional vascular risk factors have found that race is independently associated with site of atherosclerosis in the cerebrovascular circulation.[22,24]

The influence of gender on the risk of developing intracranial large-artery disease has not been systematically studied. Data from a few small series suggest that women may be more likely to develop intracranial large-artery disease than men, who tend to develop extracranial large-artery disease.[26]

Clinical Syndromes Associated with Intracranial Occlusive Disease

The neurologic ischemic syndromes associated with intracranial large-artery atherosclerotic occlusive disease are not specific. Other pathologies, such as cardioembolism or extracranial artery to intracranial artery embolism, which both cause occlusion of the major intracranial arteries, produce similar neurologic syndromes. However, review of a patient's risk factor profile, history of TIAs, and temporal course of the neurologic deficit may help to narrow the diagnostic possibilities. For example, a black male with a high burden of atherosclerotic risk factors who presents with aphasia and right hemiparesis is more likely to have carotid siphon or MCA occlusive disease than extracranial carotid disease or cardioembolism.

Recurrent, stereotypical TIAs should always suggest intrinsic large-artery disease (extracranial or intracranial) rather than cardioembolism. TIAs tend to be more common in patients with extracranial carotid disease than in patients with carotid siphon or MCA disease. In one study of patients with infarction in the territory supplied by the MCA, the rate of TIA preceding stroke in patients with MCA occlusive disease was 20 percent compared with 64 percent in patients with extracranial carotid occlusive disease.[27] TIAs in patients with MCA disease also occur over a shorter period than TIAs associated with extracranial carotid disease.[27]

The frequency of TIAs preceding stroke in patients with carotid siphon stenosis has not been well studied. In three retrospective studies, TIAs were the presenting complaint in 28 to 47 percent of patients with carotid siphon stenosis.[28–30] However, only the study with the smallest number of patients ($n = 15$) provided data on the frequency of TIA preceding stroke: one of five patients presenting with stroke had a previous TIA.[29] The frequency of TIAs preceding stroke in patients with vertebral or basilar stenosis has not been systematically evaluated in a large number of patients; however, a few small series suggest that at least 50 percent of patients with basilar artery disease have TIAs preceding stroke.[31,32]

There is evidence that race may also influence the rate of TIAs associated with MCA disease; whites with MCA stenosis present more frequently with TIAs rather than stroke, whereas blacks and Japanese with MCA disease present more frequently with unheralded stroke.[27,33–35] The character of TIA can also be also useful for distinguishing between extracranial carotid disease and carotid siphon disease. Because atherosclerotic carotid siphon disease usually occurs distal to the ophthalmic artery origin, amaurosis occurs infrequently in patients with carotid siphon stenosis, but is common in patients with extracranial carotid atherosclerotic stenosis. When amaurosis does occur in patients with carotid siphon disease, it is often a late manifestation that is related to propagation of thrombus proximally in the carotid siphon.

The temporal course of the neurologic deficit may also lead one to suspect intracranial large-artery disease. In one study by Caplan et al,[27] patients with MCA disease typically had a deficit on awakening that fluctuated and progressed over a few days. The authors suggest that this temporal profile indicates that low flow is the usual mechanism of stroke in patients with MCA disease. On the other hand, patients with an embolic mechanism (e.g., cardioembolism or artery-to-artery embolism) often have a maximal deficit at onset that occurs during normal daily activities.

An understanding of the neurologic syndromes associated with occlusive disease of the major intracranial arteries requires a knowledge of the typical location of atherosclerosis in these arteries and the territories of the brain supplied by each of these vessels. A detailed description of these vascular territories is beyond the scope of this article; however, the reader is referred to detailed descriptions of these vascular territories in the monograph by Osborn.[36] A brief summary of the common neurologic syndromes associated with occlusive disease of the major intracranial arteries follows.

Atherosclerosis of the *intracranial carotid artery* typically involves the cavernous section just distal to the origin of the ophthalmic artery (Fig. 25-1).[28] Infarcts in patients with stenosis or occlusion of the intracranial carotid artery usually involve the MCA territory in our experience. The mechanism of infarction may be carotid siphon to MCA embolus or hypoperfusion. These pa-

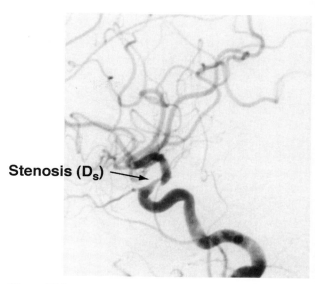

Stenosis (D$_s$) →

Figure 25-1.
Intracranial carotid artery stenosis. Black arrow *points to cavernous segment stenosis.*

tients typically present with hemiparesis, aphasia (dominant hemisphere), and anosognosia and neglect (nondominant hemisphere), hemianopia, and hemisensory loss. Partial syndromes are common depending on which division of the MCA is primarily involved. Carotid siphon disease may also cause infarction in the anterior cerebral artery (ACA) territory.[37] Patients with an infarct in this territory often have leg weakness or leg and face weakness with relative sparing of the arm.

Atherosclerosis of the *middle cerebral artery* (Fig. 25-2) typically involves the stem (M1 segment) but occasionally affects the superior division alone.[34] Infarction of the entire MCA territory causes hemiplegia, hemisensory loss, hemianopia, gaze preference, global aphasia (dominant hemisphere), or neglect syndromes (nondominant hemisphere). Infarction in the territory supplied by the *superior division of the MCA* causes hemiplegia and hemisensory loss, sometimes sparing the lower extremity, conjugate gaze preference, contralateral neglect (nondominant hemisphere), and a Broca's type of aphasia (dominant hemisphere). Vision is spared with these infarcts. Infarctions in the territory supplied by the *inferior division of the MCA* in the dominant hemisphere cause Wernicke's aphasia, hemianopia, and agitation, whereas the mirror image infarct in the nondominant hemisphere causes confusion, agitation, hemi-

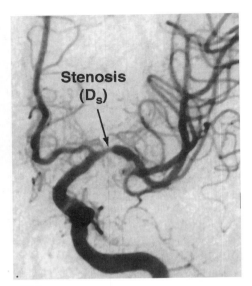

Figure 25-2.
Middle cerebral artery stenosis. Black arrow *depicts the proximal portion of the artery, which is stenotic.*

anopia, poor drawing, and copying.[38] Because infarction involving the nondominant inferior division of the MCA does not cause paralysis or aphasia, the vascular etiology of this syndrome is frequently not recognized by non-neurologists. We have seen a few patients with non-dominant inferior division MCA infarcts who were initially admitted to the psychiatry service with a diagnosis of delirium. Recognition of the hemianopia is critical for preventing this error.

Nonstenotic atherosclerotic disease of the MCA stem that involves the origins of several lenticulostriate arteries causes a moderate-sized (2 to 5 cm) infarction involving the internal capsule and basal ganglia (striato-capsular infarction) with sparing of the cortical areas supplied by the MCA. Typically, these patients present with the lacunar syndrome of pure motor hemiparesis. The clue that the vascular pathology involves the MCA and not a single small penetrating artery is the relatively large size of the subcortical infarct.[39]

The *anterior cerebral artery* is uncommonly affected by atherosclerosis. The majority of infarcts in the ACA territory is caused by emboli from the carotid siphon, extracranial carotid artery, or heart.[40] When atherosclerosis is present, it is usually distal to the stem of the ACA (A1 segment) and involves the pericallosal or callosal marginal branch.[41] These branches supply part of the corpus callosum, the medial paracentral gyrus,

and the parietal lobule. Therefore, infarcts caused by atherosclerotic occlusive disease of these two main branches of the ACA cause weakness that typically involves the foot and thigh and cortical sensory disturbances. Language dysfunction is also common after left ACA infarction. In one series, mutism was a frequent finding at presentation that was sometimes followed by mild mixed transcortical aphasia.[40] When the corpus callosum is involved, the right primary motor and sensory areas are disconnected from the language area in the left hemisphere. This results in left arm apraxia, poor naming of objects in the left hand, and aphasic writing with the left hand. When a large infarct involves most of the ACA territory because of an occlusive A1 lesion, there may be personality change such as apathy (abulia) and a gaze preference. The caudate and anterior internal capsule are supplied by the ACA through penetrating arteries that arise from the A1 segment. Most infarcts of the caudate or anterior capsule are caused by intrinsic disease of these penetrating arteries and not by ACA disease.[42]

Atherosclerosis of the *intracranial vertebral artery* usually involves the vertebral artery at the level of the posterior inferior cerebral artery (PICA) but also occurs at the craniocervical junction of the vertebral artery. The clinical syndromes produced by intracranial vertebral occlusive disease depend on the location of the obstruction, whether the vertebral artery is the source of distal embolism, and whether one or both vertebral arteries are involved. Atherothrombosis of the vertebral artery at the origin of posterior inferior cerebellar artery (PICA) causes lateral medullary infarction (Wallenburg's syndrome) that is often associated with infarction of the inferior cerebellar hemisphere.[43] Ischemia in the medial medulla has been reported much less often than has lateral medullary infarction. Medial medullary infarction is most commonly caused by atheromatous vertebral artery branch disease or embolic occlusions of the distal intracranial vertebral artery (distal to the take-off of the PICA).[44] Neurologic signs typically include Dejerine's triad of (1) contralateral hemiparesis sparing the face, (2) loss of contralateral arm and leg sensation, and (3) variable ipsilateral tongue weakness.[45] If thrombus from a vertebral dissection or an underlying atherosclerotic plaque extends from one vertebral artery to the proximal basilar artery, or if both vertebrals are occluded, the clinical syndrome will resemble that of intrinsic basilar occlusion. If the vertebral artery is a source of distal embolism, the embolus most commonly lodges at the top of the basilar artery or in the posterior cerebral arteries.[46]

The clinical syndromes associated with *basilar artery* occlusive disease depend on the location of the vascular lesion, whether unilateral or bilateral brainstem infarction has occurred, and whether distal embolism has occurred. It is commonly believed that atherosclerosis typically involves the proximal basilar artery (Fig. 25-3); however, recent studies suggest that the middle and distal segments of the basilar artery are involved as frequently as the proximal segment.[31] TIAs often precede stroke in patients with basilar occlusive disease and typically consist of diplopia, dizziness, dysarthria, perioral numbness, paraplegia, or alternating hemiplegia.[31,32,47] In patients with a proximal basilar occlusion whose distal basilar artery and superior cerebellar arteries are patent (i.e., supplied by retrograde flow from the anterior circulation through the posterior communicating arteries), the infarct is usually limited to the midline and paramedian structures in the pons.[37] The pontine tegmentum and cerebellum are usually spared because these structures are supplied by circumferential branches arising from the segment of the basilar that is patent and the PICAs. Consequently, patients with proximal basilar occlusion usually have combinations of the following signs: quadraparesis (bilateral infarction), hemiparesis (unilateral infarction), pseudobulbar palsy, abnormalities of eye movements (unilateral gaze palsy, internuclear ophthalmoplegia, the one and a half syndrome, skew deviation, ocular bobbing), pupillary abnormalities (bilateral small pupils, Horner's syndrome), and reduced level of consciousness, with sparing of sensory and cerebellar function. Occipital headache occurs frequently as well.[37]

In some patients with bilateral infarction of the basis pontis from proximal basilar occlusion, severe weakness of the limbs and horizontal eye movements permits only eye blinking or vertical gaze (i.e., the "locked-in" syndrome). Nonstenotic atherosclerotic disease of the basilar artery may occasionally cause bilateral basis pontis infarcts by occluding the orifices of paramedian-penetrating branches of the basilar artery.[48] The deficits in these patients may be similar to that of patients with proximal basilar artery occlusion. We have seen two such patients who underwent urgent vertebrobasilar angiography for consideration of intra-arterial thrombolytic therapy. In both cases, the basilar artery was widely patent, but diffuse atherosclerotic plaque was visualized in the basilar artery.

When the distal basilar artery is occluded, infarction may involve the midbrain, thalamus, medial temporal lobes, and occipital lobes. Caplan has described in detail the signs associated with "top of the basilar syndrome."[49] Midbrain involvement causes pupillary abnormalities (decreased reactivity, eccentric shape, altered size), oculomotor abnormalities (vertical gaze palsies, skew deviation, third nerve palsy, pseudo sixth nerve paresis), and behavioral abnormalities (peduncular hallucinosis). Thalamic involvement causes decreased alertness, amnesia, and sensory abnormalities depending on the size and location of the infarct. The signs associated with temporal lobe and occipital lesions are described below.

Atherosclerosis of the *posterior cerebral artery* most often affects the proximal (perimesencephalic) segment near the origins of the thalamogeniculate branches.[50] Therefore, the ventroposterolateral thalamus (VPL), medial temporal lobes, and occipital lobes are at risk of infarction from occlusive disease in this segment of the PCA. Hemianopia or hemisensory TIAs are the most common presentations.[50] Signs in patients with infarction in the territory supplied by the PCA include hemisensory loss (infarction of VPL), memory disturbance and naming difficulties (medial temporal infarction), hemianopia, hemiachromatopsia, alexia without agraphia, and visual agnosias (occipital infarction).[51] Headache associated with PCA infarction is typically felt around the ipsilateral orbit or forehead.[37] Paralysis occurs only when the orifices of the perforating branches to the cerebral peduncle are involved by an

Figure 25-3.
Basilar artery stenosis. Black arrow *points to the proximal segment stenosis.*

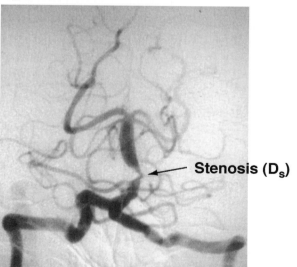

Stenosis (D$_s$)

atherosclerotic lesion in the very proximal part of the PCA. Involvement of the medial thalamoperforating branches of the PCA results in behavioral abnormalities and memory loss.[52] Bilateral PCA infarction is associated with cortical blindness, memory loss (due to medial temporal involvement), and agitation.

Prognosis of Intracranial Large Artery Disease

In patients with stroke caused by *carotid siphon* disease, the size and location of the infarct are important determinants of early outcome (Table 25-1). Patients whose infarcts involve the MCA territory typically have a more severe deficit than patients whose infarct involves the ACA territory. If an embolus from the intracranial ICA lodges in the MCA stem, the prognosis is very poor (see below), whereas an embolus to a distal branch of the MCA is usually not life threatening and may produce a relatively mild deficit.

The long-term prognosis of carotid siphon stenosis has mostly been studied retrospectively.[53] Two studies of patients with symptomatic or asymptomatic siphon stenosis showed that the rates of ipsilateral stroke from carotid siphon disease were low, but the rates of stroke from other causes (e.g., coexistent extracranial carotid stenosis) and death from CAD were high.[28,29] In one of these studies, 66 patients with carotid siphon stenosis of ≥50 percent were followed for an average of 3.9 years. Ten patients (15 percent) had a stroke, and 33 patients (50 percent) died. Eight of the 10 patients with stroke had ipsilateral siphon stenosis, and in six of these there was tandem extracranial carotid stenosis. Therefore, only two of the strokes could be attributed solely to carotid siphon stenosis. Fifty-five percent of the deaths were caused by CAD.[28] In another study of 15 patients with carotid siphon stenosis of ≥50 percent followed for a mean of 51 months, only 1 patient (7 percent) had

a stroke that could be attributed to the siphon stenosis, and 5 patients (33 percent) died (3 from CAD, 1 cerebellar hemorrhage, 1 basilar thrombosis).[29]

Another retrospective study of 58 patients found a much higher rate of stroke caused by carotid siphon stenosis.[30] Patients in this study had symptomatic or asymptomatic carotid siphon stenosis that reduced the diameter of the artery by at least one third. Only 10 percent of patients had tandem extracranial carotid stenosis of ≥50 percent. During a mean follow-up of 30 months, 17 patients (29 percent) had a stroke (11 of which were ipsilateral to the siphon stenosis), and 25 patients (43 percent) died (11 from CAD, 9 from stroke, 5 from other causes). The annual ipsilateral stroke rate was 7.6 percent per year, and there were no apparent differences in stroke rates in patients whose siphon lesions were asymptomatic at entry vs. patients whose siphon lesions were symptomatic. Additionally, the degree of siphon stenosis had no effect on outcome. These subgroup analyses, however, need to be interpreted cautiously because of the low power of this study.

The only prospective estimate of stroke risk in patients with carotid siphon stenosis comes from the extracranial-intracranial (EC-IC) bypass study.[54] One of the subgroups enrolled in this study included patients with stenosis of the internal carotid artery at or above the C-2 vertebral body. It is likely that most of these patients had carotid siphon stenosis given the typical distribution of atherosclerosis in the distal intracranial internal carotid artery. Of 72 patients with ICA stenosis of ≥70 percent at or distal to C-2 who were treated with aspirin (325 mg qid), 26 percent (36 percent) had a nonfatal or fatal stroke in any vascular distribution (ipsilateral stroke rate not provided). The follow-up period for this subgroup of patients was not specified, but the mean follow-up for all patients in the study was 55.8 months. Overall, these studies suggest that the annual rate of stroke in patients with high-grade carotid siphon stenosis is 4 to 12 percent in any vascular territory and is approximately 8 percent in the territory supplied by the diseased carotid siphon (see Table 25-1). In one study, Marzewski et al[28] found that patients with tandem extracranial and intracranial stenosis had a 22 percent risk of stroke over an average 4-year follow-up, whereas the stroke risk in isolated siphon stenosis was only 7 percent.

There are limited data on the early prognosis of patients with infarction caused by atherosclerotic *middle cerebral artery* occlusive disease. Most of the studies that have evaluated outcome in patients with infarction caused by an MCA stem occlusion did not distinguish

Table 25-1.

Risk of stroke in patients with stenosis of the major intracranial arteries

Intracranial	In any vascular territory	In same vascular territory
Carotid siphon	4%–12%[29,30,33,34]	7.6%[30]
Middle cerebral artery	4%–9.5%[34,39,74]	7.8%[74]
Vertebral artery	3%–13%[62,63]	2%–7.7%[62,63]
Basilar artery	15%[62]	11%[62]

between in situ atherothrombotic occlusion and embolic occlusion (from the heart or the extracranial carotid artery).[33,56–60] In this heterogeneous group that consists largely of patients with embolic occlusion, the prognosis is dismal. Approximately 14 to 30 percent of patients died, and 37 to 65 percent had a major residual deficit.[24,42–46] A study by Caplan et al[27] provides some data on early outcome of stroke in patients with atherosclerotic MCA occlusive disease. In this study, patients with a cardiac or carotid source of embolus were excluded. Of the 20 patients evaluated, the deficit at discharge was severe in 4 patients, moderate in 8 patients, and slight in 8 patients. None of the patients died from their stroke.

The EC-IC bypass study provides important data on the long-term outcome of patients with atherosclerotic MCA occlusive disease.[54,58] Studies prior to this were retrospective, included small numbers of patients, and did not distinguish between atherosclerotic MCA disease and embolic occlusion from the heart or carotid artery.[33,34,59] Most of these studies suggested that the long-term risk of stroke or death was low. In the EC-IC bypass study, 79 patients with MCA occlusion and 85 patients with MCA stenosis were treated with medical management of risk factors and antithrombotic therapy (aspirin or warfarin). All of these patients had a TIA or nondisabling stroke in the distribution of the diseased MCA within 3 months of study entry, and none had a cardiac source of embolus or severe extracranial carotid stenosis. In the 79 patients with MCA occlusion followed for a mean of 40.8 months, 21 patients (27 percent) had a stroke (some of whom had multiple strokes), and 7 patients (9 percent) died (2 from a cerebral hemorrhage, 3 from nonvascular causes, 2 not specified). The annual rate of stroke in any vascular territory was 10.1 percent and the annual rate of ipsilateral stroke was 7.1 percent. The mortality rate was 2.6 percent per year.[58]

In the 85 patients with MCA stenosis followed for a mean of 43.3 months in the EC-IC bypass study, 18 patients (21 percent) had a stroke, and 10 patients (12 percent) died (3 from stroke, 2 from CAD, and 5 from other causes). The annual rate of stroke in any vascular territory was 9.5 percent and the annual rate of ipsilateral stroke was 7.8 percent. The mortality rate was 3.3 percent per year. There were no apparent differences in the rates of stroke or death in patients with <70 percent stenosis vs. patients with ≥70 percent stenosis of the MCA.[58] These data suggest that the annual rate of stroke in patients with symptomatic MCA occlusive disease is 10 percent in any vascular territory and 7 to 8 percent in the territory of the diseased MCA. These rates are similar to the rates of stroke in patients with carotid siphon disease (see Table 25-1). The rate of cardiac death in patients with MCA disease, however, seems to be substantially lower than the rate associated with carotid siphon disease.[58]

The long-term prognosis of atherosclerotic *anterior cerebral artery* disease has not been studied systematically. In our limited experience with these patients, recurrent stroke in the ACA territory is uncommon during follow-up, but stroke in other territories or myocardial infarction has occurred, suggesting that these patients have widespread atherosclerosis.

Early outcome in patients with stroke from unilateral atherosclerotic vertebral artery disease is usually good unless distal embolism has occurred. Lateral medullary infarction rarely causes major disability or death unless autonomic and respiratory centers in the medulla are affected.[60] Similarly, inferior cerebellar infarction has a good prognosis unless the infarct is large and compresses the medulla. Stroke associated with bilateral intracranial vertebral artery occlusion is often severe. In one series of nine patients with stroke from bilateral vertebral artery occlusion, eight patients (89 percent) died soon after presentation.[61] The infarcts in these patients involved the pons in four patients, the right lateral medulla in one patient, and the brainstem in one patient. None of the patients died during initial hospitalization, but two were locked in, one of whom improved and could walk with a cane 2 months later. The long-term outcome of these ten patients was surprisingly benign; none had recurrent stroke during a mean follow-up of 6.8 years.

In the largest study reporting on the prognosis of patients with intracranial vertebral stenosis, 31 patients with TIA or stroke caused by ≥50 percent vertebral artery stenosis were followed for a mean of 20 months.[62] Seven (23 percent) patients had a recurrent stroke (13 percent/year), four in the territory of the stenotic vertebral artery, 3 in a different arterial territory, and two patients (6 percent) died. In another study of 25 patients with ≥50 percent of an intracranial vertebral artery (asymptomatic and symptomatic included), 5 patients (20 percent) had a stroke (3 in the vertebrobasilar distribution) during a mean follow-up of 6.1 years (3 percent per year).[63] These studies suggest that the annual rates of recurrent stroke in patients with >50 percent stenosis vertebral artery stenosis are 3 to 13 percent in any vascular territory and 2 to 7.7 percent in the territory of the vertebral artery.

In 1946 when Kubik and Adams described the clinical and pathologic features of *basilar artery* occlusion, it was thought that basilar occlusion invariably led to death.[64] Subsequently, however, other investigators have shown that patients can survive basilar artery occlusion.[32,47,65] In one series of six patients who survived stroke from basilar occlusion, four patients had minimal or no deficit, one had a moderate deficit, and one had a severe deficit at discharge from the hospital.[65] In our experience, infarction from basilar artery occlusion has usually led to severe disability or death unless recanalization of the vessel occurs, or well established collateral exists (see "Evidence").

There are limited retrospective data and no prospective data on the long-term outcome of patients with angiographically proven basilar occlusive disease.[54,66] In one study of 22 patients with angiographically proven basilar occlusion, 13 patients (59 percent) survived for longer than 3 months after angiography. During a median follow-up of 1.75 years (range 6 months to 4 years), 3 patients (23 percent) died (2 from cardiac causes, 1 from pneumonia), but none had recurrent stroke.[32] In another study of patients with ≥50 percent stenosis of the basilar artery or vertebral artery, 19 patients had isolated basilar stenosis. During a mean follow-up of 6.1 years, 3 patients (16 percent) had a stroke (1 brainstem, 1 occipital lobe, and 1 uncertain territory).[63] A third study on the prognosis of basilar artery stenosis by Pessin et al[31] showed that some patients with symptomatic stenosis (40 to 90 percent) of the middle or distal segments of the basilar artery have a relatively low risk of stroke. In this series of nine patients presenting with TIA or stroke, most of whom were treated with warfarin, only one patient (11 percent) had a stroke during a median follow-up of 2 years. This patient had a fatal brainstem stroke.

In the largest study to date, 28 patients with TIA or stroke related to ≥50 percent basilar artery stenosis were followed for a mean of 20 months. Seven patients (25 percent) had a recurrent stroke (5 in the territory of the stenotic basilar artery, 2 in a different territory), and 4 patients (14 percent) died. The annual rates of stroke were 15 percent in any vascular territory and 11 percent in the basilar artery territory.[62]

There are limited data as well on the outcome of patients with *posterior cerebral artery* stenosis. Pessin et al[50] studied six patients with symptomatic PCA stenosis of 50 to 80 percent. Five patients had unilateral PCA disease, and one had bilateral disease. Four patients presented with hemianopic or hemisensory TIAs, and two patients presented with stroke (one had a hemianopia, one had a superior quadrantanopia). All patients were treated with warfarin, and the range of follow-up was 4 months to 4 years. None of the patients had a stroke in the territory of the stenotic PCA, but

three patients died (one from a traumatic intracerebral hemorrhage, one from an MCA infarct, one sudden death).

There are limited data on the prognosis of patients with *occlusion* of a major intracranial artery. Several studies have shown that the annual rate of ipsilateral stroke in patients with atherosclerotic occlusion of the extracranial internal carotid artery (ICA) is 2 to 6 percent.[54,67–70] This rate is relatively low when compared with the rate of ipsilateral stroke in medically treated patients with symptomatic high-grade (70 to 99 percent) extracranial ICA stenosis (26 percent over 2 years).[71] Several studies reporting on the prognosis of patients with presumed atherosclerotic occlusion of a major intracranial artery were retrospective and of small sample size.[32,46,72,73] Bogousslavsky et al[74] reported the outcome of 165 patients with MCA occlusion and 187 patients with MCA stenosis who were medically treated in the EC/IC Bypass Study.[54] In patients with MCA occlusion, annual stroke rate was 10.1 percent (7.1 percent ipsilateral). In patients with MCA stenosis, the annual stroke rate was 9.5 percent (7.8 percent ipsilateral). The annual death rate was 3.3 percent in patients with MCA stenosis and 2.6 percent in patients with MCA occlusion. This study suggests that patients with atherosclerotic intracranial occlusion have a similar rate of stroke to patients with intracranial stenosis. In a recent study, Samuels et al[75] compared the annual rate of stroke in 52 patients with presumed atherosclerotic occlusion and 151 patients with stenosis (≥50 percent) of a major intracranial artery (carotid, anterior, middle or posterior cerebral, vertebral, or basilar). All patients were identified by angiography at centers participating in the WASID study.[62] In the 52 patients with intracranial occlusion, the rate of stroke (per 100 patient-years of follow-up) was 2.8 (same territory 1.9, different territory was zero), and the rate of MI/SD was 3.7 (per 100 patient-years of follow-up). Patients with intracranial stenosis had a higher rate of stroke (6.8 per 100 patient years of follow-up; same territory 4.5, different territory 2.3) and MI/SD (6.1 per 100 patient years of follow-up). Of the 52 patients with intracranial occlusion, 16 patients were treated with aspirin, and 36 patients were treated with warfarin. Three strokes occurred in patients treated with aspirin and none in patients treated with warfarin. The results of this study[75] suggest that the annual stroke rate in patients with symptomatic occlusion of a major intracranial artery is low. However, given this small sample size and retrospective design, definitive conclusions regarding the prognosis of these patients cannot be made. A larger prospective study is needed to confirm the apparent relatively benign prognosis of certain patients

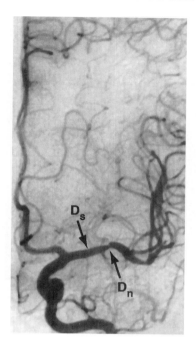
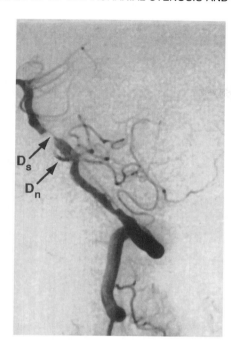

Figure 25-4.
WASID method for measuring intracranial stenosis. A, stenosis of the distal segment MCA M-1 segment. Because the proximal MCA is normal, it is taken as the measurement for D_{normal}. B, stenosis of the mid-basilar segment. Because the proximal basilar artery is normal, it is taken as the measurement of D_{normal}.

with symptomatic occlusion of a major intracranial artery and determine the most effective therapy.

Vascular Imaging of Intracranial Occlusive Disease

The "gold standard" for establishing the diagnosis of intracranial large-artery disease is conventional cerebral angiography. Angiography enables an accurate measurement of the degree of stenosis of the diseased artery, diagnosis of arterial occlusion, evaluation of collateral flow patterns, and evaluation of other intracranial and extracranial arteries. Because of the complexity of the intracranial arterial circulation, the established angiographic criteria used to measure extracranial carotid stenosis do not apply to the intracranial circulation. Therefore, Samuels and colleagues[76] established measurement criteria for determining the percent stenosis of the major intracranial arteries. They defined % stenosis of an intracranial artery as: % stenosis = $[(1 - D_{stenosis}/D_{normal})] \times 100$, where $D_{stenosis}$ = diameter of the artery at the site of the most severe stenosis, and D_{normal} = diameter of the proximal normal artery (Fig. 25-4). If the proximal segment was diseased, contingency sites were chosen to measure D_{normal}: distal artery (2nd

choice), feeding artery (3rd choice) (Fig. 25-5). Using a hand-held caliper, three neuroradiologists independently measured $D_{stenosis}$ and D_{normal} of 24 stenotic intracranial arteries. Interobserver agreement (% stenosis within 10 percent) ranged from 71 to 100 percent, and intraobserver observer agreement (% stenosis within 10 percent) ranged from 81 to 100 percent among three experienced neuro-angiographers. These agreements were comparable with those reported for measuring extracranial carotid stenosis.[77] The major drawback of angiography is the risk of stroke, which is 1 to 3 percent in patients investigated for cerebrovascular disease.[78]

The development of TCD in 1982 by Aaslid et al[79] and the more recent development of MRA have enabled noninvasive diagnosis of intracranial large-artery occlusive disease.[80–83] TCD/angiographic correlative studies show that TCD has a sensitivity of 75 to 90 percent and a specificity of 87 to 98 percent for detecting intracranial stenosis.[83–87] TCD is less reliable for detecting occlusive lesions in the vertebral or basilar arteries (sensitivity 76 percent, specificity 99 percent), especially in the distal basilar region.[83] In our experience, TCD cannot reliably detect low-grade intracranial stenosis (<50 percent), distal ACA, distal PCA, or MCA branch disease.

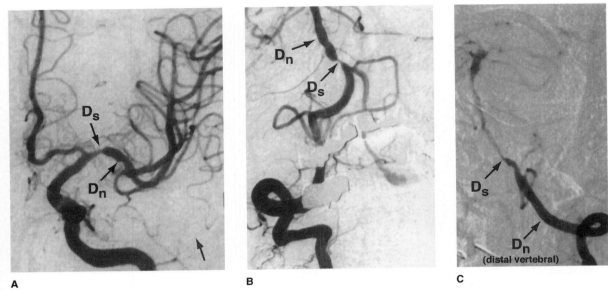

A   **B**   **C**

Figure 25-5.
WASID method for measuring intracranial stenosis. A   *stenosis of the proximal portion of the MCA;
as the proximal portion is diseased, the distal normal segment of the MCA is the measurement of*
D_{normal}. B   *stenosis of the proximal portion of the basilar artery; therefore, the distal normal segment
is used as the measurement of* D_{normal}. C   *diffuse disease of the basilar artery; therefore, the most
distal normal portion of the feeding vertebral artery is measured as* D_{normal}.

MRA is also used commonly to evaluate patients with suspected intracranial occlusive disease. There are limited MRA/angiographic correlative studies in patients with intracranial large-artery occlusive disease. MRA is reported to have a sensitivity of 82 to 97 percent and a specificity of 81 to 99 percent in several studies.[83,88–91] One recent MRA/TCD/angiographic correlative study of 41 patients with vertebrobasilar ischemia showed that the sensitivity of MRA for the detection of 34 occlusive lesions (15 occlusions, 19 stenoses) was 97 percent and the specificity was 99 percent.[83] However, the degree of stenosis could not be accurately measured by MRA. In the same group of patients, the sensitivity of TCD was 76 percent, and the specificity was 99 percent. Although TCD had a lower sensitivity than MRA, TCD provided more complete hemodynamic data (collateral supply, estimations of degree of stenosis) than MRA.[83]

Until recently, our evaluation of patients with suspected intracranial large-artery disease routinely involved conventional angiography. Currently, however, we usually proceed noninvasively by performing TCD and MRA. If these studies provide concordant results,

we do not perform cerebral angiography, but if the results of TCD and MRA are discordant, we recommend conventional cerebral angiography.[83]

EVIDENCE

Medical Management for Symptomatic Intracranial Stenosis

Despite the importance of intracranial stenosis as a cause of ischemic stroke, there have been no prospective trials evaluating antithrombotic therapy in patients with this disease. Antiplatelet agents (aspirin or ticlopidine) are frequently used in this setting based on studies that have shown a benefit of these agents for lowering the risk of stroke in patients with noncardioembolic TIA or minor stroke.[92] However, the efficacy of antiplatelet agents has not been established in patients with symptomatic intracranial large-artery disease. In fact, the high rate of stroke in patients with carotid siphon or MCA stenosis who were treated with high-dose aspirin (1300 mg per day) in the medical arm of the EC-IC bypass study (7.7 to 9.5 percent per patient-year) raises a question about the efficacy of *aspirin* in this setting.[54,58]

Ticlopidine, another antiplatelet agent, has been shown to be slightly more effective than aspirin for secondary stroke prevention in patients with non-cardioembolic TIA or minor stroke.[93] However, the efficacy of ticlopidine in patients with symptomatic intracranial stenosis has not been established either. A post hoc analysis of the Ticlopidine Aspirin Stroke Study (TASS) suggests that ticlopidine may be more effective in Blacks than in Whites.[94] As Blacks are at higher risk of intracranial large-artery stenosis, it might be inferred that ticlopidine is effective therapy for this disease. However, Blacks are also at higher risk of intracranial small vessel disease for which ticlopidine may be effective. If cerebral angiography had been performed routinely in TASS, clarification of the role of ticlopidine in patients with intracranial large-artery stenosis may have been possible. However, angiography was only performed in approximately half the patients in this study, most of whom had carotid territory symptoms. Of note is that in the subgroup of patients with extracranial carotid stenosis >70 percent, ticlopidine was significantly less effective than aspirin for preventing stroke.[95] This finding raises a question about the efficacy of ticlopidine for the treatment of intracranial large-artery stenosis.

Clopidogrel, a cogener of ticlopidine with potentially less adverse side effects, has recently been compared with aspirin (325 mg per day) in the Clopidogrel vs. Aspirin in Patients at Risk of Ischemic Events (CAPRIE) trial.[96] Although clopidogrel was slightly more effective than aspirin in preventing stroke, MI, or vascular death in patients presenting with MI, stroke, or peripheral vascular disease, clopidogrel was not significantly more effective than aspirin in the stroke cohort alone.[66] Moreover, the CAPRIE trial did not provide data on the relative efficacy of clopidogrel vs. aspirin in patients with stroke caused by intracranial arterial stenosis.

Warfarin is frequently used for the treatment of intracranial stenosis based on the results of nonrandomized, retrospective studies of patients with symptoms suggestive of vertebrobasilar disease.[97,98] In a retrospective, nonangiographic study of patients with vertebrobasilar symptoms, Whisnant et al found that patients treated with anticoagulation had a lower risk of stroke in the first 6 months of treatment compared with untreated patients; however, the rates of stroke beyond 6 months were similar in both groups.[98]

In a retrospective, nonrandomized, multicenter study, warfarin was compared with aspirin for prevention of major vascular events (stroke, myocardial infarction, or vascular death) in patients with symptomatic angiographically proven stenosis (50 to 99 percent) of a major intracranial artery (see Table 25-2).[62] Qualifying criteria for the study were (1) 50 to 99 percent stenosis of one of the major intracranial arteries, (2) a TIA or minor stroke in the distribution of the stenotic artery, and (3) therapy with aspirin or warfarin. Treatment with aspirin or warfarin was based on local physician preference. The most common dose of aspirin prescribed was 325 mg per day, and the dose of warfarin was typically adjusted to maintain prothrombin times (PT) in the range of 1.2 to 1.6 × control. Primary endpoints in this study were stroke in any vascular territory, MI, or sudden death. Recording hemorrhagic complications assessed safety of warfarin and aspirin. Hemorrhages were classified as major (fatal hemorrhage, any intracranial hemorrhage, bleeding requiring hospitalization, bleeding requiring transfusion) or minor (any other bleeding complication).

Of the 151 patients who qualified for the study, 96 (64 percent) were male, 55 (36 percent) were female, 100 (66 percent) were white, 42 (28 percent) were black, 5 (3 percent) were Hispanic, and 4 (3 percent) were Asian or Arabic. Stroke was the qualifying event in 89 patients (59 percent), and TIAs were the qualifying events in 62 patients (41 percent). The stenotic lesions at angiography involved the anterior circulation in 83 patients (55 percent) and the posterior circulation in 68 patients (45 percent). The percent stenosis of the symptomatic intracranial artery was 50 to 69 percent in 62 patients (41 percent) and 70 to 99 percent in 89 patients (59 percent).

Of the 151 patients in the study, 88 patients (58 percent) were treated with warfarin, and 63 patients (42 percent) were treated with aspirin. There were no significant differences in the frequency of risk factors for stroke between the two groups. Major ischemic events (ischemic stroke, MI, or sudden death) occurred in 26 patients on aspirin during 143 patient-years of follow-up and in 14 patients on warfarin during 166 patient-years of follow-up ($p < .01$, log rank test). Hemorrhagic complications occurred in 13 patients on warfarin (3 major, 10 minor) during 166 patient-years of follow-up and in two patients on aspirin (both minor) during 143 patient-years of follow-up ($p < .01$, log rank test).

Cox proportional hazards analysis showed that the relative risk of stroke, MI, or sudden death in patients treated with warfarin was 0.45 (95 percent CI,

Table 25-2.

Rates of endpoints and hemorrhagic complications in a retrospective study comparing warfarin vs. aspirin in patients with symptomatic intracranial arterial stenosis

	Warfarin N = 88	Aspirin N = 63
Median follow-up (months)	14.7	19.3
Stroke	6(7%)	15(24%)
Fatal	1(1%)	3(5%)
Nonfatal	5(6%)	12(19%)
Nonfatal MI or SD	5(6%)	6(10%)
Nonfatal MI	3(3%)	5(8%)
Stroke per 100 patient-years	3.6	10.4
Fatal MI or SD per 100 patient-years	3.0	4.2
Nonfatal MI per 100 patient-years	1.8	3.5
Major hemorrhage per 100 patient-years	1.8	0
Minor hemorrhage per 100 patient-years	5.9	1.4

0.23 to 0.86) compared with patients treated with aspirin. The major effect of warfarin was in preventing stroke. A Kaplan-Meier analysis that included hemorrhagic deaths as a primary endpoint (i.e., in addition to ischemic stroke, MI, or sudden death) showed that a significantly higher proportion of patients treated with warfarin survived free of these endpoints compared with patients treated with aspirin ($p = .03$, log rank test).

Patients with moderate intracranial stenosis (50 to 69 percent) had a lower risk of stroke in the same vascular territory than patients with a severe intracranial stenosis (70 to 99 percent). Of 62 patients with 50 to 69 percent intracranial stenosis, 5 patients (6 percent) had a stroke in the same territory as the stenotic artery during a median follow-up of 20 months; 4 of 28 (14 percent) on aspirin, 1 of 34 (3 percent) on warfarin. In comparison, of 89 patients with 70 to 99 percent intracranial stenosis, 9 patients (10 percent) had a stroke in the same territory as the stenotic artery during a median follow-up of 14 months; 5 of 35 (14 percent) on aspirin, 4 of 54 (7 percent) on warfarin. Patients with stenosis of the vertebral or basilar arteries had a higher rate of stroke in the same vascular territory than patients with carotid siphon or MCA stenosis basilar artery 11 percent/year, vertebral artery 8 percent/year, carotid siphon 2 percent/year, MCA 3 percent/year.[99]

In summary, the major findings in this retrospective study[62] were that (1) warfarin lowered the combined endpoint of stroke, MI, or sudden death by nearly 50 percent compared with aspirin (325 mg/day) and that the major benefit of warfarin was for preventing stroke; (2) the rate of major hemorrhagic complications in patients with symptomatic intracranial stenosis treated with warfarin (PT 1.2 to 1.6 × control) was approximately 1.8 percent annually, which is similar to the rate of major hemorrhagic complications in patients treated with warfarin in the stroke prevention in atrial fibrillation trials.[100] Despite the increased risk of major hemorrhagic complications in patients on warfarin, the overall risk/benefit strongly favored warfarin; (3) patients with 70 to 99 percent stenosis of a major intracranial artery had the highest risk of stroke in the territory of the stenotic artery. Although warfarin seems to be more effective than aspirin in patients with 70 to 99 percent intracranial stenosis, the risk of ipsilateral stroke on warfarin is still high (greater than 5 percent per year) in these patients. Although this retrospective study strongly suggests that warfarin is more efficacious than low-dose aspirin (325 mg per day) for the treatment of symptomatic intracranial arterial stenosis, definite recommendations regarding the use of warfarin vs. antiplatelet agents in this setting must await confirmation of these findings in a prospective, randomized trial.

Surgical Management for Symptomatic Intracranial Stenosis

Intracranial bypass surgery is also a therapeutic option for patients with intracranial arterial stenosis; however, enthusiasm for bypass has waned since the overall disappointing results of the EC-IC bypass study results were reported.[54] In that study, patients with extracranial carotid occlusion, distal carotid occlusive disease, or MCA stenosis were randomized to medical therapy alone (risk factor management and antithrombotic therapy, usually aspirin 325 mg qid) vs. medical therapy and EC-IC bypass. The results demonstrated that EC-IC bypass was ineffective for preventing stroke. Subgroup analyses of patients with distal carotid or MCA stenosis showed that EC-IC bypass was also ineffective in these groups.[54] In patients with carotid siphon stenosis ≥70 percent, 26 of 72 patients (36 percent) treated medically and 29 of 77 patients (38 percent) who underwent EC-IC bypass had a stroke during a mean follow-up of 55.8 months. In patients with MCA stenosis ≥70 percent, those undergoing EC-IC bypass actually had a poorer outcome than medically treated patients did: 14 of 59 (24 percent) patients treated medically and 22 of 50 (44 percent) patients treated surgically had a stroke during follow-up ($p < .05$).[54] Bypass surgery or endarterectomy has also been used occasionally for the treatment of intracranial vertebral artery occlusive disease,[101,102] but the efficacy of these procedures has not been evaluated systematically.

Interventional Radiology for Symptomatic Intracranial Stenosis

Transluminal angioplasty is another therapeutic option for the treatment of intracranial stenosis. Experience in the early 1980's suggested that intracranial angioplasty was associated with an unacceptably high risk of stroke or death, and the procedure was largely abandoned.[103,104] However, recent advances in microcatheter and balloon technology have led to renewed interest and use of angioplasty for symptomatic intracranial arterial stenosis.[105–107] Recent studies have shown that intracranial angioplasty is technically feasible and may be performed relatively safely. In one study of 27 patients with stenosis of a major intracranial artery (carotid, MCA, vertebral, or basilar) that had recurrent cerebral ischemic symptoms on anticoagulation, angioplasty was technically successful in 82 percent of cases. The average pre-angioplasty stenosis was 72 percent, and the average postangioplasty stenosis was 46 percent. There were three strokes during angioplasty for a 30-day morbidity rate of 11 percent.[106,108] During an average follow-up of 28 months, one patient (4 percent) had a fatal stroke referable to the treated vessel, and three patients (11 percent) had TIA. In another study of 19 patients with

TIA or stroke caused by stenosis of an intracranial artery, angioplasty was performed because of "unstable neurological symptoms" on antiplatelet therapy. Angioplasty was technically successful in 13 of 19 (68 percent) patients, with the average pre-angioplasty stenosis = 83 percent and the average postangioplasty stenosis = 36 percent. None of the patients had a stroke during angioplasty, though 2 had transient hemiparesis and 1 had an asymptomatic dissection. Moreover, none of the 13 patients who had successful angioplasty had recurrent stroke during follow-up ranging from 6 to 12 months, whereas 2 of the 6 patients whose angioplasty was unsuccessful had "neurological deterioration" 2 months later.[109] In a Japanese study, Hyodo et al reported 36 patients who underwent angioplasty for symptomatic >70 percent stenosis of a major intracranial artery.[110] Three patients (8 percent) had a stroke during the procedure. During a mean follow-up of 35 months, none of the patients had TIA or stroke. Cerebral angiography in 28 patients showed restenosis in five patients (18 percent) and occlusion in one patient. The long-term clinical outcome in 21 patients undergoing intracranial angioplasty has also been evaluated by Marks et al.[111] Angioplasty was technically successful in 91 percent of cases. One patient (4.5 percent) died during the procedure from rupture of the vessel, and another patient (4.5 percent) had ischemic symptoms immediately after angioplasty that resolved following thrombolytic therapy. During a mean follow-up of 31.3 months, one patient had a stroke in the territory of the treated artery, and another patient had a stroke in a different territory. The annual stroke rates were 3.8 percent in the territory of the treated artery and 5.8 percent for all strokes.[111] When thrombosis occurs at a site of severe atherostenosis, local intra-arterial thrombolysis can be combined with angioplasty. In such cases, acute reocclusion following thrombolysis and angioplasty may occur despite "therapeutic" anticoagulation with heparin. This situation has prompted the use of abciximab (ReoPro), a platelet integrin monoclonal antibody (approved during high-risk coronary angioplasty), in these high-risk patients during intracranial angioplasty.[112,113] Wallace and colleagues successfully used abciximab to prevent rethrombosis of the basilar artery after angioplasty. Mohammed et al recently reported preliminary data on the safety and potential efficacy of abciximab as adjunctive therapy for vertebrobasilar angioplasty.[113] Four patients with vertebrobasilar stenosis were treated with angioplasty and abciximab. Three patients presented with crescendo TIAs despite full anticoagulation with intravenous heparin. None of the patients suffered a new stroke or reocclusion during the procedure. At 3 months following treatment, one patient was asymptomatic, two had infrequent vertebrobasilar TIAs, and one patient died. These recent studies suggest that angioplasty is a promising therapy that is increasingly being used to treat symptomatic intracranial stenosis. However, more data on safety, long-term outcome, and restenosis rates, and adjunctive therapy(ies), in patients undergoing intracranial angioplasty are needed.

TREATMENT RECOMMENDATIONS

Absent prospective randomized trials for intracranial stenosis, an evidence-based treatment recommendation is impossible. A multicenter prospective trial, WASID, is currently under way to determine the "best" medical therapy (warfarin vs. high-dose aspirin [1300 mg]) for symptomatic patients with large-artery intracranial stenosis. Pending the results of this trial, warfarin (INR 2.0 to 3.0) is frequently recommended for the treatment of intracranial stenosis based on the results of nonrandomized, retrospective studies of patients with symptoms suggestive of vertebrobasilar disease.[97,98] The WASID retrospective study also strongly suggested that warfarin is more efficacious than low-dose aspirin (325 mg per day) for the treatment of symptomatic intracranial arterial stenosis. However, definite recommendations regarding the use of warfarin vs. antiplatelet agents in this setting must await confirmation of these findings in the prospective WASID randomized trial.

Antiplatelet treatment with aspirin, ticlopidine, clopidogrel, or dipyridamole is an alternative treatment option for these patients. Combined warfarin and an antiplatelet agent (e.g., warfarin plus aspirin) or combined antiplatelet therapy (e.g., aspirin plus dipyridamole) is also a treatment alternative in those patients who have failed monotherapy. Currently, there is no prospective and scant retrospective data to support combined therapy in this setting. Intracranial angioplasty, a promising treatment for intracranial large artery stenosis, should be reserved for those patients at the highest risk who have failed conventional medical therapy. More data on safety, long-term outcome, and restenosis rates, and adjunctive therapy(ies), in patients undergoing intracranial angioplasty are needed before this therapy can be recommended.

REFERENCES

1. American Heart Association: *Heart and Stroke Facts.* Dallas, American Heart Association, 1994.
2. National Stroke Association. *Brain Attack Statistics.* 1995.
3. Sacco R, Zamanillo C, Kargman D, Shi T: Determinants of intracranial atherosclerotic stroke: The Northern Manhattan Stroke Study (Abstract). *Stroke* 25:259, 1994.
4. Executive Committee for the Asymptomatic Carotid Atherosclerosis Study: Endarterectomy for asymptomatic carotid artery stenosis. *JAMA* 273:1421, 1995.
5. The Stroke Prevention in Atrial Fibrillation Study Group: Preliminary report of the stroke prevention in atrial fibrillation study. *N Engl J Med* 322:863, 1990.
6. Hass W, Fields W, North R, Kricheff II, Chase N, Bauer R: Joint study of extracranial arterial occlusion II arteriography, techniques, sites, and complications. *JAMA* 203:961, 1968.
7. McGarry P, Solberg L, Guzman M, Strong J: Comparisons of lesions age, sex, and race. *Lab Invest* 52:533, 1985.
8. Moosey J: Cerebral infarction and intracranial arterial thrombosis. *Arch Neurol* 14:119, 1966.
9. Gorelick P: Distribution of atherosclerotic cerebrovascular lesions: Effects of age, race, and sex. *Stroke* 24:116, 1993.
10. Bauer R, Sheehan S, Wechsler N, Meyer J: Arteriographic study of sites, incidence, and treatment of arteriosclerotic cerebrovascular lesions. *Neurology* 12:698, 1962.
11. Sacco R, Kargman D, Gu Q, Zamanillo M: Race-ethnicity and determinant of intracranial atherosclerotic cerebral infarction: The Northern Manhattan Stroke Study. *Stroke* 26:14, 1995.
12. Naylor A, Sandercock P, Sellar R, Warlow C: Patterns of vascular pathology in acute, first-ever cerebral infarctin. *Scot Med J* 38:41, 1993.
13. Passero S, Rossi G, Nardini M, et al: Italian multicenter study of reversible cerebral ischemic attacks: Part 5. Risk factors and cerebral atherosclerosis. *Atherosclerosis* 63:211, 1987.
14. Wityk R, Lehamn D, Klag M, Coresh J, Ahn H, Litt B: Race and sex differences in the distribution of cerebral atherosclerosis. *Stroke* 27:1974, 1996.
15. Bogousslavsky J, Van Melle G, Regli F: The Lausanne Stroke registry: Analysis of 10000 consecutive patients with first stroke. *Stroke* 19:1083, 1988.
16. Qureshi A, Safdar K, Patel M, Janssen R, Frankel M: Stroke in young black patients: Risk factors, subtypes, and prognosis. *Stroke* 26:1995, 1995.
17. Weisberg L: Clinical characteristics of transient ischemic attacks in black patients. *Neurology* 41:1410, 1991.
18. Heyden S, Heyman A, Goree J: Nonembolic occlusion of the middle cerebral artery and carotid arteries: A comparison of predisposing factors. *Stroke* 1:363, 1970.
19. Gorelick P, Caplan L, Hier D, Patel D, Langenberg P, Pessin M: Racial differences in the distribution of posterior circulation occlusive disease. *Stroke* 16:785, 1985.
20. Kieffer S, Takeya Y, Resch J, Amplatz K: Racial differences in cerebrovascular disease: Angiographic evaluation of Japanese and American populations. *Am J Roentgenol* 101:94, 1967.

21. Nishimaru K, McHenry L, Toole J: Cerebral angiographic and clinical differences in carotid system transient ischemic attacks between American Caucasian and Japanese patients. *Stroke* 15:56, 1984.

22. Feldmann E, Daneault N, Kwan E, Ho K, Pessin M, Lanenberg P: Chinese-white differences in the distribution of occlusive cerebrovascular disease. *Neurology* 40: 1541, 1990.

23. Brust RJ: Patterns of cerebrovascular disease in Japanese and other population groups in Hawaii: An angiographical study. *Stroke* 6:539, 1975.

24. Gorelick P, Caplan L, Langenberg P, Hier D, Pessin M, Patel D: Clinical and angiographic comparison of asymptomatic occlusive cererovascular disease. *Neurology* 38: 852, 1988.

25. Williams A, Resch J, Loewenson R: Cerebral atherosclerosis: A compartive autopsy study between Nigerian Negroes and American Negroes and Caucasians. *Neurology* 19:205, 1969.

26. Caplan L, Gorelick P, Hier D: Race, sex and occlusive cerebrovascular disease: A review. *Stroke* 17:648, 1986.

27. Caplan L, Babikian V, Helgason C, Hier D, DeWitt D, Patel D: Occlusive disease of the middle cerebral artery. *Neurology* 35:975, 1985.

28. Marzewski D, Furlan A, St Louis P, Little J, Modic M, Williams G: Intracranial internal carotid artery stenosis: Long-term prognosis. *Stroke* 13:821, 1982.

29. Wechsler L, Kistler J, Davis K, Kaminski M: The prognosis of carotid siphon stenosis. *Stroke* 17:714, 1986.

30. Craig D, Meguro K, Watridge C, Robertson J, Barnett H, Fox J: Intracranial internal carotid artery stenosis. *Stroke* 13:825, 1982.

31. Pessin M, Gorelick P, Kwan E, Caplan L: Basilar artery stenosis: Middle and distal segments. *Neurology* 37: 1742, 1987.

32. Thompson J, Simmons C, Hasso A, Hinshaw D: Occlusion of the intradural vertebrobasilar artery. *Neuroradiology* 14:219, 1978.

33. Moulin D, Lo R, Chiang J, Barnett H: Prognosis in middle cerebral artery occlusion. *Stroke* 16:284, 1985.

34. Hinton R, Mohr J, Ackerman R, Adair L, Fisher C: Symptomatic middle cerebral artery stenosis. *Ann Neurol* 5:152, 1979.

35. Naritomi H, Sawada T, Kuriyama Y, Kinugawa H, Kaneko T, Takamiya M: Effect of chronic middle cerebral artery stenosis on the local cerebral hemodynamics. *Stroke* 16:214, 1985.

36. Osborn A: *Introduction to Cerebral Angiography.* Philadelphia, Harper and Row, 1980.

37. Caplan L, Stein R: *Stroke: A Clinical Approach.* Boston, Butterworths, 1986.

38. Caplan L, Kelly M, Kase C, et al: Infarcts of the inferior division of the right middle cerebral artery: Mirror image of Wernicke's aphasia. *Neurology* 1986:1015, 1986.

39. Chimowitz MI, Furlan A, Sila C, Paranandi L, Beck G: Etiology of motor or sensory stroke: A prospective study of the predicative value of clinical and radiologic features. *Ann Neurol* 30:15, 1991.

40. Bogousslavsky J, Regli F: Anterior cerebral artery territory infarction in the Lausanne Stroke Registry. *Arch Neurol* 47:144, 1993.

41. Kazui S, Sawada T, Naritomi H, Kuriyama Y, Yamaguchi T: Angiographic evaluation of brain infarction limited to the anterior cerebral artery territory. *Stroke* 24:549, 1993.

42. Caplan L, Schmahmann J, Kase C, et al: Caudate infarcts. *Arch Neurol* 47:133, 1990.

43. Fisher C, Karnes W, Kubik C: Lateral medullary infarction: The pattern of vascular occlusion. *J Neuropathol Exp Neurol* 20:323, 1961.

44. Duffy P, Jacobs G: Clinical and pathogical findings in vertebral artery thrombosis. *Neurology* 1958:862, 1958.

45. Bogousslavsky J, Mattle H, Bernasconi A: Medial medullary stroke: Report of seven patients and review of the literature. *Neurology* 48:882, 1997.

46. Castaigne P, Lhermitte F, Gautier J, et al: Arterial occlusions in the vertebro-basilar system: A study of 44 patients with post-mortem data. *Brain* 96:133, 1973.

47. Archer C, Horenstein S: Basilar artery occlusion: Clinical and radiological correlation. *Stroke* 8:383, 1997.

48. Fisher C, Caplan L: Basilar artery branch occlusion: A cause of pontine infarction. *Neurology* 21:900, 1971.

49. Caplan L: Top of the basilar syndrome: Selected clinical aspects. *Neurology* 30:72, 1980.

50. Pessin M, Kwan E, DeWitt L, Hedges T, Gale D, Caplan L: Posterior cerebral artery stenosis. *Ann Neurol* 21:85, 1987.

51. Pessin M, Lathi E, Cohen M, Kwan E, Hedges T, Caplan L: Clinical features and mechanisms of occipital infarction. *Ann Neurol* 21:290, 1987.

52. Bogousslavsky J, Regli F, Uske A: Thalamic infarcts: Clinical syndromes, etiology, and prognosis. *Neurology* 38: 837, 1988.

53. Borozan P, Schuler J, LaRosa M, Ware M, Flanigan D: The natural history of carotid siphon stenosis. *J Vasc Surg* 1:744, 1984.

54. EC/IC Bypass Study Group: Failure of extracranial-intracranial arterial bypass to reduce the risk of ischemic stroke: Results of an international randomized trial. *N Engl J Med* 313:1191, 1985.

55. Mackey W, O'Donnell TJ, Callow A: Carotid endarterectomy in patients with intracranial vascular disease: Short-term risk and long-term outcome. *J Vasc Surg* 10:482, 1989.

56. Ogawa A, Kogure T, Yoshimoto T, Fukao N, Seki H, Suzuki J: Prognosis of middle cerebral artery occlusion: Analysis of the nationwide cooperative study in Japan, in Spetzler R, Selwan W, Carter L, Marin NA (eds): *Cerebrovascularization for Stroke.* 1985.

57. Saito I, Segawa J, Shiokawa Y, Taniguchi M, Tsutsumi K: Middle cerebral artery occlusion: Correlation of computed tomography and angiography with clinical outcome. *Stroke* 18:863, 1987.

58. Bogousslavsky J, Barnett H, Fox A, Hachinski V, Taylor W for the EC/IC Study Group: Atherosclerotic disease of the middle cerebral artery. *Stroke* 17:1112, 1986.

59. Corston R, Kendall B, Marshall J: Prognosis in middle cerebral artery stenosis. *Stroke* 15:237, 1984.

60. Currier R, Giles C, Westerberg M: The prognosis of some brainstem vascular syndromes. *Neurology* 8:664, 1958.

61. Caplan L: Bilateral distal vertebral artery occlusion. *Neurology* 33:552, 1983.

62. Chimowitz M, Kokkinos J, Strong J, et al: Warfarin-Aspirin Symptomatic Intracranial Disease (WASID) Study. *Neurology* 45:1488, 1995.

63. Moufarrij N, Little J, Furlan A, Leatherman J, Williams G: Basilar and distal vertebral artery stenosis: Long term follow up. *Stroke* 17:938, 1986.

64. Kubik C, Adams R: Occlusion of the basilar artery: A clinical and pathological study. *Brain* 69:6, 1946.

65. Caplan L: Occlusion of the vertebral or basilar artery: Follow up analysis of some patients with benign outcome. *Stroke* 10:277, 1979.

66. Ausman J, Shrontz C, Pearce J, Diaz F, Crecelius J: Vertebrobasilar insufficiency: Review. *Arch Neurol* 42:803, 1985.

67. Barnett H, Peerless S, Kaufmann J: "Stump" of internal carotid artery; A source for further cerebral embolic ischemia. *Stroke* 9, 1978.

68. Cote R, Barnett H, Taylor D: Internal carotid occlusion: A prospective study. *Stroke* 14:898, 1983.

69. Furlan A, Whisnant J, Baker Jr. H: Long-term prognosis after carotid artery occlusion. *Neurology* 30:986, 1980.

70. Fields W, Lemak N: Joint study of extracranial arterial occlusion: Internal carotid artery occlusion. *JAMA* 235:2734, 1976.

71. North American Symptomatic Carotid Endarterectomy Trial Collaborators: Beneficial effect of carotid endarterectomy in symptomatic patients with high-grade carotid stenosis. *N Engl J Med* 325:445, 1991.

72. Bogousslavsky J, Gates P, Fox A, Barnett H: Bilateral occlusion of vertebral artery: Clinical patterns and long term prognosis. *Neurology* 36:1309, 1986.

73. Caplan L: Occlusion of the vertebral of basilar artery. *Stroke* 10:277, 1979.

74. Bogousslavsky J, Barnett H, Fox A, Hatchinski V, Taylor W, for the EC/IC Bypass Study Group: Atherosclerotic Disease of the Middle Cerebral Artery. *Stroke* 17:1112, 1986.

75. Samuels O, Chimowitz M, for the Warfarin-Aspirin Symptomatic Intracranial Disease (WASID) Study Group: Long-term prognosis of atherosclerotic occlusion of a major intracranial artery (Abstract). *Stroke* 1997.

76. Samuels O, Dawson D, Joseph G, et al: A new method for measuring intracranial arterial stenosis using conventional angiography. *Neurology* 48:A157, 1997.

77. Rothwell P, Gibson R, Slattery J, Warlow C, for the European Carotid Surgery Trialist's collaborative Group: Prognostic value and reproducibility of measurements of carotid stenosis: A comparison of three methods on 1001 angiograms. *Stroke* 25:2440, 1994.

78. Dion J, Gates P, Fox A, Barnett H, Bloom R: Clinical events following neuroangiography: A prospective study. *Stroke* 18:997, 1987.

79. Aaslid R, Markwalder T, Normes H: Noninvasive transcranial Doppler ultrasound recording flow velocity in basal cerebral arteries. *J Neurosurg* 49:769, 1982.

80. Lindegaard K, Bakke S, Aaslid R, Normes H: Doppler diagnosis of intracranial occlusive disorders. *J Neurol Neurosurg Psychiatry* 49:510, 1986.

81. Mattle H, Grolimund P, Huber P, Sturzenegger M, Zurbrugg H: Transcranial Doppler sonographic findings in middle cerebral artery disease. *Arch Neurol* 45:289, 1988.

82. Ross J, Masaryk T, Modic M, Harik S, Wiznitzer M, Selman W: Magnetic resonance angiography of the extracranial carotid and intracranial vessels: A review. *Neurology* 39:1369, 1989.

83. Rother J, Wentz K-U, Rautenberg W, Schwartz A, Hennerici M: Magnetic resonance angiography in vertebrobasilar ischemia. *Stroke* 24:1310, 1993.

84. Ley-Pozo J, Ringelstein E: Noninvasive detection of occlusive disease of the carotid siphon and middle cerebral artery. *Ann Neurol* 28:640, 1990.

85. deBray J, Joseph P, Jeanvoine H, Maugin D, Dauzat M, Plassard F: Transcranial Doppler evaluation of middle cerebral artery stenosis. *J Ultrasound Med* 7:611, 1988.

86. Rorick M, Nichols F, Adams R: Transcranial Doppler correlations with angiography in detection of intracranial stenosis. *Stroke* 25:1931, 1994.

87. Camberlingo M, Casto L, Censori B, Gazzaniga G, Mamoli A: Transcranial Doppler in acute ishemic stroke of the middle cerebral artery territories. *Acta Neurol Scand* 24:1310, 1993.

88. Dagirmanjian A, Ross J, Obuchowski N, et al: High resolution, magnetization transfer saturation, variable flip angle, time-of-flight MRA in the detection of intracranial vascular stenoses. *J Comput Assist Tomogr* 19:700, 1995.

89. Stock K, Radue E, Jacob A, Bao X, Steinbrich W. Intracranial arteries: Prospective blinded comparative study of MR angiography and DSA in 50 patients. *Radiology* 195, 1995.

90. Bogousslavsky J, Regli F, Maeder P, Meuli R, Nader J: The etiology of posterior circulation infarcts: A prospective study using magnetic resonance imaging and magnetic resonance angiography. *Neurology* 43:1528, 1993.

91. Katz D, Marks M, Napel S, Bracci P, Roberts S: Circle of Willis: evaluation with spiral CT angiography, MR angiography, and conventional angiography. *Radiology* 195:445, 1995.

92. Antiplatelet Trialist's Collaboration: Secondary prevention of vascular disease by prolonged antiplatelet treatment. *Br Med J* 296:320, 1988.

93. Hass W, Easton J, Adams HJ, et al: A randomized trial comparing ticlopidine hydrochloride with aspirin for the

prevention of stroke in high risk patients. *N Engl J Med* 321:501, 1989.

94. Weisberg L, Ticlopidine Aspirin Stroke Study Group: The efficacy and safety of Ticlopidine in non-whites: Analysis of a patient subgroup from the Ticlopidine Aspirin Stroke Study. *Neurology* 43:27, 1993.

95. Grotta J, Norris J, Kamm B, TASS Baseline and Angiographic Data Subgroup: Prevention of stroke with Ticlopidine: who benefits most? *Neurology* 42:111, 1992.

96. CAPRIE Steering Committee: A randomised, blinded, trial of clopidogrel versus aspirin in patients at risk of ischaemic events (CAPRIE). *Lancet* 348:1329, 1996.

97. Millikan C, Siekert R, Shick R: Studies in cerebrovascular disease III. The use of anticoagulant drugs in the treatment of insufficiency and thrombosis within the basilar arterial system. *Mayo Clin Proc* 30:116, 1995.

98. Whisnant J, Cartlidge N, Elveback L: Carotid and vertebral-basilar transient ischemic attacks: Effect of anticoagulants, hypertension, and cardiac disorders on survival and stroke occurrence a population study. *Ann Neurol* 3:107, 1978.

99. The Warfarin-Aspirin Symptomatic Intracranial Disease (WASID) Study Group: Prognosis of patients with symptomatic vertebral or basilar artery stenosis (Abstract). *Stroke* 26:162, 1995.

100. Albers G: Laboratory monitering of oral anticoagulant therapy: Are we being misled? *Neurology* 43:468, 1978.

101. Sundt T, Whisnant J, Piepgras D, Campbell J, Hollman C: Intracranial bypass grafts for vertebral basilar ischemia. *Mayo Clin Proc* 53:12, 1978.

102. Ausman J, Diaz F, de losReyes R, Pak H, Patel S, Boulos R: Anastomosis of occipital artery to anterior inferior cerebellar artery for vertebrobasilar stenosis. *Surg Neurol* 16:99, 1981.

103. Piepgras D, Sundt T, Forbes G: Balloon catheter transluminal angioplasty for vertebral basilar ischemia, in Berguer R, Bauer R, (eds). *Vetrobasilar arterial occlusive disease.* New York, Raven Press, 1984, pp 215–224.

104. Sundt TJ, Smith H, Campbell J, Vliestra R, Cucchiara R, Stanson A: Transluminal angioplasty for basilar artery stenosis. *Mayo Clin Proc* 55:673, 1980.

105. Jensen M, Mathis J, DeNardo A, Dion J: Angioplasty of brachiocephalic and cerebral vessels in atherosclerotic disease (Abstract). *Stroke* 25:273.

106. Clark W, Barnwell S, Nesbit G, O'Neill O, Wynn M, Coull B: Safety and efficacy of percutaneous transluminal angioplasty for intracranial atherosclerotic stenosis. *Stroke* 26:1200, 1995.

107. Higashida R, Tsai F, Halbach V, et al: Transluminal angioplasty for atherosclerotic disease of the vertebral and basilar arteries. *J Neurosurg* 78:192, 1993.

108. Kellog J, Nesbit G, Clark W, Barnwell S: Percutaneous transluminal angioplasty for intracranial atherosclerotic stenosis: Long term follow-up (Abstract). *Interventional Neuroradiology* 3:39, 1997.

109. Touho H: Percutaneous transluminal angioplasty in the treatment of atherosclerotic disease of the anterior cerebral circulation and hemodynamic evaluation. *J Neurosurg* 82:953, 1997.

110. Hyodo A, Matsumaru Y, Anno I, et al: Percutaneous transluminal angioplasty for atherosclerotic stenosis of the intracranial cerebral arteries: Results with more than one year follow-up (Abstract). *Interventional Neuroradiology* 3:38, 1997.

111. Marks M, Marcellus M, Norbash A, Steinberg G, Albers G: Evaluation of long term clinical outcome in patients undergoing intracranial angioplasty (Abstract). *Interventional Neuroradiology* 3:38, 1997.

112. Wallace R, Furlan A, Moliterno D, Stevens G, Masaryk T, Perl II J: Basilar artery rethrombosis: Sucessful treatment with Platelet glycoprotein IIB/IIIA inhibitor. *Am J Neuroradiol* 18:1257, 1997.

113. Mohammed Y, Samuels O, Stern B, et al: Percutaneous transluminal angioplasty (PTA) plus abciximab for symptomatic vertebrobasilar (VB) stenosis. *Neurology* 50: A157, 1988.

Chapter 26

CORONARY ARTERY DISEASE AND STROKE

Alfredo M. Lopez-Yunez
Betsy Love
José Biller

BACKGROUND

Stroke and myocardial infarction are interrelated diseases as they share similar vascular risk factors and pathogenic mechanisms. Myocardial infarction and stroke are the first and third leading causes of death in the United States, respectively. Together, they affect over 20 million persons between 65 and 80 years of age. The coexistence of coronary atherosclerotic disease (CAD) and cerebrovascular disease (CVD) is not an unexpected finding. Postmortem studies have shown that atherosclerosis is a progressive process that affects different arterial trees at different ages. The aorta is usually the first vascular structure to show atherosclerotic changes. It is followed by the coronary arteries, peripheral vasculature, the extracranial cervical arteries, and, finally; the intracranial cephalic circulation.

Data from large randomized stroke therapy trials[1-9] as well as population studies indicate that cardiac arrhythmias and myocardial infarction are the leading causes of long-term mortality among stroke patients. It is estimated that up to 60 percent of stroke patients have underlying CAD. The association of CAD and CVD is so strong that after presentation with a threatened stroke, patients are at a higher risk for a myocardial infarction than for stroke.[10] The 5 to 6 percent annual mortality rate after a TIA is mainly due to myocardial infarction, similar to the mortality rate in patients with unstable angina pectoris. Conversely, myocardial infarc-

tion complicated by stroke occurs in approximately 1 to 5 percent of patients.

Medical therapies such as thrombolytics are available for the treatment of acute ischemic stroke and for the treatment of myocardial infarction. However, we must also consider the major cause of death in the first year after stroke, namely CAD, if we are going to impact upon long-term survival. No prospective multicenter approach for the evaluation of the coexistence of CAD and CVD has been developed.

Technologic advances in the surgical management of cardiovascular and cerebrovascular disorders have resulted in an expansion of eligibility criteria for these interventions, specifically coronary artery bypass grafting (CABG) and carotid endarterectomy (CE). Because these procedures carry risks of cardiac and cerebrovascular complications, there is a growing demand for optimal preoperative screening and improved outcomes in these patients. Challenges are greater among those patients with concomitant CAD and carotid artery disease who may require both interventions.

This chapter reviews the approach to the patient with coexistent CAD and CVD. The first part of the chapter is dedicated to the association of CAD and CVD, including both symptomatic and asymptomatic patients. The second part addresses the cardiac evaluation of patients with TIAs or ischemic strokes associated with hemodynamically significant carotid stenosis. Finally, we present a rational management approach including risk factor control, medical and surgical treatment, with special consideration to the persistent dilemma of timing of carotid endarterectomy in patients with concomitant need for coronary artery bypass grafts.

ASSOCIATION OF CORONARY ARTERY DISEASE AND STROKE

Asymptomatic Coronary Artery Disease and Stroke

Asymptomatic coronary artery disease is common among patients with TIAs and stroke. The prevalence of myocardial ischemia in this population has ranged from 26 to 60 percent. There have been few studies that have prospectively evaluated the frequency of asymptomatic CAD in patients with stroke. These studies have generally used noninvasive methods such as [201]TL-myocardial scintigraphy.

An early prospective evaluation of 34 patients with TIAs or small strokes and no history of CAD undergoing exercise-radionuclide ventriculograms and stress-[201]TL scintigraphy demonstrated abnormal tests in 41 percent.[1] Coronary angiography was performed in nine of these patients, and eight of those patients had 70 percent or greater stenosis of at least one coronary artery.[1]

Another study evaluated 506 patients with asymptomatic carotid bruits and symptomatic cerebrovascular disease and showed that approximately 40 percent of patients had severe CAD defined by coronary angiography.[11] A more traditional assessment using cardiac history and ECG enabled detection of severe CAD (defined as greater than 70 percent stenosis of one or more coronary arteries) in 46 percent of patients with a positive cardiac history or abnormal ECG. The most reliable indicator of severe correctable CAD was a convincing history of angina pectoris. Of patients with no clinical indication of CAD, abnormal coronary angiography was detected in 173 of 200 patients, of which 40 percent were classified as having advanced or severe CAD. Ventricular impairment was found in 24 percent of patients with no prior MI and 25 percent of patients with no evidence of infarction by ECG.

Another controlled study evaluated the incidence of silent myocardial ischemia in 190 patients with history of transient ischemic attacks or mild stroke.[12] Patients with no clinical or ECG evidence of previous myocardial ischemia had an exercise treadmill test. If the exercise test was positive, patients underwent exercise [201]TL-myocardial imaging. Coronary angiography was performed in selected cases. The exercise test was adequate in 140 of these patients. Thirty-six (26 percent) had a positive exercise test in the absence of angina. Exercise [201]TL-myocardial imaging showed perfusion defects in 33 of the 36 patients (26 reversible, 7 fixed). A majority had multiple defects. The cerebrovascular group was compared with a healthy control group that had a 6 percent incidence of positive exercise treadmill testing.

The same authors subsequently studied 38 patients with stroke and no prior angina or MI who were unable to exercise with [201]TL-dipyridamole testing and found that 23 (60 percent) had abnormal [201]TL tests. These results are clearly significant because the prevalence of abnormal exercise [201]TL tests in asymptomatic volunteers aged 46 to 96 (mean 60) years was 14 percent.[13] Love et al studied 45 patients with TIA or stroke with exercise [201]TL or [201]TL-dipyridamole and found that 33 percent of those with no history of CAD had an abnormal test.[14]

Because it would not be economically feasible to evaluate all patients with cerebral ischemia for asymptomatic coronary artery disease, two studies have suggested some clinical criteria that may identify those persons with symptomatic cerebral ischemia who are at greater risk of having asymptomatic CAD (Table 26-1).[5,15] Although the number of patients studied is small, some guidelines can be obtained from these studies. Persons with large artery cerebrovascular disease, particularly if combined intracranial and extracranial occlusive disease was present, had a higher frequency of asymptomatic CAD than those with penetrating artery disease or cryptogenic stroke.[5] This study involved 69 patients with TIA or stroke who had no history of overt

Table 26-1.

Variables that may identify a greater risk of detecting asymptomatic CAD in patients with TIA or stroke

Male gender
Veteran status
Tobacco use
Large artery subtype of CVD
Symptomatic carotid artery lesion >90%
Coexistence of contralateral carotid artery disease

Table 26-2.

Prevalence of asymptomatic CAD in patients with TIA or stroke

Study	No. of patients	Population	Screening test	Results
Rokey et al (1984)	34	TIA/stroke	Exercise [201]TL, exercise radionuclide ventriculography	(41%) abnormal had coronary angiography with >70% stenosis of 1 coronary artery.
Hertzer et al (1985)	200	Carotid bruit, TIA/stroke	Coronary angiography	80 (40%) severe CAD 93 (46%) mild moderate CAD 27 (14%) normal
DiPasquale et al (1986)	83	TIA/minor stroke	Exercise ECG exercise [201]TL	28% abnormal studies
DiPasquale et al (1991)	38	Cerebral ischemia (type not specified)	[201]TL-dipyridamole	23 (60%) with perfusion defects
Love et al (1992)	60	Asymptomatic carotid stenosis[15] TIA/stroke[45]	Exercise [201]TL, [201]TL-dipyridamole	33% with no history of CAD had abnormal test
Urbanati et al (1992)	106	TIA, minor stroke undergoing CE	Exercise ECG, [201]TL	Silent CAD detected in 25% of patients
Chimowitz et al (1997)	69	Nondisabling stroke,[53] TIA[16]	Exercise ECG, adenosine or dipyridamole [201]TL, or exercise [201]TL	(35%) abnormal test; 7 with severe CAD by coronary angiography

CAD and who underwent a resting ECG and cardiac stress testing (adenosine or dipyridamole thallium myocardial perfusion imaging, exercise thallium myocardial perfusion imaging, or exercise ECG). Thirty-five percent (35 percent) of patients had abnormal cardiac stress tests. Fifteen of 30 patients (50 percent) of those with large-artery cerebrovascular occlusive disease vs. 9 of 39 patients (23 percent) with other causes of brain ischemia had abnormal stress tests ($p = .04$). The rate of abnormal cardiac stress testing was 8 of 16 patients (50 percent) with isolated extracranial carotid artery stenosis, 2 of 8 patients (25 percent) with isolated intracranial stenosis of a major artery, and 5 of 6 (83 percent) with concomitant extracranial carotid and intracranial stenoses. The presence of coexisting intracranial and extracranial arterial stenosis (defined as >50 percent stenosis or occlusion) identifies a group of patients who are at even greater risk of having abnormal cardiac stress tests.[5] See Table 26-2.

There are some other factors that seem to be important in identifying patients with stroke who have a higher probability of coexisting CAD. Among patients with TIA or stroke who have abnormal adenosine or dipyridamole thallium myocardial imaging, cigarette smoking (odds ratio, 6.5; 95 percent confidence interval, 1.3 to 32.1), is a significant risk factor.[5] Among patients undergoing carotid endarterectomy for symptomatic high-grade carotid stenosis of 70 to 99 percent, a higher probability of coexisting CAD was identified in patients with carotid arterial stenosis >90 percent and with coexisting contralateral carotid disease of ≥70 percent.[15]

Stroke Complicating Acute Myocardial Infarction

The risk of ischemic and hemorrhagic stroke is increased after MI. Interestingly, after an MI, the risk of having a stroke is similar to that of having another MI. Unfortunately, this fact is not addressed often in MI trials.[16] The incidence of stroke after myocardial infarction has varied among studies dependent upon the patient populations studied, the methods used to diagnose and classify stroke and MI, and the types of treatments used. The risk of stroke after MI was approximately 1 to 10 percent in the prethrombolytic era and 0.8 to 1.1 percent in the thrombolytic era. There has been a trend toward a decrease in the incidence of MI-related stroke.[17] Early observational studies in the coronary care units in the 1970's and 1980's showed that the stroke event rate was 1 to 2 percent.[18,19] Strokes complicating MI in the prethrombolytic era were most commonly ischemic, mainly attributable to emboli.[20] Up to one-third of these strokes occurred simultaneously with the MI, and most occurred in the first 2 weeks after infarction.[21]

Some generalizations can be made about strokes occurring after MI in the prethrombolytic era. Factors that have been associated with the occurrence of stroke in various studies have included older age, prior history of stroke, a large myocardial infarction, markedly elevated creatine kinase, lactate dehydrogenase or serum glutamic-oxaloacetic transaminase levels, low cardiac output, congestive heart failure, and paroxysmal atrial fibrillation.[5,21,22] A majority of the strokes involve the cerebral cortex, usually in the distribution of a cortical branch of the middle cerebral artery. However, up to 20 percent of cardioembolic strokes affect the subcortical white matter, basal ganglia, and internal capsule.[23] In most studies, stroke was more common with anterior or apical infarctions than with inferior wall myocardial infarctions.[21] The prognosis is adversely affected when stroke occurs after MI. Studies have shown that the in-hospital mortality rate is as high as 61 percent in patients with stroke after MI compared with 13 percent in those without stroke.

In more recent trials using thrombolytic agents, the event rate of stroke in the placebo groups was 0.8 to 1.1.[24,25] Some authors have suggested that the observed decrease in the event rate is difficult to substantiate due to differing inclusion and exclusion criteria among studies and differing follow-up times. However, one study showed that the annual event rate of ischemic stroke after acute MI was reduced from 1.5 percent in 1989 to to 0.8 percent in 1994.[17] Reasons for this decline could relate to improvements in general care, in patients with acute MI early mobilization, and the routine use of thrombolytic therapy and aspirin. Evidence suggests that the types of stroke complicating MI have changed. More of the strokes are hemorrhagic events and complications of therapy, and proportionately fewer of the strokes are embolic and direct complications of the MI.[22]

Stroke-complicating acute MI is divided into early stroke, occurring within 2 to 3 months after MI, and late stroke occurring 3 or more months after MI. Approximately one-third of strokes complicating MI occur within 24 h of onset of acute MI, and about 70 percent occur within the first week.[20] The causes of early stroke after MI are different than late stroke after MI. Early strokes are more likely to be associated with anterior than nonanterior MI and are usually due to cardioembolism from a thrombus in the akinetic left ventricular apex.[26]

One study of 445 patients with MI and a high prevalence of diabetes mellitus showed that early stroke within 1 month after MI was equally likely to be associated with anterior or nonanterior MI. In the diabetic patient, severe hypotension, possibly due to poor left ventricular function, was a notable cause of stroke early after nonanterior MI.[26]

The presence of a mural thrombus on echocardiography after MI significantly increases the risk of embolization.[27] A pooled analysis of studies addressing thromboembolism after recent MI supports the use of systemic anticoagulation in patients with mural thrombus detected by echocardiography to reduce the incidence of embolic events.[28]

Some studies have indicated that left ventricular dysfunction (without the presence of documented LV thrombi) is a risk factor for stroke. In a study of 2231 patients with left ventricular dysfunction after MI, there was a 4.6 percent rate of fatal or nonfatal stroke over a mean follow-up period of 42 months (1.5 percent rate of stroke per year of follow-up).[29] For every 5 percent decrement in LV ejection fraction, there was an 18 percent increase in the stroke risk. Patients with an EF of <28 percent after MI had a relative risk of stroke of 1.9 in comparison with patients with an EF of >35 percent ($p = .01$). Other independent risk factors include older age and the absence of aspirin or anticoagulant therapy. The use of thrombolytic agents and captopril had no significant effect on the risk of stroke. More recently, the investigators from the GUSTO-I trial identified the risk factors for in-hospital nonhemorrhagic stroke in patients with acute MI treated with thrombolysis.[30] A total of 247 nonhemorrhagic strokes occurred in this trial that assigned randomly to one of four thrombolytic regimens within 6 h of cardiac symptoms' onset. Of these patients, 17 percent died and 40 percent were disabled at 30 days. The most important clinical predictors of stroke were older age, higher heart rate, history of a cerebrovascular event, diabetes, angina, and hypertension. Other factors included Killip class, coronary angiography, bypass surgery and atrial fibrillation/flutter. The authors propose that prophylactic anticoagulation in the high-risk patients may be a reasonable strategy to reduce the risk of early nonhemorrhagic stroke.

Table 26-3.
Possible causes of ischemic stroke after MI

LV thrombus

Akinetic left ventricular segment with or without LV
thrombus

Global left ventricular dysfunction

Atrial fibrillation or other cardiac arrhythmia

Hemodynamic changes such as severe hypotension

Hematologic abnormalities

Complications of treatment (CABG, cardiac catheterization)

Cerebrovascular causes (large-vessel atherosclerosis, intracranial arterial occlusive disease)

Late stroke after MI is more heterogeneous and is more likely to be related to associated risk factors than directly to the MI.[31] The Lausanne Stroke Registry studied a series of 94 patients with stroke occurring at least 3 months after MI and demonstrated a mixture of both cardiac and noncardiac causes. A compilation of possible causes of ischemic stroke after MI is detailed in Table 26-3. Other evidence that late stroke may not relate directly to MI comes from a population-based study that found a difference between the observed and expected probability of stroke within 2 months after MI. Factors that seem to be significant in persons with late stroke after MI are older age, male gender, hyper-

cholesterolemia, and a history of vascular claudication.[32] A summary of predictive factors for stroke or transient ischemic attack after MI is presented in Table 26-4.

Myocardial Infarction Accompanying Acute Stroke

Patients with cerebrovascular disease often have concomitant cardiovascular disease, and the two share similar risk factors. Patients with asymptomatic and symptomatic extracranial and intracranial occlusive disease are at high risk of stroke, myocardial infarction, or vascular death. Transient ischemic attacks are forerunners of stroke and predictors of underlying coronary artery disease. Patients with TIAs are at greater risk than normal controls of stroke or death from vascular causes. Subarachnoid hemorrhage is frequently associated with myocardial injury, left ventricular wall motion abnormalities, and electrocardiographic (ECG) changes simulating myocardial infarction. While ECG changes, such as prolongation of the Q-T interval, increased T-wave amplitude, U waves, T-wave inversion, peaked inverted T waves, and S-T segment, elevation, and depression are more common in subarachnoid hemorrhage, they also occur with some frequency in ischemic stroke. Hypokalemia, frequently observed in patients with subarachnoid hemorrhage, increases the likelihood of prolongation of the Q-T interval.[33] Among patients with acute cerebral infarction, approximately 9 percent have

Table 26-4.
Predictors of stroke/TIA after acute MI

Factor	Odds ratio	95% confidence interval
Age (10-year increments)	1.58	1.24–2.00
Chronic atrial fibrillation	3.86	1.09–13.70
History of stroke	3.45	1.89–6.30
Glutamic oxaloacetic transaminase >4 times normal	1.89	1.21–2.96
Paroxysmal atrial fibrillation	1.70	1.02–2.82
Acute myocardial infarction site (anterior)	1.60	1.03–2.51
Anterior MI plus large infarction (serum glutamic oxaloacetic transaminase >4 times normal)	2.53	1.41–4.56

Used with permission from Tanne D, Reicher-Reiss H, Boyko V, Behar S. SPRINT Study Group: Secondary prevention reinfarction Israeli Nifedipine trial. Stroke risk after anterior wall acute myocardial infarction. *Am J Cardiol* 76:825, 1995.

a myocardial infarction at the same time or within a few days.[34] There is also a high incidence of silent myocardial ischemia among these patients.[34] Arrhythmias, both supraventricular and ventricular, have been noted with ischemic stroke. Atrial fibrillation is the most common. Therefore, some suggest that continuous cardiac monitoring be done in all patients with acute ischemic stroke. If there is any question of concurrent cardiac ischemia, the patients must have cardiac monitoring and serial creatine kinase (CK) isoenzymes and ECG done. The presence of concurrent stroke and myocardial infarction affects prognosis, with 60 percent of these people dying during hospitalization.[21]

Acute Stroke As a Complication of Therapy for Acute Myocardial Infarction

Stroke-Complicating Thrombolysis Thrombolytic therapy used in patients with acute MI is associated with an increased risk of hemorrhagic stroke but reduced risk of ischemic stroke.[35] The most feared, albeit infrequent, complication of thrombolytic therapy is intracerebral hemorrhage (ICH). Most hemorrhages occur within 24 h after infusion of thrombolytics. Typically, hemorrhages are large (average volumes of 70 mL), solitary, supratentorial, and show a hematoma blood/fluid level, suggestive of fibrinolysis-related coagulopathy. Relevant identifiable risk factors for post-thrombolysis ICH include low body weight (<70 kg), age greater than 65 years old, hypertension, prior cerebrovascular disease, use of oral anticoagulation prior to thrombolysis, and underlying cerebral amyloid angiopathy. Overall, this complication occurs in 0.1 to 1.4 percent of patients receiving thrombolysis for MI and is associated with poor outcome, with two-thirds of patients dying during hospitalization. Management of these patients should include discontinuance of thrombolysis, anticoagulants or antiplatelet agents, infusion of cryoprecipitate and fresh frozen plasma, and a prompt neurosurgical consultation to evaluate possible surgical intervention.[36,37] Platelet transfusion and antifibrinolytic drugs may be required. Nonhemorrhagic stroke may also occur after thrombolysis as discussed in the previous section.

Stroke-Complicating Percutaneous Transluminal Angioplasty Primary percutaneous transluminal coronary angioplasty (PTCA) and thrombolytic therapy are alternative means of achieving reperfusion in patients with acute MI. PTCA has grown in acceptance as evidence from meta-analysis, and the Primary An-

gioplasty in Myocardial Infarction (PAMI) trial has shown better clinical outcomes with similar or reduced costs when compared with thrombolysis[38,39] and/or traditional care.[40]

Angioplasty may be complicated by ischemic stroke due to factors associated with myocardial infarction or to dislodging of protruding aortic arch atheromas.[41] The overall reported rates for all strokes associated with MI treated with PTCA range from 0.2 percent to 0.7 percent, similar to nonhemorrhagic stroke rates reported after thrombolysis and lower than stroke rates following traditional therapy. This evidence suggests that limiting the myocardial injury has a favorable effect in lowering subsequent stroke risk.

Stroke-Complicating Coronary Artery Bypass Surgery Although there is a good correlation between carotid artery disease and cerebrovascular events during CABG, no study has conclusively shown that underlying carotid artery disease is the cause of perioperative stroke. Strokes following CABG are multifactorial in nature and may be due to embolization from an atheromatous ascending aorta[42] or the carotid artery, from air or platelet aggregates formed during cardiopulmonary bypass,[43] or due to cerebral hypoperfusion.

The risk of developing a postoperative neurologic event following CABG is 0 to 9 percent in patients with carotid artery stenosis greater than 50 percent.[44] Faggioli found an overall 18.7 percent prevalence of carotid artery stenosis >50 percent and a 6.8 percent prevalence of >75 percent carotid artery lesions. In patients undergoing CABG, severe stenosis occurred more frequently among patients older than 60 years, and increased incidents of postoperative stroke were seen almost exclusively in patients with a carotid artery stenosis of >75 percent. All of these patients were asymptomatic before surgery and showed a postoperative stroke rate of 15 percent.[45] Schwartz et al also found the risk of stroke increased with greater severity of carotid stenosis. In their series, patients with bilateral carotid stenosis >80 percent[46] doubled the rate of postoperative stroke of those patients with unilateral carotid stenosis >50 percent.

DIAGNOSIS

The major cause of death in patients with cerebral ischemia treated either medically or surgically is CAD.[47] Because CAD is largely asymptomatic in the general population and in patients with CVD, a cardiac evaluation limited to those patients with clinically overt CAD will fail to identify those individuals with coexistent silent myocardial ischemia. However, evaluation for CAD is usually neglected and rarely integrated into the management of stroke patients. This section reviews the cardiologic evaluation of the stroke patient with possible coexistent CAD and the evaluation of patients considered for carotid endarterectomy. A practical algorithm is proposed.

A careful cardiac history is an essential part of the evaluation of patients with CVD. History of previous angina, myocardial infarction, congestive heart failure, arrhythmias, and coronary revascularization procedures is helpful in screening for CAD. Frequency and complexity of ventricular ectopic activity usually correlates with the severity of CAD and the extent of left ventricular function impairment. Cardiac examination may show signs suggestive of prior CAD or CHF such as dyskinetic apical impulse, presence of S3, pulsus alternans, or alternating intensity of the second sound.[48]

In the absence of lung disease, the ability to exercise is a measure of cardiac function. Performance is ideally expressed in terms of the amount of oxygen used during exercise, that is stated in multiples of the unit for an individual's basal oxygen requirement, or metabolic equivalent (MET). One MET is equal to 3.5 mL of oxygen/min/kg of body weight and is assumed to be the average basal requirement for all persons. A clinician can estimate level of fitness by questioning the patient about performance of certain activities, for which oxygen consumption values are known. For example, walking at 4 miles per hour equals 4 METs, swimming or jogging at 6 miles an hour equals 10 METs.[49] A score is assigned according to the activity that the patient is able to do routinely without developing chest pain or significant shortness of breath. Patients with cardiac ischemia who can exercise 10 METs have the same good prognosis with medical therapy or CABG.[50]

All patients with transient ischemic attack, stroke, or patients undergoing carotid endarterectomy CE should have an ECG. This is a widely available, inexpensive tool that may be predictive of cardiac events in patients with CVD. The Dutch TIA Trial Study Group investigators determined the predictive value of clinical history and ECG findings for nonfatal myocardial infarction and cardiac death.[51] Specifically, male gender, age >65 years, diabetes mellitus, peripheral vascular disease, current angina, prior myocardial infarction (especially anterior wall), inverted T wave on ECG, enlarged cardiothoracic ratio on chest roentgenogram, and left ventricular hypertrophy predicted cardiac outcome

events. Interestingly, of patients with a history of MI by ECG, approximately half were silent or unrecognized.

Stroke patients may show electrocardiographic abnormalities in 15 to 20 percent of cases. Not all of these changes are secondary to coronary artery disease. Specifically, reversible left axis deviation, QT interval prolongation, septal U waves, and repolarization changes have been described without concomitant myocardial injury. These changes have been thought to be centrally mediated through the autonomic nervous system.[52] Basic and clinical research suggest that ischemic lesions in the left insular region may increase the sympathetic tone and decrease the parasympathetic tone, predisposing to development of cardiac arrhythmias.[53,54]

It should be noted that acute strokes, both ischemic and hemorrhagic, can produce ECG changes, sometimes in the presence of normal coronary arteries and without actual acute ischemic changes. Up to 95 percent of stroke patients may show some ECG changes, compared with 50 percent of a control group. ST depression and prolongation of the QT interval occurred seven times more frequently.

The presence of atherosclerotic risk factors and comorbidities such as pulmonary disease, diabetes, liver disease, and renal insufficiency also affect the risk of coexistent CAD and have an impact in perioperative morbidity. Additional predictors have been established for the perioperative cardiovascular evaluation for noncardiac surgery.[55] Major predictors requiring aggressive treatment included unstable coronary syndromes within the past 7 to 30 days, decompensated heart failure, serious arrhythmias (high-grade atrioventricular block, supraventricular arrhythmias with rapid ventricular response, and symptomatic ventricular arrhythmias), and severe valvular disease. Intermediate risk factors that increase perioperative cardiac risk included prior myocardial infarction by ECG or history, compensated or prior heart failure, and diabetes.

Patients with an estimated high risk for CAD as determined by history, physical examination, ECG, and functional status should undergo further testing to confirm the diagnosis and to establish the extent of disease. Currently, the following diagnostic modalities are available: treadmill exercise testing, cardiopulmonary exercise testing, radionuclide determination of left ventricular function, ambulatory ECG monitoring, stress myocardial perfusion imaging, stress echocardiography, and coronary angiography. A summary of negative predictive value and positive predictive value, in detecting CAD and predicting perioperative cardiac events for these techniques, is depicted in Table 26-5.

Table 24-5.

Predictive values[a] for perioperative cardiac events of noninvasive testing

Technique	Positive predictive value	Negative predictive value
	%	
Exercise electrocardiography	8–81	91–100
Dipyridamole thallium stress test	4–20	+99
Dobutamine echocardiography	7–23	93–100

[a]Positive predictive value is defined as the proportion of individuals who test positive who truly have the disease. The negative predictive value is the proportion of individuals who test negative who truly do not have the disease.

Treadmill exercise testing is frequently used to diagnose CAD. Patients with very good exercise tolerance have a lower risk of cardiac complications and have good long-term prognosis. Conversely, patients likely to have three-vessel and/or severe left main CAD are identified by an inability to complete Bruce stage I, the attainment of a maximum heart rate of 120 per minute, the development of marked ST segment depression, or the development of hypotension during exercise. Exercise electrocardiography is contraindicated in acute MI, unstable angina, infective endocarditis, severe aortic stenosis, uncontrolled heart failure, pulmonary embolism, pericarditis or myocarditis, peripheral vascular thrombosis, renal failure, and thyrotoxicosis.[50] It is less informative when ECG interpretation is difficult, as in cases of left bundle branch block, left ventricular hypertrophy with strain, and digitalis effect. In addition, many stroke patients are unable to exercise due to their neurologic sequelae.

The cardiopulmonary exercise testing measures the oxygen uptake and carbon dioxide production during exercise. Maximum ventricular performance is estimated by calculating the anaerobic threshold from the oxygen uptake data, which is the point at which mixed venous lactate increases due to failure of the left ventricle to meet the metabolic demands of the body. Although few reports found this technique predictive of cardiac risk, more corroborative studies are needed. This technique is not widely available and presents the same limitations mentioned above for the evaluation of the stroke patient.

Radionuclide angiography has been used to determine the resting left ventricular ejection fraction as part of the preoperative assessment. It has not been uniformly valuable in predicting perioperative cardiac morbidity in patients undergoing major noncardiac surgery,

as left ventricular perioperative performance depends on coronary flow reserve and the amount of myocardium at risk, none of which is addressed by the radionuclide angiography. This technique should be reserved for patients with current or poorly controlled heart failure.[55]

Ambulatory ECG monitoring has been used prior to vascular and nonvascular surgery. Some data indicate that this technique can be useful in stratifying perioperative high-risk patients, but the evidence in vascular surgery patients has not been convincing.[56,57]

Vasodilator stress simulates the exercise-related coronary vasodilation. Stress-myocardial perfusion studies are based on the fact that the coronary bed distal to a flow-limiting coronary lesion is substantially dilated to preserve normal coronary flow and that further major increases in vasodilation are not possible in response to exercise or vasodilator drugs. Thus, a region of myocardium that is not well perfused will show little or no uptake of thallium when compared with an adjacent normal segment in which flow may increase up to five-fold. Adenosine and dipyridamole are available, but the latter is more commonly used. The risk of these agents inducing myocardial ischemia is minimal, but they may cause bronchospasm and delayed atrioventricular node conduction, which contraindicates their use in patients with obstructive pulmonary disease or AV node conduction defects. Many publications describing the use of dipyridamole thallium stress testing in the preoperative evaluation of patients have shown positive predictive value of 4 to 20 percent for myocardial infarction or cardiac death and negative predictive value close to 99 percent.[58–63] Baron and colleagues have challenged these results.[64] They reported that dipyridamole-thallium myocardial perfusion scanning using single photon emission computed tomography did not predict adverse cardiac outcome in a prospective study of 457 patients undergoing abdominal aortic surgery. Age >65 years and clinical evidence of CAD were the only predictors of cardiac complications. Patient selection bias, nonconsecutive enrollment, and detection bias by physicians (knowledge of test results) are some of the factors explaining such contradictory results.

Few studies have evaluated these techniques to stratify the risk prior to CE. In a retrospective, nonrandomized study, Ombrellaro and colleagues found dipyridamole thallium testing ineffective in predicting adverse cardiac events in patients considered for CE.[65] In 1994, Urbinati and co-workers studied 172 candidates for CE with symptomatic high-grade carotid stenosis, using exercise electrocardiography, followed by exercise thallium testing if abnormal.[66] Mean follow-up was 6.2 years. Patients with no history of CAD (who did not have further workup) and those with history of CAD and negative noninvasive cardiac testing showed no cardiac deaths at 30 days and an estimated 97 percent survival free of coronary events after CE. The remaining patients who either had silent CAD (abnormal exercise or thallium tests without prior history) or were unable to undergo exercise testing due to previous stroke and/or claudication, or patients with known CAD, showed estimated survivals free of coronary events of 51, 49, and 59 percent, respectively. There were three cardiac deaths within the first 30 days after surgery.

Dobutamine has been used preoperatively to predict cardiac risk in patients undergoing vascular surgeries. Dobutamine, a short-acting synthetic catecholamine, stimulates cardiac beta receptors producing an increase in heart rate and myocardial contractility with an associated increase in myocardial oxygen demand and coronary blood flow. A positive test is defined as a new or worsening wall motion abnormality seen by echocardiography during dobutamine infusion. All studies showed very similar results to those of vasodilator myocardial perfusion scans and concluded that dobutamine echocardiography is relatively safe and useful in predicting perioperative cardiac risk.[67-69] Overall, the positive predictive value was 7 to 23 percent, and the negative predictive value ranged from 93 to 100 percent.[59] Clinicians should be aware of the potential for inducing myocardial ischemia with this technique and the limited value in evaluating patients with left bundle branch block who may have reversible septal motion abnormalities in the absence of significant left anterior descending coronary artery disease.

Coronary angiography remains the gold standard to define coronary anatomy and determine the location and severity of CAD. Hertzer et al studied 506 patients presenting with symptomatic ($n = 288$) or asymptomatic ($n = 218$) extracranial cerebrovascular disease.[11] He found severe surgically correctable CAD in 37 percent of patients who were clinically suspected to have CAD and in 16 percent who were not, and inoperable CAD in 9.8 percent and 1.5 percent of the respective groups. Severe CAD was defined as greater than 70 percent stenosis in one or more coronary arteries serving unimpaired myocardium; inoperable CAD was defined as greater than 70 percent stenosis of multiple arteries with diffuse distal involvement or generalized ventricular impairment. Gathering these data and the available literature, coronary angiography is indicated in the following scenarios: (1) suspected or proven CAD in high-risk patients during noninvasive testing, (2) before any coronary revascularization procedure, either angioplasty or CABG, (3) angina unresponsive to medical therapy, (4) unstable angina, and (5) equivocal or nondiagnostic noninvasive test in previously determined high-risk patient. It also may be helpful as a confirmatory test when noninvasive tools provide an intermediate risk. An interesting option in patients with concomitant CAD/CVD is the performance of combined angiography. Chimowitz and colleagues studied 247 patients who had combined carotid and coronary angiography and compared them with 686 patients who underwent coronary angiography alone.[70] Complication rates were similar; there were no strokes and two TIAs at 24 h in the combined group. The carotid arteries were inadequately visualized in 11 percent of patients undergoing combined angiography. The combined procedure has the advantages of convenience for the patient and lower cost. However, carotid artery films are of lesser quality than conventional carotid angiography, and the percentage of inadequate visualization is relatively high. Therefore, combined carotid and coronary angiography cannot be recommended as a standard evaluation for combined CAD/CVD at this point.

A different and original approach to the evaluation of predictors for CAD has been proposed by ultrasonography researchers. Since the early 1990's, several structural changes of the carotid artery wall detected with B-mode ultrasonography have been associated with the risk of myocardial infarction.[71] Nowak et al compared the B-mode carotid artery findings with exercise testing, variance ECG, and coronary angiography in 184 patients with history suggestive of angina or frequent ectopic beats on resting ECG.[72] The presence of plaques, alone or with angina, and the left common carotid artery intima-media area greater than 15 to 20 mm², correlated with higher coronary scores (sum of disease in all coronary vessels). Sensitivity, specificity, and predictive values were comparable with exercise testing. This study was done in high-risk symptomatic patients, which constitutes a selection bias. The results cannot be extrapolated to an intermediate or low-risk population. Further studies will be necessary to determine the potential value of this tool in other populations and in comparison with vasodilator thallium scanning.

Finally, an algorithm for the cardiac evaluation of patients with CVD is proposed (Fig. 26-1). Several conclusions can be obtained from this section. Clinical history, physical examination, fitness determination, and ECG are the most helpful tools in stratifying the cardiac risk. Those patients with low risk do not require further evaluation. Those with high risk, including unstable coronary syndromes, should be evaluated directly with coronary angiography. Until additional prospective and blinded studies help to improve patient risk analysis, the intermediate predictors group with decreased functional capacity should undergo noninvasive testing, usually va-

Figure 26-1.
An algorithm for the cardiac evaluation of stroke patients.

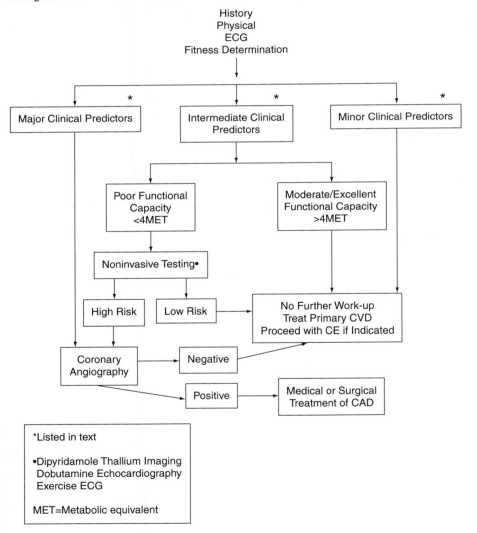

sodilator myocardium imaging in stroke patients. If results are suggestive of severe CAD, angiography is the logical next step.

MANAGEMENT OF COMBINED CORONARY ARTERY AND CEREBROVASCULAR DISEASE

Patients presenting with symptomatic atherosclerotic vascular disease including the carotid, coronary, or peripheral vascular systems are likely to have occult or manifest comorbidities in the other sites. This is particularly important in the case of CAD and carotid disease, in which the potential complications may be devastating.

Management of patients with serious concomitant carotid and coronary artery disease is usually complex and remains controversial. The clinician may be faced with one of these combinations: symptomatic cardiac and carotid disease, symptomatic carotid disease and asymptomatic cardiac disease, or symptomatic cardiac disease with asymptomatic carotid disease. Therapeutic options are medical or surgical according to the severity of involvement of the specific vascular bed. Regardless of the indicated therapy, all patients should undergo strict control of risk factors for atherosclerosis such as hypertension, hyperlipidemia, diabetes, and smoking.

Prevention

Risk factor control is the cornerstone of secondary prevention in CAD and carotid artery disease. Hypertension is the most powerful, prevalent, and treatable risk factor for stroke and CAD.[73] Treatment of isolated systolic hypertension (SBP >160 mmHg) in people older than 60 years reduces stroke incidence by 36 percent,[74] and an average reduction of 6 mmHg in diastolic blood pressure produces a 42 percent reduction in stroke incidence.[75]

Elevated serum lipid levels have clearly been associated with CAD. However, their relation to the incidence of stroke in individual population studies has not been established definitely. Although a meta-analysis of lipid-lowering trials found no stroke risk reduction,[76] more recent studies of the statins, simvastatin,[77] lovastatin,[78] and pravastatin,[79] have shown a 30 percent reduction in strokes. These last two statins have also shown slowing of the progression of carotid artery disease by ultrasound (Table 26-6).[78–80] It may be assumed that the reported benefits would be greater in patients with concomitant CAD and CVD.

Cigarette smoking substantially increases the risk of CAD and stroke. It is also a risk factor for carotid restenosis. Smoking cessation should be encouraged, as it promptly reduces the risk of stroke and MI.[81]

Medical Management

Most patients will fall in this category. As a general rule, asymptomatic CAD and CVD are treated only with risk factor control, unless there are surgical indications discussed in the next section. Symptomatic carotid artery disease of less than 50 percent stenosis associated with nonsurgical CAD is treated with platelet antiaggregant medications and risk factor modification. The Antiplatelet Trialists[82] found a 22 percent reduction in risk for nonfatal stroke, nonfatal myocardial infarction, and vascular death in patients with TIA or stroke treated with antiplatelet medications. This benefit was independent of age, gender, or common risk factors like hypertension or diabetes. Aspirin prescribed at doses ranging from 30 to 1300 mg/day reduces all vascular events by about 25 percent and remains foremost among platelet-antiaggregating agents. There is also suggestive evidence that aspirin may decrease perioperative coronary events after carotid endarterectomy.[83]

Table 26-6.
Carotid artery disease lipid trials

Carotid U.S. study	Intervention	IMT (mm/y)		Reduction in events
		Control	Treated	
ACAPS[78]	Lovastatin	+0.006	−0.009	64
PLAC II[79]	Pravastatin	+0.067	+0.059	60
KAPS[80]	Pravastatin	+0.031	+0.017	38

IMT, intima-media thickness.

Ticlopidine 250 mg twice a day is indicated for patients with TIA or stroke occurring while on aspirin or with contraindications for aspirin, and for coronary artery stents. It reduces stroke or MI by 30 percent. Ticlopidine has been associated with severe neutropenia, which mandates the monitoring of CBC with differential every 2 weeks for the first 3 months of therapy.[84] Clopidogrel is an antiplatelet agent that inhibits ADP-induced aggregation like ticlopidine. The recommended dose is 75 mg/day. Clopidogrel has a better tolerance profile and less risk of neutropenia when compared with ticlopidine. Clopidogrel showed an 8.7 percent relative-risk reduction of stroke, MI, and vascular death with respect to aspirin.[85]

Symptomatic cardiac disease associated with 60 percent stenosis of carotid arteries is treated according to the specific coronary syndrome. Review of these current therapies is beyond the scope of this chapter.

Surgical Management

The subset of patients in this group with a surgical indication for one vascular bed with nonsurgical indication for the other is the easiest to approach. Timing and type of surgery are conventional. The overall perioperative mortality and morbidity in CABG and CE are shown in Table 26-7.[8,86,87]

Patients with surgical indications for both CEA and CABG represent a therapeutic dilemma. The debate on how to treat these patients has continued for many years. The options include: CE only, CABG only, staged separate procedures with CABG first, staged separate procedures with CE first, or combined CE/CABG procedures. Numerous publications address this controversy in the literature and differ in definitions of procedures, degree of carotid disease, presence of neurologically symptomatic patients, and methods. Although the studies are difficult to compare, some conclusions can be obtained from their review.

Symptomatic Cardiac and Carotid Disease There is little doubt that surgical treatment is indicated in this group of patients. Patients with known carotid artery stenosis undergoing CABG may have an increased risk of perioperative stroke. These trials are retrospective and included both symptomatic and asymptomatic patients and varied in the method of determining stenosis. The stroke rate may be higher in these patients, especially when carotid stenosis is greater than 75 percent. Table 26-8 shows the perioperative stroke rates in patients with known carotid disease undergoing CABG, including studies with both symptomatic and asymptomatic patients[88–91] or asymptomatic[45,46,92] only.

Patients with known CAD undergoing CE only may have an increased risk of perioperative MI. Among 614 patients undergoing CE, those with history of MI, angina, or EKG abnormalities consistent with CAD had a perioperative MI rate of 4.3 percent compared with 0.7 percent of those with no evidence of CAD.[93] Perioperative stroke rates were 2.8 percent.

The dilemma is to decide whether it is better to perform simultaneous vs. sequential operations.

The first alternative, simultaneous procedure of CE and CABG was proposed by Bernhard et al in 1972.[94] CE may be performed before the institution of cardiopulmonary bypass or during bypass. Performing CE before bypass theoretically ensures higher cerebral perfusion pressures during the operation and allows increased cerebral perfusion during bypass. This concept becomes more relevant in patients with critical carotid stenosis in whom cerebral autoregulation is impaired. On the other hand, advocates of performing CE during CABG maintain that systemic hypothermia (20° C) provides cerebral protection during the period of carotid clamping, and if unexpected delays occur in the noncardiac portions of the procedure, they would not prolong aortic cross-clamping. CE is then performed after circulatory arrest has occurred. These technical aspects may have differential effects on the stroke or nonfatal MI rates, but unfortunately the available studies vary in the operatory techniques, and no conclusions favoring one or the other can be obtained.

In Bernhard's study, the reported postoperative stroke rate was 6 percent with an overall mortality rate of 6 percent. Since then, several studies have reported the mortality, nonfatal stroke rates, and nonfatal MI rates, associated with the combined procedure (Table 26-8). All of these studies are retrospective and vary on whether the patients had symptomatic or asymptomatic cerebrovascular disease and the degree of carotid stenosis. Mortality ranges from 0 to

Table 26-7.

General perioperative mortality and morbidity in CABG and CE

	Mortality	Stroke	MI
		%	
CABG[86]	3.5	1.6	2.5
CE-symptomatic[8]	0.6	5.5	0.9
CE-asymptomatic[87]	0.1	1.4	——

Table 26-8.

Perioperative stroke rates in patients undergoing CABG and known carotid disease

	Year	# Patients	Neurologically asymptomatic and/or symptomatic	Carotid stenosis	Perioperative stroke
Combined symptomatic/asymptomatic carotid disease					
Furlan[88]	1985	29	Both	>50%	%
Schultz[89]	1988	50	Both	Angio "hemodynamically significant"	3.0 6.0
Gerraty[90]	1993	203	Both	Variable	1.0
Salasidis[91]	1995	387	Both	<80% >80%	1.7 18.2
Asymptomatic					
Brener[92]	1987	64	Asymptomatic	>50% 50–75%	1.6
Faggioli[45]	1990	88	Asymptomatic	>75%	14.3
Schwartz[46]	1995	130	Asymptomatic	50–100%	3.8

12 percent, nonfatal stroke 0 to 18 percent, and nonfatal MI 0 to 8 percent.

The Multidisciplinary Consensus Statement from the AdHoc Committee of the American Heart Association reviewed the English language reports on surgical treatment of CAD and carotid disease.[95] These retrospective studies included three strategies: simultaneous CE/CABG, CE followed by CABG, and CABG followed by CE. The perioperative stroke rate was 5.3 percent if CE preceded CABG, 6.2 percent if they were performed simultaneously, and 10 percent if CABG preceded CE. The respective MI rates were 11.5, 4.7, and 2.7 percent. These findings indicate that the perioperative morbidity is increased in the arterial tree not operated on initially.

In 1998, the American Heart Association published an update of the guidelines for carotid endarterectomy.[96] Indications were outlined under the headings: proven, acceptable but not proven, uncertain, and proven inappropriate. For low-risk patients with symptomatic carotid artery stenosis greater than 70 percent who require CABG for coronary disease, CE performed by a surgeon whose combined surgical morbidity and mortality rate is less than 6 percent is considered acceptable but not proven, when performed simultaneously with CABG. Patients with 50 to 69 percent stenosis measured on arteriography also had benefit from CE when compared with medical therapy, especially for nondiabetic men with hemispheric ischemia, according to the final report of primary endpoints from NASCET.[97] However, if a patient with 50 to 69 percent carotid stenosis also requires CABG, we consider that the indication for CE still continues to be uncertain, and therapeutic decisions should be individualized (patient surgical risk, institution experience, etc.).

Some authors have proposed the use of less invasive techniques for the management of symptomatic and asymptomatic carotid disease.[98] This recommendation is based on the risk of complications from the vascular bed not operated upon first in combined surgical procedures. Carotid angioplasty without stenting has been used sporadically since 1981. More recently, the use of carotid artery stents has shown improved outcomes, specifically fewer complications, better postoperative angiographic results, and decreased incidence of restenosis than in the past. Several small series have also shown comparable complication rates with CE.[99] Although these data are appealing, formal randomized-controlled trials testing carotid angioplasty and stenting are necessary before adopting them as alternative treatments. If it proves to be successful in the management of symptomatic carotid disease without an increase in morbidity, it would offer a reasonable alternative for treatment of carotid disease before CABG. Use of carotid artery stenting is still considered to be experimental.[100]

Symptomatic Cardiac Disease and Asymptomatic Carotid Artery Disease　The Asymptomatic Carotid Atherosclerosis Study (ACAS)[85] has contributed significantly to the understanding of asymptomatic carotid disease. This study of 1662 patients showed a 2.3 percent perioperative risk of stroke or death (30 days) and a 5.1 percent risk of ipsilateral stroke or perioperative stroke or death (5-year projection) in the CE group compared with the medical group, with 0.4 and 11 percent risks, respectively, for the same time points. This study did not look at concomitant CAD and carotid disease. However, further analysis of perioperative risk in ACAS showed that some baseline variables were significant predictors of perioperative complications; prior history of stroke, contralateral internal carotid artery stenosis ≥60 percent, and abstinence from alcohol were associated with a higher risk of all complications combined (stroke, transient ischemic attack, myocardial infarction, and death). In addition to these three variables, diabetes mellitus and contralateral siphon stenosis were associated with a high risk of stroke. Of the surgical variables, the length of external carotid artery plaque was associated with stroke and all event rates; the use of local or regional anesthesia was associated with a higher risk of transient ischemic attack or myocardial infarction.[101] These findings should be interpreted with caution because of three basic reasons: the data from ACAS do not explain why these variables are significant; the selection of local vs. general anesthesia may depend on differences in the baseline characteristics of the patients, leading to differences in event rates; and the number of events in the study was small, which may have not shown the association of other significant factors. Another interesting observation from this analysis was the higher rate of complications seen in patients with a maximum systolic blood pressure (SBP) >180 mmHg in the recovery room, whereas those patients with maximum SBP <145 mmHg had significantly fewer complications ($p = .012$). Reasonably, the authors conclude that those patients with SBP >145 mmHg in the postoperative period should receive close neurologic monitoring.

Other series[45–47] have reported the perioperative stroke rate in patients undergoing CABG with asymptomatic carotid stenosis greater than 50 percent. These are retrospective studies with patient numbers ranging from 64 to 130. Perioperative stroke rates range from 0 to 3.8 percent.

A review of published reports from 1972 to 1985 included 1483 patients with asymptomatic carotid artery disease.[102] Patients underwent staged CE then CABG or simultaneous CE and CABG, but no staged CABG before CE. The perioperative rates for stroke, MI, and death were 2.9, 5.6, and 6.2 percent, respectively. Although the stroke rates were comparable between the staged CE-CABG group and the combined procedure group (3.1 percent vs. 2.8 percent, respectively), the death and MI rates were much higher in the staged group (11.1 and 11.8 percent vs. 4.7 and 3.8 percent). These findings suggest that in asymptomatic carotid stenosis patients undergoing CABG surgery, the combined procedure is superior to the staged-first CE then CABG, as the latter does not protect from stroke and increases mortality.

A valuable contribution to the topic is found in Hertzer's study of 275 patients with indications for CE and CABG. He reported the cumulative 5-year stroke rates and survival rates in three different groups, divided based on their perceived cardiac and neurologic risk. Group 1 consisted of patients with unilateral carotid stenosis and acceptable cardiac status who underwent staged procedures with CE prior to CABG. Group 2 had unilateral asymptomatic carotid stenosis patients with more unstable cardiac status who were randomized to combined CE/CABG (IIa) or staged procedures with CABG prior to CE (IIb). Group 3 consisted of patients with symptomatic or severe bilateral carotid disease and cardiac disease who were treated on an individual basis. The cumulative 5-year stroke rates were 20.3 percent for group 1, 4.6 percent for group IIa, 26.2 percent for group IIb, and 10.8 percent for group 3. The cumulative 5-year survival rates ranged from 77.2 percent in group 2A up to 90.5 percent in group IIb. Those patients undergoing combined CE/CABG had lower stroke rate, but also a lower survival at 5 years.[103]

Symptomatic Carotid Disease and Asymptomatic Cardiac Disease　This group includes patients with symptomatic carotid disease and CAD detected by the preoperative workup. Possible interventions range from nonpharmacologic, pharmacologic, and more aggressive approaches such as angioplasty or coronary artery bypass.

A simple nonpharmacologic measure is to assure normovolemia starting from the preoperative period. Pharmacologic interventions directed to prevent hemodynamic instability during surgery may be started in patients with uncontrolled hypertension or tachycardia. For omitted medications, readily parenteral substitutes may be administered.[104]

Patients with more severe CAD should have the standard intraoperative monitoring in addition to more invasive techniques like two-dimensional transesophageal echocardiography, which may detect segmental wall motion abnormalities rapidly. Use of pulmonary artery catheters is controversial and generally reserved for operations in which transesophageal echocardiography is unavailable or unsatisfactory.[104]

Percutaneous angioplasty to improve cardiac status prior to surgery has been proposed if a correctable lesion is found.[105] However, this recommendation is not based on data from controlled or randomized studies. If main or triple vessel disease is found, a combined operation is considered an acceptable approach.[96]

Recommendations

The management of combined CAD and CVD has not been tested in a properly designed and randomized multicenter trial. Therefore, the following guidelines for patients with combined coronary and carotid artery disease often fall into the category of acceptable or uncertain indication. Evidently, each patient should be evaluated on an individual basis.

Symptomatic CAD-CVD   Until results of properly designed trials become available, simultaneous CABG and CE is an acceptable indication for these patients. Risk may not be greater with this approach, and it may be more cost effective than the staged approach.[106]

Asymptomatic Carotid Disease and Symptomatic CAD   For patients with a CE surgical risk of less than 3 percent, life expectancy of at least 5 years, and >60 percent stenosis with or without ulceration of the internal carotid artery in whom CABG is otherwise indicated, simultaneous CE and CABG is an acceptable indication.[96] Patients who do not fulfill these criteria often undergo CABG only and medical therapy with antiplatelets and risk factor modification.

Symptomatic Carotid Artery Disease and Asymptomatic CAD   If left main or triple vessel CAD is found, a simultaneous revascularization procedure is considered an acceptable approach. For less severe CAD, only CE is performed. The CAD is often approached with medical therapy or angioplasty and close perioperative monitoring.

SUMMARY

Patients presenting with stroke often have severe concomitant coronary artery disease. This association has an impact on morbidity and mortality. The rational use of relevant clinical information and paraclinical studies should lead to appropriate risk stratification of patients with concomitant disease and to effective therapies directed to improve patient outcomes. Based on the data above, it is obvious that we have scarce prospective data on patients who may need CE and CABG. Prospective randomized trials addressing this question are urgently needed.

REFERENCES

1. Rokey R, Rolak L, Harati Y, et al: Coronary artery disease in patients with cerebrovascular disease: A prospective study. *Ann Neurol* 16:50, 1984.
2. Chimowitz MI, Mancini GB: Asymptomatic coronary artery disease in patients with stroke: *Curr Concepts Cerebrovasc Dis Stroke* 26:23, 1991.
3. Chimowitz M, Weiss D, Cohen S, et al: Cardiac prognosis of patients with carotid stenosis and no history of coronary artery disease. *Stroke* 25:759, 1994.
4. Howard G, Evans G, Crouse J III, et al: A prospective reevaluation or transient ischemic attacks as a risk factor for death and fatal or nonfatal cardiovascular events. *Stroke* 25:342, 1994.
5. Chimowitz MI, Poole RM, Starling MR, et al: Frequency and severity of asymptomatic coronary disease in patients with different causes of stroke. *Stroke* 28:941, 1997.
6. Koudstaal PJ, Algra A, Pop GA, et al: Risk of cardiac events in atypical transient ischaemic attack of minor stroke. *Lancet* 340:630, 1992.
7. Kaplan M, Pratley R, Hawkins W, et al: Silent myocardial ischemia during rehabilitation for cerebrovascular disease. *Arch Phys Med Rehabil* 72:59, 1991.
8. North American Symptomatic Carotid Endarterectomy Trial Collaborators: Beneficial effect of carotid endarterectomy in symptomatic patients with high grade carotid stenosis. *N Engl J Med* 325:445, 1991.
9. European Carotid Trialists' Collaborative Group: Endarterectomy for moderate, symptomatic carotid stenosis: Interim results from the MRC European carotid surgery trial. *Lancet* 347:1591, 1996.
10. Wiebers DO, Whisnant JP, O'Fallon M: Reversible ischemic neurologic deficit (RIND) in a community: Rochester, Minnesota, 1955–1969. *Neurology* 32:459, 1982.
11. Hertzer N, Young J, Beven E, et al: Coronary angiography in 506 patients with extracranial cerebrovascular disease. *Arch Intern Med* 145:849, 1985.
12. DiPasquale G, Pinelli G, Grazi P, et al: Incidence of silent myocardial ischemia in patients with cerebral ischemia. *Eur Heart J* 9:104, 1988.
13. Fleg J, Gerstenblith G, Zonderman A, et al: Prevalence and prognostic significance of exercise-induced silent myocardial ischemia detected by thallium scintigraphy

and electrocardiography in asymptomatic volunteers. *Circulation* 81:428, 1990.

14. Love BB, Grover-McKay M, Biller J, et al: Coronary artery disease and cardiac events with asymptomatic and symptomatic cerebrovascular disease. *Stroke* 23:939, 1992.

15. Urbinati S, DiPasquale G, Andreoli A, et al: Frequency and prognostic significance of silent coronary artery disease in patients with cerebral ischemia undergoing carotid endarterectomy. *Am J Cardiol* 69:1166, 1992.

16. Brass LM, Hartigan PM, Page WF, Comcato JI: Importance of cerebrovascular disease in studies of myocardial infarction. *Stroke* 27:1173, 1996.

17. Mooe T, Erikson P, Stegmayr B: Ischemic stroke after acute myocardial infarction: A population based-study. *Stroke* 28:762, 1997.

18. Puletti M, Morocutti C, Tronca M, et al: Cerebrovascular accidents in acute myocardial infarction. *Ital J Neurol Sci* 8:245, 1987.

19. Behar S, Tanne D, Abinader E, The SPRINT study group, et al: Cerebrovascular accident complicating acute myocardial infarction: Incidence, clinical significance, and short and long-term mortality rates. *Am J Med* 91:45, 1991.

20. Tanne D, Reicher-Reiss W, Boyko V, et al for the SPRINT Study Group: Stroke risk after anterior wall acute myocardial infarction. *Am J Cardiol* 76:825, 1995.

21. Komrad MS, Coffey CE, Coffey KS, et al: Myocardial infarction and stroke. *Neurology* 34:1403, 1984.

22. Hess DC, D'Cruz IA, Adams RJ, et al: Coronary artery disease, myocardial infarction and brain embolism. *Neurol Clin* 11:399, 1993.

23. Santamaria J, Graus F, Rubio F, et al: Cerebral infarction of the basal ganglia due to embolism from the heart. *Stroke* 14:911, 1983.

24. ISIS-2 (Second International Study of Infarct Survival) Collaborative Group: Randomised trial of intravenous streptokinase, oral aspirin, both, or neither among 17,187 cases of suspected acute myocardial infarction: ISIS-2. *Lancet* 2:349, 1988.

25. Maggioni AP, Franzosi MG, Farina MI, et al: Cerebrovascular events after myocardial infarction: Analysis of the GISSI trial: Gruppo Italiano per lo studio della Streptochinasi nell'Infarto Miocardico (GISSI). *Br Med J* 302:1428, 1991.

26. Pullicino P: Pathogenesis of stroke after non-anterior myocardial infarction. *J Am Coll Cardiol* 25:1476, 1995.

27. Vaitkus PT, Barnathon ES: Embolic potential, prevention and management of mural thrombus complicating anterior myocardial infarction: A meta-analysis. *J Am Coll Cardiol* 22:1004, 1993.

28. Ekery D, Benjamin E: Cardiac disease & stroke: Innocent bystander or cause & effect. *Compr Ther* 23:281, 1997.

29. Loh E, Sutton MSI, Wun C-CC, et al: Ventricular dysfunction and the risk of stroke after myocardial infarction. *N Engl J Med* 336:251, 1997.

30. Mahaffey KW, Granger CB, Sloan MA, et al: Risk factors for in-hospital nonhemorrhagic stroke in patients with acute myocardial infarction treated with thrombolysis: Results from GUSTO-I. *Circulation* 97:757, 1998.

31. Pullicino PM, Xuereb M, Aquilina J, et al: Stroke following acute myocardial infarction in diabetics. *J Intern Med* 231:287, 1992.

32. Martin R, Bogousslavsky J: Mechanism of late stroke after myocardial infarct: The Lausanne Stroke Registry. *J Neurol Neurosurg Psychiatry* 56:760, 1993.

33. Andreoli A, di Pasquale G, Pinelli G, et al: Subarachnoid hemorrhage: Frequency and severity of cardiac arrhythmias. A survey of 70 cases studied in the acute phase. *Stroke* 18:558, 1987.

34. Rolak LA, Rokey R: The patient with concomitant stroke and myocardial infarction—clinical features, in *Coronary and Cerebral Vascular Disease—A Practical Guide*. New York, Futura, 1990, pp 117–137.

35. Vaitkus PT, Berlin JA, Schwartz JS, et al: A direct comparison of tissue plasminogen activator (tPA) and streptokinase shows an excess of strokes with tPA. *Arch Intern Med* 152:2020, 1992.

36. Gebel JM, Sila CA, Sloan MA, et al: Thrombolysis-related intracranial hemorrhage: A radiographic analysis of 244 cases from the GUSTO-1 trial with clinical correlation. Intracranial hemorrhage complicating acute myocardial infarction in the era of thrombolytic therapy. *Southern Med J* 90:5, 1997.

37. Conrad AR, Feffer SE, Rajan RT, et al: Global utilization of streptokinase and tissue plasminogen activator for occluded coronary arteries. *Stroke* 29:563, 1998.

38. Stone GW, Grines CL, Rothbaum D: Analysis of the relative costs and effectiveness of primary angioplasty versus tissue-type plasminogen activator: The Primary Angioplasty in Myocardial Infarction (PAMI) trial. The PAMI Trial Investigators. *J Am Coll Cardiol* 29:901, 1997.

39. Weaver WD, Simes RJ, Betriu A, et al: Comparison of primary coronary angioplasty and intravenous thrombolytic therapy for acute myocardial infarction: A quantitative review. *JAMA* 278:2093, 1997.

40. Grines CL, Marsalese DL, Brodie B, et al: Safety and cost-effectiveness of early discharge after primary angioplasty in low risk patients with acute myocardial infarction: PAMI-II investigators. Primary Angioplasty in Myocardial Infarction. *J Am Coll Cardiol* 31:967, 1998.

41. Shmuely H, Zoldan J, Sagie A, et al: Acute stroke after coronary angiography associated with protruding mobile thoracic aortic atheromas. *Neurology* 49:1689, 1997.

42. Mills NL, Everson CP: Atherosclerosis of the ascending aorta and coronary bypass. *J Vasc Surg* 12:724, 1990.

43. Pome G, Passini L, Colucci V, et al: Combined surgical approach to coexistent carotid and coronary artery disease. *J Thorac Cardiovasc Surg* 32:787, 1991.

44. Sahlman A, Arnio P, Karumo J, et al: Carotid artery stenosis in coronary artery bypass patients. *Int J Angiol* 2:230, 1993.

45. Faggioli GL, Curl GR, Ricotta JJ: The role of carotid screen before coronary bypass. *J Vasc Surg* 12:724, 1990.

46. Schwartz LB, Bridgeman AH, Kieffer RW, et al. Asymptomatic carotid artery stenosis and stroke in patients undergoing cardiopulmonary bypass. *J Vasc Surg* 21:146, 1995.

47. Whisnant JP, Sandok DA, Sundt TM: Carotid endarterectomy for unilateral carotid system transient cerebral ischemia. *Mayo Clin Proc* 58:171, 1983.

48. Chizner MA: Classic teachings, in *Clinical Cardiology.* Cedar Grove, NJ, Leannec Publishers, 1996, pp 1475–1478.

49. Myers J, Do D, Herbert W, et al: A nomogram to predict exercise capacity from a specific activity questionnaire and clinical data. *Am J Cardiol* 73:591, 1994.

50. Fletcher GS, Balady G, Froehlicher ZS, et al: Exercise standards: A statement for healthcare providers from the American Heart Association writing group. *Circulation* 91:580, 1995.

51. Pop GAM, Koudstaal PJ, Meeder HJ, et al: Predictive value of clinical history and electrocardiogram in patients with transient ischemic attack for minor ischemic stroke for subsequent cardiac and cerebral ischemic events. *Arch Neurol* 51:333, 1994.

52. Dimant J, Grob D: Electrocardiographic changes and myocardial damage in patients with acute cerebrovascular accidents. *Stroke* 8:448, 1977.

53. Oppenheimer SM, Martin VM, Kedem J: Left insular cortex lesions perturb cardiac autonomic tone. *Clin Auton Res* 6:131, 1996.

54. Oppenheimer S: Neurogenic cardiac effects of cerebrovascular disease. *Curr Opin Neurol* 7:20, 1994.

55. American College of Cardiology-American Heart Association Task Force on Practice Guidelines: Committee on preoperative cardiovascular evaluation for noncardiac surgery: Guidelines for preoperative cardiovascular evaluation for noncardiac surgery. *J Am Coll Cardiol* 27:910, 1996.

56. McPhail NV, Ruddy TD, Barbert GG, et al: Cardiac risk stratification using dipyridamole myocardial perfusion imaging and ambulatory ECG monitoring prior to vascular surgery. *Eur J Vasc Surg* 7:151, 1993.

57. Fleisher LA, Rosenbaum SH, Nelson AH, et al: Preoperative dipyridamole thallium imaging and ambulatory electrocardiographic monitoring as a predictor of perioperative cardiac events and long-term outcome. *Anesthesiology* 83:906, 1995.

58. Kaul S, Lilly D, Gascho J, et al: Prognostic utility of the exercise thallium-201 test in ambulatory patients with chest pain: Comparison with cardiac catheterization. *Circulation* 77:745, 1988.

59. Pamelia F, Gibson R, Watson D, et al: Prognosis with chest pain and normal thallium-201 exercise scintigrams. *Am J Cardiol* 55:920, 1985.

60. Heller L, Tresgallo M, Sciacca R, et al: Prognostic significance of silent myocardial ischemia on thallium stress test. *Am J Cardiol* 65:718, 1990.

61. Eagle K, Coley C, Newell J, et al: Combining clinical and thallium data optimizes preoperative assessment of cardiac risk before major vascular surgery. *Ann Intern Med* 110:859, 1989.

62. Stanioloff H, Forrester J, Berman D, et al: Prediction of death, myocardial infarction, and worsening chest pain using thallium scintigraphy and exercise electrocardiography. *J Nuclear Med* 27:1842, 1986.

63. Boucher C, Brewster D, Darling C, et al: Determination of cardiac risk by dipyridamole-thallium imaging before peripheral vascular surgery. *N Engl J Med* 312:389, 1985.

64. Baron JF, Muntler O, Bertrand N, et al: Dipyridamole-thallium scintigraphy and gated nuclide angiography to assess cardiac risk before abdominal aortic surgery. *N Engl J Med* 330:663, 1994.

65. Ombrellaro MP, Tieter RA, Freeman M, et al: Role of dipyridamole myocardial scintigraphy in carotid artery surgery. *J Am Coll Surg* 181:451, 1995.

66. Urbinati S, DiPasquale G, Andreoli A, et al: Preoperative noninvasive coronary risk stratification in candidates for carotid endarterectomy. *Stroke* 25:2022, 1994.

67. Poldermans D, Fioretti BM, Forster T, et al: Dobutamine stress echocardiography for assessment of preoperative cardiac risk in patients undergoing major vascular surgery. *Circulation* 87:1506, 1993.

68. Eichelberger J, Schwartz KQ, Black ER, et al: Predictive value of dobutamine echocardiography just before noncardiac vascular surgery. *Am J Cardiol* 72:602, 1993.

69. Davila-Roman VG, Waggoner AD, Sicard GA, et al: Dobutamine stress echocardiography predicts surgical outcome in patients with an aortic aneurysm and peripheral vascular disease. *J Man Coll Cardiol* 21:957, 1993.

70. Chimowitz MI, Lafranchise EF, Furlan AJ, et al: Evaluation of coexistent carotid and coronary disease by combined angiography. *J Stroke Cerebrovasc Dis* 1:89, 1991.

71. Salonen JT, Salonen R: Ultrasonagraphically assessed carotid morphology and the risk of coronary heart disease. *Arterioscler Thromb* 11:1245, 1991.

72. Nowak J, Nilsson T, Sylven C, et al: Potential of carotid ultrasonography in the diagnosis of coronary artery disease: A compassion with exercise test and variance ECG. *Stroke* 29:439, 1998.

73. MacMahon S, Rodgers A: Blood pressure, antihypertensive treatment and stroke risk. *J Hypertens Suppl* 12:S5, 1994.

74. SHEP Cooperative Research Group: Prevention of stroke by antihypertensive drug treatment in older persons with isolated systolic hypertension: Final results of the systolic hypertension in the elderly program (SHEP). *JAMA* 265:3255, 1991.

75. Collins R, Peto R, MacMahon S, et al: Blood pressure, stroke and coronary heart disease, part 2: short-term reductions in blood pressure: Overview of randomized trials in their epidemiological context. *Lancet* 335:827, 1990.

76. Atkins D, Psaty BM, Koepsell TD, et al: Cholesterol reduction and the risk of stroke in men: A meta-analysis of randomized, controlled trials. *Ann Intern Med* 119:136, 1993.

77. Randomized trial of cholesterol lowering in 4444 patients with coronary heart disease: The Scandinavian Simvastatin Survival Study (4S). *Lancet* 344:1383, 1994.

78. Furberg CD, Adams HP Jr, Applegate WB, et al: Effect of lovastatin on early carotid atherosclerosis and cardiovascular events. *Circulation* 90:1679, 1994.

79. Crouse Jr III, Byington RP, Bond MG, et al: Pravastatin, lipids, and atherosclerosis in the carotid arteries (PLAC-II). *Am J Cardiol* 75:455, 1995.

80. Solomon R, Nyyssonen K, Porkkula E, et al: Kuopio Atherosclerosis Prevention Study (KAPS): A population-based primary preventive trial of the effect of LDL lowering on atherosclerotic progression in carotid and femoral arteries. *Circulation* 92:1758, 1995.

81. Wolf PA, D'Agostino RB, Kannel WB, et al: Cigarette smoking as a risk factor for stroke: The Framingham Study. *JAMA* 259:1025, 1988.

82. Antiplatelet trialists collaboration: Collaborative overview of randomized overview of randomized trials of antiplatelet therapy, I: Prevention of death, myocardial infarction, in stroke by prolonged antiplatelet therapy in various categories of patients. *Br Med J* 308:81, 1994.

83. Mayo Asymptomatic Carotid Endarterectomy Study Group: Results of a randomized controlled trial of carotid endarterectomy for asymptomatic carotid stenosis. *Mayo Clin Proc* 67:513, 1992.

84. Hass WK, Easton JD, Adams HDJ, et al: A randomized trial comparing ticlopidine hydrochloride with aspirin for the prevention of stroke in high-risk patients: Ticlopidine Aspirin Stroke Study Group. *N Engl J Med* 321:501, 1989.

85. CAPRIE Steering Committee: A randomized, blinded, trial of clopidogrel versus aspirin in patients at risk of ischaemic events. *Lancet* 348:1329, 1996.

86. Subcommittee on coronary artery bypass graft surgery of the American College of Cardiology/American Heart Association Task Force: Guidelines and indications for coronary artery bypass graft surgery. *J Am Coll Cardiol* 17:543, 1991.

87. Executive Committee for the Asymptomatic Carotid Atherosclerosis Study: Endarterectomy for asymptomatic carotid artery stenosis. *JAMA* 273:1421, 1995.

88. Furlan AJ, Craciun AR: Risk of a stroke during coronary artery bypass graft surgery in patients with internal carotid artery disease documented by angiography. *Stroke* 16:797, 1985.

89. Shultz RD, Strerpetti AV, Feldhaus RJ: Early and late results in patients with carotid disease undergoing myocardial revascularization. *Ann Thorac Surg* 45:603, 1988.

90. Gerraty RP, Gates PC, Doyle JC: Carotid stenosis and preoperative stroke risk in symptomatic and asymptomatic patients undergoing vascular and coronary surgery. *Stroke* 24:1115, 1993.

91. Salasidis GC, Latter DA, Steinmetz OK, et al: Carotid artery duplex scanning in preoperative assessment for coronary artery revascularization: The association between peripheral vascular disease, carotid artery stenosis, and stroke. *J Vasc Surg* 21:154, 1995.

92. Brenner BJ, Brief DK, Alpert J, et al: The risk of a stroke in patients with asymptomatic carotid stenosis undergoing cardiac surgery: A follow-up study. *J Vasc Surg* 5:269, 1987.

93. Mackey WC, O'Donnell TF, Callow AD: Cardiac risk in patients undergoing carotid endarterectomy: Impact on perioperative and long-term mortality. *J Vasc Surg* 11:226, 1990.

94. Bernhard VM, Johnson WD, Peterson JJ: Carotid artery stenosis associated with surgery for carotid artery disease. *Arch Surg* 105:837, 1972.

95. Moore WS, Barnett HJM, Beebe HG, et al: Guidelines. Statement from the Ad Hoc committee, American Heart Association. *Circulation* 91:566, 1995.

96. Biller J, Feinberg WM, Castaldo JE, et al: Guidelines for carotid endarterectomy: A statement for healthcare professionals from a special writing group of the stroke council, American Heart Association. *Stroke* 29:554, 1998.

97. Barnett HJM, Taylor DW, Eliasziw M, et al: Benefit of carotid endarterectomy in patients with symptomatic moderate or severe stenosis. *N Engl J Med* 339:1415, 1998.

98. Yadav JS, Roubin GS, Lyer S, et al: Elective stenting of the extracranial carotid arteries. *Circulation* 95:376, 1997.

99. Gaines PA: Carotid angioplasty. *Vasc Med* 1:121, 1996.

100. Bettman MA, Katzen BT, Whisnant J, et al: Carotid stenting and angioplasty: A statement for healthcare professionals from the Councils on Cardiovascular Radiology, Stroke, Cardio-Thoracic and Vascular Surgery, Epidemiology, and Prevention, and Clinical Cardiology, American Heart Association. *Stroke* 29:336, 1998.

101. Young B, Moore WS, Robertson JT, et al: An analysis of perioperative surgical mortality and morbidity in the asymptomatic carotid atherosclerosis study: ACAS Investigators. Asymptomatic Carotid Artheriosclerosis Study. *Stroke* 27:2216, 1996.

102. Barnes RW: Asymptomatic carotid disease in patients undergoing major cardiovascular operations: Can prophylactic endarterectomy be justified? *Ann Thorac Surg* 42(Suppl):S36, 1986.

103. Hertzer NR, Loop FD, Beven EG, et al: Surgical staging for simultaneous coronary and carotid disease: A study including prospective randomization. *J Vasc Surg* 9:445, 1989.

104. Wilke HJ, Ellis JE, McKinsey JF: Carotid endarterectomy: Perioperative and anesthetic considerations. *J Cardiothorac Vasc Anesth* 10:928, 1996.

105. Renton S, Hornick P, Taylor KM, et al: Rational approach to combined carotid and ischaemic heart disease. *Br J Surg* 84:1503, 1997.

106. Daily PO, Freeman RK, Dembitsky WP, et al: Cost reduction by combined carotid endarterectomy and coronary artery bypass grafting. *J Thorac Cardiovasc Surg* 111:1185, 1996.

Chapter 27

PRIMARY PREVENTION OF STROKE

David Lefkowitz

BACKGROUND

Asymptomatic carotid stenosis generally comes to medical attention in one of three ways: discovery of a bruit during routine auscultation of the neck, screening of patients at high risk for atherosclerosis or preoperative patients with coronary or aortoiliac atherosclerosis, or discovery of an asymptomatic stenosis during evaluation of contralateral symptomatic carotid artery disease.

Audible bruits are produced by turbulence resulting from increased flow or arterial stenosis. Therefore, they may provide a clue to an underlying hemodynamic carotid artery stenosis. Population studies performed in the early 1980's demonstrated an incidence of carotid bruits of approximately 4 percent in the general population over age 45.[1-3] Incidence increases with age, diabetes, and hypertension. Bruits are more common in women than in men. The incidence of bruits in black and white residents of Evans County, Georgia, was very similar.[2] Other population-based studies of bruits have not included sufficient numbers of minorities to validate these results. In referral-based clinical series, there is usually a strong preponderance of whites, which may represent selection bias or reflect a lower incidence of extracranial atherosclerosis in blacks.[4]

It should not be surprising that bruits are heard more frequently in patients with known atherosclerosis than in the general population. Five to six percent of patients are found to have bruits prior to coronary revascularization[5,6] and about 15 percent before aortoiliac surgery.[7,8]

Bruits may not always correlate well with the presence of carotid stenosis. Cervical bruits may arise from external carotid system atherosclerosis, nonatherosclerotic vasculopathies, or from hyperdynamic states such as pregnancy, hyperthyroidism, and anemia. As a stenosis increases, there may no longer be sufficient blood flow to produce the turbulence necessary to give rise to a bruit. Therefore, bruits may not be audible when an artery is critically stenosed or occluded. Venous hums and referred cardiac murmurs may be confused with carotid bruits. In one series of patients referred to a specialty clinic, moderate (30 to 69 percent) or severe (70 to 99 percent) stenosis was present in 37 percent of patients with a carotid bruit and in 17 percent of those without one.[9] Forty-three percent with severe carotid stenosis had no bruit, and 32 percent with bruits had normal carotid arteries by ultrasound. The positive predictive value of a bruit was only 37 percent. In the North American Symptomatic Endarterectomy Trial (NASCET), the existence of a carotid bruit was 63 percent sensitive and 61 percent specific for predicting an ipsilateral high-grade stenosis on angiography.[10] Therefore, the presence or absence of a bruit alone does not have sufficient predictive value to determine which patients are candidates for noninvasive testing or angiography.

Cervical bruits correlate better with the occurrence of myocardial infarction and mortality than with ipsilateral stroke. Mortality of patients with asymptomatic carotid atherosclerosis is usually cardiac at a rate of about 6 percent annually.

The widespread availability of noninvasive techniques to evaluate the carotid arteries has changed the emphasis from bruits to stenosis. Duplex ultrasound has been performed in 5201 male and female participants who were at least 65 years old and community dwelling at the time of their entry into the Cardiovascular Health Study. This has afforded an opportunity to assess the prevalence of carotid atherosclerosis and its relationship to traditional risk factors in a large elderly population in four geographic areas. Carotid atherosclerosis was present in 75 percent of men and 62 percent of women, but 50 percent or greater stenosis was detected in only 7 percent of men and 5 percent of women. Measures of carotid atherosclerosis increased with age and were higher in men than women at all ages.[11] The frequency of early atherosclerosis detected by Hennerici using continuous wave Doppler was 32.8 percent in patients with peripheral vascular disease compared with 6.8 percent in patients with coronary artery disease and 5.9 percent of those with atherosclerotic risk factors alone.[12] Twenty-five percent of neurologically normal patients with claudication have at least 50 percent asymptomatic carotid stenosis or occlusion.[13] Twenty to thirty percent of patients with symptomatic peripheral vascular disease have hemodynamically significant carotid stenosis.[14,15] Even when neurologically asymptomatic patients with peripheral vascular disease who do not have carotid bruits or decreased carotid pulsations are screened with duplex ultrasound, 14 percent will have at least 50 percent carotid stenosis.

There has been considerable controversy regarding the best management of asymptomatic carotid stenosis. This was partly due to uncertainty about the natural history of asymptomatic carotid stenosis. Many of the studies were retrospective or primarily contained patients with asymptomatic stenosis contralateral to an endarterectomy, which was performed for symptomatic stenosis. The initial question was whether carotid endarterectomy is effective in treating asymptomatic stenosis. Surgical management has the conceptual advantage of the immediate removal of the plaque, which is the presumed source of symptoms, but it carries angiographic and surgical risks, cannot be expected to affect coronary atherosclerosis or cardiac mortality, and is more expensive than medical therapies. Furthermore, carotid stenosis may recur after endarterectomy. After randomized studies made it clear that endarterectomy benefits symptomatic patients with hemodynamically significant carotid stenosis, the more valid question became whether endarterectomy should be performed while patients are still asymptomatic or whether to delay surgery until patients first develop symptoms. Only about half of the strokes that occur in patients with asymptomatic carotid stenosis are preceded by transient symptoms. Cerebral infarcts may occur in patients with asymptomatic stenosis without necessarily producing any symptoms.[16] Patients meeting clinical criteria for transient ischemic attacks may demonstrate areas of infarction on imaging studies in areas appropriate to their symptoms. Therefore, patients can accumulate tissue damage during follow-up without clinical evidence of cerebral infarction.

This may predispose to the development of multi-infarct dementia. Asymptomatic stenosis can also progress to occlusion over time. Evidence that the risk of endarterectomy is generally lower in asymptomatic patients than it is in symptomatic ones, and the absence of firm evidence of efficacy of medical therapies such as antiplatelet agents further fueled this debate.

The first carotid endarterectomy was performed in 1954. There was a progressive rise in the performance of endarterectomy during the 1970's and early 1980's.[17] The number of endarterectomies decreased in 1985 and 1986[18] but increased again after the publication of the results of the symptomatic endarterectomy trials (Fig. 27-1).[19]

EVIDENCE

Medical Management

Hypertension Hypertension is the most important treatable stroke risk factor. It is estimated that almost half of strokes could be prevented by treatment of blood pressure.[20] A decline in stroke mortality between the 1950's and 1980's is frequently attributed to effective antihypertensive therapy. An overview of unconfounded randomized trials of antihypertensive therapy found that treatment was associated with a highly significant 42 percent reduction of stroke and 45 percent of fatal stroke.[21] A stepped program of antihypertensive therapy with chlorthalidone and atenolol in elderly patients with systolic pressures greater than 160 mmHg and diastolic pressures below 90 mmHg reduced mean diastolic pressure by 4 mmHg and the systolic by 12 mmHg. There was a corresponding 36 percent reduction in stroke over 4.5 years of follow-up.[22] Treating the elderly with antihypertensive agents also reduces mortality.[23]

Hypertension is also a risk for carotid atherosclerosis. The Atherosclerotic Risk In Cohorts (ARIC) study investigators have examined the relationship between hypertension and subclinical atherosclerosis in multiethnic participants in four large cohorts by measuring carotid intima-media thickness using B mode ultrasound.[24] Higher levels of hypertension were associated with greater intima-media thickness for men and women of all ages and genders, regardless of the use of antihypertensive therapy. This relationship was primarily due to the effect of systolic hypertension. Diastolic pressure was not related to plaque thickness in blacks, was in-

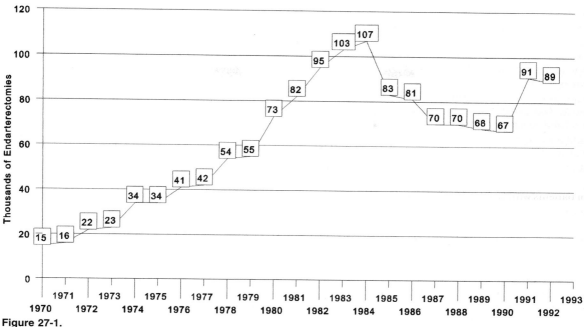

Figure 27-1.
Endarterectomies per year.

versely related in white males, and had a J-shaped relationship in white women. In patients with isolated systolic blood pressure in the Pittsburgh cohort of the Systolic Hypertension in the Elderly Program (SHEP), carotid stenosis of more than 50 percent was associated with low diastolic blood pressures.[25] Pooled data from nearly 19,000 participants in ARIC and the Cardiovascular Health Study (CHS) indicate that the magnitude of the relationship between hypertension and plaque thickness is relatively constant with increasing age over age 45 years.[26] Hypertension was inversely correlated with internal carotid artery lumen size but directly correlated with lumen diameter in the common carotid.[27] Only LDL-cholesterol was related to smaller lumen size in both the internal and external carotids. Hypertension and smoking were associated with carotid plaque and acoustic shadowing of plaque, which suggests mineralization.[28]

Furthermore, antihypertensive therapy reduces progression of carotid atherosclerosis. In an ancillary study of SHEP, the rate of progression of carotid plaque was assessed over time using ultrasound.[29] Progression occurred in 31 percent receiving placebo compared with 14 percent on active treatment. Of those patients with

a carotid stenosis at baseline, regression occurred only in treated patients. In a stepwise logistic regression model, placebo treatment was associated with a 4.3 times greater odds of progression than active medication. Arteriographic studies suggest that the antiatherogenic effect of calcium channel blockers in the coronary arteries is primarily on early lesions.[30]

Smoking Cigarette smoking is now a well-established stroke risk factor, likely due to an acceleration of atherosclerosis. Pack years of cigarette smoking[31,32] and duration of smoking[33,34] have both been shown to correlate with carotid atherosclerosis. Smoking is also a significant factor in recurrent stenosis after carotid endarterectomy.[35] In a cross-sectional study, mean plaque scores of former smokers were intermediate between those of current and never smokers, supporting the notion that smoking cessation may lead to a reversal of plaque progression.[36] There is an independent association between number of pack years of smoking and rate of plaque progression over time. Howard et al found that after controlling for demographic and lifestyle variables and other cardiovascular risk factors, current smoking was associated with a 50 percent increase in the mean progression rate over 3 years and past smoking with a 25 percent increase.[37] However, the progression rates of current and past smokers did not differ after controlling for the duration of exposure in pack years, suggesting that at least some of the adverse effects of tobacco smoke on atherosclerosis may be irreversible.

Duration of exposure to environmental tobacco smoke was associated with a significant increase in carotid intima-media thickness among nonsmoking men in the ARIC study.[32] Environmental tobacco exposure is also associated with a 20 percent increase in the rate of progression compared with those without passive exposure.[37]

Lipids Aggressive lipid lowering with diet and/or medication may also reduce the risk of stroke or progression of atherosclerosis. Atherosclerotic lesions of the carotid and aortoiliac vessels occur more frequently in patients with elevated triglycerides or cholesterol than in healthy controls.[38] LDL cholesterol is an independent predictor of carotid plaque progression, along with cardiac disease and elevated fibrinogen.[39]

Early studies of lipid-lowering drugs failed to demonstrate a clear reduction of stroke. Hepatic hydroxymethylglutaryl coenzyme A reductase inhibitors produce more marked and consistent reductions of LDL cholesterol than previously available agents. Meta-analysis of clinical trials using these agents demonstrates approximately 30 percent reduction of stroke compared with placebo.[40,41] Lipid lowering with lovastatin and pravastatin have been shown to reverse progression of plaque thickness in asymptomatic individuals with moderate levels of hypercholesterolemia and early carotid atherosclerosis.[42–44] Similar reductions have been demonstrated with a combination of colestipol, niacin, and diet.[45] Treatment with statins also reduces coronary events,[46–48] even in asymptomatic patients with modestly elevated cholesterol levels below those recommended for pharmacotherapy according to the National Cholesterol Education Program.[49] Statins may have clinical effects independent of lipid lowering.[50]

Hyperhomocysteinemia Elevated plasma homocysteine levels have recently been implicated as an independent risk factor of heart disease, stroke, and atherosclerosis. Homocysteine may contribute to atherogenesis via direct endothelial toxicity, proliferation of smooth muscle cells, or hypercoagulability. Plasma homocysteine levels are associated with carotid intimal medial wall thickness in asymptomatic individuals.[51] Selhub et al have shown that the risk of extracranial carotid artery

stenosis is directly related to plasma homocysteine levels and inversely proportional to pyridoxine and folate levels.[52] Plasma homocysteine also correlated with the severity of cerebral atherosclerosis in a Korean population with nonfatal stroke. Homocysteine was significantly higher in patients with two or more sites of stenosis detected by magnetic resonance angiography than those with one or no stenotic sites.[53] Patients with homocystinuria have markedly elevated homocysteine levels owing to a genetic defect of cystathionine synthase and are prone to premature cerebral and myocardial infarction. Moderate hyperhomocysteinemia is common in patients with vascular disease. The NHANES III investigators have recently reported that homocysteine was an independent predictor of nonfatal stroke in a large representative sample of United States adults and that homocysteine quartile was inversely related to vitamin B_{12} and folate levels.[54] Dietary supplementation with pyridoxine, folate, and vitamin B_{12} reduces plasma levels of homocysteine but has not yet been shown to reduce heart attack or stroke in patients with hyperhomocysteinemia. The ongoing Vitamin Intervention for Stroke Prevention (VISP) trial examines the effect of vitamin supplementation with vitamin B_6, B_{12}, and folate on recurrent stroke and myocardial infarction.

Antiplatelet Therapy

Despite the widespread use of antiplatelet therapy in patients with asymptomatic atherosclerosis, there is surprisingly little evidence that they are effective in asymptomatic patients. The Asymptomatic Cervical Bruit Study was a multicenter, randomized trial of aspirin vs. placebo in 372 participants with a carotid bruit, ultrasonic evidence of at least 50 percent stenosis, and selected cardiac exclusions.[55] The mean duration of follow-up was 1.9 years. The composite end point consisted of TIA, stroke, MI, and death. Annual stroke rates were 2.4 percent for aspirin-treated patients. The annual rate of the composite end point was 12.3 percent in the placebo group and 11 percent with aspirin. None of these differences was statistically significant. There was no differential effect by degree of stenosis or gender and no significant effect of aspirin on stroke severity or progression of stenosis. Nevertheless, aspirin is routinely used in high-risk asymptomatic patients with extracranial stenosis and intracranial atherosclerosis. Aspirin is generally not recommended as primary preventive therapy in low-risk asymptomatic individuals owing to the small increase in risk of intracranial hemorrhage. In the final analysis of the Physicians' Health Study, low-dose aspirin (325 mg every other day) was associated with a slightly increased incidence of both total and hemorrhagic stroke, which was not statistically significant.[56] A recent meta-analysis demonstrated a statistically significant increase in the relative risk of cerebral hemorrhage with aspirin treatment.[57]

Surgery

The Carotid Artery Stenosis with Asymptomatic Narrowing: Operation versus Aspirin (CASANOVA) study was the first clinical trial of endarterectomy in asymptomatic carotid stenosis.[58] This multicenter trial performed in Germany had an unusual design and certain flaws that make its results difficult to generalize to larger populations with asymptomatic carotid stenosis. The investigators included 410 patients with unilateral or bilateral 50 to 90 percent stenosis. Patients with more than 90 percent stenosis at baseline were excluded. All patients received 330 mg of aspirin and 75 mg of dipyridamole three times a day. Two-hundred six patients who were included in group A had unilateral or bilateral stenosis and underwent endarterectomy of one or both carotid arteries, respectively. One-hundred sixty patients were entered in group B. Patients with unilateral stenosis did not have initial surgery, whereas those with bilateral stenosis had surgery on the more stenotic side. Surgery was performed in 122 participants over the 3-year study with an operative mortality/morbidity of 6.9 percent. Indications for endarterectomy included progression to 90 percent or greater stenosis during follow-up, development of bilateral greater than 50 percent stenosis, transient ischemic attack ipsilateral to a greater than 50 percent stenosis, or restenosis greater than 50 percent. The minimal follow-up was 3 years. There were no significant differences between treatment groups for the end points of stroke or death.

The Mayo Asymptomatic Carotid Endarterectomy Study (MACE) was a single center trial of endarterectomy in patients with 50 to 99 percent carotid stenosis.[59] The study was terminated early after randomization of only 35 patients to medical therapy and 36 to endarterectomy owing to a statistically significant excess of myocardial infarction in the participants randomized to surgery, 26 percent vs. 9 percent in the medically treated group. This imbalance in myocardial infarcts has been attributed to the fact that the surgical patients were not treated with aspirin. There were no differences in major stroke or death.

In the multicenter Veterans Administration Asymptomatic Study, 444 men with 50 percent or greater carotid stenosis by angiography were randomized to medical therapy consisting of 650 mg of aspirin twice a day with or without endarterectomy.[60] Two-hundred eleven participants were randomized to endarterectomy and 233 to no surgery; perioperative mortality and morbidity were 4.4 percent. There was a 38 percent relative risk reduction for the combined end points of ipsilateral hemispheric or retinal transient ischemic attacks and stroke, which was statistically significant ($p < .001$). When the end points were analyzed individually, only transient monocular blindness was significantly reduced. There was a nonsignificant trend for reduction of ipsilateral hemispheric stroke and TIA in the surgically treated patients.

The Asymptomatic Carotid Atherosclerosis Study was another multicenter, randomized, prospective study of medical therapy (325 mg of aspirin a day and risk factor modification) with or without carotid endarterectomy.[61] To be eligible, patients had to be 40 to 79 years of age with an asymptomatic, hemodynamically significant internal or common carotid stenosis, defined as 60 percent or greater on the basis of one of three criteria. (1) Stenosis was measured on conventional or arterial digital subtraction angiography in a standardized fashion using the projection that best demonstrated the stenosis. The minimum residual lumen was measured at the smallest diameter and the distal lumen above the stenosis where the walls of the artery became parallel. Percent stenosis was calculated as $(1 - MRL/ DL) \times 100\%$. The other techniques were (2) a Doppler frequency shift or velocity "cut point" corresponding to a 95 percent positive predictive value of a 60 percent stenosis determined by regression analysis or (3) a frequency shift or velocity indicating a 60 percent stenosis with a positive predictive value of 90 percent plus a positive OPG-Gee. Patients randomized to surgery on the basis of ultrasound all underwent angiography to confirm the presence of a 60 percent stenosis. Seven percent of participants randomized to surgical management by Doppler examination alone proved to have false-positive results when they underwent angiography. Patients were excluded for confounding neurologic conditions, vertebrobasilar insufficiency and recent contralateral symptoms, uncontrolled medical conditions, contraindications to aspirin, life expectancy less than 5 years, angiographic evidence of a significant tandem lesion, vascular malformation or aneurysm requiring surgery, or a history of previous ipsilateral endarterectomy. Patients fulfilling these criteria were randomized to surgery or no surgery plus medical management. If both carotid arteries were eligible, the one with the greater degree of stenosis was randomized, and if both were equal, the left side was chosen as the study artery by convention. Participating surgeons were carefully selected on the basis of having performed a minimum of 12 endarterectomies per year with a combined mortality and morbidity less than 5 percent in their previous 50 cases and less than 3 percent in asymptomatic patients.[62]

Participants underwent follow-up at 30 days postoperatively or 42 days after randomization to medical therapy. They had telephone contacts alternating with clinic visits every 3 months for the duration of follow-up, during which they had completed a physical and neurologic examination, a TIA/stroke questionnaire, and a Folstein MiniMental State exam and were checked for drug adherence. Doppler examinations were performed at 6-month intervals for 2 years and annually thereafter. CCT was performed at entry, after documented end points, and at exit. The primary end point was any stroke or death within 30 days of surgery or 42 days of randomization to medical therapy and ipsilateral stroke thereafter. The system employed for detection and adjudication of end points was independently validated and is described elsewhere.[63] An intention to treat analysis was performed. Approximately 8 percent of participants crossed over after randomization from the treatment to which they were assigned.

Baseline characteristics were similar in the two arms of the study. Sixty-four percent had hypertension, 42 percent had previous myocardial infarction, 26 percent smoked, and 23 percent were diabetic. Seventy percent were asymptomatic on both sides, and 75 percent of patients had ipsilateral bruits. Fifteen percent of participants had silent infarcts on their baseline CCT, most of which were lacunar.[16] There was no relationship between silent stroke and the side of randomization, the degree of stenosis, the number of stenotic arteries, or the presence of contralateral carotid occlusion.

Originally, 5 years of follow-up were planned, but the study was halted early because the primary end point was reached after 2.7 years of median follow-up. Five-year outcome data were calculated using Kaplan-Meier statistics. The 5-year risk of ipsilateral stroke and any perioperative stroke or death was 5.1 percent in the surgical arm and 11.0 percent in the medical group ($p = .004$). Thus, surgery led to a 53 percent relative reduction and a 5.9 percent absolute reduction in the 5-year risk of the primary end point. The 5-year event rate was reduced by 66 percent in men ($p = .001$) and 17 percent in women ($p = .67$). Secondary analyses, including any stroke or major ipsilateral stroke and perioperative stroke or death, failed to demonstrate a statistically significant difference in outcome, although a trend existed in favor of surgical management. The treatment effect was not affected by degree of stenosis, perhaps owing to a reduction in power resulting from the relatively small number of 80 to 99 percent stenoses.

Perioperative mortality and stroke morbidity were 2.3 percent in the surgical group compared with 0.4 percent in the medical arm and included the risk of angiography. Stroke occurred as an angiographic complication in 1.2 percent of patients (5 of 414 who underwent arteriography after randomization). Thus, more than half of the perioperative mortality and morbidity could be attributed to angiography.[64] The stringent surgeon selection process probably contributed to the low complication rates seen in the trial.[65] The perioperative complication rate was twice as high in women as in men, 3.6 vs. 1.7 percent. The investigators concluded that patients with asymptomatic carotid stenosis greater than 60 percent benefited from surgery if their general health made them good candidates for surgery and perioperative morbidity and mortality were lower than 3 percent. They calculated that 19 patients would have to be treated to prevent one stroke over 5 years.

The investigators' conclusions have subsequently been scrutinized.[66] Criticisms include the short actual median follow-up of patients and the comparison of the Kaplan-Meier curves only at the 5-year time point. The lack of relationship between degree of stenosis, stroke risk, and the magnitude of therapeutic benefit of endarterectomy in ACAS is contrary to the results in symptomatic patients in NASCET.[67] It is not clear if the low perioperative complication rate in ACAS is attainable in the community setting.

The Asymptomatic Carotid Surgery Trial (ACST) is an ongoing multicenter trial of best medical management with or without carotid endarterectomy for patients with carotid stenosis who have been asymptomatic on the ipsilateral side for at least 6 months and have not had a severe contralateral infarct.[68] Participants are entered using the "uncertainty principle" rather than a fixed degree of stenosis. This technique was used previously in the European Carotid Surgery Trial (ECST) of symptomatic stenosis.[69] Investigators randomize patients only if they have a degree of stenosis for which they are uncertain of the best management. For instance, if an investigator feels that all patients with stenosis greater than 90 percent should have endarterectomy, and all patients with stenosis less than 70 percent should be treated medically, he or she would only enroll patients with 70 to 90 percent stenosis. If a sufficient number of investigators participate, the individual preferences of each should cancel each other out. Serial duplex scans are obtained at 4 and 12 months and then annually for 5 years. The main end points are stroke and death.

Cost Effectiveness of Endarterectomy for Asymptomatic Carotid Atherosclerosis

Despite evidence for the effectiveness of endarterectomy in preventing stroke in patients with hemodynamically significant asymptomatic carotid stenosis, economic considerations may affect whether surgical management is widely adopted. Endarterectomy is expensive, but so is the direct and indirect care of stroke. It is estimated that the cost of carotid endarterectomy is $8,000–15,000 per procedure. Hankey has estimated that if surgery were performed on all Australians with greater than 60 percent asymptomatic carotid stenosis, 88 strokes could be prevented annually at a cost of 1.24 billion Australian dollars.[70] The cost effectiveness of endarterectomy largely depends on a low perioperative mortality/morbidity in selected patients at high stroke risk without surgical management and adequate life expectancy. Cronenwett et al found that endarterectomy was cost effective in patients over 75 years of age with 60 percent or greater asymptomatic stenosis using assumptions based on ACAS data.[71]

Widespread screening to identify asymptomatic carotid stenoses is unlikely to be cost effective because of the low frequency in the general population, the expense of mass screening, and the complication rates of angiography and surgery.[72,73] The prevalence of asymptomatic stenosis in an enriched population with multiple atherosclerotic risk factors, cervical bruit, peripheral vascular, or coronary artery disease is higher. Screening may be cost effective in a population with a 10 to 30 percent prevalence of hemodynamically significant asymptomatic stenosis.[74] Serial screening is less cost effective than one-time evaluation.[74,75]

Timing of Endarterectomy With Other Surgeries

Asymptomatic carotid atherosclerosis is common in patients with cardiovascular disease. Likewise, coronary artery disease occurs frequently in patients with symptomatic or asymptomatic cerebrovascular disease and adversely affects their prognosis. Myocardial infarction is the most common cause of death in patients with cerebrovascular disease. This association is expected as both diseases are thought to share common pathogenic mechanisms. Stroke occurs in 1 to 2 percent of patients undergoing coronary revascularization, and coronary disease increases the risk of carotid endarterectomy. Although extracranial atherosclerosis may cause post-

operative stroke in patients undergoing coronary bypass as a result of artery-to-artery embolism or hemodynamic compromise, other potential mechanisms include arrhythmias such as postoperative atrial fibrillation, embolism from aortic cross-clamping, air embolism and nonpulsatile flow during cardiopulmonary bypass, and coagulopathy. In general, when neurologic deficit is recognized immediately or early after surgery, there is a history of intraoperative hypotension, clinical evidence of bilateral hemispheric damage, and radiographic signs of multiple strokes or watershed infarction.[76,77] Stroke occurring in the later postoperative period is usually in a single vascular distribution. Therefore, questions arise about staged or simultaneous surgeries in patients with concomitant cerebrovascular and coronary atherosclerosis. Randomized data are needed.

Many patients with cerebrovascular disease are asymptomatic from a cardiac standpoint despite having significant coronary atherosclerosis. Hertzer et al studied 200 patients with cerebrovascular disease who had no cardiac symptoms and found severe coronary atherosclerosis in 40 percent and normal coronary arteries in only 14 percent.[78] In the Veterans Affairs study of endarterectomy for asymptomatic carotid stenosis, cardiac events occurred in 43 percent of those with symptomatic coronary disease and 33 percent without symptoms during 4 years of follow-up. In the patients without previous angina or myocardial infarcts, the first symptom of coronary disease was heart attack or sudden death in 56 percent. Diabetes, peripheral vascular disease, and intracranial cerebral atherosclerosis predisposed to development of symptoms of coronary disease during follow-up[79] (see Chap. 24).

Durability of Endarterectomy: Restenosis

Frericks et al have reviewed the literature on carotid restenosis following endarterectomy and noted the heterogeneity of available data.[80] Using meta-analysis, the incidence of recurrent stenosis was approximately 10 percent in the first year, 3 percent in the second, 2 percent in the third, and 1 percent annually thereafter. The relative risk of ipsilateral stroke in patients with recurrent stenosis was 1.88. Although restenosis is relatively frequent in the first 1 to 2 years after endarterectomy, most of these early lesions are thought to be due to intimal hyperplasia, which has a better prognosis than late atherosclerosis. Because of the low prevalence of recurrent stenosis and the relative rarity of ipsilateral stroke, serial ultrasound studies to detect restenosis may result in frequent false-positive and -negative studies. The authors suggest that testing for restenosis not be performed more than 4 years after endarterectomy.

THERAPEUTIC RECOMMENDATIONS

In patients with asymptomatic atherosclerosis, risk factor modification is highly recommended. There are now substantial data that treatment of hypertension and hyperlipidemia and smoking cessation reduce subsequent stroke risk. Vitamin supplementation to reduce hyperhomocysteinemia may prove to be an effective, low-cost option for stroke prophylaxis but is not yet sufficiently proven. Treatment of other risk factors such as estrogen replacement is still unproven.

Antiplatelet therapy is generally not recommended for low-risk, asymptomatic individuals because of the small increase in hemorrhagic stroke. Its use in a high-risk, asymptomatic population seems reasonable but has been largely unstudied. There are no data on the use of antiplatelet therapies other than aspirin for primary prevention.

The low overall absolute annual risk of stroke or death (<2 percent) in asymptomatic patients treated with best medical management alone makes the identification of patient subsets at higher risk with low surgical morbidity desirable. Until such information becomes available, it is recommended that endarterectomy be reserved for asymptomatic patients who have a life expectancy of at least 5 years, whose medical condition makes them good candidates for surgery, and who have severe or progressive atherosclerotic carotid disease despite risk factor management. Minimizing operative mortality and morbidity is essential to ensure good results. In experienced hands, evaluation of patients with advanced noninvasive imaging methods such as color duplex ultrasound or magnetic resonance imaging may decrease the perioperative complication rate by decreasing the need for routine catheter angiography before surgery. Only surgeons with a documented complication rate below 3 percent should perform endarterectomy on asymptomatic patients.

REFERENCES

1. Wolf PA, Kannel WB, Sorlie P, et al: Asymptomatic carotid bruit and risk of stroke: The Framingham study. *JAMA* 245:1442, 1981.
2. Heyman A, Wilkinson WE, Heyden S, et al: Risk of stroke in asymptomatic persons with cervical arterial bruits: A population study in Evans County, Georgia. *N Engl J Med* 302:838, 1980.
3. Sandok BA, Whisnant JP, Furlan AJ, et al: Carotid artery bruits: Prevalence survey and differential diagnosis. *Mayo Clin Proc* 57:227, 1982.
4. Gil-Peralta A, Alter M, Lai SM, et al: Duplex Doppler and spectral flow analysis of racial differences in cerebrovascular atherosclerosis. *Stroke* 21:740, 1990.
5. Balderman SC, Gutierrez IZ, Makula P, et al: Noninvasive screening for asymptomatic carotid artery disease prior to cardiac operation: Experience with 500 patients. *J Thoracic Cardiovasc Surg* 85:427, 1983.
6. Skotnicki SH, Schulte BP, Leyten QH, et al: Asymptomatic carotid bruit in patients who undergo coronary artery surgery. *Eur J Cardio-Thoracic Surg* 1:11–15, 1987.
7. Carney WI Jr, Stewart WB, DePinto DJ, et al: Carotid bruit as a risk factor in aortoiliac reconstruction. *Surgery* 81:567, 1977.
8. Treiman RL, Foran RF, Cohen JL, et al: Carotid bruit: A follow-up report on its significance in patients undergoing an abdominal aortic operation. *Arch Surg* 114:1138, 1979.
9. Davies KN, Humphrey PR: Do carotid bruits predict disease of the internal carotid arteries? *Postgrad Med J* 70:433, 1994.
10. Sauve JS, Laupacis A, Ostbye T, et al: Does this patient have a clinically important carotid bruit? *JAMA* 270:2843, 1993.
11. O'Leary DH, Polak JF, Kronmal RA, et al: Distribution and correlates of sonographically detected carotid artery disease in the Cardiovascular Health Study: The CHS Collaborative Research Group. *Stroke* 23:1752, 1992.
12. Hennerici M, Aulich A, Sandmann W, et al: Incidence of asymptomatic extracranial arterial disease. *Stroke* 12:750, 1981.
13. Marek J, Mills JL, Harvich J, et al: Utility of routine carotid duplex screening in patients who have claudication. *J Vasc Surg* 24:572, 1996. Discussion: 577.
14. Gentile AT, Taylor LM Jr, Moneta GL, et al: Prevalence of asymptomatic carotid stenosis in patients undergoing infrainguinal bypass surgery. *Arch Surg* 130:900, 1995.
15. de Virgilio C, Toosie K, Arnell T, et al: Asymptomatic carotid artery stenosis screening in patients with lower extremity atherosclerosis: A prospective study. *Ann Vasc Surg* 11:374, 1997.
16. Brott T, Tomsick T, Feinberg W, et al: Baseline silent cerebral infarction in the Asymptomatic Carotid Atherosclerosis Study. *Stroke* 25:1122, 1994.
17. Dyken ML, Pokras R: The performance of endarterectomy for disease of the extracranial arteries of the head. *Stroke* 15:948, 1994.
18. Pokras R, Dyken ML: Dramatic changes in the performance of endarterectomy for diseases of the extracranial arteries of the head. *Stroke* 19:1289, 1988.
19. Gillum RF: Epidemiology of carotid endarterectomy and cerebral arteriography in the United States. *Stroke* 26:1724, 1995.

20. Gorelick PB: Stroke prevention: An opportunity for efficient utilization of health care resources during the coming decade. *Stroke* 25:220, 1994.

21. Collins R, Peto R, MacMahon S, et al: Blood pressure, stroke, and coronary heart disease: Part 2. Short-term reductions in blood pressure: Overview of randomised drug trials in their epidemiological context. *Lancet* 335:827, 1990.

22. SHEP Cooperative Research Group: Prevention of stroke by antihypertensive drug treatment in older persons with isolated systolic hypertension: Final results of the Systolic Hypertension in the Elderly Program (SHEP). *JAMA* 265:3255, 1991.

23. Mulrow CD, Cornell JA, Herrera CR, et al: Hypertension in the elderly: Implications and generalizability of randomized trials. *JAMA* 272:1932, 1994.

24. Arnett DK, Tyroler HA, Burke G, et al: Hypertension and subclinical carotid artery atherosclerosis in blacks and whites: The Atherosclerosis Risk in Communities Study. ARIC Investigators. *Arch Intern Med* 156:1983, 1996.

25. Sutton-Tyrrell K, Alcorn HG, Wolfson SK Jr, et al: Predictors of carotid stenosis in older adults with and without isolated systolic hypertension. *Stroke* 24:355, 1993.

26. Howard G, Manolio TA, Burke GL, et al: Does the association of risk factors and atherosclerosis change with age? An analysis of the combined ARIC and CHS cohorts. The Atherosclerosis Risk in Communities (ARIC) and Cardiovascular Health Study (CHS) investigators. *Stroke* 28:1693, 1997.

27. Crouse JR, Goldbourt U, Evans G, et al: Risk factors and segment-specific carotid arterial enlargement in the Atherosclerosis Risk in Communities (ARIC) cohort. *Stroke* 27:69, 1996.

28. Duncan BB, Metcalf P, Crouse JR, 3rd, et al: Risk factors differ for carotid artery plaque with and without acoustic shadowing: Atherosclerosis Risk in Communities Study Investigators. *J Neuroimaging* 7:28, 1997.

29. Sutton-Tyrrell K, Wolfson SK Jr, Kuller LH: Blood pressure treatment slows the progression of carotid stenosis in patients with isolated systolic hypertension. *Stroke* 25:44, 1994.

30. Zanchetti A: The antiatherogenic effects of antihypertensive drugs: Experimental and clinical evidence. *Clin Exp Hypertens [A]* 14:307, 1992.

31. Dempsey RJ, Moore RW: Amount of smoking independently predicts carotid artery atherosclerosis severity. *Stroke* 23:693, 1992.

32. Howard G, Burke GL, Szklo M, et al: Active and passive smoking are associated with increased carotid wall thickness: The Atherosclerosis Risk in Communities Study. *Arch Intern Med* 154:1277, 1994.

33. Whisnant JP, Homer D, Ingall TJ, et al: Duration of cigarette smoking is the strongest predictor of severe extracranial carotid artery atherosclerosis. *Stroke* 21:707, 1990.

34. Ingall TJ, Homer D, Baker HL Jr, et al: Predictors of intracranial carotid artery atherosclerosis: Duration of cigarette smoking and hypertension are more powerful than serum lipid levels. *Arch Neurol* 48:687, 1991.

35. Dempsey RJ, Moore RW, Cordero S: Factors leading to early recurrence of carotid plaque after carotid endarterectomy. *Surg Neurol* 43:278, 1995. Discussion: 282.

36. Tell GS, Howard G, McKinney WM, et al: Cigarette smoking cessation and extracranial carotid atherosclerosis. *JAMA* 261:1178, 1989.

37. Howard G, Wagenknecht LE, Burke GL, et al: Cigarette smoking and progression of atherosclerosis: The Atherosclerosis Risk in Communities (ARIC) Study. *JAMA* 279:119, 1998.

38. De Lorenzo F, De Simone B, Irace C, et al: Early signs of carotid and iliac atherosclerosis in patients with severe hyperlipoproteinemia. *Int Angiol* 11:122, 1992.

39. Grotta JC, Yatsu FM, Pettigrew LC, et al: Prediction of carotid stenosis progression by lipid and hematologic measurements. *Neurology* 39:1325, 1989.

40. Hebert PR, Gaziano JM, Chan KS, et al: Cholesterol lowering with statin drugs, risk of stroke, and total mortality: An overview of randomized trials. *JAMA* 278:313, 1997.

41. Blauw GJ, Lagaay AM, Smelt AH, et al: Stroke, statins, and cholesterol: A meta-analysis of randomized, placebo-controlled, double-blind trials with HMG-CoA reductase inhibitors. *Stroke* 28:946, 1997.

42. Furberg CD, Adams HP Jr, Applegate WB, et al: Effect of lovastatin on early carotid atherosclerosis and cardiovascular events: Asymptomatic Carotid Artery Progression Study (ACAPS) Research Group. *Circulation* 90:1679, 1994.

43. Mercuri M, Bond MG, Sirtori CR, et al: Pravastatin reduces carotid intima-media thickness progression in an asymptomatic hypercholesterolemic Mediterranean population: The Carotid Atherosclerosis Italian Ultrasound Study. *Am J Med* 101:627, 1996.

44. Hodis HN, Mack WJ, La Bree L, et al: Reduction in carotid arterial wall thickness using lovastatin and dietary therapy: A randomized controlled clinical trial. *Ann Intern Med* 124:548, 1996.

45. Mack WJ, Selzer RH, Hodis HN, et al: One-year reduction and longitudinal analysis of carotid intima-media thickness associated with colestipol/niacin therapy. *Stroke* 24:1779, 1993.

46. Holme I: Effects of lipid-lowering therapy on total and coronary mortality. *Curr Opin Lipidol* 6:374, 1995.

47. Rackley CE: Monotherapy with HMG-CoA reductase inhibitors and secondary prevention in coronary artery disease. *Clin Cardiol* 19:683, 1996.

48. Watts GF, Burke V: Lipid-lowering trials in the primary and secondary prevention of coronary heart disease: New evidence, implications, and outstanding issues. *Curr Opin Lipidol* 7:341, 1996.

49. Downs JR, Clearfied M, Weis S, et al: Primary prevention of acute coronary events with lovastatin in men and women with average cholesterol levels: Results of AFCAPS/TexCAPS. *JAMA* 279:1615, 1998.

50. Rosenson RS, Tangney CC: Antiatherothrombotic properties of statins: Implications for cardiovascular event reduction. *JAMA* 279:1643, 1998.

51. Malinow MR, Nieto FJ, Szklo M, et al: Carotid artery intimal-medial wall thickening and plasma homocyst(e)ine in asymptomatic adults: The Atherosclerosis Risk in Communities Study. *Circulation* 87:1107, 1993.

52. Selhub J, Jacques PF, Bostom AG, et al: Association between plasma homocysteine concentrations and extracranial carotid-artery stenosis. *N Engl J Med* 332:286, 1995.

53. Yoo J-H, Chung C-S, Kang S-S: Relation of plasma homocyst(e)ine to cerebral infarction and cerebral atherosclerosis. *Stroke* 29:2478, 1998.

54. Giles WH, Croft JB, Greenlund KJ, et al: Total homocyst(e)ine concentrations and the likelihood of nonfatal stroke: Results from the third National Health and Nutrition Examination Survey, 1988–1994. *Stroke* 29:2473, 1998.

55. Côté R, Battista RN, Abrahamowicz M, et al: Lack of effect of aspirin in asymptomatic patients with carotid bruits and substantial carotid narrowing: The Asymptomatic Cervical Bruit Study Group. *Ann Intern Med* 123:649, 1995.

56. Steering Committee of the Physicians' Health Study Research Group: Final report on the aspirin component of the ongoing Physicians' Health Study. *N Engl J Med* 321:183, 1989.

57. He J, Whelton PK, Vu B, et al: Aspirin and risk of hemorrhagic stroke: A meta-analysis of randomized controlled trials. *JAMA* 280:1930, 1998.

58. The CASANOVA Study Group: Carotid surgery versus medical therapy in asymptomatic carotid stenosis. *Stroke* 22:1229, 1991.

59. Mayo Asymptomatic Carotid Endarterectomy Study Group: Results of a randomized controlled trial of carotid endarterectomy for asymptomatic carotid stenosis. *Mayo Clin Proc* 67:513, 1992.

60. Hobson RWD, Weiss DG, Fields WS, et al: Efficacy of carotid endarterectomy for asymptomatic carotid stenosis: The Veterans Affairs Cooperative Study Group. *N Engl J Med* 328:221, 1993.

61. Executive Committee for the Asymptomatic Carotid Atherosclerosis Study: Endarterectomy for asymptomatic carotid artery stenosis. *JAMA* 273:1421, 1995.

62. Moore WS, Vescera CL, Robertson JT, et al: Selection process for surgeons in the Asymptomatic Carotid Atherosclerosis Study. *Stroke* 22:1353, 1991.

63. Karanjia PN, Nelson JJ, Lefkowitz DS, et al: Validation of the ACAS TIA/stroke algorithm. *Neurology* 48:346, 1997.

64. Young B, Moore WS, Robertson JT, et al: An analysis of perioperative surgical mortality and morbidity in the asymptomatic carotid atherosclerosis study. ACAS Investigators: Asymptomatic Carotid Atherosclerosis Study. *Stroke* 27:2216, 1996.

65. Moore WS, Young B, Baker WH, et al: Surgical results: A justification of the surgeon selection process for the ACAS trial: The ACAS Investigators: *J Vasc Surg* 23:323, 1996.

66. Barnett HJ, Eliasziw M, Meldrum HE, et al: Do the facts and figures warrant a 10-fold increase in the performance of carotid endarterectomy on asymptomatic patients? *Neurology* 46:603, 1996.

67. North American Symptomatic Carotid Endarterectomy Trial Collaborators: Beneficial effect of carotid endarterectomy in symptomatic patients with high-grade carotid stenosis. *N Engl J Med* 325:445, 1991.

68. Halliday AW, Thomas D, Mansfield A: The Asymptomatic Carotid Surgery Trial (ACST): Rationale and design. Steering Committee. *Eur J Vasc Surg* 8:703, 1994.

69. European Carotid Surgery Trialists' Collaborative Group: MRC European Carotid Surgery Trial: Interim results for symptomatic patients with severe (70–99%) or with mild (0–29%) carotid stenosis. *Lancet* 337:1235, 1991.

70. Hankey GJ. Asymptomatic carotid stenosis: How should it be managed? *Med J Aust* 163:197, 1995.

71. Cronenwett JL, Birkmeyer JD, Nackman GB, et al: Cost-effectiveness of carotid endarterectomy in asymptomatic patients. *J Vasc Surg* 25:298, 1997. Discussion: 310.

72. Lee TT, Solomon NA, Heicenreich PA, et al: Cost-effectiveness of screening for carotid stenosis in asymptomatic persons. *Ann Intern Med* 126:337, 1997.

73. Longstreth WT, Shemanski L, Lefkowitz D, et al: Asymptomatic internal carotid artery stenosis defined by ultrasound and the risk of subsequent stroke in the elderly: The Cardiovascular Health Study. *Stroke* 29:2371, 1998.

74. Derdeyn CP, Powers WJ: Cost-effectiveness of screening for asymptomatic carotid atherosclerotic disease. *Stroke* 27:1944, 1996.

75. Yin D, Carpenter JP: Cost-effectiveness of screening for asymptomatic carotid stenosis. *J Vasc Surg* 27:245, 1998.

76. Blossom GB, Fietsam R Jr, Bassett JS, et al: Characteristics of cerebrovascular accidents after coronary artery bypass grafting. *Am Surg* 58:584, 1992. Discussion: 589.

77. Wijdicks EF, Jack CR: Coronary artery bypass grafting-associated ischemic stroke: A clinical and neuroradiological study. *J Neuroimaging* 6:20, 1996.

78. Hertzer NR, Young JR, Beven EG, et al: Coronary angiography in 506 patients with extracranial cerebrovascular disease. *Arch Intern Med* 145:849, 1985.

79. Chimowitz MI, Weiss DG, Cohen SL, et al: Cardiac prognosis of patients with carotid stenosis and no history of coronary artery disease: Veterans Affairs Cooperative Study Group 167. *Stroke* 25:759, 1994.

80. Frericks H, Kievit J, van Baalen JM, et al: Carotid recurrent stenosis and risk of ipsilateral stroke: A systematic review of the literature. *Stroke* 29:244, 1998.

Chapter 28

STROKE IN YOUNG WOMEN

Linda A. Hershey

INTRODUCTION

Ischemic stroke is less common in young adults than it is in those over 65 years of age. The annual stroke incidence increases dramatically from 1 to 2 per 1000 in those aged 45 to 54 years, to nearly 10 per 1000 in those 65 to 74 years of age.[1] Because the prevalence of atherosclerosis rises faster in men than in women with advancing years, older men have a higher stroke risk than older women.[2] On the other hand, women in their child-bearing years are nearly equal to men in their risk for stroke.[3,4]

Even though young women are as likely as young men to experience ischemic stroke, there is laboratory evidence to show that estrogen may provide some degree of cerebral protection. For example, female gerbils with carotid occlusion have less extensive brain lesions than male gerbils treated with the same procedure.[5] This protective effect of estrogen has been attributed to its antioxidant properties. Alternative explanations include the flow-preserving effects of estrogen that could lead to the smaller infarct sizes in female animals.[6]

The diagnostic evaluation of young women with stroke is a challenge because multiple etiologies need to be considered. Table 28-1 shows that the three most common causes of ischemic stroke in young adults are the same as those found in older individuals: atherosclerosis, heart disease, and nontraumatic arterial dissection.[3,4,7–9] This chapter will concentrate on the stroke etiologies and risk factors that are more likely to be seen in young women: peripartum stroke, cranial sinus thrombosis, patent foramen ovale, oral contraceptives, migraine, etc. The clinical evidence for the various stroke subtypes will be discussed, along with currently recommended diagnostic studies and therapeutic recommendations.

CAUSES OF STROKE IN YOUNG WOMEN

Peripartum Stroke

Strokes associated with pregnancy include subarachnoid hemorrhage, intraparenchymal hemorrhage, and ischemic arterial stroke as well as intracranial venous thrombosis. Strokes occurring during pregnancy or within 6 weeks of delivery develop in women who are about 10 years younger, on average, than those whose strokes are unrelated to pregnancy.[10] In addition, women with peripartum stroke are less likely to have the same stroke risk factors as those whose strokes are unrelated to pregnancy (less hypertension, diabetes, coronary artery disease, or cigarette abuse). In a large prospective series that examined stroke in young women, 10 of the 16 peripartum infarctions occurred during the post-partum period; 5 developed in the third trimester, but none occurred during the first trimester.[10] The postpartum period probably puts women at increased risk for ischemic stroke because of rapid shifts in blood volume and hormone levels.

Four of the 16 peripartum infarcts in the American series of Kittner and colleagues[10] were related to pre-eclampsia or eclampsia, a lower percentage than the 47 percent reported in a recent French study.[11] In describing their experience in Mexico, Cantu and Barinagarrementeria found pregnancy-associated cerebral thrombosis at a younger age than nonpregnancy venous thrombosis.[13] The pregnancy-related cases also had a more abrupt onset and a better prognosis. Koch and others[14] have argued for an association between cranial sinus thrombosis (CST) and pre-eclampsia, but the one CST case in Kittner's series occurred 5 days post-partum and was not associated with symptoms of eclampsia. Lanska and Kryscio analyzed data from the National

Table 28-1.
Common causes of ischemic stroke in young adults

Authors (year)	n	Atherosclerotic	Cardioembolic	Arterial dissection
Szmanda (1994)	128	28 (22)[a]	22 (17)	10 (8)
Adams (1995)	329	58 (18)	58 (18)	20 (6)
Kristensen (1997)	107	13 (12)	35 (33)	20 (19)
Williams (1997)	116	22 (19)	16 (14)	17 (15)
Kittner (1998)	212	50 (24)	66 (31)	24 (6)
Totals	892	171 (19)	197 (22)	91 (10)

[a]Percentages are in parentheses.

Hospital Discharge Survey from a 13-year period.[12] They estimated 8918 strokes and 5723 intracranial venous thromboses were associated with 50,254,631 pregnancies. Hypertension was a highly significant risk factor for stroke but not for venous thrombosis. Women living in the South were less likely to have a stroke than those living in the West or Midwest ($p < .05$). Younger women (age 15 to 24 years) were more likely to have venous thrombosis than older women (age 25 to 34 years). No racial differences were found.

Culebras and colleagues[15] have argued that the selection of imaging studies in pregnant women with stroke should be directed by the neurologic indications themselves. Computed tomography (CT) scanners limit irradiation to a highly focused area of the brain, thereby minimizing the radiation dose to the fetus. Magnetic resonance imaging (MRI) produces no radiation at all, but its use is usually not recommended during the first trimester. Magnetic resonance angiography (MRA) is now well established as the best method to document CST or cerebral venous thrombosis.[16,17]

Transcranial Doppler (TCD) is a noninvasive method that measures blood flow velocities in medium-sized vessels of the circle of Willis. TCD studies have shown significantly higher velocities in the middle cerebral arteries of eclamptic women, compared with those measured in normotensive pregnant women.[18] This suggests that eclampsia causes moderate to severe cerebral vasospasm. Prospective studies will be needed to learn whether vasospasm is the primary event that leads to

an increased risk of cerebral infarction in women who have pre-eclampsia or eclampsia.

Because peripartum strokes are etiologically heterogeneous, the selection of therapies must be directed by the type of infarct and its cause. Warfarin is contraindicated during the first 8 weeks of pregnancy, as it crosses the placenta and is associated with developmental anomalies such as abnormal facial features, hypoplastic digits, and mental retardation.[12] If given later during the pregnancy, warfarin can cause fetal death owing to hemorrhage. Therefore, pregnant women who develop embolic strokes or CST are advised to receive standard unfractionated heparin or low molecular weight heparin, as these drugs do not cross the placenta and are not associated with significant fetal damage.[19,20]

Cranial Sinus Thrombosis

Thrombosis of the venous sinuses can be precipitated by dehydration, nephrotic syndrome, sinus infection, trauma, severe anemia, oral contraceptives, pregnancy, or the post-partum state. About 10 percent of CST cases in pregnant women are associated with pre-eclampsia or eclampsia.[14] Proteinuria in these patients, as well as in those with the nephrotic syndrome, may play an important pathogenetic role in CST (decreased levels of antithrombin III, protein S, and protein C are seen in association with proteinuria). The risk of CST is also increased in those who have mutations of the prothrombin gene and in women on oral contraceptives.[21,22] Acquired abnormalities, such as the presence of antiphospholipid antibodies, have also been associated with venous infarcts and CST.

Venous sinus thrombosis should be suspected when patients report symptoms of increased intracranial pressure (headache, nausea, and vomiting) or when signs such as papilledema or bilateral sixth nerve palsies are found on examination. Other common symptoms of CST include major motor seizures and impaired level of consciousness. Focal CST symptoms usually reflect the site of venous thrombosis, such as bilateral leg weakness in superior sagittal sinus thrombosis, dysphasia in thrombosis of the left lateral sinus, and multiple cranial nerve palsies in cavernous sinus thrombosis (III, IV, V, and VI). Cortical vein thrombosis (CVT) is less prevalent than CST and is more difficult to diagnose.[16,17] Whereas symptoms of increased intracranial pressure are not usually seen in CVT, patients can develop focal seizures and focal neurologic symptoms.

Noncontrast CT in CST is likely to show bilaterally symmetric infarcts that do not respect known arterial boundaries.[15] There are also signs of edema, such as effacement of cortical sulci and loss of the white-gray demarcation. Venous infarcts are often associated with hemorrhagic transformation, which can be identified with noncontrast CT. In the acute phases of CST, MRA may show enlarged cerebral veins and absent flow in the affected venous sinus.[14] T1-weighted MRI images in the acute stages of CST show hyperintense signal in the involved sinus (delta sign) and absence of the usual signal void (empty delta sign). As the blood clot resorbs, MRA can document resumption of blood flow in the involved sinus.

Even though venous infarcts have the potential for hemorrhagic transformation, most authors still recommend anticoagulation for patients with CST and CVT.[14,16] Before anticoagulants are prescribed, however, patients should have a detailed battery of studies to exclude a procoagulant state (protein C, protein S, antithrombin III, activated protein C resistance, lupus anticoagulant, serologic test for syphilis, and anticardiolipin antibodies). One study recommended that oral anticoagulants be given indefinitely if elevated titers of anticardiolipin antibodies persisted 6 months after an episode of venous thrombosis.[23]

Cardioembolic Stroke

Table 28-1 summarizes the results of five large studies that have examined the various etiologies of stroke in young adults (ages 15 to 50 years of age). These studies support the assertion that cardioembolic stroke is the most prevalent subtype.[3,4,7–9] Table 28-2 shows that the most common cardiac source of brain emboli in young adults is patent foramen ovale (PFO). PFO is a septal defect that functions as a conduit for emboli to travel from the venous to the arterial circulation. Mitral valve prolapse (MVP) is no longer thought to cause strokes in young people.[62,63]

Kristensen and others[4] demonstrated that when transesophageal echocardiography (TEE) is liberally applied to the young adult stroke population, as many as 30 percent of all strokes can be attributed to PFO. When TEE is used selectively, however, only 4 to 5 percent of strokes seem to be PFO-related.[3,7,8] Several authors have questioned the causal relationship between PFO and stroke, as clinical markers of paradoxical emboli are rarely seen in patients with PFO-related infarction.[24–26]

TEE is more sensitive than transthoracic echocardiography in documenting the presence of PFO and right-to-left shunt in patients with stroke of unknown origin.[27] Transcranial Doppler echocardiography (TCDE) has been used in PFO patients to demonstrate the technical effectiveness of surgical closure of the septal defect.[28] TCDE results indicate the presence of right-to-left shunting if more than three high intensity embolic signals are detected in the middle cerebral artery within 10 seconds of air-contrast injection.

The risk for recurrent stroke following PFO-related infarction is not well documented. Prolonged use of antiplatelet agents is usually employed as the first line of therapy, with anticoagulation reserved for those who experience subsequent ischemic events. Devuyst and colleagues[28] showed in a series of 30 patients with

Table 28-2.
Causes of cardioembolic stroke in young adults

Authors (year)	n	PFO[a]	AMI	PVD	IE	MVP	AF
Szmanda (1994)	128	7 (5)	6 (5)	3 (2)	—	2 (2)	2 (2)
Adams (1995)	329	13 (4)	5 (2)	12 (4)	6 (2)	5 (2)	—
Kristensen (1997)	107	32 (30)	—	—	—	1 (1)	—
Williams (1997)	116	5 (4)	—	—	3 (3)	2 (2)	1 (1)
Kittner (1998)	212	—	7 (3)	14 (7)	20 (9)	—	4 (2)
Totals	892	57 (6)	18 (2)	29 (3)	29 (3)	10 (1)	7 (1)

[a]PFO, patent foramen ovale; IE, infectious endocarditis; AMI, acute myocardial infarction; MVP, mitral valve prolapse; PVD, prosthetic valve disease; AF, atrial fibrillation.

PFO-related strokes that surgical closure of the septal defect is safe and effective for stroke prophylaxis for at least a 2-year period.

Dissection of Carotid or Vertebral Arteries

Besides cardioembolic diseases and atherosclerosis, arterial dissection is the third most common cause of stroke in young people (see Table 28-1). Although men are more likely than women to have atherothrombotic and cardioembolic infarcts, women are at equal risk with men for experiencing dissection-related strokes.[7] Arterial dissection usually begins with an intimal tear, which can be the result of such minor trauma as a quick turning of the head and neck. Blood then penetrates into the subintimal space at the site of the tear and extends longitudinally to form an intramural hematoma.

Arterial dissection should be considered in young stroke patients who have no traditional vascular risk factors and in those who experience headache or neck pain at the onset of their focal neurologic signs and symptoms.[29] Besides causing hemiparesis and hemisensory loss, carotid dissection can produce symptoms that are not usually associated with hemispheric infarction: Horner's syndrome, hemicranial pain, jaw pain, neck pain, or lower cranial nerve palsies (IX, X, XI, XII). Vertebral dissection may cause occipital headache in addition to symptoms of posterior circulation ischemia such as vertigo, nausea, and dysequilibrium.[30]

Diagnosis of arterial dissection is usually based on conventional angiographic findings: string sign, double-lumen sign, or pseudoaneurysm formation.[15] T2-weighted MRI images of the jugular foramen in carotid dissection can show intramural hematoma without compromise of the true lumen of the artery.[29] MRA lacks the sensitivity of conventional angiography for making the initial diagnosis of arterial dissection, but it is a reliable method to use in following the response of the injured vessel to anticoagulation therapy.[31]

Oral anticoagulants are usually recommended for treating arterial dissection until there is evidence on MRA for resolution of the clot.[31] Pregnant women with dissection are treated with heparin or low molecular weight heparin, as warfarin can produce fetal anomalies or fetal hemorrhage, depending on the stage of pregnancy.

Prothrombotic Strokes

Hypercoaguable states account for 6 to 15 percent of all ischemic strokes in young adults.[3,4,7,8] Table 28-3

Table 28-3.

Causes of prothrombotic strokes in young adults

Authors (year)	n	aPLA	AT III	Prot S	Prot C	Other
Szmanda (1994)	128	9 (7)	—	—	—	7 (6)
Adams (1995)	329	5 (2)	1 (0.3)	1 (0.3)	1 (0.3)	11 (3)
Kristensen (1997)	107	7 (7)	—	1 (1)	—	1 (1)
Williams (1997)	116	10 (9)	—	4 (3)	—	3 (3)
Totals	680	31 (4)	1 (0.1)	6 (1)	1 (0.1)	22 (3)

aPLA, antiphospholipid antibody syndrome; AT III, antithrombin III deficiency; Prot S, protein S deficiency; Prot C, protein C deficiency.

shows that the most prevalent of these is the antiphospholipid antibody (aPLA) syndrome, but other causes include deficiencies in antithrombin III, protein S, and protein C. In the Antiphospholipid Antibodies in Stroke Study,[32] about 10 percent of patients experiencing their first ischemic stroke had signs and symptoms of the aPLA syndrome, compared with 4 percent of age-matched stroke-free controls. Young women are more likely to have the aPLA syndrome than young men.[33]

The aPLA syndrome is defined by the presence of aPLA, lupus anticoagulant, or anticardiolipin antibody in addition to any of the following clinical symptoms and signs: recurrent strokes, dementia, deep vein thrombosis, recurrent miscarriages, livedo reticularis, or cranial sinus thrombosis.[34] Laboratory markers for the aPLA syndrome include prolonged partial thromboplastin time, thrombocytopenia, and a false-positive syphilis test. Clinical signs of aPLA syndrome are considered primary in the absence of systemic lupus erythematosis (SLE) and secondary when SLE is present (aPLAs are found in 25 to 50 percent of SLE patients).

Antithrombin III normally binds to heparin on the surface of endothelial cells to inhibit thrombin and other clotting factors. A deficiency of antithrombin III can be acquired in a number of disorders that cause protein wasting: cirrhosis, diabetes, malnutrition, nephrotic syndrome, pre-eclampsia, and eclampsia. Two young women with stroke and antithrombin III deficiency were described by Martinez and others.[35] Neither of these women had hypertension, heart disease, atherosclerosis, or arterial dissection. Nevertheless, only one stroke attributable to antithrombin III deficiency was identified in several large studies of stroke in young adults.[3,4,7,8]

Protein S deficiency is not as common as the aPLA syndrome as a cause of coagulopathy-related stroke in young people (see Table 28-3). Protein S is a vitamin K-dependent plasma protein that works as a cofactor to accelerate protein C-induced inhibition of factors V and VIII. A deficiency of protein S can be inherited in an autosomal dominant fashion, or it can be acquired (cigarette smoking, oral contraceptives, or the peripartum state). Some authors have found more strokes related to protein S deficiency in women than in men.[35,36] One prospective study showed that protein S deficiency was more prevalent as a cause of stroke in young people than either antithrombin III deficiency or protein C deficiency.[37] Longstreth and colleagues reported on 106 young women with first stroke in a case control study.[60] They found no association of factor V Leiden or prothrombin gene variant (G20210A) with stroke in young women. There were too few women with venous thrombosis to come to any conclusion between factor V Leiden and CVT. Lüdemann and colleagues, in a case-centered study of 55 patients with CVT, found factor V Leiden to be the most relevant risk factor for CVT.[61]

One retrospective study examined the clinical course of patients who experienced stroke or other thrombotic events related to the aPLA syndrome.[38] They found that recurrent stroke was a problem for 10 of the 17 patients with aPLA-related strokes. Intermediate- or high-intensity warfarin therapy (target INR of 3.0) was associated with the lowest rate of stroke recurrence in this series. If the platelet count is dangerously low, then these authors recommended immunosuppressant therapy to minimize the risk of warfarin-related hemorrhage.

Oral Contraceptives

An estimated 60 to 70 million women around the world use oral contraceptive agents. The birth control pills that are now being prescribed contain less estrogen (30 to 35 mcg each) than the 80 to 100-mcg tablets of the 1960's and 1970's. Two large U.S. studies have shown ischemic strokes to be extremely rare among users of low-dose estrogen contraceptives, as long as patients are less than 35 years of age, non-smokers, and nonhypertensives.[39,40]

European women who take low-dose estrogen birth control pills (less than 50 mcg) are 1.5 times as likely to have an ischemic stroke compared with their peers who do not take oral contraceptives.[41] Higher doses of estrogen increase stroke risk by a factor of five.

Hypertensive women who take oral contraceptives are 10 to 14 times as likely as normotensive women on the pill to have an ischemic stroke. We need to caution young women who are on the pill to have their blood pressure closely monitored and to refrain from smoking cigarettes.

Migraine

Ten to 20 percent of American women experience frequent migraine headaches. In rare situations, the vasospasm of migraine can be so severe that it causes transient or persistent symptoms of cerebral ischemia, such as hemiparesis or hemianesthesia.[42,43] Migraine-related strokes account for 1 to 5 percent of all ischemic strokes in young adults.[3,4,7–9] Stroke risk is increased 6- to 8-fold in migraineurs who experience an aura, smoke cigarettes, or take oral contraceptive agents.[44,45]

Stroke and migraine may coexist in young women who have the autosomal dominant disorder known as CADASIL, or cerebral autosomal dominant arteriopathy with subcortical infarcts and leukoencephalopathy.[46] CADASIL's most common presentation consists of transient or permanent cerebral ischemic events that simulate lacunar infarcts (no hypertension or diabetes is usually present, however). Migraine with aura is seen in 30 percent of CADASIL patients.

Hypertension

Table 28-4 outlines the evidence that hypertension, cigarette smoking, and diabetes mellitus are the most common stroke risk factors in young women.[4,39,47,48] Besides cardiac disease, hypertension is the risk factor most

Table 28-4.

Prevalence of risks in young women with stroke

Authors (year)	n	Hypertension	Smoking	Diabetes
			%	
Rohr et al (1996)	145	28 (W)[a] 59 (B)	37 (W) 48 (B)	17 (W) 25 (B)
Petitti et al (1996)	144	18	34	15
Haapaniemi (1997)	140	34	50	6
Kristensen (1997)	44	20	39	2

[a] W, white; B, black.

highly correlated with ischemic stroke for all age groups and for both sexes.[49] In the Framingham Heart Study, hypertensive women had a 3-fold increase in stroke incidence compared with normal women.[1] Because the prevalence of uncontrolled hypertension is twice as high in black women as it is in white women, it is not surprising that the risk of stroke is higher in black women.[47,50,51]

Hypertensive patients are more likely to have small, deep ("lacunar") infarcts, as chronic hypertension is associated with fibrinoid necrosis of small penetrating arterioles. The most common symptoms of lacunar infarcts are hemiparesis involving face, arm, and leg (internal capsule), hemianesthesia involving face, arm, and leg (thalamus), and clumsy hand-dysarthria (pons). If seizure, gaze preference, or hemianopsia is associated with the stroke, then it is unlikely to be caused by small vessel disease.

Unless diastolic pressures are over 120 mm, it is best not to treat hypertension in an acute ischemic stroke. After the patient has stabilized, however, it is important to bring the blood pressure under control. The good news for all hypertensive women is that consistent control of blood pressure can reduce stroke risk by 30 to 45 percent.[50]

Smoking

Women who smoke are three times as likely as nonsmoking women to experience ischemic stroke.[52,53] One way that cigarettes increase stroke risk is by facilitating atherogenesis. In fact, significant carotid stenosis is more likely to develop in cigarette smokers than in those with chronic hypertension.[54,55]

In an animal model of endothelial injury, Petrik and others[56] demonstrated that cigarette smoke produced intimal hyperplasia in the carotid arteries of rats in a dose-dependent fashion. This experiment helped us to understand the clinical findings of Wolf and others,[52] who had shown that women smoking 40 cigarettes per day were twice as likely to have a stroke as those smoking only 10 cigarettes per day. The good news for women who smoke is that risk in former smokers can fall to the same level as nonsmokers within 2 to 5 years of smoking cessation.[52,53]

Drug Abuse

Levine and colleagues[57] drew our attention to the fact that young women can develop ischemic stroke in close temporal relation to the use of "crack" cocaine. In fact, any form or route of cocaine use (intranasal, intrave-

nous, or intramuscular) can increase stroke risk in young adults.[58] In nonurban settings, the prevalence of drug-related strokes in young adults is only 1 to 2 percent.[3,7,8] In large metropolitan environments, however, as many as 9 percent of strokes in young women are associated with the use of illicit drugs.[9]

Severe headaches or seizures can occur at the onset of cocaine-related strokes, even in cases where there is no drug-induced hypertension.[57] Angiography in cocaine-related strokes often shows evidence of vasospasm and intramural clot. Only rarely are there signs of vasculitis. In contrast, amphetamine-related strokes are often associated with an inflammatory vasculopathy. Finally, cardioembolism is a third possible mechanism by which cocaine can cause ischemic stroke. In a case described by Petty and colleagues,[59] cocaine-induced cardiomyopathy was the probable source of embolus.

REFERENCES

1. Wolf PA, Cobb JL, D'Agostino RB: Epidemiology of stroke, in Barnett HJM, Mohr JP, Stein BM (eds): *Stroke: Pathophysiology, Diagnosis and Management,* 2nd ed. New York, Churchill Livingstone, 1992, pp 3–27.
2. Bonita R, Solomon N, Broad JB: Prevalence of stroke and stroke-related disability. *Stroke* 28:1898, 1997.
3. Adams HP, Kappelle LJ, Biller J, et al: Ischemic stroke in young adults. *Arch Neurol* 52:491, 1995.
4. Kristensen B, Malm J, Carlberg B, et al: Epidemiology and etiology of ischemic stroke in young adults aged 18 to 44 years in Northern Sweden. *Stroke* 28:1702, 1997.
5. Hall ED, Pazara KE, Linseman KL: Sex differences in postischemic neuronal necrosis in gerbils. *J Cereb Blood Flow Metab* 11:292, 1991.
6. Alkayed NJ, Harukuni I, Kimes AS, et al: Gender-linked brain injury in experimental stroke. *Stroke* 29:159, 1998.
7. Szmanda MT, Dulli DA, Levine RL, et al: Ischemic stroke in young adults: Results of the University of Wisconsin Stroke Registry. *J Stroke Cerebrovasc Dis* 4:188, 1994.
8. Williams LS, Garg BP, Cohen M, et al: Subtypes of ischemic stroke in children and young adults. *Neurology* 49:1541, 1997.
9. Kittner SJ, Stern BJ, Wozniak M, et al: Cerebral infarction in young adults: The Baltimore-Washington Cooperative Young Stroke Study. *Neurology* 50:890, 1998.
10. Kittner SJ, Stern BJ, Feeser BR, et al: Pregnancy and the risk of stroke. *N Engl J Med* 335:768, 1996.
11. Sharshar T, Lamy C, Mas JL: Incidences and causes of stroke with pregnancy and the puerperium: A study in public hospitals of Ile de France. *Stroke* 26:930, 1995.
12. Lanska DJ, Kryscio RJ: Stroke and intracranial venous thrombosis during pregnancy and puerperium. *Neurology* 51:1622, 1998.

13. Cantu C, Barinagarrementeria F: Cerebral venous thrombosis associated with pregnancy and puerperium: Review of 67 cases. *Stroke* 24:1880, 1993.

14. Koch CA, Robyn JA, Walz ET, et al: Cranial sinus thrombosis and preeclampsia. *J Stroke Cerebrovasc Dis* 6:430, 1997.

15. Culebras A, Kase CS, Masdeu JC, et al: Practice guidelines for the use of imaging in transient ischemic attacks and acute stroke: A report of the Stroke Council, American Heart Association. *Stroke* 28:1480, 1997.

16. Jacobs K, Moulin T, Bogousslavsky J, et al: The stroke syndrome of cortical vein thrombosis. *Neurology* 47:376, 1996.

17. Finelli PF, Iantosca MR, Goldman RL: Magnetic resonance angiography in the diagnosis of deep cerebral venous thrombosis. *J Stroke Cerebrovasc Dis* 5:29, 1995.

18. Qureshi Al, Frankel MR, Ottenlips JR, et al: Cerebral hemodynamics in preeclampsia and eclampsia. *Arch Neurol* 53:1226, 1996.

19. Stevenson RE, Burton OM, Ferlauto GJ, et al: Hazards of oral anticoagulants during pregnancy. *JAMA* 243:1549, 1980.

20. Olson JP: Venous thromboembolism, in Leppert PC, Howard FM (eds): *Primary Care for Women.* Philadelphia, Lippincott-Raven Publishers, 1997, pp 607–615.

21. Martinelli I, Sacchi E, Landi G, et al: High risk of cerebral vein thrombosis in carriers of a prothrombin gene mutation and in users of oral contraceptives. *N Engl J Med* 338:1793, 1998.

22. Ludemann P, Nabovi DG, Junker R, et al: Factor V Leiden mutation is a risk factor for cerebral venous thrombosis. *Stroke* 29:2507, 1998.

23. Schulman S, Svenungsson E, Granqvist S, et al: Anticardiolipin antibodies predict early recurrence of thromboembolism and death among patients with venous thromboembolism following anticoagulant therapy. *Am J Med* 104:332, 1998.

24. Ranoux D, Cohen A, Cabanes L, et al: Patent foramen ovale: Is stroke due to paradoxical embolism? *Stroke* 24:31, 1993.

25. Rohr-LeFloch J: Foramen ovale permeable et embolie paradoxale: Une hypothese controversee. *Rev Neurol (Paris)* 150:282, 1994.

26. Petty GW, Khandheria BK, Chu CP, et al: Patent foramen ovale in patients with cerebral infarction: A transesophageal echocardiographic study. *Arch Neurol* 54:819, 1997.

27. Homma S, DiTullio MR, Sacco RL, et al: Characteristics of patent foramen ovale associated with cryptogenic stroke: A biplane transesophageal echographic study. *Stroke* 25:582, 1994.

28. Devuyst G, Bogousslavsky J, Ruchat P, et al: Prognosis after stroke following surgical closure of patent foramen ovale. *Neurology* 47:1162, 1996.

29. Haapaniemi H, Salonen O, Hillbom M, et al: Carotid arterial dissection as a cause of severe brain infarction in young adults. *J Stroke Cerebrovasc Dis* 6:89, 1996.

30. Barinagarrementeria F, Amaya LE, Cantu C: Causes and mechanisms of cerebellar infarction in young patients. *Stroke* 28:2400, 1997.

31. Kasner SE, Hankins LL, Bratina P, et al: Magnetic resonance angiography demostrates vascular healing of carotid and vertebral artery dissections. *Stroke* 28:1993, 1997.

32. Antiphospholipid Antibodies in Stroke Study (APASS) Group: Anticardiolipin antibodies are an independent risk factor for first ischemic stroke. *Neurology* 43:2069, 1993.

33. Nencini P, Baruffi MC, Abbate R, et al: Lupus anticoagulant and anticardiolipin antibodies in young adults with cerebral ischemia. *Stroke* 23:189, 1992.

34. Levine SR, Brey RL, Sawaya KL, et al: Recurrent stroke and thrombo-occlusive events in the antiphospholipid antibody syndrome. *Ann Intern Med* 38:119, 1995.

35. Martinez HR, Rangel-Guerra RA, Marfil LJ: Ischemic stroke due to deficiency of coagulation inhibitors: Report of 10 young adults. *Stroke* 24:19, 1993.

36. Green D, Otoya J, Oriba H, et al: Protein S deficiency in middle-aged women with stroke. *Neurology* 42:1029, 1992.

37. Barinagarrementeria F, Cantu-Brito C, Pena A, et al: Prothrombotic states in young people with idiopathic stroke: A prospective study. *Stroke* 25:287, 1994.

38. Rosove MH, Brewer PMC: Antiphospholipid thrombosis: Clinical course after the first thrombotic event in 70 patients. *Ann Intern Med* 117:303, 1992.

39. Petitti DB, Sidney S, Bernstein A, et al: Stroke in users of low-dose oral contraceptives. *N Engl J Med* 335:8, 1996.

40. Schwartz SM, Siscovick DS, Longstreth WT, et al: Use of low-dose oral contraceptives and stroke in young women. *Ann Intern Med* 127:596, 1997.

41. WHO Collaborative Study of Cardiovascular Disease and Steroid Hormone Contraception: Ischemic stroke and combined oral contraceptives: Results of an international, multi-centre, case-control study. *Lancet* 348:498, 1996.

42. Buring JE, Hebert P, Romero J, et al: Migraine and subsequent risk of stroke in the physicians' health study. *Arch Neurol* 52:129, 1995.

43. Merikangas KR, Fenton BT, Cheng SH, et al: Association between migraine and stroke in a large-scale epidemiologic study of the United States. *Arch Neurol* 54:362, 1997.

44. Tzourio C, Tehindrazanarivelo A, Iglesias S, et al: Case-control study of migraine and risk of ischemic stroke in young women. *Br Med J* 310:830, 1995.

45. Carolei A, Marini C, Dematteis G, et al: History of migraine and risk of cerebral ischemia in young adults. *Lancet* 347:1503, 1996.

46. Joutel A, Vahedi K, Corpechot C, et al: Strong clustering and stereotyped nature of Notch 3 mutations in CADASIL patients. *Lancet* 350:1511, 1997.

47. Rohr J, Kittner S, Feeser B, et al: Traditional risk factors and ischemic stroke in young adults: The Baltimore-Washington Cooperative Young Stroke Study. *Arch Neurol* 53:603, 1996.

48. Haapaniemi H, Hillbom M, Juveca S: Lifestyle-associated

risk factors for acute brain infarction among persons of working age. *Stroke* 28:26, 1997.

49. Coull BM, Brockschmidt JK, Howard G, et al: Community hospital-based stroke programs in North Carolina, Oregon, and New York. *Stroke* 21:867, 1990.

50. Hypertension Detection and Followup Program Cooperative Group: Five-year findings of the Hypertension Detection and Followup Program. *JAMA* 247:633, 1982.

51. Anastos K, Charney P, Charon RA, et al: Hypertension in women: What is really known? *Ann Intern Med* 115:287, 1991.

52. Wolf PA, D'Agostino RB, Kannel WB, et al: Cigarette smoking as a risk factor for stroke: The Framingham Study. *JAMA* 259:1025, 1988.

53. Kawachi I, Colditz GA, Stampfer MJ, et al: Smoking cessation and decreased risk of stroke in women. *JAMA* 269:232, 1993.

54. Whisnant JP, Homer D, Ingall TJ, et al: Duration of cigarette smoking is the strongest predictor of severe extracranial carotid artery atherosclerosis. *Stroke* 21:707, 1990.

55. Rodman KD, Furlan AJ: Severe extracranial carotid atherosclerosis in young adults. *J Stroke Cerebrovasc Dis* 2:173, 1992.

56. Petrik PV, Gelabert HA, Moore WS, et al: Cigarette smoking accelerates carotid artery intimal hyperplasia in a dose-dependent manner. *Stroke* 26:1409, 1995.

57. Levine SR, Brust JCM, Futrell N, et al: Cerebrovascular complications of the use of the "crack" form of alkaloidal cocaine. *N Engl J Med* 323:699, 1990.

58. Klonoff DC, Andrews BT, Ohana WG: Stroke associated with cocaine use. *Arch Neurol* 46:989, 1989.

59. Petty GW, Brust JCM, Tatemichi TK, et al: Embolic stroke after smoking "crack" cocaine. *Stroke* 21:1632, 1990.

60. Longstreth WT, Rosendaal FR, Siscovick OS, et al: Risk of stroke in young women and two prothrombotic mutations: Factor V Leiden and prothrombin gene variant. *Stroke* 29:577, 1998.

61. Lüdemann P, Nabavi DG, Junker R, et al: Factor V Leiden mutation is a risk factor for cerebral venous thrombosis. A case control study of 55 patients. *Stroke* 29:2507, 1998.

62. Gilon D, Buonanno FS, Joffe MM, et al: Lack of evidence between mitral-valve prolapse and stroke in young patients. *N Engl J Med* 341:8, 1999.

63. Orencia AJ, Petty GW, Khandheria BK, et al: Mitral valve prolapse and the risk of stroke after initial cerebral ischemia. *Neurology* 45:1083, 1995.

Chapter 29

STROKE IN AFRICAN AMERICANS

Timothy G. Lukovits
Philip B. Gorelick

BACKGROUND

Introduction

African Americans are disproportionately affected by stroke.[1,2] They are about two times more likely than whites to die of cerebrovascular disease or experience stroke. This disparity is most evident in early and middle life and may rob African Americans of many productive years of life. African Americans suffer epidemic stroke rates that are unparalleled by other major ethnic or racial groups in the United States. The reason for this excess stroke morbidity and mortality remains uncertain. As epidemiologic and other clinical research efforts attempt to uncover explanations for the disproportionate stroke burden in African Americans, three main themes arise: excess of cardiovascular disease risk factors, differential susceptibility to risk factors, and delay in treatment or access to medical care. In this chapter, we review the epidemiology of stroke in African Americans, provide rationale for the excess stroke risk, and address special issues in this population that relate to diagnosis and management of intracranial occlusive disease and sickle cell disease. We also discuss the impact of vascular dementia, an important sequelae of cerebrovascular disease in African Americans.

Epidemiology

Mortality   African American men and women in the United States have almost twice the rate of death as a result of stroke when compared with their white counterparts.[3] Although African Americans also suffer higher death rates from heart disease overall and coronary heart disease specifically, the disparity in these rates is not as great as those for stroke when racial comparisons are made. Furthermore, the rate ratio for stroke mortality is most pronounced at relatively younger ages.[4] For example, African American men and women under age 55 are approximately 4 times and 3.2 times more likely to die of stroke than their white counterparts, respectively. These rate ratios for men and women, however, level off to 1.26 and 1.10, respectively, for those ≥75 years of age. In the United States, excess stroke mortality has been highest for both African Americans and whites in the southeastern portion of the country, an area referred to as the Stroke Belt.[5,6] The reason for this geographically based excess remains unknown, although some data suggest that stroke mortality rates have fallen in this region.

Secular trends in stroke mortality rates reveal an alarming trend. In the 1980's, we began to observe deceleration of stroke mortality decline when compared with the late 1960's and early 1970's.[7] This deceleration has continued into the 1990's.[8] The slowing of the absolute rate of decline of stroke mortality has been substantial for African American women.[7] The precise reason for the deceleration is uncertain, but it may relate to an increase in the prevalence of certain cardiovascular disease risk factors such as congestive heart failure, atrial fibrillation, diabetes mellitus and obesity, or less than optimal treatment and control of hypertension.

Prevalence   The prevalence of stroke is believed to be higher for African Americans.[9] The disparity for higher prevalence rates may be most pronounced for African

American women. Although case fatality rates might be expected to be higher for African Americans, such trends have not been demonstrated definitively.[10,11]

Several studies including the Lehigh Valley Stroke Register and the Stroke Data Bank have shown that African Americans tend to have more lacunar infarctions, "silent" infarctions, and infarctions of unknown cause, but less embolic infarctions than whites.[10,12–14]

Incidence The incidence of stroke is substantially higher for African Americans. Representative data from key studies of the past several decades are listed in Table 29-1.[12,13,15–17] Stroke incidence rates are approximately two times higher for African American men and women. The disparity for African Americans, however, is most pronounced at younger ages when compared with whites.[11,12,18] By taking into account the higher stroke incidence rates in African Americans, the estimate of first-ever or recurrent strokes in the United States has been revised upward from approximately 500,000–550,000 to over 730,000.[16]

When stroke subtypes are studied, African Americans have a higher incidence of cerebral infarction, intracerebral hemorrhage, and subarachnoid hemorrhage.[11,13,18–22] Again, these rates generally show a trend for disproportionate burden of risk for blacks at relatively younger ages.

In a Northern Manhattan population, the age-adjusted incidence of hospitalized cerebral infarction was 632, 488, 296, and 318 per 100,000 for African American women, African American men, white women, and white men, respectively.[13] In this same study, the incidence of intracerebral hemorrhage was 60, 64, 24, and 17 per 100,000 for these same groups, respectively. Autopsy series[23] and hospitalization rates for the Kaiser Permanente Medical Care Program[21] are concordant with these incidence figures and have found that African Americans have an increased frequency of intracerebral hemorrhage when compared with whites. In a population-based study from Cincinnati, Broderick and colleagues[20] showed that African Americans under the age of 75 years had 2.3 times the risk of intracerebral hemorrhage (95 percent confidence interval, 1.5 to 3.6), but for those over the age of 75 years, the risk was 0.23 (95 percent confidence interval, 0.1 to 0.8). Heightened risk for intracerebral hemorrhage, which is disproportionately greater for younger African Americans, has also been shown in Texas.[4]

African Americans also have a higher risk of subarachnoid hemorrhage. The age-adjusted incidence of hospitalized subarachnoid hemorrhage in a population from Northern Manhattan was 18, 11, 4, and 6 per 100,000 for African American women, African American men, white women, and white men, respectively.[13] Broderick and colleagues[20] found that African Ameri-

Table 29-1.
Stroke incidence rates

Study	Incidence rate
Lehigh Valley years[12]	2.43 black: white SMR[a] 4.50 black: white SMR for age <65
Northern Manhattan[13]	567/100,000 black men[b] 351/100,000 white men[b] 716/100,000 black women[b] 326/100,000 white women[b]
South Alabama[15]	208/100,000 blacks[b] 109/100,000 whites[b]
Greater Cincinnati/Northern Kentucky[16]	288/100,000 African Americans (first-ever stroke)[c] and 411/100,000 African Americans (first-ever and recurrent stroke)[c] vs. 179/100,000 whites (first-ever stroke in Rochester, MN)[c]
Northern Manhattan[17]	233/100,000 blacks[b] 93/100,000 whites[b]

[a] SMR, standard morbidity ratio.

[b] Age-adjusted rates.

[c] Age- and sex-adjusted rates.

cans had 2.1 times the risk of subarachnoid hemorrhage (95 percent confidence interval, 1.3 to 3.6) when compared with whites.

The explanation for the possible racial disparity in stroke subtypes remains uncertain but may be related to the occurrence and severity of select cardiovascular disease risk factors (e.g., hypertension, tobacco abuse, hypercholesterolemia) and their influence on specific cerebrovascular beds.[24] African Americans may also be more likely to demonstrate an abnormal circadian blood pressure pattern with elevations at nighttime. This pattern, called "reverse dipping," has been linked to an increased risk of small artery disease, lacunar infarctions, and intracerebral hemorrhage.[25–27]

Risk Factors Major cardiovascular disease risk factors such as hypertension, diabetes mellitus, smoking, and obesity as well as the sequelae of some of these risk factors, end-stage renal disease, left ventricular hypertrophy, and congestive heart failure, generally are more common in African Americans.[1,2] Traditional cardiovascular disease risk factors, however, may not be as prevalent in persons of rural or urban Africa. For example, Cooper and colleagues[28] described the distribution of blood pressures, hypertension prevalence, and associated risk factors among populations of West African origin (Nigeria, Cameroon, Jamaica, St. Lucia, Barbados, and the United States). There was a gradient of hypertension prevalence that rose from 16 percent in West Africa to 26 percent in the Caribbean to 33 percent in the United States. The increase in hypertension prevalence with age was two times as steep in the United States as in Africa, and environmental factors such as obesity and sodium and potassium intake varied consistently with disease prevalence for each region. This study demonstrated the role of social conditions as possible determinants in the development of hypertension. Gillum has suggested that epidemiologic changes in the patterns of cardiovascular disease among black societies that span precolonial Africa and traditional African societies, modern black populations in the West Indies, rural and inner-city black populations in the United States, and affluent suburban or urban black Americans may be determined by social influences related to acculturation, urbanization, and affluence.[29] These social influences are associated with saturated dietary fat intake, salt intake, and smoking, and their occurrence parallels hypertensive and atherosclerotic cardiovascular diseases. Thus, there may be an important window of opportunity to redouble efforts to control certain potentially modifiable behaviors that could lead to a more favorable cardiovascular disease risk profile and, subsequently, less cardiovascular disease.[30]

Cardiovascular disease risk factor burden is thought to be a possible explanation for disproportionate stroke mortality and incidence in African Americans. This makes intuitive sense as certain factors such as hypertension may not only be more prevalent among blacks but more severe as well. When these factors are studied, however, they do not account for all of the variance associated with the excess stroke risk.[31] This suggests that other factors (e.g., genetic, psychosocial) may be important. One such factor, socioeconomic status (SES), may account for a proportion of excess African American stroke mortality.[32,33] More information, however, about the behavioral, social, psychologic, and biologic pathways by which SES acts is needed.

Access to medical care is another factor that may be important in the understanding of excess stroke risk in African Americans. African Americans have traditionally had less access to medical care[1,34,35] and are more frequently Medicaid beneficiaries. Furthermore, knowledge of stroke risk factors and warning signs has been shown to be deficient among this high-risk group.[36] Thus, in addition to access to medical care, more education and awareness about stroke risk factors, warning signs, and treatments are needed in the African American community.

Despite the disproportionate stroke burden in African Americans, there has been a relative paucity of research on cardiovascular risk factors for stroke in this group.[37] Although age and hypertension seem to be firmly established risk factors for stroke in African Americans, other factors may be classified as only putative based on a paucity of focused study. The role of such factors as blood lipids, alcohol consumption, exercise, genetic factors, coagulation factors, hormone replacement therapy, markers of inflammation, stress and racism, and homocysteine needs to be better defined.[2]

Race and the Anatomic Distribution of Cerebral Atherosclerosis

Pathologic series and studies using conventional angiography and ultrasound suggest that African Americans are predisposed to intracranial large artery occlusive disease. They also suggest, but less consistently, that African Americans have less extracranial atherosclerotic disease compared with whites. The possibility of selection bias must be considered when interpreting these studies. Referral centers that report these findings may examine a select population that is not representative of the community-at-large and, thus, may not reflect the actual prevalence of intracranial and extracranial occlusive disease by race.

In an autopsy series, Resch and colleagues[38] reported that 242 middle-aged African Americans from Maryland had more severe large vessel intracranial occlusive disease when compared with 238 age-matched whites from Maryland. This study used an aggregate score for atherosclerosis from multiple locations, and site-specific information was not available.

Pathologic specimens of intracranial vessels from 234 African Americans and 129 age and gender-matched whites were compared in the International Atherosclerosis Project.[39] The patients had no history or pathologic evidence of stroke or hypertension. The African Americans were found to have three times the rate of raised atherosclerotic lesions in the intracranial vessels. The carotid siphon and the vertebral arteries were not examined. Overall, there was no difference in the extent of extradural carotid artery occlusive disease between the two groups, but 55 to 70-year-old African American women had slightly more disease at this site. In a separate analysis, this study showed that hypertension had a relatively greater effect on the extent of atherosclerosis of the intracranial circulation compared with the extradural carotid artery.

Angiography-based series also suggest that African Americans have more intracranial occlusive disease and less extracranial atherosclerosis than whites. In the Joint Study of Extracranial Arterial Occlusion, middle cerebral artery (MCA) main stem occlusion was reported in 3 percent of African Americans and 0.6 percent of whites, whereas extracranial carotid stenosis or occlusion was seen in 48 percent of African Americans and 65 percent of whites.[40]

In the early 1980's, Gorelick and colleagues observed that the anatomic distribution of occlusive cerebrovascular lesions of their African American patients did not conform to the findings described previously for whites.[24,41] They compared the clinical and angiographic features of 45 African Americans and 26 whites who were hospitalized for stroke or transient ischemic attacks (TIAs) in the anterior circulation.[41] Disease of the carotid siphon, MCA stem, and distal MCA was more common in African Americans, whereas symptomatic disease of the extracranial internal carotid artery (ICA) was more common in whites (Table 29-2).

Gorelick et al also reported their findings in patients with symptomatic posterior circulation occlusive disease.[42] African Americans had more lesions in the distal basilar artery and the intracranial branches of the

Table 29-2.

Distribution of symptomatic sites by race (right and left territories combined)

	Symptomatic sites[a]	
Artery site	Whites (N = 24)	African Americans (N = 27)
	%	
Extracranial carotid	64[b]	17
Carotid siphon	4	13
MCA stem	0	27[c]
MCA division/branch	4	14

[a]Cases were included only if a determination could be made as to the vascular site responsible for symptoms.
[b]Groups differ, $p < .001$, chi-square with Yate's correction, df = 1.
[c]Groups differ, $p < .02$, chi-square with Yate's correction, df = 1.
Reproduced with permission.[41]

basilar artery, especially the proximal portions of the posterior cerebral artery (PCA). Whites had more symptomatic lesions in the extracranial and intracranial vertebral artery (Table 29-3). Similar findings were reported for asymptomatic lesions that were detected by angiography in patients who presented with symptomatic carotid artery disease.[43]

Table 29-3.

Distribution of symptomatic lesions by race (right and left territories combined

	Symptomatic sites	
Artery site	Whites (N = 27)	African Americans (N = 24)
	%	
Vertebral origin	26	8
Extracranial vertebral	26	8
Intracranial vertebral	41	25
Proximal or middle basilar	14	12
Distal basilar	7	17
PICA	0	4
SCA	0	4
PCA	7	13
Basilar branches[a]	7	29

[a]Includes PICA, SCA, PCA, thalamoperforators, and basilar branch arteries (PICA, posterior inferior cerebellar artery; SCA, superior cerebellar artery; PCA, posterior cerebral artery.)
Reproduced with permission.[42]

In a series of 20 patients with symptomatic occlusive disease of the middle cerebral artery, 85 percent were African American.[44] In the International Cooperative Study of Extracranial-Intracranial Arterial Anastomosis (EC/IC Bypass Study), isolated MCA occlusive lesions were present in 10 percent of African Americans and 5 percent of whites, and isolated ICA lesions were present in 64 percent of African Americans and 82 percent of whites.[45] Race had a significant effect on the prediction of the location of the stenosis after controlling for the effect of other risk factors including hypertension. Whites were also more likely to have extracranial disease in other angiographic studies.[46,47]

Ultrasound-based series confirm this predilection for intracranial occlusive disease but do not support a large difference in the occurrence of extracranial carotid artery disease between African Americans and whites. These studies may have less selection bias when compared with angiographic studies because ultrasound is less invasive, may be more widely applied without selection bias, and many of these studies are community-based, rather than hospital-based.

In the Northern Manhattan Stroke Study (NOMASS), 6 percent of African Americans and 1 percent of non-Hispanic whites had strokes secondary to intracranial occlusive disease that was measured by transcranial Doppler (TCD) or conventional angiography.[48] African Americans and non-Hispanic whites had a similar frequency of stroke secondary to extracranial disease as measured by carotid ultrasound or conventional angiography (8 percent vs. 11 percent). The ratio of symptomatic extracranial to intracranial disease was 1.2 for African Americans and 9 for non-Hispanic whites. In another report from this study, African Americans and non-Hispanic whites had a similar degree of ICA plaque thickness.[49]

In the Multicenter Isradipine Diuretic Atherosclerosis Study, African Americans from Detroit had a lower frequency of carotid artery intimal-media thickness when compared with whites, but no difference was observed for those who resided in Augusta, Georgia.[50] Gil-Peralta and colleagues found that African Americans had less carotid stenosis than whites, as measured by duplex ultrasonography.[51] Other ultrasound-based studies have reported no difference in the frequency of carotid disease by race.[52-54]

One possible explanation for the differences in the distribution of atherosclerosis in African Americans is that hypertension and diabetes are more prevalent in African Americans, and these risk factors have a disproportionate potentiating effect on occlusive disease of intracranial large and small arteries as compared with extracranial arteries.[39,55] Studies, however, have shown that the increased risk of intracranial occlusive disease and certain stroke subtypes persists after controlling for the effects of hypertension and diabetes.[21,31,39,45] Thus, there must remain as yet defined genetic and environmental factors that predispose one to extracranial or intracranial occlusive cerebrovascular disease.

Outcome After Stroke and Stroke Recurrence

Several reports have shown that African Americans may have more severe strokes and a worse outcome following stroke when compared with whites. In the Joint Study of Extracranial Arterial Occlusion, African Americans were more likely to be obtunded or comatose following stroke.[40] In a study of over 12,000 patients from the Maryland Health Services Cost Review Commission, African Americans were more likely to become comatose and had longer hospitalizations following ischemic and hemorrhagic stroke when compared with whites.[56] It is unclear whether African Americans actually have more severe strokes or are less likely to seek hospitalization for less severe strokes.

There is a paucity of information on the functional outcome after stroke by race. Compared with whites, African Americans may have more residual physical impairment but a similar degree of functional impairment following stroke.[57] In the Stroke Data Bank and the NOMASS, race had no significant effect on the risk of stroke recurrence.[58-60]

Sickle Cell Disease and Stroke

Sickle cell disease (SCD) is associated with chronic disability in young African Americans. Approximately 8 percent of African Americans carry the gene for SCD, 0.03 to 0.16 percent have SCD, and up to 17 percent of children with SCD experience a stroke before adulthood.[61] Those with SCD have a markedly increased risk of ischemic brain infarction and are more likely to experience intracerebral hemorrhage and subarachnoid hemorrhage. In addition, SCD patients with subcortical lesions on magnetic resonance imaging (MRI) seem to be at risk for vascular dementia.[62]

The average age for first ischemic stroke in SCD is 7.7 years, and the incidence is highest between the ages of 2 and 5 years.[63] Recurrent ischemic stroke tends to occur within 3 years of the initial event.[64] Intracranial hemorrhage tends to occur later in life, at an average

age of 25 years.[63] Factors that have been associated with an increased risk of stroke in patients with SCD include current infection, a history of central nervous system infection, prior stroke, cardiomegaly, lower hemoglobin concentrations, hemoglobin S fraction greater than 30 percent, lower hemoglobin F concentration, higher reticulocyte counts, and more frequent SCD crises.[64,65]

Increased blood flow velocities as measured by TCD have been shown to predict brain infarction in children with SCD.[66] The Stroke Prevention Trial in Sickle Cell Anemia (STOP) demonstrated that exchange or simple red blood cell transfusion to maintain the hemoglobin S fraction at less than 30 percent substantially decreases the risk of stroke in children with elevated blood flow velocities (time-averaged mean blood flow velocities greater than 200 cm/s in the middle cerebral artery or the internal carotid artery).[67] It is now recommended that all children with SCD between the ages of 2 and 16 years have TCD screening every 6 months to determine who should be considered for transfusion therapy.[68] The risk of alloimmunization and iron overload and the inconvenience of frequent transfusion makes the management of these patients complex.

Vascular Dementia

Racial or ethnic groups with a high risk of stroke, including Japanese and African Americans, may have a risk of vascular dementia that approaches or surpasses that of Alzheimer disease.[69,70] In a community-based case control study of patients with recent ischemic stroke, non-white race increased the odds of dementia after stroke by more than a factor of 3.[71] White matter lesions on MRI have been associated with cognitive impairment.[72] In the Atherosclerosis Risk in Communities (ARIC) study, African Americans had a lower prevalence of white matter lesions on MRI but a higher prevalence of more severe white matter lesions when compared with whites.[73] Alcohol and tobacco use were associated with an increased risk of white matter lesions in African Americans only. The association of hypertension and white matter lesions was stronger for African Americans than whites.

Several studies have attempted to define the determinants of vascular dementia in African Americans. In a case-control study of mostly African American stroke patients, a history of myocardial infarction, recent cigarette smoking, lower educational attainment, and older age increased the risk of dementia.[74] In a group of 185 African American patients diagnosed with

vascular dementia, Alzheimer disease, or stroke without dementia, radiographic evidence of white matter lesions, nonlacunar infarcts, left subcortical infarcts, and enlargement of the third ventricle on MRI or computed tomography distinguished vascular dementia from the other conditions.[75]

African Americans have a high prevalence of cardiovascular disease risk factors and may have an abnormal circadian blood pressure pattern (see above), which may heighten the risk for vascular dementia. As many of the determinants of vascular dementia are modifiable, a concerted effort to diagnose and treat them could prevent this sequela of stroke.

EVIDENCE

Clinical Trials

African Americans have been under-represented in clinical trials.[76,77] Federal agencies have now mandated diversity in study populations, and with this, there have been concerted efforts to recruit women and minorities into clinical research studies. Some improvement in recruitment of African Americans for stroke clinical trials has been noted. Participation of African Americans in recent stroke trials is reviewed in Table 29-4.[78–84]

Data from clinical stroke trials suggest that the efficacy and side effects of medications for treatment and prevention of vascular disease could differ by race or ethnic group. For example, an on-treatment analysis of the Ticlopidine Aspirin Stroke Study (TASS) data showed that non-whites may benefit more from ticlopidine than aspirin and have less adverse events than whites.[78] In the TASS and the Canadian American Ticlopidine Study (CATS) combined, 21 subjects experienced moderate or severe neutropenia, and none of these were African Americans.[78,79] One-half of the 18 patients who experienced mild neutropenia in these trials were African American, but these cases may have had idiopathic cyclic neutropenia, as a similar number of cases were noted in both treatment groups. The African American Antiplatelet Stroke Prevention Study (AAASPS) is the first secondary stroke prevention study that is targeted exclusively for African Americans and is testing whether aspirin or ticlopidine is more effective in secondary stroke prevention in an entirely African American population.[84–86]

Data from the Thrombolysis and Angioplasty in Myocardial Infarction (phase 1) study suggested that African Americans may have an exaggerated fibrinolytic

Table 29-4.

Representation of blacks in recent stroke prevention studies

Study	Total # patients	% black
Ticlopidine Aspirin Stroke Study[78] (1989)	3069	16
Canadian American Ticlopidine Study[79] (1989)	1053	28 (Non-white)
North American Symptomatic Carotid Endarterectomy Trial (70–99% stenosis group)[80] (1991)	659	3
NINDS t-PA[81] (1995)	624	27
Asymptomatic Carotid Atherosclerosis Study[82] 1995	1659	2
Clopidogrel vs. Aspirin in Patients at Risk of Ischemic Events (CAPRIE)[83] (1996)	6431 (Stroke subgroup)	9
African American Antiplatelet Stroke Prevention Study (AAASPS)[84] (ongoing, as of 8/2/99)	1166	100

response to thrombolytic agents. African Americans were more likely to experience vessel patency and had lower fibrinogen concentration nadirs, higher peak fibrin degradation product concentrations, and a higher rate of transfusions following thrombolytic treatment.[87] An effect of race on outcome or risk of intracerebral hemorrhage following thrombolytic therapy for ischemic stroke, however, was not found in the NINDS t-PA study, a study that was made up of 27 percent African Americans.[81,88,89]

Explanations for Under-representation of African Americans in Clinical Trials Under-representation of African Americans in clinical trials parallels other black health care trends for lack of access to preventive and palliative medical diagnostic and treatment services.[85] Because clinical trials play a pivotal role in the development of safe and effective treatments, participation of women and minorities is crucial to guarantee sufficient information to adequately assess the safety and efficacy of new treatments.

African Americans had been subjected to medical demonstration and experimentation by reason of their slave status as early as the time period of the antebellum South.[85] It is believed that such experimentation was often brutal, and the medical establishment came to be viewed with mistrust. Such experimentation culminated in the infamous Public Health Service Tuskegee Syphilis Study, a prolonged and unethical violation of human rights that was finally terminated in the 1970's. These factors, coupled with socioeconomic hardship and racism, may have set the stage for under-representation of African Americans in clinical trials.

We have identified four key barriers for entry of African Americans into clinical trials: lack of awareness of clinical trials, economic factors, communication issues, and mistrust.[85] We believe that these barriers as well as others can be surmounted with proper pretrial planning, patient education, culturally sensitive staff, patience, flexible office hours and home study visits, travel stipends for patients who are in need, and genuine commitment. Although mistrust is a difficult and important challenge to overcome, study staff with good communication skills, honesty, and patience can overcome this barrier and be successful in their efforts to recruit and retain minority study patients.

It is important to understand why potential study patients choose to enroll in a program, refuse to enroll, or voluntarily withdraw. In an interim study that our AAASPS research group carried out, we found that persons who enrolled in the AAASPS and remained in the program did so to reduce their risk of stroke recurrence and to help find a "cure" for stroke.[86] Those who withdrew or refused to participate were fearful of "experimentation" and of possibly being used as "guinea pigs." From this experience, we conceptionalized a recruitment triangle made up of the patient, key family members and friends, and the primary medical doctor and other medical personnel. As long as these three main components of the triangle remain intact (i.e., supportive), we believe that it is likely that the study patient will enroll and remain in the program.

AAASPS AAASPS is a double-blind, randomized, multicenter study that is comparing the effectiveness and safety of ticlopidine hydrochloride (500 mg/day) and aspirin (650 mg/day) in the prevention of recurrent stroke, myocardial infarction, and vascular death in African Americans with noncardioembolic ischemic stroke within the past 90 days. AAASPS is a historic initiative, as it is first stroke prevention study that is targeted exclusively to the African American community. AAASPS participating sites are located throughout the United States at centers that serve substantial numbers of African American stroke patients.[84-86] The recruitment goal is to enroll 1800 patients and to follow each of them for 2 years.

TREATMENT

Diagnostic Considerations

For the most part, the diagnostic evaluation of African American stroke patients is similar to that of other stroke patients. Because African Americans may have a higher prevalence of intracranial large vessel disease, and because such lesions may require a different treatment strategy (see Chap. 21), the threshold for evaluation of intracranial disease is lower for African Americans. In the evaluation of African Americans with possible intracranial occlusive disease, TCD may be technically limited, as African Americans, especially older African American women, may have thickened temporal bone that interferes with insonation.[90] More penetrating 1-MegaHertz probes and contrast agents that are being developed may improve the utility of TCD in this circumstance. At the present time, magnetic resonance angiography and conventional cerebral angiography of the intracranial vessels play an important role in the diagnostic workup of African American stroke patients.

Some lacunar syndromes, such as pure motor stroke owing to infarction in the striatocapsular region or basis pontis, may be caused by cardioembolism or large artery disease rather than small vessel disease. Therefore, African American patients with lacunar syndromes should be evaluated for these underlying stroke mechanisms.

African American children with unexplained stroke should have a sickle cell prep and, if indicated, hemoglobin electrophoresis. Stroke, however, is rarely the presenting sign of sickle cell disease and sickle cell trait.

Treatment Recommendations

Although African Americans may have an exaggerated fibrinolytic response to thrombolytic agents (see above), there are no data to indicate that acute interventions including thrombolysis should be withheld from African Americans. At the present time, there are no prospective randomized trials that conclusively indicate a differential response to antiplatelet agents based on race. Until the results of the AAASPS are known, stroke prevention therapy will need to be individualized. If an African American is at high risk for recurrent stroke and cannot be entered into this trial, we recommend choosing a therapy without regard to race based on the presumed stroke mechanism. Treatments that target intracranial disease, including anticoagulation and angioplasty, may play an important role in stroke prevention in African Americans. Ongoing studies will help to better define the effectiveness and safety of these treatments in African Americans. One such program, the Warfarin-Aspirin Symptomatic Intracranial Disease (WASID) study, began in 1999.[91] Until the results of this randomized prospective trial are known, African Americans with large vessel intracranial disease may be treated with antiplatelet agents or warfarin. Although these treatments are important, aggressive control of risk factors, especially hypertension and tobacco abuse, are central to any stroke prevention program.

REFERENCES

1. Gorelick PB, Harris Y: Stroke: An excess burden on African Americans. *Chicago Med* 96:28, 1993.
2. Gaines K, Burke G, for the SECORDS Investigators: Ethnic differences in stroke: Black-white differences in the United States population. *Neuroepidemiology* 14:209, 1995.
3. National Center for Health Statistics: Health, United States, 1996–97 and Injury Chartbook. Hyattsville, Maryland, 1997.
4. Morgenstern LB, Spears WD, Goff DC, et al: African Americans and women have the highest stroke mortality in Texas. *Stroke* 28:15, 1997.
5. Pickle LW, Mungiole M, Gillum RF: Geographic variation in stroke mortality in blacks and whites in the United States. *Stroke* 28:1639, 1997.
6. Howard G, Evans GW, Pearce K, et al: Is the stroke belt disappearing? *Stroke* 26:1153, 1995.
7. Cooper R, Sempos C, Hsieh S-C, et al: Slowdown in the decline of stroke mortality in the United States, 1978-1986. *Stroke* 21:1274, 1990.

8. Gillum RF, Sempos CT: The end of the long-term decline in stroke mortality in the United States? *Stroke* 28:1527, 1997.

9. Scheoenberg BS, Anderson DW, Haerer AF: Racial differentials in the prevalence of stroke. *Arch Neurol* 43:565, 1986.

10. Sacco RL, Hauser WA, Mohr JP, et al: One-year outcome after cerebral infarction in whites, blacks and hispanics. *Stroke* 22:305, 1991.

11. Epstein A, Kittner S, Hebel JR, et al: Black-white differences in stroke risk: The Baltimore-Washington Cooperative Young Stroke Study. Abstract, 23rd International Joint Conference on Stroke and Cerebral Circulation. Orlando, FL, February 5–7, 1998.

12. Friday G, Lai SM, Alter MA, et al: Stroke in the Lehigh Valley: Racial/ethnic differences. *Neurology* 39:1165, 1989.

13. Sacco RL, Hauser WA, Mohr JP: Hospitalized stroke in blacks and hispanics in Northern Manhattan. *Stroke* 22:1491, 1991.

14. Weisberg LA: Racial differences for lacunar infarcts documented by computed tomography: A comparison of black and white patients. *J Stroke Cerebrovasc Dis* 3:157, 1993.

15. Gross CR, Kase CS, Mohr JP, Michenfelder JP: Stroke in South Alabama: Incidence and diagnostic features—A population based study. *Stroke* 15:249, 1984.

16. Broderick J, Brott T, Kothari R, et al: The Greater Cincinnati/Northern Kentucky Stroke Study. Preliminary first-ever and total incidence rates of stroke among blacks. *Stroke* 29:415, 1998.

17. Sacco RL, Boden-Albala B, Gan R, et al: Stroke incidence among white, black and hispanic residents of an Urban community: The Northern Manhattan Stroke Study. *Am J Epidemiol* 147:259, 1998.

18. Giles WH, Kittner SJ, Hebel JR, et al: Determinants of black-white differences in the risk of cerebral infarction: The National Health and Nutrition Examination Survey Epidemiologic Follow-up Study. *Arch Intern Med* 155:1319, 1995.

19. Kittner SJ, McCarter RJ, Sherwin RW, et al: Black-white differences in stroke risk among young adults. *Stroke* 24 (Suppl I): 1-13, 1993.

20. Broderick JP, Brott T, Tomsick T, et al: The risk of subarachnoid and intracerebral hemorrhage in blacks as compared with whites. *N Engl J Med* 326:733, 1992.

21. Klatsky AL, Armstrong MA, Friedman GD: Racial differences in cerebrovascular disease hospitalization. *Stroke* 22:299, 1991.

22. Cooper ES: Clinical cerebrovascular disease in hypertensive blacks. *J Clin Hypertens* 3:79S, 1987.

23. Aronson SM: Intracranial vascular lesions in patients with diabetes mellitus. *J Neuropathol Exp Neurol* 32:183, 1973.

24. Caplan LR, Gorelick PB, Hier DB: Race, sex and occlusive cerebrovascular disease: A review. *Stroke* 17:648, 1986.

25. Lip GYH, Zarifis J, Farooqi IS, et al: Ambulatory blood pressure monitoring in acute stroke: The West Birmingham Stroke Project. *Stroke* 28:31, 1997.

26. Gretler DD, Fumo MT, Nelson KS, et al: Ethnic differences in circadian hemodynamic profile. *Am J Hypertens* 7:7, 1994.

27. Yamamoto Y, Akiguchi I, Oiwa K, et al: Adverse effect of nighttime blood pressure on the outcome of lacunar infarct patients.

28. Cooper R, Rotimi, C, Ataman S, et al: The prevalence of hypertension in seven populations of West African origin. *Am J Public Health* 87:160, 1997.

29. Gillum RF: The epidemiology of cardiovascular disease in black Americans. *N Engl J Med* 335:1597, 1996.

30. Gillum RF: Secular trends in stroke mortality in African Americans: The role of urbanization, diabetes and obesity. *Neuroepidemiology* 16:180, 1997.

31. Kittner SJ, White LR, Losconczy KG, et al: Black-white difference in stroke incidence in a national sample: The contribution of hypertension and diabetes mellitus. *JAMA* 264:1267, 1990.

32. Kaplan GA, Keil JE: Socioeconomic factors and cardiovascular disease: A review of the literature. *Circulation* 88:1973, 1993.

33. Howard G, Russell GB, Anderson R, et al: Role of social class in excess black stroke mortality. *Stroke* 26:1759, 1995.

34. Ammons L: Demographic profile of health-care coverage in America in 1993. *J Natl Med Assoc* 89:737, 1997.

35. Kenton EJ: Access to neurological care for minorities. *Arch Neurol* 48:480, 1991.

36. Chaturvedi S, Femino L: A pilot study regarding knowledge of stroke risk factors in an urban community. *J Stroke Cerebrovasc Dis* 6:426, 1997.

37. Gillum RF: Stroke in blacks. *Stroke* 19:1, 1988.

38. Resch JA, Williams AO, Lemercier G, et al: Comparative autopsy studies on cerebral atherosclerosis in Nigerian and Senegal Negroes, American Negroes and Caucasians. *Atherosclerosis* 12:401, 1970.

39. Solberg LA, McGarry PA: Cerebral atherosclerosis in negroes and Caucasians. Atherosclerosis 16:141, 1972.

40. Heyman A, Fields WS, Keating RD: Joint Study of Extracranial Arterial Occlusion. *JAMA* 222:285, 1972.

41. Gorelick PB, Caplan LR, Hier DB, et al: Racial differences in the distribution of anterior circulation disease. *Neurology,* 34:54, 1984.

42. Gorelick PB, Caplan LR, Hier DB, et al: Racial differences in the distribution of posterior circulation occlusive disease. *Stroke* 16:785, 1985.

43. Gorelick PB, Caplan LR, Langenberg P, et al: Clinical and angiographic comparison of asymptomatic occlusive cerebrovascular disease. *Neurology* 38:852, 1988.

44. Caplan LR, Babikian V, Helgason C, et al: Occlusive disease of the middle cerebral artery. *Neurology* 35:975, 1985.

45. Inzitari D, Hachinski VC, Taylor W, et al: Racial differences in the anterior circulation in cerebrovascular disease. *Arch Neurol* 47:1080, 1990.

46. Heyden S, Heyman A, Goree JA: Nonembolic occlusion

of the middle cerebral and carotid arteries: A comparison of predisposing factors. *Stroke* 1:363, 1970.

47. Russo LS: Carotid system transient ischemic attacks: Clinical, racial, and angiographic correlations. *Stroke* 12:470, 1981.

48. Sacco RL, Kargman DE, Qiong G, et al: Race-ethnicity and determinants of intracranial atherosclerotic cerebral infarction: The Northern Manhattan Stroke Study. *Stroke* 26:4, 1995.

49. Sacco RL, Roberts JK, Boden-Albala B, et al: Race-ethnicity and determinants of carotid atherosclerosis in a multiethnic population: The Northern Manhattan Stroke Study. *Stroke* 28:929, 1997.

50. Prisant LM, Zemel PC, Nichols FT, et al: Carotid plaque associations among hypertensive patients. *Arch Intern Med* 153:501, 1993.

51. Gil-Peralta AG, Alter M, Lai SM, et al; Duplex Doppler and spectral flow analysis of racial differences in cerebrovascular atherosclerosis. *Stroke* 21:740, 1990.

52. Ryu JE, Murros K, Espeland MA, et al: Extracranial carotid atherosclerosis in black and white patients with transient ischemic attacks. *Stroke* 20:1133, 1989.

53. Cohen SN, Goldman C: Comparison by duplex scan of racial differences in stroke risk factors (Abstract). *Ann Neurol* 30:280, 1991.

54. Aronow WS, Schoenfeld MR: Prevalence of atherothrombotic brain infarction and extracranial carotid arterial disease, and their association in elderly blacks, hispanics and whites. *Am J Cardiol* 71:999, 1993.

55. Dyken ML, Wolf PA, Barnett HJM, et al: Risk factors in stroke: A statement for physicians by the Subcommittee on Risk Factors and Stroke and the Stroke Council. *Stroke* 15:1105, 1984.

56. Kuhlemeier KV, Stiens SA: Racial disparities in severity of cerebrovascular events. *Stroke* 25:2126, 1994.

57. Horner RD, Matchar DB, Divine GW, et al: Racial variations in ischemic stroke-related physical and functional impairments. *Stroke* 22:1497, 1991.

58. Sacco RL, Foulkes MA, Mohr JP, et al: Determinants of early recurrence of cerebral infarction: The Stroke Data Bank. *Stroke* 20:983, 1989.

59. Hier DB, Foulkes MA, Swiontoniowski M, et al: Stroke recurrence within 2 years after ischemic infarction. *Stroke* 22:155, 1991.

60. Sacco RL, Shi T, Zamanillo MC, et al: Predictors of mortality and recurrence after hospitalized cerebral infarction in an urban community: The Northern Manhattan Stroke Study. *Neurology* 44:626, 1994.

61. Pavlakis SG, Prohovnik I, Piomelli, S, et al: Neurologic complications of Sickle cell disease. *Adv Pediatr* 36:247, 1989.

62. Kugler S, Anderson B, Cross D, et al: Abnormal cranial magnetic resonance imaging scans in sickle-cell disease. *Arch Neurol* 50:629, 1993.

63. Powars D, Wilson B, Imbus C, et al: The natural history of stroke in sickle cell disease. *Am J Med* 65:461, 1978.

64. Wood DH: Cerebrovascular complications of sickle cell anemia. *Stroke* 9:73, 1978.

65. Powars DR, Schroeder WA, Weiss JN, et al: Lack of influence of fetal hemoglobin levels or erythrocyte indices on the severity of sickle cell anemia. *J Clin Invest* 65:732, 1980.

66. Adams R, McKie V, Nichols F, et al: The use of transcranial ultrasonography to predict stroke in sickle cell disease. *N Engl J Med* 326:605, 1992.

67. Adams RJ, McKie VC, Hsu L, et al: Prevention of first stroke by transfusions in children with sickle cell anemia and abnormal results on transcranial Doppler ultrasonography. *N Engl J Med* 339:5, 1998.

68. National Heart, Lung, and Blood Institute: Clinical alert: Periodic transfusions lower stroke risk in children with sickle cell anemia. September 18, 1997.

69. Udea K, Kawano H, Hasuo Y, et al: Prevalence and etiology of dementia in a Japanese community. *Stroke* 23:798, 1992.

70. Gorelick PB: Status of risk factors for dementia associated with stroke. *Stroke* 28:459, 1997.

71. Tatemichi TK, Desmond DW, Mayeux R, et al: Dementia after stroke: Baseline frequency, risks, and clinical features in a hospitalized cohort. *Neurology* 42:1185, 1992.

72. Longstreth WT, Manolio TA, Arnold A, et al: Clinical correlates of white matter findings on cranial magnetic resonance imaging of 3,301 elderly people. *Stroke* 27:1274, 1996.

73. Liao D, Cooper L, Cai J, et al: The prevalence and severity of white matter lesions, their relationship with age, ethnicity, gender, and cardiovascular risk factors: The ARIC study. *Neuroepidemiology* 16:149, 1997.

74. Gorelick PB, Brody J, Cohen D, et al: Risk factors for dementia associated with multiple cerebral infarcts. *Arch Neurol* 50:714, 1993.

75. Charletta D, Gorelick PB, Dollear TJ, et al: CT and MRI findings among African-Americans with Alzheimer's disease, vascular dementia, and stroke without dementia. *Neurology* 45:1456, 1995.

76. Svensson C: Representation of American blacks in clinical trials of new drugs. *JAMA* 261:263, 1989.

77. Bonner GJ, Miles TP: Participation of African Americans in clinical research. *Neuroepidemiology* 16:281, 1997.

78. Weisberg LA for the Ticlopidine Aspirin Stroke Study Group: The efficacy and safety of ticlopidine and aspirin in non-whites: Analysis of a patient subgroup from the Ticlopidine Aspirin Stroke Study. *Neurology* 43:27, 1993.

79. Gent M, Easton JD, Hachinski VC, et al and the CATS group: The Canadian American Ticlopidine Study (CATS) in thromboembolic stroke. *Lancet* 1:1215, 1989.

80. North American Symptomatic Carotid Endarterectomy Trial Collaborators: Beneficial effect of carotid endarterectomy in symptomatic patients with high-grade carotid stenosis. *N Engl J Med* 325:445, 1991.

81. The National Institute of Neurological Disorders and Stroke rt-PA Stroke Study Group: Tissue plasminogen acti-

vator for acute ischemic stroke. *N Engl J Med* 333:1581, 1995.

82. Executive Committee for the Asymptomatic Carotid Atherosclerosis Study: Endarterectomy for asymptomatic carotid artery stenosis. *JAMA* 273:1421, 1995.

83. CAPRIE Steering Committee: A randomized, blinded, trial of clopidogrel versus aspirin in patients at risk of ischemic events (CAPRIE). *Lancet* 348:1329, 1996.

84. Gorelick PB, Richardson D, Hudson E, et al: Establishing a community network for recruitment of African Americans into a clinical trial: The African-American Antiplatelet Stroke Prevention Study (AAASPS) Experience. *J Natl Med Assoc 88:701, 1996.*

85. Harris Y, Gorelick PB, Samuels P, et al: Why African Americans may not be participating in clinical trials. *J Natl Med Assoc* 88:630, 1996.

86. Gorelick PB, Harris Y, Burnett B, et al: The recruitment triangle: Reasons why African Americans enroll, refuse to enroll, or voluntarily withdraw from a clinical trial. An interim report from the African American Antiplatelet Stroke Prevention Study (AAASPS). *J Natl Med Assoc* 90:141, 1998.

87. Sane DC, Stump DC, Topol EJ, et al: Racial differences in responses to thrombolytic therapy with recombinant tissue-type plasminogen activator: Increased fibrinogenolysis in blacks. *Circulation* 83:170, 1991.

88. The NINDS t-PAStroke Study Group: Intracerebral hemorrhage after intravenous t-PA therapy for ischemic stroke. *Stroke* 28:2109, 1997.

89. The NINDS t-PA Stroke Study Group: Generalized efficacy of t-PA for acute stroke:subgroup analysis of the NINDS t-PA Stroke Trial. *Stroke* 28:2119, 1997.

90. Halsey JH: Effect of emitted power on waveform intensity in transcranial Doppler. *Stroke* 21:1573, 1990.

91. Chimowitz MI, Kokkinos J, Strong J, et al: The Warfarin-Aspirin Symptomatic Intracranial Disease Study. *Neurology* 45:1488, 1995.

Chapter 30

STROKE ASSOCIATED WITH CAROTID ENDARTERECTOMY

Wesley S. Moore

INTRODUCTION

Carotid endarterectomy is an interventional strategy designed to prevent new or recurrent stroke in the distribution of the diseased carotid bifurcation. The role of carotid endarterectomy has now been well defined by the results of several carefully controlled prospective randomized trials.[1-5] The benefit of carotid endarterectomy when compared with alternative methods of management is entirely dependent upon minimizing the complications associated with the procedure, including perioperative stroke and death. Thus, carotid endarterectomy, when used in asymptomatic patients with high-grade asymptomatic carotid stenosis, was shown to be beneficial over medical management only if the perioperative stroke morbidity and mortality could be kept competitive with the low rate achieved in the study, 2.6 percent.[2] Likewise, carotid endarterectomy in patients with symptomatic carotid stenosis 50 percent or greater was shown to be superior to medical management, providing the perioperative stroke morbidity and mortality could be kept less than 6.7 percent.[6]

Over the past several decades, the safety of carotid endarterectomy has steadily improved, and the rate of perioperative stroke associated with the operation has declined. Nonetheless, this complication does still occur, and the expeditious evaluation and proper management of the patient who is unfortunate to suffer a perioperative stroke will play a very large role in the patient's ultimate outcome. This chapter will address the pathogenetic mechanisms of perioperative stroke, outline optimum methods for rapid patient evaluation and management, review the results obtained, and finally address the issues of preventing the complication.

PATHOGENETIC MECHANISMS OF PERIOPERATIVE STROKE

An understanding of the specific pathogenetic mechanism for the complication of perioperative stroke is essential in establishing a course of management as well as designing techniques for prevention.

Technical Error

After many years of observation and analysis, it has become apparent that the most common cause of perioperative stroke is a technical error.[7-10] This most often presents in the form of an incomplete endarterectomy with a residual intimal flap. Usually, the intimal flap presents in the internal carotid artery and serves as both a partial obstruction as well as a nidus for thrombus formation with subsequent thrombosis or thromboembolism. A less well-recognized technical error is a similar intimal flap, but this time occurring in the external carotid artery. This is a much more pernicious problem because most surgeons view the external carotid artery as not being relevant to the overall outcome of endarterectomy. However, we have recently identified a mechanism of perioperative stroke specifically related to technical error and intimal flap in the external carotid artery. It seems that thrombus forms in the external carotid artery, and retrograde propagation occurs to the area of the bifurcation. This thrombus can be dislodged and swept into the intracranial circulation by the blood flowing past the orifice of the external carotid artery.[11,12] The final locus of technical error is in the proximal end point of the common carotid artery. At the time of carotid endarterectomy, usually there is a relatively thick portion of intima or residual atheromatous plaque that is sharply divided in the common carotid artery. If the plaque is left adherent to the adventitia, this is usually well tolerated. However, if the plaque is divided with a leading edge being nonadherent to the adventitia, this provides for an area of dead space, which is an excellent nidus for either platelet aggregation or thrombus formation with subsequent thromboembolism.

Thromboembolism

The atheromatous plaque that is the subject of concern and the object of removal as a part of the carotid endarterectomy procedure is often relatively unstable. The plaque itself may contain intraplaque hemorrhage or have loose debris on the surface. Care must be taken during mobilization of the carotid bifurcation so as to not dislodge any material that is loose on the plaque surface. Material can be dislodged, embolize, and occlude important intracranial branches.

Another source of intraoperative thromboembolism can occur in the presence of an otherwise technically satisfactory operation. The intimectomized surface of the carotid bifurcation is covered by a layer of platelet aggregate material. Usually, this is microscopically thin and of no concern. However, in some patients, the platelet aggregation response may be exaggerated, leading to a build-up of large mounds of platelet aggregate material. If this is not recognized by some perioperative imaging method, the platelet aggregates can be dislodged and embolized to the intracranial circulation.

Clamp Ischemia

Most patients have adequate intracranial collateral circulation such that temporary clamping of the carotid artery to perform carotid endarterectomy is well tolerated and well compensated for. However, approximately 10 to 15 percent of patients presenting for carotid endarterectomy who are either asymptomatic or have transient cerebral ischemia as an indication for operation will be intolerant of the temporary clamp time that is required for carotid endarterectomy.[13,14] This intolerance can be recognized by neurologic defect during regional anesthesia,[13,14] ischemic changes with electroencephalographic monitoring,[15,16] poor back flow or back pressure from the internal carotid artery,[13,14,17–20] severe drop of blood flow in the middle cerebral artery as documented by transcranial Doppler,[21] or loss of a normal somatosensory-evoked potential response on the appropriate extremity being monitored.[22] Failure to recognize cerebral ischemia associated with clamping, particularly if the clamp time is prolonged for some reason, may result in irreversible damage in a watershed region leading to a postoperative deficit.

Patients who are being operated on for an indication of prior stroke are particularly vulnerable to clamp ischemia. Because focal areas of cerebral infarction are surrounded by a zone of relatively poor perfused brain, the ischemic penumbra, maintenance of adequate blood flow during endarterectomy becomes particularly important. The ischemic penumbra will be very vulnerable to periods of temporary clamping. Failure to recognize this will result in extension of the cerebral infarction and worsening of the preoperative neurologic deficit.

Intracerebral Hemorrhage

This is a relatively uncommon cause of postoperative neurologic deficit. It can occur in two circumstances. The first circumstance is related to patients who have a relatively tight carotid stenosis and have poorly controlled hypertension preoperatively. Re-establishment of blood flow with carotid endarterectomy will be associated with hyperperfusion of the brain. Because there is a temporary loss of autoregulation after a cerebral infarction, this hyperperfusion will be seriously aggravated by elevated blood pressure and, in its most extreme form, will result in intracerebral hemorrhage. Another potential cause of postcarotid endarterectomy intracerebral hemorrhage can occur in patients who have a relatively recent and large infarct in whom there is a serious blood-brain barrier defect. Bleeding can occur into the infarct, converting an ischemic zone to a hemorrhagic zone.[23–25]

EVIDENCE

Because the event of stroke associated with carotid endarterectomy is a relatively infrequent occurrence, the evidence for the various pathogenetic mechanisms is at best anecdotal. All four mechanisms cited have been reported in individual cases, and retrospective reviews suggest that technical error and perioperative thromboembolism represent the most common etiologic mechanisms. Likewise, the proposed treatment is also based upon anecdotal evidence. As the event rate is so low, it would not be possible to validate proposed algorithms of evaluation and management with a prospective randomized trial.

PATIENT EVALUATION AND MANAGEMENT

The occurrence and detection of perioperative stroke can occur at three distinct time intervals: during operation, in the recovery room, and at an interval 24 to 72 h following operation. The mechanisms and management will be quite different for each time of presentation.

Intraoperative Stroke

Most strokes that occur intraoperatively will not be detected until the patient awakes from anesthesia. However, if the patient is being monitored during the operation with a modality such as EEG, a significant neurologic event may be detected.[26] If the neurologic change is reversed with the placement of an internal shunt, this is most likely because of clamp ischemia, and the reversibility indicates that no permanent damage took place. However, if the ischemic electrical change is not reversible with a shunt, this suggests that an intraoperative embolic event to an important branch has occurred. The embolism may either be atheromatous debris or thrombus. If it is thrombus, this may be immediately and successfully treated with thrombolytic agents. An intraoperative contrast angiogram should be immediately obtained, with imaging of the distal internal carotid artery and its branches. If there is evidence of an embolic occlusion of the branch of the middle cerebral artery, for example, lytic therapy should be immediately begun.[27,28] This could be started with a direct infusion in the internal carotid artery through a catheter or a side arm of an internal shunt, or a microcatheter can be passed up the internal carotid artery selectively to the artery involved and a direct infusion carried out. The exact dose of lytic agent and timing have not been completely worked out. Empirically, an infusion of 250,000 units of urokinase dissolved in 100 mL of saline and containing 1,000 units of heparin have been successfully used in peripheral applications. Anecdotal reports of up to 1,000,000 units of urokinase have also been described.

Neurologic Deficit Detected in the Recovery Room

A neurologic deficit may be noted when the patient first awakes in the recovery room, or may come on shortly after awaking and noted by the recovery room nurse in attendance. There are three potential mechanisms for this, which include intraoperative microembolization, clamp ischemia, or technical error leading to thromboembolism at the endarterectomy site. The management of each of these three pathogenetic mechanisms is quite different, and therefore an expeditious diagnostic workup will make the difference between a successful and adverse outcome. There are two circumstances that mandate an immediate return to the operating room for surgical correction. These include a technical problem at the endarterectomy site, leading to obstruction and thrombosis, and a build-up of platelet aggregate at the operative site, resulting in distal thromboembolism. Because elapsed time between detection and correction is critical, this has led many surgeons to advocate an immediate return to the operating room upon detection of neurologic deficit in the recovery room. This will provide the most expeditious opportunity for both a diagnosis and management. An alternative would be to obtain immediate noninvasive testing to detect whether or not a mechanical problem is present at the carotid bifurcation and return only those patients with demonstrable mechanical defect to the operating room. The noninvasive testing is best performed by carotid duplex scanning or oculopneumoplethysmography. If either of these tests, including equipment and technical personnel, is immediately available, it is not unreasonable to do that first and then to return to the operating room on a selective basis. However, if there is going to be a delay in obtaining testing, the safest thing to do is to return to the operating room and re-explore the incision and arteriotomy site as quickly as possible. An arteriogram would also provide excellent diagnostic information about the carotid bifurcation as well as the possibility of intracerebral embolization. However, much valuable time would be lost in preparing for and obtaining a contrast angiogram. Upon returning to the operating room, the wound is rapidly reopened and the carotid bifurcation mobilized. A continuous-wave, hand-held Doppler probe can be used to examine the carotid bifurcation, or an immediate contrast angiogram can also be obtained. If it is obvious that there is a mechanical problem in the bifurcation, the patient should be anticoagulated with intravenous heparin and the internal, external, and common carotid arteries clamped. The arteriotomy should be opened and inspected for either platelet aggregate or intimal flap of the partially complete thrombosis. If thrombus or platelet aggregate is found, this should be removed and an internal shunt placed carefully so as to not further aggravate a problem with intimal flap. If necessary, the arteriotomy on the internal carotid artery should be further extended. Once the obstructive material is removed and the intimal flap, if present, corrected, the arteriotomy should then be closed with a patch angioplasty. A completion angiogram is advisable to confirm the technical quality of the repair.

If upon exploration of the carotid bifurcation, no evidence of mechanical obstruction is found, an intraoperative angiogram with imaging of the intracranial circulation should be carried out. If there is evidence of intracerebral embolus, this can be treated with a urokinase infusion and preferably with selective catheterization.

Delayed Appearance of Neurologic Deficit

Patients who awake without neurologic deficit and have an uneventful course during the first 24 h and then present with a deficit somewhere between 24 and 72 h represent a distinctly unusual occurrence. The differential diagnosis for the pathogenetic mechanism includes late embolization vs. a hyperperfusion syndrome with possible intracerebral hemorrhage.

When this occurs, the first thing to do is to check the blood pressure control in the perioperative interval. If the patient is hypertensive, immediate attention to correction should be carried out. The workup should include a rapid carotid duplex scan and a contrast-enhanced CT scan of the brain. The order of these examinations will depend upon which test can be obtained with the least loss of time. If the duplex scan of the carotid bifurcation demonstrates a mechanical defect, plans should be made to return the patient to the operating room, provided that the CT scan shows no evidence of intracerebral hemorrhage. If the carotid duplex scan was normal, and there is no evidence of intracerebral hemorrhage, the differential diagnosis will include embolization vs. a less lethal version of the hyperperfusion syndrome. At this point, it would be advisable to move the patient to the intensive care unit for careful monitoring and management of blood pressure and the institution of systemic heparin anticoagulation therapy. If the patient does not show improvement within the next 30 to 60 min of observation, plans for emergency contrast angiography should be made. The angiogram should include imaging of the carotid bifurcation to rule out a technical problem, and then intracranial views in several projections should be obtained to look for the possibility of an embolic branch occlu-

sion. If this is identified, selective catheterization with a microcatheter should be carried out with direct infusion of a lytic drug.

PREVENTION

Although this chapter has been devoted to the issue of diagnosis and management of perioperative stroke, it goes without saying that all efforts should be directed toward preventing rather than treating the complication. The following will suggest several measures that have been helpful in the author's experience to prevent the complication and will be divided by the pathogenetic mechanism.

Technical Error

Technical error is clearly the most common and most easily preventable of all the pathogenetic mechanisms. It has been the author's practice to perform routine completion angiography upon restoration of blood flow following carotid endarterectomy. By making this a routine, both the operating room and the radiology department expect this to be part of the operative management and are quickly and readily available to carry out the study upon completion of closure of the arteriotomy. Thus, there is minimal time spent in setting up and obtaining the study. When this is not part of the routine, instrumentation and personnel are not readily available. Surgeons who carry out routine completion angiography find that the subsequent incidence of perioperative technical error leading to internal carotid artery thrombosis is virtually nonexistent. Intimal flap of the external carotid artery, a recently described problem that may lead to intracerebral thromboembolization, is readily visible with a completion angiogram and easily correctable. Other methods of perioperative imaging, such as B-mode duplex scan or duplex scanning in the operative field, are also quite satisfactory.

A completion angiogram may also detect the presence of a build-up in platelet aggregate on the intimectomized surface. This can be easily diagnosed by the presence of filling defects in the midportion of the endarterectomy site, a place where one would not expect an intimal flap to be present. If this is seen, the artery should be reclamped promptly, the arteriotomy opened, and the platelet aggregate material removed. Careful irrigation of the intimectomized site with heparinized saline and reclosure usually results in a satisfactory outcome.

Intraoperative Cerebral Embolization

This is probably the most difficult mechanism to prevent. Careful handling of the carotid bifurcation during mobilization, clamping of the internal carotid artery first in the sequence of clamping the carotid bifurcation vessels, and the careful insertion of the shunt, when necessary, are all helpful in reducing the incidence of intracerebral mechanization. Surgeons who use shunting on a selective basis are often less skilled in the details of shunt insertion than those who use it on a routine basis. On the other hand, instrumentation that takes place with the insertion of a shunt has been associated with a slightly higher instance of perioperative complication. If a shunt is to be employed, the distal end of the shunt must be inserted first and the internal carotid artery allowed to back bleed through the shunt. This will ensure the operator that the shunt has been properly placed and, if any atheromatous debris or air bubbles have been trapped, will allow them to back bleed through the open end of the shunt. With the shunt actively back bleeding, it is then placed into the proximal portion of the common carotid artery, at the same time allowing any material within the cul de sac of the proximal common carotid artery to be washed out. I prefer to use a Javid shunt, which is relatively long and allows for clamping of the shunt as the proximal end is secured in the common carotid artery. Once the clamp is removed from the common carotid artery, the clamp on the shunt can be slowly released. Because the shunt is translucent, if there are any trapped air bubbles or atheromatous debris present proximally, they would be seen as flow begins through the shunt. If present, the shunt can be promptly clamped and the above procedure repeated.

Clamp Ischemia

Ischemic damage to the brain during carotid endarterectomy can be prevented with either the selective or the routine use of an internal shunt. Those who advocate routine use of an internal shunt will not require perioperative cerebral monitoring. Those who use carotid shunting on a selective basis must do so on a basis of both clinical assessment and intraoperative monitoring. Patients who have had a prior stroke as an indication for carotid endarterectomy are best served by the routine use of an internal shunt during endarterectomy. This will protect the ischemic penumbra from further damage by clamp ischemia time. Patients whose indication for operation is either an asymptomatic carotid stenosis or transient cerebral ischemia without prior stroke can be successfully managed with the selective use of an internal shunt based upon evidence of clamp ischemia with perioperative monitoring. Popular monitoring techniques include electroencephalography, transcranial Doppler assessment, and somatosensory-evoked potential monitoring.

The Hyperperfusion Syndrome

Avoidance of various manifestations of the hyperperfusion syndrome, including intracerebral hemorrhage, is entirely dependent upon the careful perioperative management of a patient's blood pressure. If the patient is hypertensive at the time of initial evaluation, sufficient time and planning should include appropriate medication for blood pressure management to bring the patient into a reasonable control before considering proceeding with operation. The blood pressure should also be carefully monitored intraoperatively and immediately postoperatively to avoid hypertension. If necessary, an intravenous nitride drip may be required for the first 24 to 48 h in some patients whose blood pressure is difficult to control.

REFERENCES

1. Hobson RW II, Weiss DG, Fields WS, et al: Efficacy of carotid endarterectomy for asymptomatic carotid stenosis: The Veterans Affairs Asymptomatic Cooperative Study Group. *N Engl J Med* 328:221, 1993.
2. Executive Committee for the Asymptomatic Carotid Atherosclerosis (ACAS) Study: Endarterectomy for asymptomatic carotid artery stenosis. *JAMA* 273:1421, 1995.
3. North American Symptomatic Carotid Endarterectomy Trial Collaborators: Beneficial effect of carotid endarterectomy in symptomatic patients with high-grade carotid stenosis. *N Engl J Med* 325:445, 1991.
4. European Carotid Surgery Trialists' Collaborative Group: MRC European Carotid Surgery Trial: Interim results for symptomatic patients with severe (70–99%) or with mild (0–29%) carotid stenosis. *Lancet* 337:1235, 1991.
5. Mayberg MR, Wilson SE, Yatsu F, et al: Carotid endarterectomy and prevention of cerebral ischemia in symptomatic carotid stenosis: Veterans Affairs Cooperative Studies Program 309 Trialists Group. *JAMA* 266:3289, 1991.
6. Barnett HJM, for the NASCET Investigators: Presentation at the American Heart Association XXIII International Joint Conference on Stroke and Cerebral Circulation, Orlando, FL, February 5–7, 1998.
7. Riles TS, Imparato AM, Jacobowitz GR, et al: The cause of

perioperative stroke after carotid endarterectomy. *J Vasc Surg* 19:206, 1994.

8. Hertzer NR: Presidential address: Outcome assessment of vascular surgery: Results mean everything. *J Vasc Surg* 21:6, 1995.

9. McKinsey JF, Desai TR, Bassiouny HS, et al: Mechanisms of neurologic deficits and mortality with carotid endarterectomy. *Arch Surg* 131:526, 1996.

10. Koslow AR, Ricotta JJ, Ouriel K, et al: Re-exploration for thrombosis in carotid endarterectomy. *Circulation* 80:11173, 1989.

11. Moore WS, Martello JY, Quiñones-Baldrich WJ, Ahn SS: Etiologic importance of the intimal flap of the external carotid artery in the development of post-carotid endarterectomy stroke. *Stroke* 21:1497, 1990.

12. Pacini D, Farneti TA, Donati A, et al: Intimal flap of the external carotid and postoperative stroke in patients surgically treated with thrombo-endarterectomy of the internal carotid. *Minerva Cardio Angiol* 44:511, 1996.

13. Moore WS, Hall AD: Carotid artery back pressure: A test of cerebral tolerance to temporary carotid occlusion. *Arch Surg* 99:702, 1969.

14. Hobson RW II, Wright CB, Sublett JW, et al: Carotid artery back pressure and endarterectomy under regional anesthesia. *Arch Surg* 109:682, 1974.

15. Sundt TM, Sharbrough FW, Anderson E, Michenfelder JP: Cerebral blood flow measurements and electroencephalogram during carotid endarterectomy. *J Neurosurg* 41:310, 1974.

16. Ahn SS, Jordan SE, Nuwer MR, et al: Computed electroencephalographic topographic brain mapping: A new and accurate monitor of cerebral circulation and function for patients having carotid endarterectomy. *J Vasc Surg* 8:247, 1988.

17. Moore WS, Yee JM, Hall AD: Collateral cerebral blood pressure: An index of tolerance to temporary carotid occlusion. *Arch Surg* 106:520, 1973.

18. Hays RF, Levinson SA, Wylie EJ: Intraoperative measurement of carotid back pressure as a guide to operative management for carotid endarterectomy. *Surgery* 72:953, 1972.

19. Archie JP Jr: Technique and clinical results of carotid stump back-pressure to determine selective shunting during carotid endarterectomy. *J Vasc Surg* 13:319, 1991.

20. Hunter GC, Sieffert G, Malone JM, Moore WS: The accuracy of carotid artery back pressure as an index for shunt requirements: A reappraisal. *Stroke* 13:319, 1982.

21. Cao P, Giordano G, Zannetti S, et al: Transcranial Doppler monitoring during carotid endarterectomy: Is it appropriate for selecting patients in need of a shunt? *J Vasc Surg* 26:973, 1997.

22. Horsch S, Ktenidis K: Intraoperative use of sensory evoked potentials for brain monitoring during carotid surgery. *Neurosurg Clin NM* 7:693, 1996.

23. Mansoor GA, White WB, Grunnet M, Ruby ST: Intracerebral hemorrhage after carotid endarterectomy associated with ipsilateral fibrinoid necrosis: A consequence of the hyperperfusion syndrome? *J Vasc Surg* 23:147, 1996.

24. Lepojarvi M, Peltola T, Ylonen K, et al: Cerebral hemorrhage after carotid endarterectomy. *Ann Chir Gynaecol (Finland)* 85:23, 1996.

25. Jansen C, Sprengers AM, Moll FL, et al: Prediction of intracerebral hemorrhage after carotid endarterectomy by clinical criteria and intraoperative transcranial Doppler monitoring. *Eur J Vasc Surg* 8:303, 1994.

26. Krul JM, Ackerstaff RG, Eikelboom VC, Vermulen FE: Stroke-related EEG changes during carotid surgery. *Eur J Vasc Surg* 3:423, 1989.

27. Comerota AJ, Eze AR: Intraoperative high-dose regional urokinase infusion for cerebrovascular occlusion after carotid endarterectomy. *J Vasc Surg* 24:1008, 1996.

28. Barr JD, Horowitz MV, Mathis JM, Sclabassi RJ, Yonas H: Intraoperative urokinase infusion for embolic stroke during carotid endarterectomy. *Neurosurgery* 36:606, 1995.

Chapter 31

NEURO-OPHTHALMOLOGIC MANIFESTATIONS OF ISCHEMIC CEREBROVASCULAR DISEASE

Lynn K. Gordon

INTRODUCTION

Cerebrovascular ischemia may produce neuro-ophthalmic consequences including loss of vision, visual field alterations, and ocular motor disturbances. These manifestations may be transient or permanent and are a major cause of morbidity in patients with cerebrovascular disease. Specifically, difficulties in the visual pathways may interfere with performance of necessary activities of daily life in the home, proper use of prescribed medications, or adequate job performance.[1] It is therefore important to recognize the spectrum of ophthalmologic presentations of ischemia to promptly diagnose the ophthalmic syndrome, obtain the proper diagnostic tests, and initiate therapy for the underlying disease to minimize further ischemic episodes. Cerebrovascular ischemia may be defined as decreased blood flow ranging from transient and partial, with potentially reversible neuro-ophthalmic symptoms, to prolonged and complete, producing permanent neuro-ophthalmic and systemic morbidity. Ischemia may result from thrombosis, embolism, or insufficient vascular perfusion.[2]

Neuro-ophthalmic disorders from thrombotic events arise from involvement of the large and small, intra- and extracranial arterial circulation.[3] These types of thrombotic events are commonly associated with atherosclerosis, hyperlipidemia, hypertension, diabetes mellitus, obesity, and smoking.[2] However, there is a large differential diagnosis in the underlying etiology of thrombotic events including migraine, arteritis, arterial dissections, fibromuscular dysplasia, sickle cell disease, radiation, amyloid, neoplasia, iatrogenic misadventure, and hypercoagulable states. Emboli from the heart and major arteries and veins produce numerous neuro-ophthalmic syndromes.[4] The underlying etiologies of emboli include atheromatous plaques, infectious diseases (i.e., bacterial endocarditis), and intracardiac tumors (i.e., atrial myxoma). Insufficient systemic perfusion may result from catastrophic cardiac events, severe trauma, or intraoperative hemorrhage. This chapter will concentrate on the differential diagnosis of neuro-ophthalmic signs and symptoms of ischemic cerebrovascular disease.

NEURO-OPHTHALMOLOGIC EXAMINATION

History

The neuro-ophthalmic evaluation is necessary to accurately diagnose the ocular manifestations of cerebrovascular ischemia. A thorough history must include the usual systemic, past medical, and family histories, but the present history of visual complaints must be specifically targeted in the diagnosis of neuro-ophthalmic symptoms. If visual loss occurs, it is important to know if the loss is unilateral or bilateral, complete or partial, transient or permanent. The time course of transient visual loss is critical in establishing a differential diagnosis; for example, transient and fleeting loss lasting less than a few seconds is typical of optic nerve swelling, lasting 3 to 5 min is typical of emboli, or lasting 15 to 30 min is typical of migrainous phenomenon.[5]

Characteristics of visual scotomatas and their time course may also be helpful.[6] The patient may perceive visual field loss if it interferes with activities of daily life. However, many diseases can result in partial loss of visual field that is not recognized by the patient. Therefore, visual field testing is essential in all patients with suspected cerebrovascular ischemia affecting the visual pathways. It is important to note if the visual field disturbance is monocular, most likely implying an etiology affecting the optic nerve anterior to the chiasm, or binocular, affecting the chiasm, optic tracts, or optic radiations. Occasionally, patients will confuse binocular and monocular transient visual field disturbances; in these cases, the history must be taken with extreme care to elicit a clear and accurate response from the patient. The time course of visual field impairment may differentiate acute ischemic events with sudden loss from chronic hypoperfusion injuries with gradual and changing loss of visual field function.

Complaints of diplopia need to be specifically characterized.[5] The patient must be asked if the diplopia is present only when both eyes are open. Monocular diplopia, diplopia while using only one eye, is not indicative of a neuro-ophthalmic disease; this symptom may arise from psychological etiologies or may result from a local ocular change, for example uncorrected astigmatism or macular disease.[7] Comprehensive ophthalmologic examination including dilated funduscopy will reveal ocular causes of monocular diplopia. In the setting of binocular diplopia, it is important to note if the diplopia worsens in different positions of gaze, indicative of either a cranial nerve palsy or myopathy. Oscillopsia, jumping of images, is also an important symptom and indicates acquired nystagmus.

Ocular Examination

In the setting of cerebrovascular disease, complete ophthalmologic evaluation requires comprehensive and systematic testing. If the patient's condition is stable, it is always preferable to perform this evaluation in an appropriate facility by an ophthalmologist who is skilled in the neuro-ophthalmic evaluation. However, analysis of visual performance and pupillary function, gross examination of ocular motility, and direct and indirect ophthalmoscopy may be performed at the bedside to form a preliminary diagnosis of ocular or neuro-ophthalmic abnormality.

Measurement of the best corrected visual acuity helps in the initial definition of the ophthalmic condition. Although analysis of best corrected visual acuity requires a new refraction to be done at the time of examination, an estimate of this measurement may be obtained with the use of a pinhole screen over the patient's current refraction. Careful evaluation of the pupil and its reaction to light is an important feature of the neuro-ophthalmic examination.[8] The pupils are observed for size, regularity, and symmetry. If anisocoria is observed, then it is important to note if the anisocoria increases in dim or bright light conditions. Pharmacologic testing is indicated in cases of suspected Horner's syndrome to both confirm the diagnosis and to determine if the lesion is pre- or postganglionic (Table 31-1). Reactivity to accommodation should be checked only in cases of either a tonic or small pupil that is poorly reactive to light. The relative afferent pupillary

Table 31-1.

Evaluation of anisocoria associated with a possible Horner's syndrome

---

Anisocoria is greater in dim illumination suggestive of Horner's Syndrome

Step 1. Is the anisocoria due to a sympathetic lesion?
   Cocaine test: cocaine reduces reuptake of norepinephrine
   Instill 10% cocaine drop into each eye; repeat once; evaluate after 15 min in dim light
   Results
      Both pupils dilate equally = simple anisocoria
      Smaller pupil dilates less than larger pupil = Horner's; proceed to Step 2

Step 2. Is the Horner's preganglionic or postganglionic?
   Hydroxyamphetamine test: hydroxyamphetamine causes release of norepinephrine from postganglionic neuron
   Instill 1% hydroxyamphetamine into each eye; repeat once; evaluate after 15 min in dim light
   Results
      Both pupils dilate equally = central or preganglionic lesion
      Smaller pupil dilates less than larger pupil = postganglionic lesion

Step 3. Additional neurologic and radioneurologic imaging as directed by results in Step 2.

---

defect, abnormal swinging flashlight test or Marcus Gunn pupil, is an important sign of asymmetric optic nerve disease or extensive retinal disease.[5] Color vision abnormalities are a common feature of the optic neuropathies; consequently, formal color vision testing is indicated in patients with suspected optic nerve disease.

Motility examination must be done in all cases of complaints of binocular diplopia, blurring of vision, or oscillopsia. In some mild cases of cranial nerve palsies, misalignment may not be obvious in the primary position and may only be elicited in the field of action of the involved nerve or muscle. Therefore, ocular alignment is examined in the primary and cardinal positions of gaze using cover testing with careful measurements of alignment using a prism. Ocular pursuits and saccades are evaluated in both vertical and horizontal directions. The eyes are carefully observed for nystagmus in different fields of gaze.

The slit lamp examination reveals any changes in the anterior visual pathway that could affect visual function such as corneal opacities, lens clarity, and intraocular inflammation. A binocular view of the optic nerve and the posterior pole is obtained at the slit lamp using a high plus lens. Additional information about the optic nerve and retina is obtained through the use of the direct and indirect ophthalmoscopes. The optic nerve is examined for evidence of swelling, hemorrhage, or atrophy. The retina is examined for evidence of vascular lesions including arterial occlusion, venous occlusion, neovascularization, and intra-arterial plaques. Emboli may be observed in the retinal vascular circulation and have different appearances depending on their composition and origin.[4] Hollenhorst plaques are noted to be refractile and are usually bright, shiny, and yellow or orange in color. They are cholesterol emboli that usually will not obstruct blood flow but may lodge at sites of arterial bifurcations and may cause focal opacification of the retinal arteriole[2] (Fig. 31-1, color insert 6). Emboli composed of platelets and fibrin are usually dull, gray-white plugs that cause decreased blood flow and then move further into the peripheral circulation after the reflex vasodilation. Calcium emboli are generally chalky-white, nonrefractile particles that originate from the great vessels or heart.[9] These may be associated with retinal arteriole occlusions and subsequent retinal infarcts and may be associated with systemic stroke.[10]

Visual Field Analysis

Visual field tests range from simple bedside approximations to complex, thorough evaluations of visual field

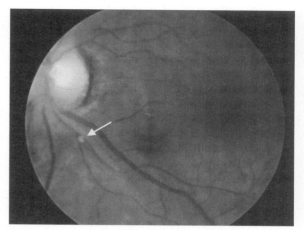

Figure 31-1.
Hollenhorst plaque. Note presence of intra-arterial plaque at a bifurcation point (arrow). (*See also color insert 6.*)

function using either Goldmann or automated perimetry. In all cases, formal visual field testing should be done when there is suspected neuro-ophthalmic consequences of cerebrovascular disease. Goldmann, or kinetic, perimetry is useful for analyzing the full field and is helpful particularly in identifying cases of the temporal crescent syndrome. The temporal crescent syndrome occurs in vascular lesions located in the parieto-occipital sulcus, resulting in a monocular defect in the far temporal periphery, an area that is not tested by the automated perimeters.[11,12] These defects are the only example of a monocular visual field disturbance arising from a lesion posterior to the optic chiasm. The monocular defect results from the normal asymmetry of visual fields where the temporal half is larger than the nasal half; in these cases, there is no nasal field in the contralateral eye that corresponds to the area of temporal field defect in this syndrome. Goldmann perimetry also allows for interactions between the patient and the examiner and is useful in patients with difficulties in concentration or mentation.

Static computerized automated perimetry is generally used in the formal evaluation of visual fields. This form of testing is usually limited to the examination of the central 30 degrees of the visual field, the most critical area for useful sight. Automated perimetry quantitates the sensitivity of vision at specific points in the visual field and documents reliability of the patient in the examination. It is particularly sensitive in cases of optic neuropathies and is useful in determining progression of field defects over time.

Homonymous visual field disturbances that respect the vertical meridian are generally associated with lesions of the optic tract or radiations and are commonly affected in cerebrovascular ischemia and stroke.[13] Greater congruity of incomplete homonymous defects helps localize the ischemic event to the optic radiations, whereas incongruity is more likely seen in tract defects. The presence of a relative afferent pupillary defect in the more affected eye is only seen in lesions anterior to the synapses of the lateral geniculate body. Lesions of the temporal lobe tend to be denser in the superior half of the visual field, whereas lesions of the parietal lobes tend to be denser in the inferior half of the visual field. Occipital lobe infarctions may cause homonymous hemianopsias or homonymous quadrantanopsias and tend to be congruous with the exception of the temporal crescent syndrome. Occipital lobe visual field defects may also spare or preferentially involve fixation. Bilateral occipital lobe infarctions may cause total or near-total loss of vision. In cases of bilateral occipital lobe infarctions with macular sparing, one can demonstrate a homonymous asymmetry in the visual field across the vertical meridian near fixation. If there is no macular sparing, then the patient will be bilaterally blind with retained pupillary reflexes.

Ancillary Tests

All ancillary testing should be performed under the direction of the consulting ophthalmologist. Fluorescein angiography and fundus photography are useful adjuncts to the ophthalmologic examination. Photographs of the fundus are taken after a peripheral intravenous injection of fluorescein dye; this identifies sites of vascular occlusion or abnormal vascular leakage in the optic nerve head and retina. Results from fluorescein angiography are used in the diagnosis of disease and, when indicated, in the treatment plans for laser therapy.

Testing of optic nerve function using visual-evoked responses (VER) or electroretinograms (ERG) are important in the diagnosis of many retinal and prechiasmal neuro-ophthalmologic diseases. In particular, the VER is a helpful test in diagnosis of demyelinating diseases. ERG is used to identify retinal degenerations. These tests are not generally used in the diagnosis of ischemic ocular disease.

Recent advances in color Doppler have allowed investigators to begin to analyze blood flow at the level of the optic nerve and choroid. These techniques require further refinement, but may be a promising new tool for the study of ocular perfusion.[14-16] In cases of suspected carotid-cavernous fistulas, auscultation of the orbit may reveal a bruit. In most cases of carotid- or dural-cavernous fistulas, orbital ultrasonography will reveal an enlargement of the superior ophthalmic vein.

NEURO-OPHTHALMIC SIGNS AND SYMPTOMS

Vascular Supply of the Eye and Orbit

The arterial blood supply of the eye and orbit primarily consists of the ophthalmic artery, originating from the internal carotid or rarely from the middle meningeal artery, and the infraorbital artery, originating from the external carotid artery.[17] The ophthalmic artery pierces the dura, becomes extradural over the course of the optic canal, and supplies the intracanalicular optic nerve.[18] Intraorbital branches of the ophthalmic artery include the central retinal artery, posterior ciliary arteries, anterior ciliary arteries, ethmoidal arteries, supraorbital arteries, recurrent meningeal artery, and lacrimal artery.[19] The arterial circulation of the eye is supplied primarily by the central retinal artery, the posterior ciliary arteries, and the anterior ciliary arteries (Table 31-2). The central retinal artery pierces the optic nerve about 10 mm posterior to the globe and forms an end artery supplying the inner two-thirds of the retina. It also may supply the superficial fibers at the optic disc. Occlusion of the central retinal artery or its branches produces severe retinal ischemic damage. The posterior ciliary arteries consist of 2 long and up to 20 short branches of the ophthalmic artery that supply the choroid, optic disc, and outer one-third of the retina.[20] In some individuals, a posterior ciliary artery produces a cilioretinal branch that appears at the disc edge and supplies a portion of the macula. The long posterior ciliary arteries proceed anteriorly, supplying the vasculature of the ciliary body, and anastomosing with the anterior ciliary arteries. The anterior ciliary arteries supply the extraocular muscles on their path to supply the vasculature of the anterior ocular segment.

Transient Monocular Loss of Vision (TMB)

Background   Often termed amaurosis fugax, this condition is the acute, painless loss of all or a portion of the vision in one eye.[21] The typical description of vision

Table 31-2.
Vascular supply of the eye

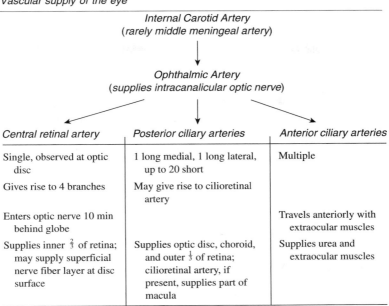

Central retinal artery	Posterior ciliary arteries	Anterior ciliary arteries
Single, observed at optic disc	1 long medial, 1 long lateral, up to 20 short	Multiple
Gives rise to 4 branches	May give rise to cilioretinal artery	
Enters optic nerve 10 min behind globe		Travels anteriorly with extraocular muscles
Supplies inner $\frac{2}{3}$ of retina; may supply superficial nerve fiber layer at disc surface	Supplies optic disc, choroid, and outer $\frac{1}{3}$ of retina; cilioretinal artery, if present, supplies part of macula	Supplies urea and extraocular muscles

loss is that of a shade or darkening that advances in the visual field, commonly from superior to inferior or inferior to superior and less commonly from the periphery to the center. The shade may involve central vision and generally lasts minutes with gradual full recovery. Although the majority of episodes of amaurosis fugax are not associated with any antecedent event or concurrent generalized neurologic symptoms, other symptoms or signs may be present. Associated ophthalmic complaints may include a sensation of color or photopsias in the affected visual field. In cases of severe carotid stenosis and chronic hypoperfusion to the eye, cases of amaurosis following bright light exposure or following ingestion of a large meal have been documented, probably on the basis of inability to keep up with metabolic demand.[22] TMB is often associated with carotid disease. Significant ipsilateral carotid stenosis is found in 27 percent to 69 percent of patients.[1,21,23] Ultrasound characteristics in carotid plaques indicative of high risk, including plaque ulceration or heterogeneous echogenicity, were found in a majority of patients with TMB.[23,24] It is important to recognize that the presence of a cervical bruit is not a reliable sign of significant carotid stenosis and may be absent in up to 33 percent of patients with high-grade stenosis.[25,26] The risk of stroke after episodes of

TMB is less than the risk of stroke with hemispheric TIAs but has been estimated to be about 2 to 8 percent per year with an additional risk of permanent visual sequelae of about 1 percent per year.[27–30]

Ocular examination performed during the time of visual disturbance may reveal a unilateral relative afferent pupillary defect or segmental pupillary changes from local ischemia. Fundus examination may reveal emboli or other abnormality in the retinal vascular circulation[31] (see Fig. 31-1). However, the majority of patients with a history of TMB will have an ophthalmologic exam that is relatively normal.[24]

Systemic neurologic evaluation is indicated, and comprehensive medical testing for cardiovascular risk factors should be performed. Initial examination of the carotid arteries should be done using noninvasive studies. Further studies will be indicated by the results of the initial testing.

Alternative etiologies for TMB need to be considered in the differential diagnosis. Other embolic sources include the heart, talc (seen in intravenous drug users), tumor, sepsis, fat (following long bone trauma), and local facial injections of medication.[32] In one study, only 2.5 percent of affected patients exhibited a cardiac source of emboli.[32] Nonembolic causes of transient visual disturbance include migraine and local ocular conditions including floaters, optic disc drusen, and papilledema. All patients with a history of TMB that seems to be of embolic etiology must undergo testing for embolic sources.

Evidence The North American Symptomatic Carotid Endarterectomy Trial reported a clear benefit of carotid endarterectomy over medical management alone in patients with 70 percent to 99 percent stenosis in the surgically accessible carotid in the neck.[138] However, a subset analysis of patients entering the study with TMB showed a much less robust, though still positive effect. In the patients with 50 percent to 69 percent carotid stenosis, the NASCET investigators found surgery had a negative effect compared with medical management alone.[139] similarly, no surgical benefit was found for TMB patients who had moderate stenosis in the European Carotid Surgery Trial.[140]

Treatment By definition, TMB is transient, and by the time he presents for medical attention, the patient either is asymptomatic or soon will be. TMB, therefore, does not need acute treatment. Treatment is geared toward finding a potential embolic source and reducing the risk of future stroke. Discussions of the diagnostic testing for cardiac and carotid sources of emboli and their treatment are covered elsewhere in this volume (see Chaps. 33–37 and Chaps. 2, 3, and 4).

For patients with TMB and a proven carotid stenosis of greater than 70 percent, who are good surgical risks and in the hands of surgical specialists who can perform the surgery with less than a 5 percent complication rate, we favor carotid endarterectomy. For patients with a stenosis of 50 percent to 69 percent, we recommend treatment with platelet antagonists and atherosclerotic risk factor reduction.

For the patient with TMB and a cardiac source of emboli identified, consideration should be given to chronic anticoagulation or surgical repair. Chronic use of platelet antagonists is appropriate for patients with TMB and no source of emboli identified. Discussion of choice of agents is beyond the scope of this chapter (see Chap. 4).

Permanent Monocular Loss of Vision

Permanent monocular loss of vision is caused by a lesion anterior to the optic chiasm. In the setting of cerebral vascular diseases, the most common causes of vision loss include ischemia at the level of the retinal arteries,

retinal veins, or optic nerve, comprising arteritic, nonarteritic, and posterior ischemic optic neuropathies.

Central or Branched Retinal Artery Occlusion

Background The central retinal artery arises in the orbit from the ophthalmic artery, has a short course in the subarachnoid space surrounding the optic nerve, and terminates in the prelaminar portion of the optic nerve, giving rise to the terminal branch retinal arteries (see Table 31-2).[33] Acute occlusion of the central retinal artery (CRAO) or its terminal branches (BRAO) results in an immediate, painless loss of vision in the territory of the involved artery.[34] In the case of CRAO, this involves the entire vision of the involved eye unless the patient has a common anatomic variant of the arterial vasculature. The cilioretinal artery arises from a short posterior ciliary artery in up to 50 percent of individuals and supplies the retina immediately adjacent to the optic nerve. In CRAO, the cilioretinal artery may be uninvolved, and consequently there may be sparing of the vision in the distribution of the cilioretinal artery, the corresponding macular retina (Fig. 31-2, color insert 7). BRAO presents with an acute loss of vision in the vascular territory of the involved arterial branch. However, ischemic involvement of the far periphery may produce a defect that is unrecognized by the patient.

Figure 31-2.
CRAO. Central retinal artery occlusion demonstrating white retinal swelling with sparring of a portion of the macular area supplied by a cilioretinal artery. (See also color insert 7.)

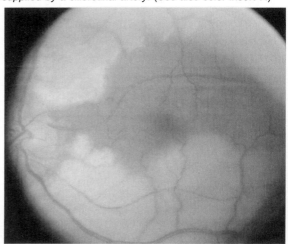

On examination of a patient with CRAO, there is an immediate loss of color of the optic nerve from local vascular attenuation. Subsequently, the retina is diffusely swollen and pale, and there is a macular "cherry red" spot from the intact choroidal circulation.[34] Occasionally, an embolus is noted lodged in the region of the lamina cribosa. In BRAO, there is an immediate attenuation of the involved vasculature with subsequent pale swelling of the corresponding retina. Emboli may be visible ophthalmoscopically in the affected artery. It is important to recognize that it may take more than 1 h of ischemic damage to produce the classic ophthalmoscopic retinal swelling and opacification after arterial occlusion.[35]

Comprehensive systemic evaluation of the patient is required. Common risk factors for the development of CRAO and BRAO include atherosclerotic disease, hypertension, diabetes mellitus, smoking, and hyperlipidemia.[34] The most common cause of retinal artery occlusions are embolic, arising from the ipsilateral carotid artery, the aortic arch, the heart, or other sources.[36-38] The embolic material commonly originates from atheromatous plaques but may be secondary to infections, intravenous drug use (talc), long bone fractures, amniotic fluid embolus, and facial or periocular steroid injections.[34] In a study of BRAO patients who were younger than 45 years, transthoracic echocardiography revealed disease in 27 percent of the patients that required either anticoagulation or cardiac surgery.[39] It is therefore critical to initiate a prompt, thorough systemic evaluation for embolic sources to limit subsequent embolic events, thereby reducing the potential for additional morbidity. Other causes of arterial occlusions include vasculitis, migraine, infection, and thrombosis.[40-45]

Prognosis for visual recovery following retinal artery occlusions is poor and probably depends on the extent and duration of ischemia.[34] The time course for permanent damage following retinal artery occlusion in the human is unknown, although animal studies of total vascular occlusion suggest a window of about 100 min before permanent damage occurs. Mechanisms of neuronal cell damage from ischemia include decreased intracellular energy stores with subsequent increase in intracellular calcium, release of glutamic and aspartic acids with subsequent increase in intracellular calcium, acidosis with lipid peroxidation, and production of toxic free radicals. An additional mechanism includes reperfusion injury from restoration of blood flow.

Evidence Although anecdotal reports have suggested visual recovery in occasional patients with pro-longed ischemic damage, most studies observe permanent loss of vision in the vast majority of these individuals.[34] Fibrinolytic therapies have been applied with success in some cases of retinal artery occlusion.[46] In a study of 14 patients with retinal artery occlusion treated either with urokinase or tissue plasminogen activator (TPA) injected via catheterization into the region of the ophthalmic artery, 4 patients with symptoms for 3.8 to 6.8 h demonstrated significant improvement, and 5 patients with symptoms for 8 to 55 h showed mild improvement in visual functioning.[47] It should be noted that all patients who improved significantly following thrombolytic therapy had at least 20/700 vision at time of treatment. This contrasted with only one of 41 control patients managed with conservative therapy who showed recovery. Although this study provides evidence for the potential benefit of thrombolytic therapy in retinal artery occlusions, the potential for significant morbidity associated with this therapy and the potential for visual recovery needs to be carefully considered prior to the therapeutic recommendation.

Therapy Traditional therapies for retinal artery occlusions include mechanisms to dislodge emboli into the peripheral arterial circulation and to reduce intraocular pressure with a theoretical improvement in retinal perfusion. These modalities include digital massage, paracentesis, and pharmacologic reduction in aqueous humor production.[46]

Central or Branched Retinal Vein Occlusion

Background Retinal venous occlusions tend to occur in individuals over the age of 50 with associated systemic diseases including hypertension, diabetes mellitus, and cardiovascular disease.[48-53] Other associations include open angle glaucoma, vasculitis, coagulopathies, and blood dyscrasias. Typically, the patient will complain of a sudden, painless loss of vision. One of the most serious consequences of central retinal artery occlusion (CRVO) is the development of neovascular glaucoma, which is associated with significant retinal ischemia. In cases of neovascular glaucoma, aggressive therapy is required to preserve remaining visual function, control pain, and prevent phthisis bulbi.[31,54,55]

Retinal vein occlusions are recognized by their characteristic ophthalmoscopic appearance of dilated tortuous veins and scattered intraretinal hemorrhages.[48] In the case of branch retinal vein occlusion (BRVO) these findings are limited to the affected quadrant or area (Fig. 31-3, color insert 8). In contrast, CRVO will exhibit these findings diffusely throughout the fundus. In addition, there may be a swollen appearance to the optic nerve head (Fig. 31-4, color insert 9). Ocular evaluation for undiagnosed open-angle glaucoma is important in all patients with a retinal vein occlusion. Fluorescein angiography of the retina demonstrates areas of retinal hypoperfusion and, where indicated, is useful in planning for laser photocoagulation. Gonioscopic evaluation allows the direct visualization of the anterior chamber angle and the diagnosis of anterior chamber neovascularization at an early stage.[56]

Systemic evaluation must include investigations for cardiovascular risk factors. Individuals who are young, have bilateral retinal vein occlusions, or have no cardiovascular risk factors should be further evaluated for hemorrheologic abnormalities.[48]

A prospective study of more than 700 patients with central retinal vein occlusion determined the natural history of the disease and to identified subgroups of patients at high risk for ocular complications.[53] Final visual acuity is found to positively correlate with the visual acuity at time of presentation. Patients with an initial visual acuity in the affected eye of better than 20/40 have a 65 percent chance of maintaining their vision at that level. In contrast, 80 percent of patients with an initial visual acuity of less than 20/200 in the

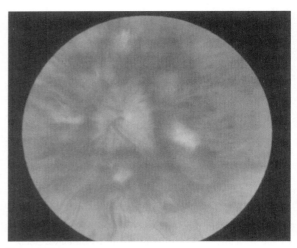

Figure 31-4.
CRVO. Typical appearance of a central retinal vein occlusion with diffuse hemorrhage. (See also color insert 9.)

affected eye will not improve. Patients with initial intermediate visual loss in the affected eye, 20/50 to 20/200, have a variable outcome with 37 percent deteriorating to less than 20/200 and only 19 percent improving to better than 20/50. Anterior segment neovascularization occurs in 16 percent of the affected eyes and correlates with poor vision at the initial visit and evidence of nonperfusion on fluorescein angiography.

Evidence Fibrinolytic agents have been used in experimental series.[48,55] The observed risks of this therapy in patients with retinal vein occlusions included fatal stroke and intraocular hemorrhage. Although 59 percent of patients with initial visual acuity of 20/100 showed improvement of at least three lines of vision following TPA administration, the significant side effects of this therapy may limit its usefulness.[55] There is no current clear consensus regarding fibrinolytic treatment of retinal vein occlusion.

Treatment There are no good data on the vascular management of this entity. Fibrinolytic therapy in this setting is experimental and cannot be recommended. Recommended local ocular therapy is well defined and consists of glaucoma management and, when indicated, laser surgery to control neovascular disease.[48,53] Underlying systemic conditions should be appropriately managed. Antiplatelet agents are often prescribed in patients with a history of retinal vein

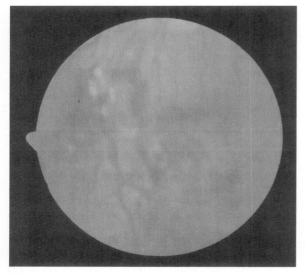

Figure 31-3.
BRVO. Branch retinal vein occlusion showing dilation of the vein and associated hemorrhage. (See also color insert 8.)

occlusion; however, there is no role for active anticoagulation in these patients.

Arteritic Anterior Ischemic Optic Neuropathy

Background   The arteritic form of ischemic optic neuropathy is generally associated with a systemic vasculitis, including Churg-Strauss vasculitis,[57] polyarteritis nodosa,[58] and giant cell or temporal arteritis (GCA).[59] In general, it is believed that interruption in blood flow at the level of the posterior ciliary arteries causes optic nerve head ischemia with resultant signs and symptoms. Typically, the patient will complain of a profound and sudden loss of visual acuity or visual field in one or both eyes.

On examination, the visual acuity may range from essentially normal to no light perception. The disease usually presents with asymmetric involvement; therefore there will be a relative afferent pupillary defect on the more involved side. The optic disc is swollen and often pale. The swelling may be profound or minimal and may be associated with cotton wool spots and peripapillary hemorrhages. Visual field testing may reveal generalized field disturbance, central scotoma, inferonasal sectorial defects, or altitudinal type of visual field loss. An associated retinal arterial occlusion is often considered to be strong evidence for an underlying vasculitis. Tests of optic nerve function using VER, which is nonspecifically affected, is not helpful in the diagnosis of this condition. Retinal function testing using the ERG is also not helpful and may actually be normal in the setting of profound optic nerve dysfunction. Prompt systemic evaluation for vasculitic etiologies is crucial in protecting the second eye from ischemic damage.

Evidence   There are numerous anecdotal reports of the use of various steroid dosages to prevent and treat ophthalmologic complications of GCA. Parsons-Smith described three cases of arteritis-induced visual loss recovering with the use of ACTH.[141] Model reported a case of recovery of vision with the use of intravenous methylprednisolone (IVMP).[142] Matzkin and colleagues reported two cases of patients with GCA with loss of vision to no light perception who recovered to baseline vision with the use of high-dose intravenous methylprednisolone (15 to 30 mg/kg/day).[143] On the other hand, Cornblath and Eggenberger reviewed cases of high-dose IVMP to treat GCA visual loss and found similar rates of visual loss to patients treated with oral steroids.[144] In a review of the topic, Swannell concluded that the dosage must be individualized and may vary from 40 mg of prednisolone to "megadose" IVMP for patients with visual symptoms.[145]

Treatment   Immunosuppressive therapy must be initiated immediately at the time of presentation of visual loss from an arteritic ischemic optic neuropathy. There is unresolved controversy about the initial recommended dose and route of administration of steroid therapy for arteritic ischemic optic neuropathy associated with GCA.[59] The potential for an increased rate of complications with the higher dose of steroids must be balanced against the risk of irreversible visual loss with inadequate or delayed treatment.[146] Although there is no large, prospective clinical trial of steroid therapy in arteritic ischemic optic neuropathy, we recommend an initial starting dose of the equivalent of 1.2 to 2.0 mg/kg/day of prednisolone. Many authors advocate an initial treatment of higher doses of intravenous steroids. The evidence for this recommendation comes from reports of more frequent steroid-associated improvement in visual functioning following intravenous as opposed to oral therapy.[59] There is also concern about maximally protecting against involvement of the second eye. Therapy must be titrated against the systemic symptoms and laboratory measurements of the disease activity.

Nonarteritic Anterior Ischemic Optic Neuropathy (NA-AION)

Background   NA-AION is the most common optic neuropathy that affects adults in the middle and older age groups. These patients complain of loss of visual acuity or visual field often noticed upon awakening in the morning.[60] Systemic associations include smoking, diabetes mellitus, and atherosclerosis.[61] In a review of over 400 patients with NA-AION, patients in the 45 to 65-year age group had an association with cerebrovascular disease.[62] NA-AION has been observed in patients following systemic surgery and is thought, in those cases, to result from profound hypotension or anemia resulting in ischemia at the level of the optic nerve head.[63,64] Hyperviscosity syndromes may be associated with this disease.[57] In the setting of renal failure requiring dialysis, NA-AION may occur secondary to ischemia from profound systemic hypotension, anemia, or generalized atherosclerotic disease.[65] The natural history of NA-AION was recently evaluated in a national prospective study that demonstrated spontaneous improvement of up to three lines of vision in 43 percent of patients and deterioration of vision in about 12 percent of patients.[66]

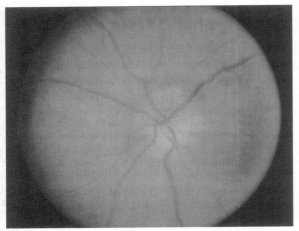

Figure 31-5.
AION. The optic disc in anterior ischemic optic neuropathy is swollen and often has associated nerve fiber layer hemorrhages. (See also color insert 10.)

Examination of visual acuity may range from normal, 20/20, to profound visual loss, no light perception. Although the classic description of visual field loss in these patients is that of an altitudinal type of scotoma, a variety of visual field abnormalities are seen in NA-AION including central scotomas, arcuate scotomas, and generalized visual field constriction. In most cases, an afferent pupillary defect will be noted on the involved side. An afferent pupillary defect may not be observed if there is bilateral symmetric involvement of the optic nerves (unusual) or if there was a previous optic neuropathy in the fellow eye. Examination of the fundus of the involved eye reveals optic nerve head swelling that may be diffuse, resembling papilledema or may be sectorial, corresponding to the defect in the visual field (Fig. 31-5, color insert 10). There may be associated splinter hemorrhages or cotton wool spots. The color may be pale or hyperemic.

It is therefore difficult to differentiate the optic nerve head swelling of NA-AION, papilledema, arteritic AION, and optic neuritis with edema. Several clues in the examination and evaluation are helpful in distinguishing these very different etiologies of optic disc edema. First, the fellow eye in NA-AION usually has a crowded appearance to the optic disc with a small cup-to-disc ratio. This is the classic "disc-at-risk" that is thought to be a predisposing factor in the development of NA-AION.[67] However, the risk of involvement of the second eye of a patient with NA-AION is high, from 15 to 40 percent.[68] It is therefore possible that the fellow optic disc may exhibit optic atrophy from a prior episode of NA-AION, mimicking a Foster Kennedy syndrome. It is also possible for the second eye to be asymptomatically involved by disc swelling prior to visual loss,[69] mimicking papilledema with optic nerve infarction. Second, color vision is usually abnormal in patients with acute NA-AION but is typically less affected than in cases of optic neuritis, where the patient typically experiences profound alterations in color perception. Third, fluorescein angiography may be helpful in distinguishing anterior ischemic optic neuropathy from other types of optic disc swelling.[70] Careful examination of the initial filling times of the prelaminar optic disc demonstrates delayed filling only in ischemic optic neuropathies and delayed filling in the adjacent peripapillary choroid only in the arteritic form of AION. The use of the pattern electroretinography (PERG) combined with careful analysis of other electrophysiologic testing has been favorably used in experimental series to differentiate between optic neuritis and ischemic optic neuropathy.[71]

Proper diagnosis of ischemic optic neuropathies directs the subsequent laboratory and radiographic analysis as well as potential therapy. For example, neuroradiologic analysis is generally not indicated in classic cases of suspected ischemic optic neuropathies. However, magnetic resonance imaging (MRI) of patients with NA-AION often reveals an increase in subcortical white matter lesions, a finding that is believed to indicate small vessel cerebrovascular disease.[72]

Evidence Multiple studies have evaluated a variety of putative therapies for NA-AION; however, they have generally failed to demonstrate a significant therapeutic response as measured by improvement in visual function when compared with an appropriate control population. A trial of hyperbaric oxygen at 100 percent and a pressure of 2 absolute atmospheres failed to produce improvement in NA-AION.[73] Although initial studies using optic nerve sheath fenestration in the treatment of NA-AION were promising, a national prospective study failed to confirm any therapeutic benefit of optic nerve surgery in this disease.[74] This study enrolled more than 240 patients with decreased vision to the level of 20/64. These patients were randomized to optic nerve surgery or careful observation. At the sixth month time period, it was noted that there was a significant risk of loss of at least three lines of vision in the surgical group as compared with the controls, 23.9 percent vs. 12.4 percent. Optic nerve sheath fenestration consequently has no role in the therapy of NA-AION.[74] Other studies with smaller numbers of enrolled patients demonstrated some improvement in visual functions after the use of either levodopa and carbidopa.[75] or HELP (heparin-induced extracorporeal LDL/fibrinogen precipitation).[76] Carefully controlled, large prospective studies are required to determine if these treatments are beneficial in the therapy of NA-AION.

Treatment   Although there is no currently accepted therapy for NA-AION, many physicians will request that the patients initiate low-dose aspirin therapy in an attempt to reduce involvement of the second eye.[68,77,78] Patients that are at risk for NA-AION involvement of their second eye may require modifications of the target levels of antihypertensive control. Less stringent control of hypertension with prevention of nocturnal systemic hypotension may be beneficial.[60] Finally, patients that have multiple risk factors for NA-AION may require special attention during surgical procedures to prevent significant hypotension or anemia and to protect the at-risk optic nerve from hypoperfusion injury and infarction.

Posterior Ischemic Optic Neuropathy

Background   Characterized by visual failure without obvious abnormality on visual examination of the fundus, posterior ischemic optic neuropathy is probably an underdiagnosed cause of neuro-ophthalmic visual loss.[79,80] This is a diagnosis of exclusion.

Early in the clinical evaluation, the patient will usually demonstrate visual loss and a relative afferent pupillary defect on the affected side. There may be no abnormal ophthalmoscopic findings. Ultimately, optic atrophy will be present, but this finding may take several weeks to develop. The likely site of ischemia is the circulation of the retrolaminar portion of the optic nerve arising from ischemia in the ophthalmic or posterior ciliary arteries or their branches. Advances in either Doppler evaluation or other analysis of blood flow to the optic nerve and choroid will be helpful in establishing this diagnosis in the future. A thorough systemic evaluation for cerebrovascular risk factors should be performed.

Treatment   Currently, there is no specific therapeutic option in the treatment of posterior ischemic optic neuropathy. Therapy must be targeted to reduce morbidity from associated systemic diseases and cardiovascular risk factors.

Ocular Motor System

Diplopia   Diplopia is a common neuro-ophthalmic complaint that may be present with neurologic and non-neurologic etiologies. It is important to note that if the diplopia is monocular, it is always ocular or psychiatric in origin, not neurologic. Diplopia or binocular blurring of vision from a neuro-ophthalmic etiology may be caused by a single peripheral cranial nerve, multiple cranial nerves, brainstem gaze pathways, supranuclear events, or abnormalities at the neuromuscular junction.[81–83]

Peripheral cranial mononeuropathies affecting the ocular motor nerves are commonly caused by ischemia to the involved nerve.[84–89] Significant risk factors include diabetes, hypertension, left ventricular hypertrophy, and elevated hematocrit. Often, there is associated pain at the time of onset of cranial mononeuropathy, and there can be early progression of the motility deficit.[84,85] In the setting of ischemic oculomotor nerve palsy, the pupillary fibers are often spared secondary to the peripheral location of the pupillary fibers with collateral circulation from pial sources. However, compressive lesions still may rarely cause partial, pupil-sparing third nerve palsies. Therefore, it is important to consider a compressive etiology in any case of third nerve palsy with the exception of a complete, pupil-sparing third nerve palsy.[90,91] Other etiologies in the differential diagnosis include vasculitides and brainstem stroke syndromes.[92–94]

Involvement of multiple cranial nerves causing neuro-ophthalmic disease may occur with ischemic lesions of the brainstem or with compressive lesions arising in the cavernous sinus.[90] Rarely, multiple cranial nerve involvement can be seen in cases of diabetic medical ischemic cranial nerve palsy.[83] Carotid-cavernous fistulas may initially present with single or multiple cranial nerve palsies, often involving the sixth or the third nerve.[90,95] Brainstem lesions may result in many neurologic and neuro-ophthalmologic syndromes including nuclear third nerve palsies, fascicular lesions, internuclear ophthalmoplegias, the one-and-a-half syndrome, and gaze palsies. Careful analysis of these patients using magnetic resonance imaging is indicated to help diagnose the underlying disease.

Nystagmus   Nystagmus is a common finding in patients with cerebellar infarctions, occurring in about 50 percent of patients with ischemia in the region of the superior cerebellar artery (SCA) and 75 percent of patients with ischemia in the region of the posterior inferior cerebellar artery (PICA).[96] Acquired pendular nystagmus is associated with brainstem stroke and demyelinating disease.[97]

SPECIFIC CONDITIONS

Giant Cell Arteritis (GCA)

GCA is a systemic disease of the medium and large-sized arteries in patients greater than 50 years of age and may affect the intracranial, extracranial, and systemic arterial circulation.[59,98] Therefore, the term "temporal arteritis" is misleading and should be abandoned. The systemic manifestations of this disease are widespread and may include weight loss, fatigue, fever, and malaise. The patients may complain of generalized muscle pain, claudication of the jaw or tongue, or localized scalp or temporal pain, swelling, and tenderness. Systemic symptoms may be absent from up to 21 percent of patients with neuro-ophthalmic signs of biopsy-proven GCA.[99] Neuro-ophthalmic mansifestations include arteritic anterior ischemic optic neuropathy, posterior optic neuropathy, choroidal ischemia, diplopia, retinal arterial occlusions, and ocular ischemic syndromes.[100] Neuro-ophthalmic involvement occurs in up to 70 percent of patients with GCA and constitutes a true ophthalmic emergency because of the significant risk of bilateral blindness from involvement of the optic nerve.[98] Simultaneous presentation of an ischemic optic neuropathy and retinal artery occlusion in the elderly patient should be considered GCA unless otherwise proven. Cases of early oculomotor involvement, estimated to occur in up to 15 percent of patients, represent a great opportunity to make the diagnosis and initiate appropriate therapy prior to the onset of visual loss.[59] It is therefore critical to consider this diagnosis in patients older than 50 with the new onset of diplopia from a cranial nerve palsy.

Diagnosis of GCA, according to the 1990 guidelines of the American College of Rheumatology, relies on the presence of a constellation of signs or symptoms and is associated with a greater than 93 percent sensitivity and 91 percent specificity.[101] These criteria depend on the presence of at least three of the following: (1) age greater than 50, (2) new onset headache, (3) reduced pulsation or tenderness of the temporal artery, (4) Westergreen erythrocyte sedimentation rate of greater than 50 mm/h, and (5) arterial biopsy demonstrating a necrotizing vasculitis with mononuclear cell infiltration or granulomatous inflammation. A positive biopsy confirms the diagnosis, but a negative biopsy does not rule out the diagnosis of GCA. Pathologic diagnosis may be difficult because only 60 to 80 percent of biopsies yield diagnostic pathology. As a result of skip lesions, the biopsy must be of sufficient size, at least 2 to 3 cm, and must be thoroughly evaluated to maximize the diagnostic yield.[102] The biopsy remains positive for at least a week after the initiation of steroid therapy; therefore, immediate initiation of high-dose steroids should be started in all cases of clinically suspected GCA followed by temporal artery biopsy to attempt a positive pathologic diagnosis.[59]

Isolated Granulomatous Angiitis of the Central Nervous System (GANS)

GANS is a recurrent, idiopathic vasculitis of the small and medium-sized blood vessels of the brain and spinal cord that occurs in children and adults.[58] Microinfarctions result from thrombotic occlusive disease in the affected vasculature. Neuro-ophthalmic manifestations include cortical visual disturbances, visual hallucinations, cranial nerve paresis, and optic neuropathy. Aggressive immunosuppressive therapy is required to cause disease remission. For a detailed discussion of this entity, please see Chapter 19.

Polyarteritis Nodosa (PAN)

PAN is a systemic vasculitis affecting small and medium-sized arteries in middle-aged individuals.[58,103] It is seen more commonly in men than women and causes constitutional changes, peripheral neuropathy, damage to the visceral organs, and may cause central nervous system disease including both hemorrhagic and ischemic stroke. The neuro-ophthalmologic consequences include homonymous hemianopsias from cerebral stroke and local ocular manifestations of ischemia. Common retinal findings include cotton wool spots and arterial occlusions of either a branch retinal artery or the central retinal artery. This may lead to profound and irreversible loss of vision. Transient monocular loss of vision may be symptomatic of transient ischemia to the retina or optic nerve in association with vasculitic involvement. Optic nerve involvement includes anterior ischemic optic neuropathy with a swollen optic disc and posterior optic neuropathy. Orbital involvement of the vasculitis may result in proptosis or orbital apex syndrome.

Diagnosis is difficult and relies on characteristic abnormalities on pathologic evaluation of biopsy specimens or angiography, demonstrating arterial narrowing or aneurysms. Immunosuppressive treatment is required to reduce the mortality and morbidity of this severe disease.

Churg-Strauss Syndrome

This systemic vasculitis causes eosinophilic granulomas, asthma, and peripheral eosinophilia.[57,104] Diagnosis is often confirmed by pathologic analysis of affected tissues. Neuro-ophthalmic manifestations are uncommon but range from transient visual loss to bilateral simultaneous blindness from optic neuropathy.[105] Additional ocular signs or symptoms may include retinal ischemia, retinal artery occlusions, and cranial mononeuropathies. Immunosuppressive therapy may be helpful in control of this vasculitis.[106]

Takayasu's Arteritis

Takayasu's arteritis is a severe occlusive disease of unknown etiology affecting the aorta and large arteries predominantly in young women, aged 10 to 30 years.[58,104,107] The resultant vascular insufficiency causes severe head, neck, and upper extremity consequences. Systemic constitutional symptoms and generalized arthralgias are prodromal and occur in the initial stages of this disease. Occlusion of the cerebral vasculature may result in stroke. Neuro-ophthalmic manifestations include the visual field consequences of stroke, retinal arteriovenous anastomes from ocular ischemia, and optic nerve ischemia with resultant infarction, loss of vision, and atrophy.[108–110] Diagnosis is suspected on the basis of the vascular ischemia, decreased or absent peripheral pulses, and bruits. Arteriography confirms the vascular abnormalities. Fluorescein angiography of the ocular fundus reveals retinal arteriovenous anastomoses that may be pathognomonic of moderate or advanced stages of Takayasu disease.[111] Therapy consists of immunosuppression and, in some cases, vascular surgery. For more detailed discussion, see Chapter 20.

Wegener's Granulomatosis

Initially characterized by a triad of systemic vasculitis, glomerulonephritis, and pulmonary involvement with granulomatous inflammation, Wegener's granulomatosis remains an uncommon but life-threatening disease. It is estimated that between 30 and 60 percent of patients exhibit neuro-ophthalmic consequences.[58,103,104,112,113] These include orbital granulomatous disease, scleritis, and retinal or optic nerve involvement from vasculitis. Retinal vasculitis may be mild and reversible, causing cotton wool spots and intraretinal hemorrhages, or severe and permanent, causing retinal artery occlusions, neovascularization, and rubeotic glaucoma. Intracranial disease consisting of meningitis, dural sinus thrombosis, and intracranial granulomas may result in papilledema. Diagnosis depends on observation of pathologic necrotizing granulomas in association with vasculitis. Laboratory analysis frequently reveals the presence of antineutrophil cytoplasmic antibodies (cANCA), IgA hypergammaglobulinemia, and leukocytosis without eosinophilia. Therapy relies on aggressive use of cytotoxic drugs to cause immunosuppression.[106] Steroid therapy is inadequate to control this potential fatal disease. (See also Chapter 19.)

Behçet's Disease

The characteristic triad of Behçet's disease is uveitis, oral ulceration, and genital ulceration.[114] This disease is now known to be a multisystem inflammatory process that may involve the central nervous system in up to 10 percent of patients. Although vaso-occlusive disease may affect all sizes of vasculature, the large vessels may develop thrombosis or aneurysmal dilation. This involvement may lead to cerebral infarction with resultant homonymous visual field deficit, papilledema from occlusion of a venous sinus with increased intracranial pressure, and retinal vasculitis. Additional neuro-ophthalmic signs, for example an internuclear ophthalmoplegia, may result from focal ischemia.[115] Diagnosis of this condition relies on the clinical findings on examination. Laboratory abnormalities are not specific for Behçet's but include elevation of the erythrocyte sedimentation rate and C-reactive protein. HLA typing may support the diagnosis because of the strong association with HLA-B51. Adequate control of the disease requires careful use of cytotoxic and immunosuppressive agents. Steroids may be useful in combination therapy. (See also Chapter 19.)

Systemic Lupus Erythematosis (SLE)

SLE is a chronic inflammatory disease of connective tissue that affects many organ systems.[58] Constitutional symptoms almost universally affect the patients causing fatigue, weight loss, and fever. Arthritis and mucocutaneous lesions are characteristic. Thromboembolic disease positively correlates with presence of circulating antiphospholipid antibodies, causing stroke, thrombophlebitis, and myocardial infarction. Cranial neuropathies, involving the facial, ocular motor, or trigeminal nerves have been associated with SLE and may be involved in the initial presentation of this disease. Transient ischemic attacks or stroke may cause transient monocular loss of vision or transient or permanent loss of visual field in affected individuals. Ischemic events may also involve the ocular motor pathways leading to an internuclear ophthalmoplegia or the vestibular system leading to nystagmus. Local ocular conditions include severe dry eye from associated Sjogren's syndrome, inflammation of the sclera or episclera, orbital inflammatory disease, optic neuropathy, and retinal vascular occlusive disease.

Retinal vascular disease is a common ophthalmic manifestation of SLE. This ranges from mild or asymptomatic to severe or vision-threatening involvement. The asymptomatic findings include cotton wool spots, intraretinal hemorrhages, dilated capillaries, and microaneurysms. These findings may be evaluated by fluorescein angiography. Retinal vascular involvement may also lead to central retinal artery occlusion, branch retinal artery occlusion, central retinal vein occlusion, and diffuse vascular occlusion. These may be an initial finding in SLE and usually result in permanent vision loss.

Optic nerve involvement may occur in 1 to 2 percent of SLE patients and may resemble optic neuritis, from demyelination, or may resemble ischemic optic neuropathy, from microangiopathy in the vascular supply of the optic nerve. In cases of possible optic nerve involvement, pupillary examination for a relative afferent pupillary defect is important in the initial evaluation. Careful analysis of the visual field is helpful in the initial workup as well as in the long-term follow-up of these individuals.

Diagnosis of SLE relies on the presence of at least 4 of a constellation of 11 clinical and laboratory criteria with a 96 percent sensitivity and specificity. Medications including hydralazine and procainamide have also been implicated as an etiology in a lupus-like disease, which is reversible upon stopping the medication. Circulating antinuclear antibodies (ANA) are positive in most patients with SLE and, in the presence of a high clinical suspicion for the disease, may be helpful in establishing the diagnosis. However, the presence of ANA is not pathognomonic for SLE and is demonstrated in a significant percentage of patients with other connective tissue diseases including scleroderma and juvenile and adult rheumatoid arthritis. Treatment may include cytotoxic agents and is targeted to control of symptoms.[106] For further discussion of SLE and stroke, see Chapter 19.

Thrombophilic States

Cerebral ischemia with resultant retinal vascular occlusions has been associated with conditions that are associated with thrombosis.[25,43,116–118] Protein S deficiency has been associated with CRAO, and, in one series, was found in about 15 percent of patients with cerebral infarctions in patients younger than 40.[117] Protein C deficiency has been associated with BRVO, BRAO, and amaurosis fugax. Antithrombin III deficiency has been linked to venous thrombosis, CRVO, and cilioretinal vascular occlusion.[43] A mutation in factor V, activated protein C resistance (APCR), which leads to decreased cleavage of factor V by protein C, has been reported in association with AION.[119] Antiphospholipid antibodies are known to be associated with multiple retinal vascular occlusions.[120,121] The linkage of retinal vascular disease with deficiency of plasminogen activator is controversial. Individuals who are younger than 45 years with retinal vascular occlusions should be evaluated for vasculitides and hematologic alterations in addition to the standard atherosclerotic risk factors including diabetes mellitus, hypertension, and atherosclerosis. For more detailed discussion, see Chapter 15.

Ocular Ischemic Syndrome

Severe ocular ischemia causes reduction in the ocular blood flow causing anterior and/or posterior segment ischemia, which ultimately results in anterior segment neovascularization with subsequent neovascular glaucoma.[122] Other signs of ocular ischemia include conjunctival injection, corneal haze, cataract, NA-AION, optic disc atrophy, increased cup-to-disc ratio, retinal hemorrhages, neovascularization, retinal arteriolar occlusion, low central retinal artery pressure, and central retinal vein occlusion. Symptoms of ocular ischemia include amaurosis fugax, ocular and orbital pain, and loss of vision. Ophthalmic etiologies of the neovascular glaucoma include central retinal vein occlusion, proliferative diabetic retinopathy, uveitis, chronic retinal detachment, or intraocular tumor. Systemic associations with the ocular ischemic syndrome include diabetes mellitus, systemic hypertension, coronary artery disease, and cerebrovascular disease. In a series of 39 eyes with the ocular ischemic syndrome, approximately 60 percent of the patients had occlusion of the ipsilateral carotid artery.[122] An additional 15 percent had severe ipsilateral carotid stenosis of 80 to 90 percent. Therefore, the presence of the the ocular ischemic syndrome should alert the clinician to the likelihood of severe carotid occlusive disease.

Susac Syndrome

This syndrome is characterized by a triad of bilateral branch retinal artery occlusions, encephalopathy, and deafness.[123] Headaches and tinnitus may be prodromal symptoms. The retinal artery occlusions vary from asymptomatic and subtle, causing no significant visual problems, to severe and extensive, involving the posterior pole. After resolution of the occlusion, the retinal artery may show silver streaks. The encephalopathy is characterized by personality changes, unusual behavior, extensor plantar reflex, pseudobulbar speech, seizures, and myoclonus. Neuroradiologic imaging with MRI demonstrates multiple gray and white matter infarcts and may be misinterpreted as consistent with multiple sclerosis. During the subacute phase of the disease, these infarcts exhibit gadolinium enhancement. EEG exhibits diffuse slowing. A subset of patients with recurrent idiopathic branch retinal artery occlusions may have a partial Susac's syndrome; these patients have a favorable outcome with only 9 percent having permanent visual loss and 28 percent with permanent, partial loss of visual field.[124]

The etiology of Susac's syndrome is obscure. It is a self-limited disease that lasts for 1 to 2 years with some resolution. Visual loss and hearing loss may be permanent, and about half of the patients may have some persistent dementia. Therapeutic options include steroids or anticoagulants, but these are not universally accepted. Anecdotal evidence suggests that aspirin and calcium channel blockers may be helpful but a prospective analysis of the therapies is needed.

Carotid Artery Dissection

Dissecting aneurysms result from a breach in the endothelium followed by the separation of arterial layers by flowing blood. They may originate in any arterial system or in any location but commonly involve the internal carotid and vertebral arteries. The blood in the false lumen may thrombose, return to the normal pathway of flow, or may rupture through the external arterial wall. Dissections may occur spontaneously, following trauma, or in association with systemic disorders of connective tissue.[125–128] Generally, the patients complain of radiating head and neck pain with a wide variety of neurologic symptoms.

Neurologic sequelae usually result from vascular occlusion, thromboembolism from the aneurysm, or contiguous compression from the acutely expanded vessel. Numerous neuro-ophthalmic associations include amaurosis fugax, AION, CRAO, ophthalmic artery occlusion, ophthalmoparesis, sixth nerve palsy, Horner's syndrome, ocular or orbital ischemic syndrome, and visual field defects.[129,130] For a detailed discussion of diagnosis and treatment, see Chapter 16.

Vertebral Artery Dissection

Dissection of the vertebral artery is associated with a wide variety of neuro-ophthalmic signs and symptoms.[131] The most common symptom in the majority of patients is neck or head pain. Other common complaints include blurred vision, transient visual dimming, vertigo, hemisensory alterations, and diplopia. Although diplopia ultimately affects a significant proportion of patients with this syndrome, it is an unusual presenting complaint. Less common complaints include oscillopsia, photophobia, dry eye, and upside-down vision.

Nystagmus is a major sign in vertebral artery dissections and may present in up to 37 percent of affected patients. The nystagmus may be horizontal, rotary, upbeat, or downbeat. Ocular misalignments are also common and occur in up to 33 percent of patients. These result from skew deviations or from cranial nerve palsies involving the abducens, oculomotor, or trochlear nerves. Horner's syndrome is observed in about 27 percent of affected patients. Decreased corneal sensation and ptosis are also common. Visual field defects in these patients result from occipital lobe infarction. Less common signs include abnormal pursuits or saccades, ocular bobbing, or anisocoria. (See also Chap. 16.)

Midbrain Infarction

Isolated infarctions of the midbrain may occur in about 6 percent of patients with stroke in the distribution of the posterior circulation.[132] These patients will present with nonspecific neurologic symptoms including dizziness, unsteadiness, and gait ataxia. Lesions affecting the upper midbrain may have impairment of vertical gaze. Lesions of the lower midbrain with dorsal involvement may demonstrate a fourth nerve palsy or Horner's syndrome. The majority of patients with infarctions involving the middle midbrain will have third nerve dysfunction. The presentations of the third nerve palsy from middle midbrain infarction include nuclear third nerve palsies, characterized by bilateral ptosis, bilateral mydriasis, and contralateral superior rectus involvement, and peripheral third nerve palsies. The unusual topography of the third nerve subnuclei allow for the unusual development of bilateral ptosis to occur in isolation with otherwise normal extraocular movements.[133]

Pontine Infarction

Isolated infarctions of the pons may comprise 6 percent of patients with acute vertebrobasilar stroke.[134] Ventral pontine infarcts may produce transient ocular motor defects. These include sixth nerve palsy, internuclear ophthalmoplegia, lateral gaze palsy, and the one-and-a-half syndrome. Tegmental pontine infarcts may also cause sixth nerve palsies as well as internuclear ophthalmoplegia and supranuclear alterations of eye movement. The lateral pontine syndrome is often associated with cranial nerve palsies and Horner's syndrome.

Migraine

Migraine with aura is often associated with an antecedent bilateral homonymous scintillating scotoma that resolves within 15 to 20 min. Migraine may also be associated with transient or permanent neuro-ophthalmologic sequelae including ophthalmoplegia, ischemic optic neuropathy, amaurosis fugax, and visual field loss.[135] Posterior ischemic optic neuropathy has also been associated with migraine.[136] Migraine is likely to be a precipitating event in retinal artery occlusions or stroke in patients who are younger than 40.[137,138] A detailed discussion of diagnosis and treatment is present in Chapter 22.

Intracranial Aneurysms

Intracranial aneurysms cause variable neuro-ophthalmologic signs and symptoms as a consequence of mass effect from an intact aneurysm or ruptured aneurysms with resultant hemorrhage.[139] Intracranial aneurysms may occur in different locations but are commonly associated with the internal carotid artery, the anterior communicating artery, or the posterior communicating artery. Their tendency to rupture depends on location and size.

Aneurysms of the internal carotid artery as it traverses the petrous bone may be associated with a sixth nerve palsy, facial weakness, or hearing loss.[140] Aneurysms of the intracavernous carotid artery may present with a cavernous sinus syndrome involving multiple cranial nerves or may present with a cranial mononeuropathy. Rupture of the intracavernous carotid aneurysms may cause a carotid cavernous fistula. Aneurysms at the junction of the ophthalmic and carotid arteries are likely to cause a compressive optic neuropathy or junctional scotoma. Supraclinoid carotid artery aneurysms may cause cranial nerve palsies or optic neuropathy. Poste-rior communicating artery aneurysms will involve the third cranial nerve in up to 40 percent of patients. Although a pupil-involving third nerve palsy is likely with a compressive lesion, partial third nerve palsies from aneurysmal pressure may initially spare the pupil. It is therefore necessary to carefully follow the patient with a cranial mononeuropathy for several weeks to identify an evolving and changing pattern of neuro-ophthalmic response.[141] Posterior cerebral artery aneurysms may cause homonymous hemianopsias. Vertebrobasilar artery aneurysms may affect multiple cranial nerves.

CONCLUSION

The spectrum of ischemic cerebrovascular disease is varied and creates a broad variety of neuro-ophthalmic consequences to the optic nerve, retinal vasculature, visual field, and ocular motor system. It is important to carefully explore the history of the patient, document the neuro-ophthalmic findings, and develop an appropriate differential diagnosis. This systematic approach will help to appropriately design the proper laboratory tests, radiologic studies, and consultations with other subspecialists to develop the finest possible treatment program to minimize additional morbidity.

REFERENCES

1. Ivers RQ, Cumming RG, Mitchell P, et al: Visual impairment and falls in older adults: The Blue Mountains Eye Study. *J Am Ger Soc* 46:58, 1998.
2. Miller NR: Cerebrovascular disease in Miller NR (ed): *Walsh and Hoyt's Clinical Neuro-ophthalmology,* 4th ed. Baltimore, Williams & Wilkins, 1991, p 2210.
3. Baglivo E, Dosso A, Pournaras C: Thrombus and branch retinal vein occlusion. *Graefes Arch Clin Exp Ophthalmol* 235:10, 1997.
4. Mitchell P, Wang JJ, Li W, et al: Prevalence of asymptomatic retinal emboli in an Australian urban community. *Stroke* 28:63, 1997.
5. Galetta SL, Liu GT, Volpe NJ: Diagnostic tests in neuro-ophthalmology. *Neurol Clin* 14:201, 1996.
6. Siatkowski RM, Lam BL, Anderson DR, et al: Automated suprathreshold static perimetry screening for detecting neuro-ophthalmic disease. *Ophthalmology* 103:907, 1996.
7. Liu GT, Volpe NJ, Galetta S: Eye movement disorders. *Curr Opin Ophthalmol* 6:27, 1995.
8. Handler JA, Ghezzi KT: General ophthalmologic examination. *Emerg Med Clin* 13:521, 1995.
9. Winterkorn JM: Calcific retinal emboli and collateral

shunting in a woman with rheumatic heart disease. *Arch Ophthalmol* 113:1464, 1995.

10. Bruno A, Jones WL, Austin JK, et al: Vascular outcome in men with assymptomatic retinal cholesterol emboli: A cohort study. *Ann Intern Med* 122:249, 1995.

11. Landau K, Wichmann W, Valavanis A: The missing temporal crescent. *Am J Ophthalmol* 119:345, 1995.

12. Chavis P, Clunie D, Hoyt WF: Temporal crescent syndrome with magnetic resonance correlation. *J Neuro-Ophthalmol* 17:151, 1997.

13. Wirtschafter JD: Anatomic basis and differential diagnosis of field defects, in Walsh, TJ (ed): *Visual Fields; Examination and Interpretation,* 2nd ed. Hong Kong, Palace Press, 1996, p 39.

14. Lee HM, Fu ER: Orbital colour doppler imaging in chronic ocular ischaemic syndrome. *Aust N Z Ophthalmol* 25:157, 1997.

15. Williamson TH, Baxter GM, Pyott A, et al: A comparison of colour Doppler imaging of orbital vessels and other methods of blood flow assessment. *Graefes Arch for Clin Exp Ophthalmol* 233:80, 1995.

16. Williamson TH, Harris A: Color Doppler ultrasound imaging of the eye and orbit. *Surv Ophthalmol* 40:255, 1996.

17. Hayreh SS, Dass R: The ophthalmic artery: 1. Origin and intracranial and intracanalicular course. *Br J Ophthalmol* 46:165, 1962.

18. Chou P-I, Sadun AA, Lee H: Vasculature and morphometry of the optic canal and intracanalicular optic nerve. *J. Neuro-Opthalmol* 15:186, 1995.

19. Bron AJ, Tripathi RC, Tripathi BJ. *Wolff's anatomy of the Eye and Orbit.* London: Chapman and Hall Medical, 1997.

20. Hayreh SS: The optic nerve head circulation in health and disease. *Exp Eye Res* 61:259, 1995.

21. Carter JE: Carotid artery disease and its ocular manifestations. *Ophthal Clin* 5:425, 1992.

22. Levin LA, Mootha VV: Postprandial transient visual loss: A symptom of critical carotid stenosis. *Ophthalmology* 104:397, 1997.

23. Muller M, Wessel K, Mehdorn E, et al: Carotid artery disease in vascular ocular syndromes. *J Clin Neuro-Ophthalmol* 13:175, 1993.

24. Perez-Burkhardt JL, Gonzalez-Fajardo JA, Rodriguez E, et al: Amaurosis fugax as a symptom of carotid atery stenosis: Its relationship with ulcerated plaque. *J Cardiovasc Surg* 35:15, 1994.

25. Newman NJ. Neuro-ophthalmology and systemic disease-Part 1. *J Neuro-Ophthalmol* 15:109, 1995.

26. Suave JS, Thorpe KE, Sackett DL, et al: Can bruits distinguish high-grade from moderate symptomatic carotid stenosis? *Ann Intern Med* 120:633, 1994.

27. Marshall J, Meadows S: The natural history of amaurosis fugax. *Brain* 91:419, 1968.

28. Hurwitz BJ, Heyman A, Wilkinson WE, et al: Comparison of amaurosis fugax and transient cerebral ischemia: A prospective clinical and arteriographic study. *Ann Neurol* 18:698, 1985.

29. Poole CJ, Russell RWR. Mortality and stroke after amaurosis fugax. *J Neurol Neurosurg Psychiatry* 48:902, 1985.

30. Easton JD, Wilterdink JL: Carotid endarterectomy: Trials and tribulations. *Ann Neurol* 35:5, 1994.

31. Van Den Berg E, Lohmann N, Friedburg D, Rabe F: Report of general temporary anticoagulation in the treatment of acute cerebral and retinal ischaemia. *Vasa* 26:222, 1997.

32. Smit RLMJ, Baarsma GS, Koudstaal PJ: The source of embolism in amaurosis fugax and retinal artery occlusion. *Int Ophthalmol* 18:83, 1994.

33. Miller NR: Anatomy and physiology of the cerebral vascular system, in Miller (ed): NR *Clinical Neuro-Ophthalmology.* 4th ed. Baltimore, Williams & Wilkins, 1991, p 1873.

34. Mangat HS: Retinal artery occlusion. *Surv Ophthalmol* 40:145, 1995.

35. Hayreh SS, Weingeist TA: Experimental occlusion of the central artery of the retina: 1. Ophthalmoscopic and fluorescein fundus angiographic studies. *Br J Ophthalmol* 64:896, 1980.

36. Kimura K, Hashimoto Y, Ohno H, et al: Carotid artery disease in patients with retinal artery occlusion. *Int Med* 35:937, 1996.

37. Rafuse PE, Nicolle DA, Hutnik CM, et al: Left atrial myxoma causing ophthalmic artery occlusion. *Eye* 11:25, 1997.

38. Sharma S, Maqvi A, Sharma SM, et al: Transthoracic echocardiographic findings in patients with acute retinal arterial obstruction: A retrospective review. Retinal emboli of cardiac origin group. *Arch Ophthalmol* 114: 1189, 1996.

39. Sharma S, Sharma SM, Cruess AF, et al: Transthoracic echocardiography in young patients with acute retinal arterial obstruction: RECO study group. *Can J Ophthalmol* 32:38, 1997.

40. Margo CE, Mack WP: Therapeutic decisions involving disparate clinical outcomes. *Ophthalmology* 103:691, 1996.

41. Hupp SL, Kline LB, Corbett JJ: Visual disturbances of migraine. *Surv Ophthalmol* 34:221, 1989.

42. Ros MA, Magargal LE, Uram M: Branch retinal artery obstruction: A review of 201 eyes. *Ann Ophthalmol* 21:103, 1989.

43. Vine AK, Samama MM: The role of abnormalities in the anticoagulant and fibrinolytic systems in retinal vascular occlusions. *Surv Ophthalmol* 37:283, 1993.

44. Beversdorf D, Stomel E, Allen C, et al: Recurrent branch retinal artery infarcts in association with migraine. *Headache* 37:396, 1997.

45. Zamora RL, del Priore LV, Storch GA, et al: Multiple recurrent branch retinal artery occlusions associated with varicella zoster virus. *Retina* 16:399, 1996.

46. Atebara NH, Brown GC, Cater J: Efficiency of anterior chamber paracentesis and carbogen in treating acute non-arteritic central retinal artery occlusion. *Ophthalmology* 102:2029, 1995.

47. Schmidt D, Schumacher M, Wakhloo AK: Microcatheter urokinase infusion in central retinal artery occlusion. *Am J Ophthalmol* 113:429, 1992.

48. Williamson TH: Central retinal vein occlusion: What's the story? *Br. J Ophthalmol* 81:698, 1997.

49. Fekrat S, Finkelstein D: Current concepts in the management of central retinal vein occlusion. *Curr Opin Ophthalmol* 8:54, 1997.

50. Clarkson JC: Central vein occlusion study: Photographic protocol and early natural history. *Trans Am Ophthalmol Soc* 92:203, 1994.

51. Mitchell P, Smith W, Chang A: Prevalence and associations of retinal vein occlusion in Australia. The Blue Mountains Eye Study. *Arch Ophthalmol* 114:1243, 1996.

52. Sperduto RD, Hiller R, Chew E, et al: Risk factors for hemiretinal vein occlusion: Comparison with risk factors for central and branch retinal vein occlusion. *Ophthalmology* 105:765, 1998.

53. Central Vein Occlusion Study Group: Natural history and clinical management of central retinal vein occlusion. *Arch Ophthalmol* 115:486, 1997.

54. Baumal CR, Brown GC: Treatment of central vein occlusion. *Ophthalmic Surg* 28:590, 1997.

55. Elman MJ: Thrombolytic therapy for central retinal vein occlusion: Results of a pilot study. *Trans Am Ophthalmol Soc* 94:471, 1996.

56. Browning DJ, Scott AQ, Peterson CB, et al: The risk of missing angle neovascularization by omitting screening gonioscopy in acute central retinal vein occlusion. *Ophthalmology* 105:776, 1998.

57. Acheson JF, Cockerell OC, Bentley CR, et al: Churg-Strauss vasculitis presenting with severe visual loss due to bilateral sequential optic neuropathy. *Br J Ophthalmol* 77:118, 1993.

58. Miller N, Vasculitis, in Miller NR, (ed): *Walsh and Hoyt's Clinical Neuro-Ophthalmology,* 4th ed. Baltimore, Williams & Wilkins, 1991, p 2575.

59. Ghanchi FD, Dutton GN: Current concepts in giant cell (temporal) arteritis. *Surv Ophthalmol* 42:99, 1997.

60. Hayreh SS, Podhajsky PA, Zimmerman B: Nonarteritic anterior ischemic optic neuropathy: Time of onset of visual loss. *Am J Ophthalmol* 124:641, 1997.

61. Jacobson DM, Vierkant RA, Belongia EA: Nonarteritic anterior ischemic optic neuropathy: A case-control study of potential risk factors. *Arch Ophthalmol* 115:1403, 1997.

62. Hayreh SS, Joos KM, Podhajsky PA: Systemic diseases associated with Nonarteritic anterior ischemic optic neuropathy. *Am J Ophthalmol* 118:766, 1994.

63. Katz DM, Trobe JD, Cornblath WT, et al: Ischemic optic neuropathy after lumbar spine surgery. *Arch Ophthalmol* 112:925, 1994.

64. Williams EL, Hart WM Jr, Tempelhoff R: Postoperative ischemic optic neuropathy. *Anesth Analg* 80:1018, 1995.

65. Haider S, Astbury NJ, Hamilton DV: Optic neuropathy in uraemic patients on dialysis. *Eye* 7:148, 1993.

66. The Ischemic Optic Neuropathy Decompression Trial Research Group: Optic nerve decompression surgery for nonarteritic anterior ischemic optic neuropathy (NAION) is not effective and may be harmful. *JAMA* 273:625, 1995.

67. Wakakura M, Ishikawa S: Neuro-ophthalmic aspects of vascular disease. *Curr Opin Ophthalmol* 5:18, 1994.

68. Kupersmith MJ, Frohman L, Sanderson M, et al: Aspirin reduces the incidence of second eye NAION: A retrospective study. *J Neuro-Ophthalmol* 17:250, 1997.

69. Miller NR: Anterior ischemic optic neuropathy, in Miller NR (ed): *Walsh and Hoyt's Clinical Neuro-Ophthalmology.* 4th ed. Baltimore, Williams & Wilkins, 1982, p 212.

70. Arnold AA, Badr MA, Hepler RS: Fluorescein angiography in nonischemic optic disc edema. *Arch Ophthalmol* 114:293, 1996.

71. Froehlich J, Kaufman DI: Use of pattern electroretinography to differentiate acute optic neuritis from acute anterior ischemic optic neuropathy. *Electroencephalogr Clin Neurophys* 92:480, 1994.

72. Arnold AC, Hepler RS, Hamilton DR, et al: Magnetic resonance imaging of the brain in nonarteritic ischemic optic neuropathy. *J Neuro-Ophthalmol* 15:158, 1995.

73. Arnold AA, Hepler RS, Lieber M, et al: Hyperbaric oxygen therapy for nonarteritis anterior ischemic optic neuropathy. *Am J Ophthalmol* 122:535, 1996.

74. Glaser JS, Teimory M, Schatz NJ: Optic nerve sheath fenestration for progressive ischemic optic neuropathy: Results in second series consisting of 21 eyes. *Arch Ophthalmol* 112:1047, 1994.

75. Johnson LN, Gould TJ, Krohel GB: Effect of levodopa and carbidopa on recovery of visual function in patients with nonarteritic anterior ischemic optic neuropathy of longer than 6 month's duration. *Am J Opthalmol* 121:77, 1996.

76. Haas A, Walzl M, Jesenik F, et al: Application of HELP in nonarteritic anterior ischemic optic neuropathy: A prospective, randomized, controlled study. *Graefes Arch Clin Exp Ophthalmol* 235:14, 1997.

77. Beck RW, Hayreh SS, Podhajsky PA, Tan ES, Moke PS: Aspirin therapy in nonarteritic anterior ischemic optic neuropathy. *Am J Ophthalmol* 123:212, 1997.

78. Botelho PJ, Johnson LN, Arnold AC: The effect of aspirin on the visual outcome of nonarteritic anterior ischemic optic neuropathy. *Am J Ophthalmol* 121:450, 1996.

79. Hayreh SS: Posterior ischemic optic neuropathy. *Ophthalmologica* 182:29, 1981.

80. Gladstone GJ: The afferent pupillary defect as an early manifestation of occult temporal arteritis. *Ann Ophthal* 14:1088, 1982.

81. Newman SA: Gaze-induced strabismus. *Surv Ophthalmol* 38:303, 1993.

82. Batocchi AP, Evoli A, Majolini L, et al: Ocular palsies in the absence of other neurological or ocular syptoms: Analysis of 105 cases. *J Neurol* 244:639, 1997.

83. Eshbaugh CG, Siatkowski RM, Smith JL, Kline LB: Simultaneous, multiple cranial neuropathies in diabetes mellitus. *J Neuro-Ophthalmol* 15:219, 1995.

84. Jacobson DM: Progressive ophthalmoplegia with acute ischemic abducens palsy. *Am J Ophthalmol* 122:278, 1996.

85. Jacobson DM, Broste SK: Early progression of ophthalmoplegia in patients with ischemic oculomotor nerve palsies. *Arch Ophthalmol* 113:1535, 1995.

86. Jacobson DM, McCanna TD, Layde PM: Risk factors for ischemic ocular motor nerve palsies. *Arch Ophthalmol* 112:961, 1994.

87. Lee JP: Paralytic and incomitant strabismus. *Curr Opin Ophthalmol* 7:19, 1996.

88. Keane JR: Fourth nerve palsy: Historical review and study of 215 inpatients. *Neurology* 43:2439, 1993.

89. Tiffin PA, MacEwen CJ, Craig EA, et al: Acquired palsy of the oculomotor, trochlear, and abducens nerves. *Eye* 10:377, 1996.

90. Cullom ME, Savio PJ, Sergott RC, et al: Relative pupillary sparing third nerve palsies: To arteriogram or not? *J Neuro-Ophthalmol* 15:136, 1995.

91. Kissel JT, Burde RM, Klingele TG, et al: Pupil sparing oculomotor palsies with internal carotid-posterior communicating artery aneurysm. *Ann Neurol* 13:149, 1983.

92. Fujioka T, Segawa F, Ogawa K, et al: Ischemic and hemorrhagic brain stem lesions mimicking diabetic ophthalmoplegia. *Clin Neurosurg* 97:167, 1995.

93. Bondeson J, Asman P: Giant cell arteritis presenting with oculomotor palsy. *Scand J Rheumatol* 26:327, 1997.

94. Miller NR: The oculomotor nerves. *Curr Opin Neurol* 9:21, 1996.

95. Acierno MD, Trobe JD, Cornblath WT, Gebarski SS: Painful oculomotor palsy caused by posterior-draining dural carotid cavernous fistulas. *Arch Ophthalmol* 113:1045, 1995.

96. Kase CS, Norving B, Levine SR, et al: Cerebellar infarction: Clinical and anatomic observations in 66 cases. *Stroke* 24:76, 1993.

97. Lopez LI, Bronstein AM, Gresty MA, Du Boulay EP, Rudge P: Clinical and MRI correlates in 27 patients with acquired pendular nystagmus. *Brain* 119:465, 1996.

98. Liu GT, Glaser JS, Schatz NJ, Smith JL: Visual morbidity in giant cell arteritis: Clinical characteristics and prognosis for vision. *Ophthalmology* 101:1779, 1994.

99. Hayreh SS, Podhajsky PA, Zimmerman B: Occult giant cell arteritis: Ocular manifestations. *Am J Ophthalmol* 125:521, 1998.

100. Hayreh SS, Podhajsky PA, Zimmerman B: Ocular manifestations of giant cell arteritis. *Am J Ophthalmol* 125:509, 1998.

101. Hunder GG, Bloch DA, Michel BA, et al: The American College of Rheumatology 1990 criteria for the classification of giant cell arteritis. *Arthrit Rheum* 33:1122, 1990.

102. Albert DM, Ruchman MC, Keltner JL: Skip lesions in temporal arteritis. *Arch Ophthalmol* 89:1111, 1976.

103. Moore PM: Neurological manifestations of vasculitis: Update on immunopathogenic mechanisms and clinical features. *Ann Neurol* 37 (Suppl):s131, 1995.

104. Hunder G: Vasculitis: Diagnosis and therapy. *Am J Med* 100:37s, 1996.

105. Vitali C, Genovesi-Ebert F, Romani A, et al: Ophthalmological and neuro-ophthalmological involvement in Churg-Strauss syndrome: A case report. *Graefes Arch Clin Exp Ophthalmol* 234:404, 1996.

106. Martin-Suarez I, D'Cruz D, Mansoor M, et al: Immunosuppressive treatment in severe connective tissue diseases: Effects of low dose intravenous cyclophosphamide. *Ann Rheum Dis* 56:481, 1997.

107. Sharma BK, Jain S, Suri S, et al: Diagnostic criteria for Takayasu arteritis. *Int J Cardiol* 54(Suppl):S141, 1997.

108. Charlton JF, Dalla K: Amaurosis and pulselessness in a young white woman: A case of Takayasu disease. *J Am Board Fam Pract* 10:227, 1997.

109. Schmidt MH, Fox AJ, Nicolle DA: Bilateral anterior ischemic optic neuropathy as a presentation of Takayasu's disease. *J Neuro-Ophthalmol* 17:156, 1997.

110. Lewis JR, Glaser JS, Schatz NJ, et al: Pulseless (Takayasu) disease with ophthalmic manifestations. *J Clin Neuro-Ophthalmol* 13:242, 1993.

111. Tanaka T, Shimizu K: Retinal arteriovenous shunts in Takayasu disease. Ophthalmology 94:1380, 1987.

112. Heathcote JG: Update in ophthalmologic and general pathology: Wegener's granulomatosis. A review of the ophthalmic manifestations. *Can J Ophthalmol* 32:149, 1997.

113. Newman NJ, Slamovits TL, Friedland S, et al: Neuro-ophthalmic manifestations of meningocerebral inflammation from the limited form of Wegener's granulomatosis. *Am J Ophthalmol* 120:613, 1995.

114. Mochizuki M, Akduman L, Nussenblatt RB: Behcet disease, in Pepose JS, Hollands GNWKR (eds): *Ocular Infection and Immunity.* St. Louis, Mosby, 1996, p 663.

115. Masai H, Kashii S, Kimura H, et al: Neuro-Behcet disease presenting with internuclear ophthalmoplegia. *Am J Ophthalmol* 122:897, 1996.

116. Schafer Al: Hypercoagulable states: Molecular genetics to clinical practice. *Lancet* 344:1739, 1994.

117. Barinagerrementeria F, Canu-Brito C, De La Pena A, et al: Prothrombotic states in young people with idiopathic stroke: A prospective study. *Stroke* 25:287, 1994.

118. Bertram B, Remky A, Arend O, et al: Protein C, protein S, and antithrombin III in acute ocular occlusive diseases. *Ger J Ophthalmol* 4:332, 1995.

119. Worrall BB, Moazami G, Odel JG, et al: Anterior ischemic optic neuropathy and activated protein C resistance. *J Neuro-Ophthalmol* 17:162, 1997.

120. Dunn JP, Noorily SW, Petri M, et al: Antiphospholipid antibodies and retinal vascular disease. *Lupus* 5:313, 1996.

121. Giorgi D, Vaccaro F: Vaso-occlusive retinopathy: Is it a classic clinical manifestation of the antiphospholipid syndrome. *Lupus* 6:617, 1997.

122. Mizener JB, Podhajsky P, Hayrey SS: Ocular ischemic syndrome. *Ophthalmology* 104:859, 1997.

123. Susac JO: Susac's syndrome: The triad of microangiopathy

of the brain and retina with hearing loss in young women. *Neurology* 44:591, 1994.

124. Johnson MW, Thomley ML, Huang SS, et al: Idiopathic recurrent branch retinal arery occlusion: Natural history and laboratory evaluation. *Ophthalmology* 118:393, 1994.

125. Opeskin K. Traumatic carotid artery dissection. *Am J For Med Pathol* 18:251, 1997.

126. Treiman GS, Treiman RL, Foran RF, et al: Spontaneous dissection of the internal carotid artery: A nineteen-year clinical experience. *J Vasc Surg* 24:597, 1996.

127. Karacagil S, Hardemark HG, Bergqvist D: Spontaneous internal carotid artery dissection. *Int Angiol* 15:291, 1996.

128. Cullom RD Jr, Cullom ME, Kardon R, et al: Two neuro-ophthalmic episodes separated in time and space. *Surv Ophthalmol* 40:217, 1995.

129. Leys D, Lucas C, Gobert M, Deklunder G, Pruvo JP: Cervical artery dissections. *Eur Neurol* 37:3, 1997.

130. Mokri B, Silbert PL, Schievink WI, et al: Cranial nerve palsy in spontaneous dissection of the extracranial internal carotid artery. *Neurology* 46:356, 1996.

131. Hicks PA, Leavitt JA, Mokri B: Ophthalmic manifestations of vertebral artery dissection. *Ophthalmology* 101:1786, 1994.

132. Bogousslavsky J, Maeder P, Regli F, et al: Pure midbrain infarction: Clinical syndromes, MRI, and etiologic patterns. *Neurology* 44:2032, 1994.

133. Martin TJ, Corbett JJ, Babikian PV, et al: Bilateral ptosis due to mesencephalic lesions with relative preservation of ocular motility. *J Neuro-Ophthalmol* 16:258, 1996.

134. Bassetti C, Bogousslavsky J, Barth A, et al: Isolated infarcts of the pons. *Neurology* 46:165, 1996.

135. Yasuda Y, Matsuda I, Namura S, Biousse V, Mendocino MA, Simon DJ, et al: The ophthalmology of intracranial vascular abnormalities. *Am J Ophthalmol* 125:527, 1998.

136. Shults WT: Intracranial aneurysms. *Ophthalmol Clin North Am* 5:475, 1992.

137. Weinberg DA: Negative MRI versus real disease. *Surv Ophthalmol* 40:312, 1996.

138. North American Symptomatic Carotid Endarterectomy Trial Collaborators: Beneficial effect of carotid endarterectomy in symptomatic paients with high grade carotid stenosis. *N Engl J Med* 325:445, 1991.

139. Barnett HJM, Taylor DW, Eliaszw M, et al: Benefit of carotid endarterectomy in patients with symptomatic moderate or severe stenosis. *N Engl J Med* 339:1415, 1998.

140. European Carotid Surgery Trialists' Collaborative Group: Endarterectomy for moderate symptomatic carotid stenosis: Interim results from the MRC European Carotid Surgery Trial. *Lancet* 347:1591, 1996.

141. Parsons-Smith G: Sudden blindness in cranial arteritis. *Br J Ophthalmol* 43:204, 1959.

142. Model DG: Reversal of blindness in temporal arteritis with methylprednisolone (Letter). *Lancet* 1:340, 1978.

143. Matzkin DC, Slamovits TL, Sachs R, et al: Visual recovery in two patients after intravenous methylprednisolone treatment of central retinal artery occlusion secondary to giant cell arteritis. *Ophthalmology* 99:68, 1992.

144. Cornblath WT, Eggenberger ER: Progressive visual loss from giant cell arteritis despite high-dose intravenous methylprednisolone. *Ophthalmology* 104:854, 1997.

145. Swannell AJ: Fortnightly Review: Polymyalgia rheumatica and temporal arteritis: Diagnosis and management. *Br Med J* 314:1329, 1997.

146. Nesher G, Sonnenblick M, Friedlander Y: Analysis of steroid related complications and mortality in temporal arteritis: A 15 year survey of 43 patients. *J Rheum* 21:1283, 1994.

Chapter 32

BIOETHICAL PRINCIPLES AND STROKE MANAGEMENT

Andrei V. Alexandrov
James C. Grotta
Stanley J. Reiser

INTRODUCTION

Ethics is a discipline that examines human actions to determine their rightness and wrongness.[1-3] In Western medicine, its most significant early documents were produced by Hippocrates and his disciples from the 5th through 3rd centuries BC. Their most influential document, the Hippocratic Oath, defined essential ethical yardsticks by which to examine the actions of physicians. The most crucial end toward which these yardsticks were directed was allowing patients to place themselves in the hands of a physician, who often was a stranger to them, and trust that they would be benefited and not harmed by the encounter. Proliferation of medical ethics explorations occurred after World War II because of the growth of medical science, new technologic innovations, and the civil and women's rights movements. A significant growth in differential access to care as a result of the federal government's regulations, Medicare and Medicaid legislation produced many ethical controversies including allocation of scarce resources, availability of kidney dialysis and organ transplant, etc. Also, the right to determine who could act on one's own body, participation in human experimentation, and the control over life and death including abortion and end of life problems are a few highlights of ethical problems in modern medicine. Analyses of the ethical issues concerning cardiopulmonary resuscitation (CPR) or caring for an elderly or a dying patient are available,[2,3] but they generally lack a disease-specific approach particular to stroke.[4] It is surprising, considering the prevalence and burden of this disease and the recent proliferation of life-sustaining technologies, vascular interventions, and pharmacologic research, that ethical issues in stroke management have received little attention.[5]

Many beliefs regarding stroke are not evidence-based, which results in variable stroke management practices. Meanwhile, the public lacks essential knowledge about stroke, and patient access to health care differs among hospitals, medical systems, and countries. The goal of this paper is to identify situations in which ethical problems may arise while caring for a patient with a stroke. Ethical problems arise when two or more ethical values come into conflict. The complexity of clinical problems, often insufficient research data, and wide individual variability of situations preclude simplistic prescriptions in dealing with ethical conflicts. We will examine bioethical principles and clinical situations when health professionals have to choose between different obligations.

PRINCIPLES OF BIOMEDICAL ETHICS

The modern medical ethics movement that began in the United States in the middle of the twentieth century derived its power in part from the civil and women's rights movements of that time. These movements were focused on asserting and defining a set of rights that allowed individuals to assert a sovereignty over themselves and to ask society for fair and equal treatment in respect to opportunities for economic and social advancements and claims on social resources. The ethical values common to the civil rights that influenced the medical ethics movement were the values of autonomy or the right to be self-governing and justice or the right to be treated similarly or fairly when it came to the need for medical care. The new medical ethics focused, therefore, on providing patients with authority for self-action and decision. However, it is linked to the older medical ethics, which were focused on ethical character traits of the physician. The physician demonstrates a fundamental respect for the patient (an ethical character trait) by honoring the patient's rights to be treated fairly and as an autonomous person.

Of the Hippocratic ethics defining the behaviors that enabled patients to place their trust in physicians, those first stated in the Hippocratic Oath have had a particularly lasting and crucial influence on medical practice: "I will use treatment to help the sick according to my ability and judgement, but never with a view to injury or wrong doing." (FN Jones, v.1, p.289) In this sentence are the polar ethical opposites that all physicians must balance in making practice decision: the benefits and harms of the therapies they use. From this sentence is derived for medicine the ethical principles of benefit or beneficence and the do no harm or nonmaleficence.

Contemporary medical ethicists[1] often single out the do no harm, benefit, justice, and autonomy principles as the most significant ones in making medical decisions. We will explore these four bioethical concepts as they apply to stroke and then show how their use can help clinicians make choices.

Principle of Respect for Autonomy

The autonomous person acts in accordance with a freely self-chosen and informed plan. To respect an autonomous person requires recognition of the person's capacities and perspectives and to treat the patient as to enable him to act autonomously. A key element to this principle is to disclose information in a way that the patient can understand and consent to one of the choices given. Recognition and honoring the value of autonomy is also to acknowledge the distinction between physicians and patients in respect to knowledge. The knowledge of the physician is basically about how diseases affect populations. Physicians study medical texts describing the typical course that a given illness takes in a given population. They read in journals about how a particular therapy affected a particular and large group of people and internalize this knowledge as sets of statistical probabili-

ties in respect to how an individual may fare if given this therapy. In contrast, the knowledge of the patient is greatest about self. The patient has had a long time to understand the needs and reactions of self. When it comes to who he or she is, the patient is an expert. The autonomy principle in medicine is a reminder that for the best care, two sets of knowledge should be joined— that of the patient as a unique being and that of the typical responses to illness and therapy that the population of which the patient is part of generally displays. The principle of respect for autonomy represents a declaration to physicians and patients that they are partners in the healing enterprise. Each partner has important knowledge to give. Each has the prerogative not to honor requests that go against their beliefs. Each partner has responsibilities to bear in the fight against illness they share. Each is an individual but should recognize that the closer and more open and respectful they are of the other, the more likely that their joint effort will prove successful.

Honoring the principle of autonomy gives individuals significant say in what happens to them therapeutically. Historically, certain limits have been placed on this right to autonomy. Autonomy should be granted to individuals who are legally empowered to make choices about themselves and also who have the mental capacity to exercise such choices competently. This does not mean that those under the age of 18 have no ethical claim to being heard but that being under legal age limits the power of the claim. The issue of whether a patient is capable of making choices is sometimes a clinically difficult judgment. It can be approached, not necessarily in absolute but relative terms, by factoring in the significance and consequences to the individual of the choice being discussed. Documenting that the patient understands the situation and agrees to the care in question is provided through the informed consent process, which we discuss below.

Information about stroke, its potential consequences to the patient, particular mechanism, and potential risks/benefits of treatment should be ascertained individually and disclosed appropriately.[4,7] Uncertainty often arises from different opinions regarding the effectiveness of therapeutic or management options and shortcomings in existing clinical trials or outcome data, which need to be applied to the individual patient. Despite many years of stroke research, there are still areas where the basis for clinical judgment lacks precision, and only vague information can be offered to the patient. Therefore, health professionals are primarily responsible for the quality of information and the way it is provided to the patient.[4,7] This aspect of professional ethics points to the need for specialized in-depth knowledge of stroke diagnosis and management for health professionals caring for stroke patients.

To handle the information, the patient must be competent. The criteria for an autonomous and competent person are very similar: a competent person is able to understand a therapy or procedure, to deliberate regarding major risks and benefits, and then make a decision regarding this deliberation.[1,8] Inadequate understanding by a patient may prevent any meaningful choice and thus diminish the autonomy. This situation is common in patients with stroke who are often incapable of informed decision making and may require a substitute decision on their behalf. For example, only 8 percent of patients with severe stroke were capable of decision making regarding the Do-Not-Resuscitate (DNR) order.[4] The determination of competence is not always easy. The modified mini-mental status exam can be used as a screening tool in determining competence to sign an informed consent.

Principle of Nonmaleficence, or Do No Harm

According to the Hippocratic Oath, not harming and helping patients were equally worthy medical objectives. The "do no harm" principle morally requires health professionals to strive to serve the well being of their patients and sets the standards of due care, risk-benefit, and detriment-benefit assessments.[9] Maximizing efforts toward patient well being is the goal that, for stroke patients, often means a recovery for the acquired deficit. The first hours after stroke onset provide an opportunity to restore brain perfusion to salvageable tissues. The standard of due care refers directly to therapies such as thrombolysis, by which there is an obvious conflict with the principle of not imposing risks of harm as well as not inflicting actual harms. Any current thrombolytic therapy for ischemic stroke bears a significant risk of intracerebral hemorrhage (ICH). This requires that the benefit of the therapy should outweigh the possible harms. In case of thrombolysis, a considerable chance for a complete recovery may outweigh the risk of devastating ICH, provided that the initial ischemic insult is of sufficient degree with debilitating consequences if left untreated. The risk-benefit ratio of intravenous thrombolytic therapy has been studied in randomized trials, and the risk of ICH depends on patient selection, treatment agent, dosage, time delays, and blood pressure management.[10]

Also progressive stroke, brain edema, reperfusion injury, and systemic complications impede recovery. If a patient arrives beyond the limited time for potentially reversing the damage with thrombolysis, this delayed admission should not preclude efforts to improve the patient's condition (i.e., adequate diagnostic workup, early and intensive rehabilitation, treatment of systemic complications, and secondary stroke prevention). For example, anticoagulation with heparin bears a risk of hemorrhagic conversion, which is real but difficult to predict while the benefit remains unclear.[11,12] Invasive procedure such as digital subtraction angiography (DSA) may cause stroke and death in 1 percent of patients, whereas benefits include diagnosis of the arterial pathology and better opportunity for recanalization after intra-arterial thrombolysis with urokinase.[13] In patients with hemorrhagic strokes, surgical interventions are associated with the risk of death, whereas the benefit of ICH evacuation has not yet been proven effective in a randomized trial, and treatment selection is often physician-dependent.

Although the risk of harm may seem disproportionately high to a potential benefit from a physician's point of view, a competent patient concerned about living with handicap may evaluate this situation very differently. It is critical to understand, however, that because the physician is a participant in the therapy being administered, the doctor must believe the risk/benefit ratio is acceptable enough for him or her to act. It is not enough for the patient to desire the therapy, if the physician believes it is inappropriate. Both must agree before a medical action can take place. An unresolvable disagreement between doctor and patient on this issue is an indication that a change of physicians may be warranted.

Principle of Beneficence

It may seem obvious that the reason to administer a therapy is to seek a benefit. But defining the meaning of benefit is sometimes difficult. One should first ask, benefit from whose perspective? As noted above, what seems a benefit to a patient may not seem one to a physician, and vice versa. Similarly, the ethical obligation to confer a benefit through therapy on a patient requires the physician to conduct research on the therapy and to demonstrate scientifically and precisely the nature of the possible benefits. Therefore, it is imperative to consider a treatment's chance of success and then to balance its probable benefits against its costs and risks to the patient.

Using intervention with recombinant tissue-type plasminogen activator (rt-PA) as an example, to ensure informed decision making, patients first should be provided with correct facts and unbiased information regarding the therapy.[10,14-16] This is followed by a professional recommendation, which may vary according to individual physician beliefs,[17,18] and the patient should be allowed to choose from available options. Both over-enthusiastic endorsement of rt-PA as a panacea for stroke and nihilistic discarding of this therapy are ethically incorrect. The key to safe and effective intravenous rt-PA therapy is appropriate patient selection according to the NINDS rt-PA Stroke Study protocol, which is aimed to minimize the risks and maximize possible benefits of thrombolysis.[19]

The majority of day-to-day decisions in all stroke patients, however, have to be made regarding blood pressure management, secondary stroke prevention, prevention of systemic complications, mechanical ventilation, rehabilitation, and discharge. It is often difficult for physicians and family to accept the fact that a patient surviving a few days following a severe stroke with inevitably fatal brain damage will not benefit from mechanical ventilation. One of the major problems lies in the uncertain prognosis in a substantial number of stroke patients, as well as vague criteria for futility of life-sustaining interventions. Thus, knowledge of stroke prognosis, the effectiveness of therapies, and the futility of life-sustaining interventions is necessary to justify any management strategy.

Principle of Justice

The weighing of alternatives involving risks, costs, and benefits is typical in circumstances of distributive justice, and several therapies for stroke and stroke prevention have been subjected to such scrutiny.[20-22] Another issue pertinent to stroke care in particular is the differential access to health care according to the patient's insurance plan (i.e., health maintenance organization (HMO), Medicare, self-paid, or nonresource). Health insurance inequality may affect the choice of a hospital, therapy, and rehabilitation and as yet has not been studied in stroke patients. In many hospitals, only fundamental needs of stroke patients such as nutrition, nursing, and life-sustaining measures are provided, whereas a neurologic consultation and a CT scan are often delayed for days along with administration of preventative medication, if any. Should this approach be considered ethical

in view of the advances made in early stroke diagnosis, treatment, and rehabilitation?

Another common situation is the race to reduce the length of hospital stay (LOHS) because of limited or "equal" reimbursement under diagnosis-related groups (DRG). Because stroke is a complex syndrome with different pathogenic mechanisms and is associated with several systemic complications, no rationale besides cost containment exists behind short LOHS under DRG for *all* stroke patients. If stroke management has to be individualized to achieve maximum benefit, the pressure on physicians to discharge stroke patients earlier without parallel changes in hospital services is not ethically sound. In this context, is a specialized stroke unit[23] an expensive and unjustified decoration?

Stroke patients face irreversible brain damage if not urgently treated. Recognition must be paid to the fact that stroke is a medical emergency similar to heart attack and trauma. Therefore, urgent access to emergency room, CT scan, neurologic consult, and early therapy for all stroke patients, regardless of economic status, should be an urgent social and medical objective.

APPLICATION OF ETHICAL PRINCIPLES TO STROKE MANAGEMENT

Issues in Access to Health Care

Patients who suffer a stroke should be able to gain urgent access to health care by calling 911 and securing direct admission to a hospital. Upon arrival at the hospital, the patient should be allowed emergent neurologic examination and a noncontrast CT scan of the head. Depending on the results of the urgent evaluation, emergency interventions for brain rescue may be appropriate. In some circumstances, there are roadblocks to this algorithm. A patient may need to get permission from a primary care physician or HMO preapproval prior to admission or initiation of therapy. This requirement by some health insurance policies creates an ethical conflict, as time delay limits reversibility of brain damage and decreases the chance of a patient to benefit from treatment.

Although often unrecognized, an ethical conflict also arises when patient registration and allocation are given priority by ER staff over immediate neurologic assessment, resulting in delayed diagnostic workup and initiation of urgent stroke treatment. The sequence of actions should be prioritized toward consults and tests that primarily determine patient diagnosis, fitting in other tests such as chest x-ray, ECG, etc. when feasible. Urgent access to CT scan should be granted to stroke patients by hospital policy and admission protocols on the same basis as for head trauma patients.

Gender and access-to-care issues may be important determinants of delay in acute stroke care.[24] Time for presentation to the hospital and to a neurologic consultation may be affected by several factors including gender, ethnicity, ambulance transport, access to primary care, as well as stroke severity and type. Time for presentation to the hospital decreases with ambulance transport and increases in patients with a primary care physician and in women. Time to a neurologic consult is decreased with ambulance arrival and hemorrhagic stroke.[24] To improve patient arrival time to the hospital and prompt neurologic evaluation, attention must be paid to factors beyond recognizing stroke warning signs and calling 911.[24] Delayed access to health care means violation of the do no harm principle as well as beneficence and justice.

Access to Tissue Plasminogen Activator Therapy

Patients who arrive within the first 3 h of ischemic stroke are potentially eligible for intravenous rt-PA therapy. Ability to benefit the patient decreases if time delays occur between arrival and informed decision to receive rt-PA due to reasons such as unavailability of staff to perform CT when the scanner is available, etc. It is the responsibility of health care providers including hospital administration, nursing staff, and technical personnel to have alert systems and clinical pathways developed to ensure adequate clinical and diagnostic workup of an acute stroke patient. Failure to establish diagnosis and to provide timely treatment will violate the do no harm principle, as the opportunity to reverse the damage will be lost.

Another ethical issue arises when a patient who meets the criteria for intravenous rt-PA therapy after adequate diagnostic workup is not offered rt-PA because of physician beliefs that rt-PA therapy is more harmful than beneficial.[18] We think the patient should be *unbiasly* informed of the *data* from the NINDS rt-PA Stroke Study regarding this FDA-approved therapy for stroke, which may then be followed by the physician's recommendation, which may be for or against rt-PA based on the physician's beliefs.[18] For example, the following two statements regarding potential risks and

benefits of rt-PA will have a different impact on patient decision making:

1. In the NINDS trial, 20 percent of patients recovered with no or minimal deficit at 3 months without rt-PA, and 11 percent more did so after rt-PA was given. The risk of worsening due to bleeding to the brain was 6.4 percent after rt-PA compared with 0.6 percent without clot busting.

2. In the NINDS trial, 50 percent more patients recovered with no or minimal deficit at 3 months after rt-PA compared with controls, whereas the risk of worsening from bleeding to the brain was 10 times higher with rt-PA.

We believe that actual data and not the relative figures should be presented to a patient or family. Also, it needs to be mentioned that despite a greater likelihood of bleeding, there is no increase in risk of severe disability and death after treatment.

Inability to provide intravenous rt-PA in a given hospital also violates bioethical principles and represents a separate issue deserving attention of health care providers and community.

An ethical dilemma also exists when the decision to receive rt-PA is being made. It refers to the risk of symptomatic ICH as a complication and requires careful weighing of potential benefits and risks. Physicians must ensure that the patient or decision maker is competent and an informed decision takes place. If the patient is incompetent, a substitute decision-maker, or proxy, needs to be urgently identified. Family members may not realize the urgency and catastrophic consequences of stroke and may replace the patient's preferences with their own. Finally, if no substitutes are available for a competent patient, the decision must be made by a physician in the patient's best interests. Once again, the urgency of the situation and stroke sequelae may justify a risk benefit ratio that is unacceptable with elective procedures. Intravenous rt-PA therapy is being further developed by exploring longer time windows, lower dosages, and a combination of intra-arterial thrombolysis with neuroprotective agents. More information on stroke pathogenesis within the first hours as well as predictors of complications are indeed necessary to establish the risk/benefit ratio of reperfusion therapies more precisely.[17,18]

Issues in Hemorrhagic Stroke

Patients who are diagnosed with hemorrhagic stroke on CT scan have a different perspective for treatment.

Patients with subarachnoid hemorrhage (SAH) have to undergo DSA to find the aneurysm for possible surgical clipping or endovascular coiling. Ethical issues in SAH management deserve a separate analysis, which is beyond the scope of this chapter. Patients who have primary intracerebral hemorrhage represent a clinical and ethical dilemma partly attributable to the lack of randomized trials comparing conservative therapy with surgical removal of the hematoma. Although surgeons prefer to operate on alert and significantly disabled patients with lesions in the nondominant hemisphere,[4] the risk-to-benefit ratio for surgical intervention is difficult to estimate. Like in patients with ischemic stroke, the issues of time delays and access to specialized neurosurgical and neurocritical care are most important to avoid violation of ethical principles of do no harm and justice.

Issues in Life-Sustaining Therapy

Proliferation of medical technology allows maintenance of living functions in patients with severe stroke. Such commonly used interventions include mechanical ventilation and CPR. Both interventions have not been systematically studied in stroke patients, and multicenter trials are lacking. Evidence derived from relatively small series of patients indicates that although stroke patients requiring intubation generally have poor prognosis, in-hospital survival can be achieved in 20 percent of patients after elective intubation[25] and in 8 percent of all intubated patients at 1 year.[26] However, the issue of quality of life after recovery from severe stroke and intubation remains unexplored. Patients may view permanent hemiplegia worse than death,[27] and therefore, their preferences may not necessarily be toward aggressive maintenance of living functions. In order not to violate the principle of autonomy, patient preferences have to be unbiasly established whenever possible. Usually, specific discussions with a proxy or relatives need to take place because patients with severe stroke are often incompetent. Also, the complications of life-sustaining interventions must be weighed against possible benefit from this perspective to satisfy the do no harm and beneficence principles.

No survivors were documented in three studies after in-hospital CPR in 46 patients suffering cardiac arrest after stroke (0–7.7 percent, 95 percent confidence intervals).[28,29] Undoubtedly, CPR may have immediate but temporary success in restoring life functions of stroke patients, and patient wishes should be paramount in decisions regarding CPR. A group of stroke neurologists regarded CPR futile in patients with severe stroke,

life-theatening brain damage, and/or significant comorbidities but suggested CPR as potentially appropriate in patients with minor or brainstem strokes with no significant comorbidities[7] (also see Appendix). Physicians should not have absolute power to withhold CPR against patient wishes, and information should be shared between all parties involved in decision making. A mechanism of recommending not to attempt CPR is called the DNR order.

Issues in DNR Orders

The DNR orders are commonplace in patients with stroke. As many as 31 percent of consecutive patients with ischemic and hemorrhagic strokes received a DNR order, and 83 percent of these patients died.[4] DNR orders were related to stroke severity, incompetency, advanced age, and conservative management of patients with ICH.[4] General guidelines for DNR orders suggested by the American Medical Association lack a disease-specific approach, and the criteria for DNR orders particular to acute stroke were recently developed.[7] These criteria include the definition of severe stroke, life-threatening brain damage, and significant comorbidities (Appendix). A consensus among 26 stroke neurologists was reached that in patients who meet at least two of these criteria, a DNR order is appropriate, and this information should be shared among physician(s), patient, and family.[7] Other reviewers suggested that the proposed criteria should be taken into consideration along with individual, professional, and societal differences in values[30] and moved into clinical practice through wider discussions among neurologists, hospitals, and legislatures.[30,31]

A DNR order is often wrongly associated with patient abandonment and discontinuation of treatment and life support.[4,31] Ethical problems may arise when stroke outcome is difficult to predict; when physicians "give up" striving to ensure survival (anticipated poor quality of life), and when the patient is incompetent.[5] Patient condition may be exacerbated by infection, seizures, or metabolic disorders, which often may be successfully treated or prevented.[5] Another common dilemma is whether or not to give fluids in a patient with a severe stroke who is unable to swallow. It was suggested that intravenous fluids, feeding with nasogastric tubes, and antibiotics may not be necessary and may not prolong life in unconscious patients and should not be continued long term.[5] Leaving aside the legal aspects of these actions, artificial feeding and prevention of painful infections has a powerful symbolic act of comfort care rather than medical intervention.[31] Under the principle of autonomy, death with dignity is an appropriate exit if fatal outcome is unavoidable and thus providing dignified care is the only acceptable solution.

Treatment limitation and avoidance of CPR are best achieved by ongoing and frank communication (ideally based on reliable prognostic data) in relationship to goals set among physician, patient, and family.[31] Physicians must be prepared to discuss these issues and negotiate when facing both medical uncertainty and inevitable plurality of values and their conflict.[31] Therefore, physicians and nurses are primarily responsible for the quality of information regarding stroke prognosis and the way it is presented to the patient and family.[7]

Issues in Compassionate Care

Not all interventions to reverse brain damage have been conclusively tested in clinical trials, and not all of them can be tested. Uncertainty begins with questions regarding optimal blood pressure management, indications, benefits and risks for intra-arterial thrombolysis, early anticoagulation, etc. Sometimes physicians, patients, and families are inclined to pursue the most aggressive plan and go beyond the current standards of therapy.[32]

After obtaining approval from our committee for the protection of human subjects and informed consent, the Stroke Team at the University of Texas–Houston has treated several patients using strategies not yet proven effective in clinical trials. These therapies and interventions were presented to patients or family as experimental procedures. For instance, intra-arterial thrombolysis, surgical decompression, and hypothermia were offered compassionately to patients with severe and inevitably devastating stroke admitted beyond the window for intravenous rt-PA. It was assumed that a risky procedure may have potential benefit to the patient based on experimental data, anecdotal successful case reports, or preliminary data from randomized trials. For example, patients with locked-in syndrome and proven basilar artery occlusion who present within the first 3 to 10 h after stroke onset received intra-arterial thrombolysis with urokinase. Although benefit was seen in only a few of these patients, the devastating consequences of remaining locked-in made even a 1 in 50 chance of improvement worth taking the risks from the patient's perspective.

The need to employ treatment with uncertain risk benefit ratio is common in stroke care. Ethical considerations should incorporate the patient's perspective expressed as prior wishes, preferences, or best interests when the possibility of helping the patient being treated, as well as current preferences, is not known. Such therapy may be justified by the goal that future patients may benefit from the experience gained through performing a new procedure or testing a new treatment in a randomized trial.

Issues in Randomized Stroke Trials

The rationale to use a randomized controlled trial (RCT) is to demonstrate the effectiveness and safety of a treatment over placebo. Before beginning an RCT, two ethical questions must be addressed. First, is the RCT as essential as the proponents say, and second, can it be used without compromising the physicians' responsibilities to their patients.[1] To avoid ethical problems, informed consent should disclose the goals of the RCT, currently available treatment options, and preliminary evidence for safety and efficacy of the proposed treatment. An RCT comparing a putative therapy with placebo is usually used in circumstances when there is genuine doubt about the merits of existing, standard, or new therapies under the promise that future patients will benefit from tested therapy and knowledge gained.

FDA approval of intravenous rt-PA as the first effective therapy for selected patients with ischemic stroke imposes a dilemma. Is it ethical to randomize rt-PA eligible patients to placebo to test an alternative reperfusion strategy or other treatment to reverse brain damage? After FDA approval in 1996, several RCTs continued to randomize patients within the first 3 h to placebo, whereas others allowed for a subgroup to be treated with rt-PA in combination with the study medication.

Those who consider randomization of stroke patients to placebo ethical indicate that rt-PA therapy is not universally accepted, the risk of symptomatic ICH may be viewed as too high compared with potential benefit, and a subgroup of patients who particularly benefit from rt-PA has not been identified. Moreover, a recent bioethical analysis indicated that no thrombolytic regimen tested so far has met all five justification criteria including safety, efficacy, effectiveness, efficiency, and outcome.[33] These criteria were derived from the ethical rules of proportionality (risk-benefit-cost) and informed consent. Major criticism of intravenous rt-PA therapy were potential variability of risk-benefit-cost ratios between physicians and patient subgroups, as well as the lack of evidence for the effectiveness and cost effectiveness of rt-PA outside of the NINDS trial.[33] Since the analysis was published, both effectiveness and cost-effectiveness studies were published.[14,15,20] Although the NINDS protocol may keep the rate of symptomatic ICH relatively low, reliable predictors of this complication are still lacking.

Those who consider randomization to placebo unethical indicate that benefit from rt-PA was seen in all subroups of eligible patients including large-vessel atherosclerosis, small vessel, and cardioembolic stroke as well as patients with advanced age, severe stroke, and early ischemic changes on CT scan.[10] Furthermore, the risk-to-benefit ratio for intravenous rt-PA takes into account complication rates, and the experience has been replicated in settings outside RCT.[14,15] Therefore, the question "Is it worth it?" and "Are benefits proportional to risk?"[33] may be positively answered by patients fearing disability more than the risk of bleeding.

In our opinion, patients who are eligible for rt-PA should receive unbiased information regarding the risks and benefits as well as information regarding other options (i.e., to participate in RCTs of new medications, including placebo-controlled trials). Patients who may reject rt-PA as unacceptably risky treatment may choose to participate in RCTs offering potentially safer alternative treatment. Patients eligible for rt-PA may be included into trials combining rt-PA with intra-arterial thrombolysis or neuroprotective agents. Patients who are ineligible for rt-PA or admitted beyond the first 3 h are, perhaps, the target population for new RCTs in ischemic stroke. Nevertheless, patient consent is often determined not only by the data presented but by the professional recommendation given regarding the available options.

Concern has been expressed regarding the ethics of phase 1 clinical studies that offer no therapeutic benefit to the patient and variable standards of care for a control group in RCTs.[34] Institutional review boards (IRB) should consider acute stroke patients as a "vulnerable population" and impose additional safeguards appropriate to the nature of RCTs (i.e., disclosure of timing of treatment, risk/benefit assessment, dose escalation monitoring).[34]

The attempts to find new and better treatments for stroke should continue. IRBs generally provide special consideration and additional protection to human subjects enrolled in the early phase toxicity studies.[35] Choosing to do nothing exposes the patients to well-known risks and no benefit, whereas development of new therapies exposes patients to uncertain risks along with possible benefits.[36] Indeed, a patient enrolled in the early phase studies may not experience any benefit.

However, these data may help to ascertain the risks and carefully plan future RCTs. By way of example, a lower rt-PA dosing schedule and blood pressure management protocol were established in the early phase trials prior to the NINDS-rt-PA Stroke Study. Future patients will benefit from a safe and effective treatment emerging from RCTs. This goal is worthy from a perspective of the entire human race, and current methods are ethically sound.

Finally, the ethical standards of clinical research should be rigorously maintained. At the same time, the effort of a large number of physicians, nurses, government agencies, and pharmaceutical companies should be acknowledged as well as the courage of patients and families who participate in these studies.[36]

CONCLUSIONS

As we have shown, the following problems in stroke care have direct ethical implications for all participants:

1. Lack of recognition of stroke as a medical emergency;

2. Inconsistent application of stroke therapies;

3. Shortcomings in clinical trials and outcome data;

4. Differences in care for a dying patient; and

5. Cost-containment and technologic advances.

It is the physician's responsibility to use the best knowledge and to approach each patient's problems individually. Examination of these ethical issues reveals that many problems remain unsolved in stroke management.

APPENDIX

Disease-Specific Criteria for Do Not Resuscitate Orders in Acute Stroke

These criteria supplement general DNR policies to aid the specific use of DNR orders in patients during the first 2 weeks after a stroke (modified from Ref. 7).

Background

Patients suffering acute stroke are facing the irreversibility of the neuronal damage if treatment is delayed. Controversial clinical attitudes toward stroke are partly grounded in effective interventions to prevent death but as yet limited effectiveness of treatment of brain damage to reduce subsequent disability. The unexpectedness of stroke and difficulties with prognosis complicate decision making.

The early mortality rate following stroke is high mainly due to brain swelling and herniation during the first week and from systemic complications thereafter.

Consent should be obtained for the use of CPR and mechanical ventilation as a treatment option. A DNR order is a secondary action that occurs after the decision not to perform CPR is made.

Ethics

Physicians and nurses are primarily responsible for the quality of information concerning stroke prognosis and the way it is presented to the patient and family. The final decision about resuscitation should be made by an informed patient (when possible) or an appropriate surrogate. Acute stroke patients are often incapable of participating in discussions regarding CPR as a result of aphasia, dementia, and impaired consciousness, thus being unable to understand and appreciate the nature and consequences of CPR. Therefore, the choice of an informed substitute increases the physician's responsibility. The decision must be made irrespective of the patient's age and according to the patient's expressed preferences or best interest (when preferences are not known).

Applicability and Institutional Issues

These criteria, suggested for patients with ischemic stroke and intracerebral hemorrhage, should be updated regularly and may be modified if new treatment strategies prove effective in severe stroke.

The criteria apply mainly to the acute phase of stroke (the first 2 weeks); general DNR policies are also applicable during and after this time.

The criteria are intended to supplement, not replace, existing DNR policies in institutions. Staff should be informed of the issues identified.

Team Issues and Management

Nurses should be informed of the prognosis and patient's preferences and best interests.

If the attending physician has doubts, it is prudent to wait and obtain a second opinion from another physician.

A DNR order should not be interpreted as a decision to discontinue patient care and treatment. The appropriateness of any treatment and nutrition should be evaluated on its own merits.

General Considerations

Dying is a natural process. An intervention is futile if it prolongs dying and brings discomfort but no improvement (i.e., if it does not alter the fatal outcome and is of no benefit). Such intervention may also be considered harmful as the risk of systemic complications of subacute stroke is high in severely disabled survivors.

Stroke is an unexpected and often irreversible event. However, warning signs (e.g., transient ischemic attack) are common, and because the major risk factor for stroke is stroke itself, prior discussions and advance directives regarding the patient's preferences on resuscitation should be encouraged.

Unless requested, CPR and mechanical ventilation should not be recommended as treatment options in patients with severe stroke, as these are often futile or not in the best interests of these patients. CPR may be appropriate in patients with minor and brainstem strokes with no significant comorbidities.

Clinical Criteria for DNR Orders

A DNR order may be written any time that two of the following clinical criteria are present and the prognosis has become clear and shared whenever possible among physician(s), patient, and family (or appropriate surrogate).

1. *Severe stroke.* Clinically, severe stroke produces persisting (more than 24 h) and sometimes deteriorating neurologic deficit, often with early impairment of consciousness leading to total dependency of the patient in activities of daily living. The patient must have little or no active movement on at least one side of the body, with impaired consciousness, global aphasia, or lack of response indicating cognition (NIH Stroke Scale Score >20, Glasgow Coma Scale score of <9, Canadian Neurologic scale score of <5.0).

2. *Life-threatening brain damage.* Life-threatening brain damage is associated with brain stem compression caused by large intracerebral hemorrhage usually with intraventricular extension, large hemispheric infarction with midline shift, infratentorial strokes involving multiple levels in the brain stem, or cerebellar le-

sions. Fatal outcome in acute stroke is associated with lesion volume >400 mL, septum pellucidum displacement >9 mm, or pineal gland displacement >4 mm. If any of these is present within 48 h, patients have a low probability of survival (OR 0.16; CI 0 to 0.32; specificity 89 percent, sensitivity 46 percent).[37]

3. *Significant comorbidities.* The following non-neurologic conditions are important risk factors for death within the first month after stroke: pneumonia, pulmonary embolism, sepsis, recent myocardial infarction, cardiomyopathy, and life-threatening arrhythmias. These comborbid factors should be considered part of the expected consequences of severe stroke pointing to an increased likelihood of death in the subacute phase of stroke.

REFERENCES

1. Beauchamp TL, Childress JF: *Principles of Biomedical Ethics.* New York, Oxford University Press, 1989.
2. Graber GC, Beasley AD, Eaddy JA: *Ethical Analysis of Clinical Medicine: A Guide to Self-Evaluation.* Baltimore, Urban & Schwarzenberg, 1985.
3. Gillon R (ed): *Principles of Health Care Ethics.* Chichester, John Wiley & Sons, 1994.
4. Alexandrov AV, Bladin CF, Meslin EM, Norris JW: Do-not-resuscitate orders in acute stroke. *Neurology* 45:634, 1995.
5. Warlow CP, Dennis MS, Van Gijn J, et al: *Stroke: A practical Guide to Management.* Oxford, Blackwell Science, 1996.
6. American Hospital Association (AHA): Statement of a patient's bill of rights. *Hospitals* 47:41, 1973.
7. Alexandrov AV, Pullicino PM, Meslin EM, Norris JW: Agreement of the disease-specific criteria for do-not-resuscitate orders in acute stroke. *Stroke* 27:232, 1996.
8. Applebaum PS, Lidz CW, Meisel A: *Informed Consent: Legal Theory and Clinical Practice.* New York, Oxford University Press, 1987.
9. Jonsen AR: Do no harm axiom in medical ethics, in Spicker SF, Englehardt HT (eds): *Philosophical and Medical Ethics: Its Nature and Significance.* Dorddecht, D. Reidel, 1977, pp 27–41.
10. NINDS rt-PA Stroke Study Group: Tissue plasminogen activator for acute ischemic stroke. *N Engl J Med* 333:1581, 1995.
11. Cerebral Embolism Study Group: Immediate anticoagulation of embolic stroke: Brain hemorrhage and management options. *Stroke* 15:779, 1984.
12. International Stroke Trial Collaborative Group: The International Stroke Trial (IST): A randomized trial of aspirin, subcutaneous heparin, both, or neither among 19,435 patients with acute ischemic stroke. *Lancet* 349:1569, 1997.
13. Del Zoppo GL, Higashida RT, Furlan AJ, et al: PROACT: A phase II randomized trial of recombinant pro-urokinase by direct arterial delivery in acute middle cerebral artery stroke. *Stroke* 29:4, 1998.
14. Chiu D, Krieger D, Villar-Cordova C, et al: Intravenous tissue plasminogen activator for acute ischemic stroke: Feasibility, safety, and efficacy in the first year of clinical practice. *Stroke* 29:18, 1998.
15. Tanne D, Mansbach HH, Verro P, et al: Intravenous rt-PA therapy for stroke in clinical practice: A multicenter evaluation of outcome (Abstract). *Stroke* 29:288, 1998.
16. Haley EC, Lewandowski C, Tilley BC: Myths regarding NINDS rt-PA Stroke Trial: Setting the record straight. *Ann Emerg Med* 30:676, 1997.
17. Grotta JC: T-PA: The best current option for most patients. *N Engl J Med* 337:1310, 1997.
18. Caplan LR, Mohr JP, Kistler JP, Koroshetz W: Thrombolysis: Not a panacea for ischemic stroke. *N Engl J Med* 337:1309, 1997.
19. NINDS rt-PA Stroke Study Group: A systems approach to immediate evaluation and management of hyperacute stroke: Experience at eight centers and implications for community practice and patient care. *Stroke* 28:1530, 1997.
20. Fagan SC, Morgenstern LB, Petitta A, et al: Cost-effectiveness of tissue plasminogen activator for acute ischemic stroke. *Neurology* 50:883, 1998.
21. Oster G, Huse DM, Lacey MJ, et al: Cost-effectiveness of ticlopidine in preventing stroke in high-risk patients. *Stroke* 25:1149, 1994.
22. Kraiss LW, Kilberg L, Critch S, Johansen DJ: Short-stay carotid endarterectomy is safe and cost-effective. *Am J Surg* 169:512, 1995.
23. Anonymous: Collaborative systematic review of the randomized trials of organized inpatient (stroke unit) care after stroke: Stroke Unit Trialists' Collaboration. *Br Med J* 314:1151, 1997.
24. Menon SC, Pandey DK, Morgenstern LB: Critical factors determining access to acute stroke care. *Neurology* 51:427, 1998.
25. Grotta JC, Pasteur W, Khwaja G, Hamel T, Fisher M, Ramirez A: Elective intubation for neurologic deterioration after stroke. *Neurology* 45:640, 1995.
26. Burtin P, Bollaert PE, Feldmann L, et al: Prognosis of stroke patients undergoing mechanical ventilation. *Intensive Care Med* 20:32, 1994.
27. Solomon NA, Glick HA, Russo CJ, Lee J, Schulman KA: Patient preferences for stroke outcomes. *Stroke* 25:1721, 1994.
28. Bedell SE, Delbanco TL, Cook EF, Epstein FH: Survival after cardioplumonary resuscitation in the hospital. *N Engl J Med* 309:569, 1983.
29. O'Keeffe STO, Lye M: DNR orders in acute stroke (Letter). *Lancet* 347:1415, 1996.

30. Plum F: Reversing the options in therapy for severely damaging stroke. *Neurol Alert* 14:61, 1996.

31. Cohen S, Germanishkis L: Agreement on disease-specific criteria for do-not-resuscitate orders in acute stroke, (Letter). *Stroke* 27:774, 1996.

32. Youngner SJ: Beyond DNR: Fine-tuning end-of-life decision-making. *Neurology* 45:615, 1995.

33. Furlan AJ, Kanoti G: When is thrombolysis justified in patients with acute ischemic stroke? A bioethical perspective. *Stroke* 28:214, 1997.

34. Styler H: Ethical challenges in stroke research. *Stroke* 29:1725, 1998.

35. Marler JR, Walker MD: Progress in acute stroke research. *Stroke* 29:1491, 1998.

36. Albers GW, Zivin JA, Choi DW: Ethical standards in phase 1 trials of neuroprotective agents for stroke therapy. *Stroke* 29;493, 1998.

37. Pullicino PM, Alexandrov AV, Shelton JA, et al: Mass effect and death from severe acute stroke. *Neurology* 49:1090, 1997.

Part 5
DIAGNOSTIC TESTING IN STROKE

Chapter 33

ULTRASOUND IMAGING IN CEREBROVASCULAR DISEASE

Edward G. Grant
Andre Duerinckx

Although atherosclerosis may affect the intracranial vessels themselves, as many as 88 percent of all major hemispheric events (stroke, TIA, or amaurosis fugax) are thought to originate at the carotid bifurcation.[1] However, the realization that extracranial carotid atherosclerosis is frequently responsible for hemispheric symptoms only took on practical meaning after it was demonstrated that such lesions could be removed from the bifurcation and reduce the incidence of stroke. The North American Symptomatic Carotid Endarterectomy Trial (NASCET) study has shown carotid endarterectomy (CEA) produces an absolute reduction of 17 percent in stroke at 2 years when compared with medical therapy in symptomatic patients with ≥70 percent stenosis.[2] More recent data from the NASCET study shows improvement in outcome with CEA in patients in the 50 to 69 percent lesion category, though to a far less dramatic degree than those with tighter stenoses.[3] The Asymptomatic Carotid Atherosclerosis Study (ACAS) also showed a reduction in stroke in asymptomatic patients with ≥60 percent lesions but by only 6 percent over 5 years.[4] Other studies, both here and abroad, confirm the benefit of CEA and assure this procedure a prominent role in the future.[5,6]

As technology has improved and confidence in the technique has grown, ultrasound has assumed an increasingly important role in the selection of patients for CEA. Although originally considered a potential screening procedure to decrease the number of negative angiograms, sonography has become the pivotal examination in the majority of patients considered for CEA in the United States. Although the ultimate imaging algorithm remains to be determined, the role of angiography is clearly decreasing. In many laboratories, ultrasound is the only imaging technique used. In others, MRA is performed in combination with sonography in cases where significant luminal narrowing is identified on the ultrasound. MRA is rapidly evolving, and which of its various techniques will prove to be the best remains to be investigated.

TECHNICAL ASPECTS OF THE CEREBROVASCULAR ULTRASOUND EXAMINATION

The accuracy of any cerebrovascular ultrasound examination is highly dependent upon a well-performed and technically excellent scan. A standardized and systematic approach must be followed in every patient. The gray-scale portion of the examination should be performed using the highest frequency transducer possible; most patients can be adequately evaluated with a 5 to 7.5 MHz center frequency, linear array transducer. The gray-scale examination should be performed in both transverse and longitudinal planes, and representative images should be documented at the proximal, mid, and distal common carotid artery (CCA), the bulb, and the bifurcation vessels bilaterally. Areas of plaque should be thoroughly investigated, internal characteristics defined, and the degree of luminal narrowing estimated whenever possible.

After the gray-scale assessment is completed, the transducer can be returned to the low CCA and the

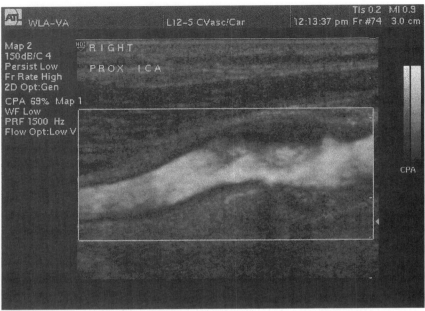

Figure 33-1.
Non-hemodynamically significant lesions. Color power Doppler image of the right proximal internal carotid artery reveals a well-defined, hypoechoic plaque that narrows the vessel lumen less than 50 percent. Non-hemodynamically significant lesions may be screened for using only power imaging in the future. Further investigation needs to confirm the efficacy of this technique prior to widespread use. (See also color insert 11.)

Doppler examination begun. Color Doppler may be used to obtain an overview of flow patterns and identify/estimate any potential regions of significant narrowing. Several investigators[7] are evaluating the possibility of accurately identifying patients with ≤50 percent lesions using color power Doppler and eliminating the need for detailed spectral evaluations in this group of patients (Fig. 33-1, color insert 11). However, until more experience is available using this technique, a detailed spectral examination should be part of *every* examination. Doppler values should be documented at the low, mid, and distal CCA, the bulb, external carotid artery (ECA) origin, and the proximal, mid, and distal internal carotid artery (ICA). Any other areas of suspected luminal narrowing should be thoroughly evaluated using Doppler. The Doppler portion of the examination is performed in the longitudinal plane where Doppler angles can be accurately measured. Doppler angles are of paramount importance in the examination of the carotid arteries, as estimation of flow velocity is the major diagnostic parameter. To ensure the highest degree of accuracy,

the *actual* angle between the Doppler beam and flow should be kept below 60°, and Doppler angle should be factored into the velocity calculation using the angle adjustment cursor on the screen (Fig. 33-2). In the past, sonographers tended to angle-adjust using the walls of the vessel on the gray-scale examination as an indicator of flow direction. As flow is often nonlaminar about bifurcations or areas of plaque, using color to define flow vectors and Doppler angle is probably a more consistent technique and should be used if color is available.

THE NORMAL EXAMINATION

Scanning is performed with the patient in the supine position; the examiner may either sit above or adjacent to the patient. Typically, the patient's neck should be hyperextended slightly and the head turned away from the side being scanned. The examination is best performed using gray-scale alone then repeated with color/spectral Doppler. The CCA is usually the first vessel identified and serves as a good landmark for orientation. Placing the transducer in the transverse plane in the mid-neck will usually provide an overview of the anatomy and, from superficial to deep, depict the jugular vein, the CCA, and the thyroid gland. Medial to the thyroid is the shadowing from the air in the trachea (Fig. 33-3, color insert 12). The CCA should be followed as far proximally as the clavicle will permit. In most patients, the origin of the right CCA can be identified as it arises from the innominate artery, although with tortuous vessels one may have to turn or angle the transducer considerably to see the innominate bifurcation. The left CCA originates directly from the aorta and is usually too low to be seen. The cervical portions of the CCA are usually easily imaged, although in some cases the CCA may follow a rather tortuous course. The CCA eventually widens somewhat as the carotid bulb is reached and alerts the sonographer to the fact that the bifurcation is immediately distal.

When scanning in the longitudinal plane (which is how the Doppler examination is usually performed), the carotid bifurcation may be approached from either anterior or posterior to the sternocleidomastoid muscle. Although variability exists, the ICA is usually located posterolateral to the ECA, and this location makes the posterior approach a better method of "opening the bifurcation" and seeing both vessels separately in most patients. From this vantage point, the ICA will lie closer to the transducer. Rocking the transducer slightly from side to side will bring each of the vessels into view separately if they cannot be imaged in the same plane, which is often the case. If the definition of two separate vessels is difficult in the longitudinal orientation, one may also follow the CCA distally in the transverse orientation and observe its division into two separate arteries. One can then rotate the transducer 90° on each of the two vessels and define them separately.

Once two vessels are identified, differentiation between ICA and ECA must be made. This may be accomplished by means of appearance (the ICA is generally larger than the ECA, has a mildly dilated ampullary region at its origin, and is located posterolaterally),

Figure 33-2.

True Doppler angle vs. angle-adjusted velocity. Angle adjustment cursor (curved arrow) *allows the operator to factor in the Doppler angle and obtain accurate velocity measurements. The actual angle formed between the Doppler beam* (represented by the white line *on the screen*) *and blood flow direction should always be less than 60 degrees. When angles greater than 60 degrees are used, the ability to obtain accurate velocities becomes compromised.*

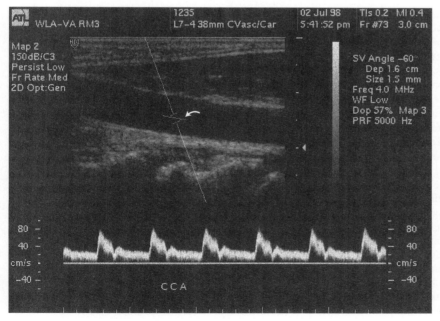

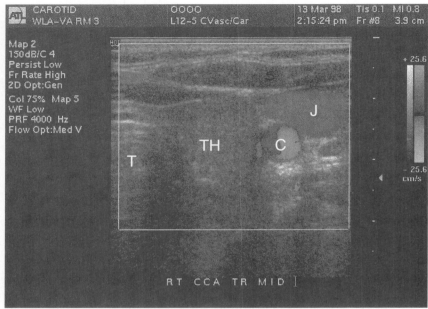

Figure 33-3.
Normal anatomy. Transverse image through mid-neck depicts normal sonographic anatomy. The trachea (T) lies in the midline adjacent to the low-level gray-scale echoes of the thyroid (TH). Lateral to the thyroid lies the common carotid artery (C) and jugular vein (J). The sternocleidomastoid muscle (S) lies anteriorly. (See also color insert 12.)

but normal variations are sufficiently common to make this inadvisable. The best method of distinguishing between the two vessels is the identification of branches. The ICA has no branches in the neck, whereas the ECA has several (beginning with the superior thyroidal artery), which are often easily identified. This task is made simpler with color Doppler. Evaluation of Doppler spectra also offers an excellent method of differentiating between ICA and ECA. The former, which supplies the brain with blood, produces a typical low resistance pattern, whereas the latter serves the muscular bed of the jaw and face and has a high resistance waveform. In cases where a question exists about the two vessels, one may also perform a temporal tap. This simple maneuver takes advantage of the fact that the temporal artery, a large branch of the ECA, courses over the temporomandibular joint. Although not infallible, tapping over this area will produce oscillations in the spectral pattern at the bifurcation if one is scanning the ECA.[8] Once the differentiation between the ICA and ECA has been accomplished, the bifurcation vessels may be interrogated for plaque/stenosis. All visualized

portions of the ICA must be thoroughly investigated; only the origin of the ECA requires evaluation (Fig. 33-4, color inserts 13–17).

The vertebral arteries must also be evaluated as part of every scan. This portion of the test need not be as exhaustive as that for the carotids. For the most part, definitive identification of the vertebral artery and assessment of flow direction and the spectral pattern are sufficient. The vertebral artery can be located by scanning in the longitudinal plane and angling laterally from the mid/proximal CCA; the vertebral artery lies deeper than the adjacent CCA. Whereas the vertebral artery is usually the only large vessel in the area, other arteries, including the costocervical and thyrocervical arteries, can be mistaken for the vertebral in patients with prominent collateral beds. For this reason, one should always identify the vertebral artery with certainty by virtue of its periodic areas of shadowing, which are caused by the lateral masses of the cervical spine. Only the vertebral vessels pass through the transverse foramen and have this appearance. Occasionally, the vertebral vessels will not enter the transverse foramen at the

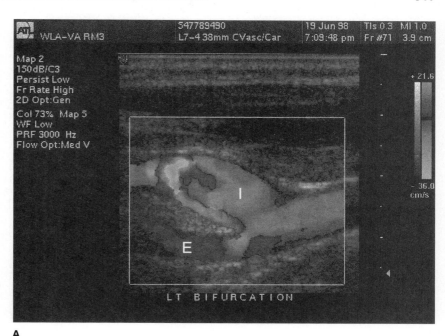

A

Figure 33-4.
Normal carotid bifurcation: A with proper angulation, images of both bifurcation vessels can often be obtained in a single plane. Note that color assignment is totally angle dependent. Flow in the external carotid artery (E) is displayed in blue beyond its immediate bifurcation as flow has turned toward the transducer. Areas of flow in the ICA (I), which are displayed in various shades of blue and shade into yellow, are likely due to the presence of boundary separation layers. Boundary separation layers are areas of flow reversal and slow flow and are normal at vascular bifurcations. The stress factors imposed by boundary separation layers on the vessel walls may be an associated factor in the development of atherosclerotic plaquing. (See also color insert 13.) B the external and internal carotid arteries frequently are scanned individually, in separate scan planes. The ECA can be differentiated from the ICA by means of identifying branches (arrows). The ICA gives off no branches in the neck. The most commonly identified branch is the superior thyroidal artery, which is typically identified at or near the origin of the ECA. (See also color insert 14.)

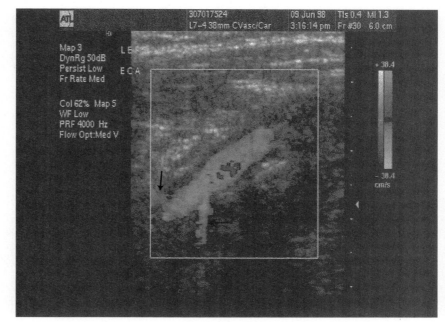

B

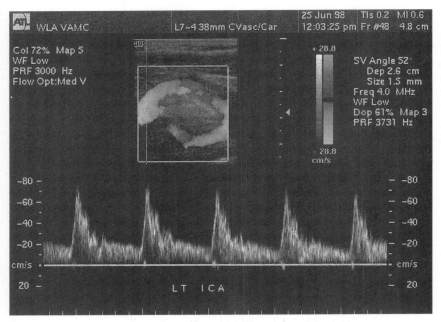

C

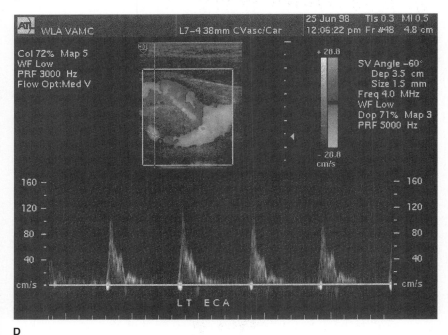

D

Figure 33-4 (*Continued*).
C   *the internal and external carotid arteries are also able to be differentiated by means of their spectral Doppler signatures. The internal carotid artery is a typical low resistance vessel with a large amount of diastolic flow. Flow continues in a forward direction throughout the cardiac cycle. (See also color insert 15.) D   the spectral pattern of the ECA can be readily differentiated from that of the ICA by virtue of a high resistance spectral signal. In this particular patient, the ECA demonstrates no diastolic flow. Note brief period of flow reversal, which is the hallmark of high resistance arteries supplying muscular beds. (See also color insert 16.)*

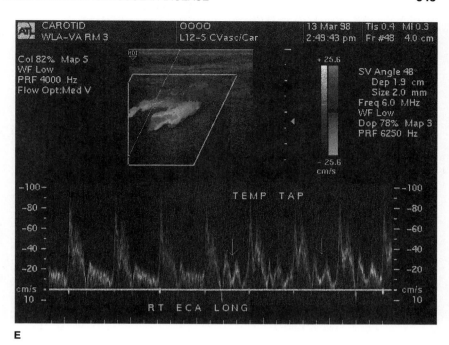

Figure 33-4 (*Continued*).
E   *a third method of differenti-ating the ICA from the ECA is* the *temporal tap. In this maneu-ver, one taps lightly over the temporomandibular joint where a large branch of the external carotid artery (the temporal ar-tery) lies in a superficial loca-tion. Tapping over the temporal artery will produce oscillations in the ECA, which are particu-larly prominent in diastole* (arrows). *This maneuver may be used as further supportive evidence that the spectral Doppler cursor is in the exter-nal carotid artery as shown.* (*See also color insert 17.*)

E

base of the cervical spine as they normally do. In this normal variant, a large vessel near the expected location of the vertebral artery will be identified but lack the expected shadowing. The vessel should be followed dis-tally and invariably enters the transverse foramen before reaching the fourth cervical vertebra. The vertebral ar-tery is accompanied by the vertebral vein, and one must be certain which of these two vessels is being insonated. As the flow in the vein runs toward the heart, a misdiag-nosis of subclavian steal syndrome can be made if the two vessels are confused. The vein tends to lie anterior to the artery and has a distinctive triphasic signal that should never be mistaken for the pattern of an artery (Fig. 33-5, color inserts 18–20).

DIAGNOSTIC CONSIDERATIONS

Plaque Characterization

Several articles have shown that as many as 80 percent of patients with clearly defined hemispheric events will have no evidence of a significant luminal narrowing at the carotid bifurcation.[9,10] Because many of the patients in these studies had no other obvious source for emboli

(atrial fibrillation, coagulopathy, etc.), one must postu-late that embolic events commonly arise from lesions in the ICA that do not cause hemodynamically signifi-cant flow alterations. In an effort to identify those pa-tients at risk for embolic phenomena and possibly those who might benefit from surgical removal of nonflow limiting lesions, high resolution real-time ultrasound has been used to evaluate the internal characteristics of carotid bifurcation plaque. Bluth et al[11] have shown that intraplaque hemorrhage can be identified within the vessel wall with an accuracy of 90 percent as evidenced by a heterogeneous internal echopattern. Reilly[12] and O'Donnell[13] also associated plaque heterogeneity with intraplaque hemorrhage. All three studies showed that homogeneous plaques never have pathologic evidence of intraplaque hemorrhage or even ulcerations.

Heterogeneous plaque typically has a mixed echo-pattern with areas of high and low-level echogenicity. The specific hallmark of intraplaque hemorrhage is the identification of prominent anechoic areas within plaque. Unfortunately, lipid-laden plaque may also cause anechoic areas, and the two may be difficult to differentiate. Homogeneous plaque has a relatively uni-form echotexture throughout and a smooth surface. Cal-cifications have no bearing upon plaque classification

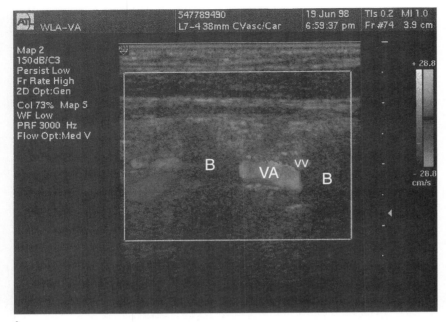

A

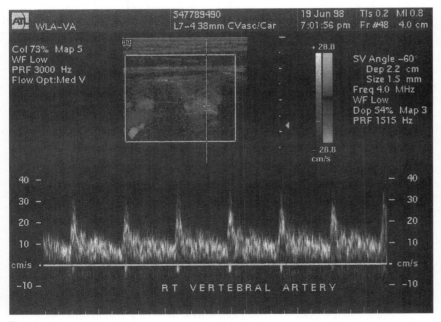

B

Figure 33-5.

Normal vertebral vessels. A
*The normal vertebral artery
courses through the transverse
foramina of the cervical spine
producing areas of periodic
shadowing as the vessel passes through bone (B). Note the
varying Doppler angle relationships as the vessel changes direction in relation to the linear
array transducer. The more inferior portion of the vertebral artery is directed toward the transducer and displayed in red
(VA). The more distal portion is
displayed in blue as flow is directed away from the transducer. The vertebral vein is displayed in the opposite colors
(VV). (See also color insert 18.)
B the spectral pattern of the
normal vertebral artery is that
of a low resistance artery; it
supplies the posterior fossa
with blood. The vertebral arteries join to form the basilar artery within the skull. (See also
color insert 19.)*

Figure 33-5 (*Continued*).
C *spectral patterns from the vertebral vein may be confused with those of the accompanying artery. The two must be carefully differentiated to avoid a misdiagnosis of subclavian steal. In this particular subject, the venous patterns are fairly similar to those from an artery. If a question exists, breath-holding and other physiologic maneuvers may allow differentiation, as arterial flow is usually unaffected. In most cases, the venous wave forms display a more typical triphasic pattern, which is present but somewhat subtle in this case. The differentiation of vein from artery can also often be made by listening to the Doppler sounds. (See also color insert 20.)*

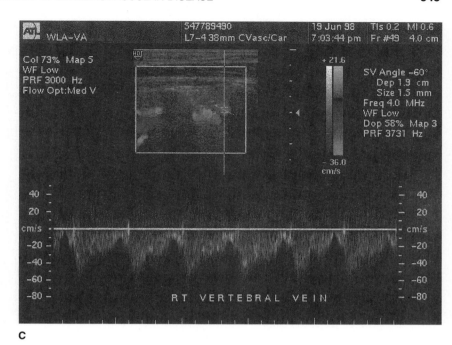

C

and may be identified in either heterogeneous or homogeneous plaques (Fig. 33-6). Several studies[14,15] have shown an increase in ipsilateral hemispheric symptoms in patients with heterogeneous plaque. Ulcerations are notoriously difficult to identify with sonography. The cross-sectional nature of the technique makes it uncertain that ulcerations will be imaged, and the differentiation between two adjacent plaques and a true ulcer is even more challenging. When large ulcers are suspected on gray-scale imaging, color can be useful in confirming the diagnosis (Fig. 33-7). With recent large trials confirming the efficacy of CEA in stenotic lesions, interest in plaque characterization and its possible role in stroke prevention have waned. Well controlled, longitudinal studies similar to those evaluating the effect of CEA on stenosis will be needed if we are ever to know conclusively whether specific types of plaque are prognostic indicators and truly deserving of close evaluation or removal.

The Doppler Evaluation of the ICA

Numerous investigations during the 1980's reported excellent results using duplex sonography in diagnosing internal carotid artery stenoses.[16–20] In these early stud-

ies, angiographic estimates of stenosis to which the Doppler data were compared often determined the degree of narrowing by estimating the size of the original ICA and comparing it with the measured residual lumen. This method is still used and serves as the basis for measurement in the European Carotid Endarterectomy Trial.[5] In the NASCET[2] and ACAS[3] studies, the smallest luminal diameter was compared with the luminal diameter of the "normal" ICA distally. Although the ACAS/NASCET method may not accurately reflect the true degree of luminal narrowing, this method has the advantage of minimizing interobserver error. Results are highly reproducible from one reviewer to the next.[21] This method is currently the standard on which the recent North American studies are based and should be used to make clinical decisions about which patients undergo CEA. As such, Doppler thresholds from earlier studies do not necessarily apply today, and the values from more recent evaluations should be substituted.

Numerous Doppler parameters have been used to diagnose ICA disease. These include both absolute velocity measurements and various ratios. Currently, most laboratories rely on one or more of the three following measurements: peak systolic velocity (PSV), end diastolic velocity (EDV), and the ratio of peak

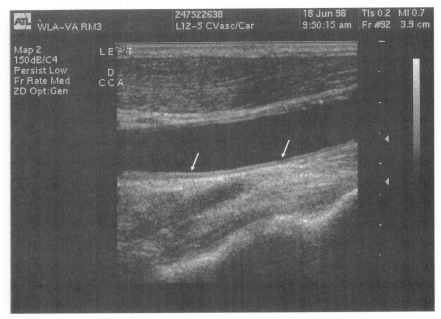

A

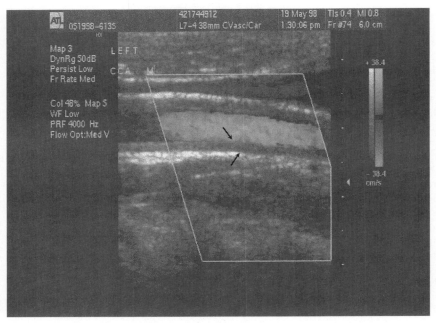

B

Figure 33-6.
Plaque characterization. A   the normal intima should be visible as a fine line paralleling the vessel wall (arrows). The intima is usually only visualized where the vessel lies at 90 degrees to the Doppler beam. Resolution is best in this region and degrades when the beam interacts with those portions of the vessels that run parallel to it. Visualization of intima in anterior or posterior carotid does not indicate early plaque deposits, although thickening has been related to the presence of atherosclerotic disease in several epidemiologic studies. B with severe atherosclerosis, intimal thickening may be observed (arrows). This may occur in scattered, patchy regions throughout the carotid system or be more diffuse as is shown in this patient.

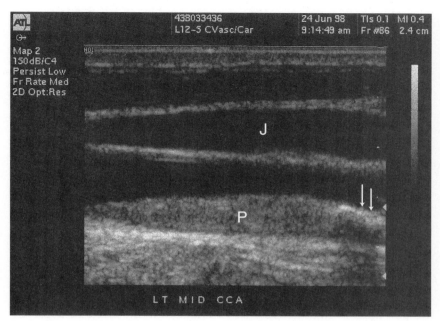

C

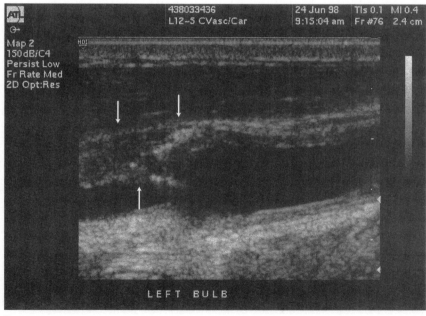

Figure 33-6 (*Continued*). C *homogeneous plaque is frequently encountered in the CCA and is typically associated with benign, fibrofatty deposits. The plaque in this case (P) exhibits relatively homogeneous echogenicity. Note area of internal calcification (arrows). J, jugular vein. D heterogeneous plaque exhibits areas of high and low level echogenicity. Heterogeneous plaque is associated with intraparenchymal hemorrhage, which may be responsible for embolic phenomenon.*

D

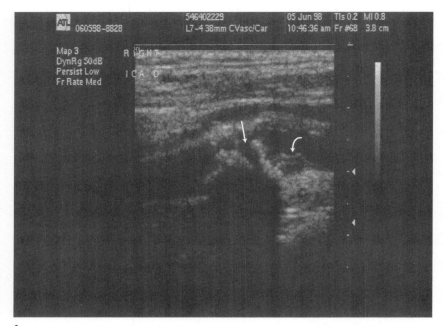

A

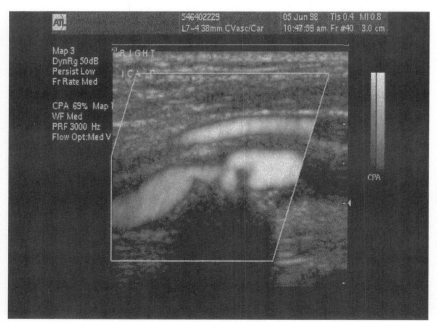

B

Figure 33-7.
Plaque ulceration. A gray-scale imaging reveals a large plaque at the internal carotid artery origin, which is densely calcified. A prominent cleft is noted on its intimal surface (arrow). *Note hypoechoic component inferiorly* (arrow). B *color power Doppler confirms a large ulceration within the cleft identified by gray scale.*

systolic velocity in the ICA to that in the ipsilateral mid/distal CCA (VICA/VCCA). Several studies[22,23] have shown PSV to be the most accurate and reproducible of the three parameters, and this measurement is by far the most commonly used. As there is variation of normal absolute velocity among individual patients, we feel the addition of a systolic ratio to PSV is advantageous and helps to identify those who, for hemodynamic reasons (hypertension, low cardiac output, arrhythmias, tandem lesions, etc.), fall outside the expected norm for PSV. For this reason, we recommend using PSV and ratio in all examinations. Low cardiac output, for example, may diminish a patient's ability to generate velocities, which are in keeping with the degree of stenosis present, and ratio may actually be more reflective of the true degree of vessel narrowing. In the above scenario, ratio will be elevated out of proportion to the PSV. Velocities in the ICA contralateral to a high-grade stenosis or occlusion may be spuriously high if the vessel is the major supplier of collateral blood flow around the circle of Willis.[24] As flow velocities are elevated throughout the contralateral carotid, again the ratio may be more indicative of the degree of stenosis than absolute flow velocities. Some authors have recommended using ratio preferentially over PSV.[25] Our own evaluation of these two parameters in our laboratory has shown their diagnostic capabilities to be almost identical (Fig. 33-8).[26]

Reviewing the recent literature in which Doppler thresholds were generated from comparison with ACAS/NASCET-measured stenosis,[23,25–34] we find there is a remarkably wide range of recommended values for a given degree of carotid stenosis (Table 33-1). All of these investigations have generated Doppler thresholds using angiographic measurements arrived at in keeping with the ACAS/NASCET technique. The method of measurement of the gold standard is, therefore, not a factor in the variation of recently published Doppler thresholds.

A comparison of results from several investigators, including our own, demonstrates that, if one chooses a specific angiographic threshold and examines accuracy of a Doppler parameter, rates are similar, with most laboratories reporting accuracy between 85 and 95 percent when compared with angiography. Similar results should be achievable by practitioners in most centers. Although accuracy is similar when comparing various laboratories, sensitivity and specificity vary for a given Doppler value. For example, at the ≥70 percent stenosis level, a threshold of 300 cm/s (PSV) in our symptomatic population produced 60.8 percent sensitivity, whereas in Moneta's[25] population, it corresponded

to a sensitivity of 84 percent. The same threshold applied to the study by Carpenter et al[29] produced a sensitivity of approximately 72 percent. The reasons for interlaboratory variations are many and include such factors as scan or measurement technique, interobserver variability of the Doppler examination,[35] or even equipment.[36] Interlaboratory variation has lead to the frequent recommendation that individual laboratories should develop, or at least validate, their own internal standards. Unfortunately, many physicians practice in settings where few arteriograms are performed and must depend on published data for their threshold selection. If threshold values are chosen from the literature, one should be aware that interlaboratory variations exist and that methods of threshold selection vary from paper to paper. One should try to choose thresholds from institutions that match those in the laboratory doing the selecting as closely as possible. Sources of variation include not only technical factors described above but also factors related to patient population such as disease prevalence, the mix of symptomatic vs. asymptomatic patients, and the operative threshold.

Although actual differences in results when comparing one laboratory with another undoubtedly account for some of the variation in literature thresholds, the most significant factor is probably the variation in methods of *selection* of Doppler criteria. For this reason, it is important to understand how individual investigators arrived at their conclusions. In Moneta's article[25] dealing with the identification of ≥70 percent stenosis, threshold values were chosen on the basis of highest accuracy (PSV = 325, VICA/VCCA = 4.0). Carpenter et al[29] examining the same degree of stenosis, selected thresholds based on maximizing sensitivity and chose far lower values (PSV = 210, EDV = 70, VICA/VCCA = 3.0).

Most authors have chosen Doppler thresholds based on an acceptable level of sensitivity, specificity, or accuracy or some combination of the three. Among the articles listed in Table 33-1, maximum accuracy was the most commonly used selection criteria. Reviewing our receiver operator curve (ROC) data and that of others, one finds that accuracy is relatively flat over a broad range of Doppler values and may not even maximize to a single point. As such, minor degrees of variation in accuracy between laboratories could potentially lead to large differences in threshold choice if this parameter is used alone.

Choosing a threshold based on an acceptable level of sensitivity or specificity has the advantage over simple peak accuracy of producing a predictable

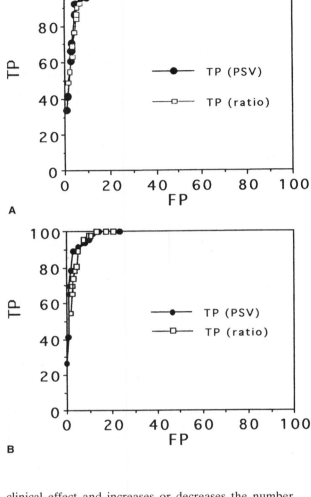

Figure 33-8.
Receiver-operator-curves (ROC) for the use of duplex ultrasound to detect carotid lesions in our own population. A ROC for the use of duplex ultrasound to detect ≥70 percent carotid lesions in a group of symptomatic patients. Changes in sensitivity (TP) and specificity (1-FP) are shown for varying detection thresholds of two duplex Doppler parameters: peak systolic velocity (PSV) in the proximal internal carotid artery and the ratio (Ratio) of PSV in the ICA and distal common carotid artery. Note that the two curves are almost identical. B ROC for the use of duplex ultrasound to detect ≥60 percent carotid lesions in a group of asymptomatic patients. Changes in sensitivity (TP) and specificity (1-FP) are shown for varying detection thresholds of two duplex Doppler parameters: peak systolic velocity (PSV) in the proximal internal carotid artery (ICA) and the ratio (Ratio) of PSV in the proximal ICA and distal common carotid artery. Again, there is minimal difference between the two parameters. TP, true positives; FP, false positives.

clinical effect and increases or decreases the number of false positives or negatives. For a given level of stenosis, as Doppler thresholds are raised, sensitivity decreases and specificity increases. In situations in which there is a large benefit, or risk reduction, from CEA (≥70 percent stenosis in symptomatic patients), one would logically choose high sensitivity to decrease the likelihood that a patient with an operative lesion will be missed. Conversely, in patients with low benefit from CEA (50 to 69 percent stenosis in symptomatic patients or ≥60 percent stenosis in asymptomatic patients), specificity may be favored over sensitivity to avoid sending patients to angiography or directly to surgery unnecessarily. The decision to favor sensitivity or specificity has undoubtedly been a major factor in

variance of recommended Doppler values in previous articles. Whether one is to be favored over the other must be considered in light of the clinical implications of the patient being examined or the imaging/surgical algorithm of an individual laboratory.

Considering the potential clinical impact of the choice of Doppler thresholds, some investigators have begun investigating their selection based on clinical outcomes or cost in terms of decreased morbidity and mortality.[33,34] The discussion above regarding the interplay of sensitivity and specificity is a simplified version of an outcome study as the clinical implication of increasing the numbers of over- or undercalls is estimated. If decreasing the number of strokes is the goal of both imaging and surgery, maximized outcome in terms of

Table 33-1

Comparison of recommended values from data in the published literature

	Lesion severity	PSV	EDV	Ratio	Method
		(cm/s)	(cm/s)		
Moneta (25)[a]	≥70%	325.0	130.0	4.0 (to 4.2)	Accuracy/sensitivity
Carpenter (29)	≥70%	210.0	70.0	3.0	Accuracy/sensitivity
Neal (30)	≥70%	270.0	110.0		Sensitivity/specificity
Hood (31)	≥70%	130.0	100.0		Accuracy/specificity
Browman (32)	≥70%	175.0			Sensitivity
Wilterdink (33)	≥70%	7 KHz			Outcome
Moneta (27)	≥60%	260.0	70.0	3.2	Accuracy/specificity
Carpenter (28)	≥60%	170.0	40.0	2.0	Accuracy/sensitivity
Derdeyn (34)	≥60%	230.0			Cost

[a]Number in parenthesis refers to the Ref. number in text.

strokes should be considered in the selection Doppler thresholds. Several methods have been used, but a basic function that can provide Doppler thresholds arrived at through a cost/outcome analysis contains three variables: (1) the cost of false-positive diagnoses (overcalls), (2) the cost of false-negative diagnoses (missed lesions/ undercalls), and (3) the prevalence of disease.[37] When considering outcomes in patients with carotid disease being evaluated with sonography who will go to angiography prior to CEA, an overcall sends a patient to an unnecessary angiogram with an estimated complication rate of 1 percent.[38] Undercalling a significant stenosis implies that a patient with a significant lesion does not get a CEA. According to NASCET data (≥70 percent stenosis), the 2-year stroke rate for medically treated patients is 26 vs. 9 percent for patients who had CEA plus medical management, yielding a 17 percent absolute risk reduction for CEA. Basically, in the symptomatic population with ≥70 percent lesions, there is a 17-fold greater cost to a missed diagnosis than to an overcall. The NASCET study (≥70 percent stenosis, symptomatic patients) results are much better than those of the ACAS study (≥60 percent stenosis, asymptomatic patients). In the ACAS study, there was a 6 percent absolute decrease in stroke over 5 years when comparing patients who underwent surgery to those who had medical treatment. The cost of a false-negative diagnosis in an asymptomatic patient at the ≥60 percent level of stenosis, therefore, is considerably less than symptomatic patients fitting NASCET criteria at the ≥70 percent stenosis level. The use of outcomes in the determination

of Doppler thresholds for patients with ≥50 percent lesions has not been undertaken to our knowledge. This may be necessary in the near future, as the results of the 50 to 69 percent cohort of the NASCET study do show benefit from CEA.

The prevalence of disease also has an effect on the outcome equation. If few patients in a given population have carotid stenosis, as Doppler thresholds are lowered, a point is reached at which the cost of the increasing number of overcalls thus generated begins to outpace the benefit of high sensitivity. Prevalence has been quoted to vary widely in the literature[39,40] and is dependent on several factors. Obviously, prevalence is directly related to the degree of stenosis being evaluated, and the higher the degree of stenosis the lower the prevalence. Additionally, clinical selection criteria affect prevalence. In a nursing home population, significant carotid disease was found to be present in 3.5 percent of the population.[39] In highly selected populations with hemispheric symptoms, prevalence of significant stenoses may be 40 percent or higher (Fig. 33-9).

Regarding selection criteria when considering carotid disease, historically, patients have been divided into symptomatic and asymptomatic cohorts. Although the actual selection criteria for "asymptomatic" patients have often been somewhat vague, one should not assume this group to be without a significant incidence of disease if patients are scanned for clinically accepted indications. Asymptomatic patients are usually selected on the basis of having markers for atherosclerotic disease (precoronary artery bypass, carotid bruit, severe

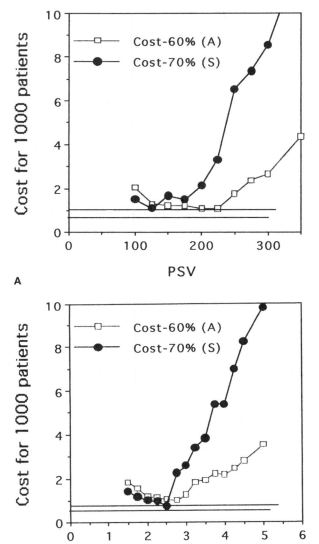

A

B

Figure 33-9.

Use of cost to determine optimum Doppler thresholds. A changes in cost (expressed as increased risk for strokes) vs. detection threshold values for Doppler parameter PSV in two groups of patients: symptomatic patients with ≥70 percent carotid lesions and asymptomatics with ≥60 percent carotid lesions. B changes in cost (expressed as increased risk for strokes) vs. detection threshold values for Doppler parameter ratio (Vicca/Vcca) in two groups of patients: symptomatic patients with ≥70 percent carotid lesions and asymptomatics with ≥60 percent carotid lesions.

peripheral vascular disease) and in our own population have only a marginally lower incidence of carotid stenosis than those selected on the basis of hemispheric symptoms. In our own population, disease prevalence in the "asymptomatic" population was 12.4 percent for ≥60 percent stenosis. This is not radically different from our neurologically symptomatic group, which had a prevalence of 16.1 percent for the same level of stenosis.[26] The prevalence of stenosis in a nonselected population (screening all patients over the age of 60 years of age, for example) would obviously be far lower, and this very low prevalence would have a considerable effect on Doppler threshold choice. Our own investigation has shown that outcome-based thresholds cannot be derived in this population, as cost remains constant over a wide range of Doppler values. Were one to screen a very low prevalence population, mathematically derived thresholds based on accuracy, specificity, or sensitivity would have to be used.[26] Of note, Derdyn's investigations[34,41] indicated it is not cost effective at all to screen low-prevalence populations of asymptomatic patients with ultrasound.

In the choice of Doppler thresholds, little attention has been given in the literature to the potential effect of segregating populations into symptomatic and asymptomatic cohorts. However, such segregation has been the basis of both the NASCET and ACAS studies. Previous authors who have used ROC data to arrive at Doppler thresholds have done so in a mixed population of symptomatic and asymptomatic patients, regardless of whether the threshold thus derived specifically applied to one or the other group. Investigations based on outcome obviously used appropriately segregated populations, as cost/benefit ratios derived from the NASCET and ACAS are directly related to the status of the patients being evaluated. We split our population into symptomatic and asymptomatic cohorts in an effort to evaluate the effect of population segregation on both the ROC analysis and outcome methodology. When compared with our mixed populations, ROC improved and shifted to the left in both the symptomatic and asymptomatic cohorts. Though variable in magnitude, this effect was encountered at both the ≥60 and ≥70 percent levels of stenosis and for both of the Doppler parameters that we evaluated (PSV and ratio). In most cases, accuracy rates improved 3 to 4 percent; sensitivity and specificity improved as well (Tables 33-2 and 33-3). The reasons for this improvement are not certain, but if this trend can be reproduced by other investigators, it would argue for segregating populations regardless of the method used to select Doppler thresholds.

Table 33-2

Carotid study: Asymptomatic population >60 percent stenosis

PSV 60%	PSV/averaged data			vica/vcca 60%	Ratio/averaged data		
	Sensitivity	Specificity	Accuracy		Sensitivity	Specificity	Accuracy
100	100	76.7	82	1.5	100	79.2	83.9
125	100	85.5	88.8	2	100	86.8	89.8
150	95.7	89.9	91.2	2.25	97.8	89.3	91.2
175	93.5	91.8	92.2	2.5	97.8	89.9	91.7
200	91.3	95	94.1	2.75	95.7	92.4	93.2
225	89.1	96.9	95.1	3	89.1	95	93.7
250	78.3	98.1	93.7	3.25	80.4	95.6	92.2
275	69.6	98.7	92.2	3.5	78.2	96.2	92.2
300	65.2	98.7	91.2	3.75	73.9	96.9	91.7
350	41.3	99.4	86.3	4	73.9	97.4	92.2
400	26.1	100	83.4	4.5	65.2	97.5	90.2
				5	54.3	98.1	88.3

The above considered, is there actually an optimum method for choosing Doppler thresholds? In Table 33-4, we have summarized PSV and ratio thresholds arrived at in our population using three different methods: peak accuracy, sensitivity and specificity ≥90 percent, and outcome. It is obvious that each of these methods produces a different value, or a range of values, and each yields reasonably good results. Having this amount of information available, however, we weighed the advantages and disadvantages of each and factored this into the final decision. As improved outcome is the goal of all patient interventions, thresholds based on maximized outcome or risk reduction should be considered as the primary directors of our choice. Although maximum accuracy is also desirable, accuracy levels for identifying both ≥60 and ≥70 percent lesions remain

Table 33-3

Carotid study: Symptomatic population >70 percent stenosis

PSV 70%	PSV/averaged data			vica/vcca 60%	Ratio/averaged data		
	Sensitivity	Specificity	Accuracy		Sensitivity	Specificity	Accuracy
100	100	82.8	85	1.5	100	83.9	86
125	100	87.6	89.2	2	100	88.5	90
150	96.1	90.5	91.2	2.5	100	91.7	92.7
175	96.1	92.5	93	2.75	92.2	93.4	93.2
200	92.2	95.1	94.7	3	90.2	94.5	94
225	86.3	95.7	94.5	3.25	86.3	94.8	93.7
250	70.6	96.8	93.5	3.5	84.3	94.8	93.5
275	66.7	97.1	93.2	3.75	76.5	95.7	93.2
300	60.8	97.4	92.7	4	76.5	95.7	93.2
350	41.2	98.6	91.2	4.5	62.7	96.8	92.5
400	33.3	99.4	91	5	54.9	97.7	92.2

Table 33-4
Doppler thresholds for ≥60 + ≥70 percent ICA stenosis

	Peak accuracy	Sensitivity specificity ≥90%	Outcome	Recommended threshold
Symptomatic >70%				
PSV	200	150–225	125–175	175
Ratio	3.0	2.5–3.0	2.5	2.5
Asymptomatic >60%				
PSV	225	150–225	125–225	200
Ratio	3.0	2.75	2.75	3.0

relatively high over a wide range of Doppler values for both PSV and ratio. Therefore, methods of threshold selection based on outcome and sensitivity/specificity can be factored into the final threshold decision without a significant sacrifice of accuracy. At the ≥70 percent level in symptomatic patients, PSV thresholds based on outcome showed an absolute nadir in the cost function at 125 cm/s. However, Doppler thresholds can be raised to 175 cm/s before an upswing in cost in terms of stroke occurs. This elevation of the Doppler threshold, which has little or no effect on outcome, improves accuracy

from 89.2 to 93 percent. The tradeoff is a decrease in sensitivity from 100 percent to 96 percent, but this is accompanied by improvement in specificity. We chose 175 cm/s for PSV, but it can be seen that potential choices could vary somewhat depending on personal preferences and the exact method of choice. Using ratio, the range of values produced by each of the three methods we evaluated was more tightly clustered and between 2.5 and 3.0. As can be seen from Fig. 33-9B, cost rises rapidly when the ratio exceeds 2.5. At this level and all lower Doppler values, sensitivity

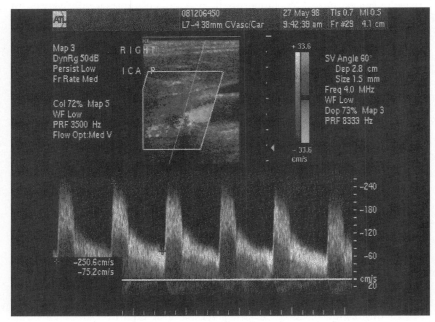

A

Figure 33-10.
Moderate (≥60 percent) internal carotid artery stenosis. A Color Doppler imaging reveals an area of intense aliasing (note mixture of color) suggesting a region of high-speed flow in association with a significant stenosis. Spectral Doppler demonstrates the peak systolic velocity was 250 cm/s; end diastolic velocity was 75 cm/s. The ratio in this case measured 2.9. (See also color insert 21.)

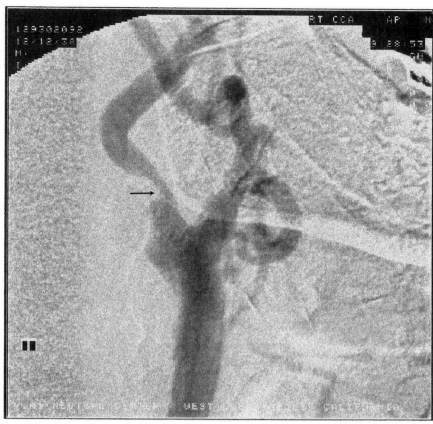

Figure 33-10 (*Continued*).
B *selective carotid arte-riogram confirms presence of significant stenosis* (arrow). *By NASCET method of mea-surement, the lesion was esti-mated at 68 percent.*

B

is 100 percent but falls rapidly if one chooses thresholds that are higher. Specificity, on the other hand, rises slowly throughout the spectrum of Doppler thresholds. Again, accuracy changes minimally throughout the range. The abrupt differences that are found in both sensitivity and outcome strongly favor a ratio threshold of 2.5.

For asymptomatic patients at the ≥60 percent level, the cost plot using PSV is relatively flat over a wide range (125 to 225 cm/s), leading one to look at other methods for direction of the eventual choice. Selection based on peak accuracy would favor the upper limit of the range defined by outcomes. Considering the small absolute risk reduction of CEA in this group, a higher threshold would reduce false positives and with it the complications of unnecessary angiograms. In the asymptomatic group, therefore, specificity should probably be favored over sensitivity. A 95 percent level of

specificity (similar to that required by the ACAS study) can be achieved by choosing 200 cm/s. This threshold causes a <1 percent sacrifice in accuracy and lies within the range dictated by optimized outcome. Regarding ratio, again the thresholds arrived at by the three different methods are tightly clustered, leaving less latitude in their selection. Based on the desire to maximize outcome and to achieve >95 percent specificity, we chose a ratio of 3.0. It is obvious that thresholds based on outcome or even the composite method we have outlined are somewhat different than those usually shown in the literature. Most remarkably, thresholds for ≥60 percent lesions are higher than those for ≥70 percent stenosis. This is the effect of looking at separate populations and of including outcome in the threshold choice. Typical examples of carotid stenoses at the ≥60 and ≥70 percent levels are provided in Figs. 33-10, color insert 21, and 33-11, color insert 22.

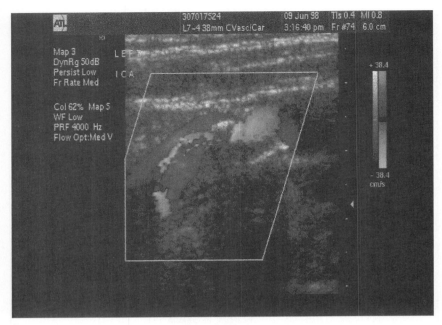

A

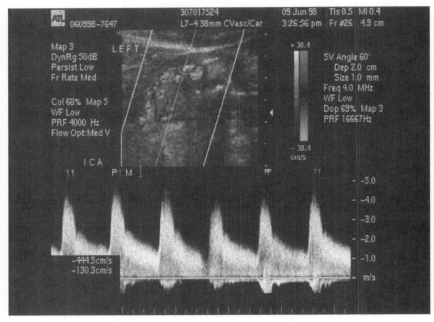

B

Figure 33-11.
Severe (≥70 percent) internal carotid artery stenosis. A color Doppler imaging reveals an area of marked vessel narrowing at the origin of the left internal carotid artery (arrow). Note aliasing and flow reversal distal to the region of stenosis. The superficial vessel (arrowheads) represents the jugular vein. (See also color insert 22.) B spectral evaluation of region of suspected lesion confirms the presence of a stenosis >70 percent. Peak systolic velocity was 444 cm/s; end diastolic velocity was 130 cm/s. Ratio was 7.2.

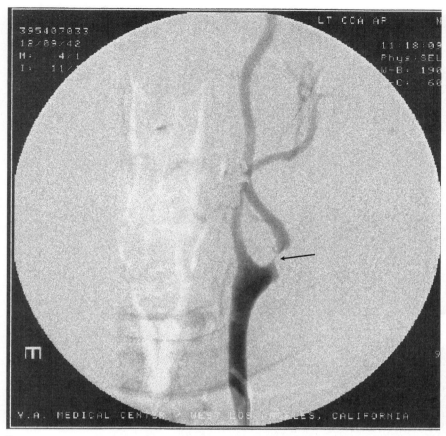

C

Figure 33-11 (*Continued*).
C *selective carotid arteriography confirms a stenosis* (arrow) *measured at 86 percent by NAS-CET methodology.*

In laboratories where patients go directly to surgery based on the ultrasound results or where MRA is the follow-up study to ultrasound, other thresholds may be more optimal. Certainly, were a study that carries no risk such as MRA used as the only follow-up study to ultrasound in symptomatic patients, thresholds could be lowered even further as cost is the only determining factor.[42] One could choose almost any acceptable combination of sensitivity specificity, or accuracy from ROC data in Tables 33-2 and 33-3 or the literature and factor in general trends based on estimated outcome depending on population and expected prevalence. Exactly how ultrasound, MRA, and angiography are used in the future in the evaluation of ICA disease will un-doubtedly continue to evolve. In most centers, the number of angiograms has decreased dramatically. The use of MRA continues to rise as equipment improves and more accurate techniques are found.

Total Occlusion

Total occlusion of the ICA has several possible sonographic appearances. In many cases, the occluded lumen will be plainly visible as a hypoechoic or anechoic structure, with no Doppler signals arising beyond the carotid bulb. Often, using today's high-resolution transducers, internal areas of echogenic or calcified plaque can be identified within the occluded lumen (Fig. 33-12, color

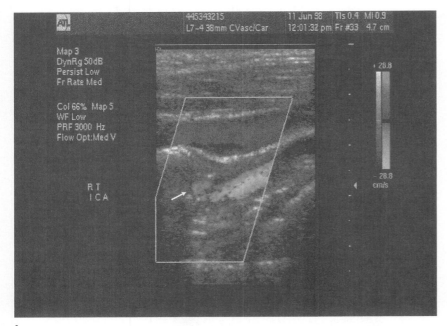

A

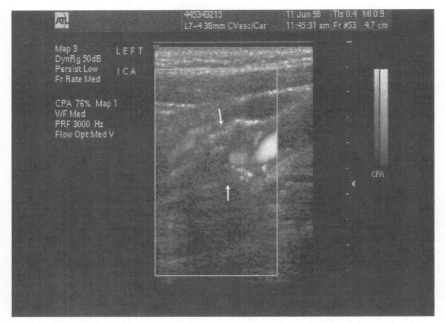

B

Figure 33-12.
*Total internal carotid occlusion.
A color Doppler imaging reveals an abrupt cessation of
flow just beyond the origin of
the internal carotid artery. Note
focal area of flow reversal*
(arrow) *as forward-moving flow
strikes occluding plaque and
direction/color are reversed.
(See also color insert 23.)*
B *color power Doppler confirms presence of complete occlusion. No evidence of a minute flow channel is depicted.
The original occluded vessel*
(arrows) *is well defined in this
patient; solid plaque fills lumen.
(See also color insert 24.)*

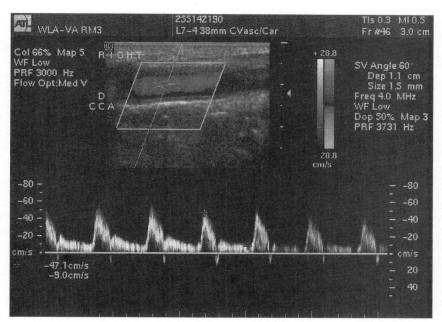

C

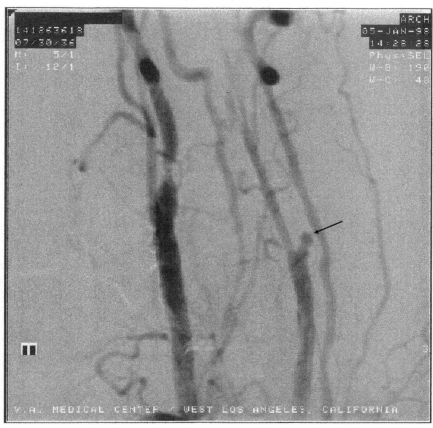

Figure 33-12 (*Continued*).
C *spectral tracing from the common carotid artery of the same patient reveals an externalized wave form typical of patients with ICA occlusion in whom all flow in the common carotid artery is directed toward the ECA. Note, typical periods of flow reversal in early diastole. (See also color insert 25.)*
D *aortic arch arteriogram confirms complete occlusion of the left ICA. Small patent stump (arrow) corresponds to the residual ICA stump demonstrated on Doppler imaging.*

D

inserts 23–25). In some cases, the occluded lumen cannot be identified distinctly and blends into the echoes of the soft tissues of the neck. The diagnosis in this situation is made on the basis of finding one vessel at the bifurcation. Pitfalls, such as mistaking a large ECA collateral for a tightly stenosed ICA, are more likely when the occluded vessel is not clearly depicted. Occasionally, a patent stump may remain at the ICA origin, but in most cases the occluded area can be found if one scans distally. In occlusions distal to the ICA origin (even at the siphon), the correct diagnosis can be suggested if diastolic flow is absent and velocity is low when compared with the opposite ICA. Secondary features of complete ICA occlusions include identification of a small area of flow reversal just before the occluding thrombus and "externalized" flow patterns in the CCA. In the latter situation, as all flow in the CCA is diverted to the external vasculature when the ICA is occluded, flow in the CCA reflects its end organ and assumes a high resistance pattern. Externalization of the CCA may not occur if the ECA has converted to a low resistance system. This physiology may be found if the ECA is serving as a major collateral around a compromised ICA. Although externalization of the CCA is suggestive of ICA occlusion, it may be seen in normal patients and should not be a cause for alarm if the ICA is clearly patent.

Although the imaging characteristics of carotid occlusion are relatively straightforward, one cannot be completely confident with this diagnosis, as a small, residual channel ("string-sign") may be present and missed by ultrasound. The differentiation between total and subtotal occlusions is clinically very important. Subtotal occlusions are operative lesions, whereas total occlusions are not. For this reason, the sonographer must search diligently for a residual lumen. One should maximize color sensitivity and use power Doppler if available (Fig. 33-13, color insert 26). As subtotal occlusions can be missed with even the best technique (they may even be missed at angiography), we do not advise making the diagnosis of total occlusion based on ultrasound alone and always recommend an alternative study. In our practice, patients with subtotal and total occlusions as a whole were identified with essentially 100% accuracy. When total occlusion was found at angiography, sonography was invariably correct in this diagnosis. Among the smaller group of patients with subtotal occlusions, approximately one-third were subtotal occlusions overcalled as being total occlusions, one-third demonstrated high velocity flow and a minute channel on color, and one-third showed very slow velocity flow or undetectable flow on spectral analysis. In the latter group, the diagnosis was made by color/power Doppler

alone. We have found that, since the introduction of power Doppler, the number of subtotal occlusions thought to be occluded has decreased. Ultrasound contrast agents may provide even better visualization of subtotal occlusions than existing technology and may be a routine method for identifying subtotal occlusions in the future.[43]

The Common Carotid Artery

The CCAs are large vessels that are usually easily found and well imaged with both gray-scale and color Doppler. The anatomy of the CCAs, however, makes their evaluation somewhat different depending on which portion of the vessel is being examined and whether or not one is dealing with the right or left. As described above, the right CCA arises from the innominate artery and should be visible in its entirety in almost every patient, although some degree of transducer manipulation may be necessary to image the origin. The left CCA, however, arises directly from the aorta. The entire innominate artery and the proximal one-third of the left CCA are unable to be seen without considerable effort (if at all) and are not imaged as part of the routine scan. Significant narrowing of any of these vessels may cause symptoms and should be identified.

Imaging of lesions in the CCA can be divided into three major categories: (1) lesions of the carotid bulb, (2) lesions in the visible portions of the arteries proximal to the carotid bulbs and distal to the clavicle, and (3) lesions in the supra-aortic trunks (innominate artery and proximal left CCA). Lesions in the carotid bulb are generally classified along with those in the ICA and need little further discussion. Worth noting in this area is the occasional apparent discrepancy between the degree of narrowing estimated by gray-scale measurement and Doppler. Typically, moderate degrees of narrowing (50 to 60 percent) at the bulb are identified using gray-scale measurement, but the Doppler velocities remain normal. This apparent mismatch can be explained by the fact that the original diameter of the bulb is wider than the more proximal parts of the vessel. Although narrowing may, indeed, have occurred within the bulb itself, the lumen remains the same diameter as the remainder of the CCA, and no hemodynamic alterations result. As might be imagined, arteriograms read using the ACAS/NASCET method will also show minimal narrowing, if any. In this case, the luminal diameter of the bulb is being compared with the diameter of the ICA. In both Doppler and arteriographic evaluations,

Figure 33-13.

Subtotal internal carotid occlusion.
A conventional color Doppler im-
aging failed to reveal evidence of
flow in the internal carotid artery;
complete occlusion was sus-
pected. Color power imaging dem-
onstrated a small vascular channel
(arrow) suggesting subtotal occlu-
sion. (See also color insert 26.)
B careful selective arteriographic
technique confirms the presence
of a subtotal ICA occlusion (arrow).
Although angiography is consid-
ered the gold standard, both
MRA with contrast and ultrasound
may occasionally identify subtotal
occlusions not found on arteriog-
raphy.

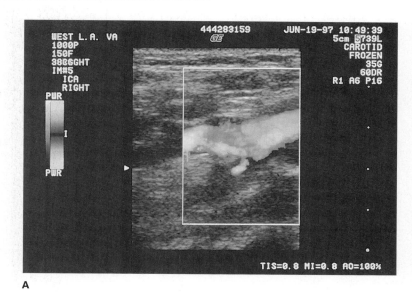

A

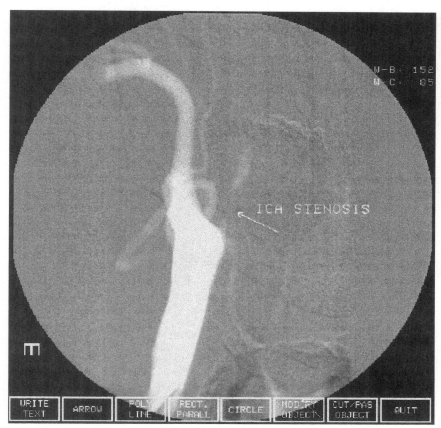

B

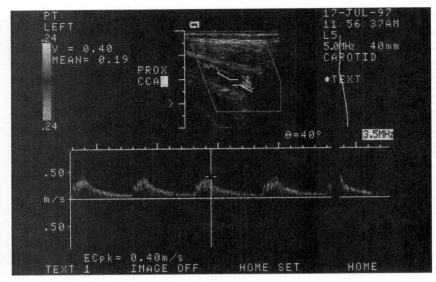

A

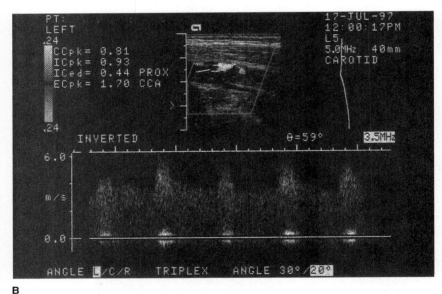

B

Figure 33-14.

Common carotid artery stenosis. A   slow flow was identified in the proximal left common carotid artery in this patient. Peak systolic velocity was 40 cm/per s. B   markedly elevated flow velocities were identified across a long segment of the mid/distal CCA. Peak systolic velocities were >6 m/s; end diastolic velocities approached 4 m/s. The ratio in this case exceeded 15.

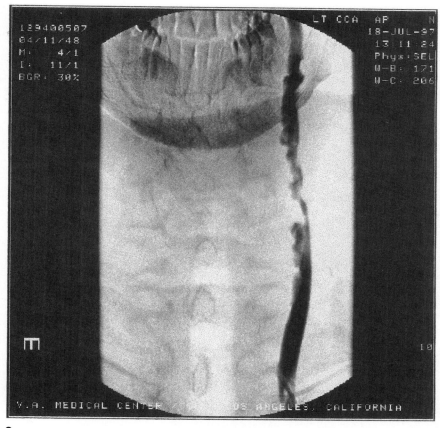

C

Figure 33-14 (*Continued*).
C   selective arteriography reveals a bizarre, long segment stenosis in the mid and distal common carotid artery of this patient. Patient underwent successful carotid endarterectomy, and TIA-like symptoms referable to the left hemisphere resolved.

the normal ectasia of the bulb is not taken into account. Luckily, this phenomenon is unlikely to produce clinically significant sequelae. Hemodynamically significant lesions behave like those in the ICA when higher degrees of stenosis occur.

Stenoses in the visible portions of the CCA proximal to the bulb are diagnosed in a similar fashion to vascular narrowings anywhere else in the body: by elevations in flow velocity or ratio. However, one must be aware that Doppler values discussed in previous sections were derived only for lesions in the ICA. They do not apply directly to CCA lesions. There is little information in the literature about normal values for the CCA and no good series providing values for stenosis prediction.

Absolute values such as PSV may be difficult to apply in the CCA, as velocity tends to decrease as one moves distally. We use a ratio of peak velocity proximal and at or distal to a presumed lesion. A ratio of 2.0:4.0 usually indicates a moderate degree of stenosis. Any ratio greater than 4.0 is suggestive of a high-grade (operative) lesion. CCA stenoses are uncommon when compared with lesions in the ICA. Although atherosclerosis is by far the most common cause of CCA disease, patients who have had trauma or head and neck irradiation have an increased incidence of stenosis and occlusion. In many of these cases, long segment or bizarre-appearing lesions may be identified and accompanied by extremely high velocities on Doppler (Fig. 33-14).

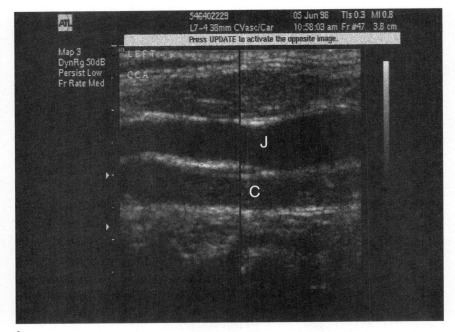

A

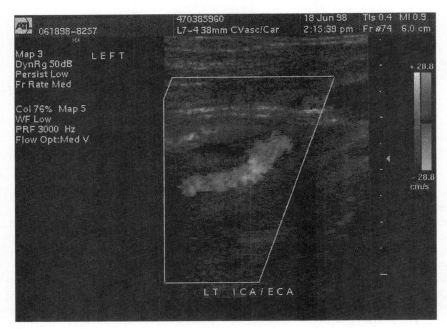

B

Figure 33-15.
Occlusion of common carotid artery. A gray-scale imaging reveals two tubular structures in the neck. The anechoic, more superficial structure (J) represents the jugular vein. CCA lumen (C) is filled with hypoechoic plaque. Complete occlusion was confirmed by color. B scanning at the carotid bifurcation reveals two patent vessels with differing color/flow direction. Flow in the ECA (shown in blue) was reversed and toward the transducer. The artery was serving as a feeding collateral to the ICA (shown in red) which maintains normally directed flow. In patents with common carotid artery occlusion, it is essential to scan at the bifurcation to identify such collateral pathways. (See also color insert 27.)

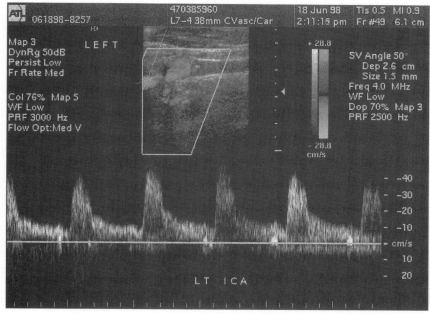

C

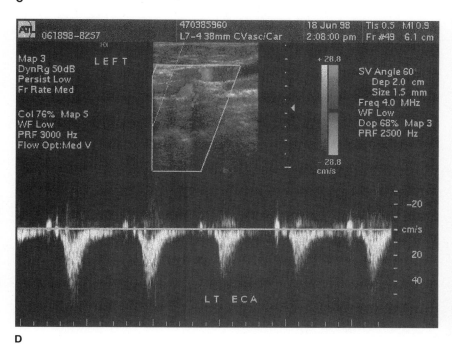

Figure 33-15 (*Continued*). C *spectral Doppler of the internal carotid artery reveals normally directed flow with a typical low resistance pattern. (See also color insert 28.) D scanning in the external carotid artery demonstrates reversed flow with a higher resistance pattern than was identified in the internal carotid. (See also color insert 29.)*

D

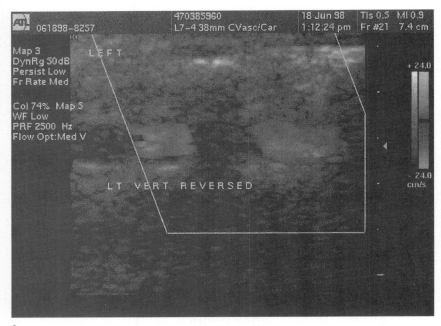

A

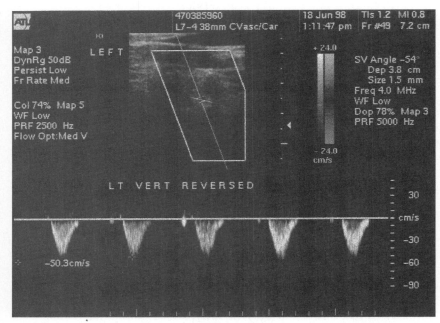

B

Figure 33-16.
Subclavian steal syndrome.
A   color Doppler imaging dem-
onstrates reversed flow in the
left vertebral artery. Flow is to-
ward the feet and displayed in
blue. Note periodic areas of
shadowing from the lateral
masses of the cervical spine
confirming that this vessel rep-
resents the vertebral artery.
(See also color insert 30.)
B   spectral evaluation of the
same vessel confirms reversal
of flow and that vessel is an ar-
tery. Note absence of diastolic
flow component. This finding is
typical of spectral patterns from
the vertebral arteries of pa-
tients with subclavian steal. It is
most likely caused by the verte-
bral artery serving the high
resistance vasculature of
the arm. (See also color
insert 31.)

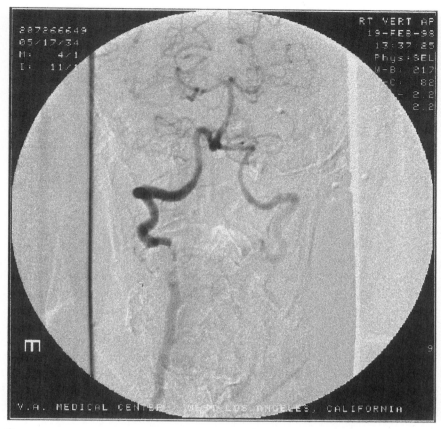

C

Figure 33-16 (*Continued*).
C   angiography confirms the presence of subclavian steal. Imaging of the vertebrobasilar confluence following injection into the right vertebral artery shows flow proceeding into the distal left vertebral artery.

Occlusions of the CCA may occur as well. CCA occlusions are usually easily identified by gray-scale and color Doppler. We have never encountered the difficulty of differentiation between total and subtotal occlusions in the CCA that is experienced at the bulb and ICA. As these occlusions are often the result of chronic, progressive vascular compromise, collaterals may be found at the bifurcation vessels. The most interesting of these configurations is found when the ECA is fed by collaterals and demonstrates retrograde flow direction, thus providing blood to the ICA, which continues to flow toward the head. In this situation, the bifurcation vessels will be displayed in different colors, and spectral waveforms will lie on opposite sides of the baseline (Fig.

33-15, color inserts 27–29). One must always scan the bifurcation vessels in patients with CCA occlusions to identify a potentially patent ICA. In symptomatic patients, a subclavian ICA graft may be constructed.

In cases where stenotic lesions affect the origin of the innominate or left CCA, the diagnosis must be made by virtue of flow alterations downstream from the lesion, as the origins of these vessels lie in the chest. Again, no good guidelines are available from the literature, but low-velocity (less than 50 cm/s) flow, which is asymmetric when compared with the opposite CCA, should raise the suspicion of origin disease. Other features of origin lesions that have been described in the CCA in the neck include diminished pulsatility, delayed

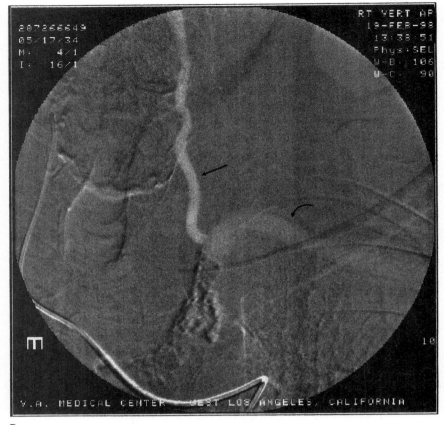

D

Figure 33-16 (*Continued*).
D   *later image at the vertebral/subclavian junction shows flow preceding inferiorly through the vertebral artery* (arrow) *and filling the subclavian artery* (curved arrow).

systolic upstroke (tardus-parvus waveform), spectral broadening implying poststenotic turbulence, and rarely, reversed flow in the right CCA.[44,45] Results of the available studies indicate that duplex sonography is quite accurate in diagnosing origin lesions on the basis of downstream abnormalities.

The Vertebral Artery

An exhaustive examination of the vertebral artery is unnecessary. A sufficient amount of information can be obtained from any clearly identified segment of the vessel. The origin of the vertebral artery need not be evaluated and is unable to be seen in a significant number of patients anyway. As mentioned under the section

dealing with scan technique above, determination of flow direction and identification of a normal spectral pattern entails an adequate vertebral examination. Direction of flow can be determined using either spectral or color Doppler. If a question exists about direction, the adjacent CCA provides an easy reference. As flow in the CCA *always* goes toward the head, the normal vertebral artery should flow in the same direction and demonstrate the same color. The spectral waveform of the vertebral artery should also be evaluated. Since the identification of stenoses is not the goal of the examination, absolute velocity measurements are not important. The spectral pattern of the vertebral artery should be low resistance and similar to what is seen in the CCA or ICA. In most cases, the vertebral artery demonstrates a lower peak velocity. Though little investigated in the literature, a high resistance pattern in the vertebral artery should be viewed with concern and may indicate early subclavian artery compromise (of insufficient severity to cause flow reversal) or distal obstruction/occlusion from either atherosclerotic disease or a blind ending, hypoplastic artery. If an unusual spectral pattern is identified in the vertebral artery, it is advisable to obtain blood pressure in both arms. A greater than 20 mmHg difference in systolic pressure is further confirmation of subclavian artery compromise. A sampling of the subclavian artery spectral pattern may also be considered. A low resistance pattern is virtually diagnostic of subclavian compromise.

With subclavian steal syndrome, flow in the vertebral artery is reversed in response to stenosis or occlusion of the proximal subclavian artery. This condition is more common on the left but may occur on the right if the stenotic subclavian segment is located between the origin of the CCA and the vertebral artery. As the vertebral artery is serving as a collateral to supply blood to the arm, the spectral pattern is usually high resistance, sometimes demonstrating normally directed flow during diastole (Fig. 33-16, color inserts 30–31). Most patients in whom reversal of flow in the vertebral artery is found do not exhibit the typical symptoms of dizziness with exercise of the affected arm. In patients with symptoms, there are several options including angioplasty, stenting, or even surgical bypass. As described above, supporting evidence of subclavian steal syndrome include the identification of low resistance flow in the affected subclavian artery and a discrepancy of greater than 20 mmHg when comparing the systolic blood pressure in the two arms.

REFERENCES

1. Eisenberg R, Nemzek W, Moore W, et al: Relationship of transient ischemic attack and angiographically demonstrable lesions of the carotid artery. *Stroke* 8:483, 1977.
2. North American Symptomatic Carotid Endarterectomy Trial Collaborators: Beneficial effect of carotid endarterectomy in symptomatic patients with high-grade carotid stenosis. *N Engl J Med* 325:445, 1991.
3. Barnett HJM, Taylor DW, Eliasziw M, et al: Benefit of carotid endarterectomy in patients with symptomatic moderate or severe stenosis. *N Engl J Med* 339:1415, 1998.
4. Executive Committee for the Asymptomatic Carotid Atherosclerosis Study: Endarterectomy for asymptomatic carotid artery stenosis. *JAMA* 273:1421, 1995.
5. European Carotid Surgery Trialists' Collaborative Group: MRC European Carotid Surgery Trial: Interim results for symptomatic patients with severe (70-99%) or with mild (0-29%) carotid stenosis. *Lancet* 337:1235, 1991.
6. Hobson RW, Weiss DG, Fields WS, et al: Efficacy of carotid endarterectomy for asymptomatic carotid stenosis. *N Engl J Med* 328:221, 1993.
7. Bluth EI, Merritt CRB, Sullivan MA, et al: A screening test for carotid stenosis: A preliminary feasibility study. *Radiology* 205:696, 1997.
8. Kliewer MA, Freed KS, Hertzberg BS, et al: Temporal artery tap: Usefulness and limitations in carotid sonography. *Radiology* 401:481, 1996.
9. Brown PB, Zwiebel WJ, Call GK: Degree of cervical carotid artery stenosis and hemispheric stroke: Duplex U.S. findings. *Radiology* 170:541, 1989.
10. Carroll BA: Duplex sonography in patients with hemispheric symptoms. *J Ultrasound Med* 8:535, 1989.
11. Bluth EI, Kay D, Merritt CRB, et al: Sonographic characterization of carotid plaque: Detection of hemorrhage. *Am J Roentgenol* 146:1061, 1986.
12. Reilly LM, Lusby RJ, Hughes L, et al: Carotid plaque histology using real-time ultrasonography: Clinical and therapeutic implications. *Am J Surg* 146:188, 1983.
13. O'Donnell TF Jr, Erodes L, Mackey WC, et al: Correlation of B-mode ultrasound imaging and arteriography with pathologic findings at carotid endarterectomy. *Arch Surg* 120:443, 1985.
14. Sterpetti AV, Schultz RD, Feldhaus RJ, et al: Ultrasonographic features of carotid plaque and the risk of subsequent neurologic deficits. *Surgery* 104:652, 1988.
15. Leahy AL, McCollum PT, Feeley TM, et al: Duplex ultrasonography and selection of patients for carotid endarterectomy: Plaque morphology or luminal narrowing? *J Vasc Surg* 8:558, 1988.
16. Garth K, Carroll B, Sommer G, et al: Duplex ultrasound scanning of the carotid arteries with velocity spectrum analysis. *Radiology* 147:823, 1983.
17. Jacobs N, Grant E, Schellinger D, et al: Duplex carotid sonography: Criteria for stenosis, accuracy, and pitfalls. *Radiology* 154:385, 1985.
18. Blackshear W Jr, Phillips D, Chikos P, et al: Carotid artery velocity patterns in normal and stenotic vessels. *Stroke* 11:67, 1980.
19. Dreisbach JN, Seibert CE, Smazal SF, et al: Duplex sonography in the evaluation of carotid artery disease. *Am J Neuroradiol* 4:678, 1983.
20. Bluth EI, Stavros AT, Marich KW, et al: Carotid duplex sonography: A multi-center recommendation for standardized imaging and Doppler criteria. *RadioGraphics* 8:487, 1988.
21. Gagne PJ, Matchett J, MacFarland D: Can the NASCET technique for measuring carotid stenosis be reliably applied outside the trial? *J Vasc Surg* 24:449, 1996.
22. Robinson ML, Sacks D, Perlmutter GS, et al: Diagnostic criteria for carotid duplex sonography. *Am J Roentgenol* 151:1045, 1988.
23. Hunnick MGM, Polak JF, Barlan MM, et al: Detection

and quantification of carotid artery stenosis: Efficacy of various Doppler parameters. *Am J Roentgenol* 160:619, 1993.

24. Beckett WW Jr, Davis PC, Hoffman JC Jr: Duplex Doppler sonography of the carotid artery: False-positive results in an artery contralateral to an artery with marked stenosis. *Am J Roentgenol* 155:1091, 1990.

25. Moneta GL, Edwards JM, Papanicolaou G, et al: Screening for asymptomatic internal carotid artery stenosis: Duplex criteria for discriminating 60% to 99% stenosis. *J Vasc Surg* 21:989, 1995.

26. Grant EG, Duerinckx AJ, El Saden S, et al: Doppler parameters for detection of carotid stenosis: Is there an optimum method for their selection? *Am J Roentgenol* 172:1123, 1999.

27. Moneta GL, Edwards JM, Chitwood RW, et al: Correlation of North American Symptomatic Carotid Endarterectomy Trial (NASCET) angiographic definition of 70% to 99% internal carotid artery stenosis with duplex scanning. *J Vasc Surg* 17:152, 1993.

28. Carpenter JP, Lexa FJ, Davis JT: Determination of sixty percent or greater carotid artery stenosis by duplex Doppler ultrasonography. *J Vasc Surg* 22:697, 1995.

29. Carpenter JP, Lexa FJ, Davis JT: Determination of duplex Doppler ultrasound criteria appropriate to the North American Symptomatic Carotid Endarterectomy Trial. *Stroke* 27:695, 1996.

30. Neale ML, Chambers JL, Kelly AT, et al: Reappraisal of duplex criteria to assess significant carotid stenosis with special reference to reports from the North American Symptomatic Carotid Endarterectomy Trial and the European Carotid Surgery Trial. *J Vasc Surg* 20:642, 1994.

31. Hood DB, Mattos MA, Mansour A, et al: Prospective evaluation of new duplex criteria to identify 70% internal carotid artery stenosis. *J Vasc Surg* 23:254, 1996.

32. Browman MW, Cooperberg PL, Harrison PB, et al: Duplex ultrasonography criteria for internal carotid stenosis of more than 70% diameter: Angiographic correlation and receiver operating characteristic curve analysis. *Can Assoc Radiol J* 46:291, 1995.

33. Wilterdink JL, Feldmann E, Easton JD, et al: Performance of carotid ultrasound in evaluating candidates for carotid

endarterectomy is optimized by an approach based on clinical outcome rather than accuracy. *Stroke* 27:1094, 1996.

34. Derdeyn CP, Powers WJ: Cost-effectiveness of screening for asymptomatic carotid artery disease. *Stroke* 27;1944, 1996.

35. Tessler FN, Kimme-Smith C, Sutherland ML, Schiller VL, Perrella RR, Grant EG: Inter- and intra-observer variability of Doppler peak velocity measurements: An in-vitro study. *Ultrasound Med Biol* 16:653, 1990.

36. Howard G, Baker WH, Chambless LE, et al: An approach for the use of Doppler ultrasound as a screening tool for hemodynamically significant stenosis (despite heterogeneity of Doppler performance): A multicenter experience. *Stroke* 27:1951, 1996.

37. McNeil B, Keeler E, Adelstein S: Primer on certain elements of medical decision making. *N Engl J Med* 293:211, 1975.

38. Hankey GJ, Warlow CP, Sellar RJ: Cerebral angiographic risk in mild cerebrovascular disease. *Stroke* 21:209, 1990.

39. Pujia A, Rubba P, Spencer MP: Prevalence of extracranial carotid artery disease detectable by echo-Doppler in an elderly population. *Stroke* 23:818, 1992.

40. Hennerici M, Aulich A, Sandmann W, et al: Incidence of asymptomatic extracranial carotid artery disease. *Stroke* 12:750, 1981.

41. Derdeyn CP, Powers WJ, Moran CJ, Cross DT, Allen BT: Role of Doppler U.S. in screening atherosclerotic disease. *Radiology* 197:635, 1995.

42. Kent KC, Kuntz KM, Mahesh RP, et al: Perioperative imaging strategies for carotid endarterectomy: An analysis of morbidity and cost effectiveness in symptomatic patients. *JAMA* 274:888, 1995.

43. Sitzer M, Furst G, Siebler M, Steinmetz H: Usefulness of an intravenous contrast medium in the characterization of high grade internal carotid stenosis with color Doppler assisted duplex imaging. *Stroke* 25:385, 1994.

44. McLaren JT, Donaghue CC, Drezner AD: Accuracy of carotid duplex examination to predict proximal and intrathoracic lesions. *Am J Surg* 172:149, 1996.

45. Ligush J Jr, Burnham CB, Burnham SJ, Owens LV, Keagy BA: Accuracy of the duplex scan of the supraaortic trunks. *J Vasc Tech* 20:81, 1996.

Chapter 34

COMPUTED TOMOGRAPHY SCANNING IN ISCHEMIC STROKE

David M. Pelz

BACKGROUND

As new therapies for acute stroke such as intravenous and intra-arterial thrombolysis become more widely available, the early diagnosis of stroke with imaging confirmation has become essential. There has long been a perception that computed tomographic (CT) scanning can only identify changes in the later stages of stroke, long after these changes have become irreversible.[1] Traditionally, the use of CT in acute stroke has been to exclude associated hemorrhage. The clinical diagnosis of stroke may be wrong in up to 13 percent of cases,[2] and CT has been used in the past to exclude these alternative pathologies such as tumor, arteriovenous malformation (AVM), or primary hemorrhage.

Despite the widespread diffusion of magnetic resonance imaging (MRI) throughout the population, CT is still the fastest, most accessible, and most practical modality to image acute stroke patients. Recent studies with the new generation of high resolution, helical scanners have shown that subtle signs on CT scans may be recognized as early as 43 min after the event.[3] These CT signs may be very subtle, yet this is when therapeutic intervention has the greatest chance of being successful. Recognition of early signs of infarction is also critical to avert complications of thrombolytic therapy. The European Cooperative Acute Stroke Study (ECASS) of alteplase (rTPA) treatment in acute stroke revealed a subgroup of patients with poor outcomes who in retrospect did show the subtle signs of major infarction on their initial CT scan.[4,5] In this chapter, the early CT signs of stroke will be described, and the temporal sequence of evolving infarction will be shown. The clinical role of CT angiography (CTA) and stable Xenon CT (XeCT) will also be discussed, followed by recommended CT-imaging protocols.

EVIDENCE

CT in Hyperacute Stroke (0 to 24 h)

The older stroke literature suggests that CT scans will show changes in only 50 to 60 percent of acute stroke patients under 24 h.[6] More recent studies with higher resolution scanners have shown that subtle changes are often seen experimentally within minutes of the event[1,3] and within hours in clinical practice.[7-9] It has been estimated that approximately 60 percent of CT scans will show changes in the first 6 to 12 h, as opposed to 80 percent of MRI scans using standard spin echo sequences.[6,7,10,11] Because the middle cerebral artery (MCA) is the vascular distribution most commonly affected, most of the early CT signs are seen in this territory (Table 34-1).

Loss of Gray-White Differentiation, Sulcal Effacement In hyperacute stroke, the first sign is often subtle cortical hypodensity, resulting in loss of gray-white matter differentiation (Fig. 34-1). This is because of the development of cytotoxic edema, induced by ischemia and may be reversible if perfusion is restored. There may be subtle mass effect with slight effacement of cortical sulci, which may only be appreciable when comparison is made with the contralateral hemisphere. This mass effect may occur before the hypodensity of edema

Table 34-1.

CT findings in hyperacute stroke

Loss of gray-white matter differentiation

Mild sulcal effacement

Obscuration of the lentiform nucleus

Loss of "insular ribbon"

Hyperdense middle cerebral artery sign (HMCAS)

appears, usually less than 6 h after ictus.[12] There may also be mild ipsilateral ventricular effacement in the first few hours.

Obscuration of Lentiform Nucleus, Loss of Insular Ribbon   The lentiform nucleus may become obscured, the result of vasogenic edema in the basal ganglia, causing hypodensity and blurring of margins with adjacent white matter (Fig. 34-2). This has been observed within 2 to 3 h of the ictus[13] and may predispose to later hemor-

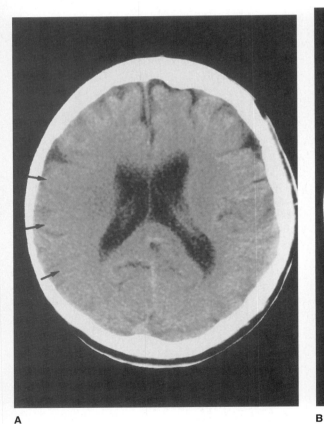
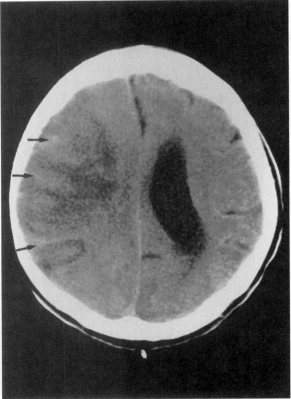

A   **B**

Figure 34-1.

A   *noncontrast CT head scan performed within 3 h of the ischemic event shows loss of gray-white matter differentiation over the right frontal and parietal convexities (arrows). There is subtle mass effect with mild effacement of cortical sulci on the right as compared with the left hemisphere.*
B   *noncontrast CT scan performed 4 days later shows the large right MCA distribution infarct with petechial hemorrhage (arrows).*

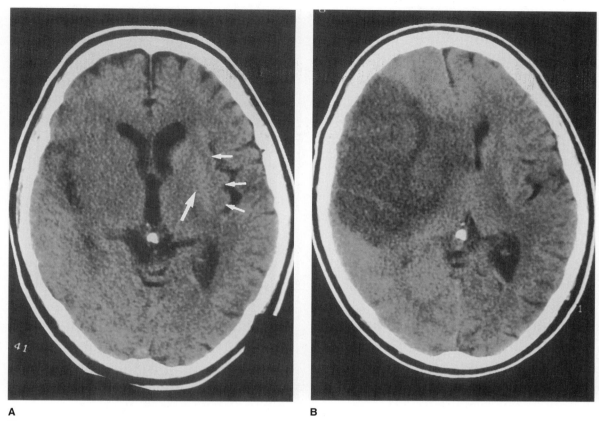

A   **B**

Figure 34-2
A   *noncontrast scan within 4 h of the ischemic event shows loss of the right lentiform nucleus and disappearance of the right insular ribbon. Note normal lentiform nucleus* (large arrow) *and insular ribbon* (small arrows) *on the left.* B   *repeat scan 3 days later shows the large deep temporal infarct with marked mass effect.*

rhagic transformation. There may be loss of gray-white matter definition in the lateral insular cortex or "insular ribbon" (Figs. 34-2, 34-3). This area is supplied by insular segments of the MCA and is far from anterior and posterior cerebral collateral channels, therefore representing a vulnerable watershed zone. Hypodensity here likely represents irreversible vasogenic edema.[14]

Hyperdense Middle Cerebral Artery Sign   The hyperdense middle cerebral artery sign (HMCAS) is often associated with large MCA distribution infarcts and represents acute thrombus in a vessel, most commonly in the M1 segment of the MCA (Fig. 34-4), less often in other vessels such as the internal carotid and posterior cerebral arteries.[6,7] When truly present, this sign is often

associated with a major neurologic deficit and a poorer response to thrombolytic therapy.[15] This sign has been shown, however, to have a relatively low sensitivity, being present in only 35 to 50 percent of MCA and 25 percent of all infarcts. Specificity is also low, with false positives most commonly due to atherosclerosis, diabetes, hypertension, or raised hematocrit, resulting in increased vascular density.[16]

CT is particularly effective for the diagnosis of acute hemorrhage, but this is an uncommon finding in the hyperacute and acute phases of stroke in normotensive patients.

33 Percent Rule   The development of vasogenic edema requires at least 3 to 6 h of diminished or absent

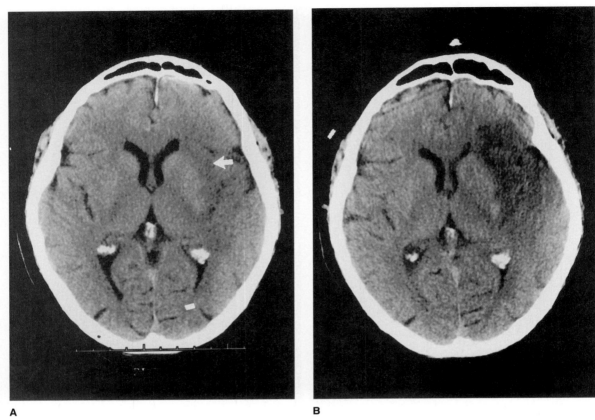

Figure 34-3.
A   noncontrast CT scan within 4 h of the event shows subtle lucency in the left insular cortex and loss of the insular ribbon (arrow). *B   a repeat scan performed 6 days later shows a well-developed insular infarct.*

cerebral blood flow, and well-defined parenchymal lucencies are difficult to identify in this stage. The extent of lucency is important to evaluate, however, as it may be a potent predictor of response to thrombolytic therapy.[1] In one study, hypodensity greater than 33 percent of the MCA territory may have been associated with an increased risk of fatal parenchymal hemorrhage when thrombolytic therapy was performed.[17] Others have shown that the 33 percent rule indicates a higher probability of a poor outcome but not necessarily an increased risk of hemorrhage.[18]

Administration of intravenous contrast material is not indicated in this stage unless the diagnosis is in doubt. The blood-brain barrier may still be intact, and parenchymal enhancement should not occur. There may be prominent enhancement in cortical vessels owing to

slow flow, but parenchymal enhancement will not be seen for at least 24 h.[9]

CT in Acute Stroke (24 h to 7 days)

By 24 h, hypodensity of the infarct becomes more visible, and cortical lesions may be wedge shaped and deeper lesions round or oval (Fig. 34-5). The size and location of the lucency can help determine etiology. If there is involvement of distal vascular territories or multiple distributions, an embolic etiology is likely. If large portions of the anterior and middle cerebral artery territories are involved, there may be an internal carotid artery occlusion present. Lucencies in the watershed zones may be hypotensive in origin.

Low density vasogenic edema and mass effect

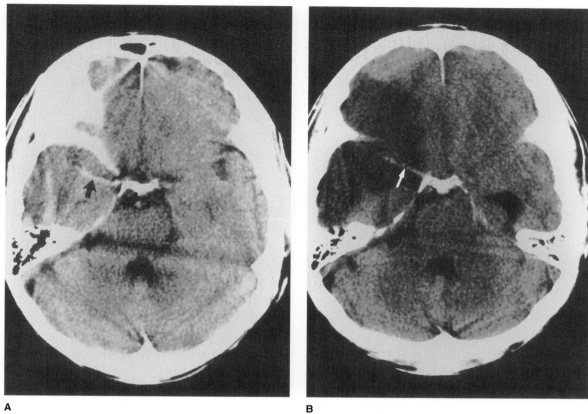

A **B**

Figure 34-4.
A   *noncontrast CT scan performed within 3 h of the ischemic event shows a hyperdense proximal middle cerebral artery* (arrow), *representing acute thrombus in the vessel.* B   *follow-up scan from 3 days later shows the large MCA infarct surrounding the hyperdense M1 segment* (arrow).

reach a maximum at 3 to 5 days and occasionally can progress up to 2 weeks. This can result in marked ventricular compression, midline shift, and uncal herniation (Fig. 34-6). Contrast enhancement is unusual before day 3 and, if it is seen early, may indicate an increased risk for hemorrhagic conversion of the infarct.

CT in Subacute Stroke (8 to 21 days)

In this stage, gyriform enhancement of the infarct is typically seen, with peak enhancement in the third week, usually after the period of maximum mass effect. The enhancement pattern can be differentiated from other causes of gyriform enhancement such as tumor or infection by the vascular distribution, the temporal sequence, and the involvement of both gray and white matter (Fig.

34-7). The enhancement is due to breakdown of the blood-brain barrier, enhanced capillary filling in affected gyri ("luxury perfusion"), reactive hyperemia, and neovascularity.

These changes should all begin to resolve by 3 weeks, and if mass effect and enhancement persist beyond 3 to 4 weeks, underlying pathology such as a neoplasm should be suspected.

Hemorrhagic transformation of the infarct occurs in 18 to 41 percent of patients in this stage.[19,20] This happens more often in embolic infarcts when there is clot lysis resulting in restoration of blood flow, and the capillary bed is then re-exposed to systemic blood pressure. These reperfusion hemorrhages are often petechial in nature and clinically silent (Fig. 34-8). They may lead to the "disappearing infarct" sign in which an infarct

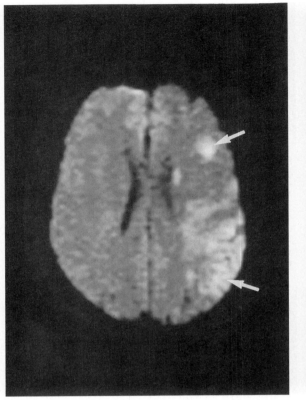
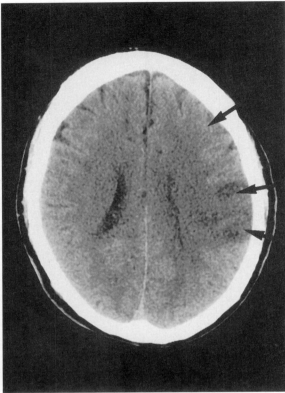

A   **B**

Figure 34-5.
A *diffusion-weighted MRI obtained within hours of the event shows multiple high-signal lesions throughout the left hemisphere consistent with ischemic injury* (arrows). *The CT scan at this stage was normal.* B *a noncontrast 5 days after the ischemic event shows well-defined left frontal cortical infarcts* (arrows).

seen in the acute phase as a lucent lesion becomes isodense with brain and is no longer well visualized. These petechial hemorrhages are more common in the cortex and deep gray matter structures, and they are different than the large gyral or lobar hemorrhages seen in the acute phase.

CT in Chronic Stroke (more than 21 days)

In the chronic phase, there is development of well-defined, sharply marginated encephalomalacic change and gliosis. Gray and white matter are usually involved but there may be a rim of preserved cortex over the lucent region as the gray matter is more resistant to ischemia (Fig. 34-9). Encephalomalacic areas will have

a density similar to CSF, although the gliotic area may be higher in density. Very rarely, gyriform enhancement may persist up to 6 weeks, but the intensity should be decreasing by 3 weeks. Other findings in this stage include dilatation of the ipsilateral ventricle and subarachnoid spaces, retraction of the midline structures, wallerian degeneration proximal to large cortical or capsular infarcts, and occasionally dystrophic calcification.

Limitations of CT

CT is usually of no help in the diagnosis of transient ischemic attacks or reversible ischemic deficits but can exclude other pathology. It is of little use in diagnosing acute posterior fossa infarcts, as these areas

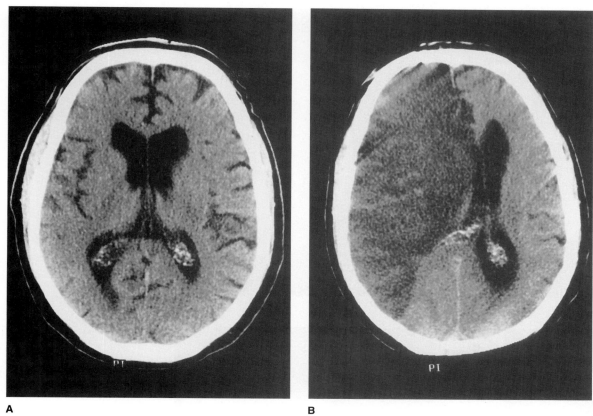

A   B

Figure 34-6.
A   *noncontrast CT scan within 4 h of the event shows subtle, diffuse loss of gray-white matter differentiation throughout the right hemisphere.* B   *a repeat scan 6 days later shows the large right MCA infarct with significant mass effect.*

are often obscured by beam-hardening artifacts from the temporal bones. MRI is currently better for the detection of acute stroke, particularly when diffusion-weighted imaging is used,[5,10,11,21] and for showing the sequelae of infarction such as hemorrhagic transformation, cystic encephalomalacia, gliosis, and wallerian degeneration.

Newer Techniques

CT has traditionally been used in acute stroke to rule out hemorrhage and to identify alternate pathologies. It may or may not show the extent of the infarct and suggest an etiology. Of critical interest in acute stroke therapy is the identification of potentially reversible ischemic tissue, the "Holy Grail" of stroke imaging.

This is the key to successful thrombolytic therapy, and newer techniques such as CTA, XeCT, and diffusion-weighted MRI (DWI) have all been applied to this problem with varying degrees of success.

CT Angiography   The new generation of helical CT scanners has made CTA widely available, and this technique has been used to image acute stroke patients.[22–25] This early work has shown promise as a method to rapidly show the site of vascular occlusion and the length of the occluded segment (Fig. 34-10). The enhancement of arteries beyond the occlusion has been used as a rough indicator of collateral flow, although its value as a predictor of ischemic injury is uncertain.[24] CTA seems to be about as sensitive to intracranial vascular stenoses and occlusions as MRI angiography and conventional

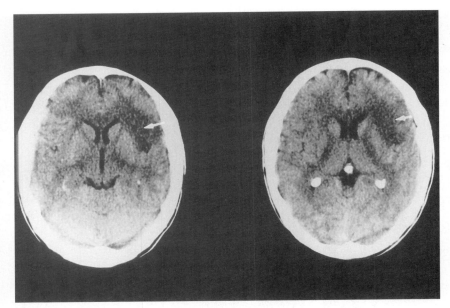

A

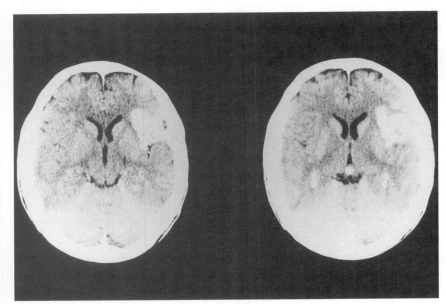

B

Figure 34-7.
A   *noncontrast CT scan shows lucency in the left frontal operculum and anterior insular cortex* (arrows). B   *a contrast-enhanced scan shows gyriform enhancement characteristic of subacute infarction.*

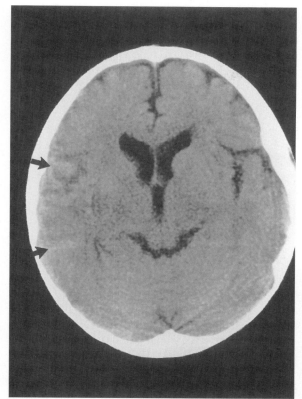

Figure 34-8.
A noncontrast CT scan shows a subtle increase in density of right insular cortical gyri (arrows) *with subcortical lucency, consistent with petechial hemorrhage in a subacute infarct.*

angiography, although extracranial vessels are not routinely seen with CTA.

Several studies have looked at using CTA and helical scan technology to rapidly measure cerebral blood flow (CBF) and to identify areas at risk of infarction.[22,23] Using standard clinical scanners, maps of CBF can be obtained, and areas of reduced perfusion and major vessel compromise can be reliably identified. Although areas of marginal perfusion may be outlined, the determination of reversible vs. irreversible ischemic damage is still not possible in most cases.

There are several limitations to these techniques. A large bolus of intravenous contrast material is required, and the effects of this contrast load are uncertain in the acute stroke patient. Although data acquisition time is very short, adding only a few minutes to the study, computer reformations and CBF determinations

may take 30 to 40 min, and this can be a critical delay if thrombolytic therapy is being considered.[26] Although CTA and CT maps of CBF are promising techniques, standard CT remains the imaging modality of choice in the acute situation[8,20] despite the fact that reliable identification of reversible ischemia is still elusive. DWI and MRI show promise for practical application in the acute setting.

Stable Xenon CT   This procedure, in which CBF maps are generated by CT scanning following inhalation of stable Xenon gas, has been available for many years and has not found wide clinical acceptance. Initial criticisms of this technique were that the machinery and performance of the test were cumbersome and time consuming, demanding compliant patients who could

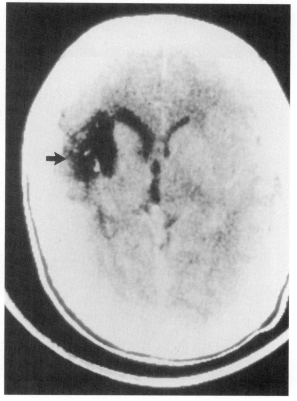

Figure 34-9.
A noncontrast CT shows a well-defined, low-density lesion in the right temporal lobe with encephalomalacic change and dilatation of the ipsilateral frontal horn, consistent with an old infarct (arrow).

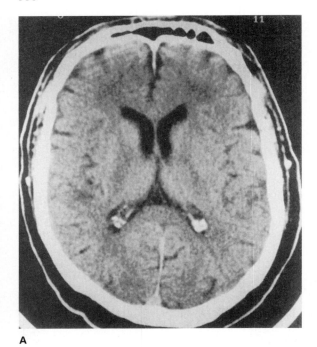

A

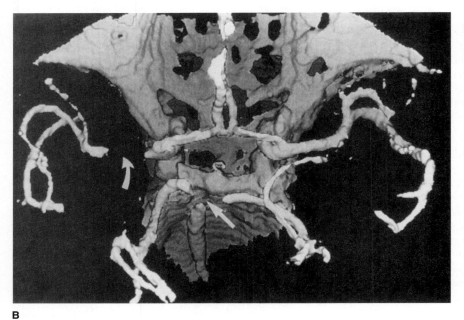

B

Figure 34-10.
A   *noncontrast CT done within hours of ictus shows no abnormality.* B   *CT angiography with three-dimensional reconstruction of the circle of Willis shows distal occlusion of the basilar artery and proximal posterior cerebral arteries* (straight arrow) *and occlusion of the left proximal MCA* (curved arrow).

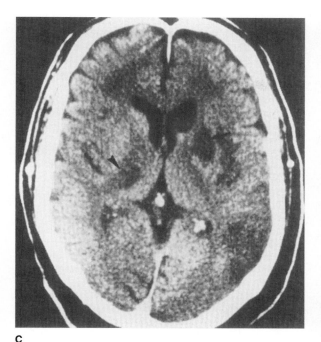

C

Figure 34-10 (*Continued***).**
C   *follow-up CT scan 1 day later shows the infarcts of the right thalamus* (arrowhead) *and left temporal lobe* (arrow). *Source: Knauth M, von Kummer R, Jansen O, et al: Potential of CT angiography in acute ischemic stroke.* Am J Neuroradiol *18:1001, 1997. Used with permission.*

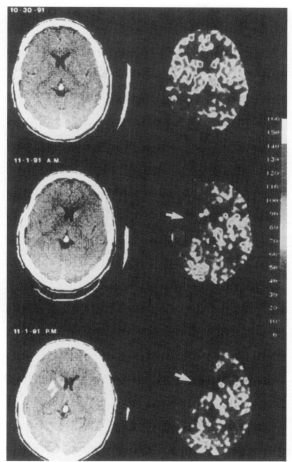

Figure 34-11.
Sequential noncontrast CT scans (left) *and XeCT CBF studies* (right) *prior to* (top) *and following elective right carotid balloon occlusion. The initial pre-occlusion CT* (top) *is normal. The XeCT study shows some decreased perfusion in the posterior temporal-occipital region. One hour after balloon occlusion, the patient developed a left hemiplegia. The CT was normal* (middle), *but the XeCT showed absence of flow in the right MCA territory* (arrow), *presumably embolic in origin. Despite attempted thrombolysis, the MCA did not reopen, and repeat studies done at 5 h* (bottom) *showed a hemorrhagic infarct in the right basal ganglia and extension of the right MCA flow defect* (arrow). *Source: Yonas H, Pindzola RP, Johnson DW: Xenon/computed tomography cerebral blood flow and its use in clinical management.* Neurosurg Clin North Am *7:605, 1996. Used with permission.*

remain motionless for at least 6 to 10 min while breathing stable Xenon gas. The gas itself has intrinsic anesthetic properties and can artificially elevate CBF values by 5 percent or more.[27] The test has been most successfully used to predict stroke risk in patients with symptomatic carotid stenoses.[28]

The new helical scanners are faster and allow up to eight sampling slices to be obtained, resulting in better correlation with anatomic images. The Pittsburgh group has used the test to assess tissue viability in acute stroke, suggesting that CBF values lower than 10 to 12 mL/100/cc/min indicate irreversibility[27,29] and probable failure of thrombolytic therapy (Fig. 34-11). Those patients were also at greater risk for development of intraparenchymal hemorrhage following thrombolysis. Although the procedure is faster and easier to perform and anesthetic properties of the gas are minimal at the concentrations currently used, XeCT is still not widely used in the acute stroke setting, and its potential remains unproven.

SUMMARY AND RECOMMENDATIONS

CT is still the fastest, most convenient, and widely available test to use for the diagnosis and early treatment of acute stroke. It can confirm the diagnosis, rule out other pathologies, and if subtle signs are searched for, it can show the extent of the lesion, suggest an etiology, and guide the use of thrombolytic agents. CT can therefore help to decide who should and who should not receive thrombolytic therapy. Scanning protocols will vary, but in general, noncontrast scans are done in the acute phase. Slices of 3-mm or 5-mm thickness can be performed through the skull base and posterior fossa to look at the Circle of Willis vessels, with 7-mm-thick images obtained to the top of the brain.

When reading a scan in the setting of a suspected hyperacute stroke, the clinician must check for the following abnormalities: (1) a nonvascular cause of a stroke-like presentation (i.e., tumor, AVM, etc.); (2) evidence of intracranial hemorrhage (acute or chronic); (3) loss of gray-white differentiation; (4) sulcal effacement; (5) obscuration of the lentiform nucleus; (6) loss of the insular ribbon; and (7) the hyperdense middle cerebral artery sign (HMCAS).

The role of CTA in this stage is uncertain, as the benefits of identifying a vascular occlusion must be weighed against the risk of intravenous contrast injection and the time delay for computer reformations. The differentiation of reversible from irreversible ischemic change cannot at present be reliably made. Techniques that measure CBF, such as three-dimensional helical CT and XeCT, are not routinely performed in the acute phase but hold promise for the future determination of those patients most likely to benefit from thrombolytic therapy.

REFERENCES

1. von Kummer R, Bozzao I, Manelfe C: Detectability, prevalence and significance of early CT signs, in *Early CT Diagnosis of Hemispheric Brain Infarction,* 1st ed. Berlin, Springer-Verlag, 1995, pp. 89-95.
2. Shuaib A, Lee D, Pelz D, et al: The impact of magnetic resonance imaging in the management of acute ischemic stroke. *Neurology* 42:816, 1992.
3. von Kummer R, Meyding-Lamade U, Forsting M, et al: Sensitivity and prognostic value of early CT in occlusion of the middle cerebral artery trunk. *Am J Neuroradiol* 15:9, 1994.
4. Fisher M, Pessin M, Furlan AJ: ECASS: Lessons for future thrombolytic stroke trials. *JAMA* 274:1058, 1995.
5. Bryan RN: Diffusion weighted imaging: To treat or not to treat? That is the question. *Am J Neuroradiol* 19: 396, 1998.
6. Leys D, Pruvo JP, Godefroy O, et al: Prevalence and significance of hyperdense middle cerebral artery in acute stroke. *Stroke* 23:317, 1992.
7. Tomsick TA: Sensitivity and prognostic value of early CT in occlusion of the middle cerebral artery trunk. *Am J Neuroradiol* 15:16, 1994.
8. Dillon WP: CT techniques for detecting acute stroke and collateral circulation: In search of the holy grail. *Am J Neuroradiol* 19:191, 1998.
9. Weingarten K: Computed tomography of cerebral infarction. *Neuroimag Clin North Am* 2:409, 1992.
10. Bryan RN, Levy LM, Whitlow WD, et al: Diagnosis of acute cerebral infarction: Comparison of CT and MR imaging. *Am J Neuroradiol* 12:611, 1991.
11. Elster AD, Moody DM: Early cerebral infarction: Gadopentetate dimeglumine enhancement. *Radiology* 177:627, 1990.
12. Horowitz SH, Zito JL, Donnarumma R, et al: Computed tomographic and angiographic findings within the first five hours of cerebral infarction. *Stroke* 22:1245, 1991.
13. Tomura N, Uemura K, Inugami A, et al: Early CT findings in cerebral infarction. *Radiology* 168:463, 1988.
14. Truwit CL, Barkovich AJ, Gear-Marten A, et al: Loss of the insular ribbon: Another early CT sign of acute middle cerebral artery infarction. *Radiology* 176:801, 1990.
15. Tomsick T, Brott T, Borsan W, et al: Prognostic value of the hyperdense middle cerebral artery sign and stroke scale score before ultra-early thrombolytic therapy. *Am J Neuroradiol* 17:79, 1996.
16. Rauch RA, Bozan C, Larsson EM, Jinkins JR: Hyperdense middle cerebral arteries identified on CT as a false sign of vascular occlusion. *Am J Neuroradiol* 14:669, 1993.
17. von Kummer R, Allen KL, Halle R, et al: Acute stroke: Usefulness of early CT findings before thrombolytic therapy. *Radiology* 205:327, 1997.
18. Roos M, Hu W, Buchan AM: Early CT signs of infarction and hemorrhagic outcomes in the treatment of acute ischemic stroke with t-PA. *Can J Neurol Sci* 25 (Suppl 2): 515, 1998.
19. Smith TP. Radiologic intervention in the acute stroke patient. *J Vasc Intervent Radiol* 7:627, 1996.
20. Horning CR, Dorndorf W, Agnoli AL: Hemorrhagic cerebral infarction: A prospective study. *Stroke* 17:179, 1986.
21. Warach S, Bosha M, Welch KMA: Pitfalls and potential of clinical diffusion-weighted MR imaging in acute stroke (Editorial). *Stroke* 28:481, 1997.
22. Hunter GJ, Hambey LM, Ponzo JA, et al: Assessment of cerebral perfusion and arterial anatomy in hyperacute stroke with three-dimensional functional CT: Early clinical results. *Am J Neuroradiol* 19:29, 1998.

23. Hambey LM, Hunter GJ, Halpern EF, et al: Quantitative, high resolution measurement of cerebral vascular physiology with slip-ring CT. *Am J Neuroradiol* 17:639, 1996.

24. Knauth M, von Kummer R, Jansen O, et al: Potential of CT angiography in acute ischemic stroke. *Am J Neuroradiol* 18:1001, 1997.

25. Shrier DA, Tanaka H, Numaguchi Y, et al: CT angiography in the evaluation of acute stroke. *Am J Neuroradiol* 18:1011, 1997.

26. Brant-Zawadzki M: CT angiography in acute ischemic stroke: The right tool for the job? *Am J Neuroradiol* 18:1021, 1997.

27. Yonas H, Pindzola RP, Johnson DW: Xenon/computed tomography cerebral blood flow and its use in clinical management. *Neurosurg Clin North Am* 7:605, 1996.

28. Yonas H, Smith HA, Durham SR, Pentheny SL, Johnson DW: Increased stroke risk predicted by compromised cerebral blood flow reactivity. *J Neurosurg* 79:483, 1993.

29. Johnson DW, Stringer WA, Marks MP, et al: Stable Xenon CT cerebral blood flow imaging: Rationale for the role in clinical decision making. *Am J Neuroradiol* 12:201, 1991.

Chapter 35

MAGNETIC RESONANCE IMAGING IN ISCHEMIC STROKE

George J. So
Suzie M. El-Saden
Jeffrey R. Alger

INTRODUCTION

In current practice, the workup of stroke begins with computed tomography (CT), which serves to evaluate for stroke as well as stroke mimics. In approximately 10 percent of patients with clinical symptoms of ischemia, the symptoms are actually due to diseases such as arteriovenous malformation, tumors, or infection. CT continues to be the first line of imaging as it is still the most sensitive modality for the detection of hemorrhage. In the early radiology literature, the sensitivity of CT in detecting acute infarct was reported to be about 50 percent in the first 48 h. At this time, CT is not sensitive enough to distinguish between a transient ischemic attack (TIA) and a fixed anatomic lesion. Magnetic resonance imaging (MRI) has further increased the sensitivity for detecting acute cerebral infarction. MRI is superior to CT in the detection of infarcts that are adjacent to bone or in the posterior fossa.

The exquisite soft-tissue contrast and multiplanar imaging capability offered by MRI have led to its wide acceptance as the method of choice for high-resolution brain imaging. Although MRI is used to evaluate a wide range of brain disorders, until recently, acute stroke has not been one of these. MRI studies of human stroke began soon after MRI units became available for clinical imaging.

ACUTE INFARCT (0 TO 6 H)

Conventional MRI using T1-weighted and T2-weighted contrast alone has proven to have relatively little value in the detection of the earliest signs of stroke.[1,2] Acutely, within the first 6 h, infarcted brain tissue demonstrates little in the way of distinct T1- and T2-weighted contrast change relative to surrounding unaffected brain tissue. Conventional T1- and T2-weighted MRI sequences are more valuable in subacute and chronic stroke, where the infarcted tissue is easily identified as hyperintense on T2-weighted and hypointense on T1-weighted images. Unfortunately, the ability of spin-echo MRI to detect these relatively late stage changes has little relevance in the setting of acute stroke therapy. These MRI signatures of infarction tend to appear well after the closing of what many consider to be the "time window of opportunity" for acute stroke intervention. Recent studies have demonstrated that acute intraparenchymal bleeding is identifiable on T2-weighted MRI.[3,4] Nevertheless, MRI has not been used extensively to rule out hemorrhagic stroke because this can be done with greater practicality and sensitivity with CT.

Since 1990, we have witnessed two technologic revolutions that have considerably altered our perception of the value of MRI in acute stroke evaluation. The first of these revolutions occurred in the early 1990's with the development of magnetic resonance angiography (MRA), which permitted the noninvasive high resolution imaging of flow through the vessels of the head and neck. At present, we are seeing a second revolution of considerable significance owing to the introduction of diffusion and perfusion MRI techniques. Progress made during the past 5 years suggests that diffusion and perfusion MRI will become indispensable tools that will be used emergently for therapeutic planning.[5] The specific goal of this section is to provide an introductory clinically oriented description of diffusion and perfusion MRI techniques as they pertain to acute stroke.

One key to developing a technically accurate understanding of diffusion and perfusion MRI is to focus on their differences. Perfusion and diffusion MRI techniques are not as closely related as they might seem. Often, the two share common MRI data acquisition techniques, but in fact, they measure quite distinct tissue parameters. Perfusion MRI provides measures of several hemodynamic parameters from the tissue within the ischemic and surrounding territory. Diffusion MRI provides an indication of the physiologic stress that the tissue experiences as a result of the ischemia. The two methods are more easily grasped if one thinks of them as being unrelated yet used in combination only because of their common physiologic relevance to stroke. For this reason, they will be presented separately.

Diffusion MRI

The signal intensity generated with MRI is inherently sensitive to the motion of the tissue water molecules that generate it. There are several different types of water molecule motion that can be exploited in MRI. For instance, MRA is sensitive to the pressure-driven flow of the water molecules within the vascular space. Similarly, the tumbling of water molecules in physiologic solution plays a major role in defining the T1 and T2 values characteristic of tissue. Diffusion MRI exploits another distinct sensitivity of MRI to the molecular motion of water. In diffusion MRI, the signal intensity reflects a sensitivity to the random motion made by tissue water molecules as they move from one place to another on a microscopic scale.[6] This translational diffusion was originally described by the English botanist, Brown, who observed in 1827 that pollen particles suspended in water seem to continuously move from place to place when viewed with a light microscope. Accordingly, the phenomenon is often referred to as "Brownian diffusion." In diffusion MRI, the image contrast depends on the rate of Brownian diffusion.

Diffusion MRI uses a slightly modified spin-echo pulse sequence similar to that used for T2-weighted

Figure 35-1.

A typical diffusion MRI pulse sequence. Only sequence elements that are directly related to the diffusion sensitization are shown. Typically, a spin-echo sequence composed of a 90-degree followed by a 180-degree radiofrequency pulse is used. Gradient pulses having a variety of different levels are played out on both sides of the 180-degree pulse to sensitize the MRI signal to Brownian diffusion. Stronger gradient pulses convey increased sensitivity to diffusion. The gradient sensitization can be performed in any number of unique anatomic directions (L/R [left/right]; A/P [anterior/posterior]; S/I [superior/inferior]). Sensitization along a chosen direction can be used to identify tissue structures (e.g., white matter fibers), which cause diffusion in particular directions to be more probable compared with other directions.

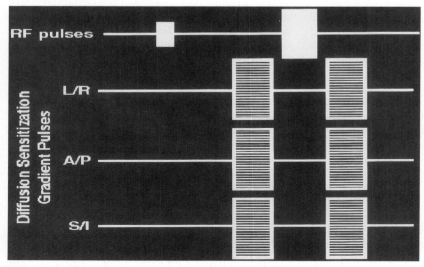

MRI (Fig. 35-1). Water molecules generate their MRI signal at a characteristic frequency that depends on the local magnetic field strength in which they are situated. Magnetic field gradients applied to the scanner hardware are used to cause the frequency generated by different water molecules to be a function of their position. For complete signal generation in sequences such as those shown in Fig. 35-1, the water molecules must have the same frequency during the entire sequence. If the molecules move because of Brownian diffusion during the sequence, their frequencies are not constant throughout the sequence and signal is lost. The extent to which signal loss occurs depends on the *rate* of Brownian diffusion. The strength of the applied magnetic field gradient, which is programmed into the pulse sequence, conveys a controlled sensitivity to motion. The extent to which the MRI signal is diffusion sensitized is expressed numerically using the "*b* value." A *b* value of 0 s/mm² connotes no motion sensitization, whereas a value of 1000 s/mm², which is about the maximum a modern human MRI scanner is capable of producing, conveys a strong sensitivity to motion occurring at rates characteristic of the Brownian diffusion of water molecules in brain tissue.

Figure 35-2 is a diffusion-weighted magnetic resonance image (DWI) obtained using $b = 1000$ s/mm² taken from a patient with acute stroke. The figure also provides several MRI scans obtained using more conventional MRI contrast characteristics. The diffusion sensitivity within the DWI becomes apparent when one compares normal parenchymal tissue signal (the left hemisphere) with cerebrospinal fluid (CSF) signal. The rate of water diffusion in tissue is relatively low compared with CSF. This is because of the presence of barriers to motion (membranes) in the tissue, whereas the CSF is mostly fluid with the exception of a small number of cells. It is also a result of the fact that the cellular fluid is more viscous because of the presence of dissolved macromolecules. On DWI, the CSF signal is, therefore, hypointense (low) relative to the parenchymal signal. The ischemic right middle cerebral artery territory appears on the DWI as a region of relative hyperintensity. Whereas the presence of ischemia in this territory might be discerned from the sulcal effacement seen on the T1-weighted image or the modest T2-weighted hyperintensity of this region, the high contrast of DWI permits one to readily appreciate the location and the extent of the ischemic territory.

The initial discovery that ischemic brain tissue produced such a remarkable contrast on DWI relative to T2-weighted spin-echo imaging grew from studies of animal models subjected to middle cerebral artery occlusion.[7] Studies with animal models have clearly demonstrated that the DWI hyperintensity delineates tissue damaged by ischemia.[7,8] More important, animal studies have demonstrated that the contrast findings

Figure 35-2.
Diagram presents a diffusion-weighted magnetic resonance image (DWI) obtained using b = 1000 *s/mm² taken from a case of acute stroke, with comparisons to other types of MR sequence (T2-weighted, T1-weighted, and proton-density weighted). The scans were taken within minutes of each other and less than 24 h from the time the patient was last known to be well.*

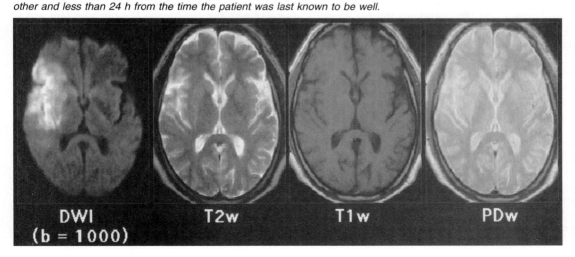

appear within a minute of the interruption of blood flow.[9] The relevance for the evaluation of acute clinical stroke is that the DWI contrast will be present as soon as the patient can be practically brought to the scanner. Subsequent studies of human stroke have demonstrated that DWI scans perfomed early in the infarction process have good potential for predicting clinical outcome.[10,11] The cause of the DWI hyperintensity associated with acute brain ischemia has been debated extensively since its discovery. A picture that is consistent with presently available information is that the hyperintense DWI signal characteristic of brain ischemia develops as a result of the movement of water from the extracellular space to the intracellular space. In the extracellular space, diffusion is relatively fast compared with the intracellular space, where the increased viscosity resulting from dissolved macromolecules and the increased density of membrane barriers serve to slow diffusion. This swelling of the intracellular space is often referred to as "cytotoxic edema"; it involves a redistribution of water between compartments rather than a net increase of water into the tissue, as occurs with "vasogenic edema." The extracellular to intracellular water redistribution occurs because of the ischemic sensitivity of brain tissue. Within seconds of interruption of oxygen and glucose delivery, brain tissue ceases to produce the energy needed to maintain the external/internal ion (Na^+,K^+) ratio and the corresponding water balance.

The concept of the diffusion sensitization of magnetic resonance signals has been understood for some time. However, it could not be achieved in human MRI scanners before 1992.[12,13] Three practical technical issues were addressed to make human DWI scans possible: (1) suppression of sensitivity to motion other than diffusion, (2) the diffusion sensitivity conveyed by the tissue structure at a somewhat more macroscopic level, and (3) the combined sensitivity of DWI to both T2 and diffusion. The following paragraphs discuss these issues.

Diffusion MRI is so sensitive to movements over small distances that larger nondiffusion motion may produce large artifacts causing degradation of image quality. The most significant of such motion is the whole head movement in patients who are unable to remain still during the scanning process. Two methods have been explored to circumvent this problem. The most well accepted is the use of echo planar imaging (EPI) to acquire the diffusion-weighted signal intensity. EPI permits the acquisition of an entire planar diffusion-weighted image in about 100 ms when modern MRI

hardware is used.[14] Such fast "snapshot" imaging serves to "freeze" any movement of the entire head. In addition to freezing large-scale motion, the imaging speed provided by EPI can be used to enable the collection of a series of images that are diffusion weighted in unique ways. This serves to add additional specificity to DWI as is described below. A complete description of EPI is beyond the scope of this chapter. However, a few key properties of the EPI technique are relevant. First, although the imaging speed attained with EPI is unsurpassed, the imaging spatial resolution is well below what is attainable when more conventional T1- and T2-weighted spin-echo imaging is used. The "fuzziness" present in the DWI scans shown in Fig. 35-2 is, in large part, derived from the use of EPI for DWI signal acquisition. EPI displays other characteristic artifacts. Signal arising in mobile lipids is displaced within the image and can, in unfavorable circumstances, produce artifacts. Characteristic EPI artifacts also appear at regions where the magnetic field homogeneity is poor because of adjacent bone or air (e.g., anteriomedial portions of the temporal lobes). Signal is "concentrated" in these regions, and they appear relatively hyperintense. EPI is not an essential ingredient for DWI scanning. The original animal studies that demonstrated the concept employed more conventional (slower) image acquisition procedures. In these early animal studies, bulk head motion was not particularly relevant because the studies were performed with anesthetized and physically restrained animal subjects. Successful clinical DWI scanning has also been achieved using alternate methods of suppressing the artifacts arising from large-scale motion.[15]

DWI is sensitive to the orientation of fibers within white matter. Water molecules diffuse more readily along or with the direction of the fibers as opposed to across and between them. Diffusion sensitization can be directionally oriented in a manner that demonstrates this sensitivity to white matter structure.[16] MRI scanners are capable of producing magnetic field gradients in three unique directions: (1) along the anterior/posterior axis, (2) along the superior/inferior axis, and (3) along the right/left axis. If only one of these diffusion sensitization directions is used for the DWI scan, white matter fibers that run parallel to the sensitization direction will appear relatively hypointense, compared with those fibers that run in other directions. Because such directional dependence of white matter intensity can lead to confusion in image interpretation,[17] it is becoming common to collect a series of three or more DWI in which diffusion sensitization in all three different directions is used. After collecting the individual images, their "average" (also referred to as a "trace" image) is formed using a computer. The white matter directional influence on the average DWI is relatively small in the trace image but still must sometimes be taken into consideration.[17] The DWI shown in Fig. 35-2 is such a trace image and, therefore, shows little in the way of white matter structure effects. When more than three diffusion sensitization directions are used, the procedure is referred to as diffusion tensor imaging because the goal is to characterize diffusion in all directions.[18] EPI greatly facilitates the collection of multiple images for this purpose because imaging is so rapid.

Diffusion-weighted image intensity does not depend solely on diffusion. There is also a strong influence of T2 relaxation on the image intensity. This is related to the fact that the pulse sequences used for DWI inherently employ T2 weighting. The combined influence of T2 and diffusion can be problematic in cases where the ischemia has been present sufficiently long enough to produce alterations in T2-weighted MRI signal. This does not occur in very acute stroke, so, in the acute setting, the DWI alone is often sufficient to identify the involved tissue. However, if ischemia persists for more than 6 h, a lengthening of T2 can also be present. Such T2 increases also produce hyperintensity on DWI scans, and, therefore, hyperintensity in DWI cannot be attrib-

uted solely to acute ischemia. The extent to which T2 alteration influences the DWI image intensity can be appreciated in one of two ways. First, one may qualitatively examine either a conventional T2-weighted image or an image acquired in the same way as the diffusion-weighted image, except with $b = 0$. The presence of hyperintensity on the T2-weighted image in the same tissue that displays hyperintensity on the DWI suggests that T2 as well as diffusion alterations contribute. A second more quantitative approach is also available. In this approach, one acquires a series of DWI using a variety of b values. These images are then subjected to computer calculation, which synthesizes an image where the image intensity conveys the value of the "apparent diffusion coefficient" (ADC). The ADC is a direct measure of the diffusion rate and, therefore, can be used to identify tissue in which diffusion has been slowed as a result of ischemia. An ADC image is shown in Fig. 35-3. Note that the ADC image contrast is reversed compared with DWI. Diffusion is slowed in the infarcted territory, so the ADC image is hypointense in this region.

Strokes evolve with time, and the key milestones in stroke evolution can be documented with diffusion MRI.[19] Most of what is now understood has been learned from studies of animal models. As was emphasized above, an abnormal diffusion signal can become appar-

Figure 35-3.
T2-weighted, DWI, and ADC images from a patient with subacute stroke demonstrating pronounced T2 prolongation. The T2W and DWI images were acquired within minutes of each other. In this setting, the hyperintensity seen on the DWI may be the result of the T2 alterations or alterations in the rate of diffusion. The T2 contribution is not present in the ADC image.

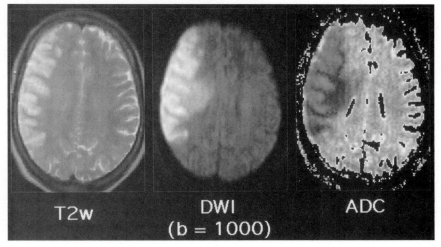

ent within minutes of the onset of ischemia. Kidwell and colleagues reported that almost half of patients with clinical transient ischemic attacks will have abnormality on DWI scan.[8a] About half of those with abnormal DWI scans had normal MRI scans at follow-up. Animal studies have demonstrated that the abnormal diffusion signal can return to normal if early and complete reperfusion occurs.[9] However, the time course of recovery is much slower than is the development of the abnormal signal. As the infarction evolves over a period of days, the diffusion abnormality undergoes an apparent normalization, which may be attributed to the enlargement of the extracellular space through vasogenic edema.[8] After one or more weeks, the tissue in the infarcted area disintegrates and becomes filled with CSF in which the diffusion is fairly rapid. At this late stage, the DWI scan shows a hypointense lesion, and the ADC image shows a hyperintense lesion. DWI studies of human stroke have demonstrated that substantial enlargement of ischemic volumes over time can be detected.[20,21] These studies suggest that DWI can document the evolution of clinical stroke in humans. Given that halting this evolution is a valid therapeutic goal, DWI may well prove to be a useful diagnostic technique to evaluate therapeutic effectiveness.

Perfusion MRI

Direct perfusion measurements using MRI would be of distinct value. This has been a goal of much research during the past ten years. Although established methods, such as xenon-computed tomography or $^{15}H_2O$ positron emission tomography, can accurately quantify cerebral blood flow (CBF), these imaging modalities are often not practical for acute stroke evaluation. They require a separate neuroimaging study and are not as readily available as MRI in most medical centers. MRI provides much of the information needed for the initial evaluation of the acute stroke victim. Older infarcts and other complicating pathologic features are visualized with conventional T1- and T2-weighted MRI. MRA provides excellent images of intracerebral and neck vascular anatomy. Diffusion MRI can be used to visualize physiologically damaged tissue, and although not widely exploited, MRI can also identify intracerebral hemorrhage. These factors argue in favor of using MRI to measure perfusion in preference to performing a separate study using another technique.

Diffusion MRI does not directly measure perfusion. It does, however, provide an indication of the tissue's physiologic response to ischemia. Our present understanding of diffusion MRI suggests that only the ischemic core produces signal alterations apparent on DWI or ADC imaging. Our understanding of stroke hemodynamics suggests that the ischemic core is surrounded by an unstable penumbra receiving reduced (but nonzero) blood flow and that this penumbral tissue may eventually become ischemic. The observed volumetric growth of DWI hyperintense regions in stroke victims over a period of days following stroke onset has been interpreted within this context. The penumbra, therefore, represents a therapeutic target. Interventions may stabilize penumbral blood flow, saving this tissue from eventual ischemia. These factors have encouraged the development of MRI examination procedures aimed at identifying the "mismatch" between the tissue volume displaying abnormal diffusion and that displaying abnormal perfusion.[11,22] To do so, it is necessary to use an MRI perfusion measure.

Two broad classifications of MRI perfusion-imaging approaches have been explored. As is the case with diffusion MRI, neither approach has yet to see widespread use except in specialized centers. The two approaches are distinguished by whether or not an intravenous MRI contrast agent is used. Approaches using intravenous MRI contrast agents are referred to by a variety of names including "dynamic susceptibility scanning" and "bolus tracking." Approaches that do not use intravenous MRI contrast are often referred to as "arterial spin labeling" or "arterial spin tagging."

In arterial spin labeling, the signal-producing characteristics of water in vessels that feed the region of interest are altered.[23,24] This can be done in a variety of ways using well-established techniques. The flow (or absence thereof) of the magnetically labeled water into the region of interest is then detected to obtain the perfusion information. In principle, this approach enables the quantitative measurement of CBF. The arterial spin-labeling technique, although new, has a firm basis in animal studies. Exploratory human studies are now under way. Because there is little definitive information available on their use for the evaluation of human stroke, they will be discussed no further here.

The bolus tracking method is based on earlier radiographic procedures for imaging blood perfusion of tissues.[25] Here, a tight bolus of paramagnetic contrast agent is intravenously administered, and a sequence of rapid MRI scans is used to detect the temporal passage of the agent through the brain tissues. The passage can be detected because the contrast agent produces a local magnetic field distortion that reduces the image intensity as long as the agent is present. Figure 35-4 illustrates the process.

A key requirement for perfusion MRI is rapid

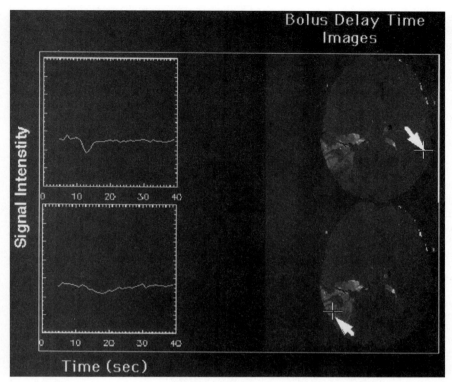

Figure 35-4.

Perfusion MRI study using the bolus tracking method in a stroke patient. A tight bolus of contrast is administered at time zero. The left panels display the time course of the signal intensity changes from the image regions displayed on the right panels (arrows and crosses). The top row demonstrates the pattern in the well-perfused left hemisphere territory. A transient drop in the signal intensity as the bolus passes is apparent. The bottom row provides data from the ischemic right hemisphere. The signal intensity drop is delayed and broadened as a result of the ischemia. The right panels are the perfusion images. In these images, the grayscale is used to display how much time passed before the bolus arrived in each volume element with more intense image intensity representing slower contrast appearance.

image acquisition for which EPI technology is well suited. EPI also provides scans that have the appropriate sensitivity to the magnetic field distortions produced by the presence of paramagnetic contrast agent in the vasculature. The distortions occur over reasonably large distances so that parenchymal signal is affected even though the material remains within the vascular space.

Bolus tracking perfusion MRI is limited in its quantitative accuracy. Even proponents of the technique have been critical of its ability to accurately measure CBF,[26] although they have repeatedly demonstrated meaningful measures of cerebral blood volume (CBV). The principal limitations to CBF quantification

have been twofold: (1) the exact relationship between the vascular concentration of contrast agent and the parenchymal signal alterations is not known with certainty, and (2) quantitative CBF determination requires knowledge of the arterial input function, which is also an unknown. Several computational techniques for dealing with these limitations are available. One of these is to measure the "residual" time evolution function for each image volume element using the assumed linear relationship between the MRI signal intensity and tracer concentration. This function is then fitted to a "gamma-variate" function. The mean transit time (MTT) and the CBV are determined from the fitted function, and the CBF is determined from their ratio. A further refinement involves tracking the changes in image intensity in the large vessels in the vicinity of the circle of Willis as a means of estimating the arterial input function.[27] When this is done, reasonably accurate CBF images of normal subjects can be obtained.[28,29] Thus far the emphasis in stroke studies has been to obtain a more qualitative picture of perfusion. In most cases, this has been obtained by forming a synthesized image in which the gray scale intensity conveys the time at which the contrast bolus arrived in each image volume element (Fig. 35-4).

Figure 35-5 provides a bolus arrival time image obtained from the time course data displayed in Fig. 35-4. An ADC image from the same tissue section is also displayed for comparison. Comparison of the two images illustrates the extent of mismatch between the tissue volume displaying a diffusion defect and that

showing a perfusion defect. This case illustrates that large regions of relatively subtle perfusion defects can be qualitatively identified using the bolus tracking method and that these regions extend beyond stressed tissue demonstrated with ADC or DWI. The regions of perfusion-diffusion "mismatch" may well represent the ischemic penumbra.

Contrast-Enhanced MRI

Although conventional spin-echo MRI may not be as sensitive as diffusion imaging in the acute setting (0 to 6 h), there may be findings suggestive of early infarction when contrast is administered. These include focal intravascular enhancement signaling, vascular stasis, or slow flow within the affected arterial segment(s) (Fig. 35-6). Additionally, one may see enhancement of the meninges

Figure 35-5.
ADC, DWI, and perfusion images from a patient with a right hemisphere stroke. DWI and ADC images indicate physiologic stress in the anterolateral portions of the vascular territory. Perfusion images display a prominent region of abnormal perfusion, which coincides with the ADC and DWI defects. However, the perfusion image suggests that there is additional abnormal perfusion throughout the more posterior aspects of the territory (arrows).

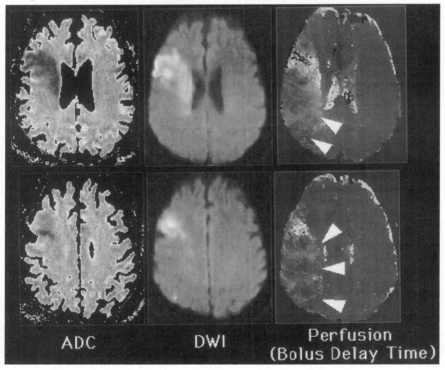

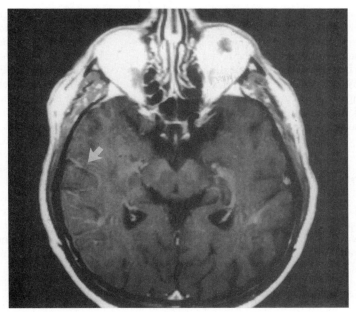

A

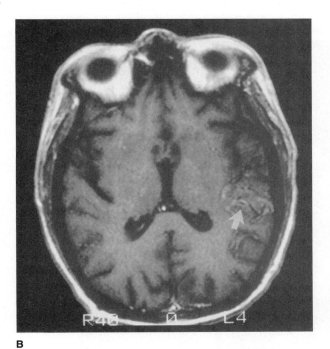

B

Figure 35-6.
Two different examples (A and B) of intravascular enhancement in early infarctions (arrow). This phenomenon is thought to be due to sluggish flow of the arterial supply in the infarcted area. It is believed that this sign is associated with severe ischemia and poor prognosis. This may also be the earliest sign in conventional MRI reflecting changes in the macrocirculation of vascular stenosis or occlusion, before infarction has occurred.

adjacent to the infarcted tissue, owing to leptomeningeal collateral flow to the infarcted area or reactive inflammation within the dura. These enhancement patterns may continue beyond the first few hours of infarction and are also discussed in the next section. On the conventional T2W images, one should always look for corroborating signs such as absence of a normal flow void within a major artery of the circle of Willis (Fig. 35-7). Usually in such cases, MRA will further characterize the vascular occlusion.

SUBACUTE INFARCT (6 TO 72 h)

Subacute infarct is defined as infarction that is older than 6 h beyond symptom onset. MRI usually shows prolongation of both T1 and T2 relaxation times without significant mass effect. On the T1W images, there will be decrease in signal intensity in the territory affected, and on the T2W and proton density-weighted (PDW) images, marked hyperintensity is observed (Fig. 35-8). Gadolinium-enhanced studies may increase the sensitivity of detection. Three types of infarct-related enhancement have been described; intravascular, meningeal, and parenchymal enhancement. As mentioned in the previous section, intravascular enhancement is due to stasis of flow within the vessels supplying the area of infarct. Parenchymal enhancement is thought to be due, in part, to breakdown of the blood-brain barrier. It can be gyriform, wedge-shaped or geographic in appearance (Fig. 35-9). Enhancement in subacute infarcts usually begins 3 to 6 days after onset and is typically gone by 3 months.[30,31] Parenchymal enhancement has a better prognosis for clinical improvement than intravascular enhancement. Meningeal enhancement or enhancement of the dura adjacent to the area of infarct usually appears

Figure 35-7.
MRI examination of a 55-year-old man with left-sided weakness of face, arm, and leg. The T2-weighted study (A) *demonstrates absence of the normal flow void in the right intracranial internal carotid artery* (arrow).

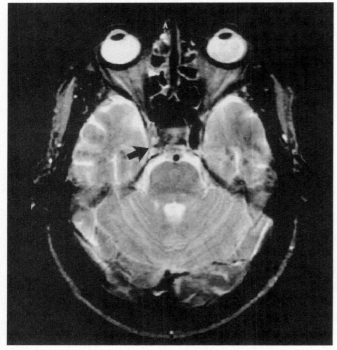

A

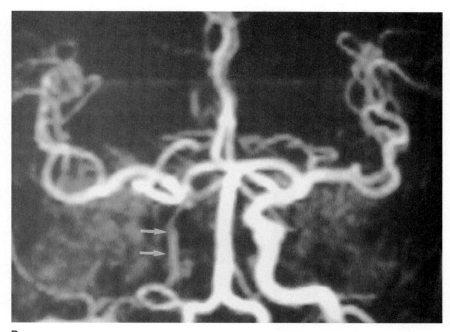

B

Figure 35-7 (*Continued*).
MRA (B) *shows no signal in the right ICA* (thin arrows). *There is cross-filling from the left intracranial vessels via the anterior communicating artery.*

from day 2 to day 6 after infarction but may occur earlier. It is thought to be due to reactive hyperemia and local inflammatory response within the meninges. Occasionally, T1W hyperintensity in a gyriform pattern can be seen prior to contrast administration in the infarcted cortex. This is due to cortical laminar necrosis. The etiology of this T1W hyperintensity has been reported to be the result of lipid-laden macrophages (Fig. 35-10). Laminar necrosis can become apparent as early as a few days after the ischemic stroke and may last for months.

CHRONIC INFARCT

Eventually, some degree of encephalomalacia ensues after a vascular insult. Tissue loss typically results in focal enlargement of cerebral sulci and/or adjacent ventricles. There is often a thin rim of T2-weighted hyperintensity surrounding the area of encephalomalacia that is thought to be due to gliosis (Fig. 35-11).

MR APPEARANCE
OF HEMORRHAGIC INFARCTS

The first imaging study of patients who develop acute stroke-like symptoms is usually CT partly due to availability and partly to rule out recent hemorrhage. This distinction is critical for planning therapy. Also, hemorrhagic infarcts usually carry a poorer prognosis. There may be a large parenchymal hematoma within the infarcted area or the hemorrhage may be confined to the peripheral cortex in a petechial pattern of bleeding, forming a ribbon-like appearance.

The appearance of blood on MRI changes dramatically depending on the stage of the blood product (Table 35-1). Because of oxidative denaturation of hemoglobin within the red blood cell, the paramagnetic effect upon the adjacent proton molecules is different at different stages of breakdown. Oxidative denaturation of hemoglobin begins with oxyhemoglobin, which is a nonparamagnetic substance. The breakdown of oxyhemoglobin to deoxyhemoglobin changes the configu-

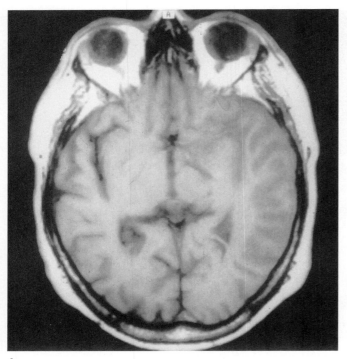

A

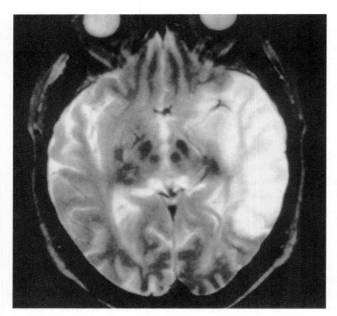

B

Figure 35-8.
Figure (A) *depicts a subacute
infarct, with decrease in T1-
weighted signal intensity due to
vasogenic edema of the parenchyma. In this patient, there are
flattened and swollen cerebral
gyri and blurring of the gray-
white matter demarcation due to
edema in the left temporal lobe
and insular cortex. On the T2-
weighted image* (B), *marked hyperintensity of the corresponding
area is present.*

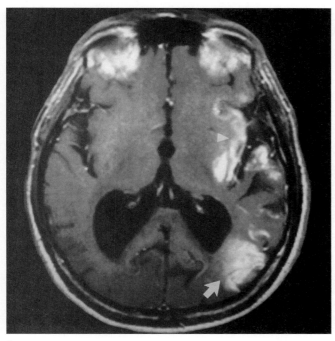

A

Figure 35-9.
Four patterns of contrast enhancement in subacute infarcts. In A, *three types of enhancement are present: (1) gyriform enhancement* (arrowhead), *(2) wedge-shaped enhancement* (arrow) *(which are thought to be due to necrosis and disruption of the blood-brain barrier), and (3) intravascular enhancement, which can be seen between the areas of wedge-shaped and gyriform enhancement.*

ration around the heme iron. In deoxyhemoglobin, there are four unpaired electrons, hence it is paramagnetic. In time, deoxyhemoglobin forms methemoglobin when the heme iron converts to the ferric state.

Oxyhemoglobin is the predominant component in the hyperacute hematoma (Fig. 35-12). The T1W sequence reveals its nonparamagnetic state and has a long T1 relaxation time. Hence, it is hypointense or isointense to gray matter on the T1W images. Because of the high fluid content, T2W images show hyperintensity. There may be a thin rim of low T2W intensity around the hematoma. This is thought to be due to the rapid transformation of oxyhemoglobin to deoxyhemoglobin in the periphery of the denaturing clot.

Approximately 24 h after the blood has extravasated outside the vessel, most of the oxyhemoglobin has transformed into deoxyhemoglobin. The hemoglobin molecule is still located within the intact red blood cell. Although deoxyhemoglobin is paramagnetic, the effect

upon proton molecules outside of the intact red cell is small. Hence, there is no significant T1 shortening. There is, however, T2 shortening during this time due to diffusion of water molecules into the cell as well as hemoconcentration of the clot from thrombosis and clot retraction. On T2W images, the clot will exhibit decreased signal intensity. This process usually lasts for about 3 days after the insult.

From 3 to 7 days, deoxyhemoglobin, which is still located in the intact red cell, will transform into methemoglobin. There is marked T1 relaxation time shortening due to dipole-dipole interactions. This causes marked increase in signal intensity on T1W images. If the hematoma is large, this process will be observed at the periphery of the clot and will proceed toward the center of the clot. This is due to the fact that oxygen is needed to oxidate the deoxyhemoglobin heme iron. There is higher oxygen concentration at the periphery of the clot than at the center. Hence, a hyperintense rim

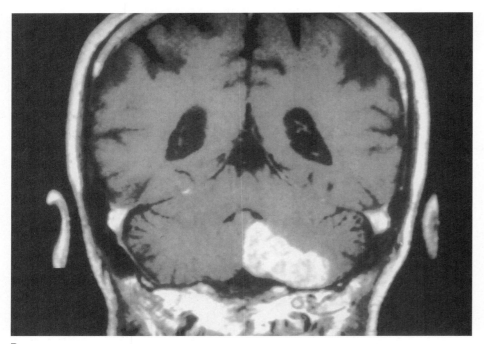

B

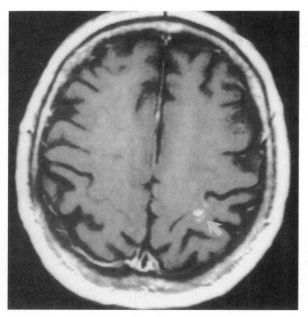

C

Figure 35-9 (*Continued***).**
In B   geographic enhancement of the infarcted tissue is confined to the left posterior inferior cerebellar artery (PICA) territory. In C   a small infarct (arrow) located in the high precentral and postcentral gyri is enhanced by contrast. This patient presented with focal right arm weakness, and the lesion was missed without the contrast-enhanced sequence.

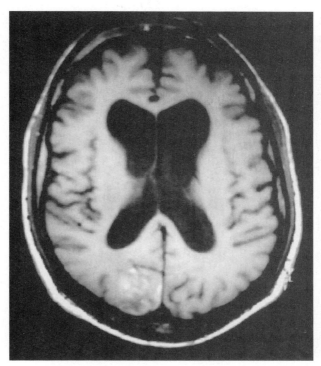

A

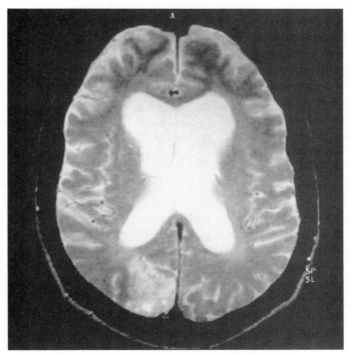

Figure 35-10.
This unenhanced T1-weighted image (A) shows ribbon-like hyperintensity along the right mesial occipital lobe; the appearance is typical for laminar necrosis. T2-weighted (B) and diffusion-weighted (C) images demonstrate a slightly larger area of involvement.

B

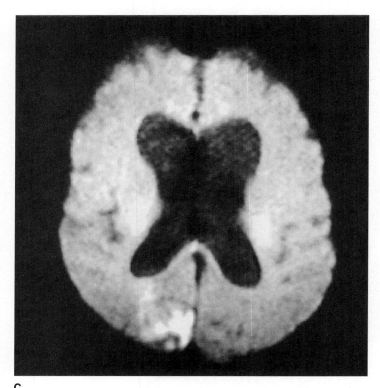

C

Figure 35-10 (*Continued*).

will be seen surrounding the clot. There is corresponding persistent and progressive T2 shortening, which will be reflected as low-signal intensity on T2W images (Fig. 35-13).

As time progresses, the red blood cells within the clot lyse. The T2 shortening due to the methemoglobin that was contained within the red cell is no longer seen due to breakdown of the red cell membrane. There is also an increase in water content within the clot. The combined effect will lead to increase in T2W signal intensity with little effect on the T1 relaxation time. Hence, the clot will appear bright on both T1W and T2W images.

Beyond 7 days, there will develop a rim of dark T2W signal around the periphery of the hematoma. This is due to the formation of hemosiderin and ferritin (Fig. 35-13). There are large numbers of macrophages ingesting and transforming the methemoglobin into hemosiderin and ferritin at the periphery of the clot. Some de-

gree of hemosiderin staining can be seen on the T2W images for years after the hematoma has been removed.

MAGNETIC RESONANCE ANGIOGRAPHY

Techniques

Techniques to image blood vessels using magnetic resonance angiography (MRA) can generally be divided into black blood or white blood methods. In black blood methods, the signals from the water molecules in a particular imaging volume or slice leave that volume/slice before they have recovered from their excitation pulse and therefore offer no signal. This results in a signal void. Hence, patent blood vessels appear dark. White blood MRA techniques can be acquired using time-of-flight technique, phase contrast (PC) technique, or most recently contrast-enhanced MRA.

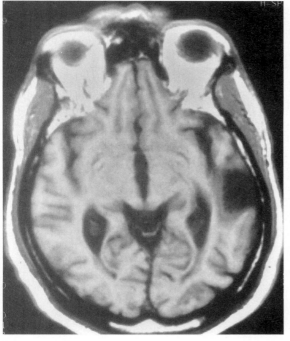

A

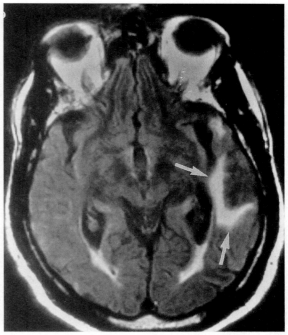

B

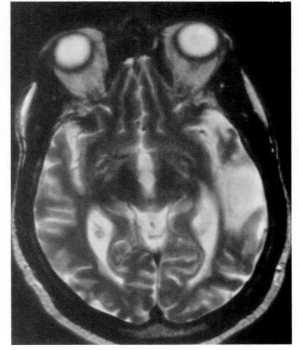

Figure 35-11.
T1W (A), *FLAIR* (B), *and T2W*
(C) *axial images throughout the
brain in a patient with an old infarct of the left temporal lobe cortex. On the T1W image, cystic
encephalomalacia can be seen
centrally, whereas the T2W image does not distinguish encephalomalacia from surrounding gliosis. With the FLAIR technique,
water is suppressed, and the
area of encephalomalacia (CSF)
is easily distinguished from the
surrounding gliosis* (arrows)
within the brain.

C

Table 35-1.
Appearance of hemorrhage (basic concepts for a 1.5T magnet)

Time	Blood product	T1W signal	T2W signal
0–24 h	Oxyhemoglobin	Hypo or isointense	Hyperintense
24–72 h	Deoxyhemoglobin	Hypo or isointense	Hypointense
3–7 days	Intracellular MET-HGB	Hyperintense	Hypointense
3–7 days	Extracellular MET-HGB	Hyperintense	Hyperintense
>7 days	Hemosiderin	Hypo or isointense	Hypointense

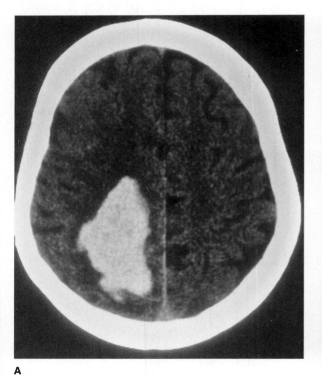

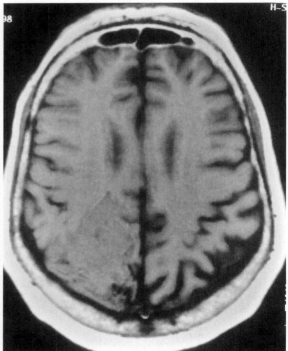

A   **B**

Figure 35-12.
CT scan (A) and MR images with T1W (B), T2W (C), and FLAIR (D) sequences demonstrating a hematoma in the right parietal region within hours of ictus. The signal characteristics of this acute hematoma (isointense on T1W images and hyperintense on T2W images) are consistent with the blood breakdown product oxyhemoglobin. Note the relative lack of surrounding edema at this early stage.

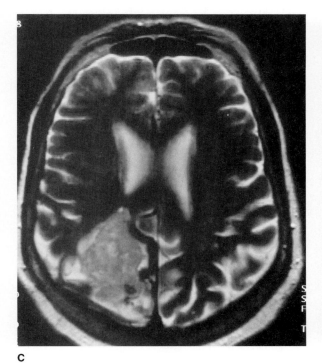

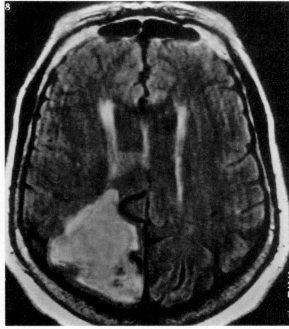

C   D

Figure 35-12 (*Continued*).

Time-of-Flight MRA

Time-of-flight (TOF) MRA is the most commonly used technique for MR vascular imaging in clinical practice. TOF technique is based on the repeated excitation of protons within a particular slice of interest. The stationary protons within the slice such as those from the surrounding soft tissues will be saturated by the rapidly repeated radiofrequency pulses. These stationary protons will, therefore, contribute very little to the overall signal. When protons from flowing, nonstationary water molecules enter the slice of interest, a relatively large fraction of their signal is detected, whereas only a small fraction of signal is detected from the stationary tissues. The technique is heavily dependent on the T1 relaxation time of the tissues imaged. Therefore, in addition to flowing blood, substances with short T1 relaxation times will appear bright on the TOF technique. This includes fat, proteineous fluid, hemorrhage-containing methemoglobin, and MRI contrast agents (Fig. 35-14). Because these substances will appear bright on the MRA, they may mimic signal from flowing blood. Time-of-

flight technique can be applied in two dimensions (2D-TOF) or three dimensions (3D-TOF). There are different advantages for each of the two techniques.

Using the 3D-TOF technique, partition thickness can be much thinner, (0.7 mm compared with 1.2 mm for 2D-TOF), yielding higher spatial resolution, an advantage when imaging a complex vascular lesion. 3D-TOF technique requires a shorter echo time (TE), which decreases spin-dephasing and loss of signal, a common problem at sites of turbulent flow (e.g., stenoses and aneurysms). A drawback of 3D-TOF is saturation effect. Because the data acquisition requires excitation of a volume of tissue, blood remaining in the volume for a long period of time will become saturated and stop giving off signal. In arterial imaging, this will occur toward the top of the slab where the signal from flow will fade. 3D-TOF is used primarily in the evaluation of the circle of Willis where vessels are tortuous and the slab thickness required to cover the area is not prohibitively large (Fig. 35-15).

2D-TOF is commonly used in the evaluation of the extracranial common carotid bifurcation. With the

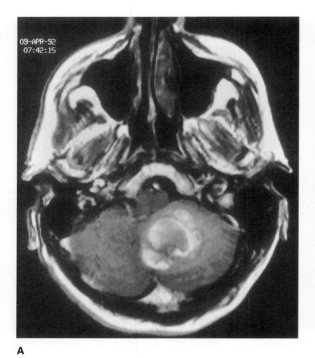

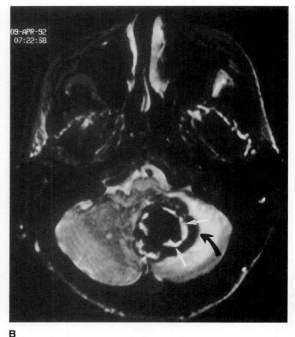

A   B

Figure 35-13.
Axial T1W (A) *and T2W* (B) *MR images through the posterior fossa in a patient with a hemorrhage secondary to a cavernous angioma. This lesion exhibits the classic target configuration of a hematoma with central deoxyhemoglobin* (isointense on T1 and hypointense on T2), *surrounding extracellular methemoglobin* (bright on T1 and T2) (arrows) *and peripheral hemosiderin* (isointense on T1 and hypointense on T2) (curved arrow).

2D-TOF technique, there is little saturation effect because each slice is acquired separately, maximizing sensitivity to flow and minimizing saturation of protons. 2D-TOF is more sensitive to slow-flowing blood than 3D-TOF. In the CCA bifurcation, this is advantageous when trying to image very tight stenoses where flow may be very slow through the lesion and easily susceptible to saturation effect. Additionally, because the slices are acquired individually, a larger area can be covered, making 2D-TOF ideal for studying the cervical vessels.

Phase Contrast MRA

Phase contrast (PC) technique is fundamentally different from time-of-flight technique. The signal is generated by velocity-induced phase shifts. The technique uses the principle that the proton will generate a phase shift when traveling along a magnetic field gradient. In contrast to the TOF technique, PC MRA is not influenced by the T1 relaxation time of protons. Hence, tissues with a short T1 relaxation time such as methemoglobin, fat, and proteineous fluid will not be confused for vascular structures. When using this technique, one must select an optimal velocity for the vessels to be imaged. By selecting slower velocities, the venous system may be imaged; by selecting faster velocities, the arterial system may be selectively imaged. However, the need for velocity encoding is also a serious limitation of this technique. For example, the optimal velocity for imaging the normal vessels of the circle of Willis may omit visualization of a small aneurysm containing much slower blood flow (Fig. 35-16). Additionally, the velocity must be encoded in all three directions to accurately detect flow in a three-dimensional structure such as the circle of Willis. Acquisition times are much longer for PC than TOF technique, and post-processing is long

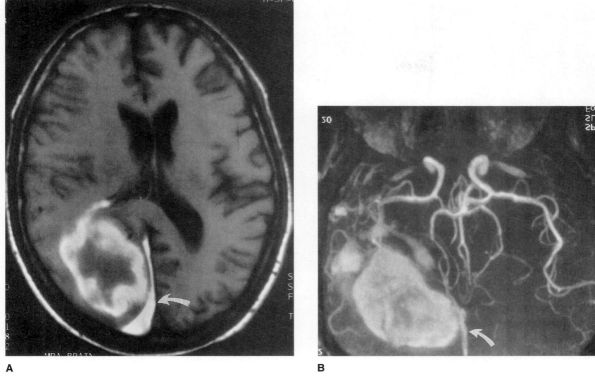

A   B

Figure 35-14.
Axial T1W image (A) *through a right occipital hematoma. In* B, *there is "shine through" of the hematoma on the 3D-TOF axial image through the circle of Willis due to the T1-shortening effect of the extracellular methemoglobin. Note also the small subdural hematoma* (curved arrow).

and laborious, often tying up valuable scanner time. For these reasons, this technique is rarely used in clinical practice. One advantage of using PC MRA is that the gradients can be adjusted so that not only velocity but also the acceleration of the flowing protons can be measured quantitatively. The technique is direction sensitive so that the direction of flow within a vessel can be determined and velocities measured.

Contrast-enhanced MRA

As mentioned previously, TOF MRA is largely limited by saturation effects. In other words, the longer the protons being imaged remain within the slab of interest, the more likely they will become saturated and no longer give off signal. This limits the volume or length of vessel that can be imaged. Contrast-enhanced MRA is an ex-

tension of the conventional TOF technique. This technique uses a timed injection of a contrast bolus of a paramagnetic agent and subtraction technique to maximally enhance flowing blood. The technique also helps to reduce signal loss due to turbulent flow and to eliminate slice misregistration and in-plane saturation. Because a snapshot of the contrast bolus can be obtained in a relatively short examination time, arterial, mixed arterial-venous, and venous phase images can be obtained (Fig. 35-17). There is also improved visualization of the more distal arterial branches intracranially. There are several disadvantages of the technique. It is highly dependent on the accurate determination of time of arrival of the contrast bolus to the area of interest. It also suffers from the same susceptibility artifact at the skull base and around the air-filled paranasal sinuses that TOF MRA does.

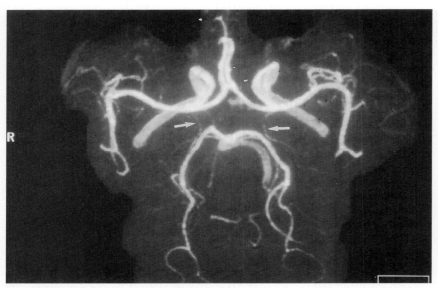

Figure 35-15.
MRA of the circle of Willis using time of flight technique. The small arrows *are pointing to the anterior choroidal arteries.*

Maximum Intensity Projection

In TOF MRA, the data are acquired in multiple contiguous slices. It is currently a common practice to post-process these source data using a computer algorithm called maximum intensity projection (MIP) method to reconstruct and display the data in a three-dimensional format. The brightest pixels on any slice or those pixels with the maximum intensity are stacked on one another to yield the three-dimensional image of the vessel. This three-dimensional representation of the data can then be infinitely rotated interactively. Certain surrounding unwanted structures can also be excluded to allow optimal viewing of a vascular stenosis or other pathology.

CLINICAL APPLICATIONS

Extracranial Carotid Artery

Disease of the extracranial carotid artery accounts for approximately 30 percent of strokes. The North American Symptomatic Carotid Endarterectomy Trial (NASCET) has shown clinical effectiveness of carotid endarterectomy in the treatment of symptomatic high-grade carotid stenosis. The accurate determination of

such stenosis is important not only for diagnosis but also for surgical planning.

Both MRA and Doppler ultrasonography are very useful in the evaluation of carotid bifurcation disease. Advantages of noninvasive studies over conventional angiography include lack of invasive intra-arterial catheterization, radiation to the patient, and in-house recovery time following the procedure. There are pitfalls associated with both of these noninvasive techniques. Duplex sonography, which is described in more detail elsewhere is this book, suffers from inability to distinguish a subtotal from a total occlusion, an important distinction for planning therapy. On the other hand, TOF MRA is known to overestimate the degree and length of a stenosis. It is thought that this overestimation is due to turbulence of flow in the area of stenosis causing a loss of signal. Complete signal void, the "flow gap," on TOF MRA may be interpreted as a total occlusion in cases where there may be only severe focal stenosis. If a long enough segment of artery is imaged, the flow distal to the area of stenosis should be visible, indicating that this is not an occclusion but only a severe stenosis. Stenoses resulting in "flow gaps" have been shown to have high correlation (>85 percent specificity) with stenoses that are greater than 70 percent, allowing for noninvasive determination of a surgical lesion. How-

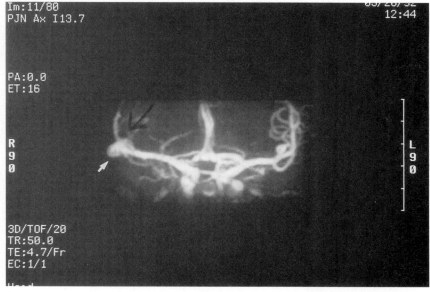

A

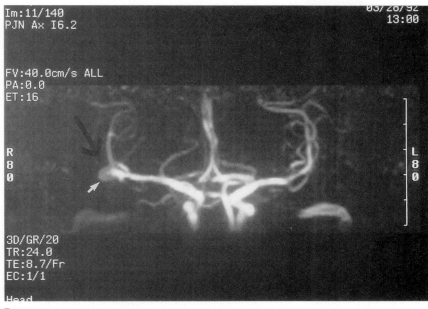

B

Figure 35-16.

Three-dimensional time-of flight (3D-TOF) (A) and three-dimensional phase contrast (3D-PC) (B) MRA images through the circle of Willis in a patient with a right MCA bifurcation aneurysm (arrow). Due to a selected velocity encoding value of 40 cm/s, the flow in the aneurysm is less well demonstrated on the 3D-PC than on the 3D-TOF technique, which is not as sensitive to the varying velocities encountered in vascular lesions.

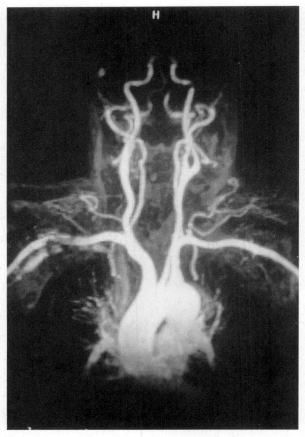

A

Figure 35-17.
Contrast-enhanced MRA during the arterial (A) *and venous* (B) *phases of the contrast bolus in the same patient. The early images are desirable for CCA bifurcation anatomy without obscuration by the jugular veins.*

ever, the lack of good anatomic data over the stenotic segment will typically prompt the surgeon to order a conventional angiogram for better delineation of the lesion prior to surgery. Enhanced MRA is a promising newer, noninvasive technique that may eventually allow for better assessment of the morphology of high-grade stenoses. One should not forget that all MRA techniques are, in fact, imaging flow rather than true anatomy of the vessel. Conventional angiography is still required in patients who cannot undergo MRA due to a pacemaker or claustrophobia or who have suboptimal

ultrasound studies because of heavily calcified plaque that limits visualization.

In older studies,[32-35] carotid bifurcation stenosis was correctly detected with high sensitivity (>90 percent) and specificity (>90 percent). In the study from Masaryk et al, correlation of $R = 0.94$ was obtained when comparing the 3D-TOF technique with conventional angiography. When comparing MRA with color Doppler ultrasound examination, one small prospective study suggested that the accuracy of MRA was the same as ultrasound Doppler studies.[36] Furthermore, if both

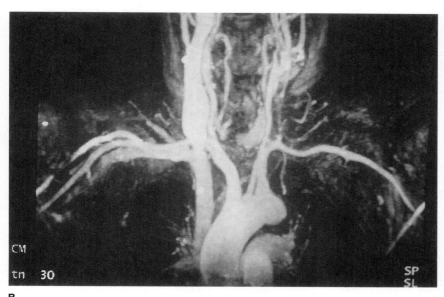

B

Figure 35-17 (*Continued*).

MRA and Doppler are performed, the sensitivity of detecting disease improves.[33]

Vertebrobasilar System

MRA can reliably detect disease in the verterobasilar system. Using 3D-TOF technique, studies have shown a high sensitivity (97 percent) and high specificity (98.9 percent) in detecting distal stenoses.[37,38] As with the carotid bifurcation, MRA tends to overestimate the degree of stenosis. Conventional MRA cannot be used to detect proximal (origin) vertebral artery stenosis, but contrast-enhanced MRA may eventually replace conventional MRA in studying this area (Fig. 35-18).

Dissection

Dissection of the carotid artery or the vertebrobasilar system can be spontaneous or related to hypertension, trauma, or vasculopathies such as fibromuscular dysplasia and cystic medial necrosis. The most common site of extracranial ICA dissection is the cervical portion, whereas the supraclinoid portion is the most common site intracranially. For the vertebral artery, the most common area affected is the C1–C2 vertebral level. Intramural hematoma is a common feature of carotid

or vertebral dissection. MRI findings include a T1-weighted hyperintensity partially surrounding and narrowing the vessel[39,40] (Fig. 35-19). In a small series, MRI was found to have a high degree of sensitivity and specificity (>90 percent) in the detection of dissection for larger vessels such as the carotid arteries. However, in smaller vessels such as the vertebral artery, the sensitivity of detecting disease drops to 60 percent.[41,42] MRI and MRA have also been shown in a small series to be a safe and effective tool for following up patients with ICA or vertebral artery dissection receiving anticoagulation or antiplatelet therapy.[43]

Intracranial Aneurysms

MRA has become a major tool in detecting intracranial aneurysms. MRA has the advantage over conventional angiography that overlapping structures can be eliminated in postprocessing. In addition, conventional angiography may not be able to detect a thrombosed aneurysm because there may no longer be a patent lumen. MRI will still depict the aneurysm containing mural thrombus even if the aneurysm is no longer patent. Studies have suggested that there is a 95 percent accuracy of MRA in demonstrating aneurysms when compared with conventional angiography.[44] However, TOF

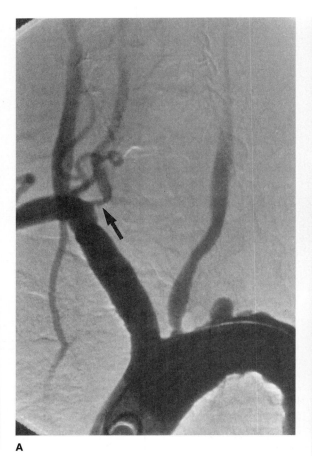

A

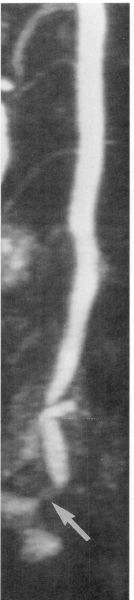

B

Figure 35-18.
A *conventional arteriogram following aortic arch injection demonstrating a right vertebral artery origin stenosis* (arrow). B *cropped image from a contrast-enhanced MRA showing the right vertebral artery origin in the same patient* (arrow).

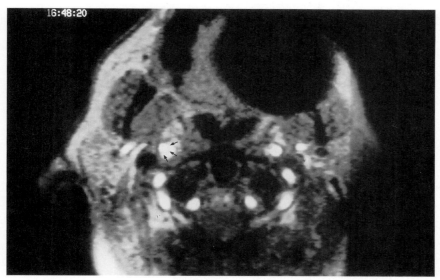

Figure 35-19.
Source image from a two-dimensional time-of-flight MRA through the skull base in a patient with a right ICA dissection demonstrating the crescentic intimal flap within the lumen (arrows).

technique may not be able to detect aneurysms measuring 3 mm or less in diameter.[45] MRA in conjunction with MRI is a major tool in the evaluation of unruptured aneurysms. Screening of unruptured aneurysms in high-risk groups such as patients with polycystic kidney disease and collagen vascular disease may be useful.[46,47] However, MRA screening of unruptured aneurysms is controversial here in the United States but is widely used in other countries.[48] Using a simulated model, the number of lives saved by MRA screening was found to be significantly larger than that without MRA screening. Another study has advocated screening of patients less than 30 years old with a positive family history of intracranial aneurysms.[49] MRI and MRA can delineate not only the presence of an intracranial aneurysm of 3 mm diameter or greater, it will also show the associated mass effect, the presence of intraluminal thrombus, and the presence of any blood breakdown products implying previous hemorrhage.

Recent developments in spiral CT scanning with timed bolus injection of contrast and postprocessing registration subtraction technique have also become a competing modality in the detection and characterization of intracranial aneurysms.

Vasculitis

Intracranial vasculitis can be divided into primary or secondary. MRI findings are usually nonspecific and are an indirect manifestation of disease of the vessels. These findings include foci of T2-weighted hyperintensity in the white matter, intraparenchymal hemorrhage, large infarcts, and diffuse leptomeningeal enhancement.[50,51] MRA has insufficient resolution to diagnose vasculitis affecting small intracranial branch vessels beyond the third segment. Conventional catheter angiography is often low yield and has been reported to have a false-negative rate of 20 to 30 percent when compared with biopsy. Therefore, a negative angiogram does not exclude the disease, and often, tissue diagnosis with brain or meningeal biopsy is required. A normal MRI brain study excludes intracranial vasculitis more definitively than a normal conventional angiogram.[50]

Venous Thrombosis and Sinus Occlusive Disease

Venous and dural sinus occlusion can be secondary to a wide variety of diseases, both local and systemic. MRI

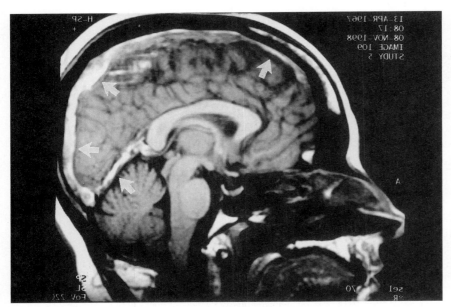

Figure 35-20.
Sagittal T1W image in a patient with superior sagittal sinus thrombosis (arrows).

is very useful in the workup and follow-up of sinus thrombosis and has virtually replaced conventional angiography except when direct intervention is anticipated. The most commonly involved site of dural sinus occlusion is the superior sagittal sinus. The MRI appearance of the brain in dural sinus thrombosis is very different from that of arterial occlusion. Unlike arterial occlusion, vasogenic edema and abnormal parenchymal enhancement usually do not occur. Instead, there may be subtle diffuse swelling of the brain parenchyma lasting up to 2 years. This finding may not be appreciated on T2-weighted images.[52] There are relatively distinct stages of parenchymal change as a result of dural sinus thrombosis. These changes correlate with the intradural sinus pressure.[53] As the pressure in the sinus rises (venous hypertension), there may be persistent CSF production with a decrease in absorption, as the normal route of absorption is through the arachnoid granulations and back to the superior sagittal sinus. This in turn will cause dilatation of the ventricular system. Intraluminal clot may be detected as high T1W signal within the sinus instead of the usual flow void that results from relatively fast-flowing blood (Fig. 35-20). There may also be abnormal enhancement of the venous structure due to stasis of flow and delayed passage of the contrast. If pressure within the sinus exceeds the inherent com-

pensation mechanisms of the small venules and capillaries, rupture occurs and intraparenchymal hemorrhage will ensue. Thus, venous infarctions are typically hemorrhagic and bilateral when the superior sagittal sinus is involved.

REFERENCES

1. Bryan RN, Willcott MR, Schneiders NJ, et al: Nuclear magnetic resonance evaluation of stroke: A preliminary report. *Radiology* 149:189, 1983.
2. Mohr JP, Biller J, Hilal SK, et al: Magnetic resonance versus computed tomographic imaging in acute stroke. *Stroke* 26:807, 1995.
3. Ebisu T, Tanaka C, Umeda M, et al: Hemorrhagic and nonhemorrhagic stroke: Diagnosis with diffusion-weighted and T2-weighted echo-planar MR imaging. *Radiology* 203:823, 1997.
4. Patel MR, Edelman RR, Warach S: Detection of hyperacute primary intraparenchymal hemorrhage by magnetic resonance imaging. *Stroke* 27:2321, 1996.
5. Siewert B, Patel MR, Warach S: Stroke and ischemia. *Magn Res Imag Clin North Am* 3:529, 1995.
6. Le Bihan D: Molecular diffusion nuclear magnetic resonance imaging. *Magn Reson Q* 7:1, 1991.
7. Mintorovitch J, Moseley ME, Chileuitt L, et al: Comparison

of diffusion- and T2-weighted MRI for early detection of cerebral ischemia and reperfusion in rats. *Magn Reson Med* 18:39, 1991.

8. Knight RA, Dereski MO, Helpern JA, et al: Magnetic resonance imaging assessment of evolving focal cerebral ischemia. *Stroke* 25:1252, 1994.

8a. Kidwell CS, Alger JR, DiSalle F, et al: Diffusion MRI in patients with transient ischemic attacks. *Stroke* 30:1174, 1999.

9. Pierpaoli C, Alger JR, Righini A, et al: High temporal resolution diffusion MRI of global cerebral ischemia and reperfusion. *J Cerebr Blood Flow Metab* 16:892, 1996.

10. Lovblad KO, Baird AE, Schlaug G, et al: Ischemic lesion volumes in acute stroke by diffusion-weighted magnetic resonance imaging correlate with clinical outcome. *Ann Neurol* 42:164, 1997.

11. Warach S, Gaa J, Siewert B, et al: Acute human stroke studied by whole brain echo planar diffusion-weighted magnetic resonance imaging. *Ann Neurol* 37:231, 1995.

12. Warach S, Chien D, Li W, et al: Fast magnetic resonance diffusion-weighted imaging of acute human stroke. *Neurology* 42:1717, 1992.

13. Moseley ME, Butts K, Yenari MA, et al: Clinical aspects of DWI. *Nmr Biomed* 8:387, 1995.

14. Reiser M, Faber SC: Recent and future advances in high-speed imaging. *Eur Radiol* 7 (Suppl 5): 166, 1997.

15. Marks MP, de Crespigny A, Lentz D, et al: Acute and chronic stroke: Navigated spin-echo diffusion-weighted MR imaging. *Radiology* 199:403, 1996.

16. Pierpaoli C, Jezzard P, Basser PJ, et al: Diffusion tensor MR imaging of the human brain. *Radiology* 201:637, 1996.

17. Ulug AM, Beauchamp N, Jr, Bryan RN, et al: Absolute quantitation of diffusion constants in human stroke. *Stroke* 28:483, 1997.

18. Basser PJ, Pierpaoli C: Microstructural and physiological features of tissues elucidated by quantitative-diffusion-tensor MRI. *J Magn Reson Ser B* 111:209, 1996.

19. Lutsep HL, Albers GW, DeCrespigny A, et al: Clinical utility of diffusion-weighted magnetic resonance imaging in the assessment of ischemic stroke. *Ann Neurol* 41:574, 1997.

20. Baird AE, Benfield A, Schlaug G, et al: Enlargement of human cerebral ischemic lesion volumes measured by diffusion-weighted magnetic resonance imaging. *Ann Neurol* 41:581, 1997.

21. Schlaug G, Siewert B, Benfield A, et al: Time course of the apparent diffusion coefficient (ADC) abnormality in human stroke. *Neurology* 49:113, 1997.

22. Sorensen AG, Buonanno FS, Gonzalez RG, et al: Hyperacute stroke: Evaluation with combined multisection diffusion-weighted and hemodynamically weighted echo-planar MR imaging. *Radiology* 199:391, 1996.

23. Ye FQ, Pekar JJ, Jezzard P, et al: Perfusion imaging of the human brain at 1.5 T using a single-shot EPI spin tagging approach. *Magn Reson Med* 36:217, 1996.

24. Wong EC, Buxton RB, Frank LR: Implementation of quantitative perfusion imaging techniques for functional brain mapping using pulsed arterial spin labeling. *NMR Biomed* 10:237, 1997.

25. Warach S, Li W, Ronthal M, et al: Acute cerebral ischemia: Evaluation with dynamic contrast-enhanced MR imaging and MR angiography. *Radiology* 182:41, 1992.

26. Weisskoff RM, Chesler D, Boxerman JL, et al: Pitfalls in MR measurement of tissue blood flow with intravascular tracers: Which mean transit time? *Magn Reson Med* 29:553, 1993.

27. Rempp KA, Brix G, Wenz F, et al: Quantification of regional cerebral blood flow and volume with dynamic susceptibility contrast-enhanced MR imaging. *Radiology* 193:637, 1994.

28. Ostergaard L, Weisskoff RM, Chesler DA, et al: High resolution measurement of cerebral blood flow using intravascular tracer bolus passages: Part I. Mathematical approach and statistical analysis. *Magn Reson Med* 36:715, 1996.

29. Ostergaard L, Sorensen AG, Kwong KK, et al: High resolution measurement of cerebral blood flow using intravascular tracer bolus passages: Part II. Experimental comparison and preliminary results. *Magn Reson Med* 36:726, 1996.

30. Yuh WTC, Crain MR, Loes DJ, et al: MR imaging of cerebral ischemia: Findings in the first 24 hours. *Am J Neuroradiol* 12:621, 1991.

31. Virapongse C, Mancuso A, Quisling R: Human brain infarcts: Gd-DTPA enhanced MR imaging. *Radiology* 161:785, 1986.

32. Masaryk TJ, Laub GA, Modic T, et al: Carotid CNS flow imaging. *Magn Reson Med* 14:308, 1990.

33. Mattle HP, Kent KC, Edelman RR, et al: Evaluation of the extracranial carotid arteries: Correlation of magnetic resonance angiography, duplex ultrasonography, and conventional angiography. *J Vasc Surg* 13:838, 1991.

34. Riles TS: The role and risks of carotid endarterectomy, in *Stroke Symposium Proceedings*. New York, Excerpta Media, 1990.

35. White JE, Russell WL, Greer MS, et al: Efficacy of screening MR angiography and Doppler ultrasonography in the evaluation of carotid artery stenosis. *Am Surg* 60:340, 1994.

36. Houston J III, Lewis BD, Weibers DO, et al: Carotid artery: Propertive blinded comparison of two dimensional time of flight MR angiography with conventional angiography and duplex US. *Radiology* 186:339, 1993.

37. Rother J, Wentz KU, Rautenberg W, et al: Magnetic resonance angiography in vertebrobasilar ischemia. *Stroke* 24: 1310, 1993.

38. Wentz KU, Rother J, Schwartz A, et al: Intracranial vertebrobasilar system: MR angiography. *Radiology* 190:105, 1994.

39. Klufas RA, Hsu L, Barnes PD, et al: Dissection of the carotid and vertebral arteries: Imaging with MR angiography. *Am J Roentgenol* 164:673, 1995.

40. Provenzale JM: Dissection of the internal carotid and verte-

bral arteries: Imaging features. *Am J Roentgenol* 165:
1099, 1995.

41. Bui LN, Brant-Zawadzki M, Verghese P, et al: Magnetic resonance angiography of cervicocranial dissection. *Stroke* 24:126, 1993.

42. Levy C, Laissy JP, Raveau V, et al: Carotid and vertebral artery dissections: Three-dimensional time-of-flight MR angiography and MR imaging versus conventional angiography. *Radiology* 190:97, 1994.

43. Jacobs A, Lanfermann H, Neveling M, et al: MRI- and MRA-guided therapy of carotid and vertebral artery dissections. *J Neurol Sci* 147:27, 1997.

44. Ross JS, Masaryk TJ, Modic MT, et al: Intracranial aneurysm: Evaluation by MR angiography. *Am J Roentgenol* 155:159, 1990.

45. Houkin K, Aoki T, Takahashi A, et al: Magnetic resonance angiography (MRA) of ruptured cerebral aneurysm. *Acta Neurochir* 128:132, 1994.

46. Ruggieri PM, Poulos N, Masaryk TJ, et al: Occult intracranial aneurysms in polycystic kidney disease: Screening with MR angiography. *Radiology* 191:33, 1994.

47. Huston J, Torres VE, Sulivan PP, et al: Value of magnetic resonance angiography for the detection of intracranial aneurysms in autosomal dominant polycystic kidney disease. *J Am Soc Nephrol* 3:1871, 1993.

48. Takahashi E, Haku M, Suzuki Y, et al: Effectiveness of magnetic resonance angiography for mass screening of unruptured intracranial aneurysms. *Jpn J Public Health* 44:509, 1997.

49. Obuchowski NA, Modic MT, Magdinec M: Current implications for the eficacy of noninvasive screening for occult intracranial aneurysms in patients with a family history of aneurysms. *J Neurosurg* 83:42, 1995.

50. Harris KG, Tran DD, Cornell SH, et al: Diagnosing intracranial vasculitis: The roles of MRI and angiography. *Am J Neuroradiol* 15:317, 1994.

51. Negishi C, Sze G: Vasculitis presenting as primary leptomeningeal enhancement with minimal parenchymal findings. *Am J Neuroradiol* 14:26, 1993.

52. Yuh WTC, Simonson TM, Wang AM, et al: Venous sinus occlusive disease: MR findings. *Am J Neuroradiol* 15:309, 1994.

53. Tsai FY, Wang AM, Matovich VB, et al: MR staging of acute dural sinus thrombosis: Correlation with venous pressure measurements and implications for treatment and prognosis. *Am J Neuroradiol* 16:1021, 1995.

Chapter 36

CEREBRAL ANGIOGRAPHY IN ISCHEMIC STROKE

Suzie M. El-Saden
Marc Garant

INTRODUCTION

Although emerging noninvasive imaging techniques continue to challenge the role of arteriography, catheter angiography (CA) remains the gold standard examination in patients with cerebrovascular disease, by which all newer modalities are measured. CA is still the preferred method for quantifying carotid artery stenosis. However, with rare exception, CA is used only to confirm findings made by less invasive studies rather than being a primary diagnostic tool as it once was. The exception to this rule is suspected intracranial vasculitis, where catheter angiography may be the only imaging technique currently able to demonstrate the presence of a vasculopathy in small vessels.

Internal carotid artery (ICA) stenosis and occlusion are most commonly secondary to atherosclerosis in the adult population. However, dissection and vasculitis should be considered when ICA stenosis occurs in children or young adults.[1-6] Clinical history is helpful in suggesting an etiology of dissection. Previous radiation therapy can lead to accelerated arterial occlusive disease in young or old patients.[7-9]

The role of arteriography in the assessment of vascular occlusive disease at the common carotid artery (CCA) bifurcation is (1) to measure the precise degree of stenosis, (2) to look for tandem intracranial stenoses, and (3) to assess the collateral circulation to the brain. Because a tandem intracranial stenosis that is greater in severity than the cervical lesion may preclude surgical endarterectomy, views of the siphon should be routinely obtained. Similarly, as a contralateral intracranial ICA stenosis or occlusion increases the risk of surgical morbidity, routine views of the contralateral ICA, both intracranial and extracranial, should also be obtained.[10] Alternatively, a technically adequate normal magnetic resonance angiogram (MRA) of the circle of Willis can exclude significant intracranial vascular stenosis/occlusion, and this technology will likely reduce the need for routine intracranial angiographic views. Routine MRA will not provide information on transit times through collaterals or on direction of flow-through collaterals unless special directionally encoded sequences are obtained.

In patients with cerebral ischemic syndromes, CA often provides definitive information critical to appropriate clinical management. CA is the only modality by which leptomeningeal collaterals and collateral flow from external carotid artery (ECA) branches to the ICA (Fig. 36-1) can be assessed in patients with ICA or other intracranial vascular occlusion. Without adequate collaterals, there may be insufficient flow to the hemisphere during surgical cross-clamping of the ICA. CA is the only modality currently able to offer physiologic, temporal, and anatomic data. Knowledge of collateral flow may assist the surgeon in deciding whether or not to perform intraoperative bypass of the extracranial ICA during carotid endarterectomy.

In subclavian steal syndrome, ultrasound may demonstrate reversal of flow within one of the vertebral arteries, but conventional angiography is indicated to define the extent and nature of the underlying stenosis or occlusion and to assess the exact pattern of blood flow (Fig. 36-2). Additionally, an underlying subclavian artery stenosis can often be treated definitively with angioplasty or stent placement at the time of evaluation.

CLINICAL CONSIDERATIONS

Angiography can be performed in virtually all patients. Relative contraindications include renal insufficiency,

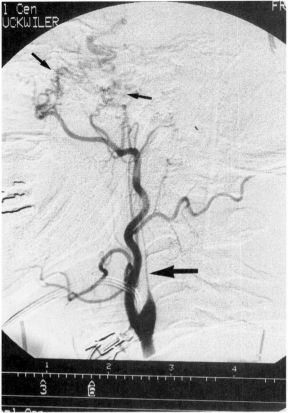

Figure 36-1.
Lateral common carotid injection demonstrating very high-grade stenosis of the ICA with the lumen appearing as a thread of contrast (large arrow). *Note the collaterals* (small arrows) *from the external carotid artery reconstituting the intracranial segments of the ICA.*

contrast allergy, and clotting disorders. Preoperative laboratory studies should include blood urea nitrogen, creatinine, hemoglobin, hematocrit, platelet count, partial thromboplastin time, and prothrombin time. Patients should be kept NPO past midnight the night before the procedure except for medications. This is mainly to avoid risks of aspiration should conscious sedation be administered for the study. Oral hypoglycemics should be held until the patient is eating again. Patients who have had breakfast may be studied in the afternoon if oral intake is discontinued from breakfast on.

All patients should be well hydrated prior to the study with fluids continued for the 24 h following angiography (oral or intravenous). This is especially true in patients with renal insufficiency (creatinine >1.5). For patients with an elevated creatinine, mannitol can be administered intravenously at the onset of the procedure to aid in the diuresis of the contrast load. The contrast load should be kept to a minimum. For patients with renal failure on dialysis, dialysis should be performed prior to the arteriogram for maintenance of volume status and electrolyte balance and immediately following the procedure for removal of the iodinated contrast. Although there is reportedly no difference in the incidence of nephrotoxicity between high osmolarity ionic contrast and the more expensive low osmolarity nonionic contrast, there is typically less discomfort associated with the administration of the latter.

Contrast reactions occur in approximately 2 to 3 percent of patients undergoing cerebral angiography and can range from minor (hives) to severe (anaphylaxis).[11] For patients with severe allergies, asthma, or a history of previous contrast reaction, we premedicate with corticosteroids and Benadryl. Several premedication protocols can be used; we typically administer 50 mg of oral prednisone or its equivalent at 8-h intervals for a total of three doses, with the last dose given on call to the angiography suite. When the patient arrives, 50 mg of Benadryl are administered intravenously (IV) at the onset of the procedure. It has been shown that a single dose of steroids given at the beginning of the procedure is inadequate to achieve membrane stabilization of mast cells, which are largely responsible for the allergic reaction.[12]

For patients with a prolonged bleeding time, platelets, fresh frozen plasma, or the deficient clotting factor can be given immediately prior to the procedure to avoid bleeding complications. In older atherosclerotic patients who are taking aspirin, we do not discontinue aspirin but anticipate a longer groin hold for hemostasis. Patients on coumadin should be admitted and converted to intravenous heparin. On the morning of the procedure, heparin is discontinued 2 h prior to the procedure and restarted without bolus injection 1 to 2 h following hemostasis at the site of arterial puncture. If needed, the procedure may be performed without discontinuation of anticoagulation. In patients with severe catheter or wire-induced vasospasm or severe atherosclerotic narrowing of the punctured common femoral artery, we often give 3000 to 5000 units of IV heparin during the procedure to avoid thrombus formation and potential arterial occlusion.

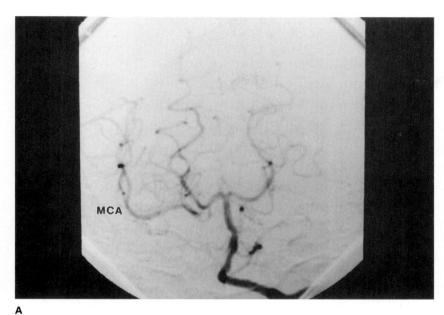

A

Figure 36-2.
A 46-year-old male with suspected subclavian steal syndrome based on ultrasound demonstrating reversal of flow in the right vertebral artery. A   AP view of the head following injection of the left vertebral artery fails to demonstrate reversal of flow down the right vertebral artery. Note filling of the right MCA via a patent posterior communicating artery.

TECHNICAL CONSIDERATIONS

As with angiography elsewhere in the body, cervical and cerebral angiography are usually performed via a transfemoral arterial approach. The groin is prepped and draped in a sterile fashion. Local anesthesia and mild intravenous sedation are sufficient for most patients. General anesthesia may be required for less cooperative patients and for patients undergoing endovascular therapy (i.e., angioplasty or embolization).

Puncture of the femoral artery is done using the Seldinger technique. We routinely place a no. 5 or no. 6 French sheath to protect the artery at the puncture site and to facilitate torque control of the catheter, especially in patients with aortic and great vessel tortuosity from hypertension or atherosclerotic disease.

Several catheters can be used, usually 4 or 5F in size and 90 to 100 cm in length. The cervical common carotid arteries (CCA) and usually one vertebral artery (VA) are selectively catheterized, and at least two or-

thogonal views are obtained, usually the frontal and lateral views. Additional projections are obtained to further evaluate areas of abnormality detected on routine biplane images or to search for lesions suggested on previous noninvasive imaging studies such as magnetic resonance angiography (MRA) or duplex carotid ultrasound. In our practice, arch angiography is not routinely performed. Contrast-enhanced MRA has become our screening procedure for suspected aortic arch disease (Fig. 36-3).

We use nonionic contrast media in all patients. Hand injections are performed in the CCAs, ICAs, and vertebral arteries. A power injector is used when large volumes of contrast must be delivered at high rates (i.e., in the aortic arch or subclavian arteries). Images are typically acquired using digital subtraction angiography (DSA) with a matrix size 1024 × 1024. DSA acquisitions are significantly faster than cut-film acquisitions, and DSA offers the advantage of subsequent image manipulation. Cut-film radiography is rarely used except per-

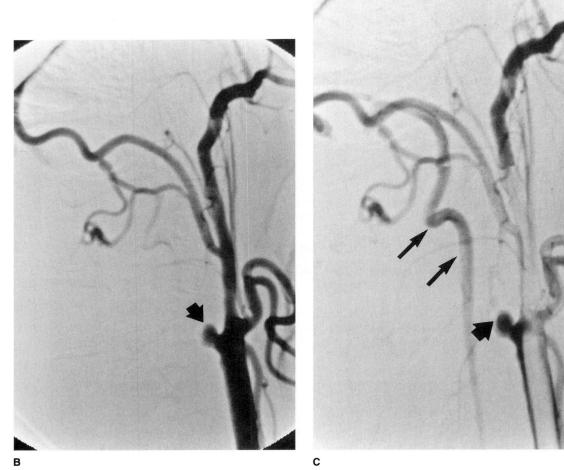

B   C

Figure 36-2 (*Continued*).
B, C,   *sequential lateral images from a right common carotid injection demonstrating occlusion of the internal carotid artery* (arrowhead) *and eventual reversal of flow in the right vertebral artery* (arrows). *Note that the ultrasound correctly suggested steal, but only the arteriogram reveals that the steal is from collateral flow from the occipital branch of the external carotid artery rather than the basilar artery.*

haps in the setting of a vasculitis workup; even this has fallen out of favor with the high resolution of newer DSA units.

    In the workup of atherosclerotic carotid artery stenosis, images of the CCA bifurcation are obtained in frontal, lateral, and oblique projections to include the cervical and intracranial ICA to assess the degree of cervical stenosis and to exclude the presence of a possible tandem lesion intracranially. Long injections with

slow film rates may be required to visualize patency in patients with high grade stenosis or the so called "string sign" (Fig. 36-4).

    For the workup of extracranial carotid disease, views of the intracranial circulation are adequately obtained from CCA injections. Selective ICA injections are reserved for the workup of specific intracranial vascular disease processes only if it is felt safe to traverse the carotid bulb with the catheter tip. This determination is

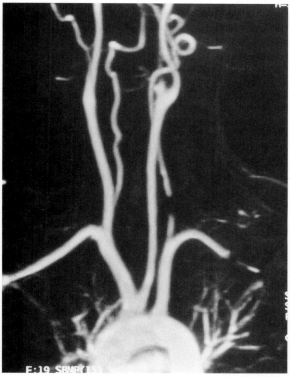

Figure 36-3.
Contrast-enhanced MRA of the aortic arch and great vessel origins in a young female. (TURBO MRA FLASH 3D single slab sequence: TR, 4.5 ms; TE, 1.7 ms; FA, 30; FOV, 380; matrix 200 × 512; slab thickness, 108 mm; effective slice thickness, 3 mm.)

made by first assessing the CCA bifurcation for patency at least fluoroscopically. For intracranial vascular evaluation, lateral and AP projections of the head are routinely obtained. Additional projections are obtained depending on the indication for the study and any questionable findings made on conventional views. Manual compression of the cervical carotid is sometimes performed to better assess patency of the circle of Willis (i.e., the anterior (ACoA) and posterior (PCoA) communicating arteries). Magnification views are helpful when assessing areas of suspected stenosis and should always be obtained in patients suspected of vasculitis. Selective external carotid artery injections should always be included in the workup of vasculitis or suspected vascular malformation, as branches of the ECA are frequent sites of disease in temporal arteritis and often supply feeders to arteriovenous fistulae and large pial arteriovenous malformations.

For vertebral artery catheterization, the tip of the catheter is advanced into the proximal subclavian artery, and the vertebral artery origin and cervical portion are assessed fluoroscopically before the vessel is selected. Abnormalities are documented on film. Orthogonal views are obtained of the posterior fossa; the frontal view is usually obtained with the x-ray tube angled craniocaudally (Towne's view) so as to maximize visualization of the intracranial course of the posterior cerebral and superior cerebellar arteries. If basilar artery disease is suspected, a true AP view or a Water's view must be obtained to avoid foreshortening of the basilar artery. The posterior circulation is assessed from injection of a single vertebral artery. Bilateral vertebral artery injections are needed only to determine the integrity of both vertebral arteries themselves (e.g., vertebral dissection) or both posterior inferior cerebellar arteries (PICA) (e.g., aneurysm workup) in the absence of adequate reflux from one injected vertebral artery down the contralateral vertebral artery. Manual compression of the cervical carotid arteries can be performed to demonstrate the patency of the PCoAs.

After completion of the procedure, manual digital pressure is applied at the puncture site for 15 to 20 min to achieve hemostasis. Compression devices and hemostatic plugs are available but are not without complication and are not routinely used at our institution. The patient is then kept flat in bed and observed for 6 h.[13,14] Studies have shown that if rebleeding occurs following compression of the artery, it will happen typically within the first 4 h. Peripheral pulses in the punctured leg should be monitored closely in the first few hours (i.e., every 15 min for the first hour and every half hour for the second hour) following the procedure. If previously palpable peripheral pulses are no longer present, arterial occlusion or embolus to the lower leg should be suspected and prompt clinical assessment and diagnostic evaluation begun to avoid limb threat.

COMPLICATIONS

Relatively minor complications of CA include local discomfort or numbness in the groin or leg related to local anesthesia (1% lidocaine), and this resolves over the course of a few hours. Groin hematoma, which occurs when there is persistent bleeding under the skin, is another minor complication. Groin hematomas usually occur within the first few hours after the

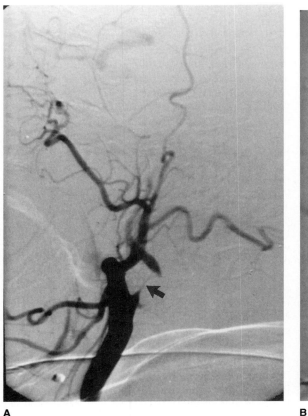
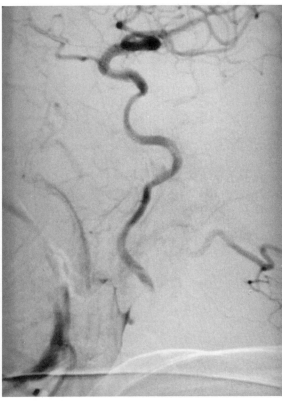

A   **B**

Figure 36-4.
Lateral common carotid injection demonstrating focal eccentric high grade atherosclerotic stenosis
(arrow) of the ICA origin (A) *with delayed filling of the patent ICA* (B) *distal to the stenosis.*

procedure and require further manual compression. A groin hematoma may go unnoticed by the patient, and for this reason all patients should have close postprocedural observation for the first 1 to 2 h whether in the holding area of the radiology department or in a recovery room. Rarely, a high arterial puncture may result in bleeding into the retroperitoneal cavity and go unnoticed until blood loss is so severe that hypotension occurs, requiring transfusion and surgical intervention. Another relatively minor complication is pseudoaneurysm of the punctured artery, which occurs if bleeding from the puncture site is confined to the periarterial region. These patients will develop a pulsatile mass in the groin, which can occur immediately after the procedure or after days. Most (more than 80 percent) of pseudoaneurysms can

be treated using ultrasound with compression of the pseudoaneurysm.[15] The success rate in this setting is dependent on the size of the pseudoaneurysm (smaller than 4 cm is better), the configuration (uniloculated do better), the age of the pseudoaneurysm (the more recent the better), and the coagulation state of the patient (anticoagulated patients have a lower success rate). If manual compression is unsuccessful, surgical correction is required. A rarer but more serious complication is the development of an arteriovenous fistula between the femoral artery and vein, which requires surgery for correction in all cases. Arterial occlusion and dissection can also occur following arteriography and may lead to lower extremity ischemic or thromboembolic complications, manifesting as lower extremity pain or loss of pulses in the foot. The incidence of local complications increases with increasing catheter size, age of patient, and degree of atherosclerosis.

The most serious complication of CA is that of disabling stroke or death. The rate of permanent neurologic deficit is quoted at 0.6 to 2.4 percent, whereas the risk of mortality is on the order of less than 0.1 percent,[11,16,17] The Asymptomatic Carotid Atherosclerosis Study (ACAS) reported a complication rate of 1.2 percent, for stroke or death.[18] Factors that increase the risk of neurologic complication include known cerebrovascular disease, number of transient ischemic attacks, experience of the angiographer, length of the procedure, amount of contrast used, number of vessels studied, number of catheters used, and age of the patient.

RADIOGRAPHIC FINDINGS

Cervical Arteries

Atherosclerotic Vascular Disease (ASVD) At angiography, ASVD can appear as concentric or eccentric irregularity of the lumen, smooth stenosis, occlusion, elongation and tortuosity of the vessels, and rarely even as dilation and ectasia of the vessels, the so called arteria magna form of the disease. As is true elsewhere in the vasculature, ASVD most often occurs at the CCA bifurcation and at other sites of branching along the intracranial circulation. Dense calcifications, when present, may degrade the angiographic resolution of a stenosis and are, themselves, not well delineated by CA because the process of digital subtraction removes the calcifications from the images. The degree of ICA stenosis is determined with the method popularized by the ACAS and the North American Asymtomatic Carotid Endarterctomy Study (NASCET) (Fig. 36-5).[16,16a,19] Measurements are taken from the view that demonstrates the narrowest patent lumen. Be aware that a preliminary visual comparison between the diameter of the normal upstream portion of the diseased ICA and the diameter of the ipsilateral ECA should be made before measurements are taken. A distal ICA in a diseased carotid artery with a lumen smaller than that of the ipsilateral ECA is thought to be an artery that is approaching occlusion. The progressive collapse of the lumen is thought to result from inadequate forward flow (pressure and volume) to maintain the normal diameter of the vessel. Because of the elasticity of the arterial wall, the lumen gets narrower with severely diminished flow, but the lumen can "re-expand" if the stenosis is cor-

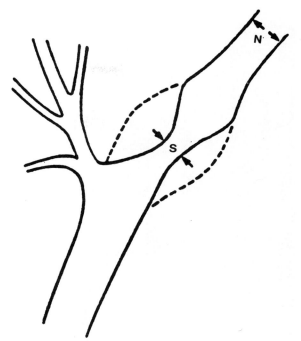

Figure 36-5.
Diagram depicting the method of quantifying an ICA stenosis as first described in the ACAS and NASCET studies.[19] The diameter measured at the site of stenosis (S) is compared with the diameter of the normal distal ICA (N) without accounting for the original configuration of bulb. Note that this measurement underestimates the true degree of atherosclerotic narrowing at the bulb but is easy to reproduce. Adapted from ref. 19 with permission.

rected and forward flow is restored. In this setting, the ACAS/NASCET method of measurement cannot be applied, as it would falsely underestimate the actual degree of stenosis (Fig. 36-6). These lesions are reported as severe arterial narrowing approaching occlusion.

Radiation therapy-related changes can be similar in appearance to ASVD. History of prior radiation therapy and atypical location (i.e., the mid-cervical CCA rather than bifurcation) will suggest the correct etiology of the changes (Fig. 36-7).

Vasculitis The most common etiologies of vasculitis in the extracranial cerebral vasculature include Takayasu's arteritis, giant cell arteritis, and fibromuscular dysplasia (FMD).[20] FMD occurs in approximately 1 percent of the population and is more common in females (>90 percent of cases). Takayasu's arteritis is a disease in

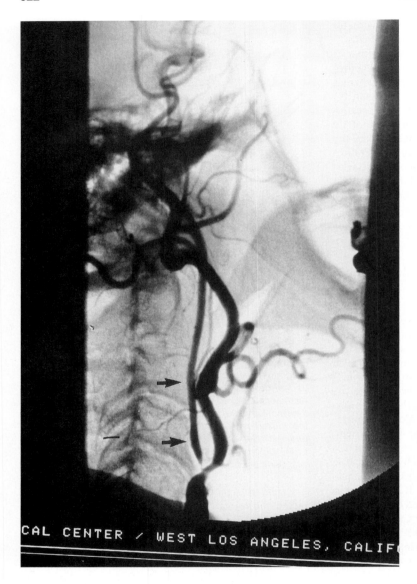

CAL CENTER / WEST LOS ANGELES, CALIF

Figure 36-6.
Lateral view from a common carotid arteriogram with the bony landmarks visible demonstrating an internal carotid artery that is approaching occlusion. The method of quantifying the stenosis described in Fig. 36-5 cannot be used as the distal lumen of the ICA is collapsed from lack of flow (arrows) and would yield a falsely small diameter for the measurement.

women between the ages of 15 and 45. Both FMD and Takayasu's arteritis typically result in narrowing and irregularity of the lumen, but ectasia and aneurysm formation may also occur.

In Takayasu's arteritis, stroke occurs in up to 15 percent of patients and may be due to ischemia or hypertensive hemorrhage from renal artery involvement. The disease tends to involve large arteries, characteristically the aorta itself and the origins of the great vessels off of the aortic arch. Though vertebral artery involvement is less common, the ostium can be occluded as part of the subclavian artery disease. Intimal proliferation, fibrosis, and smooth muscle cell destruction result in luminal narrowing, thrombosis, or occlusion. The common occurrence of intrathoracic and intra-abdominal vascular involvement makes angiography helpful in the diagnosis. The angiographic diagnosis is based more on the distribution and location of the lesions rather than

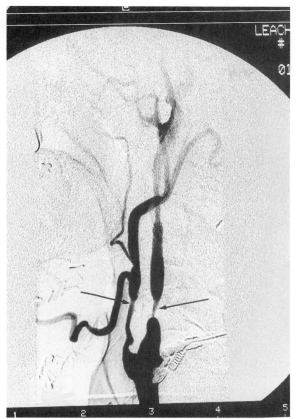

Figure 36-7.
Lateral view from a common carotid arteriogram obtained in a patient who had received radiation therapy for squamous cell carcinoma of the base of tongue. The stenosis is not significantly different in appearance from a routine atherosclerotic stenosis, but note that the ECA is stenotic at the exact same level as the ICA (arrows) and that both stenoses are remote from the origins at the branch point of the CCA, a finding that would be unusual for atherosclerosis.

on the appearance, as the latter by itself is not specific. The degree of stenosis is variable, but progression to occlusion is the natural course (Fig. 36-8).

FMD can involve, to varying degrees, the intima, the media, and the adventitia. It differs from Takayasu's in that it tends to involve the cervical ICAs rather than the CCAs. Involvement is typically distributed in the cervical ICA (75 percent of cases) distal to the carotid bulb and distal to the proximal ICA, thereby distinguishing it from atherosclerosis. The vertebral arteries are the next most common cerebral vessel to

be involved (15 to 25 percent of cases). Bilateral involvement is seen in over 50 percent of cases. At angiography, the characteristic appearance of the more common form, medial FMD, is the classical "string of beads" sign, where the lumen of the involved artery is beaded in appearance (Fig. 36-9). The areas of luminal dilatation are larger in diameter than the normal lumen, thereby distinguishing it from the catheter-related flow phenomenon of standing waves. The area of involvement may be 1 to 5 cm in length. When the intimal form of the disease predominates, the vessel may be smoothly narrowed. Dissection, spontaneous or traumatic, aneurysm formation, and occlusion may complicate FMD. Although rare, intracranial arterial involvement has been described with

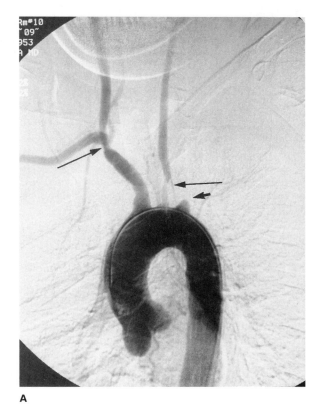

A

Figure 36-8.
Two different cases of Takayasu's arteritis. A left anterior oblique projection from an aortic arch injection in a 44-year-old female demonstrating proximal occlusion of the left subclavian artery (short arrow) and focal stenoses of the proximal left and right common carotid arteries (long arrows).

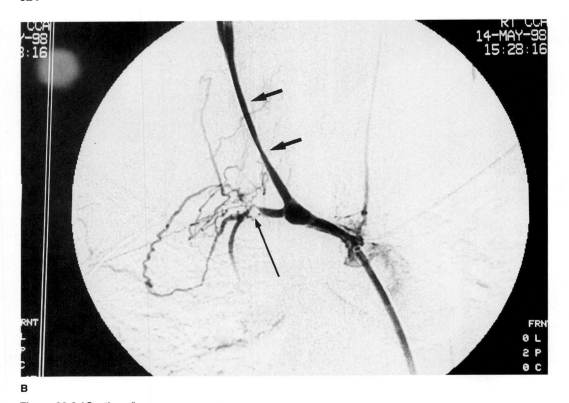

B

Figure 36-8 (*Continued*).
B *frontal view from a selective right innominate artery injection demonstrating occlusion of the right subclavian artery* (long arrow) *proximal to the origin of the right vertebral artery and the development of small collaterals. Note the long smooth stenosis of the right common carotid artery* (short arrows).

angiographic appearances ranging from the classic string of beads' luminal irregularity to a moyamoya-like pattern.

The diagnosis of these arteritides is still typically made at conventional angiography; however, newer contrast-enhanced MRA techniques for studying the aortic arch and great vessels are emerging. Angiography is being used increasingly as a treatment option in both FMD and Takayasu's arteritis, with many of the lesions amenable to angioplasty, with or without stent placement.

Whereas Takayasu's arteritis and FMD are diseases of the younger population, giant cell arteritis (GCA) or temporal arteritis, as it is also known, occurs almost exclusively in patients over the age of 50. The superficial temporal artery is the vessel most commonly involved with angiography, demonstrating smooth seg-

mental narrowings or vascular occlusion. The most serious sequela of the disease is blindness secondary to involvement of the posterior ciliary and retinal arteries, vessels that are beyond the resolution of conventional angiography.[21] The definitive diagnosis is easily achieved by biopsying the superficial temporal artery, thereby obviating the need for angiography.

Arterial Dissection   Dissection occurs when there is disruption of the intimal layer of the vessel wall allowing an intramural hematoma to form. It has been described in association with multiple conditions, classically following trauma.[3,22] Dissection has been reported to occur in 0.4 percent of patients following blunt injury to the head and neck.[23] Internal carotid artery dissection usually occurs distal to the carotid bulb with rapid smooth tapering of the distal cervical ICA lumen (Fig. 36-10).

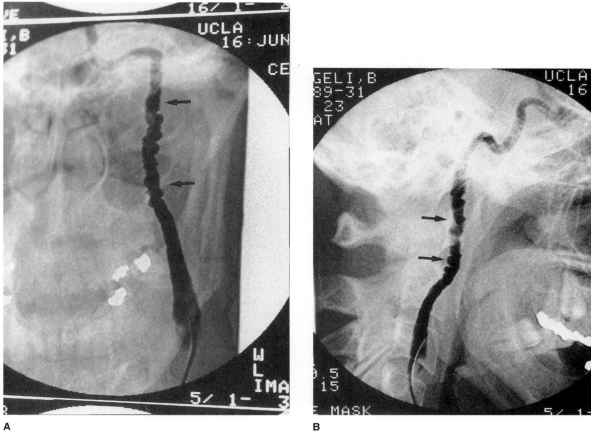

A   B

Figure 36-9.
Frontal (A) *and lateral* (B) *views from a left ICA injection in a 57-year-old male with fibromuscular dysplasia. Note the sparing of the bulb and the long segment of involvement* (arrows). *This is the classic "string of beads" appearance.*

It is thought that hyperextension and lateral flexion of the neck may stretch the ICA over the transverse processes of the upper cervical vertebrae. Vertebral artery dissection usually involves the distal cervical segment near the craniocervical junction and is also thought to be secondary to stretching of the vertebral artery wall. Dissection may result in either partial luminal narrowing or complete occlusion. Intimal flaps are rarely demonstrated. The false lumen may fill only on the delayed images (Fig. 36-11). Luminal irregularity with persistent patency may predispose to thrombus formation and subsequent embolic infarction. Therefore, stroke may occur either as a result of low flow (stenosis/occlusion) or embolic phenomena.

Conventional magnetic resonance imaging (MRI) with T1W images is often adequate to make the diagnosis of cervical carotid artery dissection, as with demonstration of both the false and true lumen as well as any pseudoaneurysm formation. MRA is also typically acquired in the setting of suspected dissection, and the source images are often better than the reformatted images at demonstrating the channels of the true and false lumen cross-sectionally (see Fig. 36-11). Arteriography is indicated when the diagnosis is in question or when patients are symptomatic from thromboembolic phenomena while fully anticoagulated or unable to undergo anticoagulation. In this setting, arteriography may be performed also for therapeutic intervention with bal-

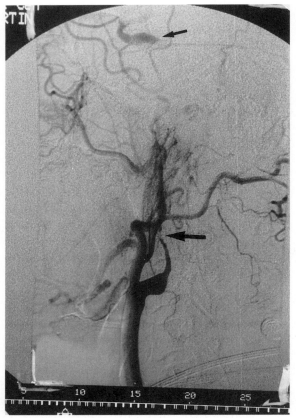

Figure 36-10.
Lateral view from a left common carotid injection in a 42-year-old male demonstrating dissection of the internal carotid artery due to hyperextension of the neck during a surfing accident. Long arrow denotes site of ICA occlusion. Note distal reconstitution of the cavernous segment of the ICA (short arrow).

lopathies with a predisposition to carotid dissection. Although the angiogram will demonstrate the dissection, the underlying disease is not always identifiable.

Intracranial Arteries

ASVD   When ASVD involves the intracranial circulation, it typically involves the carotid siphon and vertebrobasilar junction. It may also involve the proximal cerebral artery branches (Fig. 36-13). ASVD results in luminal narrowing of varying degrees, eccentric or concentric. The stenoses are usually irregular but may be focal and smooth. As previously mentioned, views of the carotid siphon should be obtained in all patients undergoing angiographic evaluation for cervical carotid artery stenosis to detect a possible tandem lesion of the intracranial ICA, which may have an impact on patient management.

Thromboembolic disease of the cerebral vasculature may have a variable appearance. In the acute setting, the arteriogram will usually demonstrate an abrupt arterial cut-off (Fig. 36-14). Sometimes the thrombus can be seen within the lumen of the vessel, and if there is only partial obstruction rather than complete occlusion of the vessel lumen, flow may be seen distal to the intraluminal filling defect (Fig. 36-15). Follow-up studies may demonstrate nonspecific residual luminal narrowing, persistent occlusion, or complete recanalization. Thromboemboli may originate from more proximal cerebrovascular arterial disease, including arterial dissection and CCA bifurcation atheromatous plaque. Therefore, these areas should be included in the evaluation. Indications for performing arteriography in the setting of suspected thromboembolic disease to the intracranial vasculature include confirmation of the disease process, follow-up of abnormalities (especially to guide further anticoagulation therapy), and treatment of the thrombus with intra-arterial thrombolytics, which is the subject of another chapter. Although the more recent literature discusses the aortic arch as a potential source of thromboemboli, transesophageal echocardiography is probably more sensitive at detecting small intimal plaques than aortography, and routine arch angiography is not typically performed. Therefore, if desired, aortography should be specifically ordered when the cerebral arteriogram is ordered.

Dissection   Dissection rarely occurs intracranially. When it does occur, it is usually related to trauma

loon occlusion of the parent vessel. MRA is less sensitive than CA at detecting vertebral artery dissection. Conventional angiography is still considered the method of choice in the diagnosis of vertebral artery dissection.[24]

Pseudoaneurysm, usually of the prepetrous or distal cervical ICA segments, may complicate dissection. In a series of 60 patients with a history of blunt trauma and resultant cervical internal carotid artery injury, 11 of the patients had pseudoaneurysm formation with or without dissection (Fig. 36-12).[25]

Fibromuscular dysplasia, Marfan disease, Ehlers-Danlos disease, and homocysteinuria are known vascu-

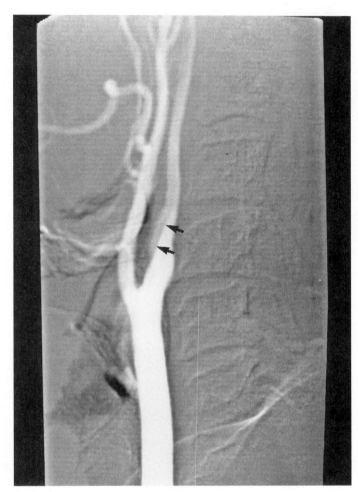

Figure 36-11.
*Delayed image from a lateral
right common carotid angiogram
(A) showing filling of false lumen
(arrows). Corresponding source
image (B) from MRA showing an
intimal flap (crescentic line)
within the right ICA lumen.*   **A**

and involves the supraclinoid segment of the ICA where the artery is relatively mobile. Rarely, dissection occurs along the petrous or cavernous segments of the ICA and is usually associated with a skull base fracture.[26]

Vasculitis   Acute stroke syndromes may be the result of segmental arterial narrowing or occlusion related to vasculitis. One study showed that angiography was positive in only 50 percent of patients with biopsy-proven vasculitis.[27] Angiography may not be able to

demonstrate the presence of abnormalities in patients with pathologically proven CNS vasculitis, probably because the vessels involved are beyond the resolution of angiography. High-resolution magnification DSA is probably sufficient to exclude angiographic abnormalities in patients undergoing investigation for suspected CNS vasculitis and has largely replaced cut-film angiography.

On angiogram, vasculitis is suggested by the presence of segmental arterial narrowing, sometimes alternating with areas of arterial dilatation or beading. Vas-

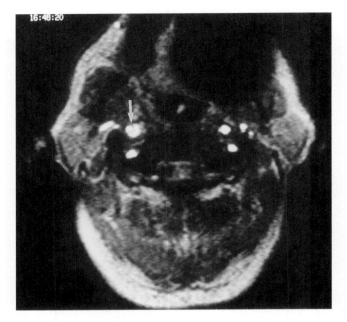

B

Figure 36-11 (*Continued*).

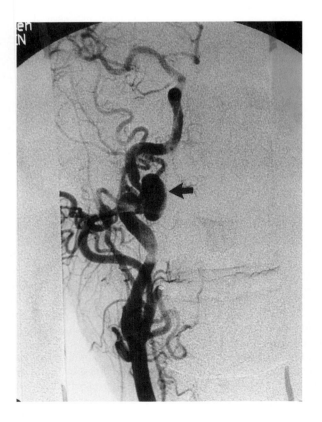

Figure 36-12.
Frontal view from a right common carotid injection in the same patient as Fig. 36-10 demonstrating pseudoaneurysm formation (arrow) along the distal right cervical internal carotid artery. There is a short segment stenosis of the ICA just distal to the pseudoaneurysm.

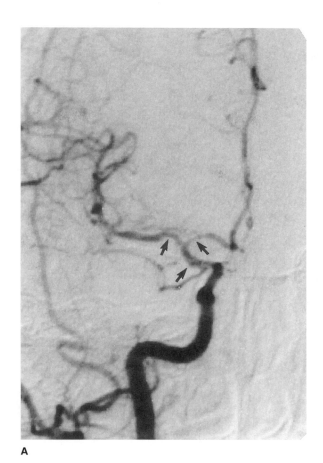

Figure 36-13.
Frontal views from right (A) *and left* (B) *common carotid injections in two different patients with intracranial atherosclerotic narrowing. In A there is disease of the distal ICA and proximal anterior and middle cerebral arteries; in B there is disease of the left MCA origin and the mid-ACA (arrows).*

A

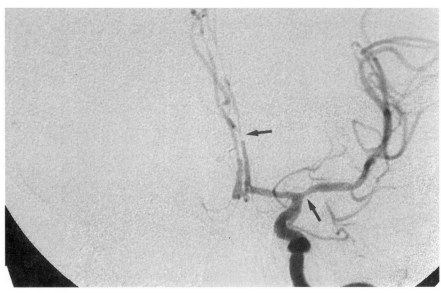

B

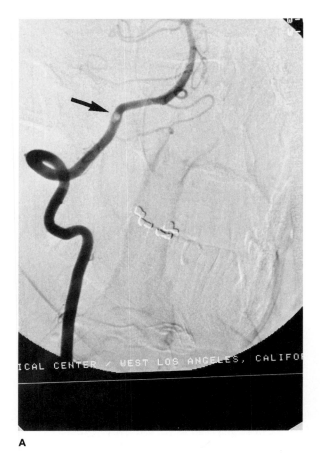

A

Figure 36-14.
Left vertebral arteriograms obtained 2 months apart in a 43-year-old male with thromboembolic disease of unknown etiology. In A there are occlusions of both posterior cerebral arteries (PCA) (arrows). B obtained 2 months later, demonstrating recanalization of the right PCA and interval development of a new embolus to the left PCA origin, causing complete occlusion (small arrow).

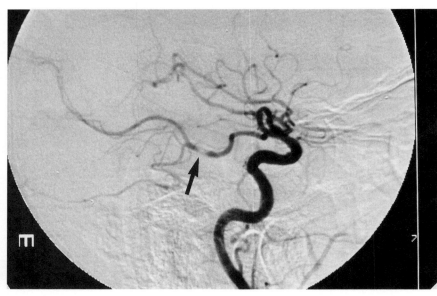

B

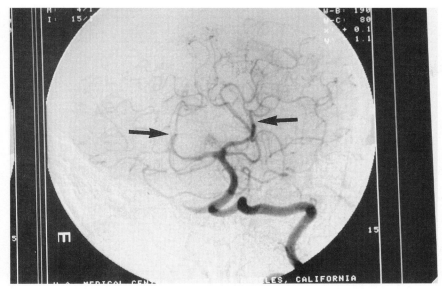

A

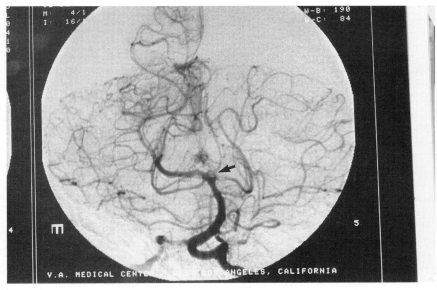

B

Figure 36-15.
Two different patients with thromboembolic disease. Frontal view from a right vertebral artery injection (A) and lateral view from a right common carotid artery injection (B) in the first patient, demonstrating clots in the right vertebral artery and right posterior cerebral artery, respectively (arrows). The second patient (C) had partial thrombosis of the basilar artery seen as filling defects within the main basilar trunk (small arrows).

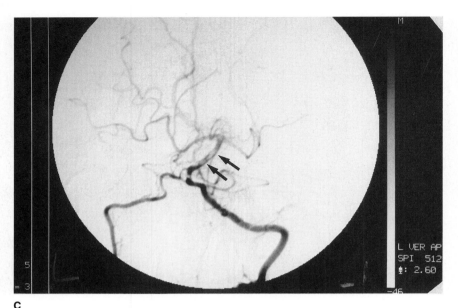

C

Figure 36-15 (*Continued*).

culitis can result from infectious and noninfectious inflammation. Noninfectious vasculitis may be primary or more commonly secondary to systemic vasculitis. The differential diagnosis for CNS vasculitis is quite extensive, and in most cases, the exact etiology of vasculitis cannot be determined from the angiographic appearance alone.

If the vasculitis is isolated to the proximal basal arteries, involving the circle of Willis and the proximal cerebral artery branches, the disease may be related to underlying disease of the leptomeninges themselves (e.g., infectious or carcinomatous meningitis). Infectious meningitis can occur secondary to bacterial, tuberculous, fungal, viral, and syphilitic infections.[28] Sickle cell anemia with vasculopathy can also have a similar pattern of proximal involvement. The differential diagnosis also includes atherosclerosis, moyamoya disease (which is discussed later), radiation therapy, and connective tissue disorders. Because imaging findings are frequently not specific for the diagnosis, clinical and laboratory correlation is always needed to confirm the etiology of the arteriopathy (Fig. 36-16). In suspected vasculitis secondary to infectious meningitis, arteriography is usually not necessary for diagnosis. The disease should be considered in the patient with suspected meningitis whose

cross-sectional images demonstrate enhancement of the basal meninges or infarcts in various vascular distributions (Fig. 36-17).

The noninfectious inflammatory vasculitides often involve the more distal arteries of smaller caliber and include vasculitis associated with lupus erythematosis, polyarteritis nodosum, rheumatoid arthritis, and primary CNS vasculitis or granulomatous vasculitis of the CNS.[29]

Moyamoya Moyamoya disease refers to progressive narrowing and occlusion of the distal ICA and/or the proximal middle (M1) and anterior (A1) cerebral arterial segments. The etiology of moyamoya disease is unknown. Although the angiographic appearance of moyamoya is quite characteristic, a similar angiographic pattern of supraclinoid ICA occlusion can be seen in severe intracranial atherosclerosis (Fig. 36-18), neurofibromatosis type I, Down syndrome, sickle cell disease, and prior radiation therapy to the brain.

Idiopathic moyamoya typically but not exclusively occurs in childhood or adolescence and is usually bilateral. Following progressive stenosis and occlusion of the distal ICA or proximal M1/A1 segments, numerous small collaterals enlarge, the lenticulostriates and

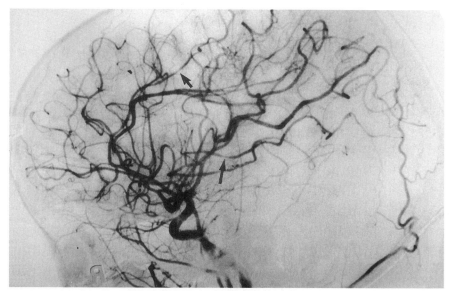

Figure 36-16.
Lateral CCA injection showing focal areas of short segmental narrowing involving distal intracranial arteries (arrows).

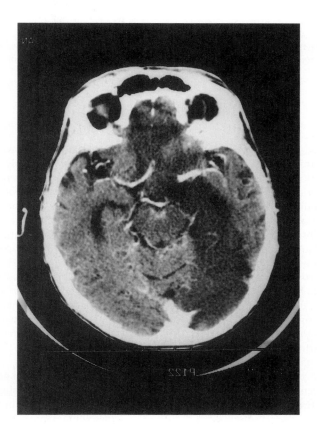

Figure 36-17.
CT image showing bilateral ACA and left PCA infarcts in a patient with basal fungal meningitis (as- pergillus).

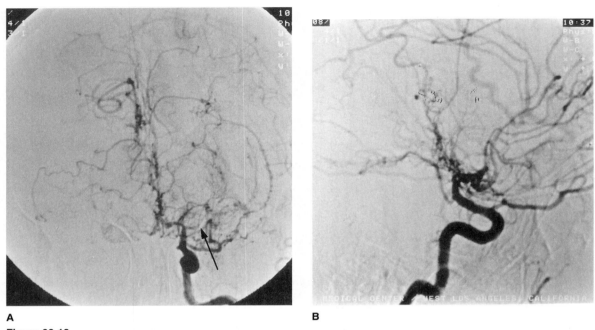

A   **B**

Figure 36-18.
Frontal (A) and lateral (B) left CCA angiograms in a patient with intracranial atherosclerotic disease resulting in a moyamoya-like pattern. Note that there is proximal occlusion of the left MCA (arrow).

the thalamoperforators, giving rise to the characteristic "puff of smoke" appearance on arteriography (Fig. 36-19). Conventional arteriography is necessary for the definitive diagnosis. Arteriography will also demonstrate the collaterals maintaining flow to the brain, vessels beyond the resolution of MRA. These include leptomeningeal collaterals from the posterior cerebral arteries and transdural collaterals from the external carotid artery (ECA) in addition to the above-mentioned perforators. Conventional arteriography is also necessary to study the ECA, and its branches as treatment options include bypass grafting of one of the ECA branches to the MCA or encephalomyosynangiosis, a surgical bypass technique where the temporalis muscle with the superficial temporal artery is placed onto the brain's surface for ingrowth of transdural collaterals to the MCA branches. In the postoperative patient in whom symptoms recur, conventional arteriography is necessary to evaluate the integrity of the anastomosis and to assess for interval progression of disease.

Vasospasm Following aneurysmal subarachnoid hemorrhage, clinically significant vasospasm occurs between 4 and 12 days out from the initial bleed.[30] It is a potential cause of stroke following subarachnoid hemorrhage. Ideally, patients at risk are followed with bedside transcranial Doppler for evidence of increasing MCA velocities. If the patients do not respond to medical management with hypervolemia, hemodilution, and hypertension ("triple H" therapy), arteriography is performed. This is done to assess the extent and degree of vasospasm and to treat with angioplasty if the spasm involves the proximal arteries (e.g., the supraclinoid ICA or M1 or A1 segments) or to infuse intra-arterial papaverine if the spasm involves more distal vessels (Fig. 36-20).

Veno-occlusive Disease The diagnosis and follow-up of major venous sinus occlusion is now readily available by noninvasive imaging using MR venography and conventional spin echo MRI (Fig. 36-21). Arteriography

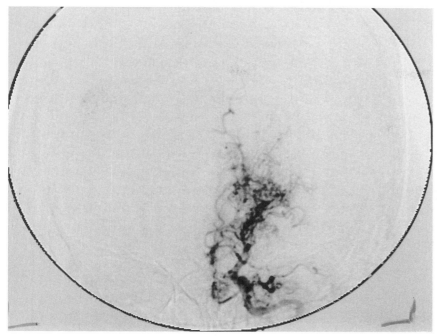

A

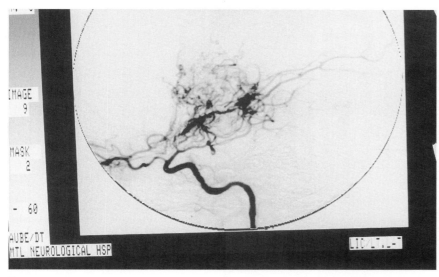

B

Figure 36-19.
Frontal (A) *and lateral* (B) *left ICA angiograms in a young patient with idiopathic moyamoya disease showing the typical "puff of smoke" appearance.*

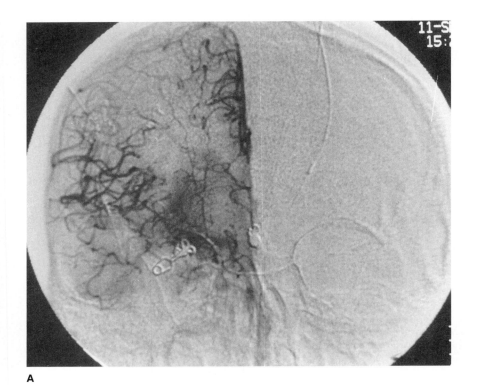

A

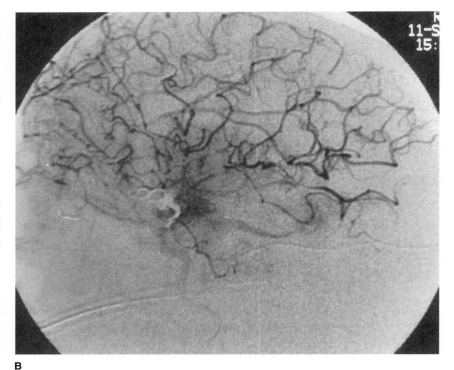

B

Figure 36-20.
Frontal (A) *and lateral* (B) *angiograms in a patient with distal vasospasm. The spastic vessels are too small to discern, but there is delayed transit time of the contrast injection through the ACA and MCA circulation indicative of spasm. This finding reversed following papaverine infusion.*

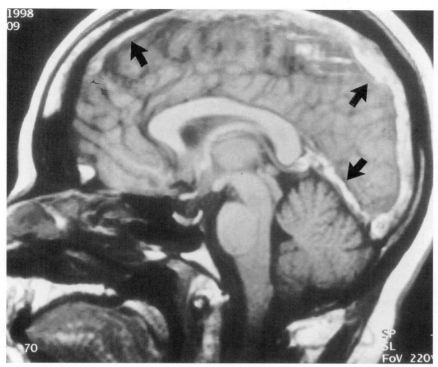

Figure 36-21.
Sagittal midline SE T1W image showing high signal intensity clot (arrows) *in the superior sagittal sinus and straight sinus in this patient with thrombosis.*

is rarely indicated unless intervention is anticipated for direct thrombolysis.[31]

REFERENCES

1. Russo CP, Smoker WRK: Nonatheromatous carotid artery disease. *Neuroimag Clin North Am* 6:811, 1996.
2. Desfontaines P, Despland PA: Dissection of the internal carotid artery: Aetiology, symptomatology, clinical and neurosonological follow up and treatment in 60 consecutive cases. *Acta Neurol Belg* 95:226, 1995.
3. Klufas RA, Hsu L, Barnes PD, et al: Dissection of the carotid and vertebral arteries: Imaging with MR angiography. *Am J Radiol* 164:673, 1995.
4. Furie DM, Tien RD: Fibromuscular dysplasia of the arteries of the head and neck: Imaging findings. *Am J Radiol* 162:1205, 1994.
5. Taniguchi N, Itoh K, Honda M, et al: Comparative ultrasonographic and angiographic study of carotid arterial lesions in Takayasu's arteritis. *Angiology* 48:9, 1997.
6. AbuRrahama AF, Thaxton L: Temporal arteritis: Diagnostic and therapeutic considerations. *Am Surg* 62:449, 1996.
7. Zidar N, Ferluga D, Hval A, et al: Contribution to the pathogenesis of radiation-induced injury to large arteries. *J Laryngol Otol* 111:988, 1997.
8. Sinsawaiwong S, Phanthumchinda K: Progressive cerebral occlusive disease after hypothalamic astrocytoma radiation therapy. *J Med Assoc Thailand* 80:338, 1997.
9. Chung TS, Yousem CM, Lexa FJ, et al: MRI of carotid angiopathy after therapeutic radiation. *J Comput Assist Tomogr* 18:533, 1994.
10. Young B, Moore WS, Robertson JT, et al: An analysis of perioperative surgical mortality and mobidity in Asymptomatic Carotid Atherosclerosis Study. *Stroke* 27:2216, 1996.
11. Pryor JC, Setton A, Nelson PK, et al: Complications of diagnostic cerebral angiography and tips on avoidance. *Neuroimag Clin North Am* 6:751, 1996.
12. Goss JE, Chambers CE, Heupler FA, et al: Systemic anaphylactoid reactions to iodinated contrast media during cardiac catherization procedures: Guidelines for prevention, diagnosis and treatment: *Cathet Cardiovasc Diag* 34:99, 1995.

13. Huber P: *Cerebral Angiography,* 2d ed. Thieme Verlag, 1982, p 585.

14. Osborn AG: *Introduction to Cerebral Angiography.* New York, Harper & Row, 1980, p 436.

15. Coley BD, Roberts AC, Fellmeth BD: Postangiographic femoral artery pseudoaneurysms: Further experience with US-guided compression repair. *Radiology* 194:307, 1995.

16. Chaturvedi S, Policherla PN, Femino L: Cerebral angiography practices at US teaching hospitals: Implications for carotid endarterectomy. *Stroke* 28:1895, 1997.

16a. Asymptomatic Carotid Atherosclerosis Study: Study design for randomized prospective trial of carotid endarterectomy for asymptomatic atherosclerosis. *Stroke* 20:844, 1989.

17. Heiserman JE, Dean BL, Hodak JA, et al: Neurologic complications of cerebral angiography. *Am J Neuroradiol* 15:1401, 1994.

18. Executive Committee for the Asymptomatic Carotid Atherosclerosis Study: Endarterectomy for asymptomatic carotid artery stenosis. *JAMA* 273:1421, 1995.

19. North American Symptomatic Carotid Endarterectomy Trial Steering Committee: North American Symptomatic Carotid Endarterectomy Trial. *Stroke* 22:711, 1991.

20. Hurst RW: Angiography of non-atherosclerotic occlusive cerebrovascular disease. *Neuroimag Clin North Am* 6:651, 1996.

21. Caselli R, Hunder G: Neurologic aspects of giant cell (temporal) arteritis. *Rheum Dis Clin North Am* 19:941, 1993.

22. Osborn AG: *Diagnostic Neuroradiology.* St Louis, Mosby-Year Book, 1994.

23. Laitt RD, Lewis TT, Bradshaw JR: Blunt carotid arterial trauma. *Clin Radiol* 51:117, 1994.

24. Levy C, Laissy JP, Raveau V, et al: Carotid and vertebral artery dissections: Three-dimensional time-of-flight MR angiography and MR imaging versus conventional angiography. *Radiology* 190:97, 1994.

25. Coghill Th, Moore EE, Meissner M, et al: The spectrum of blunt injury to the carotid artery: A multicenter perspective. *J Trauma* 37:473, 1994.

26. O'Sullivan RM, Robertson WD, Nugent RA, et al: Supraclinoid carotid artery dissection following unusual trauma. *Am J Neuroradiol* 11:1150, 1990.

27. Chu CT, Gray L, Goldstein LB, et al: Diagosis of intracranial vasculitis: A multi-disciplinary approach. *J Neuropathol Exp Neurol* 57:30, 1998.

28. Gerber O, Roque C, Coyle PK: Vasculitis owing to infection. *Neurol Clin* 15:903, 1997.

29. Younger DS, Hays AP, Brust JC, et al: Granulomatous angiitis of the brain: An inflammatory reaction of diverse etiology. *Arch Neurol* 45:514, 1988.

30. Setton A, Davis AJ, Bose A, et al: Angiography of cerebral aneurysms. *Neuroimag Clin North Am* 6:705, 1996.

31. Wang AM: MRA of venous sinus thrombosis. *Clin Neurosci* 4:158, 1997.

Chapter 37

TRANSESOPHAGEAL ECHOCARDIOGRAPHY IN THE EVALUATION OF STROKE

Benjamin J. Cohen

BACKGROUND

It has been estimated that 15 to 20 percent of all strokes are of a cardioembolic origin.[1] The use of echocardiography has greatly facilitated rapid and safe imaging of the heart and aorta in pursuit of definite and potential sources of thromboembolism (Table 37-1). Two-dimensional transthoracic echocardiography (TTE) affords an opportunity to visualize the heart and assess hemodynamic function. However, various important structures implicated as potential causes of stroke are not optimally visualized secondary to signal attenuation caused by the chest wall and lung. In contrast, transesophageal echocardiography (TEE) allows the physician to evaluate every part of the heart in exquisite detail, including structures inadequately examined by TTE (interatrial septum, left atrial appendage, and ascending aorta) or not visualized at all (aortic arch). Besides visualizing structures hidden from TTE, transesophageal probes, which routinely operate at higher frequencies (5.0 to 7.0 MHz) than standard surface echo probes (2.5 to 3.5 MHz), offer improved resolution. Only the cardiac apex is not routinely visualized with the clarity of transthoracic imaging. New ultrasound technology that employs faster computers, new methods of ultrasound beam formation, higher frequency surface echo transducers (5.0 MHz), and new imaging modalities (harmonics and contrast) are pushing the envelope of TTE. However, published comparisons to old technology and TEE in the evaluation of stroke are not available at this time. Recent technological improvements specific to TEE include the ability to image in multiple planes, although

the advantage as measured in patient outcome and cost compared with single and biplane TEE in the stroke patient is not well defined.

Technique

The transesophageal procedure can be performed using topical anesthesia alone or in combination with conscious sedation. Use of the latter approach may be gauged according to the patient's anxiety level,[2] requires strict adherence to conscious sedation protocols, and increases the expense of the procedure. A complete interrogation of the heart and aorta should take no more than 15 min; recovery from conscious sedation usually requires about 2 h, and outpatients must be driven home. Patients may experience some discomfort in the form of gagging but should not have pain in a properly performed procedure. Patients with dysphagia should undergo consultation by a gastroenterologist before having a transesophageal echocardiographic examination. A complete TEE study in the stroke patient requires routine evaluation of the aorta (ascending, descending, and arch), color Doppler interrogation of the interatrial septum, and injection of contrast during spontaneous respiration and during Valsalva, cough, or manual compression of the abdomen. These maneuvers are indicated to generate a transient elevation in right atrial pressure and thereby effect right-to-left shunting should a patient foramen ovale (PFO) be present. Patients who are too heavily sedated or who have had a large stroke may not be able to fully cooperate with the Valsalva maneuver. In such patients, the author has found it

Table 37-1.
Sources of thromboembolism

Definite sources of embolism
  Left atrial and left atrial appendage thrombi
  Left ventricular thrombus
  Rheumatic mitral stenosis with atrial fibrillation
  Left atrial myxoma
  Valvular vegetations
  Highly mobile aortic atheroma or thrombi

Potential sources of embolism
  Atrial fibrillation
  Spontaneous echo contrast
  Left ventricular apical dyskinesis
  Severe cardiomyopathy (ejection fraction <20%)
  Atrial septal aneurysm/patent foramen ovale
  Mechanical prosthetic valves
  Protruding/complex aortic atheroma
  Mitral valve prolapse
  Valvular strands
  Mitral annular calcification

useful to perform an abdominal compression maneuver to cause a transient elevation in right atrial pressure and therefore facilitate a right-to-left shunt. Contrast echocardiography is usually achieved by the agitation of saline mixed with air. Two 10-cc Luer lock syringes are connected to a three-way stopcock and then a mixture of saline (9.0 cc) and air (1.0 cc) is rapidly injected from one syringe to the other and back again several times before injection into a forearm vein during continuous recording of echocardiographic images. A successful injection requires complete opacification of the right atrium. The right-to-left movement of micro bubbles, even in the setting of a frank atrial septal defect, is not known to cause stroke or other clinically apparent systemic embolism.

TEE probes in current use tend to be either biplane (the operator can toggle between longitudinal and transverse imaging planes) or multiplane (the operator electronically changes the angle of imaging from 0 to 180 degrees). The latter technology allows for subtle changes in imaging angle, thereby affording the echocardiographer a more complete interrogation of the heart.

Risks of Transesophageal Echocardiography

The risks of TEE in 10,419 patients undergoing the procedure as part of the European Multicenter Study were found to be very low.[3] Insertion was unsuccessful in 1.9 percent (uncooperative patient or inexperienced operator, 98.5 percent, anatomical problems, 1.5 percent). Examinations were not completed in 0.9 percent of patients who underwent successful insertion because of the patient's inability to tolerate the procedure (65 cases); because of pulmonary, cardiac, or bleeding problems (18 cases); and other reasons in the remainder (10 cases). Fatality secondary to hemorrhage (0.01 percent) occurred in one patient with esophageal infiltration of a malignant lung tumor. Conscious patients were not sedated in this study.

EVIDENCE

Several trials have evaluated the diagnostic yield of TEE compared with that of TTE in stroke and TIA (transient ischemic attack) patients stratified according to the presence or absence of clinical heart disease as assessed by history, physical, ECG, and occasionally chest x-ray. It is difficult to compare results because of variations in selection of patients (consecutive stroke admissions versus echo lab referral to rule out a cardiac source of embolism), methodology (lack of adequate controls, failure to use standardized definitions, varying contrast protocols, and failure to use contrast at all), and reporting of results. Although the published literature shows that TEE compared with TTE detects a greater number of definite and potential embolic sources, this simple accounting does not necessarily relate to improved cost-effectiveness or patient outcome. For example, the finding of a thrombus in the left atrial appendage and/or spontaneous echo contrast in a patient with atrial fibrillation will not change management. There are no randomized trials evaluating the two imaging techniques using patient outcome as an endpoint. A few studies have retrospectively attempted to evaluate the effect of TEE on the decision to treat with warfarin or aspirin. Such studies are no more than anecdotes and only highlight the need for randomized trials. Nonetheless, much can be gained by reviewing these papers.

Patients with Clinical Heart Disease

Transthoracic echocardiography has been established to be of low yield for detection of definite or highly probable embolic sources in consecutive patients with stroke. Detection rates for definite or potential embolic sources are no greater than 3 percent for patients without clinical heart disease. In patients with clinical evidence of heart disease, detection rates may be as high as 22 percent.[4-6] TTE will easily identify enlargement of the left atrium and ventricle, valvular heart disease, regional wall motion abnormalities, and left ventricular thrombus (usually seen in the setting of apical dyskinesis) with accuracy comparable to TEE. In the case of the left ventricular apex, TTE offers better visualization.[7] Patients with significant obesity and obstructive lung disease may have suboptimal acoustic windows rendering less helpful surface echo. In these situations, TEE is clearly superior for the evaluation of the above mentioned structural abnormalities.

Left Ventricular Thrombi, Vegetations, and Prosthetic Valves

Left ventricular thrombi are seen in the setting of dyskinetic myocardial segments and in dilated cardiomyopathy with severely depressed ejection fraction (<20 percent). TEE has not been shown to detect left ventricular thrombi any better than TTE and, in fact, may be inferior for the assessment of apical thrombi (Fig. 37-1). Although both imaging modalities are equivalent for the diagnosis of valvular heart disease in stroke patients, improved detail is offered by TEE. Small vegetations are visualized with greater sensitivity by TEE.[8] Stroke secondary to endocarditis happens in the setting of active infection that is usually suspected on the basis of fever and positive blood cultures. Studies of TEE in the evaluation of stroke rarely include patients with endocarditis. This is probably due to selection bias, the low stroke rate of patients with endocarditis (5%), and the relatively low frequency of endocarditis compared with stroke. Distinguishing endocarditis as the cause of stroke is important because management does not include anticoagulation. Larger vegetations are felt to pose an increased risk for embolization (Fig. 37-2, color insert 32). The thromboembolic risk of mechanical valves is 1 to 2 per 100 patient years for aortic valves and 2 to 3 per 100 patient years for mitral valves.[9] Although hemodynamic function of prosthetic valves can readily be evaluated by TTE, visualization of valve structure is far better with TEE. The numbers of patients with prosthetic valves in studies of TEE and stroke are too low to draw meaningful conclusions about the routine use of TTE versus TEE in the absence of clinically suspected prosthetic valve dysfunction. Mitral valve prolapse (MVP) has been implicated as a cause of stroke in young people. When clinically evident (click-murmur), it will usually be detected by TTE (see discussion of the role of mitral valve disorders).

Left Atrial Thrombi and Atrial Fibrillation

It is well established that atrial fibrillation (AF) is a strong risk factor for stroke, especially in the setting of hypertension, congestive heart failure, previous arterial embolism, left atrial enlargement, and left ventricular dysfunction. Warfarin reduces this risk by 58 to 86 percent, as shown in several large randomized trials.[10-13] Although AF tends to occur in an older population that is already at increased risk of stroke due to generalized atherosclerotic disease, thrombi are occasionally detected in the left atrium and especially in the left atrial appendage (LAA). Although the appendage may occasionally be visualized by TTE using modified parasternal short axis views, the ability to detect clot is markedly inferior to TEE both in patients with critical mitral valve disease and patients with stroke.[14-20]

Left atrial thrombi (LAT) have been detected by TEE in 3 to 8 percent of consecutive stroke and TIA patients (mean age, 62 years); the prevalence of AF in these studies was 12 to 33 percent.[18,20-22] A similar prevalence of LAT (8.4 percent) was seen in a series of consecutive patients younger than 60 years old (mean age, 42 years), although 30 percent had severe clinical heart disease, including many with native mitral valve disease or mitral prosthetic valves.[7] For patients presenting with atrial fibrillation of at least 2 days duration (mean, 2 to 5 weeks), TEE will detect LAT in 11 to 13 percent of patients.[23,24] The reported incidence of LAT in chronic AF varies from 2.5 percent to 27 percent and may be as high as 50 percent for atrial fibrillation with recent clinical thromboembolism.[25-28] Failure to find a

Figure 37-1.
Markedly reduced left ventricular ejection fraction with apical thrombus.

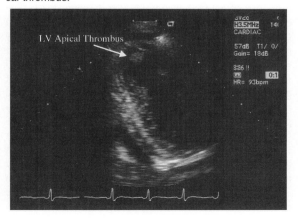

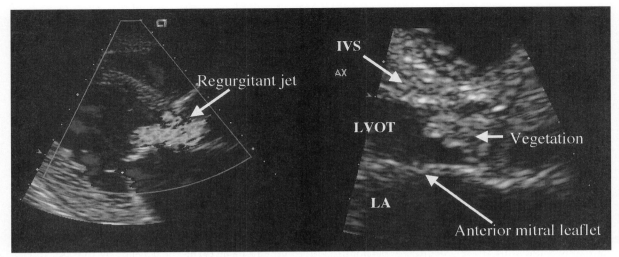

Figure 37-2.
Large aortic vegetation detected by two-dimensional transthoracic echocardiography in patient with endocarditis and cerebral embolism. LVOT = left ventricular outflow tract; IVS = interventricular septum; LA = left atrium. (See also color insert 32.)

left atrial appendage thrombus (LAAT) with TEE in a patient with atrial fibrillation and cerebral ischemia may be due to competing causes for stroke, failure to visualize the left atrial appendage in multiple planes, pretreatment with anticoagulants, or embolization of the thrombus.

In the setting of AF, LAAT (Fig. 37-3, color insert 33) are significantly associated with congestive heart failure, reduced left ventricular systolic function, diabetes, and spontaneous echo contrast.[25,26,29,30] Although one would expect a strong relationship between the presence of thrombus or thromboembolism and left atrial size, this has not been consistently demonstrated.[25,26,29,31] The reasons for this may include small sample sizes, heterogeneous patient population, and selection bias. Although patients with documented LAAT tend to have larger left atria, enlargement of the atrium may not predict future development of thromboembolism in the setting of chronic atrial fibrillation. Using pulsed Doppler sonography during the performance of TEE, one can assess left atrial appendage function by measurement of peak filling and emptying velocities (Fig. 37-4, color inserts 34–35). Patients with atrial fibrillation and LAAT or suspected embolism have significantly lower velocities (<0.25 m/s) compared with control patients with AF and no suspicion or evidence of thromboembolism.[29,31,32] Although resolution of LAAT occurs during warfarin therapy, there is no evidence that this needs

to be routinely documented in the individual patient. Some investigators have shown persistence of small LAAT in both rheumatic and nonrheumatic AF on adequate anticoagulation.[33,34]

Spontaneous Echo Contrast The introduction of TEE has led to the detection of spontaneous echo contrast (SEC) in the left atrium (Fig. 37-5). It appears as slow-moving swirls of echos and is thought to be caused by sluggish flow leading to rouleau formation. SEC is strongly associated with the presence of LAT and/or a history of arterial thrombi.[35] Rarely seen on surface echocardiography, even with harmonic imaging, SEC in the left atrium is readily demonstrated by TEE in many patients with atrial fibrillation and dilated atria, with or without mitral stenosis or a mitral prosthetic valve.[17,35–37] In atrial fibrillation, SEC is strongly associated with left atrial enlargement and is inversely correlated to mitral regurgitation.[38] Mean left atrial diameter has been reported to be significantly larger in the presence of SEC (56 mm with SEC versus 43 mm without SEC).[36] Over time, the prevalence of SEC is stable for patients with mitral stenosis and may increase in patients with chronic atrial fibrillation.[33,39] Although the presence of SEC in AF indicates an increased risk of stroke, the absence of it does not indicate a lower long-term risk of stroke because SEC may develop over time.

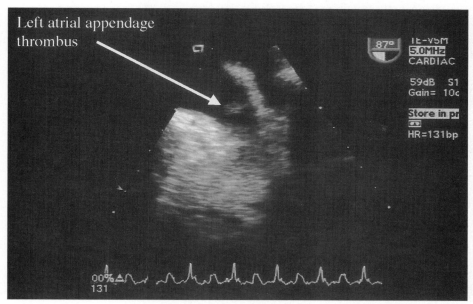

Figure 37-3.
Left atrial appendage thrombus in patient with atrial fibrillation. Left atrial and ventricular enlargement and ejection fraction of 15 percent. (See also color insert 33.)

Other Sources of Embolism in Patients with Clinical Heart Disease

Patients with acquired structural heart disease with or without atrial fibrillation may have other findings that are considered potential sources of embolism, including PFO, atrial septal aneurysm (ASA), and atherosclerotic disease of the aorta. Abnormalities of the interatrial septum have been reported in 12 to 15 percent of stroke patients with clinical heart disease and in 14 percent of patients who have an abnormal TTE and/or atrial fibrillation.[18,20] The Stroke Prevention in Nonrheumatic Atrial Fibrillation (SPINAF) investigators used TEE to evaluate the prevalence of PFO and ASA in a small cohort of chronic AF patients who, at the end of the study, had not had a stroke.[34] PFO was present in 54 percent and ASA (associated with PFO in all cases) in 7.3 percent. Complex aortic atheromas, predominantly found in those patients older than age of 60, have been detected by TEE in as many as 17 percent of patients with an abnormal TTE* and/or atrial fibrillation.[20,40] Competitive potential stroke causes could make it difficult to assign a cause in a particular patient who does not have a thrombus visualized on TEE. In favor of atrial fibrillation as the cause of stroke would be impaired left ventricular systolic function, severe SEC, and markedly impaired LAA filling and emptying velocities.

Patients without Clinical Heart Disease

The low yield of TTE in stroke patients without clinical heart disease has been confirmed in several studies comparing TTE with TEE in patients with stroke and TIA.[6,16,20,41] The Berlin Stroke Data Bank showed that TTE detects high-risk sources of emboli in 1.6 percent of patients without clinical heart disease compared with 4.2 percent for TEE.[6] TTE may occasionally detect potential sources of embolism: clinically unsuspected MVP,[16,18,19,37] atrial septal aneurysm, and patent foramen ovale.[18,42,43] It is in patients without clinical heart disease, who tend to be young, that TEE has been most useful in identifying these potential sources of embolism. Transesophageal echo findings in stroke patients without clinically apparent cardiac disease include PFO, ASA, MVP, aortic plaques, valvular strands, and isolated atrial appendage thrombi. Specific case-control

---

*Normal TTE was defined as follows: normal LV systolic function without left ventricular hypertrophy, no prosthetic valve, no significant native valve disease, left atrium <40 mm, no vegetations or thrombi.[21]

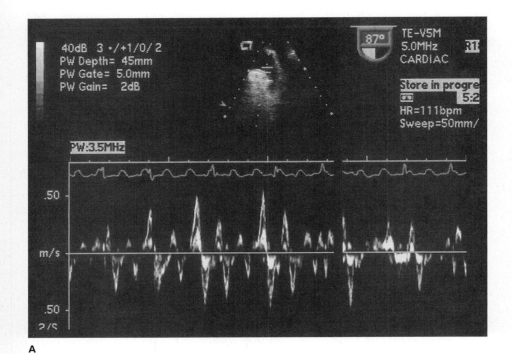

A

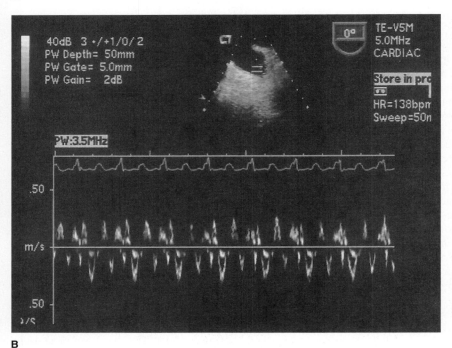

B

Figure 37-4.
A *pulsed Doppler of the left atrial appendage in a patient with atrial fibrillation and no atrial appendage thrombus; velocities vary from 0.25 to 0.50 m/s. (See also color insert 34.) B atrial fibrillation with atrial appendage flow velocities less than 0.25 m/s in patient with left atrial appendage thrombus. (See also color insert 35.)*

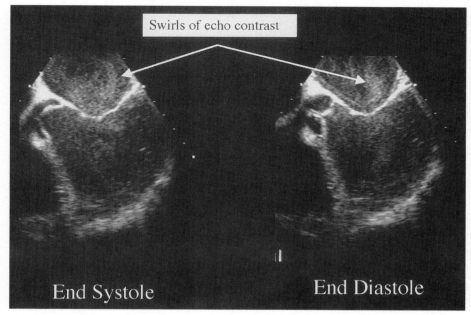

Figure 37-5.
Dilated left ventricle with poor ejection fraction and dense spontaneous echo contrast.

studies have been done to evaluate the relationship of these abnormalities to stroke.

Isolated Atrial Appendage Thrombi   Some studies report the presence of isolated left appendage echodensities.[7,16,19,21,41] It must be kept in mind that overdiagnosis of left atrial appendage thrombus may occur because of the confusion occasionally caused by pectinate muscles or by the promontory between the appendage and the left upper pulmonary vein. The interobserver variability for the diagnosis of LAA "masses" is greatest for structures <15 mm.[44] The only plausible mechanism for definite isolated atrial thrombus is a recent bout of initially undetected, spontaneously remitting atrial fibrillation. Twenty-four-hour electrocardiographic monitoring has detected AF in 3 to 11 percent of stroke patients.[45–48] Further evidence that LAAT requires an underlying substrate of heart disease comes from a study of 824 patients with stroke and TIA.[20] TEE detected LAT (predominantly LAAT) in 7 percent of 588 patients with abnormal TTE* and in none of 236 patients with sinus rhythm and normal TTE.

Abnormalities of the Interatrial Septum: Patent Foramen Ovale and Atria Septal Aneurysm   Autopsy series have shown the foramen ovale to be at patent in 14 to 35 percent of cases studied (Fig. 37-6).[49–51] Foramen size was reported varying from 1 to 10 mm in most cases. Early case descriptions of paradoxical embolism were typically postmortem and emphasized the presence of venous thrombosis.[50] A presumptive clinical diagnosis of paradoxical embolism can be made when the following are present: (1) venous thrombosis; (2) pulmonary hypertension; (3) arterial embolism without apparent left-sided source; and (4) right-to-left shunt (intracardiac or pulmonary arteriovenous malformation).[52] The potential for transient elevation of right heart pressure with the Valsalva maneuver has been emphasized.[53] TEE has allowed antemortem documentation of thrombi traversing or trapped in patent foramina (Fig. 37-7).[54–59] Diagnosing paradoxical embolism is problematic for patients without evidence of venous thrombosis or elevated right atrial pressures. Several echocardiographic case-control studies have assessed the associa-

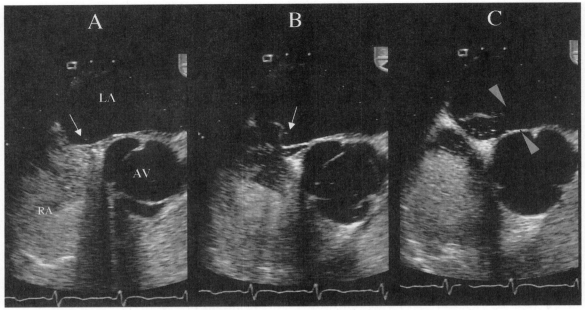

Figure 37-6.

Forty-year-old man with a cerebral embolism. Frames A, B, and C are from a single injection of agitated saline. A and B are during normal respiration; note small shunt (arrow). C is during Valsalva, which markedly increases the right to left shunt. Note increased separation of ostium primum from the secundum (arrowheads).

tion between cerebral ischemia and the presence and/or size of PFO (Table 37-2).

The initial case-control studies that examined the association between PFO and cerebral ischemia used transthoracic echocardiography and saline contrast injections. In young stroke patients without clinical heart disease PFO was found in 40 to 50 percent compared with 10 to 15 percent of controls.[60,61] When patients with cryptogenic stroke were considered separately, the prevalence of PFO was even higher. Although 18 percent of patients referred to an echo lab for stroke evaluation had PFO, patients with cryptogenic stroke had a higher prevalence of PFO compared with patients with a known cause of stroke (42 percent vs. 7 percent).[62] In this series, PFO was found to be independently associated with cryptogenic stroke, whereas hypertension was inversely related. However, PFO was not more frequent for patients older or younger than 55 years of age. This has been confirmed by both autopsy studies and subsequently performed investigations using TEE.[47,63,64]

Transesophageal studies of relatively unselected patients have shown PFO to be present in 5 to 23 percent

of patients.[18,20,21,64,65] Studies focusing on cryptogenic stroke have confirmed a significantly higher prevalence of PFO in cryptogenic stroke patients compared with controls and patients with known cause of stroke.[66–69] PFO may be present in as many as 66 to 78 percent of patients with cryptogenic stroke.[68,69] Varying detection rates may in part be related to contrast injection technique and type of contrast used. The failure to mix air with saline will lead to a less echogenic injectate. Use of specially formulated echo contrast may be more sensitive in detecting right-to-left shunts, although comparisons with properly done saline contrast are lacking.[68] Prompt and complete opacification of the right atrium is aided by the use of a large-bore intravenous needle, which facilitates rapid injection. As TEE is usually performed in the left lateral decubitus position (with left arm dependent), contrast injected via the left arm will result in less opacification than contrast injected via the right arm, which can be elevated and massaged. Finally, heavily sedated patients may not be able to perform a satisfactory Valsalva maneuver, which may lead to a lower detection rate. Several of these mechanisms may

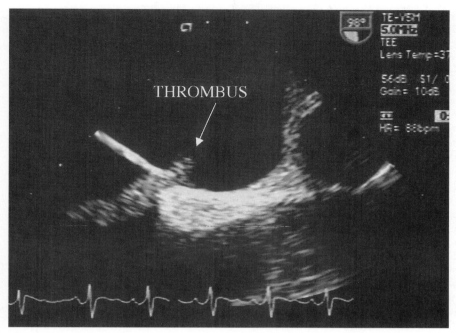

Figure 37-7.
Patent foramen ovale: thrombus-in-transit.

Table 37-2.
Published case-control studies

Author	Size	Entry criteria	Age (mean)	Technique	Control	All stroke	Cryptogenic	Known cause
Lechat[60]	60	Age <55	38.9	TTE	10	40	54	21
Webster[61]	40	Age 40	31.6	TTE	15	50	56	
DiTullio[62]	146	Consecutive echo referrals	61.8	TTE		18	42	7
Homma[66]	74	Consecutive echo referrals	46.7[a] 62.9[b]	TEE		31	44	18
Klotsch[68]	111	Consecutive stroke	58.9	TEE			71.5	27
Chen[67]	34	Age <55	39	TEE	18	44		
Ditullio[79]	49	Cryptogenic	63.6	TEE			39	
Ranoux[74]	68	Consecutive stroke, age <55		TEE		47		
Job[69]	137		36	TEE	43		66	33
Laussane[75]		Consecutive stroke, age <60				41		

[a]Cryptogenic stroke.
[b]Known cause of stroke.

have been operative in a retrospective review of 1000 patients having TEE for a variety of indications.[64] In this study PFO was not more frequent in stroke versus nonstroke patients, but the overall incidence (9.2 percent) was lower than has been reported at autopsy and in other large trials. Indeed, one would not expect PFO to be more prevalent in the general stroke population than in patients undergoing TEE for other reasons.

Studies in which the size of PFO and the degree of right-to-left shunt were measured suggest that it is the larger defects that are associated with stroke. By TTE, severe shunting (>20 micro bubbles) was detected only in young stroke patients and in no controls. Small shunts (1 to 5 micro bubbles) were distributed equally between patients and controls.[61] Using biplane TEE, the amount of shunt was greater for patients with cryptogenic stroke (who were also younger) compared with patients with other causes (13.9 vs. 1.6 micro bubbles).[66] A monoplane TEE study showed that large shunts (>20 micro bubbles) were more common in stroke patients (21 percent) than in controls undergoing TEE for other reasons (0 percent). Severe shunting was more prevalent in stroke patients younger than 45 years of age (80 percent) than in patients older than 45 (8 percent).[70] Shunt severity as measured by the percentage of left atrial area occupied by bubbles is greater for patients with strong evidence for paradoxical embolism compared with other patients with unexplained ischemia and patients with no events at all.[71] Separation of the ostium primum from the secundum is greater in stroke patients than in controls. In cryptogenic stroke patients it has been measured to be 2.1 ± 1.7 mm compared with 0.57 ± 0.78 mm for patients with known cause of stroke.[66] Other investigators have found that the opening of the PFO may be as large as 7.1 ± 3.6 mm in patients with likely paradoxical embolism compared with patients without ischemic events, in whom the PFO was measured as 3.0 ± 2.0 mm.[71] Patients with large shunts (>20 micro bubbles) are also less likely to have other potential sources of embolism compared with patients with small shunts (25 percent vs. 50 percent).[72] Brain imaging suggestive of embolism is found significantly more often in patients with medium and large PFOs (separation of septum primum from secundum >2.0 mm) than in patients with small PFOs (separation <2 mm).[73]

Paradoxical embolism is presumed to originate from either the deep veins of the legs or the pelvic veins. Most studies evaluating the role of PFO in stroke have not systematically evaluated the venous system for a source of thrombus. Using duplex sonography or venog-raphy, deep venous thrombosis has been estimated to be present in 0 to 15 percent of cases.[68,74–76] In a series of 42 patients with systemic embolism and PFO bilateral venography was abnormal in 24 patients.[77] Of the 17 patients who had venography performed within 1 week before or after the embolic event, 15 (without another cause of ischemia) had abnormal venograms. Clearly, some patients were admitted with clinically suspected deep venous thrombosis and had their systemic embolism while under observation. In a study of 227 patients with stroke or TIA, 56 were found to have a PFO.[78] Fifty-three of these patients underwent bilateral venography within 8 ± 3 days after the presenting event. Fresh venous thrombosis was found in 5 of 53 patients (9.5 percent) undergoing venography. Because all patients were treated with intravenous heparin before venography, it is unlikely that these thrombi developed as a result of hospitalization. It is conceivable that small (1 to 2 mm) venous thrombi may go undetected by all imaging techniques of the lower extremities and deep pelvic veins. Although the lung may be able to filter small emboli without sequelae, entry into the arterial system could cause clinically detectable cerebral ischemia. Furthermore, this study did not focus on cryptogenic stroke. As may be the case for atrial appendage thrombi, small deep venous thrombi may not be detectable after embolization. Besides searching for a source of embolism, several investigators have explored a possible mechanism for right-to-left shunting in the setting of normal pulmonary pressure. The detection of PFO is clearly aided by use of the Valsalva maneuver, which causes a marked, although transient, increase in right heart pressures. Unfortunately, TEE studies of PFO have not been able to show a difference in the occurrence of a Valsalva strain just before cerebral ischemia in cryptogenic stroke populations compared with patients with a known cause of stroke.[74,75] The increase in heart rate and blood pressure (increased shear forces) that occur with release of strain may be a mechanism for embolization of left-sided thrombi. Although recall of an activity that produces a Valsalva maneuver may be impaired in a stroke patient, it should not be different for patients with cryptogenic versus known cause of stroke.

Large stroke series using both TEE and TTE have consistently shown the former to be superior in the detection of PFO. Using TEE as the gold standard, studies directly comparing the two techniques have found TTE to have a sensitivity of about 44 to 47 percent.[68,79] TTE was shown in one study to detect 86 percent of large interatrial shunts identified by TEE, al-

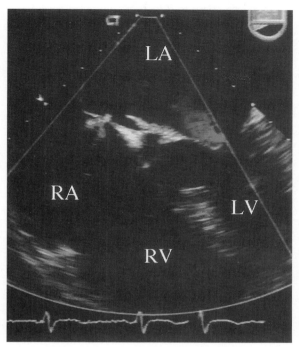

Figure 37-8.
Color flow jet across the interatrial septum demonstrating the presence of a patent foramen ovale. (See also color insert 36.)

though the authors did not have a preset definition of shunt severity.[71] Transcranial Doppler (TCD) has also been evaluated for its ability to detect PFO in stroke patients using TEE as a gold standard. TCD detected 68 to 96 percent of PFOs identified by TEE.[68,79] TCD tends to miss only small shunts that are probably of no clinical relevance. Color Doppler can also be used in conjunction with TTE and TEE to evaluate the interatrial septum (Fig. 37-8, color insert 36).[80] Its sensitivity compared with TEE contrast is variable and definition dependent. Furthermore, quantification of the right-to-left shunt, which appears to be prognostically important, cannot be done with color Doppler.

Atrial septal aneurysm (Fig. 37-9) and PFO are closely related, as shown by both autopsy and echocardiographic studies. Autopsy studies have found an ASA prevalence of 1 percent associated with probe patency of the foramen in 50 percent of subjects.[81] ASA is characterized by a severely redundant interatrial septum that may have tiny tags of fibrin or thrombus, causing there to be a roughened appearance on the convex side and a thrombus in the pit of the aneurysm on the concave side. It is diagnosed when there is a hypermobile atrial septum with a base of at least 15 mm and total excursion of at least 11 mm. A classification scheme has been suggested by Hanley et al and modified by Pearson et al (Table 37-3).[82,83]

Figure 37-9.
Excursion of interatrial septum from right atrial to left atrial in a patient with a patent foramen ovale (see Figure 37-8).

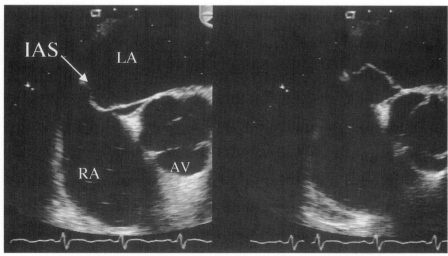

Table 37-3.
Morphologic classification of atrial septal aneurysms

Type IA	Continual protrusion into the right atrium
Type IB	Predominant protrusion into the right atrium with phasic excursion into the left atrium
Type IC	Similar to type IB aneurysm but with left atrial excursion on every beat
Type II	Continual protrusion into the left atrium

After Hanley[82] and Pearson.[83]

Diagnosis of ASA by TTE has been made in 0.5 percent of patients; 90 percent were associated with interatrial shunting.[43] In a retrospective analysis of TTE and TEE, ASA was found in 20 of 12,137 patients by TTE (0.16 percent), whereas ASA was seen in 3 percent of 765 patients by TEE.[42] Interatrial shunts were found in 41 percent of 17 patients by TTE and in 77 percent by TEE. Atrial fenestrations and thrombus were exclusively visualized by TEE. Similar results have been reported by other investigators.[84] In a monoplane TEE study of patients with unexplained cerebral ischemia, ASA was found in 15 percent of stroke patients referred for echo to rule out an embolism and in 4 percent of patients without cerebral ischemia.[83] TTE detected only 37.5 percent of the aneurysms. Interatrial shunting was found in 70 percent of stroke patients with ASA and in 75 percent of nonstroke patients with ASA. Using a liberal definition of ASA (>6 mm excursion), a young cohort of patients was examined by monoplane TEE.[85] ASA and PFO were present more frequently in patients with cryptogenic (39.1 percent) than with known cause of stroke (8.3 percent) and controls (8 percent). Corroborating other studies, there was a high prevalence of interatrial shunting in stroke patients with ASA (72 percent) versus stroke patients and controls without it (24.6 percent). Using stepwise logistic regression, PFO and ASA were both significantly associated with stroke (the relationship was even stronger for cryptogenic stroke). The strongest association, however, was for the combination of PFO and ASA. Atrial septal excursion <10 mm was not associated with stroke. In patients with PFO and unexplained stroke, morphological abnormalities (two or more of the following: hypermobility, discontinuity, distension with bulging <15 mm, duplication of the foramen) were present in 69 percent of patients with significant early shunting compared with 2 percent of patients with late shunting.[70] Other work suggests that aneurysm length, extent of bulging, and frequency of spontaneous oscillations are not associated with stroke.[84]

Interatrial Abnormalities and the Risk of Stroke Recurrence   Several investigators have evaluated the risk of recurrent stroke associated with interatrial septal abnormalities. In a small cohort of 51 patients, follow-up was available at 59 ± 12 months. Treatment was not randomized and was divided among surgical closure (3 patients), warfarin (31 patients), and aspirin (17 patients). Three patients (7 percent) had recurrent embolic events. Two of the recurrences were TIAs; one patient was on aspirin and the other was on warfarin, although the international normalized ratio (INR) at the time of recurrence was not reported. The third event was a stroke in a patient receiving aspirin.[71] In another small cohort of patients whose PFOs were detected by TEE, recurrent events occurred in 5 of 16 patients with a large shunt (average of 51 ± 29 micro bubbles; mean follow-up, 22 ± 14 months) and in none of the patients with a small shunt (7 ± 4 micro bubbles; mean follow-up, 19 ± 13 months). Three of the five patients with subsequent TIA or stroke were on warfarin and two were on aspirin; INRs at the time of the events were not reported. Only one of these patients had an alternative cause of stroke.[72]

The Laussane group evaluated 340 patients with TIA or stroke and age younger than 60 years. Forty-one percent of the patients had PFO and were followed for a mean of 36 months. Sixteen percent had an alternative cause of stroke. Treatment (aspirin, 66 percent; oral anticoagulation, 26 percent; and surgical closure, 8 percent), was not randomized but was selected according to preset criteria. Surgical closure was performed for patients without an alternative cause of stroke and two of the following: (1) ASA; (2) major right-to-left shunt (>50 micro bubbles); (3) multiple cerebral infarcts; (4) multiple clinical events; and (5) Valsalva maneuver preceding the neurologic event. Warfarin was administered to patients who were surgical candidates who declined operation and to patients without an alternative cause of stroke and only one of the above listed factors. Aspirin was given to all other patients unless an alternative cause of stroke mandated another treatment. Patients with deep venous thrombosis or pulmonary embolism received 3 months of oral anticoagulation before aspirin therapy. After a mean follow-up of 36 months, the risk of recurrent brain infarct was 1.9 percent per year. Multivariate analysis identified PFO, coexisting cause of stroke, recent migraine, and posterior circulation infarct as independent predictors of recurrence. Two or more of these factors increased the risk of recurrence to 50 percent.[75] How the latter three would predict the recurrent stroke from PFO is not clear, especially as 16 percent of patients had competing causes for stroke.

Recurrence rates in 132 patients with PFO (52.3 percent), ASA (18.9 percent), or both (28.8 percent) detected by TEE and in whom no other cause of stroke was found were analyzed retrospectively.[86] The actuarial risk of recurrent stroke was 2.3 percent at 2 years, whereas the risk of recurrent stroke and TIA was 6.7 percent at 2 years. Using a proportional-hazards model only two variables were independently associated with recurrent cerebral ischemia: systemic hypertension and the combination of PFO and ASA. For patients with both interatrial abnormalities, the actuarial risk of recurrence at 2 years was 9.0 percent for stroke and 22.0 percent for stroke and TIA. Therapy was not controlled but all first recurrent events occurred in patients who were either taking aspirin or not on therapy at all.

The Laussane group continued to explore surgical closure of PFO for patients without an alternative cause of stroke who met the criteria given above.[87,88] Thirty-two patients underwent surgery without significant complication and were then followed for a mean of 18.8 months. No patient had recurrent clinical or radiographic neurologic events. Medical therapy during follow-up was neither mandated by protocol nor mentioned by the authors.

The results of surgical closure of PFO were reported for 28 patients with cryptogenic stroke and no other potential causes. The indications for operation were refusal to take warfarin (23 patients), contraindication to the use of warfarin (3 patients), inability to maintain a therapeutic protime (1 patient), and stroke recurrence on warfarin therapy. There were no significant surgical complications. Patients were followed for a mean of 19 months (range, 1 to 52 months). Eleven patients received aspirin at the discretion of the referring physician and 17 received no medical therapy for stroke prevention. Three patients experienced recurrent TIA and one patient had a recurrent stroke. Of interest is that none of the 17 patients younger than 45 years of age experienced a recurrence, whereas 3 of the 11 patients older than 60 years had a recurrence. The fourth recurrent event was TIA in a 45-year-old man with left posterior circulation ischemia. Factors such as PFO size and associated ASA were not different between patients with and without recurrence.[89]

Other investigators have evaluated the possibility of transcatheter closure of PFOs. A "double umbrella" device was used to close PFOs in 36 patients with cryptogenic stroke or TIA and presumed paradoxical embo-

lism. There were no recurrent events after a mean follow-up of 8.4 months.[90] Subsequent device failures have led to a modification of the device, which is now under investigation. Atrial septal defects and PFOs have also been closed successfully with other devices, but to date the Food and Drug Administration has not approved any of them for clinical use.[91–94]

The mechanism of embolization from ASA has been debated. Certainly, the strong association of ASA with PFO implicates paradoxical embolism.[43,83] Autopsy and TEE have documented the presence of thrombus and fibrin tags in the aneurysm, suggesting another mechanism for embolization.[81,83,84] Although ASA can be detected with TTE, the superior imaging quality and unique spatial vantage point of TEE make it the procedure of choice for detection and morphologic definition. Although large and clinically relevant PFOs can be detected with TTE, transesophageal imaging offers improved sensitivity and may be more cost effective.[95]

The Aorta As a Source of Emboli It has long been recognized that cerebral or peripheral embolism may result from atherosclerotic disease of the aorta (Figs. 37-10 and 37-11).[96] Thrombi, fibrinous material, and cholesterol crystals may dislodge from a complex, ulcerated atherosclerotic plaque, or atheroma in the ascending or transverse aorta. This may lead to TIA, stroke, or retinal artery embolism, whereas involvement of the descending aorta has been associated with gastrointestinal embolism, renal failure, and acute lower extremity ischemia, including the blue toe syndrome.[97] Embolization may be spontaneous or provoked by disturbance of the aorta during catheterization or cardiac surgery.[98]

After protruding, freely mobile plaques in the aortic arch and descending aorta were reported in three patients with cerebral and/or systemic embolism, TEE was recognized for its potential to image the aorta in pursuit of an embolic cause of stroke.[97] Although smooth aortic plaques would not be expected to be a source of embolization, aortic ulcerations were postulated to be emboligenic. This was investigated by autopsy of 500 consecutive patients with neurologic disease.[40] The prevalence of aortic ulcerations adjusted for the presence of cerebrovascular disease was 16.9 percent in stroke patients versus 5.1 percent of controls. Patients for whom no cause of stroke was otherwise found had an adjusted prevalence of 58 percent compared with 20 percent for patients with a known cause of stroke. Ulcerations were present in 1 percent of patients younger than age 60, in 31 percent older than age 60, and in 36 percent older than age 80. They were generally found

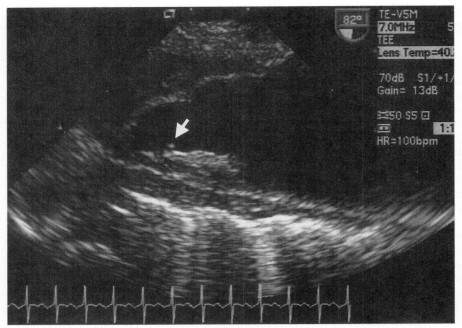

Figure 37-10.
Six-mm plaque in aortic arch near junction with descending aorta. Arrow indicates mobile component. Two-dimensional transthoracic echocardiography showed no other cardiac source of embolism (see Figure 37-11).

near the origins of the cerebral vessels. Eighty-one percent of patients had ulcerations in the arch, whereas only 44 percent had them in the ascending aorta. Ninety-four percent involved the superior wall of the arch (which is not completely imaged by TEE) and 38 percent involved the caudal wall. Of particular interest is that there was no correlation to the presence or absence of carotid stenosis > 75 percent.

Transesophageal echocardiography has been used to further describe plaque morphology. Aortic plaques are described as simple or complex. The former are smooth and tend to protrude into the lumen less than 4 to 5 mm. Complex plaques have an irregular appearance, may have ulceration or mobile debris (clot or atheroma), and/or have a thickness > 4 to 5 mm. Several case-control TEE studies demonstrated protruding plaques in 17 to 31 percent of stroke patients and 3 to 4 percent of controls.[96,98–101] Mobile components are extremely rare in control patients.[102] Protruding atheromas appear to be independent predictors of embolic events even after control for hypertension and diabetes.[99] Patients with cryptogenic stroke (mean age in the 60s) are not more likely than controls to have protuding plaque but do seem to have a higher frequency of ulcerations.[101,102] As one would expect for an older population, atrial fibrillation and carotid stenosis (>60 percent diameter reduction) are also strongly predictive of stroke.[101] Unless there are mobile atheromas/thrombi, assigning causation may be difficult for patients with other potential sources of embolism.

The French Aortic Plaque Study is remarkable for its size, data set, and follow-up.[103] It systematically assessed plaque thickness in 250 stroke patients and 250 control subjects undergoing TEE for other clinically indicated reasons (mean ages, 76 and 73 years, respectively). Plaques of 1.0 to 3.9 mm thickness were found in 46 percent of patients and 22 percent of controls. Patients with plaques measuring <1.0 mm were assigned an odds ratio (OR) of 1.0 for risk of cerebral infarction. In comparison, patients with plaques measuring 1.0 to 3.9 mm had an OR for the risk of cerebral infarction of 4.4 ($p < .001$; adjusted for age, gender, and other stroke risk factors). Plaques >3.9 mm were associated with a higher frequency of hypercholesterolemia and

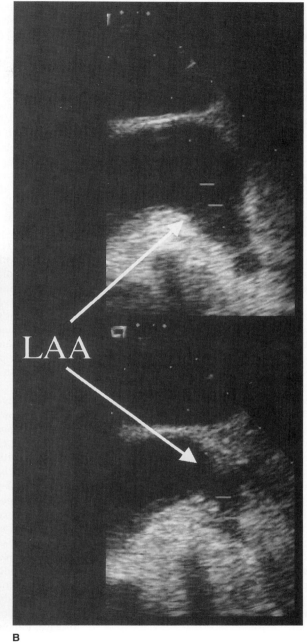

Figure 37-11.
Atrial appendage ejection velocity (arrow) *is 0.5 m/s in normal sinus rhythm* (A). *Appendage ejection fraction is excellent and LV size and function are normal. Top image shows diastole; bottom shows systole* (B). *Saline contrast echo is negative for patent foramen ovale. The aortic arch had significant plaque with mobile components (see Figure 37-10).*

smoking and less atrial fibrillation. Such plaques were present in 14.4 percent of patients and only 2 percent of controls, yielding an even higher adjusted odds ratio for risk of stroke of 9.1 ($p < .001$). The mean plaque thickness in this group of patients was 5.8 mm. Twenty-eight percent of patients without another likely cause of stroke had plaques >3.9 mm compared with 5.4 percent of patients with a known cause, 11.1 percent of patients with another possible cause, and 9.1 percent of patients with lacunar infarcts. The adjusted odds ratio for stroke associated with plaque <4.0 mm was 4.7 for the 78 patients with no known cause of stroke compared with the 172 patients with likely, possible, or lacunar causes.

One might be concerned that protruding aortic plaques detected by TEE would simply be markers for generalized atherosclerosis and would indicate patients with an overall higher risk of stroke. If this were the case there should be a strong correlation between the presence of protruding aortic atheroma and carotid stenosis. A very small study using multiplane TEE showed that 39 percent of patients with cryptogenic stroke had ulcerated aortic plaques compared with 8 percent of patients with known cause of stroke ($p < .001$).[102] Despite this difference, the severity of carotid disease was similar in the two groups. In the French Aortic Plaque Study, the prevalence of plaques measuring 1.0 to 3.9 mm was directly correlated with the severity of carotid stenosis. Plaques >4 mm were present with equal prevalence at all grades of carotid stenosis.[103] Other workers have shown that despite a strong association between the severity of aortic atheromas and carotid stenosis, the former maintained a strong independent association with stroke on multivariate analysis.[101]

Although one would expect to find mobile intra-aortic debris in patients with aortic atheromas of 4 mm or greater, mobile thrombi are rarely found in the aortic arch of younger patients. In a review of 27,855 TEE scans at 15 academic cardiology centers in France, 23 patients (mean age, 45 $\pm$ 8.4 years) had mobile thrombi attached to a small atherosclerotic plaque (<4 mm).[104] This study supports the need to assiduously evaluate the aorta in all patients with embolic stroke when the cause is not readily apparent from other clinical information.

Future Risk of Stroke in Patients with Aortic Atheromas   The risk of future embolization is higher for patients with protruding atheromas compared with controls matched for age, gender, and hypertension (mean follow-up, 13 months).[105] Thirty-three percent of cases

(37.6 events per 100 person-years) had an embolic event compared with 6 percent for controls (5.9 per 100 person-years) ($p < .003$). Of 14 patients with protruding atheroma and no prior embolism, 43 percent had events during follow-up. Even after controlling for age, gender, coronary artery disease, hypertension, smoking history, atrial fibrillation, and antithrombotic drug use, protruding atheromas independently predicted future events with an OR of 4.6 ($p = .01$). There was no significant correlation to any other variables.

In the larger French Aortic Plaque Study, recurrent embolism was predicted by plaque thickness ≥ 4 mm (11.9 per 100 person-years vs. 3.5 and 2.8 for patients with plaque thickness 1.0 to 3.9 mm and >1.0 mm, respectively; $p < .001$ for the three different Kaplan-Meier curves).[106] Furthermore, any vascular event was also strongly predicted by plaque thickness >4.0 mm (26.0 per 100 person-years vs. 9.1 and 5.9, respectively; $p < .001$). Although plaque thickness ≥ 4.0 mm would appear to indicate more severe generalized atherosclerosis, it continued to predict an increased risk of recurrent stroke even after controlling for atrial fibrillation, carotid stenosis, peripheral vascular disease (PVD), type of therapy, and other confounding factors. Similar results were found in the patients with cryptogenic stroke. The authors point out that these rates of events are higher than in atrial fibrillation and carotid endarterectomy trials.

Patients with severe atheroma identified by TEE were followed prospectively for a mean duration of 16 months.[107] Those with plaque ≥ 5.0 mm or mobile components had 13.7 vascular events per 100 person-years compared with 4.1 for patients with plaques <5 mm. Prior events had occurred in 70 percent of the severe group and 52 percent of the others. Independent predictors of embolic events were complex plaques in the aortic arch, coronary artery disease, and history of prior embolism.

In stroke patients with aortic plaque ≥ 4.0 mm, ulcerations had no independent predictive value for future events, although absence of calcification seemed to markedly increase the risk.[108] It has been postulated that a noncalcified plaque may be softer and more prone to rupture, analogous to the situation in coronary artery disease. Patients with morphologic abnormalities tend to be older and have a higher prevalence of peripheral vascular disease than patients without abnormalities. Those patients with plaque thickness >4.0 mm were more frequently smokers, but otherwise there were no differences in the distribution of atherosclerotic risk factors in patients with and without morphologic abnormalities. Although rarely detected even in stroke patients, mobile aortic debris (thrombus or atherosclerotic plaque) tends to be found only in patients with embolic events.

Randomized trials to establish the optimal treatment for stroke patients with aortic atheroma have not been done. A prospective, observational follow-up of 31 patients with systemic embolism and mobile aortic atheroma revealed that plaque mobility and not dimension predicted recurrent stroke. Patients receiving warfarin had a much lower incidence of recurrence (5 percent vs. 45 percent, $p = .006$). Forty-seven percent of patients with small, mobile plaque were not treated with warfarin and the recurrence rate was 38 percent.[109] In a more recent study in which treatment was also left to the treating physicians, future events were more likely the more severe the aortic atheroma and were highest for patients with mobile debris. Patients with plaques ≥ 4 mm thick had a relative risk of stroke of 5.9 when treated with antiplatelet therapy compared with oral anticoagulants. When aortic debris was considered, patients treated with aspirin had a relative risk of 7.1 compared with those who received oral anticoagulants.[110]

Mitral Valve and Stroke

Mitral Valve Prolapse (Fig. 37-12)   MVP has been associated with the occurrence of cerebral embolism. Classically, in MVP the leaflets appear to be thickened and irregular. Pathologic findings include collagen degeneration and regions of endothelial disruption, which may promote thrombus formation.[111,112] Thrombi attached to myxomatous leaflets have been reported by echocardiography.[113,114] Early m-mode studies suggested that MVP was present in 20 to 61 percent of young patients with unexplained cerebral ischemia compared with 6 to 8 percent of control subjects.[115] Subsequent TTE studies found MVP in 24 to 34 percent of young patients with unexplained cerebral ischemia.[116,117] Studies comparing TEE and TTE in consecutive stroke patients with an average age of 60 years reported MVP in 2 to 8 percent of patients[18,21,22,37,65]; the prevalence was 9 to 11 percent for patients younger than 60 years.[8,66] Detection of MVP by TEE was only slightly better than with TTE. Both TTE and TEE have shown that patients with cerebral ischemia and MVP tend to have diffusely thickened valves.[118,119] Abnormalities of leaflet motion and morphology are more frequently detected by TEE.[120]

Using updated diagnostic criteria the prevalence of MVP and PFO was evaluated in a series of young

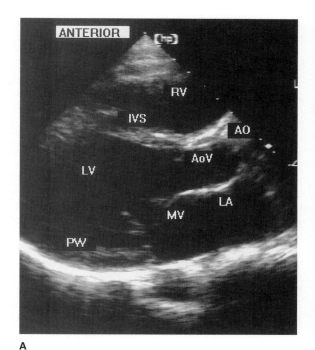

A

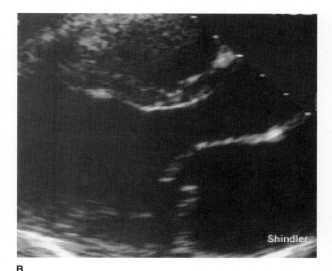

B

Figure 37-12.
A   *anterior leaflet prolapse. (Courtesy of University of Kansas Medical Center, www.kumc.edu.)* B   *posterior mitral leaflet prolapse. (Courtesy of Daniel Shindler, M.D., www2.umdnj. edu.)*

patients with stroke.[60,121] The prevalence of MVP in young patients with unexplained cerebral ischemia was 22 percent compared with 4 percent of controls. Eighteen percent of PFO patients had MVP compared with 6 percent of patients without PFO. Controlling for the presence of PFO, MVP lost its association with cerebral ischemia. Conversely, controlling for MVP did not weaken the association of PFO and ischemia. A re-evaluation of 18 patients (younger than 45 years) with stroke and MVP on echocardiography was performed 3 to 7 years after the initial event to determine the prevalence of PFO. Of 11 patients available for contrast TTE and/or TEE, 9 were found to have PFO. Four were reclassified as not having MVP.[122] PFO but not MVP was found to be more prevalent in patients without a traditional embolic source.[123]

A case-control study of 213 consecutive patients 45 years of age or younger with ischemic stroke or TIA used rigorous echocardiographic criteria to diagnose MVP, which was found in 1.9 percent of subjects and 2.8 percent of controls. Such results would appear to refute any previously established association between cerebral ischemia and MVP. Unfortunately, this study included 142 patients with other, less controversial potential sources of embolism (93 with carotid or vertebral disease and 49 with another potential cardiac source of embolism). This study would have been more useful had it been done on patients with cryptogenic stroke.[123a]

In summary, MVP may be detected with increased frequency in highly selected very young patients with cerebral ischemia compared with healthy volunteers. A strong association between PFO and lax diagnostic criteria (early studies) confounds its etiologic role except in rare cases in which thrombus is seen attached to myxomatous leaflets and there is no other potential cause of stroke evident. Although clinical examination and TTE can generally make the diagnosis of MVP, TEE is slightly better than TTE for the evaluation of leaflet morphology and motion and for the presence and severity of mitral regurgitation.

Strands (Fig. 37-13) "Fine, threadlike" echodensities seen on TEE were first reported in 1991.[17] They were detected on the atrial surface of the mitral valve and the ventricular surface of the aortic valve in 11 of 50 patients with stroke or TIA who had essentially normal TTE. Pathologic evaluation of strands obtained from the native valve of 1 patient who underwent mitral valve replacement revealed Lambl's excrescences (filiform valve excrescences with a core of either collagen, elastic fibers, or acellular hyaline material covered by endothelium). Case-control studies have been used to evaluate whether or not strands are associated with cerebral ischemia.

The frequency of strands in 1559 patients undergoing TEE (biplane or multiplane) for a variety of reasons (suspected embolism, 38 percent, nonstroke, 62 percent) was found to be 5.5 percent (86 patients).[124] Within this group, 41 patients had strands and no other source of embolism. They were more likely than an age- and gender-matched control group without strands to have had emboli (83 percent vs. 29 percent, OR = 10.0, $p = .00001$). Mitral strands were apparent in 2.3 percent of 968 native mitral valves studied with clinically indicated TEE.[125] The rate was 6.3 percent for patients undergoing TEE evaluation of cerebral ischemia and 0.3 percent for patients being studied for other indications. Sixteen percent of patients younger than 50 years of age with likely cardioembolic stroke or TIA were found to have strands; in 9 percent of patients there were no other causes of stroke found on TEE studies that included saline contrast to rule out PFO. Strands are also detected by TEE on prosthetic valves and appear to be more frequent in patients referred for detection of a cardioembolic source versus patients having TEE to evaluate valve function.[126] They were more frequent on mitral versus aortic valves and mechanical versus bioprosthetic valves. Finally, strands were found more often in 73 patients with ischemic stroke or TIA compared with 73 control subjects undergoing TEE for other reasons (47 percent vs. 16 percent, OR = 4.4, $p = .0002$). Casting doubt on this statistic was the finding that the frequency of strands was not greater in the patients with cryptogenic versus other causes of stroke.[127]

In contrast to the retrospective data, prospective follow-up of patients with strands does not support their role as a cause of stroke. In a study of subjects younger than 60 years old in whom multiplane TEE was used in nearly half of the patients, the frequency of strands was not different in healthy volunteer controls (38 percent), patients undergoing TEE for reasons other than cerebral ischemia (47 percent), and patients with cerebral ischemia (41 percent).[128] The prevalence was similar across age ranges and was higher for mitral than for aortic valves. Twenty-four percent of the patients without cerebral ischemia underwent follow-up TEE at a mean of 31 months and were found to have no change in the appearance of the strands. There was no difference in the risk of stroke for patients with and without strands. The one patient with strands who had a stroke had other definite causes of cerebral embolism. The frequency of strands was not different in aspirin and warfarin users versus those on no therapy. Eighty-five percent of patients with strands undergoing TEE for suspected embolic stroke had other sources of embolism.

In summary, TEE can detect filiform excrescences on the atrial side of mitral valves and the ventricular side of aortic valves in patients with and without evidence of cerebral ischemia. Retrospective studies point to a higher prevalence of strands in patients being evaluated for cerebral ischemia compared with patients undergoing TEE for other reasons. However, prospective follow-up of patients with strands does not reveal an increased likelihood of cerebral ischemia over 2.5 years.

Mitral Annular Calcification Mitral annular calcification can be readily diagnosed from transthoracic m-mode and two-dimensional echocardiographic imaging even in technically difficult studies. It tends to occur in older patients who usually have other risk factors for stroke.[129,130] Apparent thrombi attached to a calcified mitral annulus have been reported by TEE.[131]

EVALUATION AND TREATMENT GUIDELINES

Diagnostic Considerations

Transesophageal echocardiography is superior to transthoracic echocardiography in the detection of definite and potential sources of embolism in the evaluation of patients with stroke and TIA. Some of the "new" findings (found by TEE but not by TTE) are of unclear benefit to the clinician and may not effect a change in decision making. For example, a patient with atrial fibrillation may be found to have spontaneous contrast echo and even a left atrial appendage thrombus. Because the majority of patients with atrial fibrillation have a clear indication for anticoagulation, the new findings have no impact on clinical decision making. Similarly, the additional finding of a small PFO, valvular strands, mitral valve prolapse, or mitral annular calcification has no bearing on the treatment of the patient with atrial fibrillation at risk for stroke. On the other hand, a patient with lone atrial fibrillation has such a low risk of stroke that anticoagulation is not recommended for the prophylaxis of stroke and TIA. The finding of another stroke cause may lead to a change in treatment strategy. Such a patient with a large PFO should receive anticoagulation or be considered for mechanical closure. A patient with dilated cardiomyopathy, markedly reduced ejection fraction, and a low likelihood of aortic thromboembolism who has a cardioembolic stroke should be anticoagulated whether or not the echocardiogram actually shows a residual thrombus.

Unfortunately, there are no prospective trials evaluating the impact of TEE, alone or in comparison with TTE, on clinical decision making or outcome for

Figure 37-13.
Mitral valve strand. (Courtesy of N. Nighoghossian et al, Course of Valvular strands in patients with stroke: Cooperative study with transesophageal echocardiography. Am Heart J 136(6): 1065–1069, 1998.)

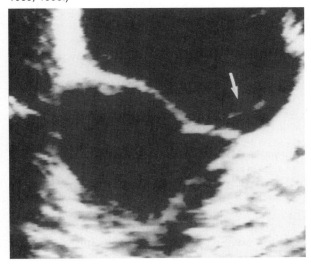

patients with suspected cardioembolic stroke. Retrospective data in limited patient subsets suggest that TEE does not have a significant impact on the management of patients with clinical heart disease.[37,41,132] Many of the patients for whom TEE is reported to have had an impact on management had atrial fibrillation.

In the absence of large, randomized trials, decision models have been employed to compare the impact of TEE and TTE on stroke outcome. The Markov decision model is useful for clinical problems with ongoing risk.[133] Hypothetical patients are allowed to transition from one state of health to another at different rates over extended periods of time. The time horizon of the analysis is divided into increments called Markov cycles. The Markovian assumption is that prior health states do not affect the prognosis of future health states. For example, a patient with a PFO is placed on anticoagulation. If the patient has a gastrointestinal hemorrhage, the prognosis then depends only on the state of bleeding and not on the fact that he or she has a PFO that requires anticoagulation. The reader is encouraged to refer to the references for a more detailed explanation of Markov models in medical decision making.

A Markov model has been used to analyze the cost-effectiveness of various echocardiographic imaging strategies in a hypothetical cohort of patients who are 65 years old, in normal sinus rhythm, and with no obvious, clinically determined cause of stroke.[95] Nine possible diagnostic strategies were analyzed for cost-effectiveness. Seven echocardiographic imaging strategies were analyzed with and without regard to cardiac history (for comparison sake, strategies of "treat-all" and "treat-none" were also analyzed). For all imaging sequences, anticoagulation was given only if thrombi were identified by echocardiography. Data were derived largely from general populations of stroke patients. Data on contrast TTE were not considered, nor were the papers on aortic plaque. Although the hypothetical cohort used for this analysis may not reflect the complexity of real-time clinical decision making (decisions to anticoagulate are frequently made without thrombus visualization), the model gives an idea of which imaging strategies may be most cost effective. The treat-none group was used as the reference (cost of recurrent events, $4740; 4.854 quality-adjusted life-years). The "selective TEE" and "all TEE" strategies cost $9000 and 13,000, respectively, relative to the treat-none group. In comparison, sequential strategies that used TTE cost $24,000 to $32,000 per quality-adjusted life-year. Strategies that used only TTE cost $36,000 to $57,000 per quality-adjusted life-year. Although the dollar amounts used for Medicare reimbursement for TEE and TTE are similar, they may not reflect actual costs, especially if conscious sedation is used. Although this paper cannot be used to guide real-time clinical decision making, it is a worthwhile exercise in our attempts to understand the impact of clinical decisions on outcome. Clearly, further study is required.

What follows is the author's recommendation for the echocardiographic evaluation and management of patients with suspected cardioembolic stroke. As with all guidelines, they do not purport to cover all clinical scenarios, and clinical judgment must prevail above all else. Although previous guidelines have used age cutoffs, disease entities do not rigidly adhere to such boundaries.[104,134,135] In our own population we have seen two patients older than 60 years whose only abnormal findings were large PFOs. Therefore, we have chosen to approach patients from the perspective of whether or not cardiovascular disease is detectable from history, physical examination, ECG, and chest radiography.

Patients with Clinical Heart Disease

Clinical heart disease is determined from history, physical examination, chest x-ray, and ECG. In patients with suspected cardioembolic stroke and clinically apparent heart disease known to be associated with stroke, the advantage of TEE over TTE is usually due to its improved ability to detect left atrial appendage thrombus, spontaneous echo contrast, and aortic atheromas. By far, these findings occur in the setting of clinically evident cardiac disease, including atrial fibrillation, mitral stenosis, prosthetic valves, dilated cardiomyopathy (ejection fraction <20 percent), large anterior infarcts with akinetic/dyskinetic segments, and risk factors for atherosclerosis.

Most patients with clinically apparent heart disease and suspected cardioembolic stroke require transthoracic echocardiography as part of the evaluation and management of their heart disease. If anticoagulation can be recommended based on clinical data and TTE, there is no need for TEE. Anticoagulant therapy would not be withheld if a thrombus were not identified. The benefit of identification by TEE of left atrial appendage thrombus, spontaneous echo contrast, patent foramen ovale, or aortic atheromas is unproven if the decision to treat with anticoagulants can be made on clinical grounds. TEE should be performed if the decision to anticoagulate is not apparent from the combination of clinically available information and TTE. In addition, TEE should be performed in the patients with recurrent stroke while on adequate anticoagulant. The result can serve as a guide to operative intervention.

Although it is beyond the scope of this chapter to review the assessment of prosthetic valve dysfunction, patients who have mechanical prostheses and minor cerebral ischemia in the absence of other correctable causes should have optimization of anticoagulant therapy. If the INR is in the target range, antiplatelet therapy can be safely added.[136] INR for mechanical aortic valves is 2.0 to 3.0; for mitral and double valves it is 3.0 to 4.0. For patients with cerebral ischemia and prosthetic valves, the benefit of TEE in the absence of clinical or TTE evidence of valve dysfunction is uncertain.

Patients without Clinical Heart Disease

Cardioembolic stroke in patients without clinically apparent heart disease may be due to patent foramen ovale, atrial septal aneurysm (usually in association with PFO), clinically silent MVP with myxomatous degeneration of the leaflets, or disease of the aortic arch. Rarely, one may find isolated LAAT secondary to undetected atrial fibrillation, thrombus attached to a heavily calcified mitral annulus, or a left atrial myxoma. PFO, ASA, and MVP are usually seen in the young stroke patient, whereas aortic ulcerations do not tend to appear until age 60, but overlap can occur. The simplest recommendation, which is supported by Markovian decision analysis as discussed above, is to perform contrast TEE on all patients. This eliminates the need for complicated algorithms.

Because TEE is more labor intensive, more uncomfortable for the patient, and may actually cost more despite similar reimbursement (Medicare) than TTE, it is of interest to explore the use of contrast TTE in patients younger than 60 years of age without atherosclerotic risk factors. The following discussion assumes an excellent acoustic window such that superior images are obtained from surface imaging. As can be seen from the earlier analysis of the literature, PFO may be present in up to 70 percent of patients with cryptogenic stroke. Up to 50 percent of all PFOs can be detected by contrast TTE. Because only large PFOs are likely to be associated with stroke, it is conceivable that an even greater percentage of clinically relevant PFOs could be detected by TTE. One study showed that 86 percent of patients identified as having large PFOs by TEE (using the author's arbitrary definition) were detected by TTE. The overall detection rate of PFO by TTE may actually be better than has been shown if current-generation echo machines are employed. Visualization of the separation

between the ostium primum and secundum can be made only by TEE, but this information is of unclear benefit and there is considerable overlap between patients with and without stroke. Thrombus-in-transit is rare and may be seen from the surface echo image. Until further data are available, patients who may be chosen for intervention with surgery or percutaneous closure should undergo TEE to rule out other causes of stroke.

Patients with risk factors for atherosclerosis are at risk for embolization of debris of thrombus from the aortic arch. These patients tend to be older than 60 years. Patients younger than 60 years with evidence of peripheral vascular disease or who have aortic calcification on chest radiography should also be considered at risk for aortic embolization.[137] As discussed previously, large studies have not demonstrated an association with PFO and stroke in this population, although isolated cases may occur. Therefore, TEE is preferable to TTE in this patient population because of its clear advantage for visualizing the aorta. Alternative imaging strategies using MRI or CT to evaluate the aorta at the time of initial brain imaging are discussed below.

Treatment of Cardioembolic Stroke in Patients without Clinical Heart Disease

Randomized treatment trials of patients with PFO have not been done. Based on the presumption that stroke related to isolated PFO is secondary to right-to-left shunting of thrombus formed in the venous system, the appropriate therapy is systemic anticoagulation. Alternative treatment is surgical closure and, pending the results of ongoing trials, percutaneous closure. Observational studies suggest that recurrences tend to occur in those patients who receive either aspirin or no treatment. The recurrence rates are low, and predicting who will have a recurrence is difficult. Risk estimates were established in patients who received nonrandomized therapy. Furthermore, the duration of anticoagulant therapy has not been established. Small, isolated PFOs, which may or may not be related to stroke, could be treated with a short course of warfarin followed by indefinite aspirin, especially if there is no evidence by history or MRI of multiple prior events. Patients with larger PFOs (>20 micro bubbles), which have a stronger association with stroke, warrant a longer duration of therapy regardless of the presence of prior events. Patients with uncomplicated initial deep venous thrombosis and pulmonary embolism are usually treated for 3 to 6 months. This analogy may not be appropriate, even for larger PFOs, if one has a zero tolerance for stroke recurrence. An alternative approach to this latter group of patients is surgical or percutaneous closure of the PFO.

Unfortunately, factors that predict stroke recurrence are not necessarily related to PFO. As discussed previously, the Laussane study showed that four independent items were associated with stroke recurrence: the presence of interatrial communication, a coexisting cause of stroke, recently active migraine headaches, and infarct in the distribution of the posterior cerebral artery. ASA was not shown to increase the risk of recurrence in this study, as it was in the French study. Complicating the prediction of recurrence is the fact that 16 percent of patients with stroke and PFO have other potential causes. The aforementioned risk factors may not actually predict the risk of recurrence from the PFO itself.

In the absence of a randomized trial, one can gain insight from Markovian decision analytic techniques.[138] When the risk of stroke recurrence was less than 0.7 percent or less, the best 5-year survival was achieved with no therapy. Above this level, treatment with anticoagulation or surgical closure of the PFO was clearly better than no therapy. Above an annual risk of recurrence of 7 percent, surgical closure prevailed over anticoagulant therapy. Risk was calculated using the four variables found to predict stroke recurrence as outlined above. Three of the four were factors not clearly related to PFO. It is not clear that one can use these factors to predict recurrent stroke from an isolated PFO. Nonetheless, surgery is attractive for selected patients because it offers closure of the atrial defect and freedom from anticoagulation and its attendant risks. In recognition of the limitation of their risk score in predicting recurrent stroke associated with PFO, the Laussane group chose selection criteria for surgical closure that were more realistic than those variables shown to predict risk in the multivariate analysis. High risk was empirically defined as the occurrence of cerebral ischemia (TIA or stroke) in a patient younger than 60 years of age, a PFO proven by contrast TEE, and no associated cause of stroke. Two or more of the following were also required: (1) Valsalva strain before stroke, (2) multiple clinical events, (3) multiple infarcts on MRI, (4) atrial septal aneurysm, and (5) large left-to-right shunt (>50 micro bubbles). The Columbia group operated only on patients unwilling or unable to take warfarin. Both series demonstrated that surgery to close a patent foramen is achievable with no mortality and minimal morbidity. The risk of recurrence in the Laussane group was zero for a follow-up period of 601 patient-months.[88] These patients would otherwise be recommended for life-long anticoagulant therapy. Recurrences in the Columbia group were largely limited to older patients. Both studies show that surgery to close a PFO is a safe alternative to anticoagulation in appropriately selected patients. Although transcatheter closure devices have not yet been approved, their availability will likely change decision making by offering a greater number of patients a nonsurgical alternative to warfarin.

Isolated atrial septal aneurysms are rarely associated with stroke. The finding by TEE of definite thrombus would warrant anticoagulation. Treatment of the patient with cerebral ischemia and isolated ASA without thrombus is unclear.

Treatment of isolated, protruding aortic has also not been evaluated by randomized trials. The available data suggest that patients with small (<4.0 mm) without mobile components should do well with aspirin in the absence of a competing etiology that compels the use of warfarin. Clearly such patients who have recurrent events on aspirin therapy can either be treated with more potent antiplatelet therapy such as clopidogrel or ticlopidine, or with oral anticoagulants. Patients in whom mobile, disrupted plaque is found should receive systemic anticoagulants and antiplatelet therapy followed by long-term oral anticoagulation. While most patients with mobile aortic debris can be successfully managed with anticoagulation, surgical excision can be considered if the mobile components are large, have a tenuous attachment, or embolize despite medical therapy.[104,135,139,140] In addition, all patients with aortic atherosclerosis require aggressive management of serum lipids, normalization of blood pressure (beta-blockers may be preferable to decrease shear forces), smoking cessation, and tight control of diabetes. New data suggesting a role for angiotensin converting enzyme inhibitors will soon be available (the HOPE trial).

Future Imaging Scenarios

Ultrafast CT, electron beam CT, and MRI have the potential to detect aortic atherosclerosis as well as intra-aortic thrombus. Preliminary work suggests that dual-helical CT has the ability to detect aortic atheroma with a sensitivity of 87 percent compared with TEE.[141] If this were done at the time of initial brain imaging, TEE expressly to evaluate the aorta would be obviated in most patients at risk for aortic atherosclerosis. In younger patients without clinical heart disease, transcranial Doppler with saline contrast (with and without Valsalva strain) would detect clinically relevant PFOs. TEE would then be reserved for the following patients: (1) those with clinical heart disease with unclear decision to anticoagulate, and (2) those with negative evaluation (or lack of availability) with noninvasive aortic imaging and TCD, (3) those in whom patent foramen ovale is documented by TCD or TTE and surgical or transcatheter closure is being considered (the latter is not yet FDA approved), and (4) those with recurrent embolization on medical therapy who are treated empirically.

Acknowledgement

The author wishes to thank Dr. Ravinder Singh for his critical editorial input and Dr. Alberta Warner who was instrumental in helping me review and digitize numerous echo tapes. All uncredited images were from our files at the VA West Los Angeles Healthcare Center.

REFERENCES

1. Cardiogenic brain embolism: The second report of the Cerebral Embolism Task Force. *Arch Neurol* 46:727, 1989.
2. Pereira SP, Hussani SH, Hanson PJV, et al: Endoscopy: Throat spray or sedation? *J R Coll Physicians London* 28:411, 1994.
3. Daniel WG, Mugge A: Transesophageal echocardiography. *N Engl J Med* 332:1268, 1995.
4. Good D, Frank S, Verhulst S, et al: Cardiac abnormalities in stroke patients with negative arteriograms. *Stroke* 17:6, 1986.
5. Sansoy V, Abott RD, Jayaweera AR, et al: Low yield of transthoracic echocardiography for cardiac source of embolism. *Am J Cardiol* 75:166, 1995.
6. Marx P, Schumacher HC, Hartmann A, et al: Diagnostic advantage by transthoracic and transesophageal echocardiography in acute ischemic infarct: A contribution to indications for transesophageal echocardiography. *Fortschr Neurol Psychiatr* 64:307, 1996.
7. Hoffmann T, Kasper W, Meinhertz T, et al: Echocardiographic evaluation of patients with clinically suspected arterial emboli. *Lancet* 336:1421, 1990.
8. Daniel WG, Mugge A, Grote J, Nonnast-Daniel B: Evaluation of endocarditis and its complications by biplane and multiplane transesophageal echocardiography. *Am J Card Imaging* 9:100, 1995.
9. Turina J, Hess OM, Turina M, Krayenbuehl HP: Cardiac bioprostheses in the 1990s. *Circulation* 88:775, 1993.
10. Petersen P, Boysen G, Godtfredsen J, et al: Placebo-controlled, randomized trial of warfarin and aspirin for prevention of thromboembolic complications in chronic atrial fibrillation: The Copenhagen AFASAK study. *Lancet* 1:175, 1989.
11. The Stroke Prevention in Atrial Fibrillation Study: Final results. *Circulation* 84:527, 1991.
12. The Boston Area Anticoagulation Trial for Atrial Fibrillation Investigators: The effect of low dose warfarin on the risk of stroke in patients with nonrheumatic atrial fibrillation. *N Engl J Med* 323:1505, 1990.
13. Ezekowitz MD, Bridgers SL, James KE, et al: VA cooperative study of warfarin in the prevention of stroke associated with nonrheumatic atrial fibrillation. *N Engl J Med* 327:1406, 1992.
14. Herzog CA, Bass D, Kane M, Asinger R: Two-dimensional echocardiographic imaging of the left atrial appendage thrombi. *J Am Coll Cardiol* 3:1340, 1984.
15. Aschenberg W, Schulter M, Kremer P, et al: Transesophageal two-dimensional echocardiography for the detection of left atrial appendage thrombus. *J Am Coll Cardiol* 7:163, 1986.
16. Pop G, Sutherland GR, Koudstaal PJ, et al: Transesophageal echocardiography in the detection of intracardiac embolic sources in patients with transient ischemic attacks. *Stroke* 21:560, 1990.
17. Lee RJ, Bartzokis T, Yeoh TK, et al: Enhanced detection of intracardiac sources of cerebral emboli by transesophageal echocardiography. *Stroke* 22:734, 1991.
18. Pearson AC, Labovitz AJ, Tatineni S, Gomez CR: Superiority of transesophageal echocardiography in detecting cardiac source of embolism in patients with cerebral ischemia of uncertain etiology. *J Am Coll Cardiol* 17:66, 1991.
19. Shyu KG, Chen JJ, Huang ZS, et al: Role of transesophageal echocardiography in the diagnostic assessment of cardiac sources of embolism in patients with acute ischemic stroke. *Cardiology* 85:53, 1994.
20. Leung DY, Black IW, Cranney GB, et al: Selection of patients for transesophageal echocardiography after stroke and systemic embolic events. *Stroke* 26:1820, 1995.
21. Comess KA, De Rook FA, Beach KW, et al: Transesophageal echocardiography and carotid ultrasound in patients with cerebral: Prevalence of findings and recurrent stroke risk. *J Am Coll Cardiol* 23:1598, 1994.
22. Jones EF, Calafiore P, Donnan GA, Tonkin AM: Transesophageal echocardiography in the investigation of stroke: Experience in 135 patients with cerebral ischemic events. *Aust NZ J Med* 23:477, 1993.
23. Klein AL, Grimm RA, Black IW, et al: Cardioversion guided by transesophageal echocardiography: The ACUTE study. A randomized, controlled trial. *Ann Intern Med* 126:200, 1997.
24. Manning WJ, Silverman DI, Gordon SPF, et al: Cardioversion from atrial fibrillation without prolonged anticoagulation with the use of transesophageal echocardiography to exclude the presence of atrial thrombi. *N Engl J Med* 328:75, 1993.
25. Stollberger C, Chnupa P, Kronik G, et al: Embolism in left atrial thrombi (ELAT study). *Wien Med Wochenschr* 147:46, 1997.

26. Tsai LM, Lin LJ, Teng JK, Chen JH: Prevalence and clinical significance of left atrial thrombus in nonrheumatic atrial fibrillation. *Int J Cardiol* 58:163, 1997.

27. Stoddard MF, Dawkins PR, Prince CR, Ammash NM: Left atrial appendage embolic event: A transesophageal echocardiographic study. *J Am Coll Cardiol* 24:452, 1995.

28. Manning WJ, Silverman DI, Keighley KS, et al: Prevalence of residual let atrial thrombi among patients with acute thromboembolism and newly recognized atrial fibrillation. *Arch Intern Med* 155:2193, 1995.

29. Rubin DN, Katz SE, Riley MF, et al: Evaluation of left atrial appendage anatomy and function in recent-onset atrial fibrillation by transesophageal echocardiography. *Am J Cardiol* 78:774, 1996.

30. Dragulescu SI, Petrescu L, Ionac A, et al: Left atrial spontaneous echo contrast as a predictor of systemic arterial embolism in rheumatic mitral valve disease: A transesophageal echocardiographic study (Abstract). *Rom J Intern Med* 34:33, 1996.

31. Mugge A, Kuhn H, Nikutta P, et al: Assessment of left atrial appendage function by biplane TEE in patient with nonrheumatic atrial fibrillation: Identification of a subgroup at increased embolic risk. *J Am Coll Cardiol* 23:599, 1994.

32. Verhorst PJ, Kamp O, Visser CA, Verheught FWA: Left atrial appendage flow velocity assessment using TEE in nonrheumatic atrial fibrillation and systemic embolism. *Am J Cardiol* 71:1922, 1993.

33. Tsai LM, Chen JH, Lin LJ, Teng JKL: Natural history of left atrial spontaneous contrast echo contrast in nonrheumatic atrial fibrillation. *Am J Cardiol* 80:897, 1997.

34. Archer SL, James KE, Kvernen RN, et al: Role of transesophageal echocardiography in the detection of left atrial thrombi in patients with chronic nonrheumatic atrial fibrillation. *Am Heart J* 130:287, 1995.

35. Daniel W, Nellessen U, Schroder E, et al: Left atrial spontaneous echo contrast in mitral valve disease: An indicator for an increased thromboembolic risk. *J Am Coll Cardiol* 11:1204, 1988.

36. Black IW, Hopkins AP, Lee LC, et al: Left atrial spontaneous echo contrast: A clinical and echocardiographic study. *J Am Coll Card* 18:398, 1991.

37. de Belder MA, Lovat LB, Tourikis L, et al: Limitations of transesophageal echocardiography in patients with focal cerebral ischemia. *Br Heart J* 67:297, 1992.

38. Mitusch R, Lange V, Stierle U, et al: Transesophageal echocardiographic determinants of embolism in nonrheumatic atrial fibrillation. *Int J Card Imaging* 11:27, 1995.

39. Peverill RE, Gelman J, Harper RW, Smolich JJ: Stability of left atrial spontaneous echo contrast at repeat transesophageal echocardiography in patients with mitral stenosis. *Am J Cardiol* 79:526, 1997.

40. Amarenco P, Duyckaerts C, Tzourio C, et al: Prevalence of ulcerated plaques in the aortic arch in patients with stroke. *N Engl J Med* 326:221, 1992.

41. Cujec B, Polasek P, Voll C, Shuaib A: Transesophageal echocardiography in the detection of potential cardiac source of embolism in stroke patients. *Stroke* 22:727, 1991.

42. Schneider B, Hanrath P, Vogel P, Meinertz T: Improved morphologic characterization of atrial septal aneurysm by transesophageal echocardiography: Relation to cerebrovascular events. *J Am Coll Cardiol* 16:1000, 1990.

43. Belkin RN, Hurwitz BJ, Kisslo J: Atrial septal aneurysm association with cerebrovascular and peripheral embolic events. *Stroke* 18:856, 1987.

44. Kronik G, Stollberger C, Schuh M, et al: Interobserver variability in the detection of spontaneous echo contrast, left atrial thrombi and left atrial appendage thrombi by transesophageal echocardiography. *Br Heart J* 74:80, 1995.

45. Hornig CR, Habaerbosch W, Lammers C, et al: Specific cardiological evaluation after focal cerebral ischemia. *Acta Neurol Scand* 93:297, 1996.

46. Richardt G, Ensle G, Schwarz F, et al: Diagnosis of cardiac causes of cerebral embolism: A contribution to 2D echocardiography and long-term ECG. *Z Kardiol* 78:598, 1989.

47. Ferrari E, Sarzotti S, Gibelin P, et al: Echocardiographie transesophagienne dans le bilan etiologique des accidents vasculaires cerebraux ischemiques. Interet chez les sujets jeunes (Abstract). *Presse Med* 23:469, 1994.

48. Corbalán R, Arriagada D, Braun S, et al: Risk factors for systemic embolism in patients with paroxysmal atrial fibrillation. *Am Heart J* 124:149, 1992.

49. Thompson T, Evans W: Paradoxical embolism. *Q J Med* 23:135, 1930.

50. Hagen PT, Scholz DG, Edwards WD: Incidence and size of patent foramen ovale during the first 10 decades of life: An autopsy study. *Mayo Clin Proc* 59:17, 1984.

51. Penther P: Patent foramen ovale: An anatomical study. Apropros of 500 consecutive autopsy studies. *Arch Mal Coeur Vaiss* 87:15, 1994.

52. Meister SG, Grossman W, Dexter L, Dalen JE: Paradoxical embolism during life. *Am J Med* 53:292, 1972.

53. Jones HR, Caplan LR, Come PC, et al: Cerebral emboli of paradoxical emboli. *Ann Neurol* 13:314, 1983.

54. Schreiter SW, Phillips JH: Thromboembolus traversing a patent foramen ovale: Resolution with anticoagulation. *J Am Soc Echocardiogr* 7:659, 1994.

55. Missault L, Trouerbach J, Vanmeerhaeghe X, et al: Trapped venous embolus in a patent foramen ovale causing recurrent paradoxical embolism. *Cardiology* 86:86, 1995.

56. Hust MH, Staiger M, Braun B: Migration of paradoxic thrombus through a patent foramen ovale diagnosed by echocardiography: Successful thrombolysis. *Am Heart J* 129:620, 1995.

57. Caes FL, Van Belleghem YV, Missault LH, et al: Surgical treatment of impending paradoxical embolism through patent foramen ovale. *Ann Thorac Surg* 59:1559, 1995.

58. Zerio C, Canterin F, Pavan D, Nicolosi GL: Spontaneous closure of a patent foramen ovale and disappearance of impending paradoxical embolism after fibrinolytic ther-

apy in the course of massive pulmonary embolism. *Am J Cardiol* 76:422, 1995.

59. Srivastava TN, Payment MF: Images in clinical medicine: Paradoxical embolism-thrombus in transit through a patent foramen ovale. *N Engl J Med* 337:681, 1997.

60. Lechat PH, Mas JL, Lascault MD, et al: Prevalence of patent foramen ovale in patients with stroke. *N Engl J Med* 318:1148, 1988.

61. Webster MW, Chancellor AM, Smith HJ, et al: Patent foramen ovale in young stroke patients. *Lancet* 2:11, 1988.

62. DiTullio M, Sacco R, Gopal A, et al: Patent foramen ovale as a risk factor for cryptogenic stroke. *Ann Intern Med* 117:461, 1992.

63. Jones EF, Calafiore P, Donnan GA, Tonkin AM, et al: Evidence that patent foramen ovale is not a risk factor for cerebral ischemia in the elderly. *Am J Cardiol* 74:596, 1994.

64. Fisher DC, Fisher EA, Budd JH, et al: The incidence of patent foramen ovale in 1000 consecutive patients: A contrast echocardiographic study. *Chest* 107:1504, 1995.

65. Labovitz AJ, Camp A, Castello R, et al: Usefulness of transesophageal echocardiography in unexplained cerebral ischemia. *Am J Cardiol* 72:1448, 1993.

66. Homma S, Di Tullio MR, Sacco RL, et al: Characteristics of patent foramen ovale associated with cryptogenic stroke. *Stroke* 25:582, 1994.

67. Chen WJ, Lin SL, Cheng JJ, Lien WP: The frequency of patent foramen ovale in patients with ischemic stroke: A transesophageal echocardiographic study. (Abstract). *J Formos Med Assoc* 90:744, 1991.

68. Klotzsch C, Janben G, Berlit P: Transesophageal echocardiography and contrast-transcranial Doppler in the detection of patent foramen ovale. *Neurology* 44:1603, 1994.

69. Job FP, Ringelstein EB, Grafen Y, et al: Comparison of transcranial contrast Doppler sonography and transesophageal contrast echocardiography for the detection of patent foramen ovale in young stroke patients. *Am J Cardiol* 74:381, 1994.

70. Van Camp G, Schulze D, Cosyns B, Vandenbossche JL: Relation between patent foramen ovale and unexplained stroke. *Am J Cardiol* 71:596, 1993.

71. Hausmann D, Mugge A, Daniel WG: Identification of patent foramen ovale permitting paradoxic embolism. *J Am Coll Cardiol* 26:1030, 1995.

72. Stone DA, Goddard J, Corretti MC, et al: Patent foramen ovale: Association between the degree of shunt by contrast transesophageal echocardiography and the risk of future neurologic events. *Am Heart J* 131:158, 1996.

73. Steiner MM, Di Tullio MR, Rundek T, et al: Patent foramen size and embolic brain imaging findings among patients with ischemic stroke. *Stroke* 29:944, 1998.

74. Ranoux RD, Cohen A, Cabanes L, et al: Patent foramen ovale: Is stroke due to paradoxical embolism? *Stroke* 24:31, 1993.

75. Bogousslavsky J, Garazi S, Jeanrenaud X, et al: Stroke recurrence in patients with patent foramen ovale: The Laussane Study. *Neurology* 46:1301, 1996.

76. Hanna JP, Sun JP, Furlan AJ, et al: Patent foramen ovale and brain infarct (echocardiographic predictors, recurrence and prevention). *Stroke* 25:782, 1994.

77. Stollberger C, Slany J, Schuster I, et al: The prevalence of deep venous thrombosis in patients with suspected paradoxical embolism. *Ann Intern Med* 119:461, 1993.

78. Lethen H, Flachskampf FA, Schneider R, et al: Frequency of deep vein thrombosis in patients with patent foramen ovale and ischemic stroke or transient ischemic attack. *Am J Cardiol* 80:1066, 1997.

79. Di Tullio M, Sacco R, Venketasubramanian N, et al: Comparison of diagnostic techniques for the detection of a patent foramen ovale in stroke patients. *Stroke* 24:1020, 1993.

80. Belkin RN, Pollack BD, Ruggiero ML, et al: Comparison of transesophageal and transthoracic echocardiography with contrast and color flow Doppler in the detection of patent foramen ovale. *Am Heart J* 128:520, 1994.

81. Silver MD, Dorsey JS: Aneurysms of the septum primum in adults. *Arch Pathol Lab Med* 102:62, 1978.

82. Hanley PC, Tajik AJ, Hynes JK, et al: Diagnosis and classification of atrial septal aneurysm by two-dimensional echocardiography: Report of 80 consecutive cases. *J Am Coll Cardiol* 6:1370, 1985.

83. Pearson AC, Nagelhout D, Castello R, et al: Atrial septal aneurysm and stroke: A transesophageal echocardiographic study. *J Am Coll Cardiol* 18:1223, 1991.

84. Mugge A, Daniel WG, Angermann C, et al: Atrial septal aneurysm in adult patients: A multicenter study using transthoracic and transesophageal echocardiography. *Circulation* 91:2785, 1995.

85. Cabanes L, Mas JL, Cohen A, et al: Atrial septal aneurysm and patent foramen ovale as risk factors for cryptogenic stroke in patients less than 55 years of age: A study using transesophageal echocardiography. *Stroke* 24:1865, 1993.

86. Mas JL, Zubre M: French Study Group on Patent Foramen Ovale and Atrial Septal Aneurysm. Recurrent cerebrovascular events in patients with patent foramen ovale, atrial septal aneurysm, or both and cryptogenic stroke or transient ischemic attack. *Am Heart J* 130:1083, 1995.

87. Devuyst G, Bogousslavsky J, Ruchat P, et al: Prognosis after stroke followed by surgical closure of patent foramen ovale. *Neurology* 47:1162, 1996.

88. Ruchat P, Bogousslavsky J, Hurni M, et al: Systematic surgical closure of patent foramen ovale in selected patients with cerebrovascular events due to paradoxical embolism: Early results of a preliminary study. *Eur J Cardiothorac Surg* 11:824, 1997.

89. Homma S, Di Tullio MR, Sacco RL, et al: Surgical closure of patent foramen ovale in cryptogenic stroke patients. *Stroke* 28:2376, 1997.

90. Bridges ND, Hellenbrand W, Latson L, et al: Transcatheter closure of patent foramen ovale after presumed paradoxical embolism. *Circulation* 86:1902, 1992.

91. Rao PS, Ende DJ, Wilson AD, et al: Follow-up of results of transcatheter occlusion of atrial septal defects with the buttoned device. *Can J Cardiol* 11:69, 1995.

92. Ende DJ, Chopra PS, Rao PS: Transcatheter closure of atrial septal defect or patent foramen ovale with the buttoned device for prevention of recurrence of paradoxical embolism. *Am J Cardiol* 78:233, 1996.

93. Rao PS, Chandar JS, Sideris EB: Role of the inverted buttoned device in transcatheter occlusion of atrial septal defects or patent foramen ovale with right-to-left shunting associated with previously operated complex congenital heart cardiac anomalies. *Am J Cardiol* 80:914, 1997.

94. Magni G, Hijazi ZM, Pandian NG, et al: Two and three-dimensional transesophageal echocardiography in patient selection and assessment of atrial septal defect closure by the new DAS-Angel Wings: Initial clinical experience. *Circulation* 96:1722, 1997.

95. McNamara RL, Lima JOAC, Whelton PK, Powe NR: Echocardiographic identification of cardiovascular sources of emboli to guide clinical management of stroke: A cost-effectiveness analysis. *Ann Intern Med* 127:775, 1997.

96. Karalis DG, Chandrasekaran K, Victor MF, et al: Recognition and embolic potential of intraaortic atherosclerotic debris. *J Am Coll Cardiol* 17:73, 1991.

97. Tunick PA, Kronon I: Protruding atherosclerotic plaque in the aortic arch of patients with systemic embolization: A new finding by transesophageal echocardiography. *Am Heart J* 120:658, 1990.

98. Davila-Roman VG, Barzilai B, Wareing TH, et al: Atherosclerosis of the ascending aorta: Prevalence and role as an independent predictor of cerebrovascular events in cardiac patients. *Stroke* 24:2010, 1994.

99. Tunick PA, Perez JL, Kronon I: Protruding atheromas of the thoracic aorta and systemic embolization. *Ann Intern Med* 115:423, 1991.

100. Rubin DC, Plotnick GD, Hawke MW: Intraaortic debris as a potential source of embolic stroke. *Am J Cardiol* 69:819, 1992.

101. Jones EF, Kalman JM, Calafiore P, et al: Proximal aortic atheroma: An independent risk factor for cerebral ischemia. *Stroke* 26:218, 1995.

102. Stone DA, Hawke MW, LaMonte M, et al: Ulcerated atherosclerotic plaque in the thoracic aorta are associated with cryptogenic stroke: A multiplane TEE study. *Am Heart J* 130:105, 1995.

103. Amarenco P, Cohen A, Tzourio C, et al: Atherosclerotic disease of the aortic arch and the risk of ischemic stroke. *N Engl J Med* 331:1474, 1994.

104. Laperche T, Roudaut R, Steg PG: Mobile thromboses of the aortic arch without aortic debris: A TEE finding associated with unexplained arterial embolism. *Circulation* 96:288, 1997.

105. Tunick PA, Rosenzweig BP, Katz ES, et al: High risk for vascular events in patients with protruding aortic atheromas: A prospective study. *J Am Coll Cardiol* 23:1085, 1994.

106. The French Study of Aortic Plaques in Stroke Group: Atherosclerotic disease of the aortic arch as a risk factor for recurrent ischemic stroke. *N Engl J Med* 334:1216, 1996.

107. Mitusch R, Doherty C, Wucherpfennig H, et al: Vascular events during follow-up in patients with aortic arch atherosclerosis. *Stroke* 28:36, 1997.

108. Cohen A, Tzourio C, Bertrand B, et al: Aortic plaque morphology and vascular events: A follow-up study in patients with ischemic stroke. *Circulation* 96:3838, 1997.

109. Dressler FA, Craig WR, Castello R, Labovitz AJ: Significantly reduced incidence of stroke during coronary artery bypass grafting using transesophageal echocardiography. *Eur J Cardio Thorac Surg* 11:234, 1997.

110. Ferrari E, Vidal R, Chevallier T, Baudoy M: Role of echocardiography in perioperative management of patients undergoing open heart surgery. *Am Heart J* 131:162, 1996.

111. Davies MJ, Moore BP, Braimbridge MV: The floppy mitral valve: Study of incidence, pathology and complications in surgical, necropsy and forensic material. *Br Heart J* 40:468, 1978.

112. Stein PD, Wanf CH, Riddle JM: Scanning electron microscopy of operatively excised severely regurgitant floppy mitral valves. *Am J Cardiol* 64:392, 1989.

113. Egeblad H, Hesse B: Mitral valve prolapse with mobile cul-de-sac thrombus and embolism to brain and lower extremity. *Am Heart J* 114:649, 1987.

114. Gross VM, Nichols FT, von Dohlen TW, D'Cruz IA: Mitral valve prolapse and stroke: Echocardiographic evidence for a missing link. *J Am Soc Echocardiogr* 2:94, 1989.

115. Hart RG, Easton JD: Mitral valve prolapse and cerebral infarction. *Stroke* 13:429, 1982.

116. Kouvras G, Bacoulas G: Association of mitral valve leaflet prolapse with cerebral ischaemic events in the young and early middle-aged patient. *Q J Med* 219:387, 1985.

117. Gagliardi R, Benvenuti L, Frosini F, et al: Frequency of echocardiographic abnormalities in patients with ischemia of the carotid territory: A preliminary report. *Stroke* 16:118, 1985.

118. Barletta GA, Gagliardi R, Benvenuti L, Fantini F: Cerebral ischemic attacks as a complication of aortic and mitral valve prolapse. *Stroke* 16:219, 1985.

119. Zenker G, Erbel R, Kramer G, et al: Transesophageal two-dimensional echocardiography in young patients with cerebral ischemic events. *Stroke* 19:345, 1988.

120. Zamorano J, Erbel R, Mackowski T, et al: Usefulness of transesophageal echocardiography for diagnosis of mitral valve prolapse. *Am J Cardiol* 69:419, 1992.

121. Perloff JK, Child JS, Edwards JE: New guidelines for the clinical diagnosis of mitral valve prolapse. *Am J Cardiol* 57:1124, 1986.

122. Besson G, Bogousslavsky J, Hommel M, et al: Patent

foramen ovale in young stroke patients with mitral valve prolapse. *Acta Neurol Scand* 89:23, 1994.

123. Kucherer H, Ratz K, Junger E, et al: Recognition of cardiac normal variants as the cause of cerebral ischemia: Significance of transesophageal echocardiography (Abstract). *Z Kardiol* 85:917, 1996.

123a. Gibon D, Buonanno FS, Joffe MM, et al: Lack of evidence of an association between mitral valve prolapse and stroke in young patients. *N Eng J Med* 341:8, 1999.

124. Freedberg RS, Goodkin GM, Perez JL, et al: Valve strands are strongly associated with systemic embolization: A transesophageal echocardiographic study. *J Am Coll Cardiol* 6:1709, 1995.

125. Tice FD, Slivka AP, Walz ET, et al: Mitral valve strands in patients with focal cerebral ischemia. *Stroke* 27:1183, 1996.

126. Orsinelli DA, Pearson AC: Detection of prosthetic valve strands by transesophageal echocardiography: Clinical significance in patients with suspected cardiac source of embolism. *J Am Coll Cardiol* 26:1713, 1995.

127. Roberts JK, Omarali I, Di Tullio MR, et al: Stroke 28:2185, 1997.

128. Roldan CA, Shively BK, Crawford MH: Valve excrescences: Prevalence, evolution and risk for cardioembolism. *J Am Coll Cardiol* 30:1308, 1997.

129. Furlan AJ, Cracium AR, Salcedo E, Mellino M: Risk of stroke in patients with mitral annular calcification. *Stroke* 15:801, 1984.

130. Aronow WS, Koenigsberg M, Kronzon I, Gutstein H: Association of mitral annular calcification with new thromboembolic stroke and cardiac events at 39 month follow-up in elderly patients. *Am J Cardiol* 65:1511, 1990.

131. Stein JH, Soble JS: Thrombus associated with mitral valve calcification: A possible mechanism for embolic stroke. *Stroke* 26:1697, 1995.

132. Hata JS, Ayres RW, Biller J, et al: Impact of transesophageal echocardiography on the anticoagulation management of patients admitted with focal cerebral ischemia. *Am J Cardiol* 72:707, 1993.

133. Sonnenberg FA, Beck JB: Markov models in medical decision making: A practical guide. *Med Deois Making* 13:322, 1993.

134. Wells KE, Alexander KK, et al: Massive aortic thrombus detected by transesophageal echocardiography as a cause of peripheral emboli in young patients. *Am Heart J* 132:882, 1996.

135. ACC/AHA guidelines for the clinical application of echocardiography. *Circulation* 82:2323, 1990.

136. Turpie AG, Gent LA, Laupacis A, et al: A comparison of aspirin with placebo in patients treated with warfarin after heart-valve replacement. *N Engl J Med* 329:524, 1993.

137. Toyoda K, Yasaka M, Nagata S, Yamaguchi T: Aortogenic embolic stroke: A transesophageal approach. *Stroke* 23:1056, 1992.

138. Nendaz MR, Sarasin FP, Junod AF, Bogousslavsky J: Preventing stroke in patients with patent foramen ovale: Antithrombotic therapy, foramen closure, or therapeutic abstention? A decision analytic perspective. *Am Heart J* 135:532, 1998.

139. Belden JR, Caplan LR, Bojar RM, et al: Treatment of multiple cerebral emboli from an ulcerated, thrombogenic ascending aorta with aortectomy and graft replacement. *Neurology* 49:621, 1997.

140. Swanson SJ, Cohn LH: Excision of focal arch atheroma using deep hypothermic circulatory arrest. *Ann Thorac Surg* 60:457, 1995.

141. Tenebaum A, Garniek A, Shemesh J, et al: Dual-helical CT for detecting aortic atheromas as a source of stroke: Comparison with transesophageal echocardiography. *Radiology* 208:153, 1998.

INDEX

Note: Page numbers in italic indicate figures; those followed by t indicate tables.

ISBN 0-07-012045-5